The Essential Guide to Primary Care Procedures

The Essential Guide to Primary Care Procedures

Editor

E.J. Mayeaux, Jr., MD
Professor of Family Medicine
Professor of Obstetrics and Gynecology
Louisiana State University Health Science Center
Shreveport, Louisiana

Wolters Kluwer Health | Lippincott Williams & Wilkins
Philadelphia • Baltimore • New York • London
Buenos Aires • Hong Kong • Sydney • Tokyo

Acquisitions Editor: Sonya Seigafuse
Managing Editor: Kerry Barrett
Project Manager: Alicia Jackson
Senior Manufacturing Manager: Benjamin Rivera
Marketing Manager: Kimberly Schonberger
Creative Director: Doug Smock
Production Service: Aptara

530 Walnut Street
Philadelphia, PA 19106 USA
LWW.com

Printed in China

Library of Congress Cataloging-in-Publication Data

The essential guide to primary care procedures / edited by E.J. Mayeaux Jr.
p. ; cm.
Includes bibliographical references and index.
ISBN-13: 978-0-7817-7390-4
ISBN-10: 0-7817-7390-3
1. Surgery, Minor—Handbooks, manuals, etc. 2. Primary care (Medicine)—Handbooks, manuals, etc. I. Mayeaux, E. J.
[DNLM: 1. Primary Health Care—methods—Handbooks. 2. Surgical Procedures, Minor—methods—Handbooks. W 49 E78 2009]
RD111.E77 2009
617'.91—dc22

2008041087

To purchase additional copies of this book, call our customer service department at (800) 638-3030 or fax orders to (301) 223-2320. International customers should call (301) 223-2300.

Visit Lippincott Williams & Wilkins on the Internet: at LWW.com. Lippincott Williams & Wilkins customer service representatives are available from 8:30 am to 6 pm, EST.

10 9 8 7 6 5 4 3 2 1

Since this book and all of my previous books came about through efforts toward excellence in teaching, it is appropriate that I dedicate this edition to those who have been my greatest teachers. I would like to thank my family who taught me to strive for things beyond myself, to do things that may make this world a better place. I also wish to thank my wife, who constantly teaches me to see beyond the mundane into the infinite. I remember my fifth grade teacher Ms. Grubbs who taught me to love reading. To the teachers at Baton Rouge High and Louisiana State University in Baton Rouge who taught me to love science and approach learning and education with discernment and enthusiasm. To my teachers at Louisiana State University Health Sciences Center, from whom I learned my best teaching skills, including Dr. Robert Clawson, Dr. David DeShay, Dr. Joe Bocchini, and Dr. Michael Harper. To my friends and teachers who have taught me and been with me around the country and the world, including Dr. Don DeWitt, Dr. Cynda Johnson, Dr. Gary Newkirk, and Dr. Richard Usatine. And finally, I would like to especially thank my friend and previous co-author Dr. Tom Zuber. He taught me much about teaching and writing, and set me firmly on the path that led to this book. Tom, thanks.

CONTENTS

PREFACE

"We love the way you teach procedures, why don't books teach this way?" This comment and many others like it finally led me and Dr. Tom Zuber, my coauthor on the *Atlas of Primary Care Procedures*, to first write our lessons down in book form. Our goal was to break down each procedure into its component parts and illustrate each step to most effectively teach it. This method can be extremely useful to both novice practitioners learning a procedure and to refresh the memory of those who have not recently performed a particular procedure. In this book, *The Essential Guide to Primary Care Procedures*, I used the same approach and expanded its useful and practical format with almost twice as many procedures. Over 1,400 full-color photographs, augmented by full-color illustrations, have been used to further enhance instruction of the procedures. Procedure "Pearls" have been included along with the popular "Pitfalls" to help the provider perform the procedures more effectively and avoid the mistakes that are most commonly made. The new Complications section succinctly provides complication information, and the new Postprocedure and Pediatric Considerations sections provide valuable information to assist the provider in performing each procedure.

This atlas is designed to provide primary care and emergency health care providers with a step-by-step instructional reference for common office procedures. The information incorporates standard methodology with practical suggestions developed by the authors during their practice and teaching of procedural medicine. Providers-in-training and teachers should benefit from a deeper comprehension of techniques incorporated in these procedures. Seasoned practitioners will appreciate the concise summary of each procedure's CPT coding, pitfalls, and complications. The 123 procedures covered in this atlas range from the basic (cerumen removal and simple interrupted sutures) to the complex (colonoscopy and chest tube placement). These procedures incorporate the vast majority of skills required of primary care and emergency practitioners, and far exceed the number performed by most practicing physicians.

Each chapter begins with an overview of background information regarding each procedure. Indications and contraindications (both relative and absolute) are listed, providing a framework for evaluating patients being considered for a particular procedure. The Procedure section provides sequential instructions, pictures, and illustrations of the performance of the procedure. Bulleted pitfalls and pearls are included to demonstrate common, helpful hints, errors, or difficulties that practitioners historically have encountered. The Coding section includes suggested CPT codes, descriptors, reported 2008 average 50% fees charged for the selected codes, and global periods. The Instruments and Materials section provides source information (phone numbers and Web site addresses) for ordering the materials mentioned in the chapter. The Bibliography section includes references used in the chapter, as well as information of interest when considering a procedure. Many chapters also have patient education materials that appear on the book's Website and may be reproduced and provided to the patient.

Modern health delivery offices and clinics must report services to third party payers using national coding resources. The CPT codes are developed by the American Medical Association and generally accepted by most national insurers. The codes listed in each chapter are suggestions; other codes may be selected that more appropriately describe the procedure performed or services rendered. In addition, certain insurers may incorporate local reporting rules that take precedence. Readers should constantly update their knowledge of annual coding changes.

This atlas includes 2008 average 50th percentile fees for listed CPT codes. These fees are provided to demonstrate national information, and not to serve as a recommendation for practices to set a specific charge for services. This information is derived from the *2008 Physicians' Fee and Coding Guide* published by MAG Mutual Healthcare Solutions, Inc., Duluth, Georgia. This annual survey of fees provides invaluable national data on fees and coding information, which can help practitioners interact with the health delivery system. Being equipped with national fee data can help medical practices counter inappropriate accusations of "overcharging" by third-party payers. To obtain a full copy of the Guide, visit www.coderscentral.com.

The resources listed in the Instruments and Materials section are not comprehensive. Materials may be included because they have historically demonstrated effectiveness or ease of use in primary care practices. Many of the instruments are listed because they provide accurate and cost-effective information. Readers should use materials that they believe are superior.

No book can replace experience. When learning any new procedural skill, it is recommended that the practitioner receive proctoring from someone skilled in the procedure. Precepted experience is strongly urged for more complex procedures to reduce patient complications and medicolegal liability. Formal procedural training courses also are available through specialty societies (such as the American Academy of Family Physicians), medical interest societies (such as the American Society of Colposcopy and Cervical Pathology), or local or regional medical societies. It is hoped that this reference will serve as an invaluable resource in the provision of high-quality procedural services.

Finally, it is the hope of the authors that this reference will prove extremely *useful*. It is meant to be a book that is kept in the procedure room of the practice, not on a book shelf. To see a copy, worn and stained from extensive use during procedures, indicates to this author and editor that it was a job well done.

E.J. Mayeaux, Jr., MD
Professor of Family Medicine
Professor of Obstetrics and Gynecology
Louisiana State University Health Science Center, Shreveport, Louisiana

CONTRIBUTING AUTHORS

Ya'aqov M. Abrams, MD
Assistant Professor
Department of Family Medicine
University of Pittsburgh
Chief of Service
Department of Family Medicine
Magee Women's Hospital
Pittsburgh, Pennsylvania

Thomas C. Arnold, MD
Associate Professor and Chairman
Department of Emergency Medicine
Louisiana State University Health Sciences Center
University Hospital
Shreveport, Louisiana

Doug Aukerman, MD, FAAFP
Assistant Professor
Department of Orthopaedics, Rehabilitation and Sports Medicine
Assistant Professor
Department of Family and Community Medicine
Penn State Milton S. Hershey Medical Center
Hershey, Pennsylvania
Team Physician
Penn State University
State College, Pennsylvania

Vinay Bangalore, MD, MPH
Fellow
Department of Critical Care Medicine
Louisiana State University and the
Louisiana State University Health Sciences Center
Shreveport, Louisiana

Ken Barrick, MD
Senior Resident
Department of Emergency Medicine
Louisiana State University Health Sciences Center
Shreveport, Louisiana

Jay M. Berman, MD, FACOG
Assistant Professor
Wayne State University School of Medicine
Department of OB/GYN
Hutzel Women's Hospital
Detroit, Michigan

Nancy R. Berman, MSN, APRN, BC
Nurse Practitioner
Northwest Internal Medicine Associates
Division of the Millennium Medical Group, PC
Southfield, Michigan

Anne Boyd, MD
Assistant Professor
Department of Family Medicine
University of Pittsburgh School of Medicine
Director
Primary Care Sports Medicine Fellowship Program
University of Pittsburgh Medical Center
Pittsburgh, Pennsylvania

Danielle Cooper, MD
Assistant Professor of Obstetrics and Gynecology
Louisiana State University Health Sciences Center
Shreveport, Louisiana

Paul D. Cooper, MD
Assistant Professor of Clinical Pediatrics
Louisiana State University Health Sciences Center
Shreveport, Louisiana

Alessandra D'Avenzo, MD
Resident
St. Joseph's Family Medicine Residency
Syracuse, New York

Sean Denham, MD
Resident
Emergency Medicine Residency
Louisiana State University Health Sciences Center
Shreveport, Louisiana

Brian Elkins, MD, DABFM, FAAFP
Associate Professor of Clinical Family Medicine
Louisiana State University Health Sciences Center
Shreveport, Louisiana

Jeffrey A. German, MD
Associate Professor
Department of Family Medicine
Louisiana State University Health Sciences Center
Shreveport, Louisiana

Laurie Grier, MD, FCCM, FCCP, FACP
Professor of Clinical Medicine
Emergency Medicine and Anesthesia
Louisiana State University Health Sciences Center
Shreveport, Louisiana

Michael B. Harper, MD, DABFM
Professor of Clinical Family Medicine
Louisiana State University Health Sciences Center
Shreveport, Louisiana

George D. Harris, MD, MS
Professor of Medicine
Department of Community and Family Medicine
University of Missouri Kansas City, School of Medicine
Kansas City, Missouri

Jeff Harris, MD
Instructor of Family Medicine
Louisiana State University Health Science Center
Shreveport, Louisiana

Edward A. Jackson, MD, DABFM, FABFM
Chair and Program Director
Synergy Medical Education Alliance
Professor
Department of Family Medicine
Michigan State College of Human Medicine
East Lansing, Michigan

Naomi Jay, RNC, NP PhD
Co-Director HPV Research Studies
Department of Medicine
University of California
San Francisco, California

Stacy Kanayama, MD, ATC
Resident
Family Medicine
Louisiana State University Health Sciences Center
Shreveport, Louisiana

Steven Kitchings, MD
Chief Resident
Family Medicine
Louisiana State University Health Sciences Center
Shreveport, Louisiana

Michael G. Lamb, MD
Clinical Associate Professor of Medicine
University of Pittsburgh Medical Center
UPMC Community Medicine, Inc.
Department of Internal Medicine
Pittsburgh, Pennsylvania

T.S. Lian, MD, FACS
Associate Professor
Department of Otolaryngology–Head & Neck Surgery
Louisiana State University Health Sciences Center
Shreveport, Louisiana

Simon A. Mahler, MD
Assistant Professor
Department of Emergency Medicine
Louisiana State University Health Science Center
Shreveport, Louisiana

E.J. Mayeaux, Jr., MD, DABFP, FAAFP
Professor of Family Medicine
Professor of Obstetrics and Gynecology
Louisiana State University Health Sciences Center
Shreveport, Louisiana

Paul McCarthy, MD
Department of Critical Care Medicine
Louisiana State University Health Sciences Center
Shreveport, Louisiana

Daniel E. Melville, MD, ABFM
Bourbon Medical Center
Paris, Kentucky

Sonya C. Melville, MD
Assistant Professor of Emergency Medicine
University of Kentucky Medical Center
Lexington, Kentucky

Samantha E. Montgomery, MD
Resident
Department of Obstetrics and Gynecology
Wayne State University School of Medicine
Detroit, Michigan

David L. Nelson, MD, LAc
Associate Professor of Clinical Family Medicine
Louisiana State University Health Sciences Center
Shreveport, Louisiana

Thomas Boone Redens, MD
Director
Cornea/External Disease/Refractive Surgery
Program Director
Department of Ophthalmology
Louisiana State University Health Sciences Center
Shreveport, Louisiana

Mary M. Rubin, RNC, NP, PhD
Associate Clinical Professor
Department of Nursing
Coordinator, GYN Oncology and Dysplasia Research
Department of OB/GYN and Medicine
University of California
San Francisco, California

Larry S. Sasaki, MD, FACS
Assistant Clinical Professor
Department of Surgery
Louisiana State University Health Sciences Center
Shreveport, Louisiana

Wayne Sebastianelli, MD
Professor
Department of Orthopaedics and Rehabilitation
Pennsylvania State University
Assistant Chief of Staff
Mount Nittany Medical Center
State College, Pennsylvania

Amber Shaff, MD
Resident
St. Joseph's Family Medicine Residency
Syracuse, New York

Valerie I. Shavell, MD
Resident
Department of Obstetrics and Gynecology
Wayne State University School of Medicine
Detroit, Michigan

Rebecca Small, MD
Assistant Clinical Professor
Director, Medical Aesthetics Training Program
Department of Family and Community Medicine
University of California, San Francisco School of Medicine
Capitola, California

Albert Lee Smith, III, MD
Chief Resident
Family Medicine
Louisiana State University Health Sciences Center
Shreveport, Louisiana

Robert W. Smith, MD, MBA, FAAFP
Vice Chair For Education
Department of Family Medicine
University of Pittsburgh School of Medicine
Pittsburgh, Pennsylvania

Jeannette E. South-Paul, MD
Andrew W. Mathieson Professor and Chair
Department of Family Medicine
University of Pittsburgh School of Medicine
Pittsburgh, Pennsylvania

Jennifer M. Springhart, M.D.
Assistant Professor of Clinical Emergency Medicine
Department of Emergency Medicine
Louisiana State University Health Sciences Center
Shreveport, Louisiana

Daniel L. Stulberg, MD FAAFP
Associate Professor
Department of Family and Community Medicine
University of New Mexico Health Sciences Center
Albuquerque, New Mexico

Sandra M. Sulik, MD, MS, FAAFP
Associate Professor
Department of Family Medicine
SUNY Upstate and St. Joseph's Family Medicine Residency
Fayetteville, New York
Department of Family Medicine
St. Joseph's Family Medicine
Syracuse, New York

Stephen Taylor, MD, FAAFP
Associate Professor of Family Medicine
North Caddo Medical Center
Vivian, Louisiana

Mandy Ton, MD
Third-Year Family Medicine Resident
Louisiana State University Health Sciences Center
Shreveport, Louisiana

Paul Trisler, MD
Chief Resident
Emergency Medicine Residency
Louisiana State University Health Sciences Center
Shreveport, Louisiana

Sean Troxclair, MD
Clinical Fellow
Critical Care Medicine
Department of Internal Medicine
Louisiana State University Health Sciences Center
Shreveport, Louisiana

Racheal Whitaker, MD
Assistant Professor of Obstetrics and Gynecology
Louisiana State University Health Sciences Center
Shreveport, Louisiana

Russell D. White, MD
Professor of Medicine
Director
Sports Medicine Fellowship Program
Department of Community and Family Medicine
University of Missouri Kansas City, School of Medicine
Kansas City, Missouri

Clint N. Wilson, MD
Chief Resident
Family Medicine Residency
Louisiana State University Health Sciences Center
Shreveport, Louisiana

Heidi Wimberly, PA-C
Clinical Instructor
Department of Emergency Medicine
Louisiana State University Health Sciences Center
Shreveport, Louisiana

Dennis R. Wissing, PhD, RRT, CPFT, AE-C
Professor of Cardiopulmonary Science
Assistant Dean for Academic Affairs
School of Allied Health Professions
Louisiana State University Health Science Center
Shreveport, Louisiana

Scott Wissink, MD
Assistant Professor
Department of Orthopaedic Surgery
University of Pittsburgh
Monroeville, Pennsylvania

Christopher James Wolcott, MD
Assistant Clinical Professor of Emergency Medicine
Department of Emergency Medicine
Louisiana State University Health Sciences Center
Shreveport, Louisiana

Lauren Moonan Yorek, MD
Assistant Clinical Professor
Department of Emergency Medicine
Louisiana State University Health Sciences Center
Shreveport, Louisiana

ACKNOWLEDGMENTS

I would like to acknowledge all of the authors that have put so much time and effort into the creation of this book. This is truly a labor of love by teachers who love what they do. I would like to especially acknowledge Dr. Larry Sasaki who enthusiastically agreed to write several chapters and Dr. Rebecca Small who at first agreed to write 1 chapter and ended up writing most of the Aesthetics section.

SECTION ONE

URGENT AND EMERGENCY CARE

CHAPTER 1

Local Anesthesia Administration

E.J. Mayeaux, Jr., MD, DABFP, FAAFP
Professor of Family Medicine, Professor of Obstetrics and Gynecology
Louisiana State University Health Sciences Center, Shreveport, LA

Most minor or office operations are performed after injection of local anesthesia. Proper administration technique can reduce patient discomfort, improve patient satisfaction with the service, and improve the procedure's outcome. Unfortunately, the techniques for minimizing discomfort during local anesthetic administration are often overlooked in modern clinical practice.

Table 1-1 shows available drugs commonly used as local anesthetics. The two main classes of injectable local anesthetics are amides and esters. The amides are more widely used and include lidocaine (Xylocaine) and bupivacaine (Marcaine). The esters, represented by procaine (Novocain), have a slower onset of action than the amides and a higher rate of allergic reactions. Individuals with an allergy to one class of anesthetics generally can receive the other class safely. Administration of the esters is limited to individuals with a prior allergic reaction to amide anesthetics.

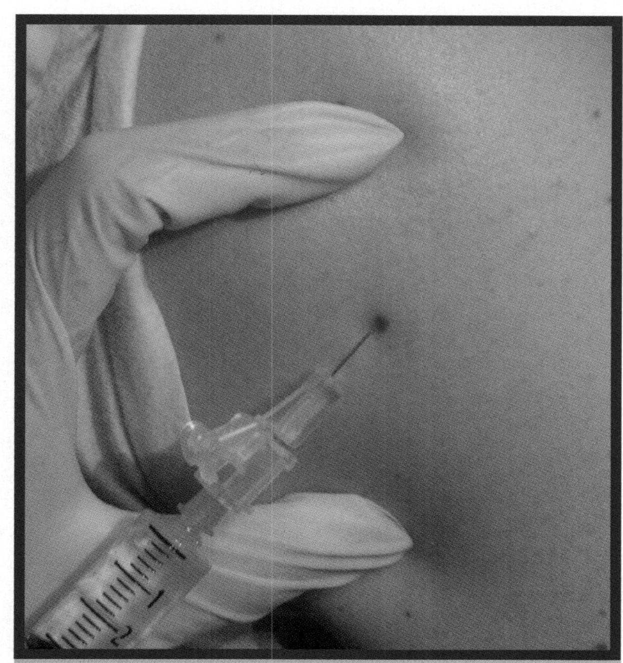

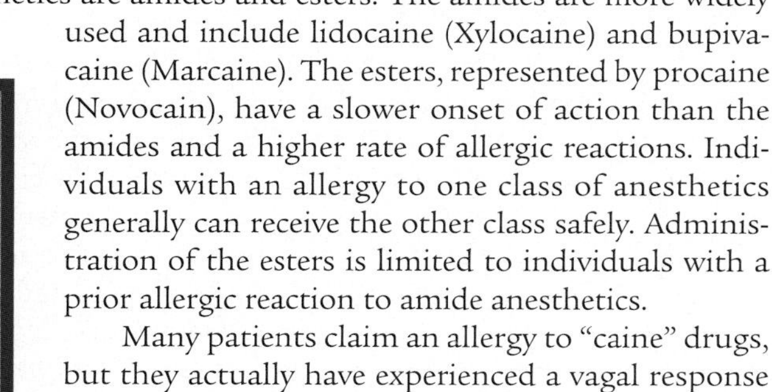

Many patients claim an allergy to "caine" drugs, but they actually have experienced a vagal response or other systemic response to receiving an injection. If the exact nature of the prior reaction cannot be ascertained, administration of diphenhydramine hydrochloride (Benadryl) can provide sufficient anesthesia for small surgical procedures. Between 1 and 2 mL of diphenhydramine (25 mg/mL) solution is diluted with 1 to 4 mL of normal saline for intradermal (not subdermal) injection.

Epinephrine in the local anesthetic solution prolongs the duration of the anesthetic and reduces bleeding by producing local vasoconstriction. The use of epinephrine also permits use of larger volumes of anesthetic. An average-sized adult (70 kg) can safely receive up to 28 mL (4 mg/kg) of 1% lidocaine and up to 49 mL (7 mg/kg) of 1% lidocaine with epinephrine.

Historically, physicians have been taught to avoid administering solutions with epinephrine to body sites served by single arteries, such as fingers, toes, penis, and the end of the nose. The safety of administering epinephrine to the tip of the nose or to the digits has been documented in some reports, but limiting the use of epinephrine in these sites is prudent in the current medicolegal climate.

TABLE 1-1. Commonly Available Local Anesthetics

	Common Local Anesthetics	Concentration	Maximum Total Adult Dose	Onset (min)	Duration (hr)
Amides	Lidocaine (Xylocaine)	1%–2%	4.5 mg/kg, max 300 mg	<2	0.5–1
	Lidocaine with epinephrine	1%–2% with epi 1:100,000 or 1:200,000	7 mg/kg, max 500 mg	<2	2–6
	Bupivacaine (Marcaine, Sensorcaine)	0.25%	2.5 mg/kg, max 175 mg	5	2–4
	Bupivacaine with epinephrine	0.25% with epi 1:200,000	Max 225 mg	5	3–7
	Mepivacaine (Carbocaine, Polocaine)	1%	Max 400 mg	3–5	0.75–1.5
Esters	Procaine (Novocain)	0.25%–0.5% (via dilution)	350 to 600 mg	2–5	0.25–1
	Chloroprocaine (Nesacaine)	1%–2%	Not to exceed 800 mg	6–12	0.5
	Diphenhydramine (Benadryl)	1%	Uncertain	<2	0.5

Local anesthetics can be injected intradermally or subdermally. Intradermal administration produces a visible wheal in the skin, and the onset of action of the anesthetic is almost immediate. Intradermal injection of a large volume of solution can stretch pain sensors in the skin, aiding in the anesthetic effect. This volume effect is believed to explain the benefit of normal saline injections into trigger points. Other strategies to reduce the discomfort of injection are shown in Table 1-2. Intradermal injection is especially useful for shave excisions, because the anesthetic solution effectively thickens the dermis, elevates the lesion, and prevents inadvertent penetration beneath the dermis.

Subdermal injections take effect more slowly but generally produce much less discomfort for the patient. Some physicians recommend initial administration of an anesthetic into a subdermal (less painful) location and then withdrawing the needle tip for intradermal injection. The initial subdermal administration often reduces the discomfort of the intradermal injection.

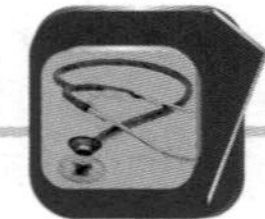

Equipment

- Syringes (TB, 5 mL, or 10 mL), anesthetic solutions, and needles (18 or 20 gauge, 1 inch long for drawing up anesthetic; 25 or 27 gauge, 1.25 inch long for delivering anesthetic) can be ordered from surgical supply houses or pharmacies. A suggested anesthesia tray that can be used for this procedure is listed in Appendix F.

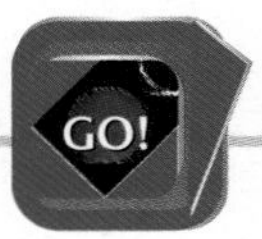

Indications

- Local or regional anesthesia for minor procedures

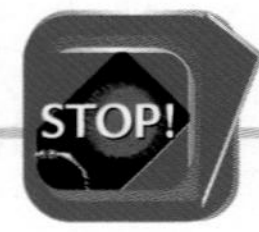

Contraindications

- Allergy to local anesthetics

The Procedure

Step 1. Prep the skin with alcohol if it is not already prepped with povidone/iodine or chlorhexidine solution. Stretch the skin with your nondominant hand before inserting the needle into the skin. Patients dread having the needle inserted; the discomfort is reduced if the pain sensors in the skin are stretched.

- PITFALL: Replace the needle used for drawing the anesthetic from the stock bottle with a smaller (30-gauge) needle before injection into the patient. A sharp needle decreases pain.

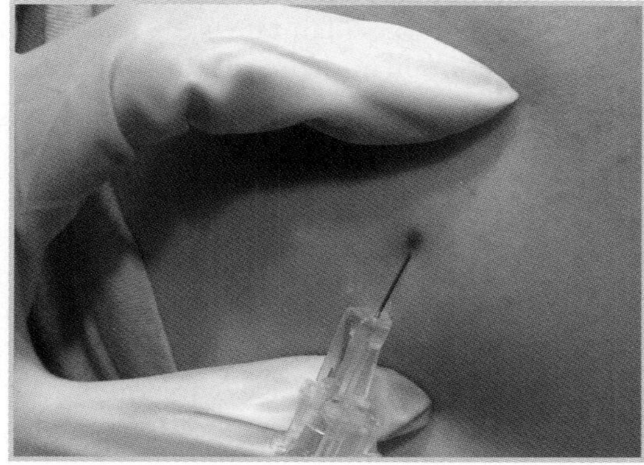

Step 1

Step 2. The syringe is held in your dominant hand in the position ready to inject. Your thumb should be near (but not on) the plunger. After the needle is inserted into skin, some physicians prefer to withdraw the plunger to ensure that the needle tip is not in an intravascular location. The thumb can be slipped under the back edge of the plunger and pulled back, watching for blood to enter the syringe to ensure that the needle tip is not in a blood vessel. The thumb then slips onto the plunger for gentle injection. However, it is very unlikely that a short, 30-gauge needle tip will enter a significant vessel, and many physicians prefer to inject without withdrawing, because pulling back on the plunger moves the needle tip and causes discomfort for the patient.

- PITFALL: Avoid movement of the needle after it enters the skin. Many physicians hold the syringe like a pencil for needle insertion. After insertion, they stop stretching the skin with the nondominant hand and grab the syringe, shift the dominant hand back onto the plunger, and pull back on the plunger to check for vascular entry of the needle tip. They then shift the hands again and move the dominant hand into a position for injection. All of these shifts cause movement of the needle tip in the skin and substantially increase the discomfort for the patient.

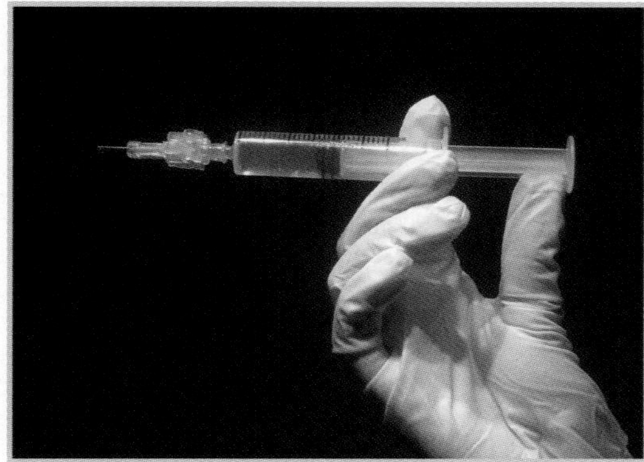

Step 2

Step 3. Insert the needle into skin at a 15- or 30-degree angle. The depth of the needle tip is more difficult to control at a 90-degree angle of entry.

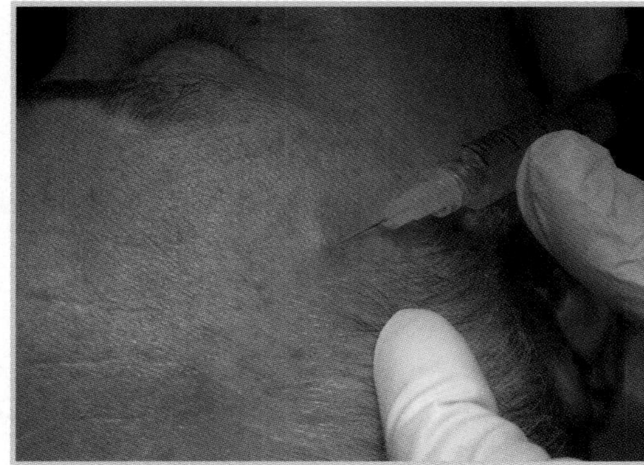

Step 3

Step 4. When injecting laceration sites for repair, insert the needle into the wound edge, rather than intact skin. Insertion of a needle into a wound edge produces less discomfort.

Step 5. Pause after the needle enters the skin. Try to make the patient talk or laugh. Patients fear the needle entry, and after they realize that the discomfort was less than anticipated, they often relax. Maintain skin stretch with the nondominant hand for the injection.

- **PITFALL:** Plunging in anesthetic immediately after needle entry causes continued discomfort and anxiety. Most vagal or syncopal episodes are related to the catecholamine storm produced by the patient's anxiety. Pausing after needle insertion and slow administration allow patients to relax, reducing their catecholamine production and reducing complications.

Step 6. Intradermal injection creates a wheal in the skin. Administer the local anesthetic for a shave excision below the center of the lesion to be removed. The anesthetic fluid effectively increases the depth of the dermis, reducing chances for subdermal penetration at shave excision. The fluid also floats the lesion upward, facilitating removal by shave technique.

- **PEARL:** When the needle tip is correctly placed, there is resistance to injecting the anesthetic within the skin.

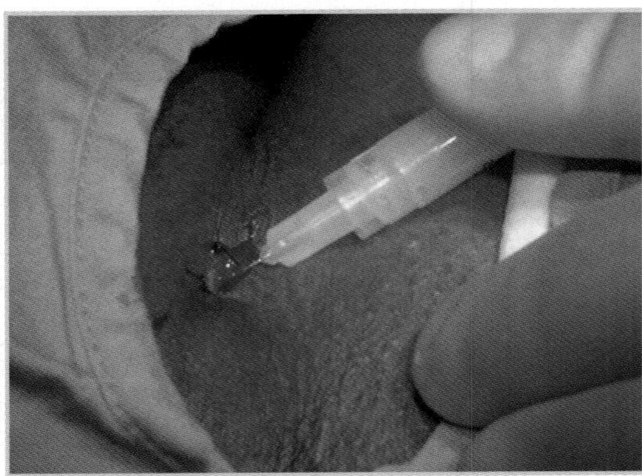

Step 4

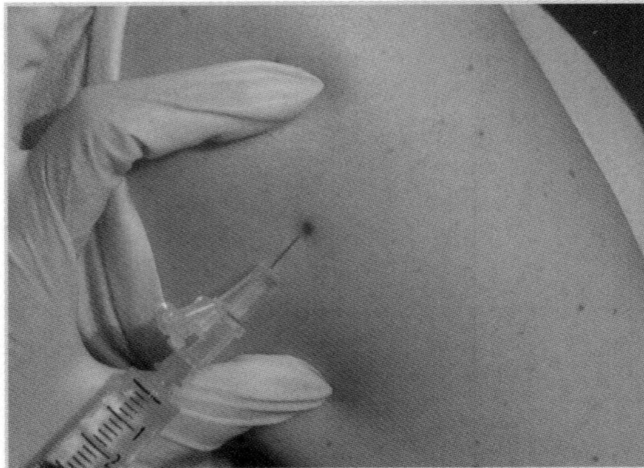

Step 5

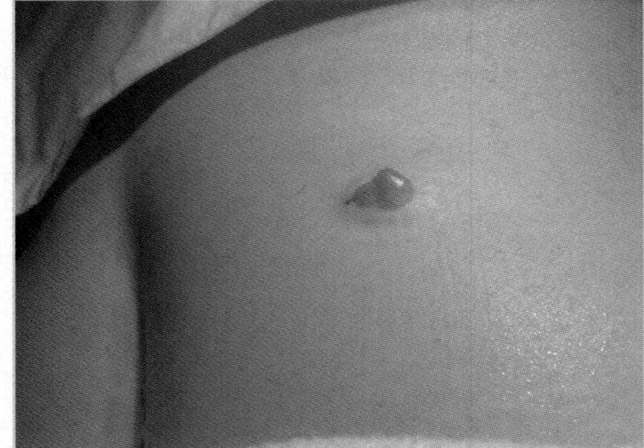

Step 6

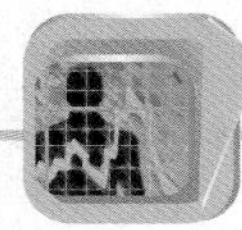

Complications

- Bleeding and hematoma formation.
- Allergic reaction is rare. Patients who believe they are allergic to lidocaine are more likely allergic to the preservative methylparaben. Preservative-free lidocaine is available.
- Infection.
- Palpitations or feelings of warmth (due to epinephrine component).

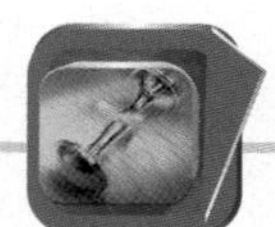

Pediatric Considerations

Children older than 6 years are dosed like adults except that the maximal dose is based on weight. The recommended maximal dose for lidocaine in children is 3 to 5 mg/kg, and 7 mg/kg when combined with epinephrine. Remember that 1% lidocaine is 10 mg/mL. Children 6 months to 3 years have the same volume of distribution and elimination half-life as adults. Neonates have an increased volume of distribution, decreased hepatic clearance, and doubled terminal elimination half-life (3.2 hours).

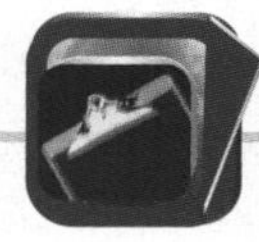

Postprocedure Instructions

Have the patient report any postprocedure local rashes or blistering that may indicate an adverse reaction or infection.

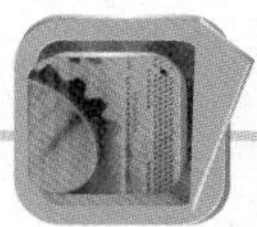

Coding Information

Anesthesia codes (00100 to 01999) are usually limited to anesthesiologists providing patient services for surgical procedures. Local anesthesia is not reported in addition to the surgical procedure. Some insurance providers permit billing of regional or general anesthesia by the physician or surgeon performing the procedure. If reporting additional anesthesia services, the -47 modifier is attached to the surgical code. It is unlikely that additional reimbursement will be provided for field blocks; the service is considered part of the reporting of the surgical procedure.

Patient Education Handout

A patient education handout, "Local Anesthetic Use in Children," can be found on the book's Web site.

Bibliography

Avina R. Office management of trauma: Primary care local and regional anesthesia in the management of trauma. *Clin Fam Pract.* 2000;2:533–550.

Baker JD, Blackmon BB. Local anesthesia. *Clin Plast Surg.* 1985;12:25–31.

Brown JS. *Minor Surgery: A Text and Atlas.* 3rd ed. London: Chapman & Hall Medical; 1997. deJong RH. Toxic effects of local anesthetics. *JAMA* 1978;239:1166–1168.

Dinehart SM. Topical, local, and regional anesthesia. In: Wheeland RG, ed. *Cutaneous Surgery.* Philadelphia: WB Saunders; 1994:102–112.

Grekin RC. Local anesthesia in dermatologic surgery. *J Am Acad Dermatol.* 1988;19:599–614.

Kelly AM, Cohen M, Richards D. Minimizing the pain of local infiltration anesthesia for wounds by injection into the wound edges. *J Emerg Med.* 1994;12:593–595.

Scarfone RJ, Jasani M, Gracely EJ. Pain of local anesthetics: Rate of administration and buffering. *Ann Emerg Med.* 1998;31:36–40.

Smith DW, Peterson MR, DeBerard SC. Local anesthesia. *Postgrad Med.* 1999;106:57–66.

Stegman SJ, Tromovitch TA, Glogau RG. *Basics of Sermatologic Surgery.* Chicago: Year Book Medical Publishers; 1982:23–31.

Swanson NA. *Atlas of Cutaneous Surgery.* Boston: Little, Brown; 1987:156–162.

Winton GB. Anesthesia for dermatologic surgery. *J Dermatol Surg Oncol.* 1988;14:41–54.

Yagiela JA. Oral-facial emergencies: Anesthesia and pain management. *Emerg Med Clin North Am.* 2000;18:449–470.

Zuber TJ, DeWitt DE. The fusiform excision. *Am Fam Physician* 1994;49:371–376.

2008 MAG Mutual Healthcare Solutions, Inc.'s Physicians' Fee and Coding Guide. Duluth, Georgia. MAG Mutual Healthcare Solutions, Inc. 2007.

Table 1-2. Recommendations to Reduce the Discomfort of Local Anesthesia

- Stretch the skin using your nondominant hand during administration.
- Encourage the patient to talk as a distraction and to monitor vagal responses.
- Talk to the patient during administration; silence increases patient discomfort.
- Use the smallest gauge needle possible (preferably 30 gauge).
- Consider spraying aerosol refrigerant onto the skin before needle insertion.
- Consider vibrating nearby skin or patting distant sites to distract during administration.
- Administer anesthetic at room temperature (i.e., nonchilled solutions).
- Insert the needle through enlarged pores, scar, or hair follicles (i.e., less sensitive sites).
- Pause after the needle penetrates the skin to allow for patient recovery and relaxation.
- Inject a small amount of anesthetic and pause, allowing the anesthetic to take effect.
- Empower the patient by temporarily stopping the injection when burning is detected.
- Inject anesthetics slowly.
- Begin the injection subdermally and then withdraw the needle tip for intradermal injection.
- Consider addition of bicarbonate to buffer the acidity of the anesthetic.
- Permit adequate time for the anesthetic to take effect before initiating a surgical procedure.

CHAPTER 2

Field Block Anesthesia

E. J. Mayeaux, Jr., MD, DABFP, FAAFP

Professor of Family Medicine, Professor of Obstetrics and Gynecology
Louisiana State University Health Sciences Center, Shreveport, LA

Field block anesthesia describes the infiltration of local anesthetic in a circumferential pattern around, and often under, a surgical site. Like nerve blocks, field blocks are used to anesthetize large areas of skin. Field blocks differ from nerve blocks in that more than one nerve experiences interruption of the nerve transmission. The technique permits large areas to be anesthetized, and it is useful for large dermatologic procedures. The field block does not disrupt the architecture of the surgical site and often is administered for facial or cosmetic repairs. However, it does require more time to work than intradermal blocks. It is not unusual for a block to require more than 5 minutes to reach full effect.

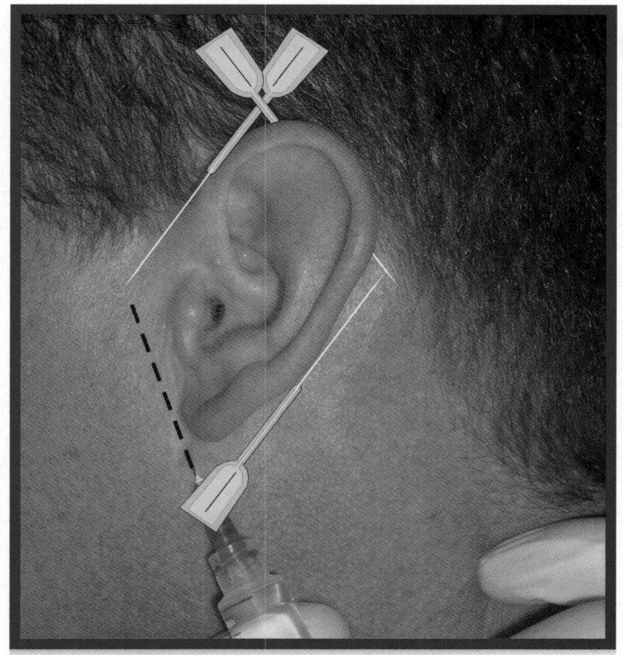

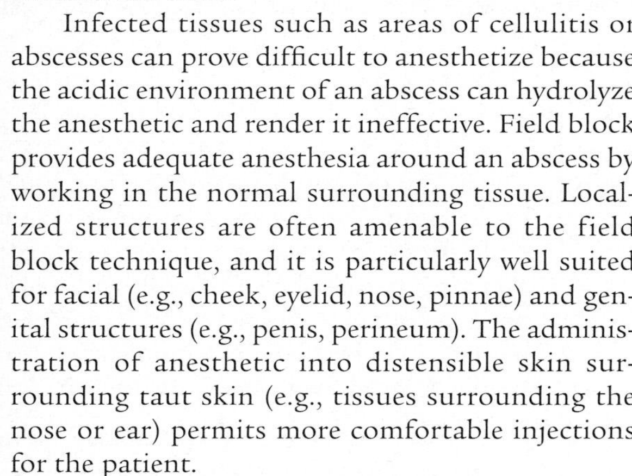

Infected tissues such as areas of cellulitis or abscesses can prove difficult to anesthetize because the acidic environment of an abscess can hydrolyze the anesthetic and render it ineffective. Field block provides adequate anesthesia around an abscess by working in the normal surrounding tissue. Localized structures are often amenable to the field block technique, and it is particularly well suited for facial (e.g., cheek, eyelid, nose, pinnae) and genital structures (e.g., penis, perineum). The administration of anesthetic into distensible skin surrounding taut skin (e.g., tissues surrounding the nose or ear) permits more comfortable injections for the patient.

Epinephrine can be added to lidocaine for some field blocks if the vasoconstrictive or anesthetic-prolonging action of epinephrine is desired. Epinephrine permits safe use of larger amounts of lidocaine because it prevents clearance of the anesthetic from the tissue. Epinephrine should be avoided in areas where vascular compromise could prove problematic, especially in individuals with vasculitis or vasoconstrictive disorders such as Raynaud's phenomenon. Many authorities discourage the addition of epinephrine for field blocks on digits, around the ear, on the nasal tip, or surrounding the penis.

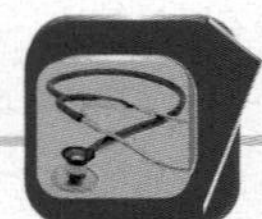

Equipment

- Syringes (TB, 5 mL, or 10 mL), anesthetic solutions, and needles (18 or 20 gauge, 1 in long for drawing up anesthetic; 25 or 27 gauge, 1.25 in long for delivering anesthetic) can be ordered from surgical supply houses or pharmacies. A suggested anesthesia tray that can be used for this procedure is listed in Appendix F.

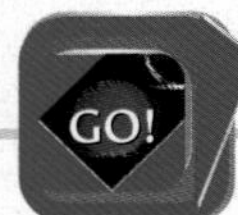

Indications

- Surrounding large lesions that would provide a large area of anesthesia
- Around infected cysts or abscesses
- To prevent distortion of skin landmarks from administration of local anesthesia
- Around facial structures (e.g., nose, pinnae, forehead, cheek, eyelids, upper lip)
- Digital blocks (see Chapter 3)
- Surrounding localized structures (e.g., penis, perineum)

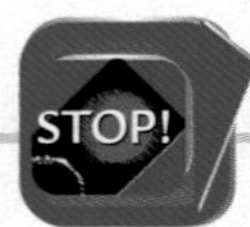

Contraindications

- Allergy to anesthetics
- Cellulitis in the injection area (relative)

The Procedure

Step 1. The field block can be performed in a square- or diamond-shaped pattern around a wound. Only two skin punctures are required. After prepping with alcohol, the needle passes along one side of the proposed excision under the dermis, and anesthetic is administered as the needle is withdrawn without exiting the skin.

- PITFALL: Make sure to anesthetize enough area to allow for undermining.

Step 2. The needle is then redirected to the other side of the proposed excision, and anesthetic is administered as the needle is withdrawn without coming out of the initial puncture site.

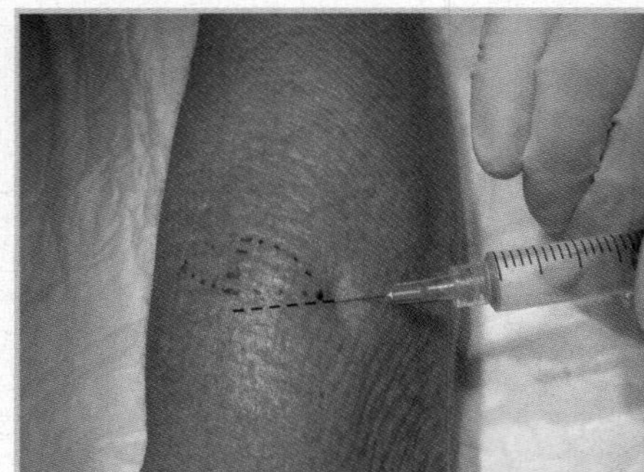

Step 1

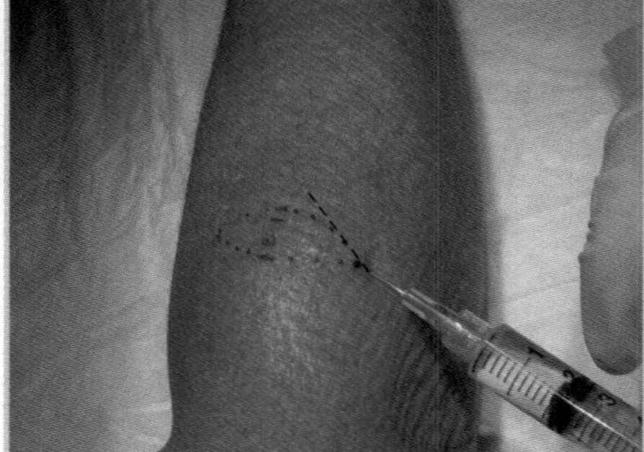

Step 2

Step 3. For large lesions and subcutaneous lesions (such as cysts and abscesses), the needle may also be redirected below the lesion in case deep dissection is required. This entire technique is repeated on the opposite site of the wound.

- **PITFALL:** Be very careful not to inject anesthetic into cystic lesions because this may cause them to rupture, either below the skin or upward toward the provider.

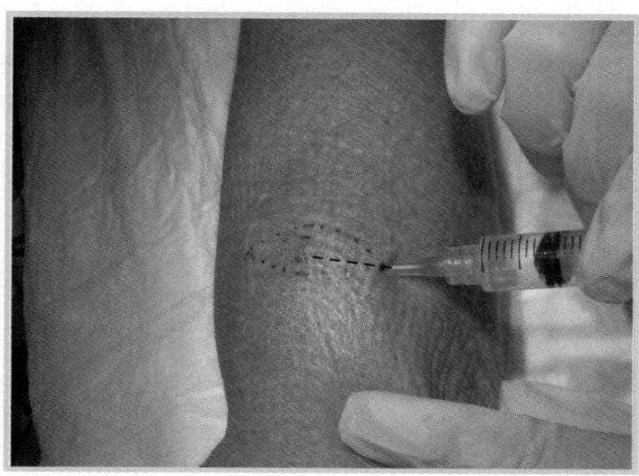

Step 3

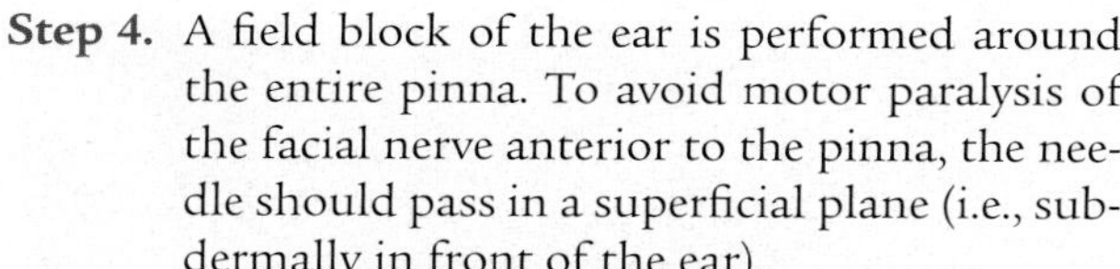

Step 4. A field block of the ear is performed around the entire pinna. To avoid motor paralysis of the facial nerve anterior to the pinna, the needle should pass in a superficial plane (i.e., subdermally in front of the ear).

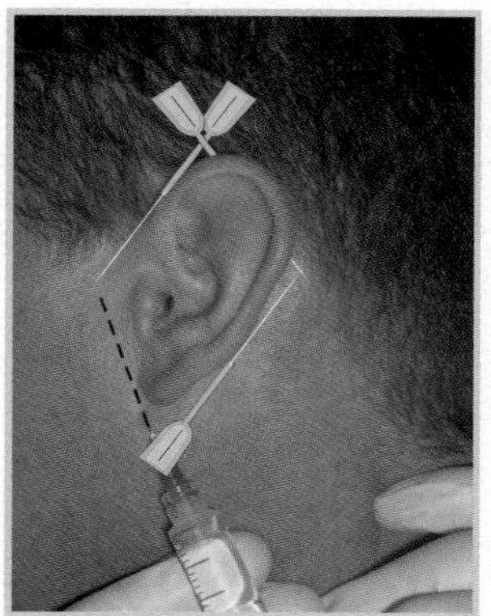

Step 4

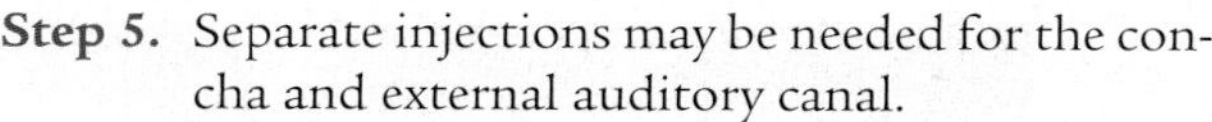

Step 5. Separate injections may be needed for the concha and external auditory canal.

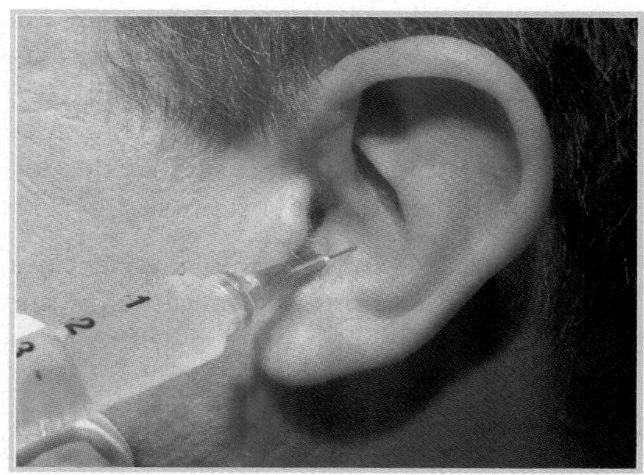

Step 5

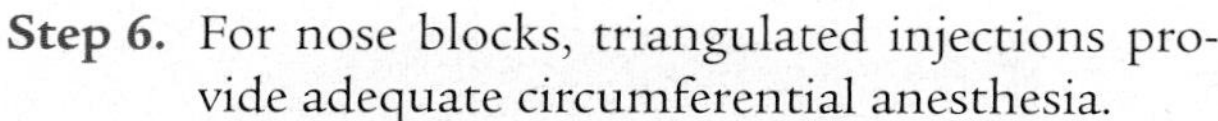

Step 6. For nose blocks, triangulated injections provide adequate circumferential anesthesia.

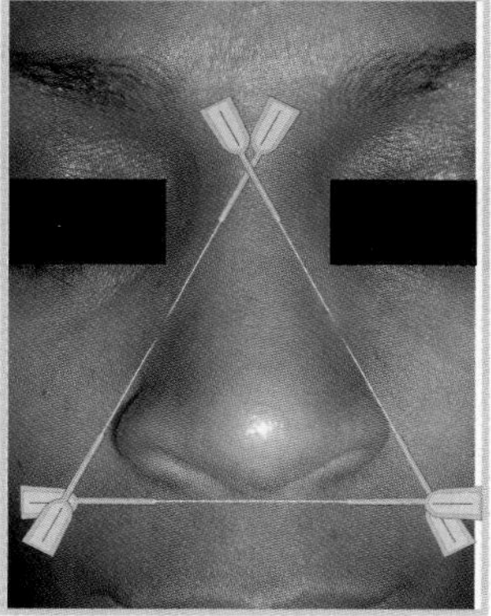

Step 6

Step 7. Additional lidocaine (usually without epinephrine) must be administered to the tip of the nose to anesthetize the external nasal nerve, which arises from the deep tissues. This nerve is usually not blocked by the circumferential injections.

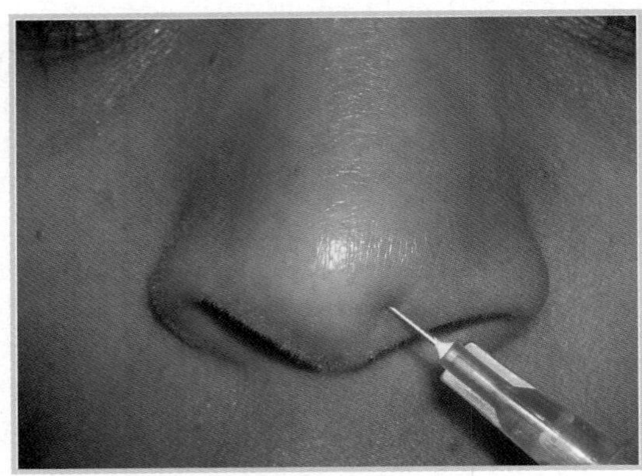

Step 7

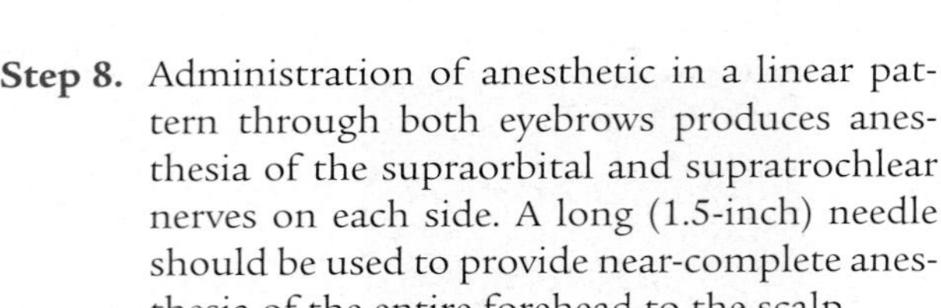

Step 8. Administration of anesthetic in a linear pattern through both eyebrows produces anesthesia of the supraorbital and supratrochlear nerves on each side. A long (1.5-inch) needle should be used to provide near-complete anesthesia of the entire forehead to the scalp.

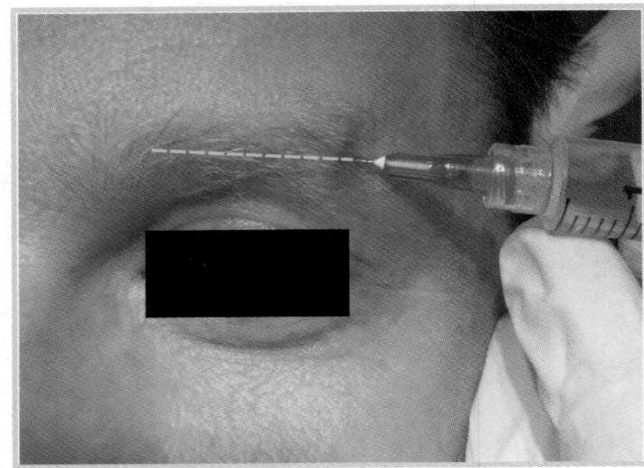

Step 8

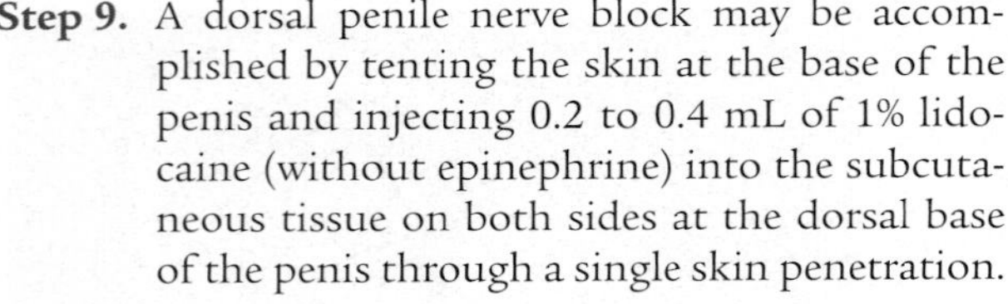

Step 9. A dorsal penile nerve block may be accomplished by tenting the skin at the base of the penis and injecting 0.2 to 0.4 mL of 1% lidocaine (without epinephrine) into the subcutaneous tissue on both sides at the dorsal base of the penis through a single skin penetration.

- PITFALL: To avoid inadvertent intravascular injection, apply negative pressure to the syringe immediately before injection to check for a backflow of blood.

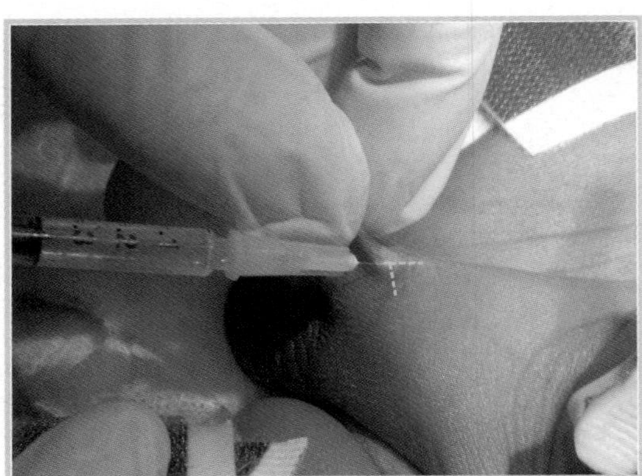

Step 9

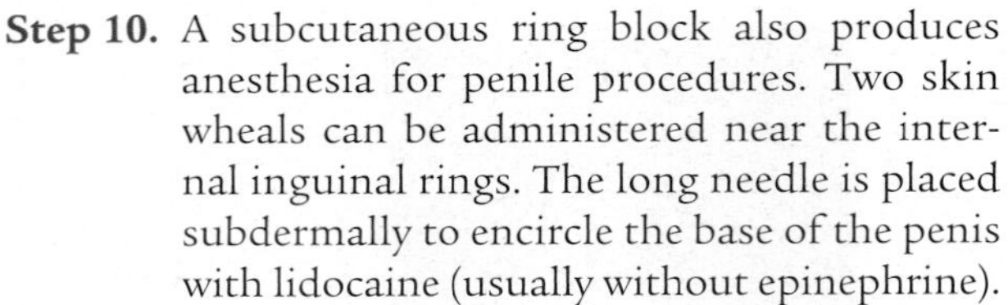

Step 10. A subcutaneous ring block also produces anesthesia for penile procedures. Two skin wheals can be administered near the internal inguinal rings. The long needle is placed subdermally to encircle the base of the penis with lidocaine (usually without epinephrine).

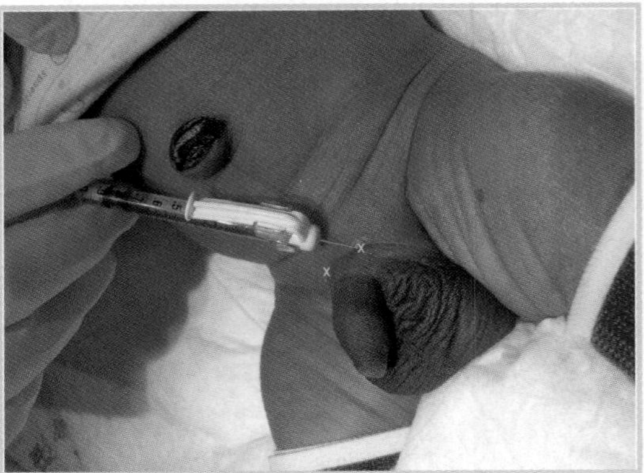

Step 10

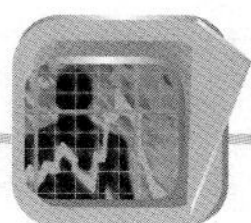

Complications

- Bleeding and hematoma formation.
- Allergic reaction is rare. Patients who believe they are allergic to lidocaine are more likely allergic to the preservative methylparaben. Preservative-free lidocaine is available, usually in single-use vials.
- Infection.
- Palpitations or feelings of warmth (due to epinephrine component).
- Temporary weakness or paralysis when large nerves are involved.
- If a large volume (10 to 20 mL) of local anesthetic is injected into a vein, it may produce convulsions, arrhythmias, or cardiac arrest. The plasma levels are usually 3 to 5 mcg/mL with regional nerve blocks. Toxicities may be observed at 6 mcg/mL but are more common at levels >10 mcg/mL.

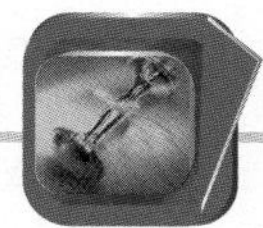

Pediatric Considerations

Children older than 6 years are dosed like adults except that the maximal dose is based on weight. The recommended maximal dose for lidocaine in children is 3 to 5 mg/kg, and 7 mg/kg when combined with epinephrine. Remember that 1% lidocaine is 10 mg/mL. Children 6 months to 3 years have the same volume of distribution and elimination half-life as adults. Neonates have an increased volume of distribution, decreased hepatic clearance, and doubled terminal elimination half-life (3.2 hours).

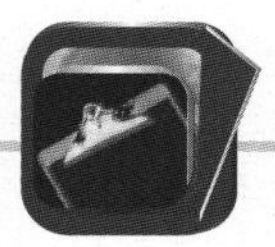

Postprocedure Instructions

Have the patient report any postprocedure local rashes or blistering that may indicate an adverse reaction or infection.

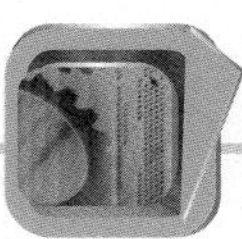

Coding Information and Supply Sources

Anesthesia codes (00100 to 01999) are usually limited to anesthesiologists providing patient services for surgical procedures. Local anesthesia is not reported in addition to the surgical procedure. Some insurance providers permit billing of regional or general anesthesia by the physician or surgeon performing the procedure. If reporting additional anesthesia services, the -47 modifier is attached to the surgical code. It is unlikely that additional reimbursement will be provided for field blocks; the service is considered part of the reporting of the surgical procedure.

Patient Education Handout

Patient education handouts, "Anesthesia for Circumcision" and "Local and Regional Anesthesia," can be found on the book's Web site.

Bibliography

Avina R. Primary care local and regional anesthesia in the management of trauma. *Clin Fam Pract.* 2000;2:533–550.

Bennett RG. *Fundamentals of Cutaneous Surgery.* Boston: Little, Brown; 1987:156–162.

Dinehart SM. Topical, local, and regional anesthesia. In: Wheeland RG, ed. *Cutaneous Surgery*. Philadelphia: WB Saunders; 1994:102–112.
Gmyrek R. Local anesthesia and regional nerve block anesthesia. Emedicine. http://www.emedicine.com/DERM/topic824.htm. Accessed August 13, 2008.
Grekin RC, Auletta MJ. Local anesthesia in dermatologic surgery. *J Am Acad Dermatol*. 1988;19:599–614.
Stegman SJ, Tromovitch TA, Glogau RG. *Basics of Dermatologic Surgery*. Chicago: Year Book Medical Publishing; 1982:29–30.
Swanson NA. *Atlas of Cutaneous Surgery*. Boston: Little, Brown; 1987:156–162.
Usatine RP, Moy RL. Anesthesia. In: Usatine RP, Moy RL, Tobinick EL, et al., eds. *Skin Surgery: A Practical Guide*. St. Louis: Mosby; 1998:20–30.
Williamson P. *Office Procedures*. Philadelphia: WB Saunders; 1957:325–339.
Winton GB. Anesthesia for dermatologic surgery. *J Dermatol Surg Oncol*. 1988;14:41–54.
Zuber TJ. Field block anesthesia. In: *Advanced Soft-Tissue Surgery*. Kansas City: American Academy of Family Physicians; 1998:22–26.
2008 MAG Mutual Healthcare Solutions, Inc.'s Physicians' Fee and Coding Guide. Duluth, Georgia. MAG Mutual Healthcare Solutions, Inc. 2007.

CHAPTER 3

Digital Nerve Block Anesthesia

E. J. Mayeaux, Jr., MD, DABFP, FAAFP

Professor of Family Medicine, Professor of Obstetrics and Gynecology
Louisiana State University Health Sciences Center, Shreveport, LA

Digital nerve block is commonly performed to provide anesthesia to an entire digit. Digital nerve block simultaneously anesthetizes the four digital nerves that traverse the sides of the digit. This technique provides longer duration of anesthesia than local infiltration and does not distort anatomic landmarks for digital surgery.

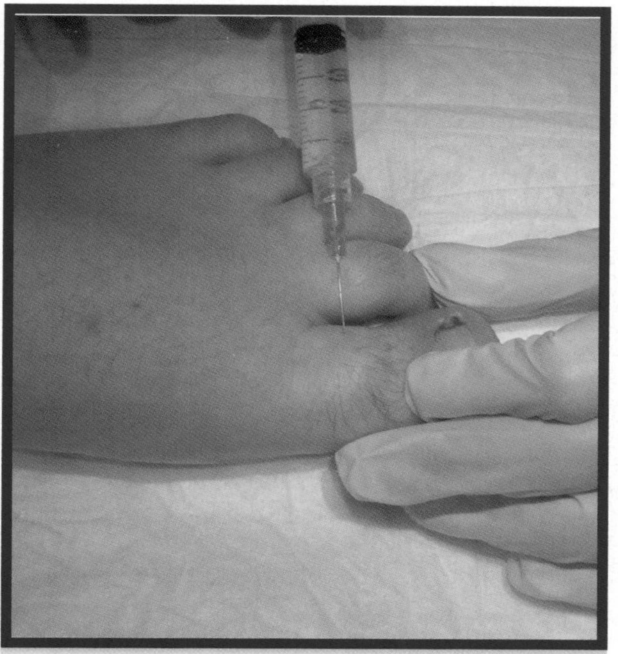

Because multiple nerves are affected during the technique, this anesthesia would be more appropriately labeled "digital field block" rather than the commonly used "nerve block." It has historically been called a "ring block" because of the circumferential infiltration of anesthetic. Administration of 1 to 3 mL of 2% lidocaine provides adequate anesthesia without use of a large volume. The great toe or thumb can also receive some additional superficial inervation proximally, and a slightly larger volume of solution may be needed for these digits. All digital blocks require some time for the anesthetic to take effect through the nerve sheath.

Historically, physicians were instructed to insert the needle into the web space to perform digital block. The advantage of a web space injection is that the nerve can be injected at the site of bifurcation between adjoining digits. However, the blood vessels of the web space are larger than on the digit, and intravascular injection of anesthetic can more easily occur with the web space technique.

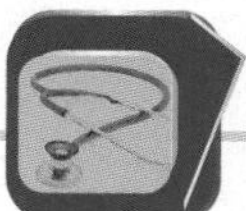

Equipment

- Syringes (3 or 5 mL), 2% lidocaine without epinephrine, and 25- or 27-gauge, 1.25-inch needles can be obtained from local surgical supply houses or pharmacies.
- A suggested anesthesia tray that can be used for this procedure is listed in Appendix F.

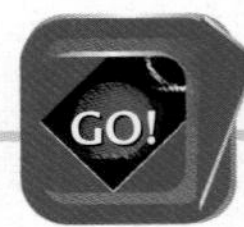

Indications

- Repair of digital lacerations
- Nail procedures (e.g., ingrown nail surgery, nail bed biopsy, nail removal)
- Incision and drainage of abscesses (e.g., felon surgery, paronychia surgery)
- Anesthesia for fracture or dislocation manipulation of digital orthopedic injuries
- Tumor or cyst removal or ablation (e.g., digital mucous cysts, giant cell tumors of sheaths, warts)

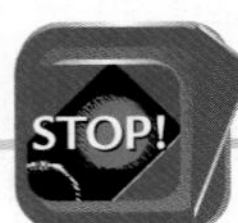

Contraindications

- Use of epinephrine added to lidocaine, especially in patients with peripheral vascular disease.
- Use of volumes >7 mL, especially in individuals with peripheral vascular disease, Raynaud disease or the phenomenon, digital vasculitis, or impaired circulation (e.g., diabetes, scleroderma).

The Procedure

Step 1. Cross section of the digit reveals the nerves traversing laterally on each side of the digit. One nerve travels on the plantar or palmar aspect, and one is more dorsal.

- PITFALL: The needle should be placed just below the dermis. Injecting the anesthetic into the dermis will not produce a satisfactory nerve block.

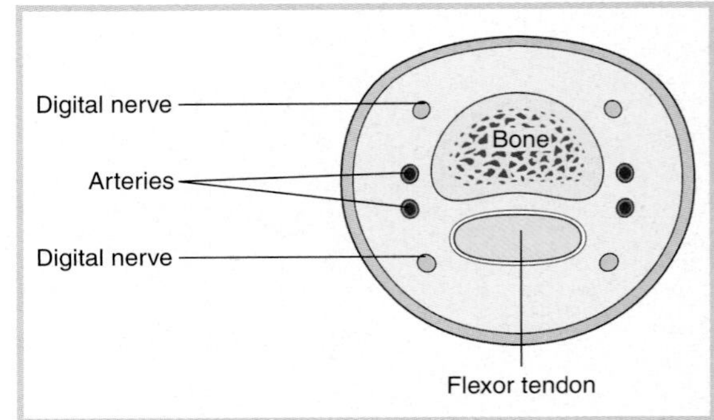

Step 1

Step 2. Prep the area with alcohol. Insert the needle near the junction of the dorsal and lateral surfaces of the digit. Slide the needle along the lateral surface, injecting as the needle tip is withdrawn back to the insertion site.

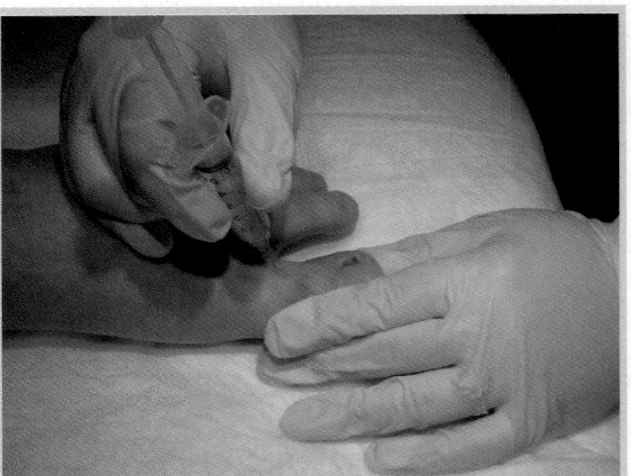

Step 2

Step 3. Without pulling the needle tip out of the skin, redirect the needle tip along the dorsum of the digit and again administer the anesthetic as the needle is withdrawn.

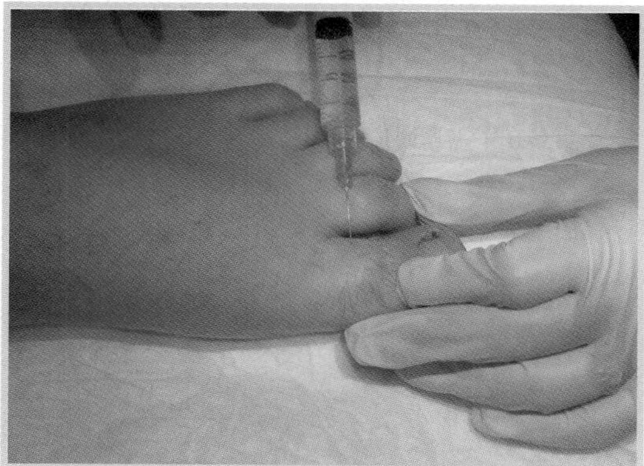

Step 3

Step 4. Administer the anesthetic along the opposite sides of the digit in a similar manner.

- PITFALL: In large digits or digits that do not develop good anesthesia at the tip, insert the needle near the junction of the volar and lateral surfaces of the digit and inject additional lidocaine along the volar surface.
- PITFALL: Do not attempt any assessment of anesthetic efficacy or the actual procedure until the block has had 5 minutes to work. Many novice and impatient physicians continue to add volume when a few more minutes of time would produce the desired effect, and the additional volume does not hasten the anesthesia.

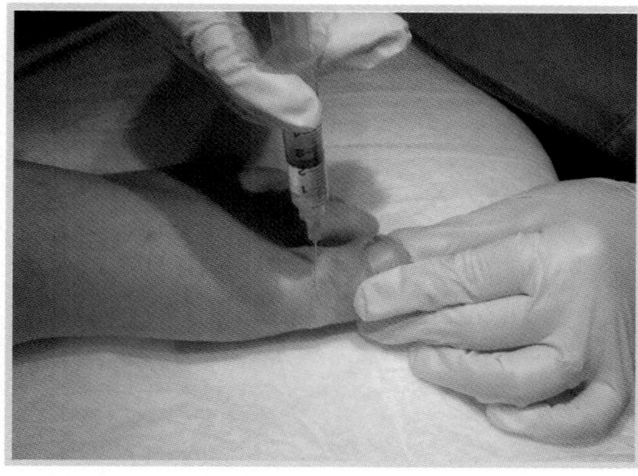

Step 4

Step 5. Smaller digits can be injected through a single insertion site. Enter the skin at the midline of the digit distal to where the toe joins the foot. Slide the needle down one lateral surface, injecting as the needle tip is withdrawn back to the insertion site. Without pulling the needle tip out of the skin, redirect the needle tip down the opposite side of the digit and administer the anesthetic as the needle is withdrawn.

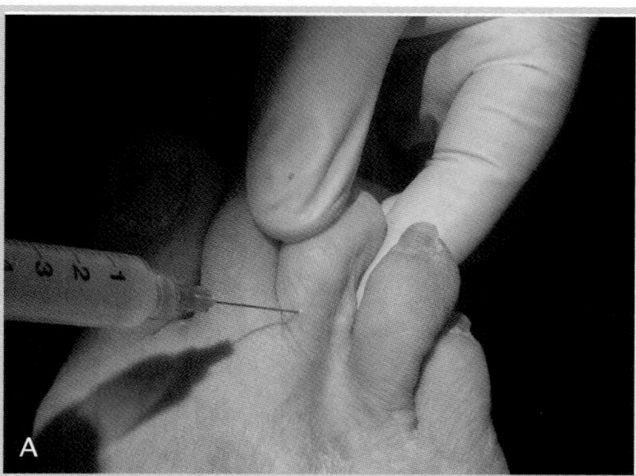

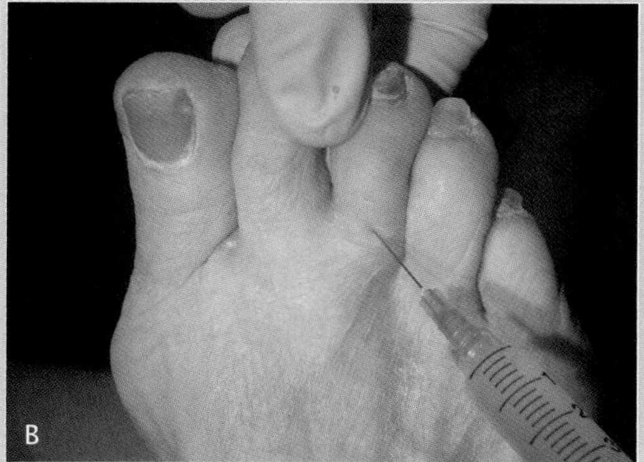

Step 5

Step 6. An alternate technique of digital block inserts the needle laterally into the base (proximal portion) of the digit, about halfway between the proximal interphalangeal joint and metacarpal interphalangeal joint.

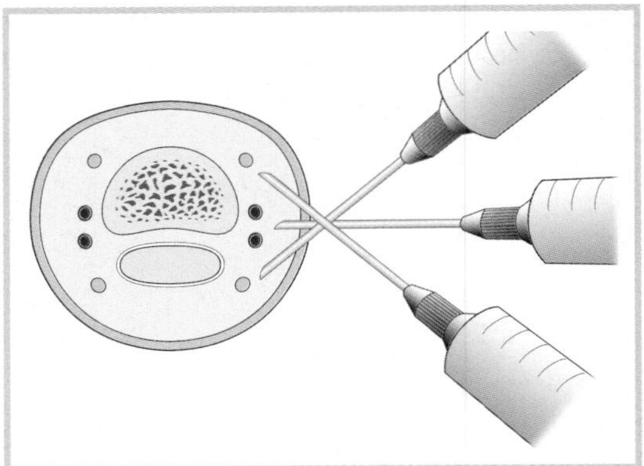

Step 6

Step 7. Insert the needle to the bone, and infuse anesthetic. Angle the needle volarly and dorsally. Repeat this technique on the opposite side.

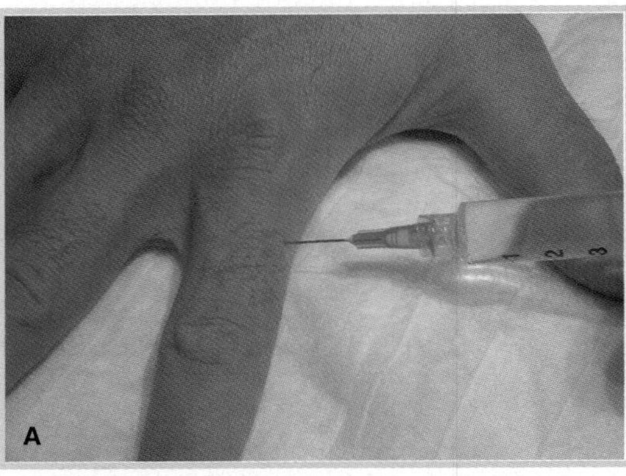

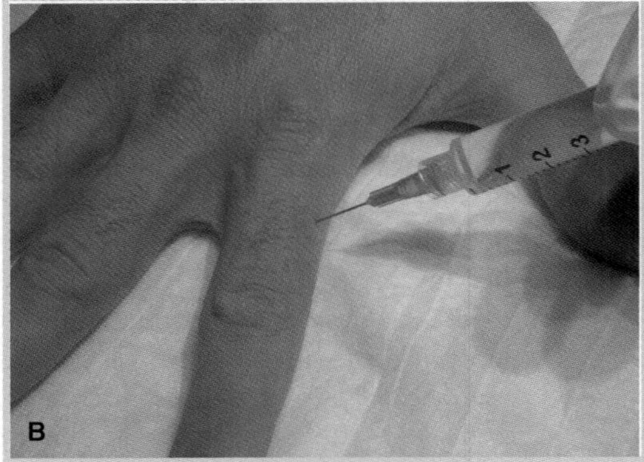

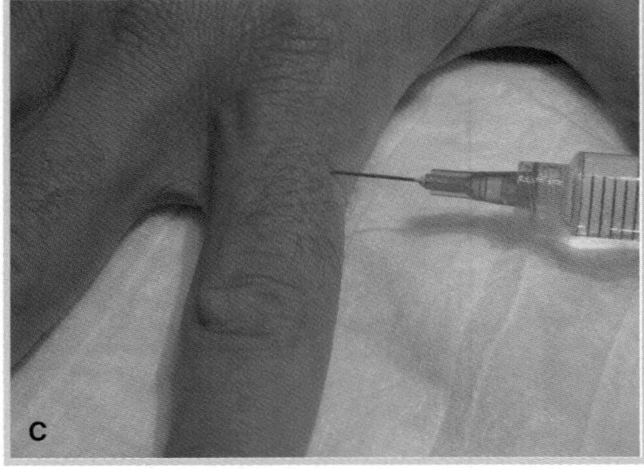

Step 7

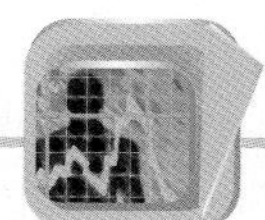

Complications

- Increasing rates of vascular compromise can be observed with circumferential infiltration, especially if volumes >7 to 8 mL are administered to the smaller digits. Use of 3- or 5-mL syringes can help avoid the temptation to deliver larger volumes.
- Impaired digital circulation can also occur if an individual suffers from vasospastic disease such as the Raynaud phenomenon or if the digit is markedly swollen before infiltration.
- Despite evidence for the safety of the practice, it is still advisable to avoid the addition of epinephrine to lidocaine for use on the digits.

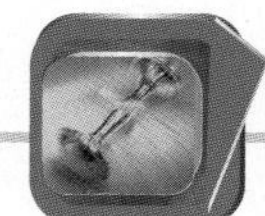

Pediatric Considerations

Children older than 6 years are dosed like adults except that the maximal dose is based on weight. Children 6 months to 3 years have the same volume of distribution and elimination half-life as in adults. Neonates have an increased volume of distribution, decreased hepatic clearance, and doubled terminal elimination half-life (3.2 hours). The recommended maximal dose for lidocaine in children younger than 6 years is 3 to 5 mg/kg, and 7 mg/kg when combined with epinephrine.

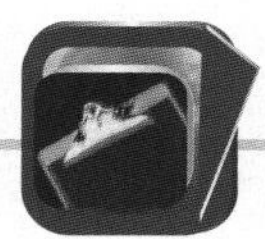

Postprocedure Instructions

Have the patient report redness, itching, or shortness of breath, which may signal an allergic reaction to lidocaine.

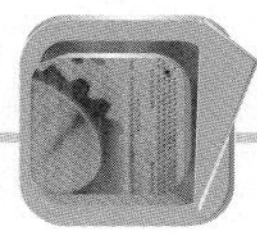

Coding Information and Supply Sources

No current procedural terminology (CPT) code exists for digital nerve block. The service is included in the reporting for the procedure for which it is performed (e.g., laceration repair, biopsy service).

Patient Education Handout

A patient education handout, "Digital Nerve Block," can be found on the book's Web site.

Bibliography

Avina R. Primary care local and regional anesthesia in the management of trauma. *Clin Fam Pract.* 2000;2:533–550.

Bartfield JM, Ford DT, Homer PJ. Buffered versus plain lidocaine for digital nerve blocks. *Ann Emerg Med.* 1993;22:216–219.

Brown JS. *Minor Surgery: A Text and Atlas.* 3rd ed. London: Chapman & Hall; 1997:52–62.

Dinehart SM. Topical, local, and regional anesthesia. In: Wheeland RG, ed. *Cutaneous surgery.* Philadelphia: WB Saunders; 1994:102–112.

Grekin RC, Auletta MJ. Local anesthesia in dermatologic surgery. *J Am Acad Dermatol.* 1988;19:599–614.

Knoop K, Trott A, Syverud S. Comparison of digital versus metacarpal blocks for repair of finger injuries. *Ann Emerg Med.* 1994;23:1296–1300.

Randle D, Driscoll CE. Administering local anesthesia. In: Driscoll CE, Rakel RE, eds. *Patient Care Procedures for Your Practice.* 2nd ed. Los Angeles: Practice Management Information Corporation; 1991:269–282.

Stegman SJ, Tromovitch TA, Glogau RG. *Basics of Dermatologic Surgery.* Chicago: Year Book Medical Publishing; 1982:23–31.

Usatine RP, Moy RL. Anesthesia. In: Usatine RP, Moy RL, Tobinick EL, Siegel DM, eds. *Skin Surgery: A Practical Guide*. St. Louis: Mosby; 1998:20–30.

Valvano MN, Leffler S. Comparison of bupivacaine and lidocaine/bupivacaine for local anesthesia/digital nerve block. *Ann Emerg Med.* 1996;27:490–492.

Waldbillig DK. Randomized double-blind controlled trial comparing room-temperature and heated lidocaine for digital nerve block. *Ann Emerg Med.* 1995;26:677–681.

Wardrope J, Smith JAR. *The Management of Wounds and Burns*. Oxford, UK: Oxford University Press, 1992:50–52.

Winton GB. Anesthesia for dermatologic surgery. *J Dermatol Surg Oncol.* 1988;14:41–54.

Woodside JR. Local and regional anesthesia of the upper extremity. In: Rakel RE, ed. *Saunders Manual of Medical Practice*. Philadelphia: WB Saunders; 1996:754–755.

Zuber TJ. Digital nerve block. In: *Advanced Soft-Tissue Surgery*. Kansas City: American Academy of Family Practice; 1998:34–38.

2008 MAG Mutual Healthcare Solutions, Inc.'s Physicians' Fee and Coding Guide. Duluth, Georgia. MAG Mutual Healthcare Solutions, Inc. 2007.

CHAPTER 4

Procedural (Conscious) Sedation

Thomas C. Arnold, MD

Associate Professor and Chairman, Department of Emergency Medicine
Louisiana State University Health Sciences Center, Shreveport, LA

Sean Denham, MD

Resident, Emergency Medicine Residency
LSU Health Sciences Center—Shreveport, Shreveport, LA

In the practice of medicine today, allowing a patient to experience unnecessary pain is unacceptable. In fact, the Joint Commission's recent attention to this issue has promoted the concept of pain as the "fifth vital sign" as we attempt to quantify and manage pain more aggressively. In no place is the anticipation of pain more acutely experienced by patients than in the application of many routine office-based, urgent care, or emergency department procedures that health-care providers are expected to provide on a daily basis. Although local and regional analgesia are very effective in a number of situations, there are many scenarios in which these techniques are not adequate, as a greater degree of analgesia and control are necessary to assure optimum results.

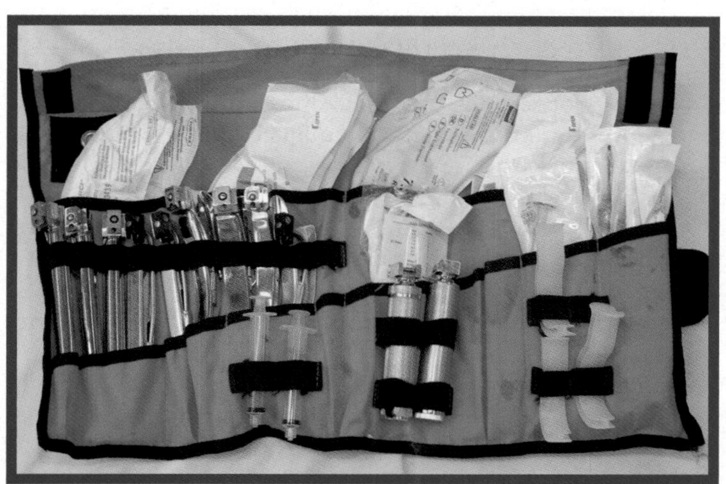

"Conscious" sedation is a misnomer commonly applied to this procedure. It is imprecise because the patient really is not conscious if the sedation is performed properly. The anesthesia term for the actual sedation level is *deep sedation*. In the acute care setting, *procedural sedation* is now the accepted terminology and more accurately describes what we are performing. The implication is that the depth and length of the sedation will be specific and tailored to the procedure to be performed.

The skill of applying procedural sedation safely and effectively requires practice and vigilance. The prudent practitioner will always focus on the patient during the sedation process while someone else attends to the procedure for which the sedation was required. Modern physiologic monitors have tremendously improved the safety of procedural sedation and should always be utilized to the extent available. Although blood pressure, heart rate, and pulse oximetry monitors are important, these physiologic parameters change late in the course of an apneic episode and may give the practitioner a false sense of security until emergent intervention is required. Conversely, monitors of respiratory effort such as capnography (end tidal CO_2 detection) have proven useful in detecting depressed respiratory effort and apnea quickly and allow intervention or adjustments to be made earlier in the process. These adjuncts are valuable safety enhancements and are slowly becoming standard practice for all procedural sedations.

Procedural sedation should be considered a complete procedure separate from the procedure for which the sedation is required. Informed consent with a clear explanation of risks and alternative options should be documented. It is helpful to have a procedural sedation packet containing all the required forms for consent, monitoring of induction, maintenance and recovery periods, and a checklist of equipment. Choice of agent(s) should be individualized to the needs of the patient and the experience and comfort of the practitioner. Procedural sedation has been performed safely by a large variety of practitioners in many practice settings and should become a routine tool for a variety of indications.

The modern practitioner has a myriad of choices concerning the agents for procedural sedation. To give a complete listing of all available agents would be beyond the scope of this text; therefore, we focus on three different drugs or drug combinations: an opiate and benzodiazepine combination (fentanyl [Actig]/midazolam [versed]), a sedative/hypnotic (propofol [Diprivan]), and a dissociative agent (ketamine).

Fentanyl is a very common opioid used for procedural sedation. Its popularity can be attributed to several factors including its rapid onset, brief duration of action, rapid reversibility by naloxone (Narcan), and lack of histamine release. Fentanyl is approximately 100 times more potent than morphine and has no intrinsic anxiolytic or amnestic properties. The effects of fentanyl can be rapidly and completely reversed with opioid antagonists (naloxone). Because anxiolysis and sedation do not occur at low doses of fentanyl (1 to 2 mcg/kg), the concurrent administration of a benzodiazepine, commonly midazolam is recommended. The combination of fentanyl and midazolam remains one of the most popular procedural sedation regimens in children, with a strong safety and efficacy profile when both drugs are carefully titrated to effect. Any necessary level of mild to deep sedation can be achieved using these agents.

Ketamine is a dissociative agent that provides sedation, analgesia, and amnesia. It has been demonstrated to be a safe and effective anesthetic dissociative in a variety of settings. It has been widely used worldwide since its introduction in 1970 and has demonstrated a remarkable safety profile in a variety of settings. Ketamine differs from all other procedural sedation agents in several important ways. First, it uniquely preserves cardiopulmonary stability. Upper-airway muscular tone and protective airway reflexes are maintained. Spontaneous respiration is preserved, although when administered intravenously (IV), ketamine must be given slowly (over 1 to 2 minutes) to prevent respiratory depression. Second, it differs from other agents in that it lacks the characteristic dose-response continuum to progressive titration. However, practitioners administering ketamine must be especially knowledgeable about the unique actions of this drug and the numerous contraindications to its use.

Propofol is a sedative-hypnotic agent that is unrelated to barbiturates or benzodiazepines. Given by IV bolus or by using an infusion pump, this drug can induce deep sedation or general anesthesia within 1 minute. Recovery following discontinuation averages 5 to 15 minutes, even after prolonged administration. Propofol exhibits inherent antiemetic and perhaps euphoric properties, and patient satisfaction is typically high. The adverse effects of this drug are potent respiratory and cardiovascular depression. However, recent studies continue to add to propofol's already growing body of evidence of its strong safety profile. Propofol has become quite popular with practitioners who frequently perform procedural sedation, primarily because of the rapid patient recovery when this agent is used.

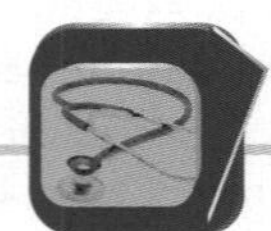

Equipment

Noninvasive monitoring equipment to monitor oxygenation (pulse oximetry), hemodynamics (blood pressure), and ventilation (capnography) should be utilized during the sedation procedure to the extent available.

- Airway management devices:
  - Oxygen source
  - Bag-valve mask
  - Equipment for rapid sequence intubation (see Chapter 17, Endotracheal Intubation)
  - Suction apparatus
- Agent(s) for sedation

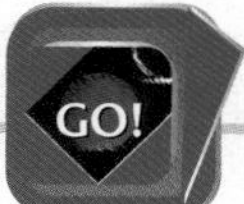

Indications

- Foreign-body removal: ears of children, rectum of adults
- Incision and drainage of an abscess: if local anesthesia is inadequate
- Imaging in children
- Complicated laceration repair in children
- Simple reduction of dislocated joints
- Closed reduction of fractures
- Reduction of fracture dislocations
- Wound management: debridement, significant pain, large surface area, severe burns

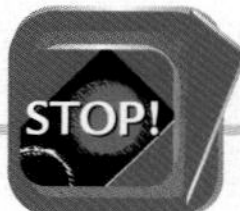

Contraindications

- Patient refusal in a competent individual
- Severe clinical instability requiring immediate attention
- Hemodynamic or respiratory compromise
- Altered sensorium or inability to monitor side effects

Although safely sedating patients at the extremes of age is challenging and requires additional care, age is not a contraindication to procedural sedation.

The Procedure

Step 1. Preparation. Written informed consent should be obtained and documented in the patient record (see Appendix A). Obtain intravenous access. Assemble appropriate patient monitoring devices including heart rhythm (electrocardiographic), blood pressure, oximetry, and backup airway management devices such as a bag-valve mask and oral airways and intubating equipment.

- **PEARL:** Peripheral access is usually sufficient with a catheter size large enough to provide resuscitation fluids if necessary.

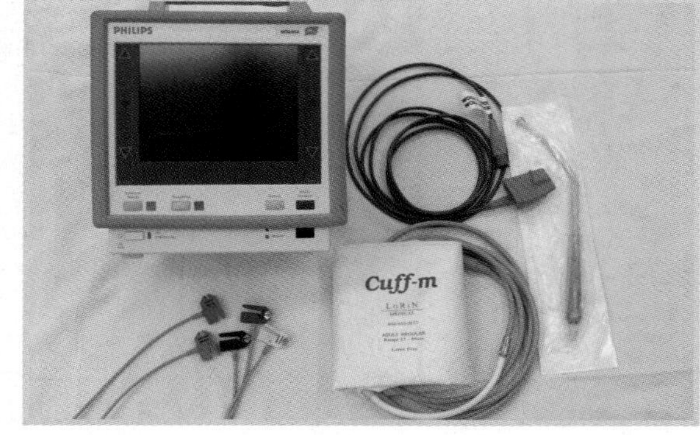

Step 1

■ **PEARL:** Recent studies have shown support for preoxygenation and capnography, which may add to the safety of procedural sedation by detecting hypoventilation earlier than clinical assessment and pulse oximetry alone.

Step 2. Administer sedation agents while monitoring the patient. Recommended doses are shown in Table 4-1. Administration of the sedating agents should proceed slowly with gradual titration to the desired depth depending on the procedure being performed and length of time sedation will be necessary. The practitioner administering the procedural sedation should maintain vigilant observation of respiratory effort, airway patency, and vital signs while not becoming distracted by the procedure being performed.

■ **PEARL:** Titrate the procedural sedation to the point that the patient's pain is relieved. This point will vary between procedures and during different parts of procedures.

■ **PITFALL:** The most common clinical errors are delayed recognition of respiratory depression and respiratory arrest, inadequate monitoring, and inadequate resuscitation.

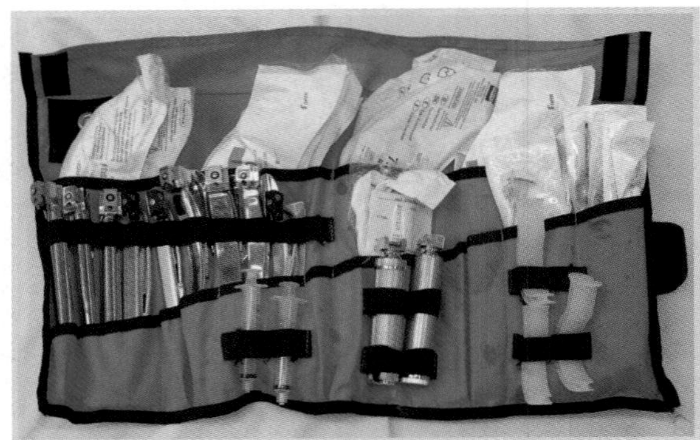

Step 1

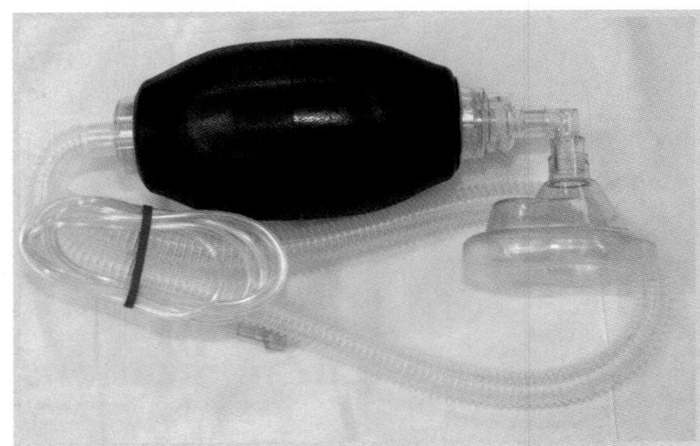

Step 1

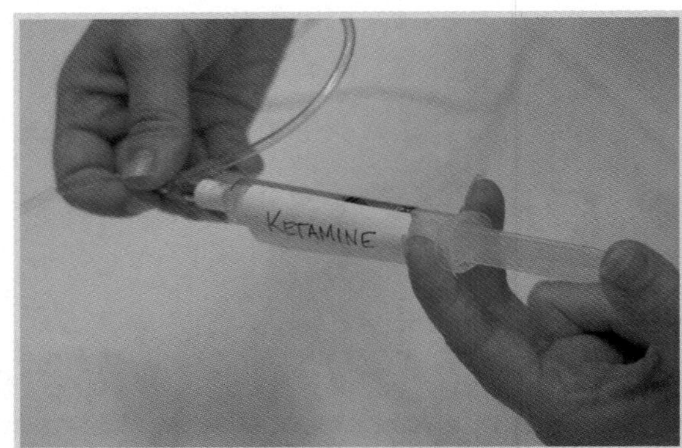

Step 2

TABLE 4-1. Drugs Used and Doses for Procedural Sedation and Analgesia

Agent	Adult Dose	Pediatric Dose
Propofol	1 mg/kg bolus, then 0.5 mg/kg every 3 min as needed IV	1 mg/kg IV
Ketamine	1–2 mg/kg IV	1–1.5 mg/kg IV; 3 mg/kg IM
Fentanyl[a]	1–2 mcg/kg IV	2 mcg/kg IV/IM
Midazolam[a]	0.01 mg/kg IV	0.05–0.1 mg/kg IV (max dose of 2 mg)

[a]Used in tendem.

Step 3. The postprocedure management phase is critical and includes close observation of all monitoring parameters until the patient is fully conscious.

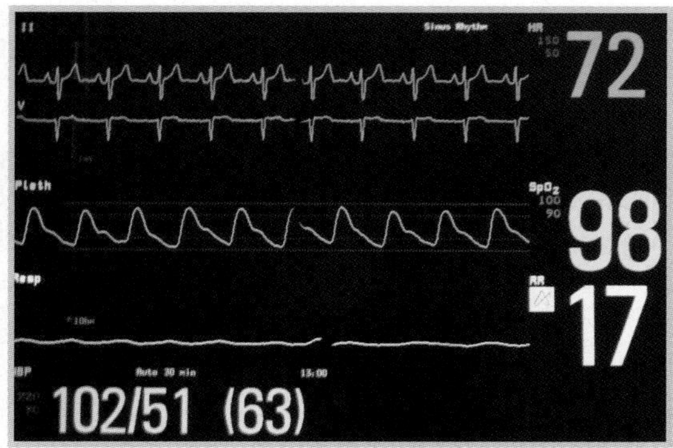

Step 3

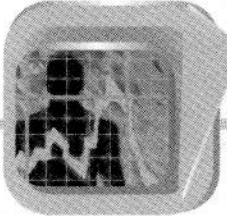

Complications

- Delayed awakening.
- Agitation.
- Nausea and vomiting.
- Cardiorespiratory events.
- Tachycardia.
- Bradycardia.
- Hypoxia.
- Respiratory depression: Like all opioids, fentanyl can cause respiratory depression. When respiratory depression occurs with fentanyl/midazolam procedural sedation, usually it is due primarily to fentanyl. As the opioid effect is most pronounced on the central nervous system respiratory centers, apnea can precede loss of consciousness. Caution must be exercised when using benzodiazepines and opioids together, because the risks of hypoxia and apnea are significantly greater than when either is used alone.
- Hallucinatory "emergence reactions": These have been reported in up to 30% of adults receiving ketamine (although rare in children) and can be fascinating and pleasurable or alternatively unpleasant and nightmarish. Concurrent benzodiazepines are believed to blunt but not entirely eliminate such reactions in adults, and apprehension regarding such unpleasant recoveries has limited the popularity of ketamine.

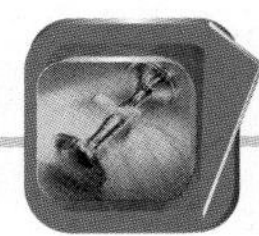

Pediatric Considerations

See pediatric doses in Table 4-1. Because children cannot reliably judge how impaired they are after the procedure, they should be monitored closely for 2 hours after the procedure by responsible adults.

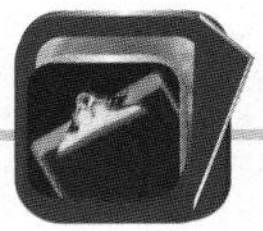

Postprocedure Instructions

All patients receiving procedural sedation should be monitored until they are no longer at risk for cardiorespiratory depression. To be discharged, they should be alert and oriented (or returned to age-appropriate baseline), and vital signs should be stable. All patients should leave the hospital with a reliable adult who will observe them after discharge for postprocedure complications. It is desirable to document the name of the individual on the hospital record. Even though patients may appear awake and able to comprehend instructions, they may not remember details once they leave the facility.

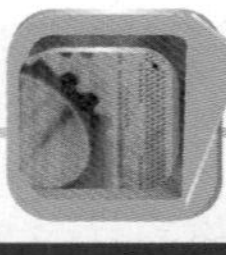

Coding Information and Supply Sources

CPT Code	Description	2008 Average 50th Percentile Fee	Global Period
99143	Moderate conscious sedation services provided by the same physician performing the diagnostic or therapeutic service—first 30 minutes	$118.00	0
99144	Age 5 or older—first 30 minutes of intraservice time	$115.00	0
99145	Each additional 15 minutes of intraservice time	$53.00	0
99148	Moderate conscious sedation services by a physician other than the healthcare professional performing the service	$183.00	0
99149	Age 5 years or older—first 30 minutes of intraservice time	$166.00	0
99150	Each additional 15 minutes of intraservice time	$64.00	0

2008 average 50th Percentile Fees are provided courtesy of 2008 MMH-SI's copyrighted Physicians' Fees and Coding Guide.

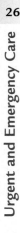

- Physiologic monitors and laryngoscope devices can be ordered directly from Welch Allyn at http://www.welchallyn.com/ or through their corporate headquarters at 4341 State Street Road, Skaneateles Falls, New York, 13153-0220. Phone: 1-800-535-6663.
- Other airway supplies can be ordered from Mallinckrodt at http://www.mallinckrodt.com/ or their corporate headquarters, 675 McDonnell Blvd. Hazelwood, MO 63042. Phone: 314-654-2000.

Patient Education Handout

Two patient education handouts, "Adult Disposition Instructions after PSA" and "Pediatric Disposition Instructions after PSA," can be found on the book's companion Web site.

Bibliography

Cote CJ, Karl HW, Notterman DA, et al. Adverse sedation events in pediatrics: a critical incident analysis of contributing factors. *Pediatrics* 2000;105:805.

Chudnofsky CR, Wright SW, Dronen SC, et al. The safety of fentanyl use in the emergency department. *Ann Emerg Med.* 1989;18:635.

Gottschling S, Meyer S, Reinhard H, Furtwangler R, Klotz D, Graf N. Intraindividual propofol dosage variability in children undergoing repetitive procedural sedations. *Pediatr Hematol Oncol.* 2006;23(7):571–578.

Green SM, Clem KJ, Rothrock SG. Ketamine safety profile in the developing world—survey of practitioners. *Acad Emerg Med.* 1996;3:598.

Mensour M, Pineau R, Sahai V, et al. Emergency department procedural sedation and analgesia: a Canadian Community Effectiveness and Safety Study (ACCESS). *Can J Emerg Med Care* 2006;8(2):94–99.

Pena BMG, Krauss B. Adverse events of procedural sedation and analgesia in a pediatric emergency department. *Ann Emerg Med.* 1999;34:483.

Sacchetti A, Senula G, Strickland J, et al. Procedural sedation in the community emergency department: initial results of the ProSCED registry. *Acad Emerg Med.* 2006;14(1):41–46.

2008 MAG Mutual Healthcare Solutions, Inc.'s Physicians' Fee and Coding Guide. Duluth, Georgia. MAG Mutual Healthcare Solutions, Inc. 2007.

CHAPTER 5

Arterial Puncture and Line Placement

E. J. Mayeaux, Jr., MD, DABFP, FAAFP
Professor of Family Medicine, Professor of Obstetrics and Gynecology
Louisiana State University Health Sciences Center, Shreveport, LA

Clint N. Wilson, MD
Chief Resident, Family Medicine Residency
Louisiana State University Health Sciences Center, Shreveport, LA

Arterial puncture is a commonly employed procedure to obtain arterial blood for analysis. For most single-time samples in emergent and urgent situations, the single arterial puncture (stick) is adequate. Intra-arterial line placement is often used in situations that require access for frequent blood sampling and for real-time blood pressure monitoring.

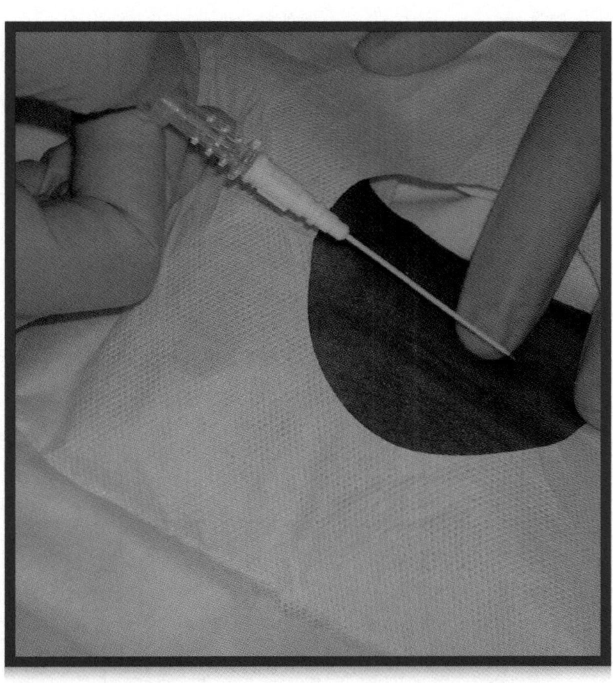

Arterial puncture is usually done using the radial artery and is performed by physicians and physician extenders, respiratory therapists, and other trained personnel. Arterial blood samples can be used for blood gas analysis, including measurement of the partial pressures of oxygen (PaO_2) and carbon dioxide ($PaCO_2$) and the pH of arterial blood. These values help the physician assess pulmonary function, establish diagnoses, direct further interventions, and determine the required intensity of monitoring in critically ill patients.

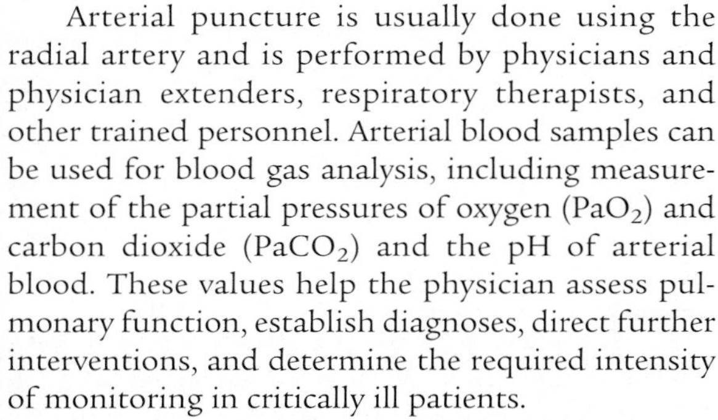

Intra-arterial lines (arterial line, art-line, or a-line) are used as an invasive blood pressure monitoring method and for continuous access to blood vessels for frequent blood sampling. Blood pressure must be monitored closely when the patient is in shock, during a hypertensive emergency, and during vasopressor use. No data exist to support a specific site, but arterial lines are most commonly placed in the radial, brachial, or femoral arteries (a radial insertion is illustrated). A guidewire may be used during placement of an arterial line, or a direct puncture approach may be taken.

Prior to radial artery puncture or arterial line insertion, an Allen test should be performed to assess collateral blood flow of the hand. To perform the Allen test, wrap your fingers around the patient's wrist and compress both the ulnar and radial arteries. As you are doing this, have the patient elevate and then open and close his or her hand several times to allow blood to drain from the hand. Afterward, open the patient's hand and see that it has blanched white. Release pressure from the ulnar artery, keeping the radial artery occluded. Within 2 to 3 seconds, normal skin color should return to first the ulnar side of the palm and then the entire palm shortly thereafter. If the hand remains white, collateral circulation is inadequate and radial artery puncture or arterial line is contraindicated.

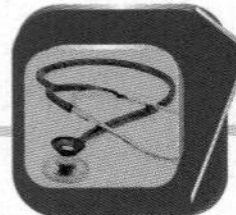

Equipment

- Arterial line kit
- Arterial line monitoring equipment (as needed)
- Pulse Doppler (as needed)

See Appendix E for skin cleansing recommendations and Appendix F for local anesthetic recommendations.

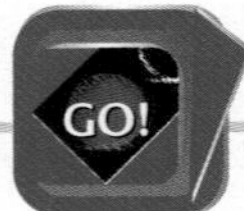

Indications

- Close monitoring of blood pressure (e.g., intensive care unit setting)
- Access to arterial blood (frequent arterial blood gasses)
- Frequent blood draws for laboratory tests
- Continuous monitoring of oxygen saturation

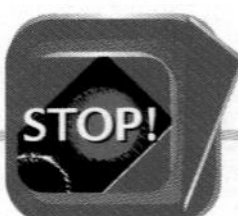

Contraindications (Relative)

- Dermatitis or cellulitis at insertion site
- Absence of palpable pulse at chosen arterial site
- Severe coagulopathy or platelet count <50,000
- Uncooperative patient
- Poor collateral circulation at proposed site (absolute contraindication)

The Procedure

Step 1. Obtain informed consent from the patient or proxy (see Appendix A). Perform the Allen test to assess adequate collateral arterial flow. Flush the arterial line tubing with normal saline to reduce risk of an air embolus. Check the kit to make sure all of the necessary components are present. Place the patient's hand in anatomical position (palm up) and secure the wrist at a gentle extension (approximately 30 to 45 degrees).

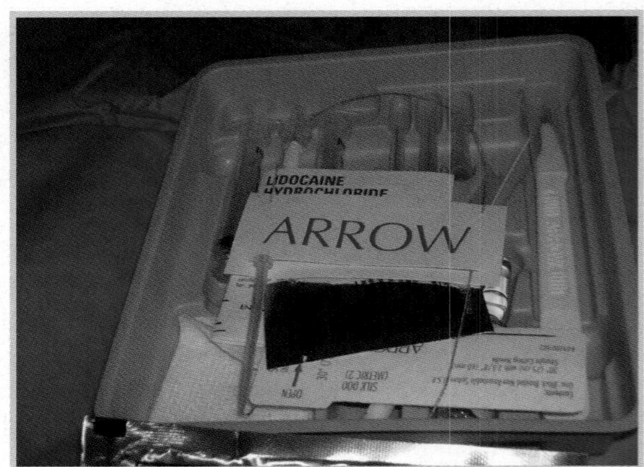

Step 1

Step 2. Prep the skin over the proposed puncture site. Arterial line kits usually will come with skin cleaning supplies, but a separate chlorhexidine swab can be used instead (see Appendix E).

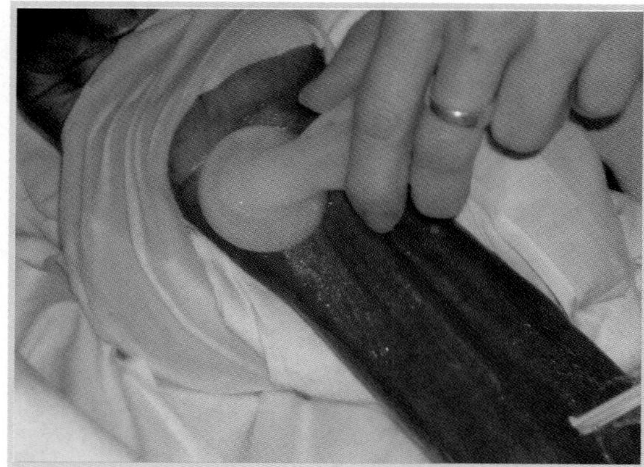

Step 2

Step 3. Drape the area per proper aseptic technique. Again, arterial line kits will usually provide a paper drape, but some practitioners prefer to use sterile towels or cloths.

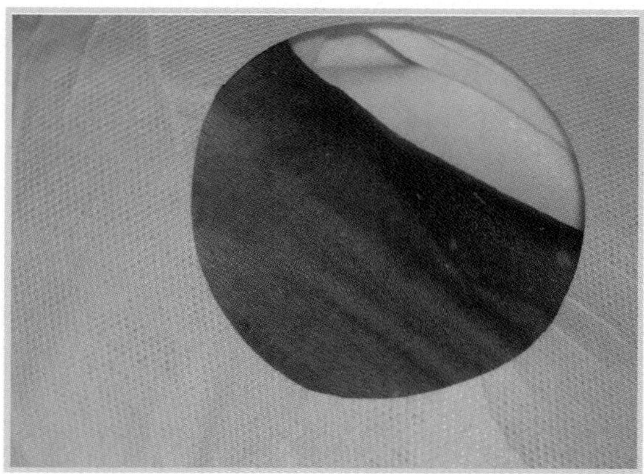

Step 3

Step 4. Anesthetize the skin over the site with 3 to 5 mL of 1% to 2% lidocaine. (Be aware that excess fluid can diminish the pulse strength and/or distort anatomy.)

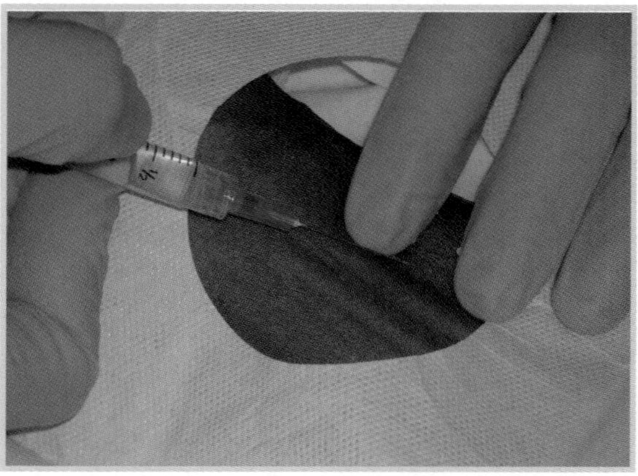

Step 4

Step 5. With the nondominant hand, gently palpate the artery. With the dominant hand, hold the intravascular catheter (an outer guidewire over a needle) with the needle bevel up and at a 30- to 45-degree angle.

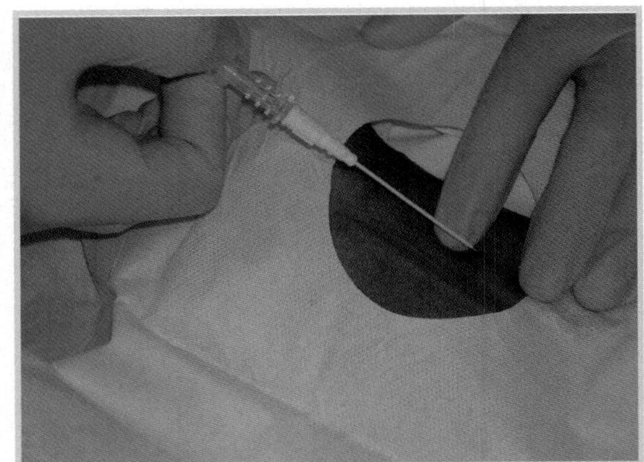

Step 5

Step 6. Puncture the skin and advance the needle slowly at the site of arterial pulsation.

- **PEARL:** At this point, some physicians like to make a superficial nick in the skin at the site of insertion to ease the passage of the intravascular catheter, but this is not necessary.

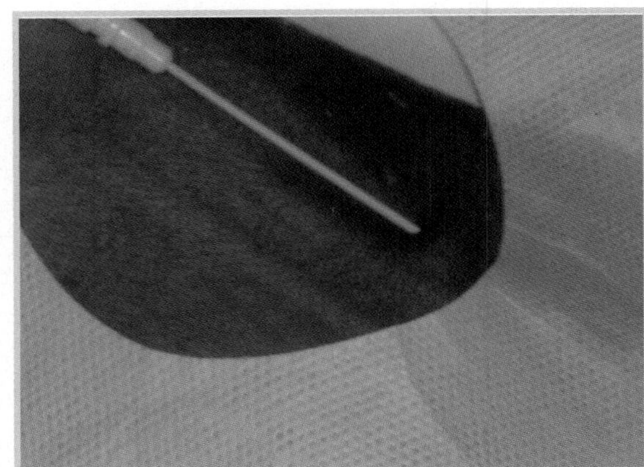

Step 6

Step 7. Advance until a flash of blood appears in the syringe. Once this flash is obtained, slowly advance the outer catheter into the artery, simultaneously removing the needle. If the arterial puncture was for a one-time arterial blood draw, the needle and catheter would be removed at this point, with a dressing placed on the site after appropriate pressure is held at the site for approximately 5 minutes.

- **PEARL:** The arterial line kit will come with a guidewire that can be used to assist in placement, especially in arterial lines not placed in the radial artery.

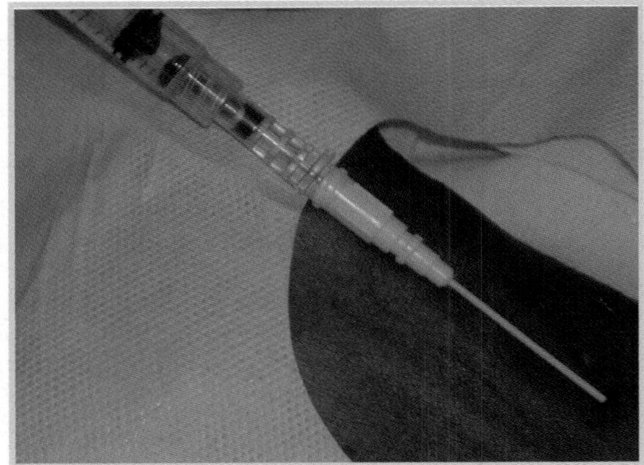

Step 7

Step 8. Upon removing the needle, pulsatile blood return should be observed. At this point, connect the arterial line transducer tubing to the tip of the catheter. After ensuring the line is in a good place and a good waveform is seen on the arterial line monitors, secure your line to the skin with the suture provided. Once it is secure, place an occlusive dressing at the site.

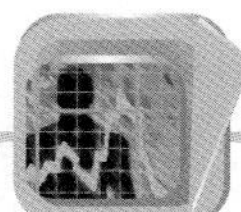

Complications

- Local infection, pain, and bleeding
- Blood clotting in the catheter
- Nerve injury
- Ischemic changes to the hand and wrist

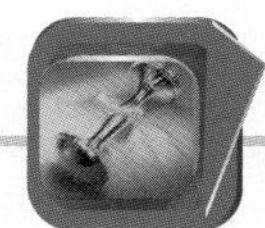

Pediatric Considerations

In the pediatric population, the ulnar artery may be used as a primary site as long as the Allen test for good radial collateral circulation is checked first. The patient's ability to cooperate also should be considered before deciding to attempt any procedure.

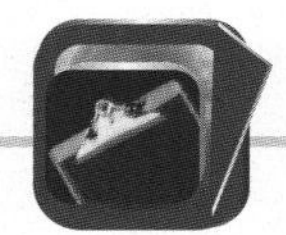

Postprocedure Instructions

Arterial line catheters are not changed on a routine basis; rather, the site is monitored closely for signs of infection and changed based on clinical judgment. However, all arterial lines placed in emergent situations should be replaced. The dressing should be kept clean, dry, and intact and be changed as necessary.

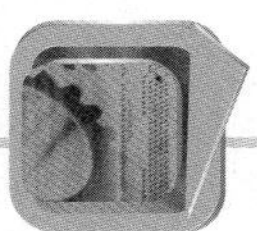

Coding Information and Supply Sources

CPT Code	Description	2008 Average 50th Percentile Fee	Global Period
36600	Arterial puncture, withdrawal of blood for diagnosis	$84.00	0
36620	Arterial catherization or cannulation for sampling, monitoring, or transfusion (separate procedure); percutaneous	$307.00	0

CPT is a registered trademark of the American Medical Association.
2008 average 50th Percentile Fees are provided courtesy of 2008 MMH-SI's copyrighted Physicians' Fees and Coding Guide.

Supplies may be purchased from these companies:

- Arrow Medical Products Ltd., 2400 Bernville Road, Reading, PA 19605. Phone: 1-800-233-3187. Web site: http://www.arrowintl.com/.
- Baxter, 1 Baxter Pkwy., Deerfield, IL, 60015-4625. Phone: 847-948-2000. Fax: 847 948-3642. Web site: http://www.baxter.com.
- American Hospital Supply. Phone: 407-475-1168. Web site: http://www.americanhospitalsupply.com/.
- Cardinal Health, Inc., 7000 Cardinal Place, Dublin, OH 43017. Phone: 800-234-8701. Web site: http://www.cardinal.com/.
- Owens and Minor, 4800 Cox Road, Glen Allen, VA 23060-6292. Phone: 804-747-9794. Fax: 804-270-7281.

Patient Education Handout

A patient education handout, “Arterial Puncture,” can be found on the book’s Web site.

Bibliography

Beards SC, Doedens L, Jackson A, Lipman J. A comparison of arterial lines and insertion techniques in critically ill patients. *Anaesthesia* 1994;49:968.

Gabel-Hughes KS, Geelhoed, GW. Methods of arterial site skin preparation and dressing. *Critical Care Nurse* 1990;10(5):90–96.

Lightowler JV, Elliot MW. Local anaesthetic infiltration prior to arterial puncture for blood gas analysis: a survey of current practice and a randomised double blind placebo controlled trial. *J R Coll Physicians Lond.* 1997;31:645.

Shiver S, Blaivas M, Lyon M. A prospective comparison of ultrasound-guided and blindly placed radial arterial catheters. *Acad Emerg Med.* 2006;13(12):1275–1279.

Ventriglia WJ. Arterial blood gases. *Emerg Med Clin N Am.* 1986;4:235–251.

Weiss BM, Galtiker RI. Complications during and following radial artery cannulation: a prospective study. *Intensive Care Med.* 1986;14:424.

2008 MAG Mutual Healthcare Solutions, Inc.’s Physicians’ Fee and Coding Guide. Duluth, Georgia. MAG Mutual Healthcare Solutions, Inc. 2007.

CHAPTER 6

Central Venous Catheter Placement

Daniel E. Melville, MD, ABFM
Bourbon Medical Center, Paris, KY

Sonya C. Melville, MD
Assistant Professor of Emergency Medicine
University of Kentucky Medical Center, Lexington, KY

Stephen Taylor, MD, FAAFP
Associate Professor of Family Medicine
North Caddo Medical Center, Vivian, LA

Central venous catheters are often inserted for a variety of clinical indications. In 1953, Sven-Ivar Seldinger introduced the technique of placing a central venous catheter by threading the catheter over a guidewire. This process, known as the Seldinger technique, is currently the most common and accepted method of facilitating cannulation of large vessels. Several advantages to using the Seldinger technique include the use of a smaller and safer needle for insertion, the ability to use a venodilator to establish large-bore catheters if higher flow rates are needed, the flexibility to exchange different catheters without repeated punctures, and the use of a J-wire, reducing risk of perforation.

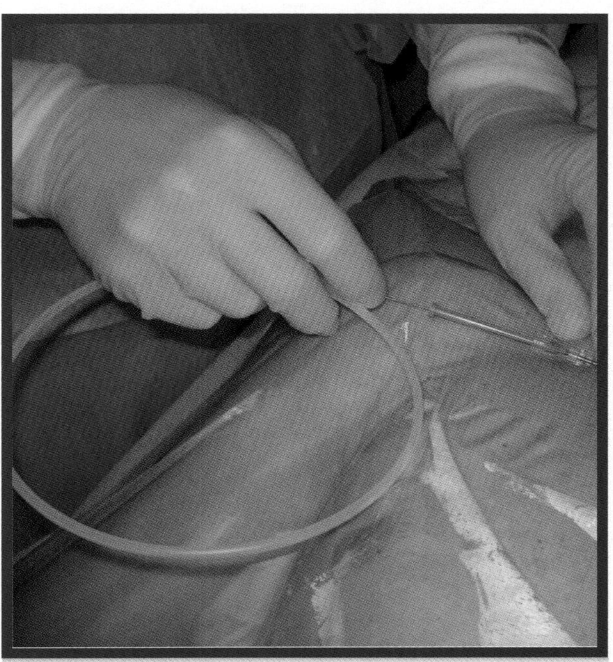

Central venous catheters can be inserted into the internal jugular, external jugular, subclavian, femoral, or brachial veins. The optimal site of insertion is influenced by operator preference, experience, patient anatomy, and clinical circumstances. The subclavian vein is the most commonly used site for central venous access. The femoral vein is the second most commonly used site and is used when access is required distally from an injury, during resuscitative measures so that cardiopulmonary resuscitative measures do not need to be stopped while venous access is established, or when the vessels of the upper body are not suitable for cannulation. Therefore, subclavian and femoral venous line placements are discussed in further detail later in this chapter.

An important concept to establishing vascular access lines is to understand the indication. At times a large-caliber peripheral intravenous catheter is preferred. For example, when a rapid bolus of large quantities of fluids is required to correct a hypovolemic shock state, a shorter length of a peripheral catheter with a large-bore radius is imperative. This concept follows the Poiseuille law, which can be summarized to state that the rate of flow is proportional to the fourth power of the radius of the cannula and inversely related to its length. Simply stated, short catheters with large diameters are more appropriate for rapid infusion rates.

Of note, ultrasound visualization of the central vein while puncture is attempted is becoming more readily available to ease cannulation. Ultrasound assistance reduces the number of punctures necessary for cannulation to establish central access and reduces the incidence of complications. It should be considered particularly if vascular anomalies or body habitus impede identification of traditional landmarks.

Standard precautions and preparation should be followed universally by all operators to prevent complications and reduce risk of infection. All providers should use an alcohol-based hand sanitizer or antimicrobial soap immediately prior to donning sterile gloves. The skin of the patient should be properly prepped with a chlorhexidine solution by rubbing back and forth with a sponge or gauze for a minimum of 30 seconds (see Appendix E). Once applied, the chlorhexidine solution should be allowed to air dry for at least 2 minutes and should not be wiped or blotted. If chlorhexidine cannot be applied because of an allergy or unavailability, a povidone-iodine solution can be applied in a similar fashion. Ideally, a sterile full-body drape should be placed on the patient. The Centers for Disease Control and Prevention recommend abiding by standard precautions of wearing a face mask, eye protection, cap, sterile and water-impervious gown, and sterile gloves prior to beginning procedures.

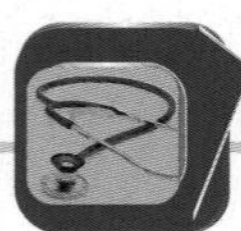

Equipment

- One multilumen indwelling catheter: size varies depending on location and reason
- One spring-wire guide: straight soft tip on one end with a J-tip on the other end
- One fastener: catheter clamp
- One introducer needle: 18-gauge with a 12-mL syringe
- One injection needle: 22-gauge with a 5-mL syringe
- One injection needle: 25-guage with a 3-mL syringe
- Skin prep materials (see Appendix E)
- One 5-mL ampule of HCL, 1% lidocaine solution
- One tissue dilator
- One drape: 24 × 36 inches with 4-inch fenestration
- Two gauze pads: 2 × 2 inches
- Five gauze pads: 4 × 4 inches
- One no. 11 scalpel
- One suture: 3-0 silk with cutting needle

The instruments can be ordered individually or in a prepackaged sterile kit from companies such as Arrow International, Inc., Reading, Pennsylvania.

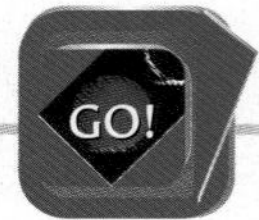

Indications

- To allow administration of numerous medications simultaneously, such as total parenteral nutrition, chemotherapy, and pressor agents
- To administer drugs that have a higher risk of causing phlebitis when given through a peripheral intravenous catheter
- To establish access to the central circulation if a pulmonary artery catheter or pacemaker placement is necessary
- To gain access to central circulation if peripheral veins cannot be cannulated

- To gain access for hemodynamic monitoring, such as to facilitate measurement of central venous pressure and venous oxyhemoglobin saturation
- To facilitate plasmapheresis, apheresis, hemodialysis, or continuous renal replacement therapy

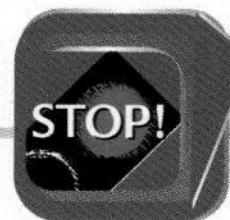

Contraindications

- Injury distal to the vessel to be cannulated
- Wounds directly over the cannulation site
- Infection or overlying cellulitis in area around vessel to be cannulated
- If the vessel to be cannulated has a known thrombus

Caution should be used when establishing a central venous access site in an area in which hygiene or a clean field would be compromised. For instance, avoid femoral line placement in a patient with fecal or urinary incontinence to avoid potential contamination and subsequent infection, or if a patient has a poor body habitus and excess pannus could potentially cover the cannulation site, again raising concerns of infection.

A patient who is on warfarin (Coumadin), or other blood-thinning agents, or has a known coagulopathy can still have a central line established, although the patient should be approached cautiously, recognizing the potential complications of excessive bleeding.

The Procedure

Subclavian Venipuncture (Infraclavicular Approach) using the Seldinger Technique

Step 1. Place the patient in a supine position. Prep the skin with povidone-iodine or chlorhexidine solution well around the venipuncture site and drape the area (see Appendix E). Standard precautions of sterile gloves, sterile gown, mask, cap, and eye protection should be followed.

- **PEARL:** Place the patient in a Trendelenburg position of at least 15 degrees down to distend the neck veins and reduce the risk of an air embolism.

Step 2. Apply a local anesthetic subcutaneously and deep at the venipuncture site. Usually 1% lidocaine without epinephrine is the anesthetic agent used.

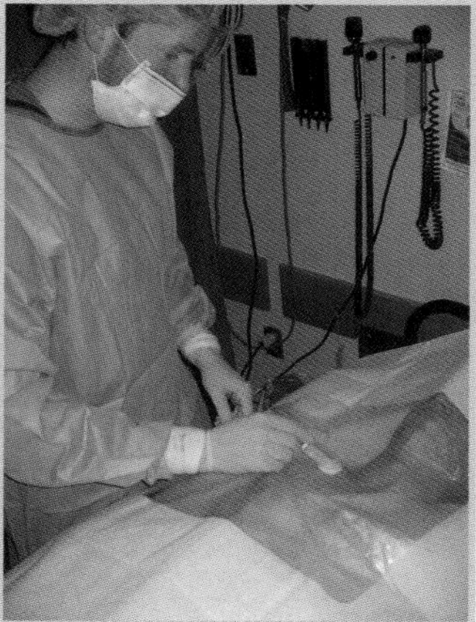

Step 1

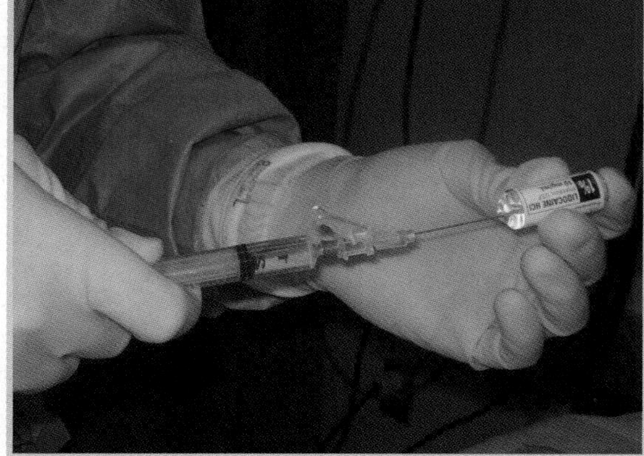

Step 2

Step 3. Identify your landmarks, remembering that the subclavian vein is a continuation of the axillary vein and typically runs a fixed course along the undersurface of the clavicle. The insertion site should be at the bisection of the middle and medial thirds of the clavicle.

- **PEARL:** The subclavian artery usually lies deeper than the vein; to reduce risk of subclavian artery puncture, avoid deep penetration by the probe needle.

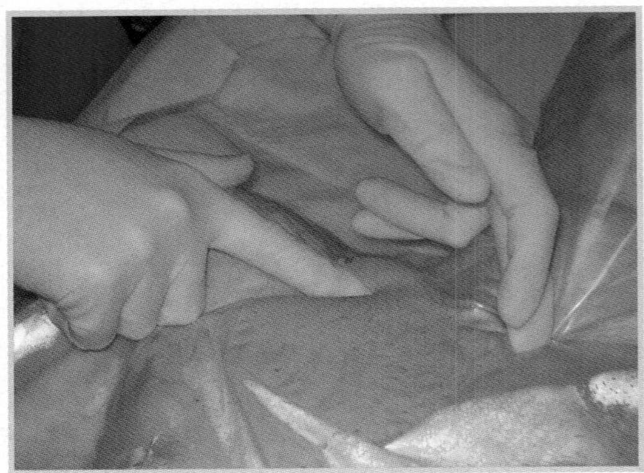

Step 3

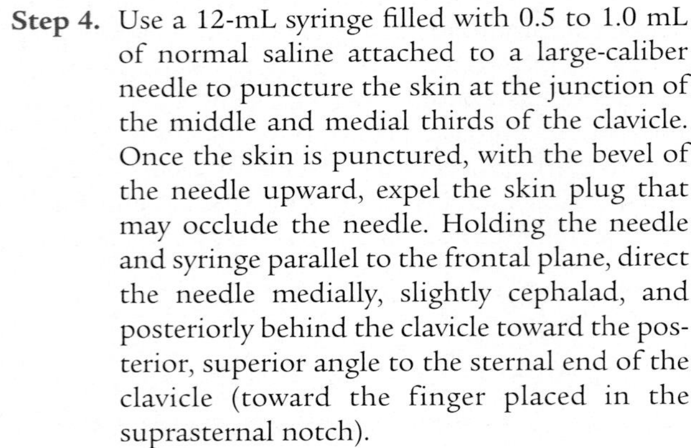

Step 4. Use a 12-mL syringe filled with 0.5 to 1.0 mL of normal saline attached to a large-caliber needle to puncture the skin at the junction of the middle and medial thirds of the clavicle. Once the skin is punctured, with the bevel of the needle upward, expel the skin plug that may occlude the needle. Holding the needle and syringe parallel to the frontal plane, direct the needle medially, slightly cephalad, and posteriorly behind the clavicle toward the posterior, superior angle to the sternal end of the clavicle (toward the finger placed in the suprasternal notch).

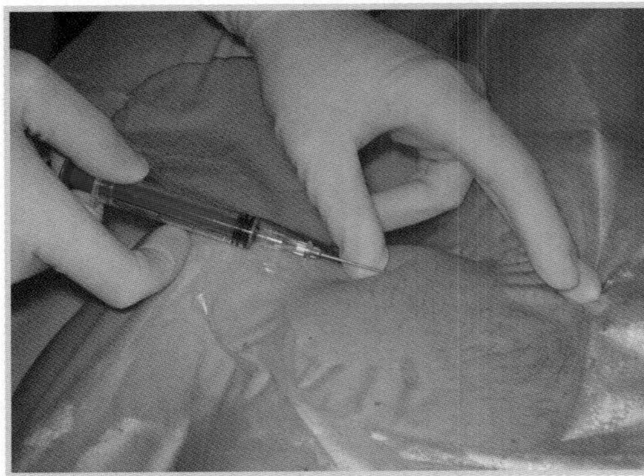

Step 4

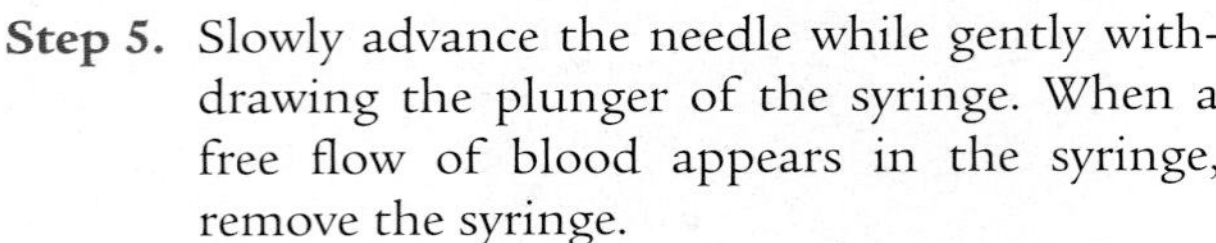

Step 5. Slowly advance the needle while gently withdrawing the plunger of the syringe. When a free flow of blood appears in the syringe, remove the syringe.

- **PEARL:** To lessen risk of air embolism, occlude the needle with a finger.

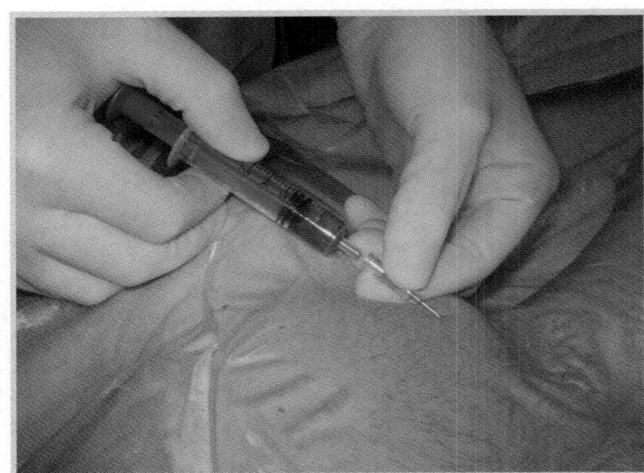

Step 5

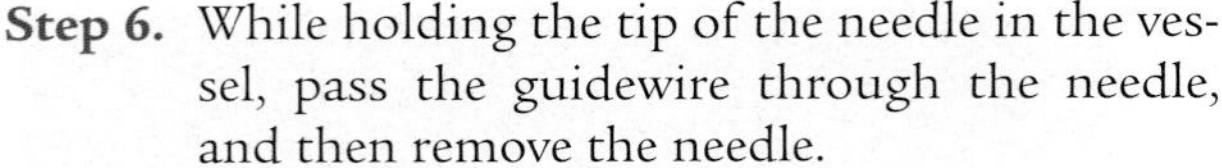

Step 6. While holding the tip of the needle in the vessel, pass the guidewire through the needle, and then remove the needle.

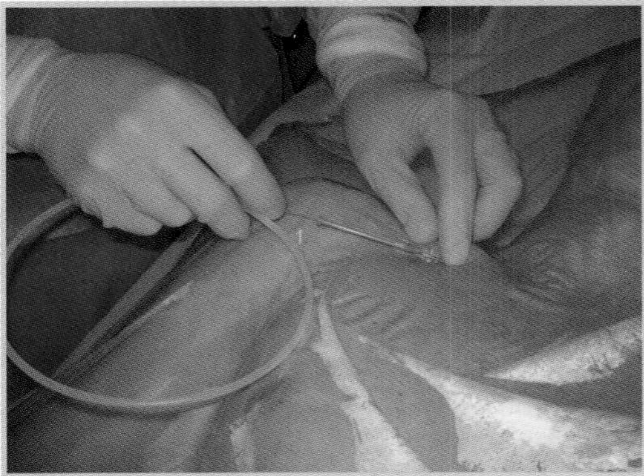

Step 6

Step 7. With a scalpel (no. 11 blade), puncture the skin at the insertion point of the guidewire to facilitate cannulation and lessen resistance when dilating the vessel. Thread the dilator catheter over the guidewire, creating a larger tract for catheter placement. Remove the dilator, keeping the guidewire in place.

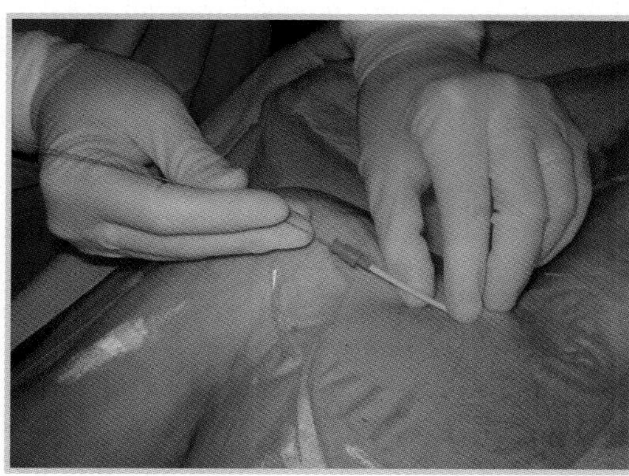

Step 7

Step 8. Advance the catheter over the guidewire into the blood vessel, and if possible, monitor for rhythm abnormalities with an electrocardiogram. Insert the catheter over the guidewire to a predetermined depth (the tip of the catheter should be above the right atrium for fluid administration).

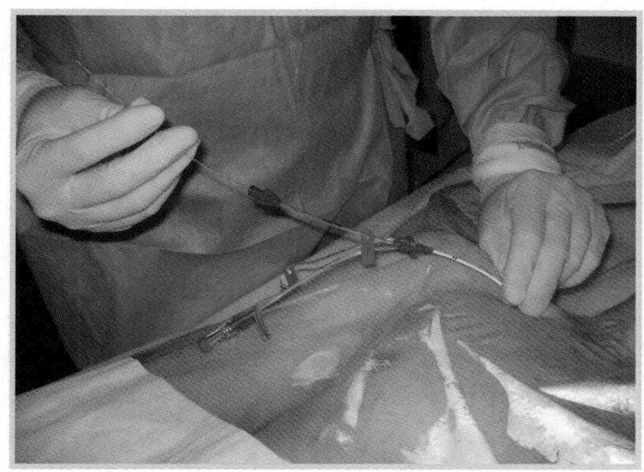

Step 8

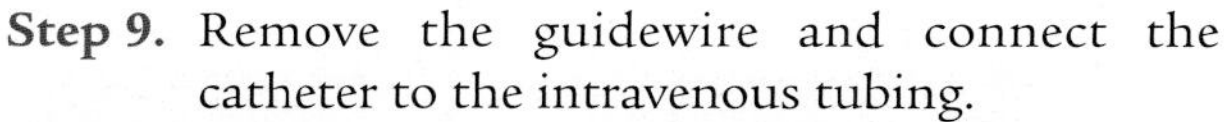

Step 9. Remove the guidewire and connect the catheter to the intravenous tubing.

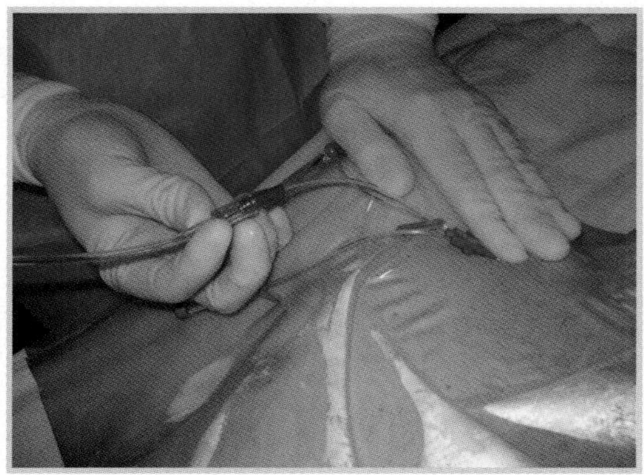

Step 9

Step 10. Affix the catheter in place with a suture, apply an antibiotic ointment, and dress the area with a hydrocolloid dressing (Tegaderm) transparent seal to reduce risk of infection and to allow monitoring for potential bleeding.

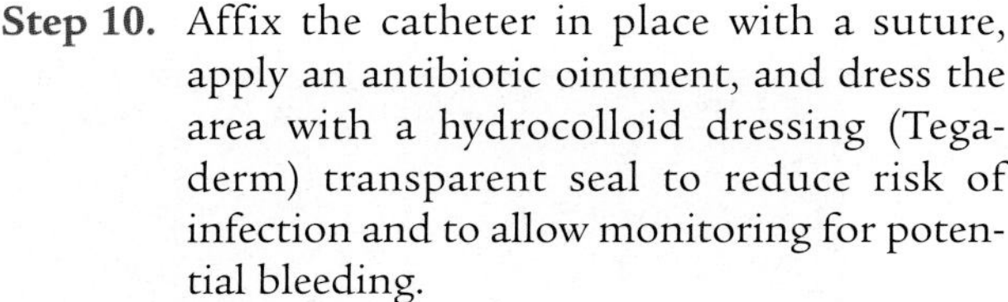

- **PEARL:** For extra security, tape the intravenous tubing in place.
- **PITFALL:** Obtain a chest x-ray to identify the position and placement of the intravenous catheter and a possible pneumothorax.

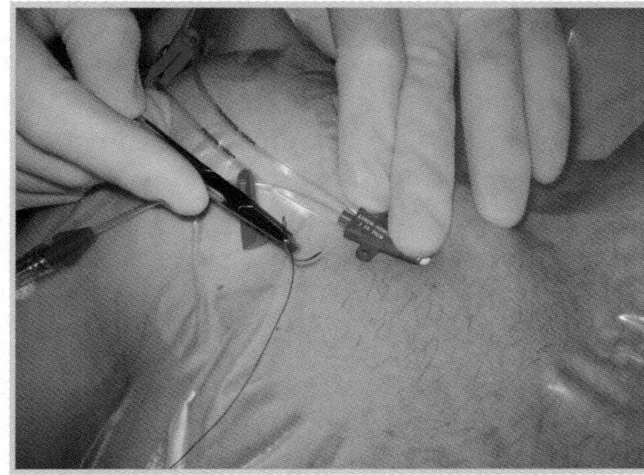

Step 10

Femoral Venipuncture using the Seldinger Technique

Step 1. Place the patient in a supine position. The ipsilateral hip should be in a neutral or slightly externally rotated position. Then cleanse the skin well around the venipuncture site and drape the area. Standard precautions of sterile gloves, sterile gown, mask, cap, and eye protection should be followed.

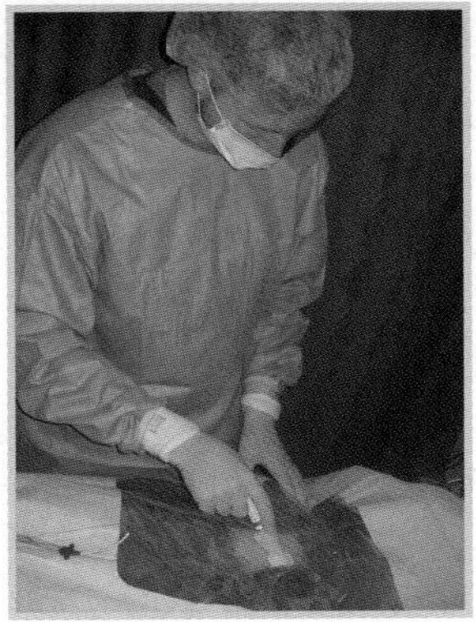

Step 1

Step 2. Palpate the femoral artery as your primary landmark. The femoral vein typically lies directly medial to the femoral artery (nerve, artery, vein, empty space, lymphatics). The insertion site should be approximately 1.5 cm medial to a palpable femoral pulse and approximately 1.5 cm below the inguinal ligament. To lessen risk of cannulation of the femoral artery, keep a finger on the artery to verify anatomical location during the procedure.

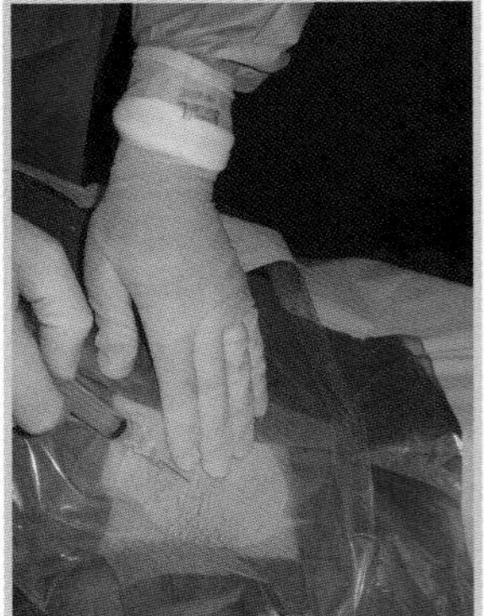

Step 2

Step 3. Apply a local anesthetic subcutaneously and deep at the venipuncture site. Usually 1% lidocaine without epinephrine is the anesthetic agent used.

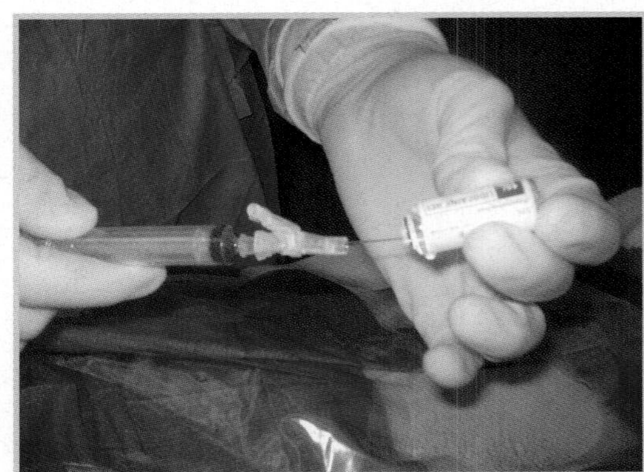

Step 3

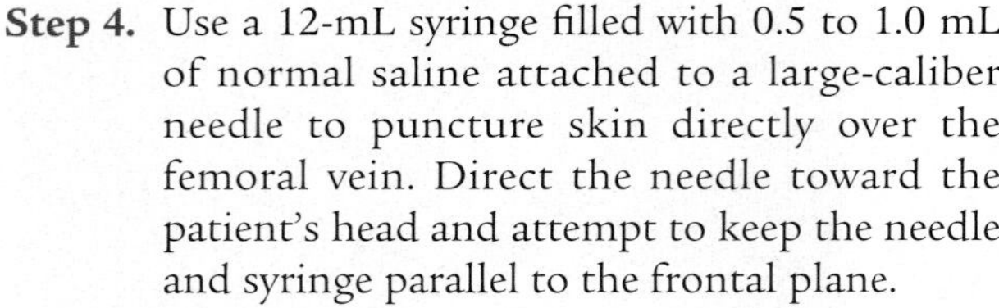

Step 4. Use a 12-mL syringe filled with 0.5 to 1.0 mL of normal saline attached to a large-caliber needle to puncture skin directly over the femoral vein. Direct the needle toward the patient's head and attempt to keep the needle and syringe parallel to the frontal plane.

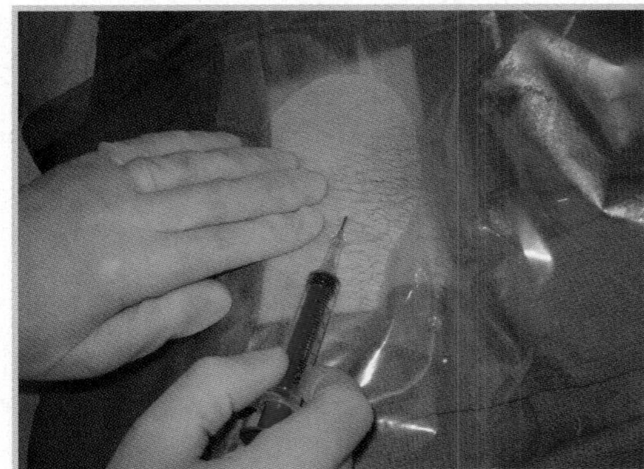

Step 4

Step 5. Slowly advance the needle in a cephalad and posterior direction while gently withdrawing the plunger of the syringe. When a free flow of blood appears in the syringe, remove the syringe.

- **PEARL:** To lessen risk of air embolism, occlude the needle with a finger.

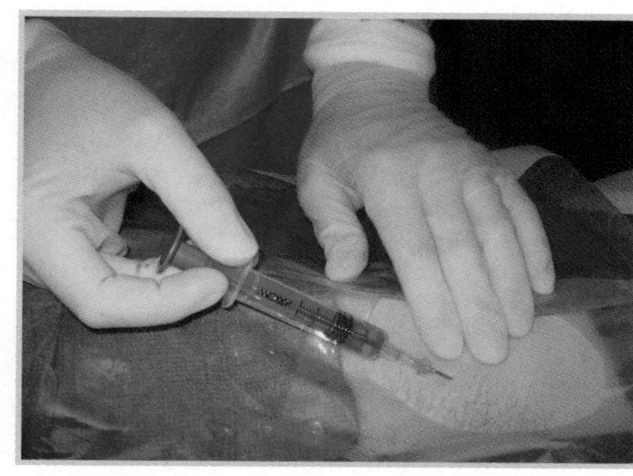

Step 5

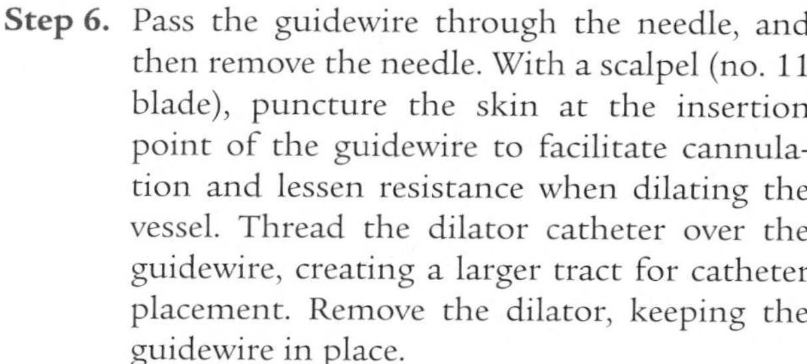

Step 6. Pass the guidewire through the needle, and then remove the needle. With a scalpel (no. 11 blade), puncture the skin at the insertion point of the guidewire to facilitate cannulation and lessen resistance when dilating the vessel. Thread the dilator catheter over the guidewire, creating a larger tract for catheter placement. Remove the dilator, keeping the guidewire in place.

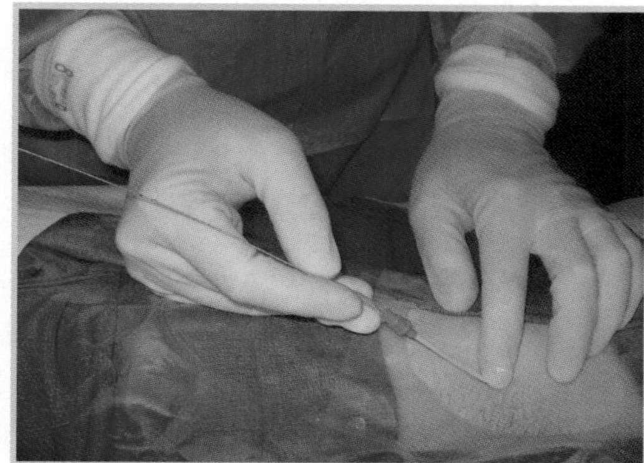

Step 6

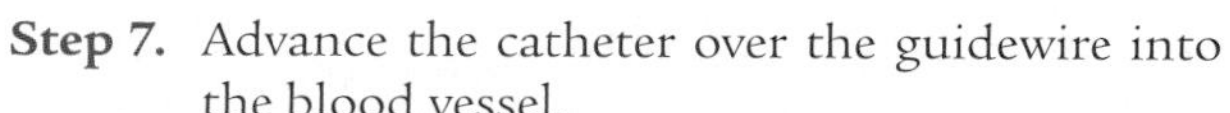

Step 7. Advance the catheter over the guidewire into the blood vessel.

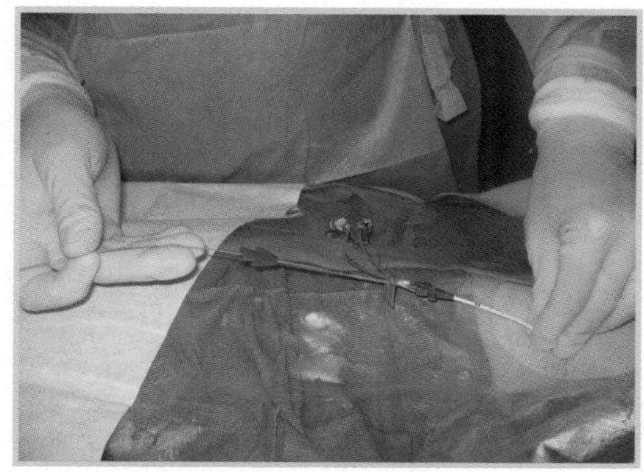

Step 7

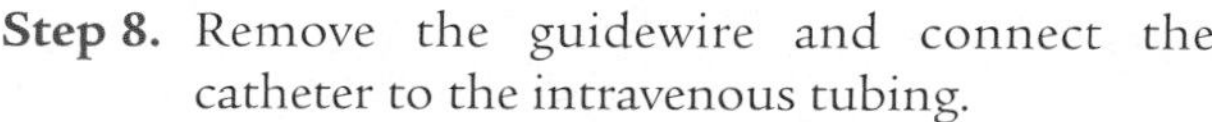

Step 8. Remove the guidewire and connect the catheter to the intravenous tubing.

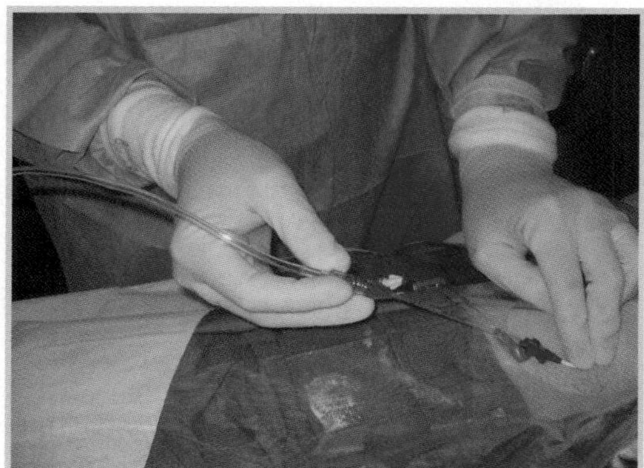

Step 8

Step 9. Affix the catheter in place with a suture, apply an antibiotic ointment, and dress the area with a hydrocolloid dressing (Tegaderm) transparent seal to reduce the risk of infection and to allow monitoring for potential bleeding.

- **PEARL:** For extra security, tape the intravenous tubing in place.
- **PITFALL:** Obtain chest and abdominal x-rays to identify the position and placement of the intravenous catheter.
- **PITFALL:** Remember that the catheter should be changed as soon as practical to reduce complications of infection and thrombosis.

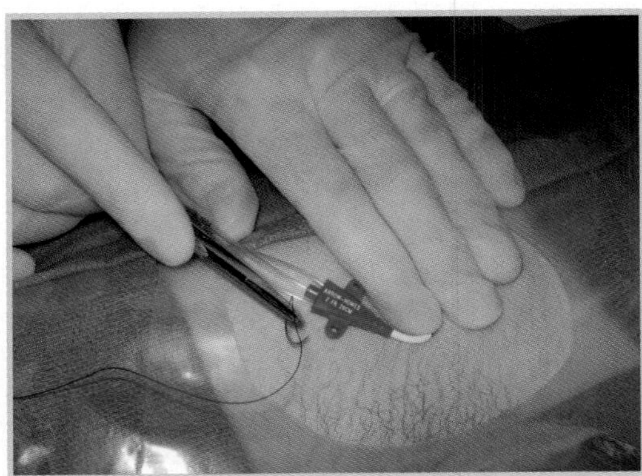

Step 9

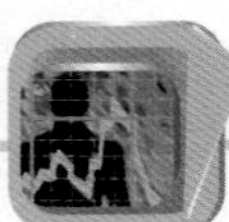

Complications

Subclavian Venous Access

- Pneumothorax or hemothorax
- Venous thrombosis
- Arterial or neurologic injury
- Arteriovenous fistula
- Chylothorax
- Infection
- Air embolism
- Malpositioning

Femoral Venous Access

- Deep venous thrombosis
- Arterial and neurologic injury
- Infection
- Arteriovenous fistula
- Malpositioning

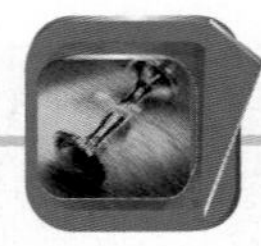

Pediatric Considerations

Pediatric patients may not cooperate with placement of the catheter. Because of the risks of damage to vessels, nerves, etc., consider conscious sedation with intramuscular injections or oral administration of sedating medications, such as midazolam (Versed) or ketamine.

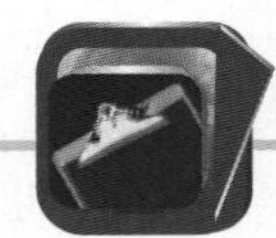

Postprocedure Instructions

The central venous catheter should be removed as soon as possible to avoid potential complications. When removing the catheter, use a 4- × 4-inch piece of gauze and apply it directly over the catheter site. Cut and remove all securing devices and then pull gently on the catheter. It should come out easily. Once removed, firm pressure should be applied directly to the area for at least 1 minute, longer if bleeding is still appreciable. Dress the wound with a dry, sterile gauze.

A potential serious complication during removal of a catheter is a venous air embolism; it can occur during insertion, while the catheter is in place, and during removal of the catheter. To decrease risk of an air embolism, the patient should be placed in a supine position and the catheter should be removed during exhalation or during a Valsalva maneuver. This is believed to be better because during exhalation, the intrathoracic pressure is greater than the atmospheric pressure, lowering the risk of air entering the venous circulation.

If there is clinical suspicion of a catheter or bloodstream infection, the tip of the catheter should be removed sterilely and sent for culture.

The patient should be instructed to monitor the bleeding of the area and to return if any abnormal bleeding is noted. The patient should also be educated to call with questions or concerns regarding pain, numbness, or discomfort in the area. The patient should also monitor for evidence of infection. Lastly, the patient should be advised to clean the area with warm soap and water and to pat the area dry.

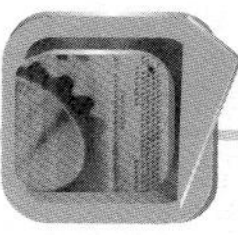

Coding Information and Supply Sources

CPT Code	Description	2008 Average 50th Percentile Fee	Global Period
36555	Insertion of nontunneled centrally inserted central venous catheter; younger than 5 years of age	$515.00	0
36556	Insertion of nontunneled centrally inserted central venous catheter; age 5 years or older	$500.00	0

CPT is a registered trademark of the American Medical Association.
2008 average 50th Percentile Fees are provided courtesy of 2008 MMH-SI's copyrighted Physicians' Fees and Coding Guide.

Supplies may be purchased from these companies:

- American Hospital Supply. Phone: 407-475-1168. Web site: http://www.americanhospitalsupply.com/.
- Arrow Medical Products Ltd., 2400 Bernville Road, Reading, PA 19605. Phone: 800-233-3187. Web site: http://www.arrowintl.com/.
- Baxter, 1 Baxter Pkwy., Deerfield, IL, 60015-4625. Phone: 847-948-2000. Fax: 847-948-3642. Web site: http://www.baxter.com.
- Cardinal Health, Inc., 7000 Cardinal Place, Dublin, OH 43017. Phone: 800-234-8701. Web site: http://www.cardinal.com/.
- Owens and Minor, 4800 Cox Road, Glen Allen, VA 23060-6292. Phone: 804-747-9794. Fax: 804-270-7281.

Patient Education Handout

A patient education handout, "Central Venous Catheter," can be found on the book's Web site.

Bibliography

American College of Surgeons Committee on Trauma: Advanced Trauma Life Support, Student Course Manual. 7th ed. Chicago; American College of Surgeons, 2004.

Marino PL. *The ICU Book*. 3rd ed. Philadelphia: Lippincott Williams & Wilkins; 2007:107–128.

Merrer J, Jonghe BD, Golliot F, et al. Complications of femoral and subclavian venous catheterization in critically ill patients: a randomized controlled trial. *JAMA*. 2001; 286:700.

McGee WT, Gould MK. Preventing complications of central venous catheterization. *N Engl J Med*. 2003;348:1123.

Seneff MG. Central venous catherization: a comprehensive review. *Intensive Care Med*. 1987;2:163–175,218–232.

Tintinalli JE, Kelen GD, Stapczynski JS. *Emergency Medicine: A Comprehensive Study Guide*. 6th ed. New York: McGraw-Hill; 2004:124–131.

2008 MAG Mutual Healthcare Solutions, Inc.'s Physicians' Fee and Coding Guide. Duluth, Georgia. MAG Mutual Healthcare Solutions, Inc. 2007.

CHAPTER 7

Pulmonary Artery Catheter Placement

Paul McCarthy, MD
Critical Care Medicine
Louisiana State University Health Sciences Center,
Shreveport, LA

Laurie Grier, MD, FCCM, FCCP, FACP
Professor of Clinical Medicine,
Emergency Medicine and Anesthesia
Louisiana State University Health Sciences Center,
Shreveport, LA

Pulmonary catheterization is a diagnostic procedure in which a balloon-tipped catheter is placed into a central vein and directed to the right side of the heart to obtain pressures and other measurements for hemodynamic monitoring. Pulmonary artery catheterization, also referred to as Swan-Ganz catheterization, is an invasive procedure usually performed in the intensive care unit, cardiac catheterization laboratory, or operating room.

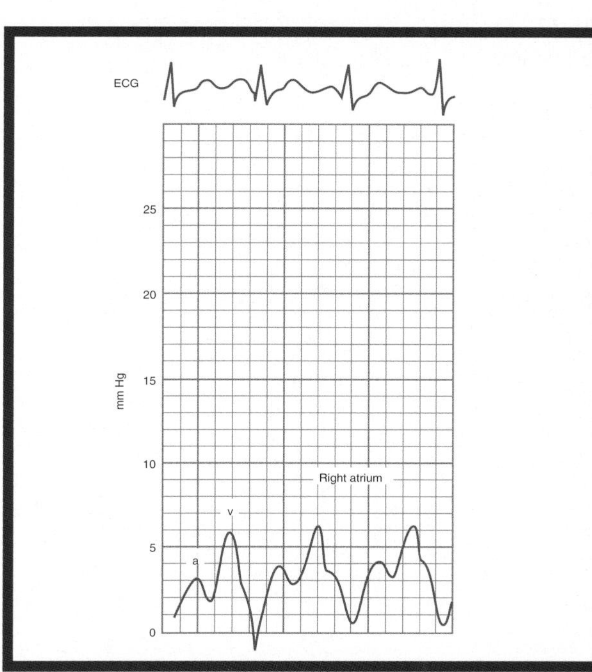

Once the catheter is in place, a small balloon is inflated to momentarily block blood flow and allow pressure measurements in the pulmonary artery system. This pressure is called a *wedge pressure* and is an indirect measurement of left ventricular filling pressure. The catheter can measure mixed venous oxygenation and can also measure cardiac output via thermodilution. The catheter is generally left in place for periods of 24 to 72 hours.

Because of the invasiveness of the procedure and lack of randomized controlled trials showing improved outcomes in patients with pulmonary artery catheters, their utility is being questioned more and more. Over the past decade, the use of the pulmonary artery catheter has steadily decreased.

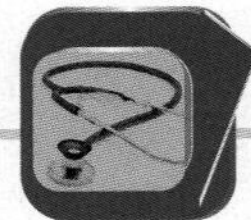

Equipment

- Sterile towels, drapes, gloves, and gowns
- Sterile saline for flushes
- Gauze pads
- Pulmonary artery catheter kit
  - Introducer
  - Pulmonary artery catheter
  - Dilator
  - Guide wire
  - Syringes
  - Scalpel
  - Suture

Most experts agree that whenever possible, the venous cannulation should be done with ultrasound guidance and the catheter should be advanced with the assistance of fluoroscopy.

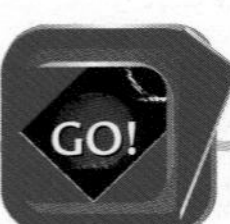

Indications

- Diagnosis of type of shock
- Diagnosis of pulmonary hypertension
- Assessment of hemodynamic response to therapies
- Diagnosis of cardiac tamponade or constrictive myopathies
- Diagnosis of intracardiac shunt
- Differentiating high-pressure versus low-pressure pulmonary edema
- Assessment of valvular heart disease
- Continuous measurement of mixed venous oxygen saturation

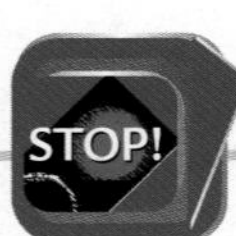

Contraindications

- Right-sided heart mass
- Tricuspid or pulmonary valve prosthesis
- Tricuspid or pulmonary valve endocarditis
- Cyanotic heart disease
- Latex allergy
- Previous pneumonectomy
- Arrhythmia (relative)
- Anticoagulation (relative)

The Procedure

Step 1. Obtain informed consent for the procedure and make sure electrolytes and clotting disorders are corrected. Check the components of the kit. Inflate and deflate the balloon and view for any malfunctions. Flush all lumens with sterile saline solution. Connect the distal lumen to the pressure monitoring system and zero the pressure transducer.

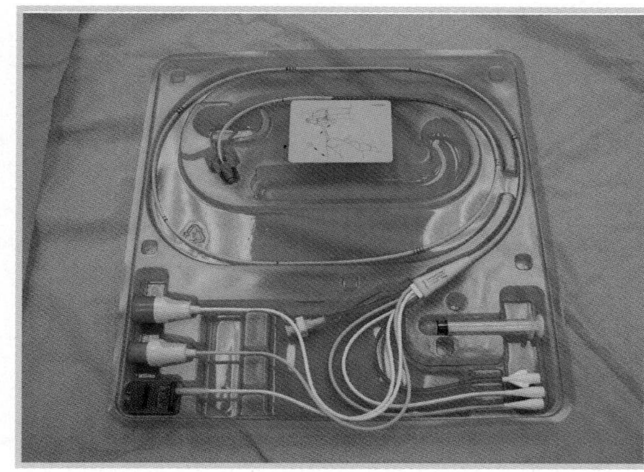

Step 1

Step 2. Place the patient in a supine position. Cleanse the skin well around the venipuncture site and drape the area (see Appendix E). Standard precautions of sterile gloves, sterile gown, mask, cap, and eye protection should be followed.

- **PEARL:** When possible, place the patient in a Trendelenburg position of at least 15 degrees down to distend the neck veins and reduce the risk of an air embolism.

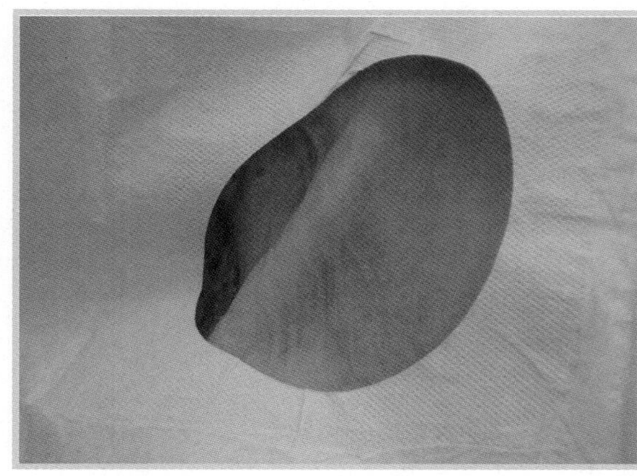

Step 2

Step 3. Apply a local anesthetic subcutaneously and deep at the venipuncture site. Usually 1% lidocaine without epinephrine is the anesthetic agent used. Identify the landmarks, remembering that the subclavian vein is a continuation of the axillary vein and typically runs a fixed course along the undersurface of the clavicle. The insertion site should be at the bisection of the middle and medial thirds of the clavicle. Use a 12-mL syringe filled with 0.5 to 1.0 mL of normal saline attached to a large-caliber needle to puncture the skin at the junction of the middle and medial thirds of the clavicle.

- **PEARL:** The subclavian artery usually lies deep under the vein; to reduce the risk of subclavian artery puncture, avoid deep penetration by the probe needle.

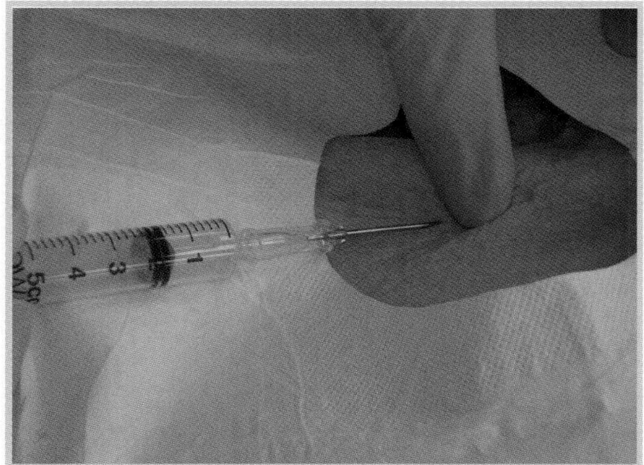

Step 3

Step 4. Holding the needle and syringe parallel to the frontal plane, direct the needle medially, slightly cephalad, and posteriorly behind the clavicle toward the posterior, superior angle to the sternal end of the clavicle (toward finger placed in the suprasternal notch). Slowly advance the needle while gently withdrawing the plunger of the syringe. When a free flow of blood appears in the syringe, remove the syringe. Pass the guidewire through the needle.

- **PEARL:** To lessen risk of air embolism, occlude the needle with a finger.

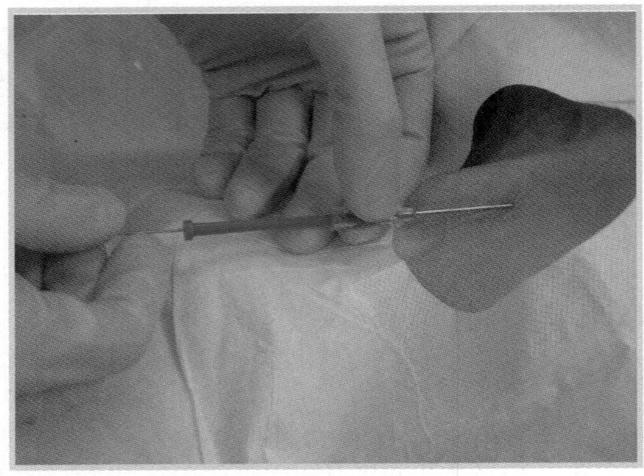

Step 4

Step 5. Remove the needle, leaving the wire in place in the vein.

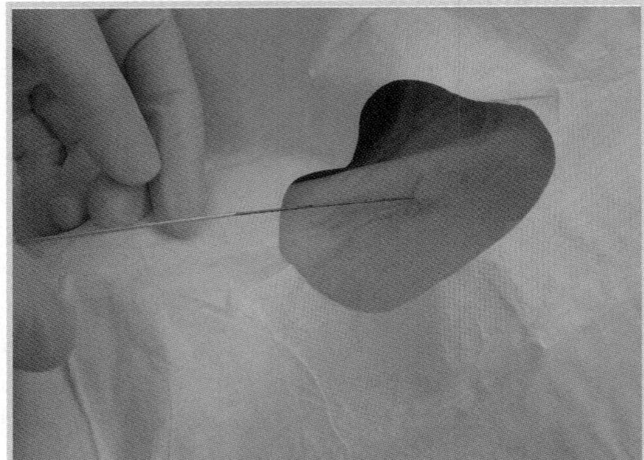

Step 5

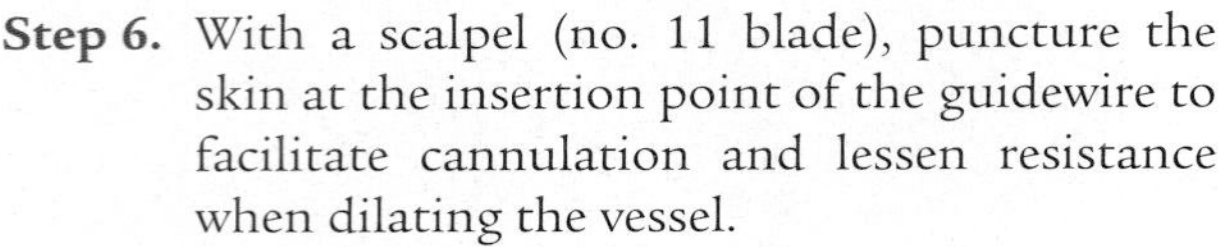

Step 6. With a scalpel (no. 11 blade), puncture the skin at the insertion point of the guidewire to facilitate cannulation and lessen resistance when dilating the vessel.

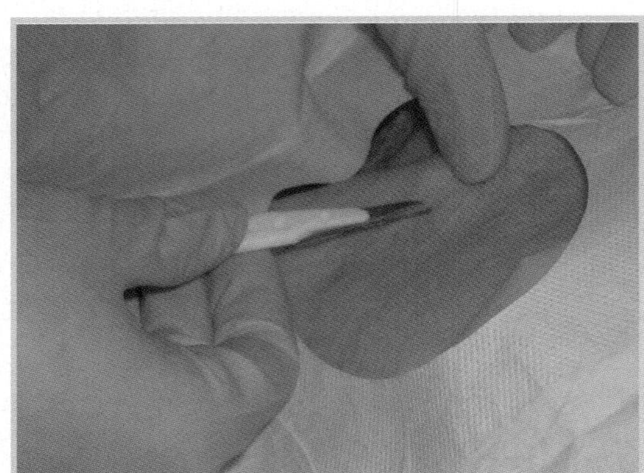

Step 6

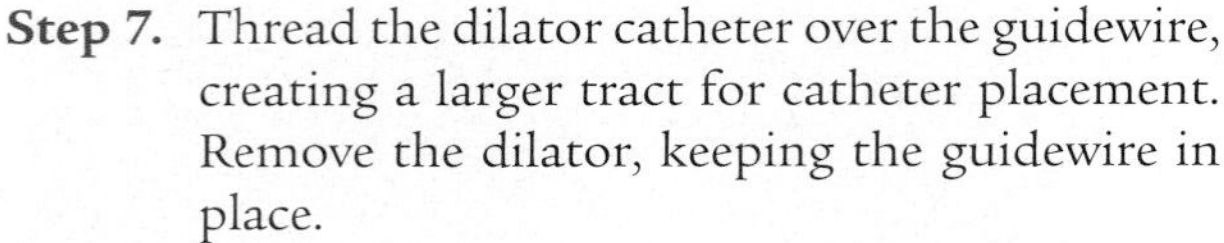

Step 7. Thread the dilator catheter over the guidewire, creating a larger tract for catheter placement. Remove the dilator, keeping the guidewire in place.

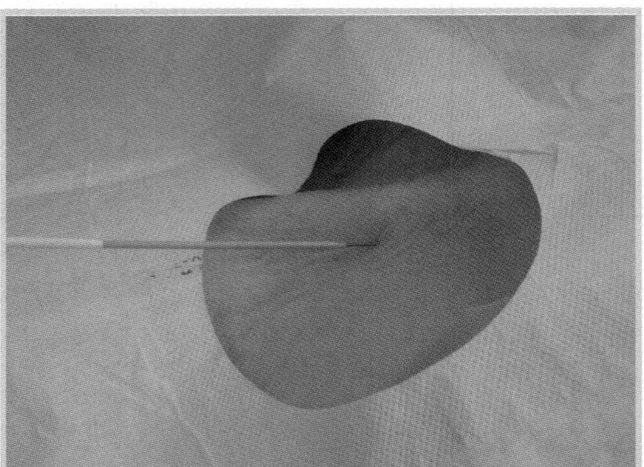

Step 7

Step 8. Advance the introducer over the guidewire into the blood vessel, and if possible, monitor for rhythm abnormalities with an electrocardiogram. Remove the guidewire.

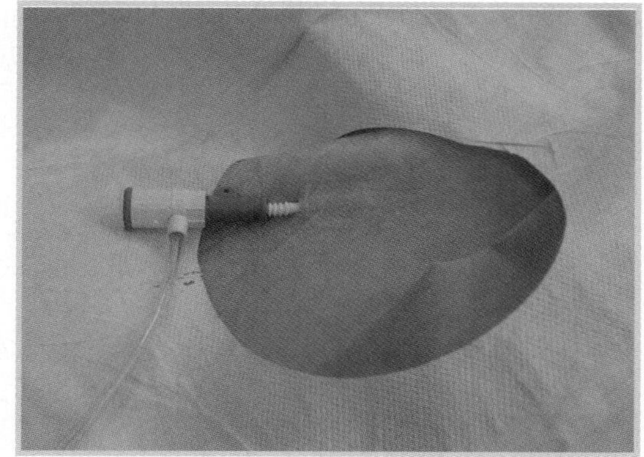

Step 8

Step 9. Pass the pulmonary artery catheter past the introducer.

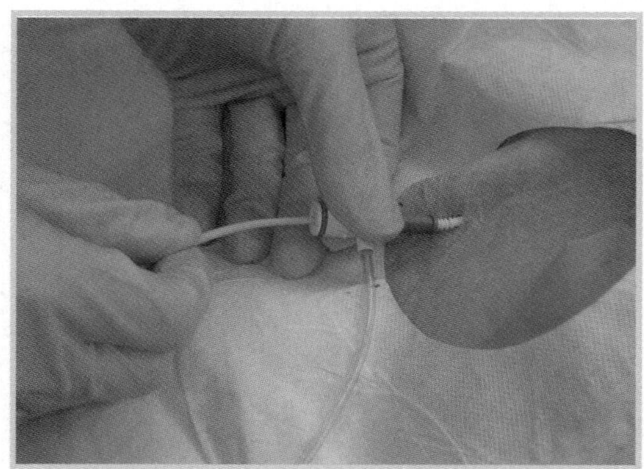

Step 9

Step 10. Inflate the balloon once the catheter tip has traveled past the end of the inducer. Advance the catheter. A right atrial waveform should be seen after advancing 15 to 20 cm if the subclavian or internal jugular approach is used. For the femoral approach, the catheter will be advance approximately 30 cm before a right atrial waveform is seen.

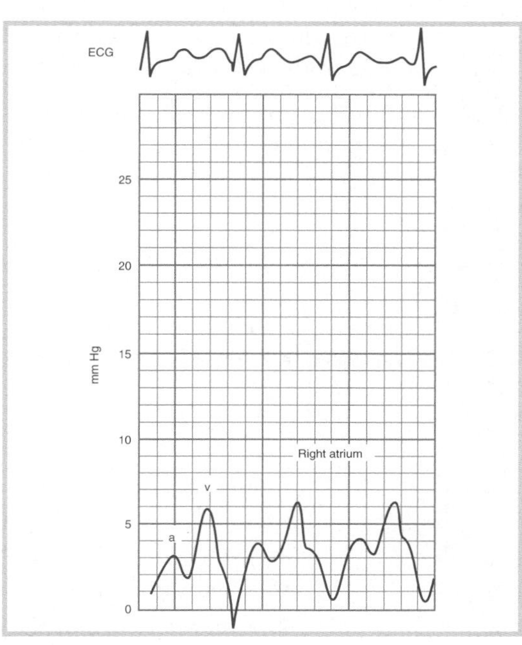

Step 10

Step 11. Continue to advance the catheter approximately 10 cm, and a right ventricular waveform will be seen.

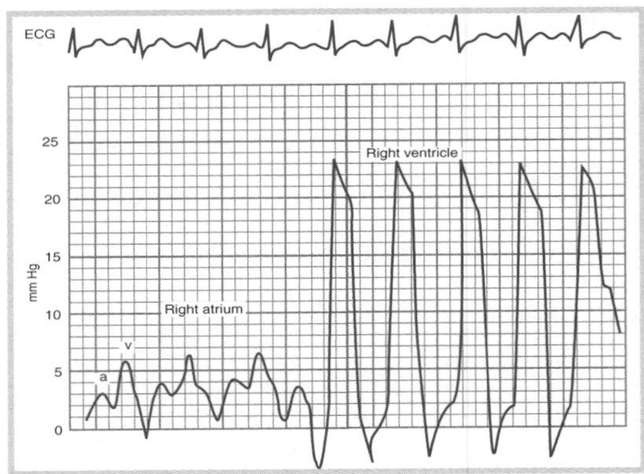

Step 11

Step 12. Continue to advance the catheter approximately 10 cm to visualize a pulmonary artery waveform. Continue to advance the catheter until a pulmonary artery wedge pressure waveform is seen.

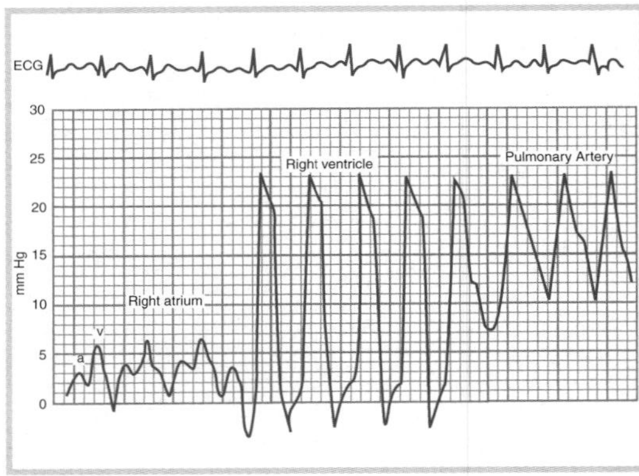

Step 12

Step 13. Deflate the balloon and confirm the presence of a pulmonary artery waveform. Extend the protective sleeve and lock to proximal and distal ends. Confirm placement of the catheter with a chest x-ray. The catheter tip should be about 2 cm from the cardiac shadow. Usually the catheter is in the right lung; however, the left side is acceptable.

- **PEARL:** Pressures should be measured at end expiration.

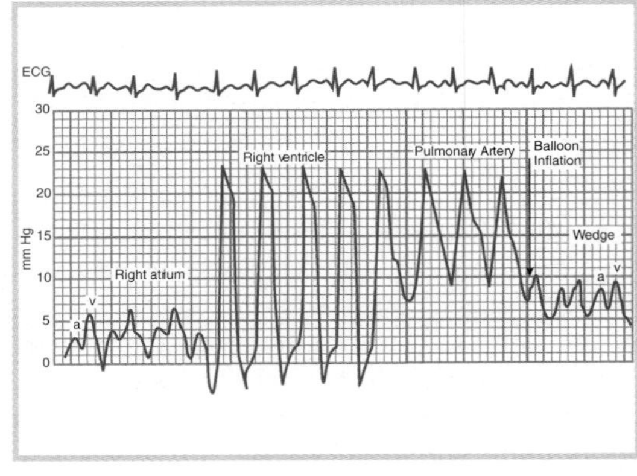

Step 13

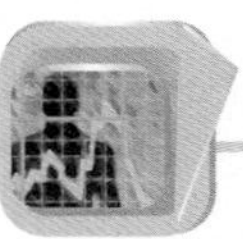

Complications

- Standard risks of central venous cannulation
- Pneumothorax
- Pulmonary hemorrhage
- Pulmonary infarction

- Pulmonary artery rupture
- Arrhythmias
- Infection
- Valvular damage
- Thrombosis
- Balloon rupture

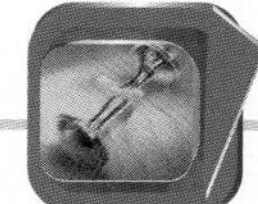

Pediatric Considerations

Pulmonary artery catheterization is performed with much less frequency in children than in adults. When used in children, it is usually in patients undergoing cardiac surgery. If the catheter is being placed in a patient with cyanotic heart disease, the lumens must be de-aired and carbon dioxide should be used for balloon inflation.

The pulmonary catheter may be difficult or impossible to place in patients with certain congenital cardiac pathology. For this and several other reasons, echocardiography is used more often in the pediatric population.

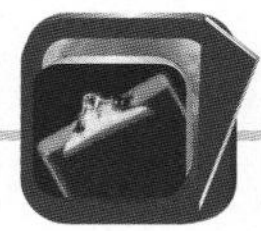

Postprocedure Instructions

Once the catheter is in place, several measurements can be made. Cardiac output can be monitored via thermodilution, and left ventricular pressure can be approximated by measuring the pulmonary artery occlusion pressure (wedge pressure). Mixed venous oxygenation, stroke volume, and systemic and pulmonary vascular resistance can all be measured.

When the catheter is in place, daily monitoring is required, and steps should be followed to safely manage the catheter. The trace display should always be on the monitor when the catheter is in place. The catheter should not be withdrawn unless the balloon is deflated; always look for pressure changes when repositioning the catheter. The catheter should be removed as soon as it is not needed or if it is not working. The catheter should also be removed in the event of unexplained fever or apparent infection.

The pulmonary artery catheter should be removed from the insertion catheter after the balloon is deflated. Once the pulmonary artery catheter is removed, the insertion catheter should be removed in a fashion similar to the removal of a standard central venous catheter. Once the insertion catheter is removed, pressure may be held for a few minutes to control bleeding, and a small dressing can be placed.

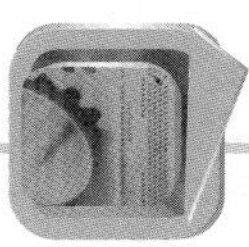

Coding Information and Supply Sources

CPT Code	Description	2008 Average 50th Percentile Fee	Global Period
93503	Pulmonary artery catheter	$718.00	0
36556	Central venous catheter	$500.00	0
76937	Ultrasound guidance for venous cannulation	$136.00	ZZZ
77001	Fluoroscopic guidance for procedure	$254.00	ZZZ

ZZZ, Code related to another service and is always included in the global period of the other service.

CPT is a registered trademark of the American Medical Association.

2008 average 50th Percentile Fees are provided courtesy of 2008 MMH-SI's copyrighted Physicians' Fees and Coding Guide.

ICD-9 Codes

Cor pulmonale, acute	415.0
CHF	428.0
Shock NOS	785.50
Cardiogenic shock	785.51
Septic shock	785.59
Anaphylactic shock	995.0

Supplier

- Edwards Lifesciences, 1 Edwards Way, Irvine, CA 92614. Phone: 1-800-424-3278. Web site: http://www.edwards.com.

Bibliography

Harvey S, Harrison DA, Singer M, et al. Assessment of the clinical effectiveness of pulmonary artery catheter in the management of patients in intensive care (PAC-Man): a randomized controlled trial. *Lancet.* 2005;366(9484):472–477.

Marino PL. The pulmonary artery catheter. In: *The ICU Book.* 3rd ed. Philadelphia: Lippincott Williams & Wilkins; 2007:163–177.

Rubenfeld GD, McNamara-Aslin E, Rubinson L. The pulmonary artery catheter, 1967–2007. *JAMA.* 2007;298(4):458–461.

Wiener RS, Welch HG. Trends in the use of the pulmonary artery catheter in the United States, 1993–2004. *JAMA.* 2007;298(4):423–428.

2008 MAG Mutual Healthcare Solutions, Inc.'s Physicians' Fee and Coding Guide. Duluth, Georgia. MAG Mutual Healthcare Solutions, Inc. 2007.

CHAPTER 8

Chest Tube Insertion

E. J. Mayeaux, Jr., MD, DABFP, FAAFP
Professor of Family Medicine
Professor of Obstetrics and Gynecology
Louisiana State University Health Sciences Center, Shreveport, LA

Sean Troxclair, MD
Critical Care Medicine
Louisiana State University Health Sciences Center
Shreveport, LA

Chest tube insertion is a common therapeutic procedure used to provide evacuation of abnormal collections of air or fluid from the pleural space. Chest tube insertion is often required in a setting of trauma and can be a medical emergency. Chest trauma is a common cause of emergency department visits and may result in pneumothorax, hemothorax, or secondary infection. Patients with chest trauma should be assessed for signs of respiratory insufficiency, such as restlessness, agitation, altered or absent breath sounds, or respiratory distress. In severe cases, patients may exhibit cyanosis, deviated trachea, and paradoxical chest wall segment motion or shock. Coagulation studies and a chest radiograph should be available. In addition, tube thoracostomy may be indicated for pleural effusions associated with malignancy or infection. In these situations, drainage is imperative to allow for lung re-expansion.

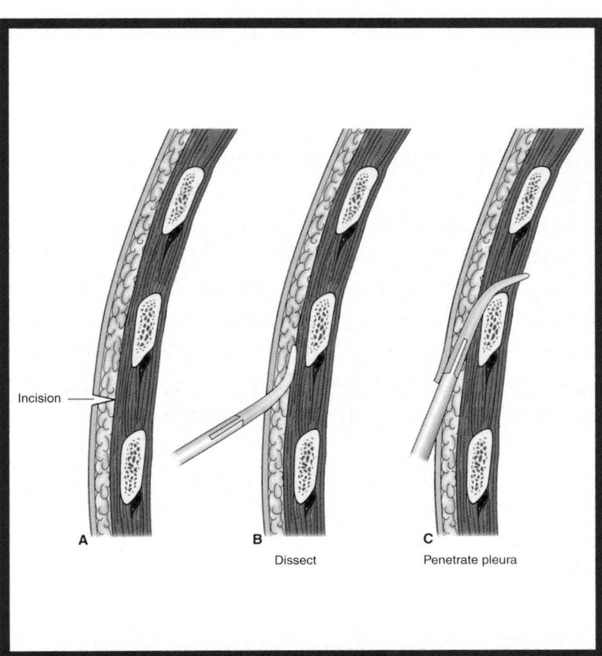

Sedation may be used if the patient is not in severe respiratory distress because of the procedural discomfort. Placement requires universal precautions for body fluids, and use good sterile technique, including a face mask and sterile gown whenever possible. Selection of the proper chest tube size is important. An 18- to 24-Fr chest tube typically is used for a pure pneumothorax. For a hemothorax, empyema, or other fluid accumulation, a 28- to 40-Fr catheter is more commonly employed.

The classic technique for chest tube insertion has remained the same for many years. Some practitioners opt to perform a percutaneous tube thoracostomy with the Seldinger approach. The patient positioning and preparation is the same as the conventional method. An introducer needle is used to place a guidewire into the pleural space. Then serial dilators are passed over the guidewire to create an adequately dilated tract. The chest tube is then passed. A disadvantage to this technique is that the chest cavity cannot be digitally explored for adhesions; however, with careful consideration of the location of the guidewire, this can be performed after the last dilation. Some advantages to this technique are that an improved hemostatic barrier exists, which may be especially advantageous to pneumothoraces and patients prone to bleeding complications. This technique can take longer than traditional techniques and may not be optimal in emergency situations. There are references in literature indicating that when used for empyema, the percutaneous drains are more likely to become obstructed and stop draining. Thus far, this is only observational data, and no large-scale studies are available.

Re-expansion pulmonary edema is a potentially life-threatening complication of chest tube placement. It usually occurs after rapid re-expansion in patients with a pneumothorax but may follow evacuation of large pleural effusions. It is related to the rapidity of lung re-expansion and to the severity and duration of lung collapse. Patients typically present soon after lung re-expansion and may range from simple radiographic changes to complete cardiopulmonary collapse. Treatment is supportive, mainly consisting of supplemental oxygen and, if necessary, mechanical ventilation. It is usually self-limited and may be prevented by limiting initial drainage to 1 to 1.5 L in the first 24 hours.

The chest tube may be removed if the lung remains fully expanded on a chest radiograph performed on a water seal or after the tube is clamped for 4 to 6 hours. Traditionally, experts recommended that a chest tube be removed when the patient reached full inspiration, often with a concomitant Valsalva maneuver. The theory is that this is the point when intrathoracic pressure and lung volume are maximal. The involuntary reflex while the tube is removed is a quick inspiratory effort because of the pleural pain. In theory, this could allow air to reaccumulate just as the tube is being removed, necessitating reinsertion of another tube. However, research indicates that discontinuation of chest tubes at the end of inspiration or at the end of expiration has a similar rate of pneumothorax after removal and that both methods are equally safe. With all other things being equal, the end-inspiration timing remains the preferred technique.

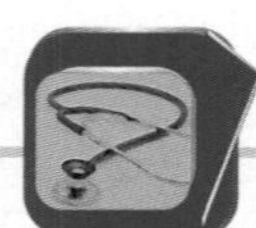

Equipment

Kits, thoracostomy trays, and suction-drainage system are available from Arrow Medical Products Ltd., 2400 Bernville Road, Reading, PA 19605. Phone: 1-800-233-3187. Web site: http://www.arrowintl.com/products/critical_care/.

Many kits and supplies from various companies (including Baxter and American Hospital Supply) can be obtained from Cardinal Health, Inc., 7000 Cardinal Place, Dublin, OH 43017 (phone: 1-800-234-8701); Allegiance Healthcare Corp., McGraw Park, IL 60085 (phone: 847-689-8410; Web site: www.cardinal.com/allegiance), and Owens and Minor, 4800 Cox Road, Glen Allen, VA 23060-6292 (phone: 804-747-9794; fax: 804-270-7281).

Chest tubes that are equipped with an intraluminal trocar are not recommended, because they are associated with a higher incidence of intrathoracic complications.

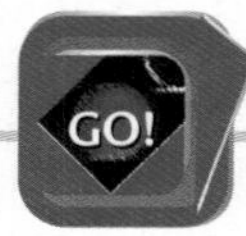

Indications

- Pneumothorax (especially if it is large or progressive or if the patient is symptomatic)
- Tension pneumothorax
- Penetrating chest trauma
- Hemothorax
- Chylothorax
- Empyema
- Drainage of recurrent pleural effusion
- Prevention of hydrothorax after cardiothoracic surgery
- Bronchopleural fistula

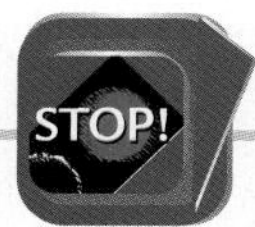

Contraindications (Relative)

- Anticoagulation or a bleeding dyscrasia
- Systemic anticoagulation
- Small, stable pneumothorax (may spontaneously resolve)
- Empyema caused by acid-fast organisms
- Loculated fluid accumulation

The Procedure

Classic Technique

Step 1. Identify the insertion site, which is usually at the fourth or fifth intercostal space in the anterior axillary or midaxillary line (just lateral to the nipple in males) immediately behind the lateral edge of the pectoralis major muscle. Direct the tube as high and anteriorly as possible for a pneumothorax. For a hemothorax, the tube is usually inserted at the level of the nipple and directed posteriorly and laterally. Elevate the head of the bed 30 to 60 degrees, and place (and restrain) the arm on the affected side over the patient's head.

- **PITFALL:** Do not direct the tube toward the mediastinum because contralateral pneumothorax may result.
- **PITFALL:** The diaphragm, liver, or spleen can be lacerated if the patient is not properly positioned or the tube is inserted too low.

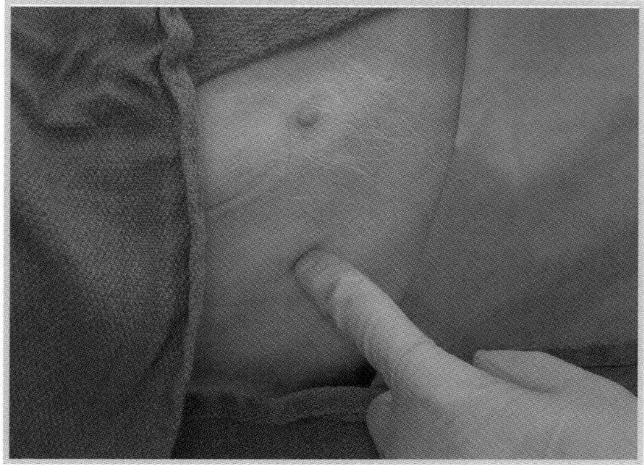

Step 1

Step 2. Assemble the suction-drain system according to manufacturer's recommendations. Connect the suction system to a wall suction outlet. Adjust the suction as needed until a small, steady stream of bubbles is produced in the water column.

- **PEARL:** If a suction-drain system is not immediately available, place a Penrose drain at the end of the chest tube to act as a one-way valve until an appropriate system is available.

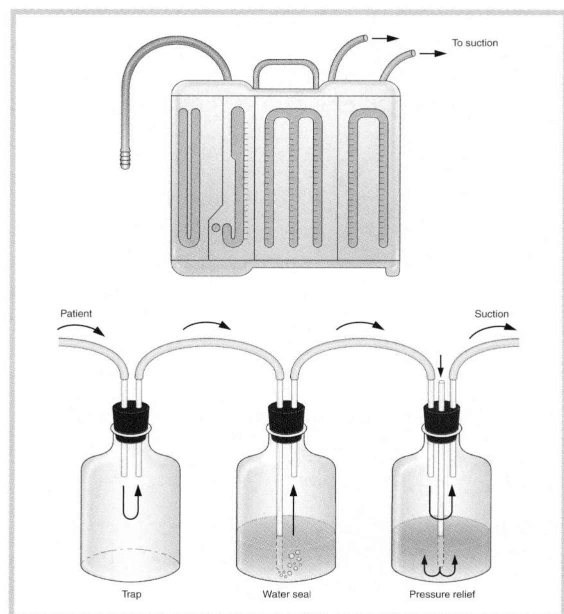

Step 2

Step 3. Prep the skin with povidone-iodine or chlorhexidine solution and allow it to dry (see Appendix E). Drape the site with a fenestrated sheet. Using the 10-mL syringe and 25-gauge needle, raise a skin wheal at the incision area (in the interspace one rib below the interspace chosen for pleural insertion) with a 1% solution of lidocaine with epinephrine.

- **PEARL:** Prep a wide area so that an undraped area is not inadvertently exposed if the drape slides a little.

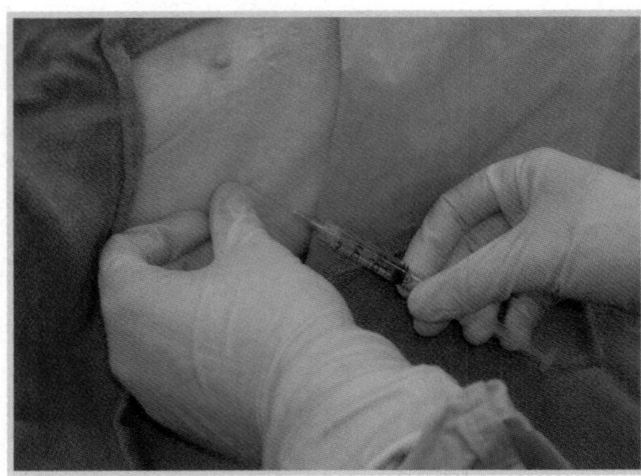

Step 3

Step 4. Liberally infiltrate the subcutaneous tissue and intercostal muscles, including the tissue above the middle aspect of the inferior rib to the interspace where pleural entry will occur and down to the parietal pleura. Using the anesthetic needle and syringe, aspirate the pleural cavity, and check for the presence of fluid or air. If none is obtained, change the insertion site.

- **PITFALL:** Use <7 mL/kg of lidocaine with epinephrine to avoid toxicity.
- **PITFALL:** Be careful to keep away from the inferior border of rib to avoid the intercostal vessels.

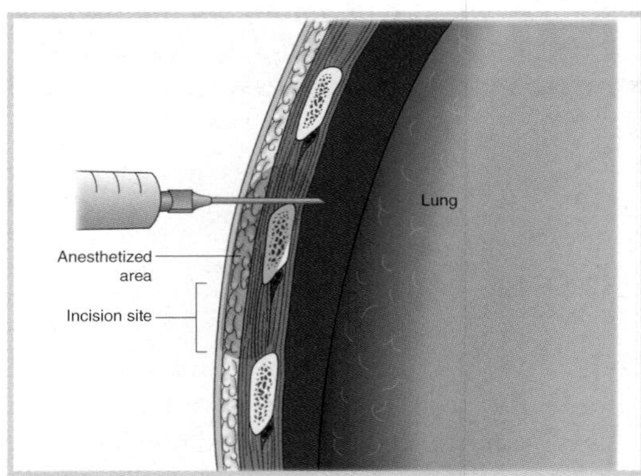

Step 4

Step 5. Make a 2- to 3-cm transverse incision through the skin and the subcutaneous tissues overlying the interspace. Extend the incision by blunt dissection with a Kelly clamp through the fascia toward the superior aspect of the rib above. After the superior border of the rib is reached, close and turn the Kelly clamp, and push it through the parietal pleura with steady, firm, and even pressure. Open the clamp widely, close it, and then withdraw it.

- **PITFALL:** Be careful to prevent the tip of the clamp from penetrating the lung, especially if no chest radiograph was obtained or if the x-ray film does not clearly show that the lung is retracted from the chest wall.
- **PITFALL:** Avoid being contaminated by the air or fluid that may rush out when the pleura is opened.

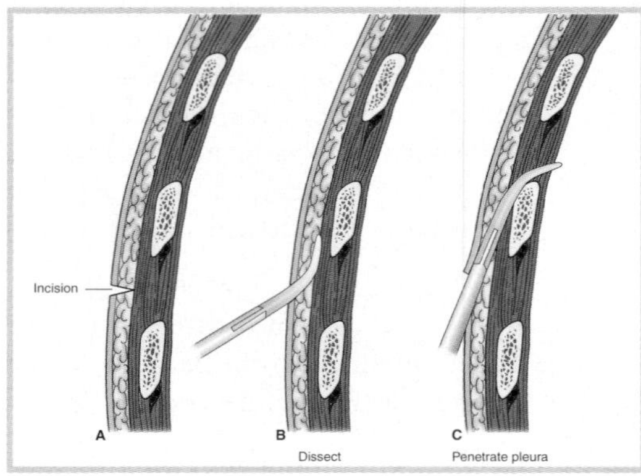

Step 5

Step 6. Insert an index finger to verify that the pleural space, not the potential space between the pleura and chest wall, has been entered. Check for unanticipated findings, such as pleural adhesions, masses, or the diaphragm.

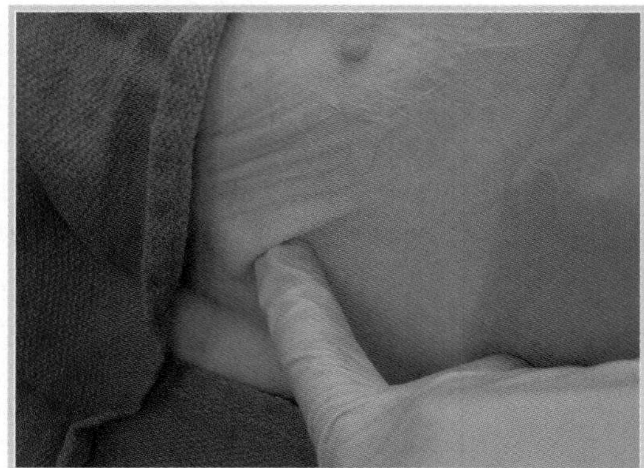

Step 6

Step 7. Grasp the chest tube so that the tip of the tube protrudes beyond the jaws of the clamp, and advance it through the hole into the pleural space using your finger as a guide. Direct the tip of the tube posteriorly for fluid drainage or anteriorly and superiorly for pneumothorax evacuation. Advance it until the last side hole is 2.5 to 5 cm (1 to 2 inches) inside the chest wall. Attach the tube to the previously assembled suction-drainage system. The chest tube should be inserted with the proximal hole at least 2 cm beyond the rib margin. Position of the chest tube with all drainage holes in the pleural space should be assessed by palpation. Confirm the correct location of the chest tube by the visualization of condensation within the tube with respiration or by drained pleural fluid seen within the tube. Ask the patient to cough, and observe whether bubbles form at the water-seal level. If the tube has not been properly inserted in the pleural space, no fluid will drain, and the level in the water column will not vary with respiration.

- **PEARL:** If a significant hemothorax is present, consider collecting the blood in a heparinized autotransfusion device so that it can be returned to the patient.

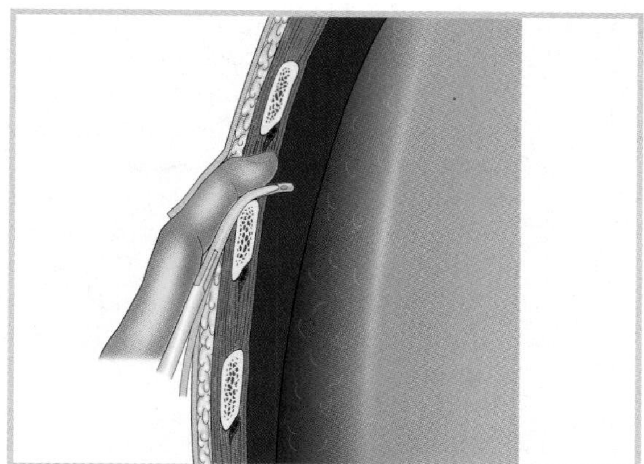

Step 7

Step 8. Suture the tube in place with 1-0 or 2-0 silk or other nonabsorbent sutures. The two sutures are tied so as to pull the soft tissues snugly around the tube and provide an airtight seal. Tie the first suture across the incision, and then wind both suture ends around the tube, starting at the bottom and working toward the top. Tie the ends of the suture very tightly around the tube, and cut the ends.

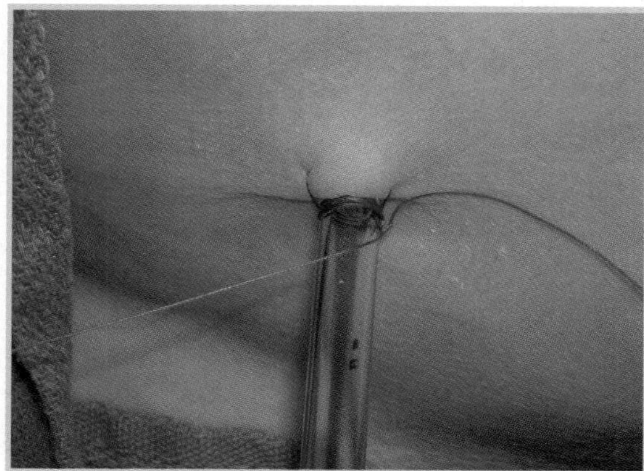

Step 8

Step 9. Place a second suture in a horizontal mattress or purse-string stitch around the tube at the skin incision site. Pull the ends of this suture together, and tie a surgeon's knot to close the skin around the tube. Wind the loose ends tightly around the tube, and finish the suture with a bow knot. The bow can be later undone and used to close the skin when the tube is removed. Alternatively some choose to only use the purse-string stitch to secure the chest tube. This usually involves wrapping the suture around the tube several more times than in the other method to ensure the tube does not slip from location.

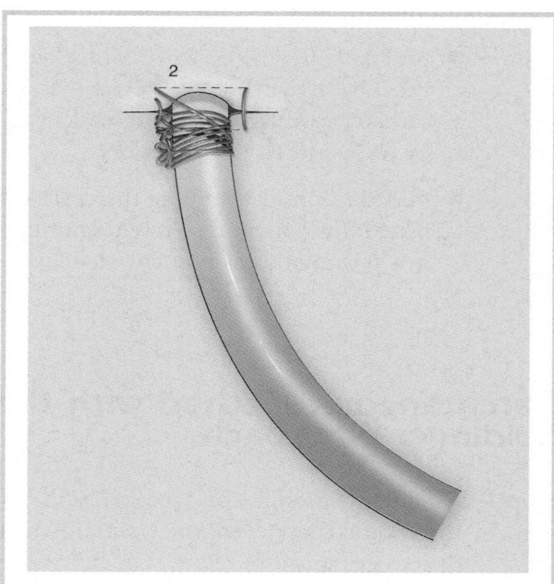

Step 9

Step 10. Place petroleum gauze around the tube where it meets the skin. Make a straight cut into the center of two additional 4 × 4-inch sterile gauze pads, and place them around the tube from opposite directions. Tape the gauze and tube in place, and tape together the tubing connections. Obtain posteroanterior and lateral chest radiographs to check the position of the chest tube and the amount of residual air or fluid as soon as possible after the tube is inserted.

- **PEARL:** Silastic chest tubes contain a radiopaque strip with a gap that serves to mark the most proximal drainage hole.
- **PITFALL:** A bedside, portable x-ray device is preferable to sending the patient to another location, because the suction usually must be removed and the tube may become displaced.
- **PITFALL:** If the patient is sent to another location for radiographs, do not clamp the chest tube, because any continuing air leakage can collapse the lung or produce a tension pneumothorax. Keep a water-seal bottle 1 to 2 feet lower than the patient's chest during transport. If a significant air leak develops, perform chest films.

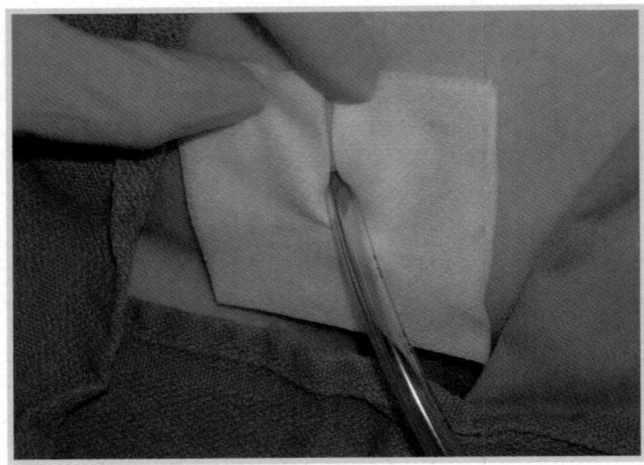

Step 10

Step 11. Use serial chest auscultation, chest radiographs, volume of blood loss, and amount of air leakage to assess the functioning of chest tubes. If a chest tube becomes blocked, it usually may be replaced through the same incision. Chest tubes are generally removed when there has been air or fluid drainage of <100 mL/24 hours for more than 24 hours.

- **PITFALL:** Trying to open a blocked chest tube by irrigating or passing a smaller catheter through it seldom works well and increases the risk of infection.
- **PEARL:** Consider keeping the chest tube in place if the patient is on a ventilator in case a new pneumothorax suddenly develops.

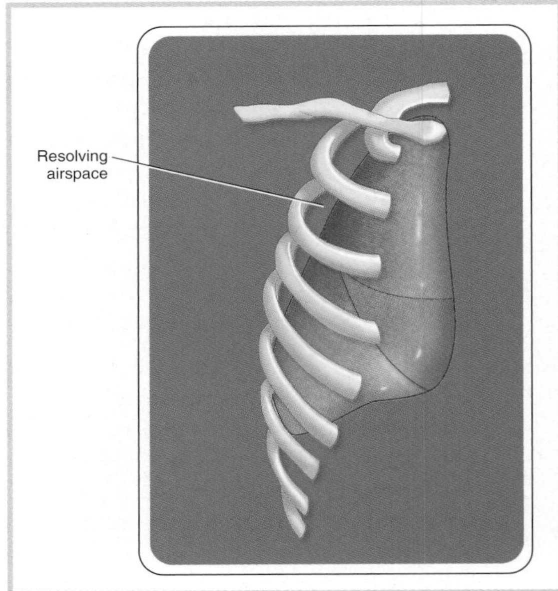

Step 11

Percutaneous Method with the Seldinger Approach

Step 1. Patient positioning and preparation remain the same as the conventional method. An introducer needle is inserted over a rib in a similar manner to needle thoracentesis.

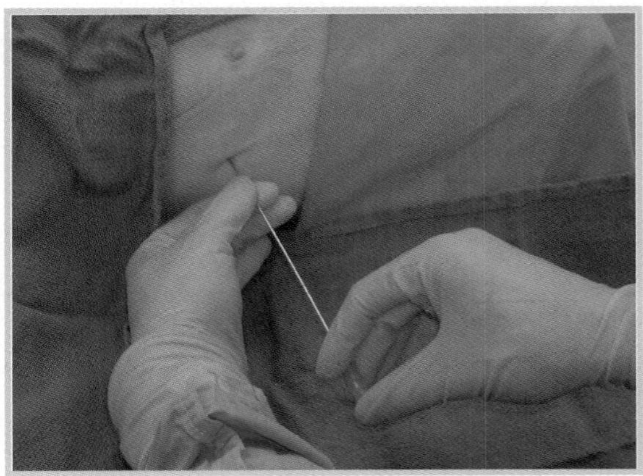

Step 1

Step 2. The obturator is removed, and a guidewire is placed through the needle into the pleural space.

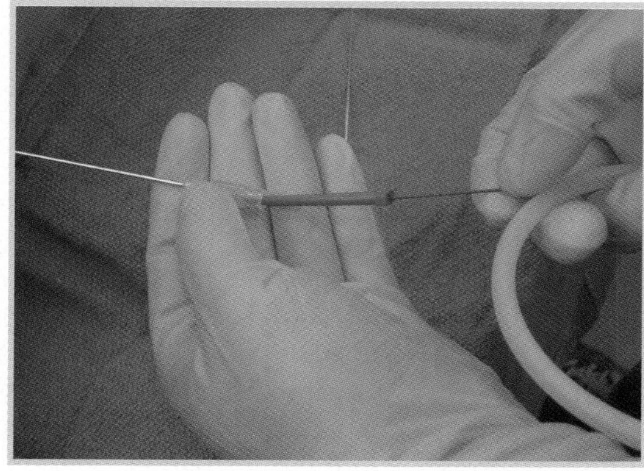

Step 2

Step 3. Serial dilators are passed over the guidewire to create an adequately dilated tract.

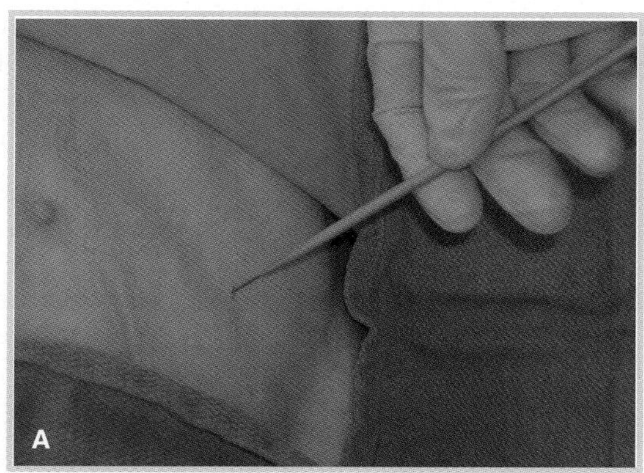

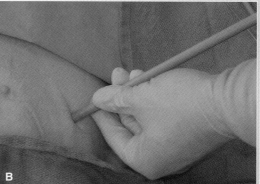

Step 3

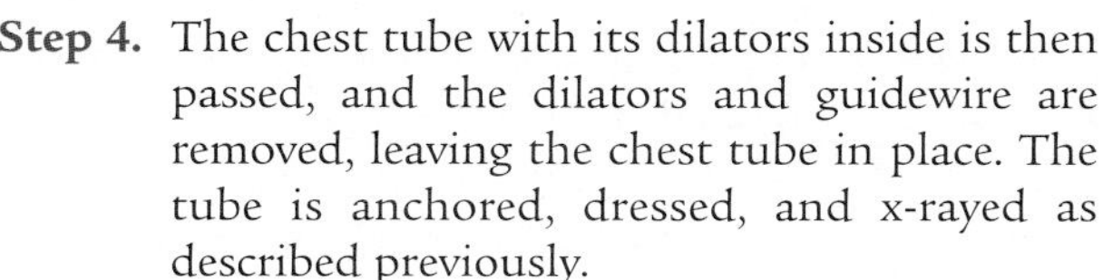

Step 4. The chest tube with its dilators inside is then passed, and the dilators and guidewire are removed, leaving the chest tube in place. The tube is anchored, dressed, and x-rayed as described previously.

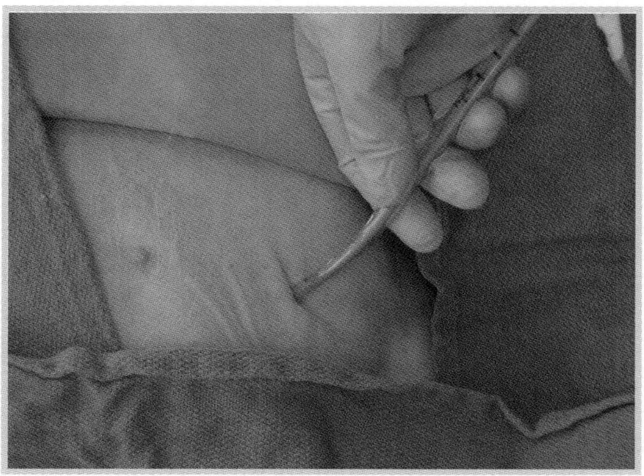

Step 4

Removal

Step 1. For chest tube removal, place the patient in the same position in which the tube was originally inserted. Prep the area, untie the suture with the bow knot, loosen the purse-string stitch, and cut the other suture near the skin. Clamp the chest tube, and disconnect the suction system. Ask the patient to take a deep breath and perform a Valsalva maneuver. Place a gauze over the insertion site, and remove the tube with a swift motion. Tie the purse-string suture. Apply petroleum gauze or antibiotic ointment on gauze, and tape securely. Obtain a chest radiograph immediately and at 12 to 24 hours to rule out a recurrent pneumothorax.

- **PEARL:** If the patient is on a ventilator, pause the ventilator during chest tube removal.

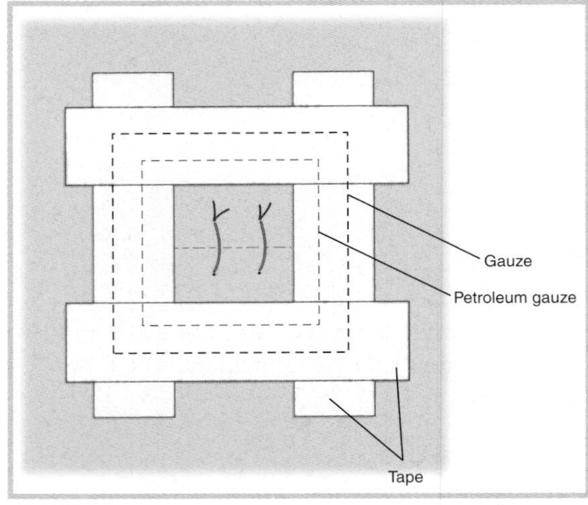

Step 1

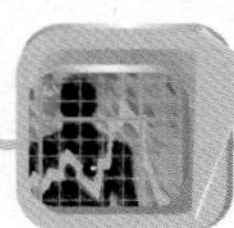

Complications

- Injury to the heart, great vessels, or lung
- Diaphragmatic perforation
- Subdiaphragmatic placement of the tube
- Open or tension pneumothorax
- Subcutaneous emphysema
- Unexplained or persistent air leakage
- Hemorrhage (especially from intercostal artery injury)
- Recurrent pneumothorax
- Empyema
- Lung parenchyma perforation
- Subcutaneous placement
- Cardiogenic shock (from chest tube compression of the right ventricle)
- Infection

There continues to be controversy concerning the need for prophylactic antibiotics in patients requiring a chest tube. Most trials show no benefit, although some have shown a reduction in infection in patients with penetrating chest trauma.

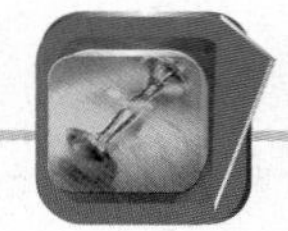

Pediatric Considerations

Chest tubes usually come in two standard lengths. Either length is appropriate for use in adults, but the shorter length should be used in pediatric patients.

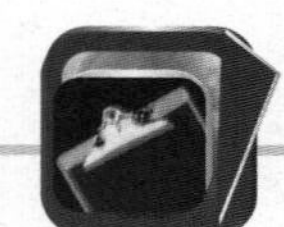

Postprocedure Instructions

Patients are rarely discharged immediately after chest tube removal. Have the patient report any shortness of breath or other symptoms of disease recurrence immediately. The bandage should be left in place for at least 24 hours, and petroleum gauze should be kept on the wound for 2 to 3 days. The sutures should be removed in about 1 week.

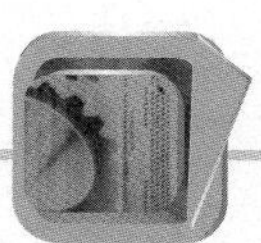

Coding Information and Supply Sources

CPT Code	Description	2008 Average 50th Percentile Fee	Global Period
32551	Tube thoracostomy with or without water seal (e.g., abscess, hemothorax, empyema)	$740	0
32422	Thoracentesis, with insertion of tube, includes water seal (e.g., for pneumothorax) when performed (separate procedure)	$508	0
76942-26	Ultrasound guidance for needle placement	$496	XXX
77002-26	Fluoroscopic guidance for needle placement	$396	XXX
77012-26	CT guidance for needle placement	$277	XXX

XXX = Global concept does not apply.

CPT is a registered trademark of the American Medical Association.

2008 average 50th Percentile Fees are provided courtesy of 2008 MMH-SI's copyrighted Physicians' Fees and Coding Guide.

Bibliography

Baldt MM, Bankier AA, Germann PS, et al. Complications after emergency tube thoracostomy: assessment with CT. *Radiology.* 1995;195:539–543.

Bell RL, Ovadia P, Abdullah F, et al. Chest tube removal: end-inspiration or end-expiration? *J Trauma.* 2001;50:674–677.

Chan L, Reilly KM, Henderson C, et al. Complication rates of tube thoracostomy. *Am J Emerg Med.* 1997;15:368–370.

Collop NA, Kim S, Sahn SA. Analysis of tube thoracostomy performed by pulmonologists at a teaching hospital. *Chest.* 1997;112:709–713.

Dalbec, DL, Krome, RL. Thoracostomy. *Emerg Med Clin North Am.* 1986;4:441.

Daly, RC, Mucha, P, Pairolero, PC, et al. The risk of percutaneous chest tube thoracostomy for blunt thoracic trauma. *Ann Emerg Med.* 1985;14:865.

Gilbert TB, McGrath BJ, Soberman M. Chest tubes: indications, placement, management, and complications. *J Intensive Care Med.* 1993;8:73–86.

Graber RE, Garvin JM. Chest tube insertion. *Patient Care.* 1988;9:159.

Grover, FL, Richardson, JD, Fewel, JG, et al. Prophylactic antibiotics in the treatment of penetrating chest wounds: a prospective double-blind study. *J Thorac Cardiovasc Surg.* 1977; 74:528.

Hesselink DA, Van Der Klooster JM, Bac EH, et al. Cardiac tamponade secondary to chest tube placement. *Eur J Emerg Med.* 2001;8:237–239.

Horsley A, Jones L, White J, et al. Efficacy and complications of small-bore, wire-guided chest drains. *Chest.* 2006;130:1857–1863.

Jones PM, Hewer RD, Wolfenden HD, et al. Subcutaneous emphysema associated with chest tube drainage. *Respirology.* 2001;6:87–89.

Mahfood S, Hix WR, Aaron BL, et al. Reexpansion pulmonary edema. *Ann Thorac Surg.* 1988;45:340.

Maxwell RA, Campbell DJ, Fabian TC, et al. Use of presumptive antibiotics following tube thoracostomy for traumatic hemopneumothorax in the prevention of empyema and pneumonia—a multi-center trial. *J Trauma.* 2004;57:742.

Millikan JS, Moore EE, Steiner E, et al. Complications of tube thoracostomy for acute trauma. *Am J Surg.* 1980;140:738.

Nahum E, Ben-Ari J, Schonfeld T, et al. Acute diaphragmatic paralysis caused by chest-tube trauma to phrenic nerve. *Pediatr Radiol.* 2001;31:444–446.

Parulekar W, Di Primio G, Matzinger F, et al. Use of small-bore vs large-bore chest tubes for treatment of malignant pleural effusions. *Chest.* 2001;120:19–25.

Rashid MA, Wikstrom T, Ortenwall P. Mediastinal perforation and contralateral hemothorax by a chest tube. *Thorac Cardiovasc Surg.* 1998;46:375–376.

Schmidt U, Stalp M, Gerich T, et al. Chest tube decompression of blunt chest injuries by physicians in the field: effectiveness and complications. *J Trauma.* 1998;44:98–101.

Symbas, PN. Chest drainage tubes. *Surg Clin North Am.* 1989;69:41.

2008 MAG Mutual Healthcare Solutions, Inc.'s Physicians' Fee and Coding Guide. Duluth, Georgia. MAG Mutual Healthcare Solutions, Inc. 2007.

CHAPTER 9

Percutaneous Cricothyrotomy

Vinay Bangalore, MD, MPH

Critical Care Medicine
Louisiana State University Health Sciences Center, Shreveport, LA

Laurie Grier, MD, FCCM, FCCP, FACP

Professor of Clinical Medicine, Emergency Medicine and Anesthesia
Louisiana State University Health Sciences Center, Shreveport, LA

The protection and maintenance of a patent airway is extremely important. Airway maintenance procedures are highly useful skills to possess for all clinicians. They permit ventilation and oxygenation and prevent further complications in an emergency.

Oral endotracheal intubation is the most common method of obtaining a secure airway. However, in certain situations, definitive airway control by means of intubation may be contraindicated or extremely difficult to perform. In such situations, cricothyrotomy may be the best way to establish an airway.

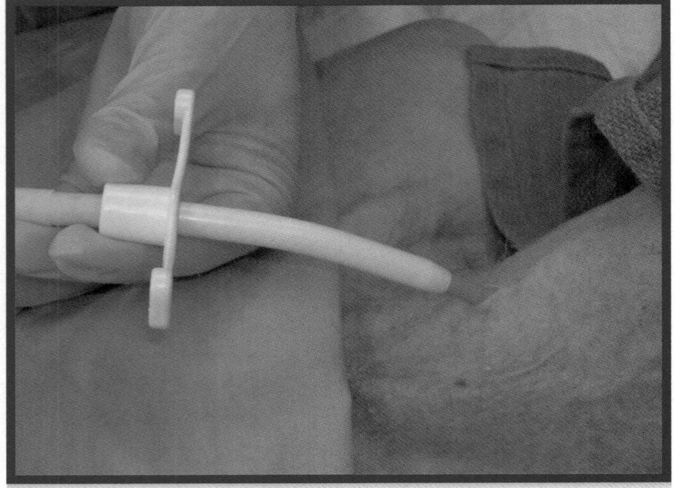

Cricothyrotomy is a procedure that makes an opening in the cricothyroid membrane to obtain an airway. It differs from a tracheostomy, which is a procedure that makes an opening in the trachea between the second and fourth tracheal rings. The cricothyroid membrane is immediately subcutaneous in location. There are no overlying muscles and no major arteries, veins, or nerves in the region. These anatomic considerations make the cricothyroid membrane an ideal choice for gaining access to the airway when endotracheal intubation is not possible.

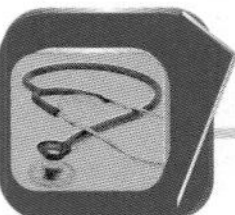

Equipment

- Melker emergency cricothyrotomy catheter set (Cook Medical), which includes these items:
  - Cricothyrotomy tube
  - Tapered curved dilator

- Syringe
- Disposable scalpel
- Polytetrafluoroethylene (Teflon, PTFE, TFE) coated catheter needle
- Guidewire with flexible tip
- Trach tape

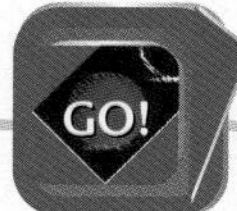

Indications

- Inability to perform oral or nasal endotracheal intubation
- Massive oral, nasal, or pharyngeal hemorrhage
- Massive emesis
- Laryngospasm
- Mass effect (cancer, tumor)
- Structural deformities of the oropharynx
- Upper airway stenosis
- Oropharyngeal edema
- Foreign-body obstruction
- Maxillofacial injuries
- Cervical spine instability

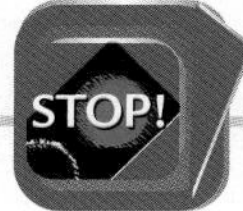

Contraindications

- Fractured larynx or significant damage to the cricoid cartilage (absolute contraindication)
- Endotracheal intubation can be accomplished easily and quickly
- Infants and children younger than 5 years old (relative contraindication)
- Bleeding diathesis (relative contraindication)
- Massive neck edema (relative contraindication)

The Procedure

Step 1. Place the patient in a supine position. Prep and drape the anterior neck using usual sterile precautions if time permits. Open the Melker emergency cricothyrotomy catheter set.

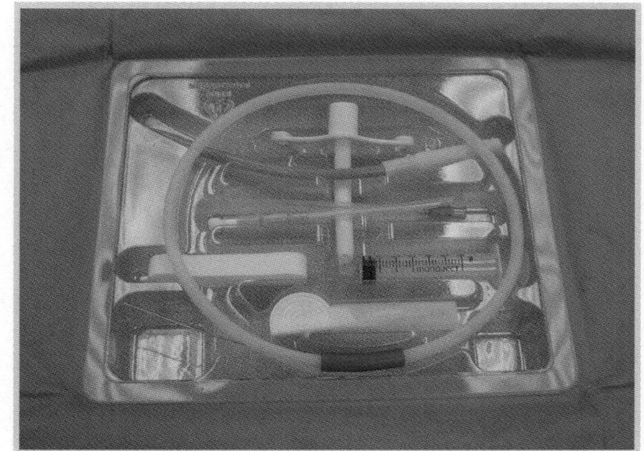

Step 1

Step 2. Advance the tapered end of the curved dilator into the connector end of the provided cricothyrotomy tube until the handle of the dilator stops against the connector. Lubrication may be used on the surface of the dilator to facilitate this step.

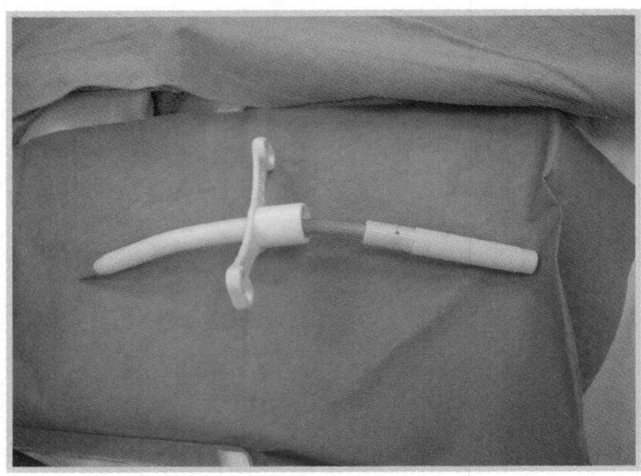

Step 2

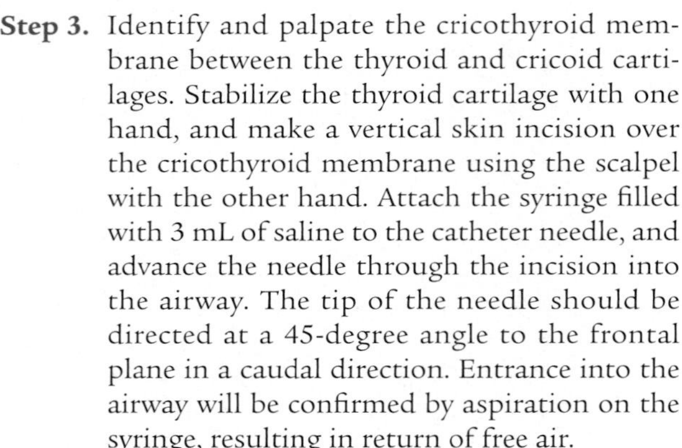

Step 3. Identify and palpate the cricothyroid membrane between the thyroid and cricoid cartilages. Stabilize the thyroid cartilage with one hand, and make a vertical skin incision over the cricothyroid membrane using the scalpel with the other hand. Attach the syringe filled with 3 mL of saline to the catheter needle, and advance the needle through the incision into the airway. The tip of the needle should be directed at a 45-degree angle to the frontal plane in a caudal direction. Entrance into the airway will be confirmed by aspiration on the syringe, resulting in return of free air.

- **PEARL:** Make sure that the incision is large enough to allow passage of the dilator and the cricothyrotomy tube.

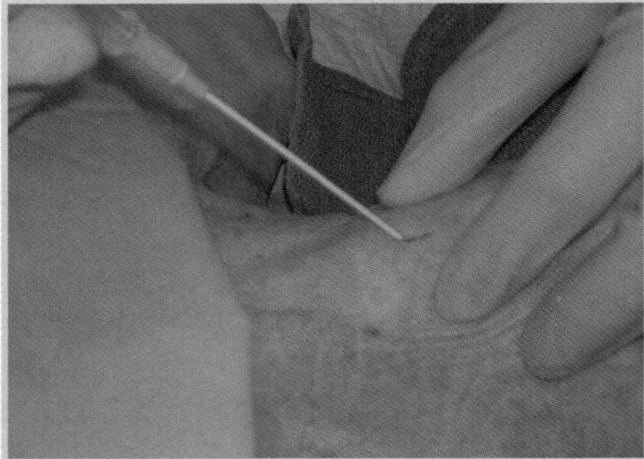

Step 3

Step 4. Once in the airway, remove the syringe and needle, leaving the catheter in place. Advance the flexible end of the guidewire through the catheter into the airway.

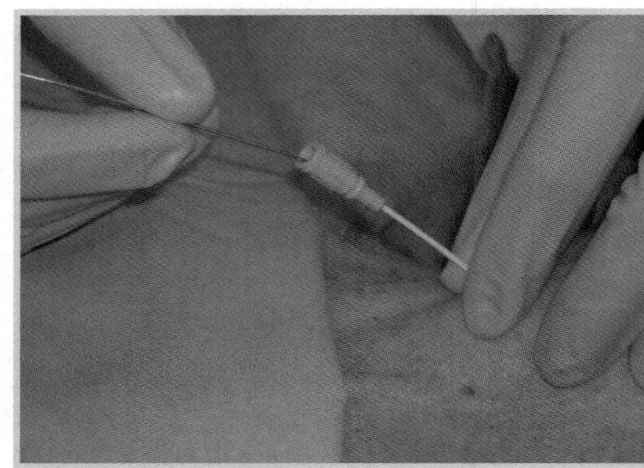

Step 4

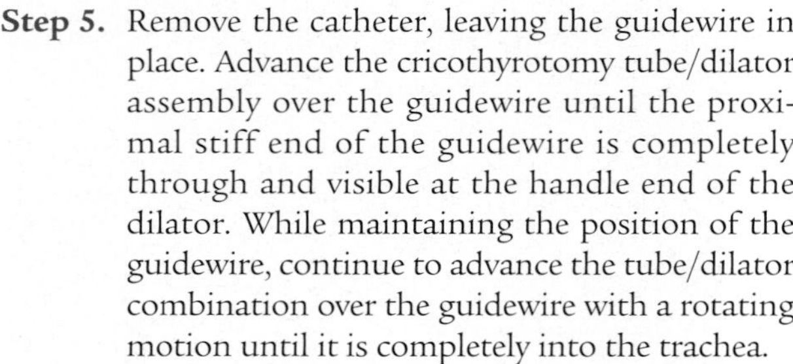

Step 5. Remove the catheter, leaving the guidewire in place. Advance the cricothyrotomy tube/dilator assembly over the guidewire until the proximal stiff end of the guidewire is completely through and visible at the handle end of the dilator. While maintaining the position of the guidewire, continue to advance the tube/dilator combination over the guidewire with a rotating motion until it is completely into the trachea.

- **PEARL:** Make sure to have control of the guidewire at all times to prevent its inadvertent loss into the trachea.

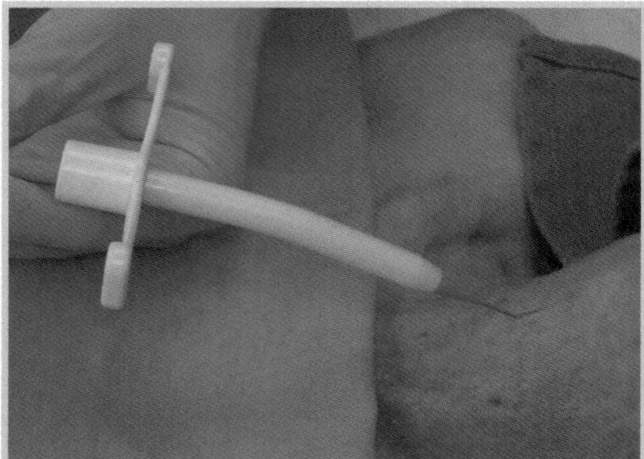

Step 5

Step 6. Remove the guidewire and dilator simultaneously. Connect the airway catheter to a ventilator using its standard 15-mm connector.

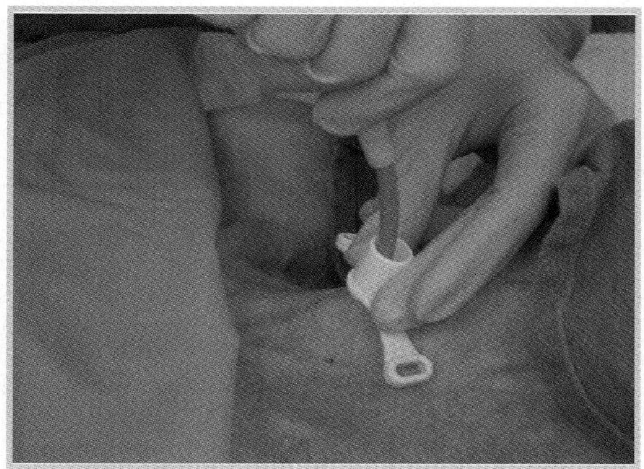

Step 6

Step 7. Fix the cricothyrotomy catheter in place with tracheostomy tape strip in the standard fashion.

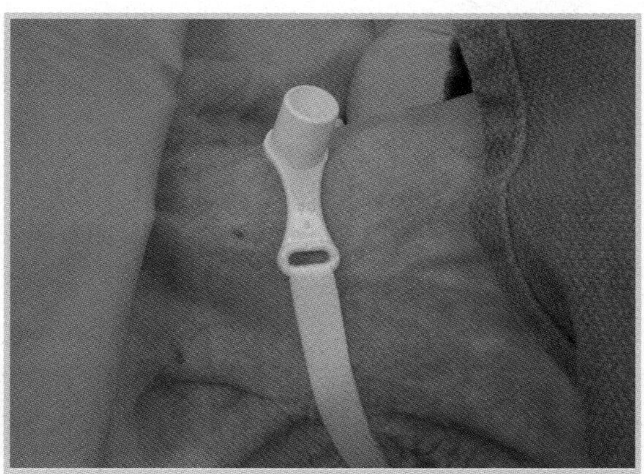

Step 7

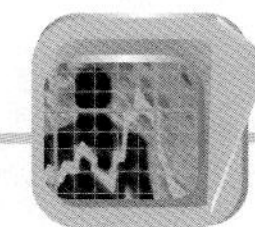

Complications

Immediate or Early Complications

- Common
  - Bleeding, hematoma
  - Incorrect/unsuccessful tube placement
  - Subcutaneous emphysema
- Infrequent
  - Esophageal perforation
  - Mediastinal perforation
  - Pneumothorax, pneumomediastinum
  - Vocal cord injury

Late Complications

- Common
  - Dysphonia
  - Persistent stoma

- Infrequent
    - Subglottic or glottic stenosis
    - Tracheoesophageal fistula
    - Tracheomalacia

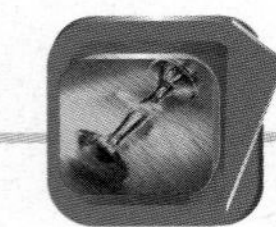

Pediatric Considerations

Although not an absolute contraindication, the procedure is not recommended in infants and children younger 10 years of age because of the difficulty in palpating and identifying important neck landmarks.

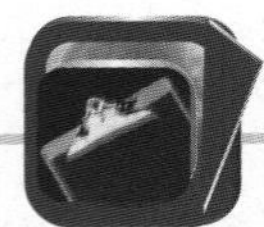

Postprocedure Instructions

General tracheostomy care is given as for regular tracheostomy and consists of suctioning respiratory secretions and keeping the stomal wound and tube flanges clean with sterile saline. Tube ties that have been contaminated with secretions should be changed.

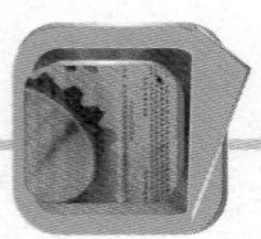

Coding Information and Supply Sources

CPT Code	Description	2008 Average 50th Percentile Fee	Global Period
31605	Tracheostomy emergency procedure, cricothyroid membrane	$1,058.00	0

CPT is a registered trademark of the American Medical Association.
2008 average 50th Percentile Fees are provided courtesy of 2008 MMH-SI's copyrighted Physicians' Fees and Coding Guide.

ICD-9 Codes

Acute respiratory failure	518.81
Acute and chronic respiratory failure	518.84
Acute respiratory distress	518.82
Chronic respiratory failure	518.83
Respiratory arrest	799.1

Supplier

Cook Medical, Inc., P.O. Box 4195, Bloomington, IN 47402-4195. Phone: 1-800-457-4500. Web site: http://www.cookmedical.com/.

Patient Education Handout

A patient education handout, "Tracheostomy," can be found on the book's companion Web site.

Bibliography

Cook Medical. Melker universal cricothyrotomy catheter set: instructions for use. http://www.cookmedical.com/cc/content/mmedia/C-T-UTCCSB304.pdf. Accessed January 2008.

Goldenberg D, Bhatti N. Management of the impaired airway in the adult. In: Cummings CW, ed. *Otolaryngology: Head and Neck Surgery*. 4th ed. Elsevier, Mosby; Philadelphia 2005. http://www.mdconsult.com. Accessed January 2008.

Mace SE, Hedges JR. Cricothyrotomy and translaryngeal jet ventilation. In: Roberts JR, ed. *Clinical Procedures in Emergency Medicine*. 4th ed. Saunders; Philadelphia 2004. http://www.mdconsult.com. Accessed January 2008.

Walls RM. Airway. In: Marx JA, ed. *Rosen's Emergency Medicine: Concepts and Clinical Practice*. 6th ed. Mosby; Philadelphia 2006. http://www.mdconsult.com. Accessed January 2008.

2008 MAG Mutual Healthcare Solutions, Inc.'s Physicians' Fee and Coding Guide. Duluth, Georgia. MAG Mutual Healthcare Solutions, Inc. 2007.

CHAPTER 10

Incision and Drainage of Abscesses

Heidi Wimberly, PA-C

Clinical Instructor, Department of Emergency Medicine
Louisiana State University Health Sciences Center, Shreveport, LA

An abscess is a confined collection of pus surrounded by inflamed tissue. Most abscesses are found on the extremities, buttocks, breast, axilla, groin, and areas prone to friction or minor trauma, but they may be found in any area of the body. Abscesses are formed when the skin is invaded by microorganisms. Cellulitis may precede or occur in conjunction with an abscess. The two most common microorganisms leading to abscess formation are *Staphylococcus* and *Streptococcus*. Perianal abscesses are commonly caused by enteric organisms. Gram-negative organisms and anaerobic bacteria also contribute to abscess formation.

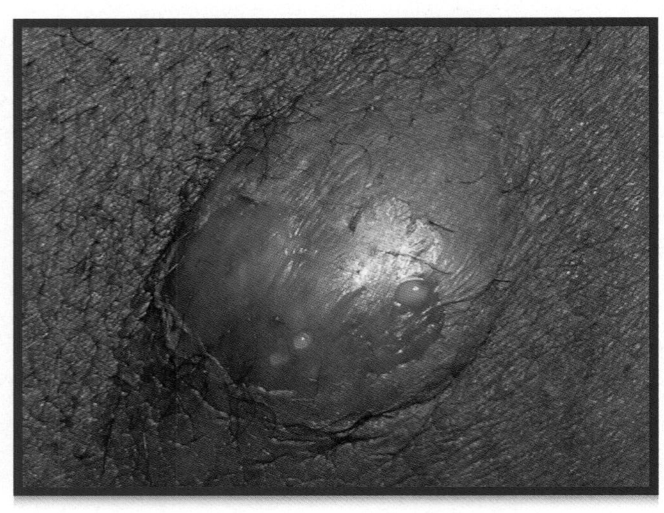

Treatment of an abscess is primarily through incision and drainage (I&D). Smaller abscesses (<5 mm) may resolve spontaneously with the application of warm compresses and antibiotic therapy. Larger abscesses will require I&D as a result of an increase in collection of pus, inflammation, and formation of the abscess cavity, which lessens the success of conservative measures.

Untreated abscesses may follow one of two courses. The abscess may remain deep and slowly reabsorb, or the overlying epithelium may attenuate (i.e., pointing), allowing the abscess to spontaneously rupture to the surface and drain. Rarely, deep extension into the subcutaneous tissue may be followed by sloughing and extensive scarring. Conservative therapy for small abscesses includes warm, wet compresses and anti-*Staphylococcal* antibiotics. I&D is a time-honored method of draining abscesses to relieve pain and speed healing. Routine cultures and antibiotics are usually unnecessary if an abscess is properly drained.

After I&D, instruct the patient to watch for signs of cellulitis or recollection of pus. Train patients or family to change packing, or arrange for the patient's packing to be changed as necessary. Cellulitis occurs most commonly in patients with diabetes or other diseases that interfere with immune function. I&D of a perianal abscess may result in a chronic anal fistula and may require a fistulectomy by a surgeon.

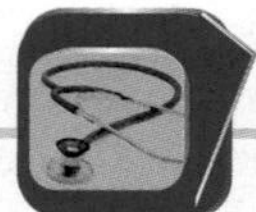

Equipment

- Universal precaution materials (gown, gloves, protective eyewear)
- Sterile draping towels and sterile gloves
- Local anesthetic (1% or 2% lidocaine with or without epinephrine)
- 10-cc syringe and 25- to 30-gauge needle
- Skin prep material (chlorhexidine [Hibiclens] or iodine swabs)
- No. 11 or 15 blade and scalpel
- Curved hemostats
- Scissors
- Packing (plain or iodoform) ribbon gauze
- Dressing (4- × 4-inch gauze pads and tape)

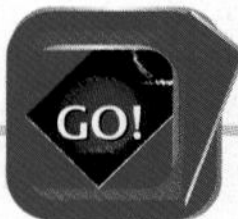

Indications

- Palpable, fluctuant abscess
- An abscess that does not resolve despite conservative measures
- Large abscess (>5 mm)

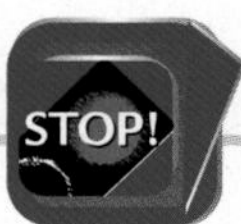

Contraindications

- Extensively large or deep abscesses or perirectal abscesses that may require surgical debridement and general anesthesia
- Facial abscesses in the nasolabial folds (risk of septic phlebitis secondary to abscess drainage into the sphenoid sinus)
- Hand and finger abscesses should receive surgical or orthopedic consultation

Use caution with immunocompromised patients and diabetic patients; these populations may require more aggressive measures and follow-up.

The Procedure

Step 1. Prep the surface of the abscess and surrounding skin with povidone-iodine or chlorhexidine solution (see Appendix E) and drape the abscess with sterile towels. Perform a field block by infiltrating local anesthetic around and under the tissue surrounding abscess.

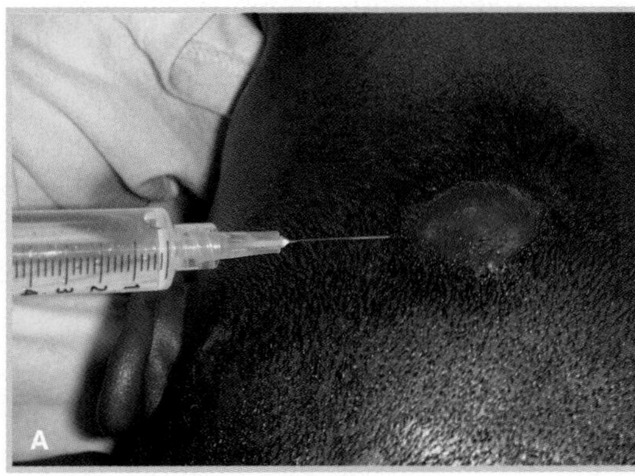

- PITFALL: The environment of an abscess is acidic, which may cause local anesthetics to lose effectiveness. Use an appropriate amount of anesthetic, and allow adequate time for anesthetic effect.
- PITFALL: Avoid injecting into the abscess cavity, because it may rupture downward into the underlying tissues or upward toward the provider.

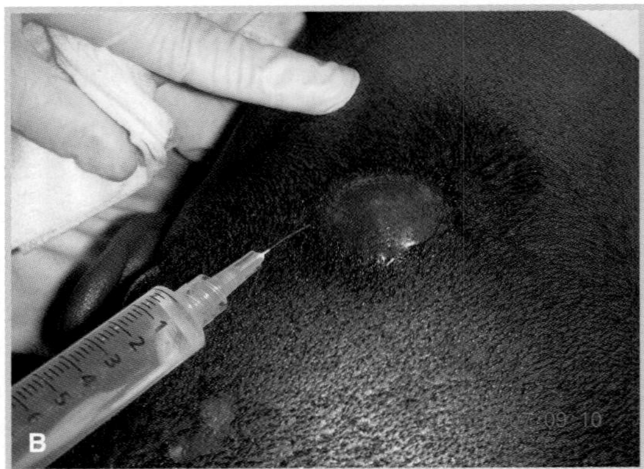

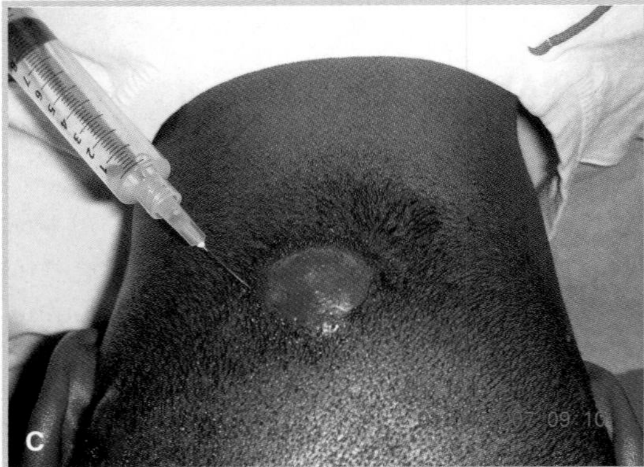

Step 1

Step 2. Make a linear incision with a no. 11 or 15 blade into the abscess.

- PITFALL: The most common cause of abscess reoccurrence is an incision not wide enough to promote adequate drainage.
- PITFALL: Inform the patient before the procedure that scarring is possible.
- PITFALL: Contents of the abscess may project upward and outward when it is incised, especially if local anesthetic was inadvertently injected into (instead of around) the abscess. Use personal protective equipment to avoid self-contamination.

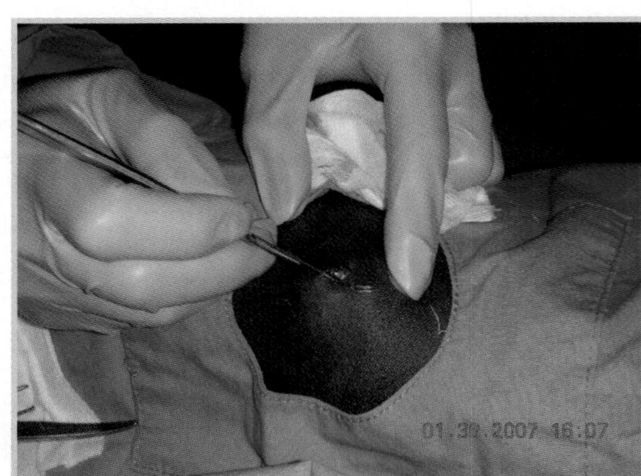

Step 2

Step 3. Allow purulent material from the abscess to drain. Gently probe the abscess with the curved hemostats to break up loculations. Attempt to manually express purulent material from the abscess.

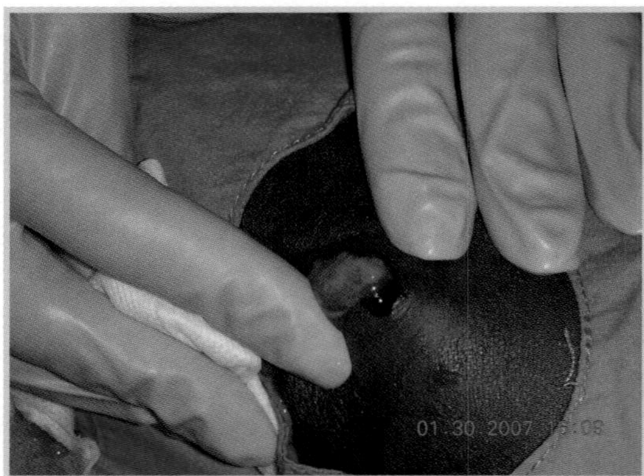

Step 3

Step 4. Insert packing material into the abscess with hemostats or forceps. Dress the wound with sterile gauze and tape.

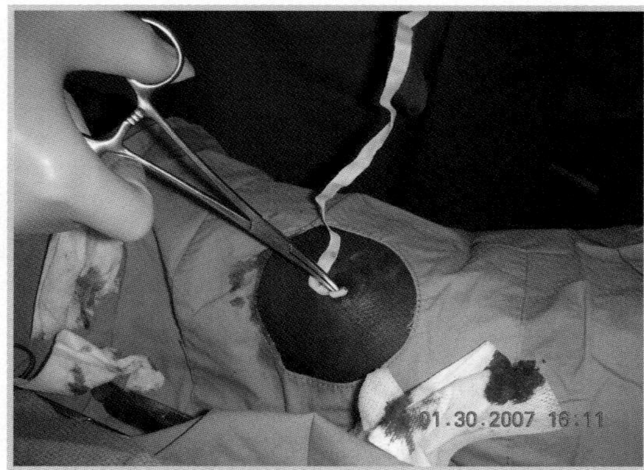

Step 4

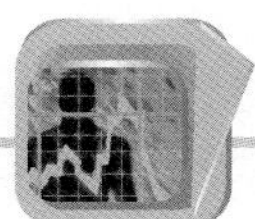

Complications

- Inadequate anesthesia
- Pain during and after the procedure
- Bleeding
- Reoccurrence of abscess formation
- Septic thrombophlebitis
- Necrotizing fasciitis
- Fistula formation
- Damage to nerves and vessels
- Scarring

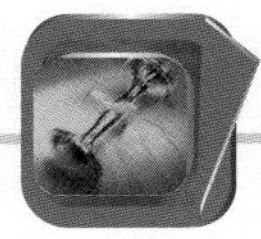

Pediatric Considerations

Skin abscesses in children should be approached the same way as for adults. Consideration should be given to pediatric antibiotic dosing if choosing to treat the abscesses with conservative measures.

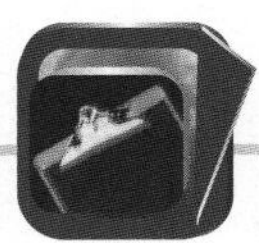

Postprocedure Instructions

The patient should be instructed to keep the wound clean, dry, and covered with absorbent material. If the abscess contains packing gauze, instruct the patient to remove packing material and repack the abscess every 1 to 2 days until the abscess cavity has resolved and packing materials can no longer be inserted into the abscess. If the patient does not feel comfortable with repacking, direct the patient to a medical facility for repacking of the abscess every 1 to 2 days. Instruct the patient to change the overlying dressing once a day. Inform the patient that he or she may take over-the-counter pain relievers or prescription pain relievers as directed for pain.

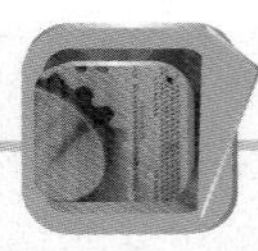

CPT Code	Description	2008 Average 50th Percentile Fee	Global Period
10040	Acne surgery	$124.00	10
10060	I&D of single or simple abscess	$167.00	10
10061	I&D of multiple or complex abscesses	$293.00	10
10080	I&D of pilonidal cyst, simple	$191.00	10
10081	I&D of pilonidal cyst, complicated	$350.00	10
10140	I&D of hematoma, seroma, or fluid collection	$195.00	10
10160	Puncture aspiration of abscess, hematoma, bulla, or cyst	$155.00	10
10180	I&D, complex, of postoperative wound infection	$531.00	0
21501	I&D of deep abscess of neck or thorax	$820.00	90
23030	I&D of deep abscess of shoulder	$764.00	10
23930	I&D of deep abscess of upper arm or elbow	$694.00	10
23931	I&D of deep abscess of upper arm or elbow bursa	$594.00	10
25028	I&D of deep abscess of forearm or wrist	$1,257.00	10
26010	I&D of simple abscess of finger	$356.00	10
26011	I&D of complicated abscess of finger or felon	$723.00	10
26990	I&D of deep abscess of pelvis or hip joint area	$1,265.00	90
26991	I&D of infected bursa of pelvis or hip joint area	$1,279.00	90
27301	I&D of deep abscess of thigh or knee region	$1,428.00	90
27603	I&D of deep abscess of leg or ankle	$1,292.00	90
28001	I&D of bursa of the foot	$423.00	10
40800	I&D of abscess, cyst, or hematoma in the vestibule of the mouth, simple	$249.00	10
40801	I&D of abscess, cyst, or hematoma in the vestibule of the mouth, complicated	$568.00	10
41000	Intraoral I&D of abscess, cyst, or hematoma of tongue or floor of the mouth, lingual	$309.00	10
41005	Intraoral I&D of abscess, cyst, or hematoma of tongue or floor of the mouth, sublingual, superficial	$339.00	10

CPT Code	Description	2008 Average 50th Percentile Fee	Global Period
41006	Intraoral I&D of abscess, cyst, or hematoma of tongue or floor of the mouth, sublingual, deep	$676.00	90
41800	I&D of abscess, cyst, or hematoma from dentoalveolar structures	$337.00	10
54015	I&D of deep abscess of penis	$644.00	10
54700	I&D of abscess of epididymis, testis, or scrotal space	$663.00	10
55100	I&D of abscess of scrotal wall	$575.00	10
56405	I&D of abscess of vulva or perineum	$311.00	10
56420	I&D of abscess of the Bartho lin gland	$340.00	10
67700	I&D of abscess of eyelid	$493.00	10
69000	I&D of abscess of external ear, simple	$265.00	10
69005	I&D of abscess of external ear, complicated	$586.00	10

CPT is a registered trademark of the American Medical Association.
2008 average 50th Percentile Fees are provided courtesy of 2008 MMH-SI's copyrighted Physicians' Fees and Coding Guide.

Standard skin tray supplies are shown in Appendix G. A suggested anesthesia tray that can be used for this procedure is listed in Appendix F. Skin preparation recommendations appear in Appendix E.

Patient Education Handout

A patient education handout, "Skin Abscess Treatment," can be found on the book's Web site.

Bibliography

Blumstein H. Incision and drainage. In: Roberts JR, Hedges JR, eds. *Clinical Procedures in Emergency Medicine*. 3rd ed. Philadelphia: Saunders, an imprint of Elsevier; 1998:634.

Halvorson GD, Halvorson JE, Iserson KV. Abscess incision and drainage in the emergency department (part 2). *J Emerg Med.* 1985;3:295.

Llera JL, Levy RC. Treatment of cutaneous abscess: a double-blind clinical study. *Ann Emerg Med.* 1985;14:15–19.

2008 MAG Mutual Healthcare Solutions, Inc.'s Physicians' Fee and Coding Guide. Duluth, Georgia. MAG Mutual Healthcare Solutions, Inc. 2007.

CHAPTER 11

Lumbar Puncture

Lauren M. Yorek, MD

Assistant Clinical Professor, Department of Emergency Medicine
Louisiana State University Health Sciences Center, Shreveport, LA

Lumbar puncture (LP) is a common diagnostic and therapeutic procedure. It is most commonly performed to obtain a sample of cerebrospinal fluid (CSF) to help establish neurological diagnoses. LP is the most accurate method for diagnosing central nervous system infection.

CSF is produced by the choroid plexus in the brain and circulates around the brain and spinal cord within the subarachnoid space. During an LP, the spinal needle penetrates the skin, subcutaneous tissue, spinal ligaments, dura, and arachnoid before entering the subarachnoid space. Four samples of CSF are usually obtained. Usual studies include bacterial culture and Gram stain from tube 1, protein and glucose from tube 2, blood cell counts and differential cell counts from tube 3, and optional tests such as viral cultures, fungal cultures, countercurrent immunoelectrophoresis, India ink studies, or latex agglutination tests from tube 4. Common CSF findings are shown in Table 11-1. There are some CSF findings that suggest a diagnosis of bacterial meningitis. A CSF absolute white blood count (WBC) value of >500 μL, a blood glucose ratio of ≤0.4, a lactate level of ≥31.5, and the presence of bacteria on Gram stain can assist with diagnosis of bacterial meningitis. However, the absence of bacteria on Gram stain does not rule out bacterial meningitis.

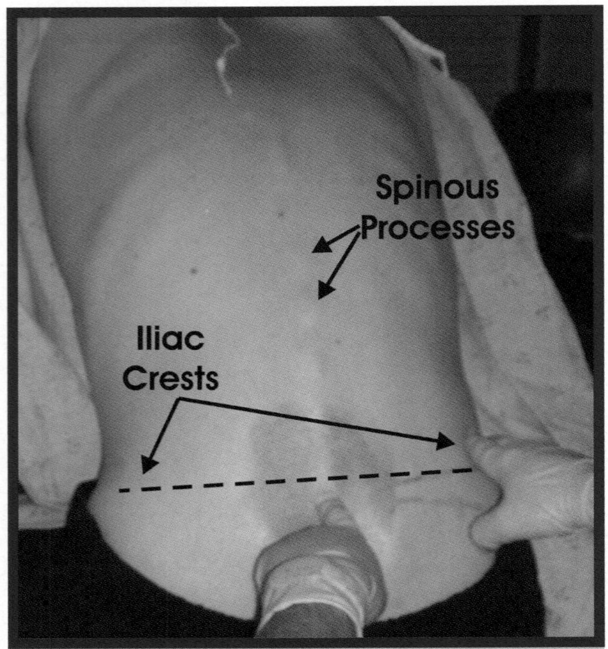

The indications for LP in neonates are not as clear as they once were. The once common practice of performing an LP in all ill newborns with suspected sepsis or respiratory distress is no longer recommended unless other findings suggest meningitis. LP is often reserved for babies who demonstrate hypothermia, hyperthermia, poor feeding 24 hours after birth, coma, or seizures. Bedside ultrasound scanning has largely replaced LP for the diagnosis of intracranial hemorrhage. Only about one half of LPs in newborns are successfully completed, and traumatic (bloody) taps are common.

The most common complication is the post-LP (spinal) headache, which occurs in 10% to 25% of patients. The headache often persists for days. Using smaller-diameter nontraumatic needles and ensuring adequate hydration can help prevent postprocedure headache. Traditionally, it has been believed that keeping patients in the supine position after an LP would prevent headache. New data now suggest that patients should be mobilized soon after LP. When the headache is persistent, an epidural blood patch may be applied by an anesthesiologist. Traumatic (bloody) taps result from inadvertent puncture of the spinal

TABLE 11-1. Common Properties of Cerebrospinal Fluid

Cerebrospinal Fluid Characteristic	Normal Values	Acute Bacterial Meningitis	Subacute Meningitis	Viral Infection	Pseudotumor Cerebr	Cerebral Hemorrhage
Opening pressure (cm H_2O)	5–20	>20	Normal to increased	Normal to increased	Increased	Increased
White blood cell count (cells/mm^3)	<5	100–700	500–5,000	100–2,000	Normal	Bloody sample
Glucose (mg/dL)	50–100 (or 60%–70% of blood glucose)	Decreased	Decreased	Normal	Normal	Normal
Protein (mg/dL)	15–45	≈100	Increased	Normal or increased	Normal or decreased	Increased

venous plexuses and may rarely lead to spinal hematoma. Other temporary complications include shooting pains in the lower extremities and local pain in the back.

A more serious potential complication is brain herniation from elevated intracranial pressure that often is caused by a supratentorial mass. However, research has shown that severe meningitis also may cause elevated intracranial pressure and herniation. Before performing an LP, always check the optic fundi for papilledema. If increased pressure from a tumor or an intracranial bleed is suspected, an emergency noncontrast computed tomography (CT) scan should be obtained before LP to reduce the potential of herniation. Altered mentation and focal neurological findings are also indications for CT prior to performing an LP. Focal neurological findings include but are not limited to gaze palsy, facial palsy, arm or leg drift, and abnormal language function. Inadvertent aspiration of nerve roots on needle withdrawal can be prevented by replacing the stylet before needle removal. Meningitis as a result of the procedure is a theoretical complication. Epidermoid spinal cord tumors have been associated with the performance of LP in infants with unstyletted needles.

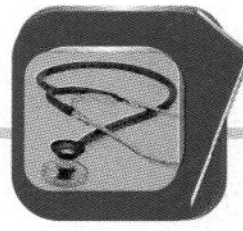

Equipment

- Lumbar puncture tray:
  - Atraumatic (Sprotte or Pajunk) needle (which has an opening on the side at the end or the needle) or the standard (Quincke) needle (which has a standard bevel) with introducer, 22 to 26 gauge
  - Local anesthesia for injection
  - Povidone-iodine or chlorhexidine (Hibiclens) for sterilization of field
  - Four sterile collection tubes with labels one through four
  - Manometer for measurement of CSF pressure if needed
  - Dressing to apply after procedure

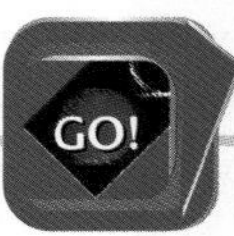

Indications

- Suspected central nervous system infection
- Suspected subarachnoid hemorrhage

- Suspected neurosyphilis
- Suspected Guillain-Barré syndrome
- Support for the diagnosis of pseudotumor cerebri (i.e., increased CSF pressure without infection)
- Serial removal of CSF
- Support for the diagnosis of multiple sclerosis (i.e., elevated IgG level and oligoclonal banding on electrophoresis)

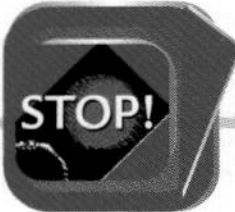

Contraindications

- Dermatitis or cellulitis at insertion site
- Raised intracranial pressure
- Supratentorial mass lesions (evaluate with CT scan first)
- Severe bleeding diathesis (relative)—increased risk of epidural hematoma
- Lumbosacral deformity (relative)
- Uncooperative patient

The Procedure

Step 1. Position the patient in the left lateral decubitus position, with the back near the edge of the bed or examination table and with the spine flexed and knees drawn toward the chest. Ensure the shoulders and back are perpendicular to the table. Place a pillow under the patient's head to keep the spine as straight as possible. An alternative method is to place the patient in the sitting position, leaning on a bedside table or with two large pillows in the patient's lap, with the spine flexed anteriorly.

- **PEARL:** Topical lidocaine (EMLA cream) has been studied in infants and found to decrease the pain response during the procedure. EMLA cream was applied in a topical dose of 1 g with an occlusion dressing placed over the site for 60 to 90 minutes before the procedure.
- **PITFALL:** Avoid forced flexion of the neck during the procedure because cardiorespiratory arrest may occur if a child's neck is excessively flexed.
- **PITFALL:** Rotation of the patient beyond perpendicular can distort the appearance of the vertebral processes and make it more difficult to insert the needle in a midline position. If the patient is rotated, then

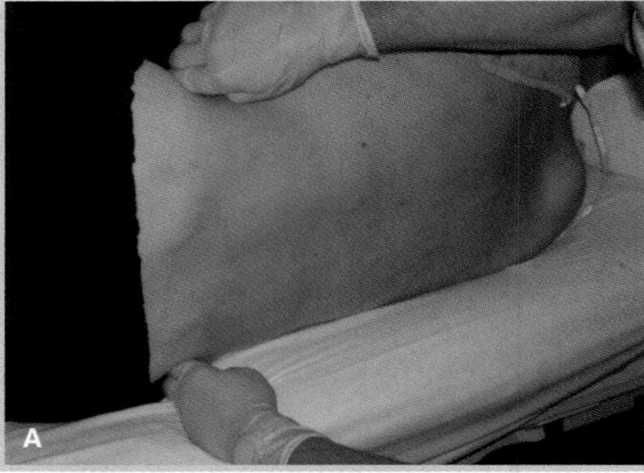
A

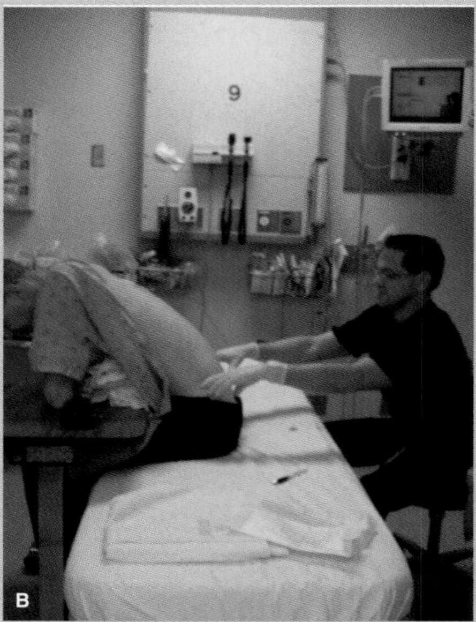

B

Step 1

insertion of the needle may be lateral and not penetrate the subarachnoid space.

Step 2. Prep the skin with povidone-iodine or chlorhexidine solution, and allow it to dry (see Appendix E). Most lumbar puncture kits include povidone-iodine swabs for sterilization of the procedure site. Set up the sterile tray, remove the tops of the sample tubes, and don a mask and sterile gloves while the povidone-iodine dries on the skin. Sterile draping typically is used for adult patients, but it can be omitted for the infant in favor of a wide prep to maximize landmark exposure and proper positioning. Inject a small amount (1 to 3 mL) of 1% lidocaine subcutaneously and into the area between the spinous processes.

- **PEARL:** Chlorhexidine may be used for patients allergic to iodine.
- **PEARL:** It can be helpful to palpate the back and identify landmarks before the patient is sterilely prepped and draped. Once the patient is draped, vertebral landmarks can be more difficult to identify. It can be useful to make an indention in the skin with the end of a retractable pen that has the tip retracted. This indention will not be washed away like ink when the patient is prepped with povidone-iodine or chlorhexidine.

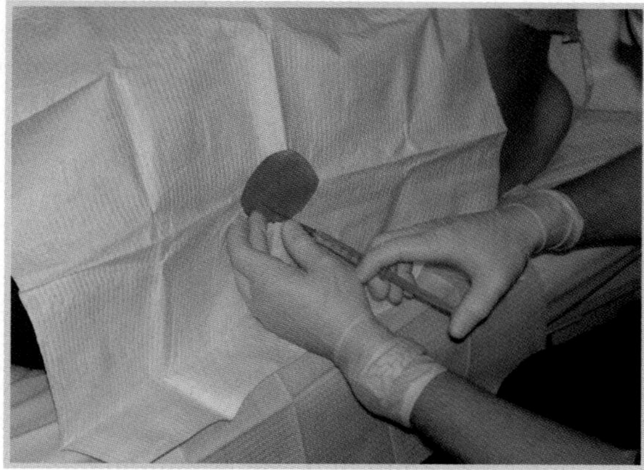

Step 2

Step 3. The optimal needle insertion site is in the center of the spinal column, as defined by the spinous processes. The L3–4 interspace can be found where the line joining the superior iliac crests meets the spinous process of L4. Insertion is usually at the L3–4 interspace, but it may be performed one space above or below.

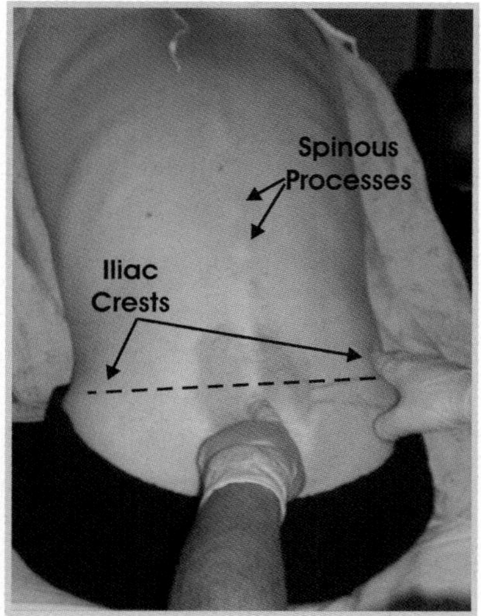

Step 3

Step 4. With the stylet in place, slowly insert the 22- or 20-gauge spinal needle midway between the two spinous processes. The correct angle for the needle is approximately toward the umbilicus, along the sagittal midplane of the body. If bone is encountered, withdraw the needle and change its angle. It is important to fully retract the needle because many kits include "cutting needles," which may destroy tissue if moved within the soft tissue space. Feel for a loss of resistance, a give, or a "pop" as the needle enters the subarachnoid space, and then advance the needle 1 to 2 mm farther. The pop may not be felt in younger children. Withdraw the stylus, and check the hub for fluid. If there is no fluid, replace the stylus, and advance another fraction before repeating.

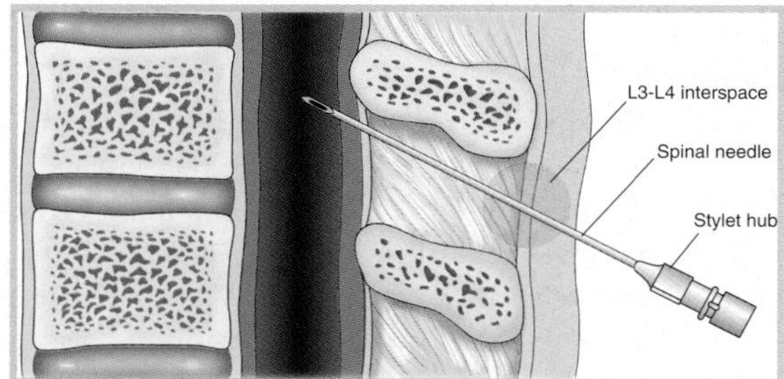

Step 4

- **PEARL:** If bone is encountered, withdraw the needle and change the angle. Bone is usually encountered when the needle has been directed away from the midline. It can also be beneficial to palpate bony landmarks again and ensure that patient position is optimal. Patient movement during the procedure can alter the physician's perception of the midline.

- PITFALL: Make sure the bevel of the needle enters and exits the dura parallel to the long axis of the spinal column. This may lower the incidence of spinal nerve root damage and postprocedure headache.
- PITFALL: Once the pop is felt, allow several seconds for the flow of CSF. The flow of CSF may not be immediate in some patients. This is especially true in dehydrated patients.

Step 5. After fluid is obtained, obstruct the passage of fluid with the stylet or your thumb. Place the stopcock and manometer onto the hub of the needle. As the CSF rises in the manometer, observe the color of the fluid and the opening pressure (Table 11-1).

- **PEARL:** The CSF opening pressure normal value is 6 to 14 mm Hg.
- PITFALL: Have the patient relax his or her legs to prevent falsely elevating the opening pressure.
- PITFALL: Accurate pressure measurements can only be made in the lateral decubitus position.

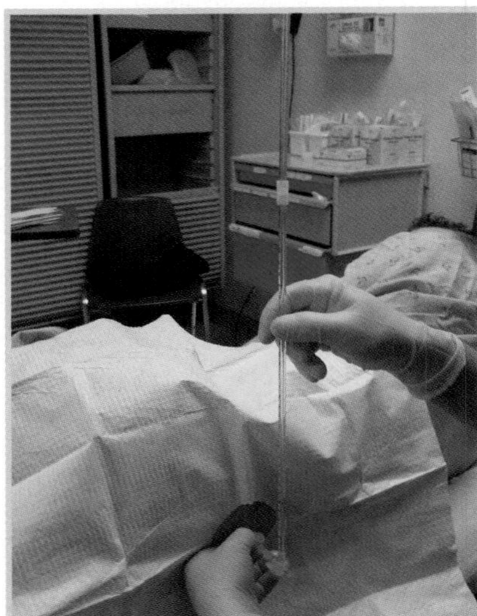

Step 5

Step 6. Turn the stopcock to allow 2 to 3 mL of the CSF in children or 4 to 5 mL in adults to flow into each test tube. If desired, measure the closing pressure, but this has little value and removes additional CSF. Replace the stylus, and withdraw the needle. Wash off the povidone-iodine, and cover the puncture site with a sterile dressing. A small bandage is included in most kits to cover the procedure site.

- **PEARL:** Allow the fluid in the manometer tube to flow into the tubes first to decrease the amount of CSF removed.
- PITFALL: If the tubes are not prelabeled, make sure to place the tubes in order so that you can easily identify and label each tube after the procedure.

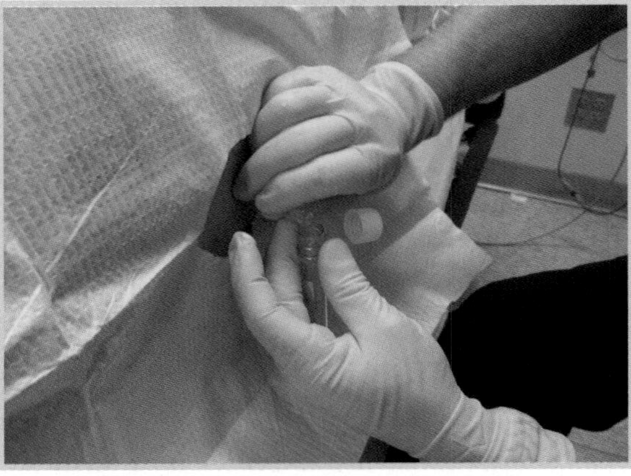

Step 6

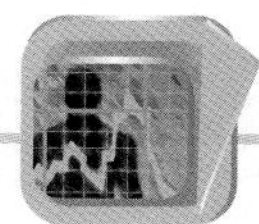

Complications

- Implantation of epidermoid tumors, which occur when epidermoid tissue is implanted into the spinal canal during a lumbar puncture: This occurs with the use of unstyletted needles or with needles that have poorly fitting stylets. These tumors cause pain to the back and lower extremities years after spinal puncture.
- Aspiration of a nerve root into the spinal space, which occurs when the needle is withdrawn without the stylet in place.
- Postprocedure headache:
  - Headache occurs in 5% to 40% of all lumbar punctures.
  - Headaches can start up to 48 hours after the procedure and usually last 1 to 2 days (sometimes up to 14 days).
  - Headache is associated with sitting upright and ceases with lying down.
  - They are thought to be caused by leakage of fluid through the dural puncture site.
  - Incidence of headache may be higher with "cutting needles" and larger-diameter needles.
  - Epidural blood patch may be performed to alleviate a persistent headache. This procedure is usually performed by an anesthesiologist.
- Infection of CSF:
  - Infection on CSF may occur if local tissue infection is present over the LP site. Overlying cellulitis is a contraindication to LP.
  - It has also been suggested that infection may be caused by introduction of bacteria from infected blood (sepsis or bacteremia) during an LP. This has not been proven, and reported cases most likely represent CSF infection that was not yet detectable at the time of LP.
- Postprocedure herniation:
  - This occurs in 2% to 3% of patients after LP.
  - Onset of symptoms is noted within 12 hours of procedure and manifested by loss of consciousness.
  - Many of these patients have a normal CSF opening pressure.
  - Most patients improve within 48 hours of symptom onset.
  - Risk of this complication can be decreased with the use of small-caliber spinal needles and ICP-lowering agents when needed.
- Backache and radicular symptoms: Minor backache occurs in up to 90% of patients because of local trauma of the spinal needle.

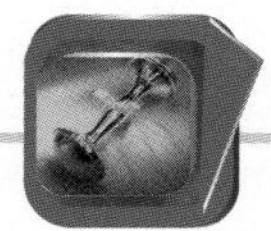

Pediatric Considerations

Topical lidocaine (EMLA cream) has been studied in infants and found to decrease the pain response during the procedure. EMLA cream was applied in a topical dose of 1 g with an occlusion dressing placed over the site for 60 to 90 minutes before the procedure.

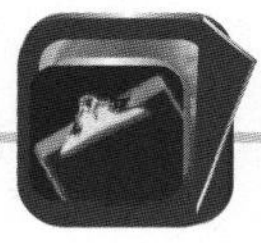

Postprocedure Instructions

Once the procedure has been successfully performed, ensure that all four collection tubes are sealed and labeled in order of CSF collection. CSF can then be sent to the laboratory for pertinent testing. Always ask the laboratory to keep the CSF available in case further studies become necessary.

Evaluation of Suspected Meningitis

- Use Gram stain, culture, glucose, protein, and lactate dehydrogenase (LDH).
- Other tests that may be performed are CSF counterimmunoelectrophoresis (CIE), CSF latex agglutination (LA), and coagulation immunoelectrophoresis.
- Commercial kits are available to detect the many common organisms that cause meningitis.
- All of these tests have a low sensitivity for bacterial meningitis; however, they have a much higher specificity. False-negative antigen tests may be seen with elevated rheumatoid factor and complement levels.
- Polymerase chain reactions hold promise for future rapid diagnosis of infection and may be available in some hospital settings.

Subarachnoid Hemorrhage

- CSF should be examined for xanthochromia, which is produced by the lysis of red blood cells (RBCs) in the CSF. RBC lysis begins to occur approximately 2 hours after exposure to CSF. The CSF is centrifuged and then examined for clarity. Collection of CSF within 12 hours of symptom onset of suspected subarachnoid hemorrhage may reveal false-negative results as a result of this phenomenon.

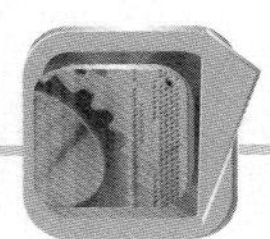

Coding Information and Supply Sources

CPT Code	Description	2008 Average 50th Percentile Fee	Global Period
62270	Spinal puncture, lumbar, diagnostic	$311.00	0
62272	Spinal puncture, therapeutic, for drainage of spinal fluid	$401.00	0

Spinal tray sets may be obtained through Arrow Medical Products, Ltd., 2400 Bernville Road, Reading, PA 19605. Phone: 1-800-523-8446. Web site: http://www.arrowintl.com/products/all/.

Many kits and supplies from various companies, including Baxter and American Hospital Supply (http://www.americanhospitalsupply.com/), can be obtained from Cardinal Health, Inc., 7000 Cardinal Place, Dublin, OH 43017 (phone: 1-800-234-8701; http://www.cardinal.com/) and from Owens and Minor, 4800 Cox Road, Glen Allen, VA 23060-6292 (phone: 804-747-9794; fax: 804-270-7281).

Patient Education Handout

A patient education handout, "Lumbar Puncture," can be found on the book's Web site.

Bibliography

Chordas C. Post-dural puncture headache and other complications after lumbar puncture. *J Pediatr Oncol Nurs.* 2001;18:244–259.

Errando CL, Peiro CM. Postdural puncture upper back pain as an atypical presentation of postdural puncture symptoms. *Anesthesiology*. 2002;96:1019–1020.

Flaatten H, Thorsen T, Askeland B, et al. Puncture technique and postural postdural puncture headache: a randomised, double-blind study comparing transverse and parallel puncture. *Acta Anaesthesiol Scand*. 1998;42:1209–1214.

Grande PO, Myhre EB, Nordstrom CH, et al. Treatment of intracranial hypertension and aspects on lumbar dural puncture in severe bacterial meningitis. *Acta Anaesthesiol Scand*. 2002;46:264–270.

Hasbun R, Abrahams J, Jekel J, et al. Computed tomography of the head before lumbar puncture in adults with suspected meningitis. *N Engl J Med*. 2001;345:1727–1733.

Holdgate A, Cuthbert K. Perils and pitfalls of lumbar puncture in the emergency department. *Emerg Med*. 2001;13:351–358.

Levine DN, Rapalino O. The pathophysiology of lumbar puncture headache. *J Neurol Sci*. 2001; 192:1–8.

Marton KI, Gean AD. The spinal tap: a new look at an old test. *Arch Intern Med*. 1986;104:840–848.

Nigrovic LE, Kupperman N, Macias CG, et al. Clinical prediction rule for identifying children with cerebrospinal fluid pleocytosis at very low risk for bacterial meningitis. *JAMA*. 2007;297(1):52–60.

Roberts J, Hedges J. *Clinical Procedures in Emergency Medicine*. 4th ed. Philadelphia: Saunders, An Imprint of Elsevier; 2004:1197–1219.

Straus S, Thorpe K, Holroyd-Leduc J. How do I perform a lumbar puncture and analyze the results to diagnose bacterial meningitis? *JAMA*. 2006;296:2012–2022.

Thoennissen J, Herkner H, Lang W, et al. Does bed rest after cervical or lumbar puncture prevent headache? A systematic review and meta-analysis. *Can Med Assoc J*. 2001;165:1311–1316.

Thomas SR, Jamieson DR, Muir KW. Randomised controlled trial of atraumatic versus standard needles for diagnostic lumbar puncture. *BMJ*. 2000;321:986–990.

Van Creval H, Hijdra A, de Gans J. Lumbar puncture and the risk of herniation: When should we first perform a CT? *J Neurol*. 2002:249(2):129–137.

Van de Beek D, de Gans J, Tunkel AR, et al. Community-acquired bacterial meningitis in adults. *N Engl J Med*. 2006;354:44–53.

Weise KL, Nihata MC. EMLA for painful procedures in infants. *J Pediatr Health Care*. 2005;19(1):42–49.

2008 MAG Mutual Healthcare Solutions, Inc.'s Physicians' Fee and Coding Guide. Duluth, Georgia. MAG Mutual Healthcare Solutions, Inc. 2007.

CHAPTER 12

Bone Marrow Biopsy

Lauren M. Yorek, MD
Assistant Clinical Professor
Emergency Department
Louisiana State University Health Sciences Center, Shreveport, LA

Bone marrow biopsy is an elective procedure that can be performed in an outpatient setting. Evaluation of bone marrow samples can be important in the diagnosis of many hematologic and malignant processes. In adults, bone marrow is usually obtained from the pelvis, which is the major site of cellular production after childhood. In infants, the tibia is also a possible site of bone marrow aspiration.

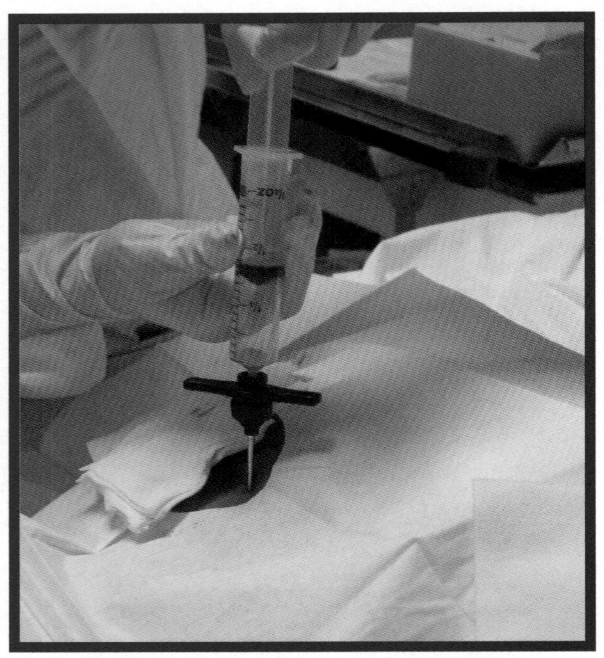

Be sure to obtain informed consent from the patient. Many practices employ standard procedure consent forms with detailed information specific to bone marrow biopsy. The listed procedural risks should include bleeding, bone fracture, infection, and pain. Before starting the procedure, consent forms should be signed by physician, patient, and a witness.

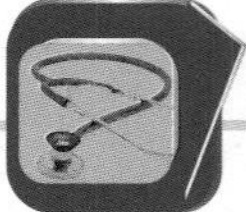

Equipment

- Bone marrow biopsy needle
- Sterile collection tubes for both aspirate and marrow biopsy
- Scalpel blade size no. 10 or 15

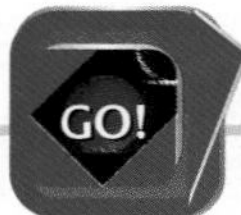

Indications

- Unexplained anemia—can determine both iron stores and underlying etiology
- Metastatic disease
- Lymphoma and leukemia diagnosis, staging, and response to treatment
- Evaluation of cytopenias
- Bone marrow transplant
- Chromosomal analysis
- Immunocompromised states, to evaluate for infection or white cell line deficiencies
- Thrombocytopenia, to assist in differentiation of bone marrow disorders from splenic sequestration and increased peripheral platelet destruction
- Infection, particularly fungal and tubercular infections
- Fever of unknown origin, to evaluate for malignancy or infection

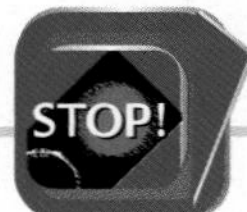

Contraindications

- Bleeding diathesis.
- Thrombocytopenia—platelet levels of $<$20,000 to 50,000 usually require platelet transfusion prior to invasive procedure. Assistance from a hematologist or other qualified specialist is advised in this situation.
- Severe osteoporosis—evaluate for risk of fracture due to procedure.
- Previous radiation at the site—marrow site may be sclerotic and may not provide good sample material.
- Infection or osteomyelitis at or near the puncture site.

The Procedure

Step 1. If an intravenous (IV) line for conscious sedation is desired to augment local anesthetic, establish IV access. See Chapters 4 and 122. Place the patient in the prone position and identify the iliac crests bilaterally. Then follow the iliac crests to the posterior superior iliac spine.

- PITFALL: Medical personnel with expertise in the use of conscious sedation should be present.
- **PEARL:** The use of conscious sedation with intravenous propofol, midazolam, and fentanyl has been studied in the outpatient setting. This conscious sedation is in addition to local anesthesia. The use of

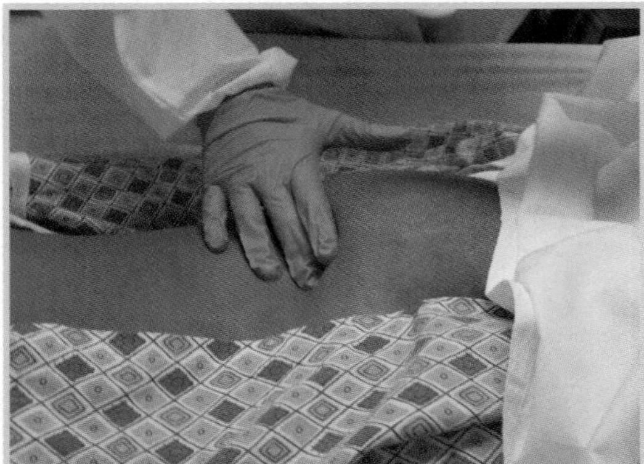

Step 1

conscious sedation has been shown to be as safe as using local anesthesia alone.

- **PEARL:** The use of oral premedication may be helpful in some patients.

Step 2. Sterile technique should be employed including the use of sterile gloves. Prep the area (see Appendix E). Place a fenestrated drape over the biopsy site.

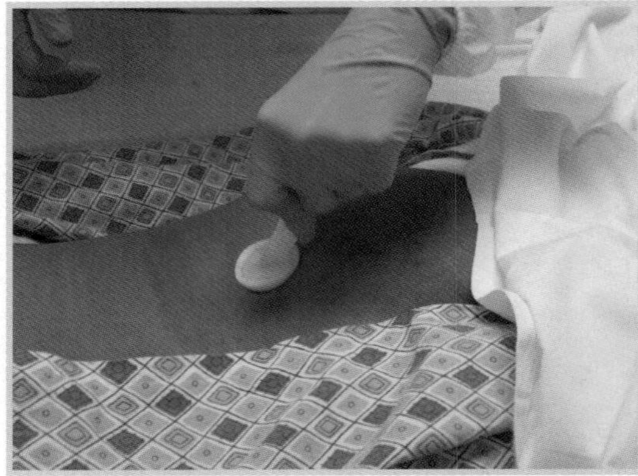

Step 2

Step 3. Inject 1% lidocaine to anesthetize the area. Make an initial wheal in the skin with a 25-gauge needle.

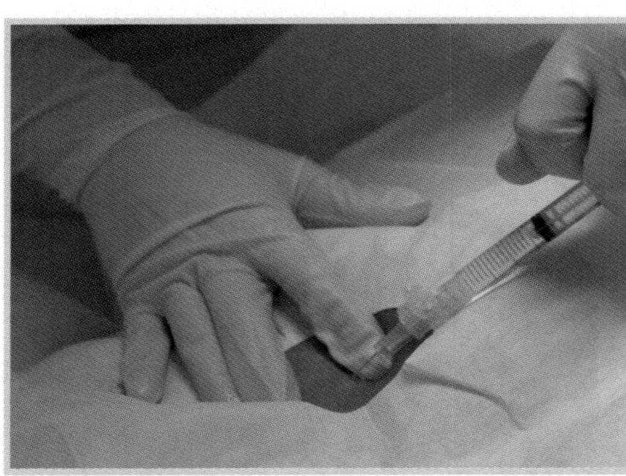

Step 3

Step 4. A 22-gauge needle should then be advanced through the area to the level of the periosteum. The periosteum will feel solid with some porous "give" to it. Up to 10 to 20 cc of lidocaine may be used to anesthetize the periosteum. It is important to adequately anesthetize the periosteum prior to the procedure.

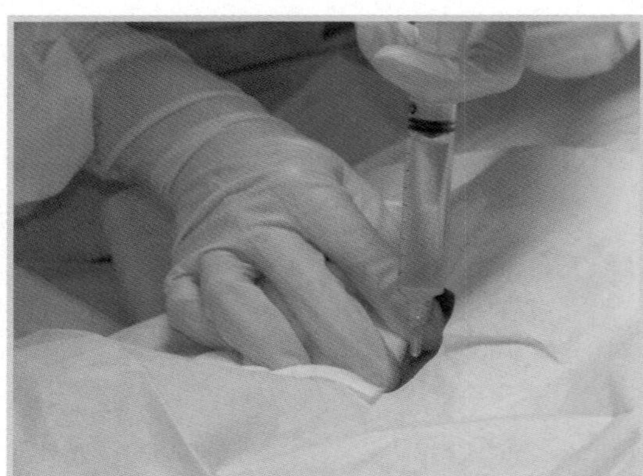

Step 4

Step 5. Once the lidocaine is injected, make a small stab wound at the site with a no. 11 scalpel blade.

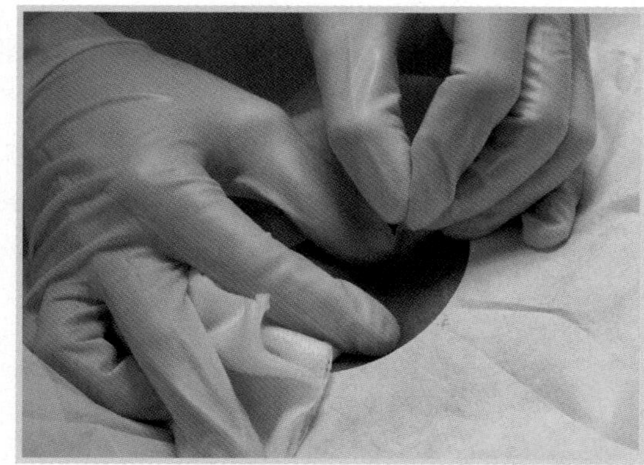

Step 5

Step 6. Examine the biopsy needle to ensure that the obturator is locked into place. Most biopsy needles will have a cap that is screwed on to secure the obturator.

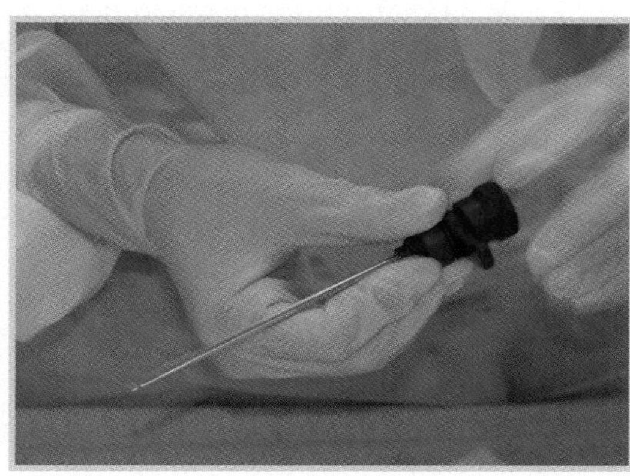

Step 6

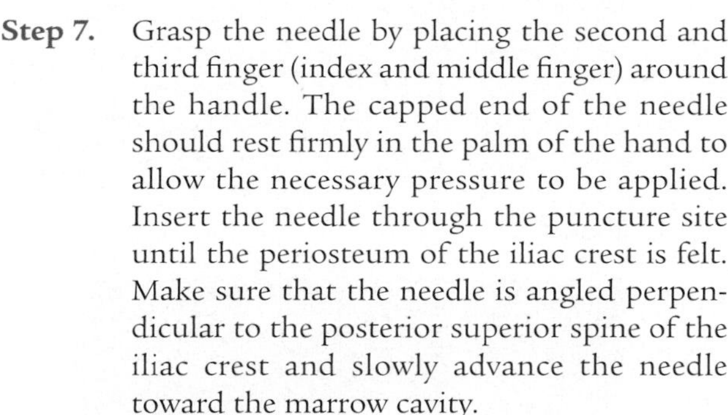

Step 7. Grasp the needle by placing the second and third finger (index and middle finger) around the handle. The capped end of the needle should rest firmly in the palm of the hand to allow the necessary pressure to be applied. Insert the needle through the puncture site until the periosteum of the iliac crest is felt. Make sure that the needle is angled perpendicular to the posterior superior spine of the iliac crest and slowly advance the needle toward the marrow cavity.

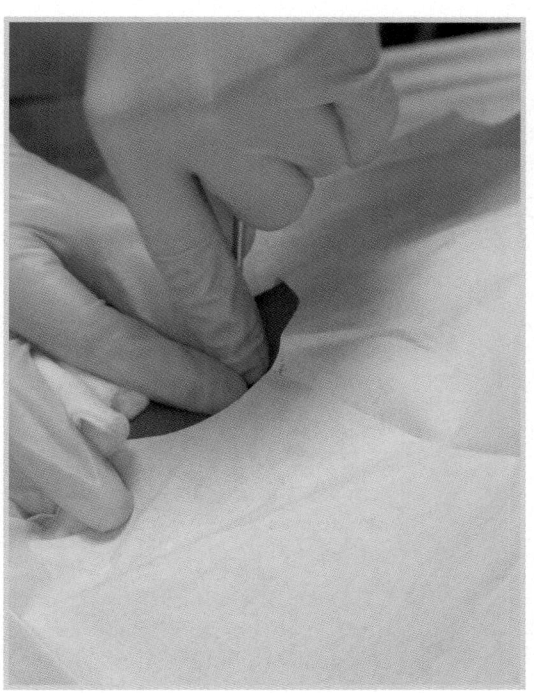

Step 7

Step 8. To advance the needle to the marrow cavity, rotate it alternately in a clockwise and counterclockwise manner while exerting firm pressure. Continue the pressure to penetrate the bony cortex, which is approximately 1 cm thick. Once the marrow cavity is entered, the needle will advance much more easily. Then advance the needle approximately 1 to 2 more mm.

- **PEARL:** The amount of pressure required often requires the full use of upper body strength rather than just arm strength (as with chest compressions during cardiopulmonary resuscitation).
- **PITFALL:** If the needle is not angled correctly, it may slip down the iliac crest and not enter the marrow cavity.

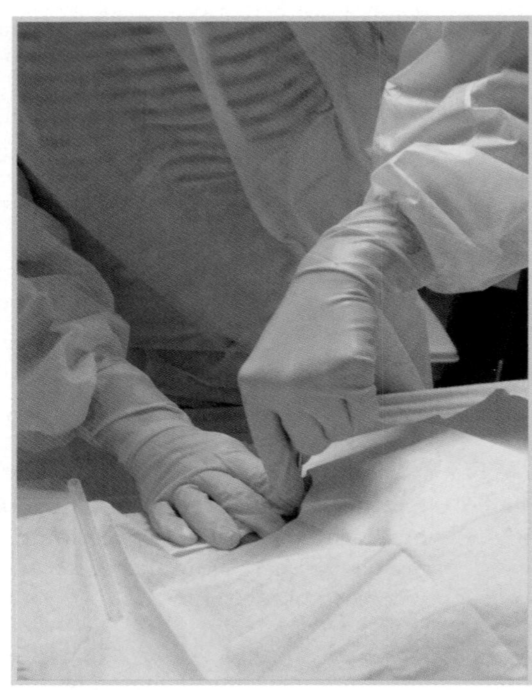

Step 8

Step 9. Remove the obturator.

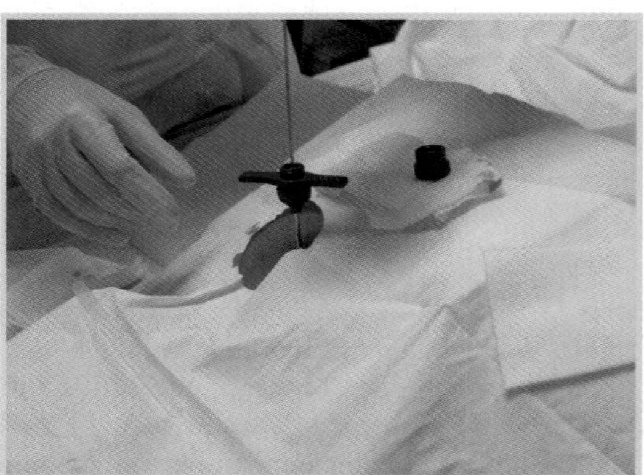

Step 9

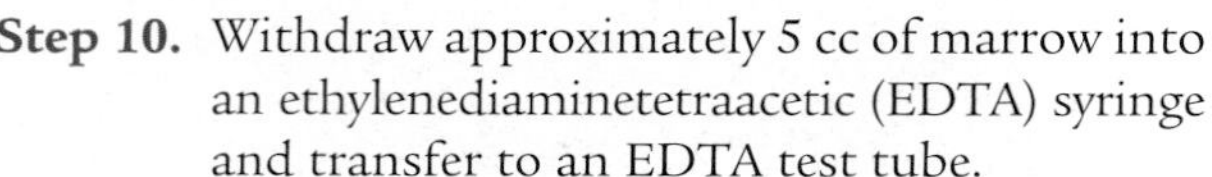

Step 10. Withdraw approximately 5 cc of marrow into an ethylenediaminetetraacetic (EDTA) syringe and transfer to an EDTA test tube.

- **PITFALL:** The aspiration process is painful. Warn the patient before the actual aspiration is performed.
- **PITFALL:** If no marrow is aspirated, replace the obturator and advance the needle 1 to 2 more mm and attempt aspiration again.
- **PITFALL:** If the needle is advanced without the obturator in place it may become clogged with bony material.
- **PEARL:** If no marrow is obtained, then change biopsy sites.

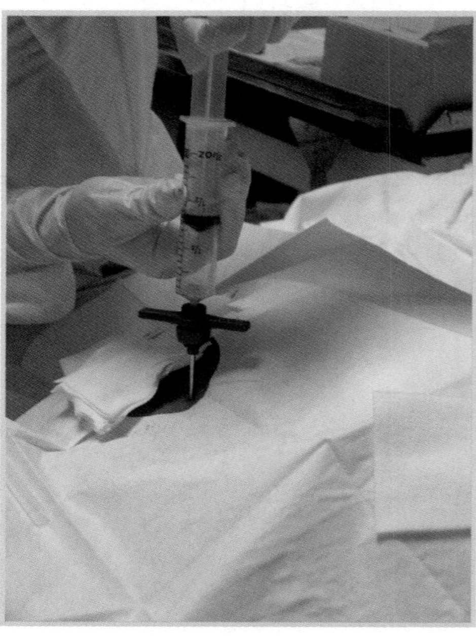

Step 10

Step 11. To obtain a biopsy after marrow aspiration has been performed, replace the obturator and withdraw the needle to the level of the cortex. Angle the needle anteriorly within the iliac spine and advance it to the marrow cavity. The resistance will decrease as the marrow cavity is entered as before.

- **PEARL:** This forward motion within the marrow cavity should be performed with the same clockwise and counterclockwise rotation used to penetrate the bony cortex.

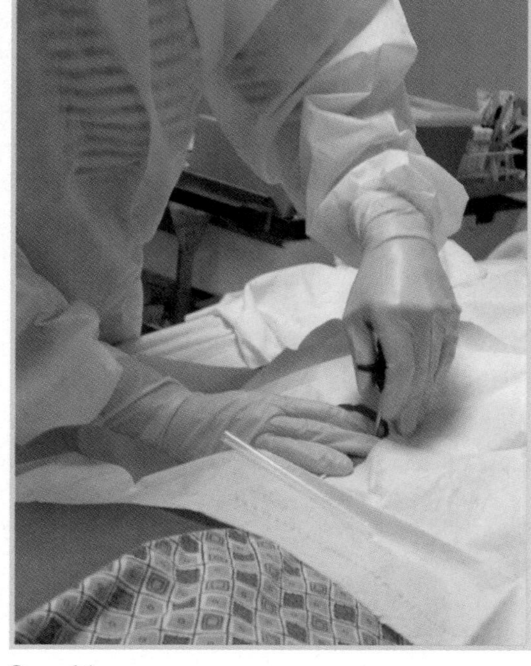

Step 11

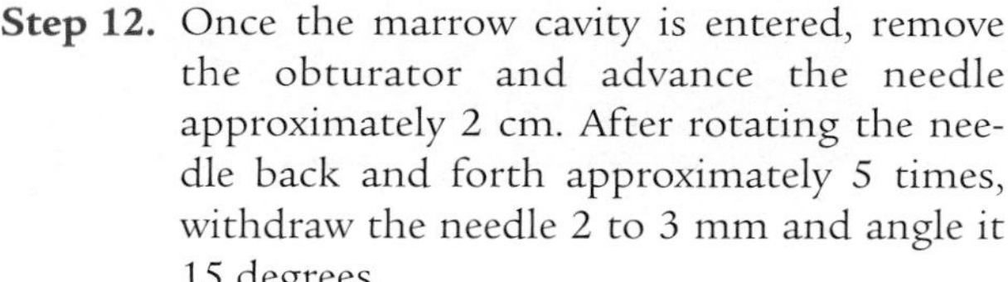

Step 12. Once the marrow cavity is entered, remove the obturator and advance the needle approximately 2 cm. After rotating the needle back and forth approximately 5 times, withdraw the needle 2 to 3 mm and angle it 15 degrees.

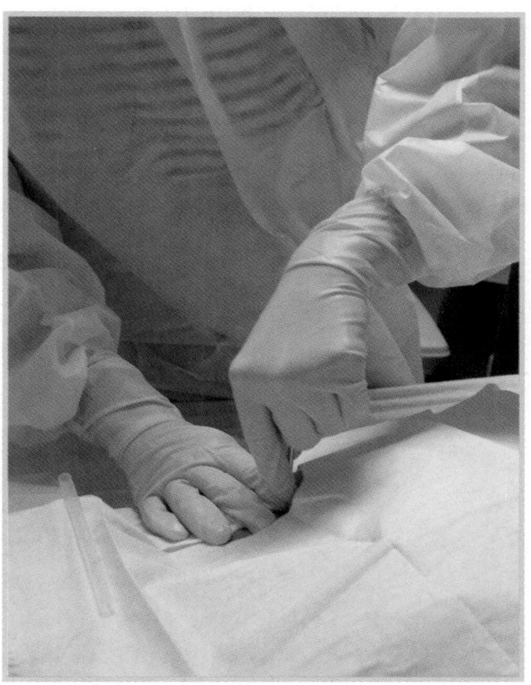

Step 12

Step 13. Advance the needle approximately 2 to 3 mm at this angle. This maneuver will dislodge the marrow. Once the marrow has been dislodged within the cavity, withdraw the biopsy needle with your thumb covering the hub of the needle. After the needle is fully withdrawn, place the obturator into the needle and push the specimen into a specimen container.

- **PITFALL:** Do not replace the obturator until the needle is fully withdrawn.

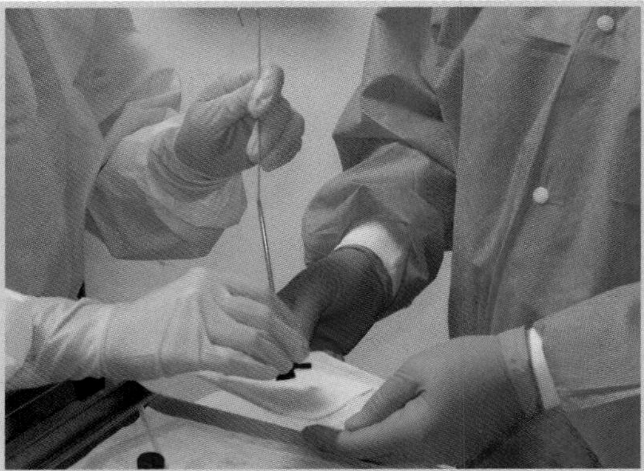

Step 13

Step 14. Place a pressure dressing over the biopsy site. Allow the patient to lie supine for 1 hour to assist with direct pressure.

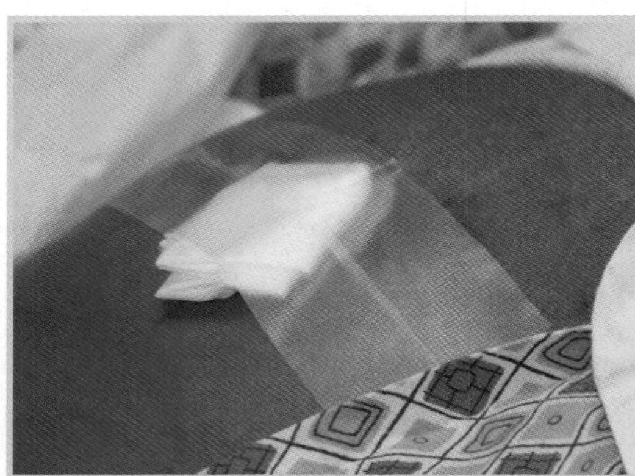

Step 14

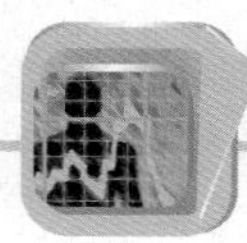

Complications

- The bone marrow needle can break and must be retrieved with either a hemostat or with the assistance of a surgeon.
- Hemorrhage may occur at the biopsy site and is treated with local pressure at the biopsy site. (This is more of a risk in patients with thrombocytopenia.)
- Retroperitoneal hematoma from bleeding complication.
- Pulmonary emboli can occur after sternal aspiration.
- Infection of bone marrow aspiration sites. (This is more of a risk in immunocompromised patients.)
- Fracture of bone.

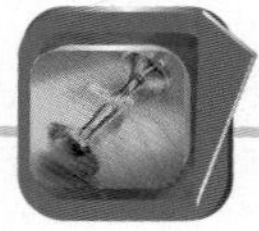

Pediatric Considerations

In many premature infants and some full-term infants, the iliac bone has not completely ossified, and an alternative bone such as the anterior tibia is used. In children, conscious sedation has been successfully used to reduce pain and distress.

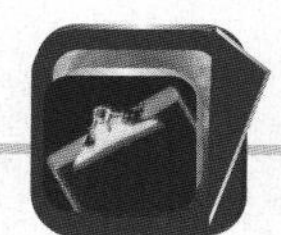

Postprocedure Instructions

After applying a pressure dressing to the site, have the patient lie supine for 1 hour. If sedation was administered, then appropriate monitoring should be performed until the patient has reached the presedation level of consciousness. Before patient discharge, examine the biopsy site for any bleeding.

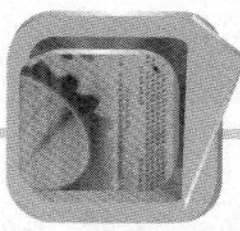

Coding Information and Supply Sources

CPT Code	Description	2008 Average 50th Percentile Fee	Global Period
38221	Bone marrow biopsy diagnostic	$486.00	0

Note that Medicare may not reimburse the cost of a bone marrow biopsy if it is not done at an approved facility.

ICD-9 Codes

Anemia	285.9
Leukemia	208.9
Lymphoma	202.8
Malignancy (unspecified)	202.9

Patient Education Handout

A patient education handout, "Bone Marrow Biopsy," can be found on the book's Web site.

Bibliography

Burkle CM, Harrison BA, Koenig LF, et al. Morbidity and mortality of deep sedation in outpatient bone marrow biopsy. *Am J Hematol.* 2004;77(3):250–256.

Hertzog JH, Dalton HJ, Anderson BD, et al. Prospective evaluation of propofol anesthesia in the pediatric intensive care unit for elective oncology procedures in ambulatory and hospitalized children. *Pediatrics.* 2000;106(4):742–747.

Lutehr JM, Lakey DL, Larson RS, et al. Utility of bone marrow biopsy for rapid diagnosis of febrile illness in patients with human immunodeficiency virus. *South Med J.* 2000;93(7):692–697.

Riley RS, Hogan TF, Pavot DR, et al. A pathologist's perspective on bone marrow aspiration and biopsy: performing a bone marrow examination. *J Clin Lab Anal.* 2004;18(2):70–90.

Ryan DH, Cohen HJ. Bone marrow examination. In: Hoffman R, Benz EJ Jr, Shattil SJ, et al., eds. *Hoffman Hematology: Basic Principles and Practice.* 4th ed. New York: Churchill Livingstone; 2005.

Ryan DH, Felgar RE. Examination of the marrow. In: Lichtman MA, Beutler E, Kipps TJ, et al., eds. *Williams Hematology.* 7th ed. New York: McGraw-Hill; 2006.

Von Heijne M, Bredlov B, Soderhall S, et al. Propofol or propofol-alfentanil anesthesia for painful procedures in the pediatric oncology ward. *Paediatr Anaesth.* 2004;14(8):670–675.

Wolanskyj AP, Schroeder G, Wilson PR, et al. A randomized, placebo-controlled study of outpatient premedication for bone marrow biopsy in adults with lymphoma. *Clin Lymphoma.* 2000;1(2):154–157.

2008 MAG Mutual Healthcare Solutions, Inc.'s Physicians' Fee and Coding Guide. Duluth, Georgia. MAG Mutual Healthcare Solutions, Inc. 2007.

CHAPTER 13

Cardioversion

Lauren M. Yorek, MD

Assistant Clinical Professor, Department of Emergency Medicine
Louisiana State University Health Sciences Center, Shreveport, LA

Cardioversion is the use of electric shock to alter the cardiac rhythm of a patient. The energy is measured in joules and is delivered to the patient via paddles or adhesive pads designed for this purpose.

Cardioversion is implemented in many cardiac rhythm disturbances and can be delivered either as synchronized or unsynchronized. When the cardiac rhythm has its origin in the atria, then synchronized cardioversion is performed to prevent deterioration to a less stable rhythm originating in the ventricle (see Table 13-1). Synchronized cardioversion can also be performed for ventricular tachycardia with a pulse.

When the patient's abnormal rhythm is not of atrial origin and the patient does not have a palpable pulse, then unsynchronized cardioversion is performed. The amount of energy or joules used for cardioversion varies upon the particular situation.

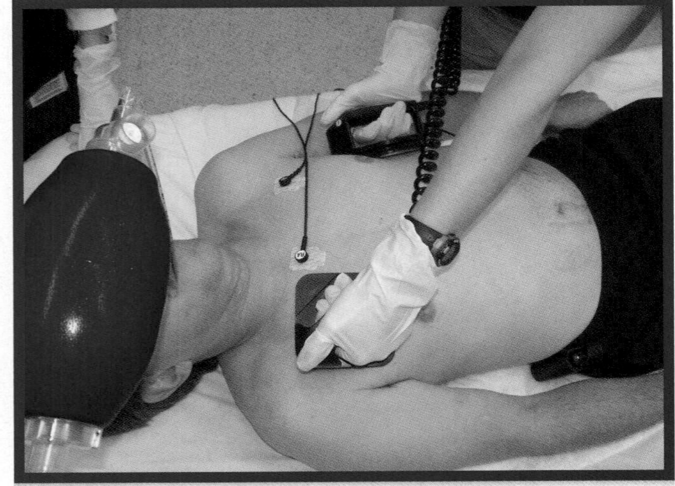

An antiarrhythmic medication is often begun on patients with atrial fibrillation or atrial flutter to increase the chances of success with electric cardioversion. If patients are placed on antiarrythmic medications, they may require a longer period of observation and continuation of medication if the cardioversion is successful. Procedural sedation can be achieved with intravenous (IV) sedatives such as diazepam, midazolam, or propofol (see Chapter 4). Analgesics may also be added for patient comfort such as IV fentanyl or meperidine. Medical staff experienced in conscious sedation techniques should be present.

A recent study in the *American Heart Journal* demonstrated a better outcome with biphasic shock than monophasic shock for patients undergoing cardioversion for atrial fibrillation. Successful cardioversion with biphasic current also required less energy delivery to the patient (fewer joules required). Patients who underwent cardioversion with biphasic current reported less pain at 1 and 24 hours postprocedure. Life Pack cardioversion models produced within the past few years are designed to deliver biphasic shocks.

Atrial flutter does have good response rates to monphasic cardioversion. However, cardioversion at lower energy levels has been successful with atrial flutter. In addition, cardioversion of atrial flutter with biphasic current has been shown to require less antiarrythmic medication to sustain sinus rhythm. The risk of skin burns is also decreased with decreased energy requirements.

TABLE 13-1. Recommended Energy Settings for Cardioversion

CONDITION	SETTINGS	NOTES
Atrial fibrillation, atrial flutter, paroxysmal supraventricular tachycardia, ventricular tachycardia with a pulse	100 J, 200 J, 300 J, 360 J	May need to resynchronize after each cardioversion attempt
Atrial flutter and paroxysmal supraventricular tachycardia	50 J, 100 J, 200 J, 300 J, 360 J	

The electrodes may be placed anteroposterior (AP) or anterolateral (AL) in biphasic conversion for atrial fibrillation. The number of shocks required and needed energy delivery is comparable with both electrode configurations.

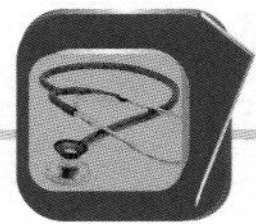

Equipment

- An automatic external defibrillator (AED) device with or without manual control option is useful in smaller clinics and urgent care centers where the cost and maintenance of a larger fully manual device may be prohibitive.
- A manual defibrillator device, which usually has manual control options, may have the option to also function automatically as an AED.
- The newer defibrillator devices (such as Life Pack 12) include pads rather than paddles, which may also be used for cardiac pacing.

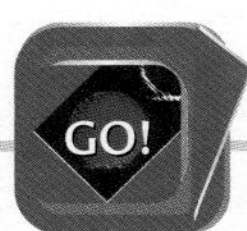

Indications

SYNCHRONIZED CARDIOVERSION

- Unstable supraventricular tachycardia with a pulse. In the absence of a pulse, unsynchronized cardioversion is performed.
- Patient with serious signs or symptoms due to arrhythmia including
  - Acute coronary syndrome.
  - Decreased level of consciousness.
  - Chest pain.
  - Dyspnea.
  - Pulmonary edema.
  - Hypotension.
- Unstable atrial fibrillation with acute presentation.
- New onset atrial fibrillation, if known to have begun within the past 48 hours:
  - Note that when attempting to restore sinus rhythm in a patient with atrial fibrillation, the presence or absence of an atrial clot must be determined. It is often recommended that patients undergo cardiac echo to determine the absence of an atrial clot, which may embolize after conversion to sinus rhythm.
- Ventricular tachycardia with a pulse that is not responsive to pharmacologic therapy.

UNSYNCHRONIZED CARDIOVERSION

- Used in cardiac arrhythmias of ventricular origin without a palpable pulse:
  - Ventricular tachycardia.
  - Ventricular fibrillation.

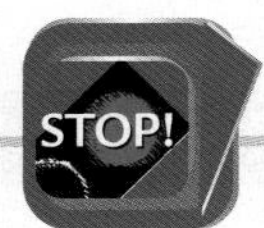

Contraindications: Synchronous Cardioversion

Elective Cardioversion

- Electrolyte disturbances
- Atrial tachycardias that do not respond to cardioversion: [comp: nested
  - Multifocal atrial tachycardia, which is usually a supraventricular tachycardia with an irregular rhythm and is not usually responsive to cardioversion
  - Sinus tachycardia, which is a response to underlying pathology (shock, pulmonary embolus, etc.) and not a primary rhythm disturbance
- Digitalis toxicity
- Patients with little proven symptomatic improvement with sinus rhythm
- Left atrial diameter >4.5 cm (relative)
- Patients who have a low probability of maintaining sinus rhythm and readily return to atrial fibrillation (relative)
- Patients who require a pacemaker for maintenance of stable rhythm after cardioversion such as patients with sick sinus syndrome or sinoatrial (SA) nodal blockade

Urgent Cardioversion

- Absence of electrocardiographic wave (QRS) complex on electrocardiogram (EKG) monitor
- Absent pulse

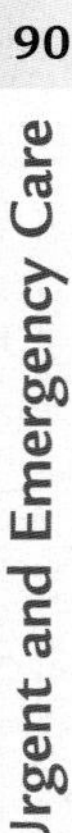

The Procedure

Step 1. For elective procedures, the anticoagulant therapy must be at therapeutic levels for patients in atrial fibrillation at risk or producing emboli from an atrial thrombus. Also evaluate the electrolyte and serum digoxin levels. The patient should be held on nothing by mouth (NPO) status for 8 hours. Informed consent must be obtained and documented if the procedure is elective. Insert an IV line for sedation and necessary medication in the event that the patient decompensates.

- **PEARL:** A general procedure form with the benefits and risks of the procedure described is acceptable and must be signed by the patient or guardian, the provider, and a witness.

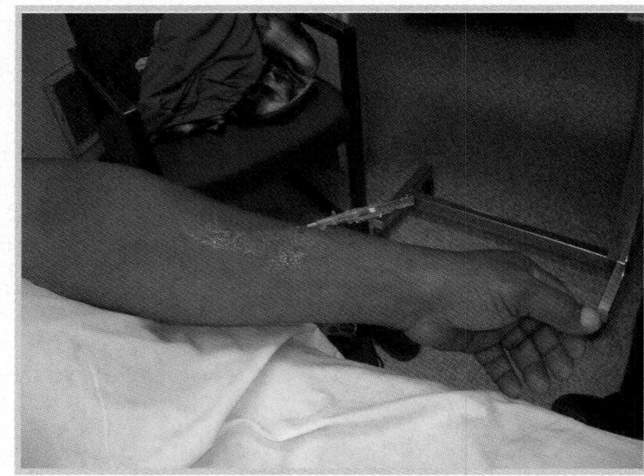

Step 1

Step 2. Place the patient under full cardiac and respiratory monitoring, lying flat on a dry surface. Supplemental oxygen should be given with ventilatory support available in the event of respiratory suppression. IV sedation should be given prior to the procedure. Electrode pads or paddles should be applied. Defibrillator pads are placed on the sternum and the skin over the apex of the heart.

- **PITFALL:** Skin burns can occur if inadequate gel is applied to the patient's skin.
- **PEARL:** Urgent cardioversion in the unstable patient may not allow time for sedation. If possible in the conscious patient, adequate sedation should be administered.

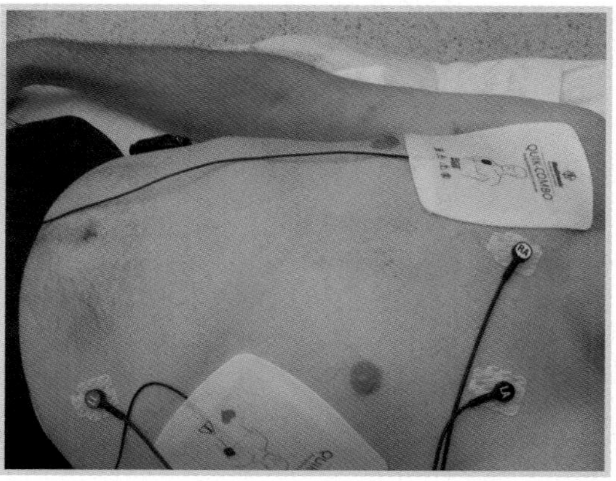

Step 2

Step 3. Turn on the defibrillator and select the appropriate energy level (see Table 13-1). Ensure that synchronization mode is selected if necessary. Check for proper electrode placement. Synchronization will be indicated by markers above R-waves on the EKG monitor.

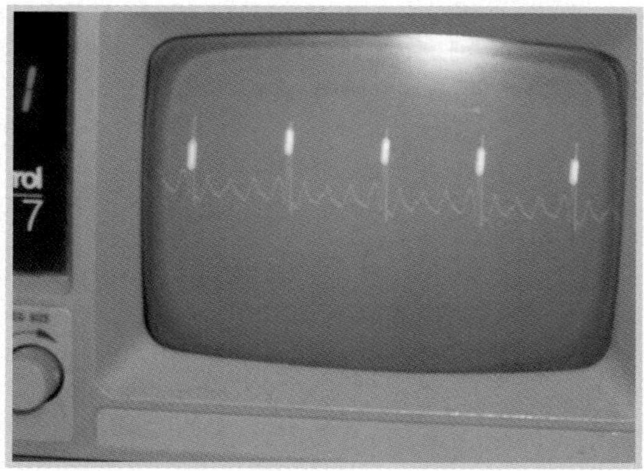

Step 3

Step 4. Call "all clear," and ensure all personnel are clear before discharging electrodes. Deliver shock with approximately 25 pounds of pressure if paddles are applied. Evaluate cardiac rhythm after the shock is delivered. Start with the lower end of the recommended range and increase as needed to obtain a response.

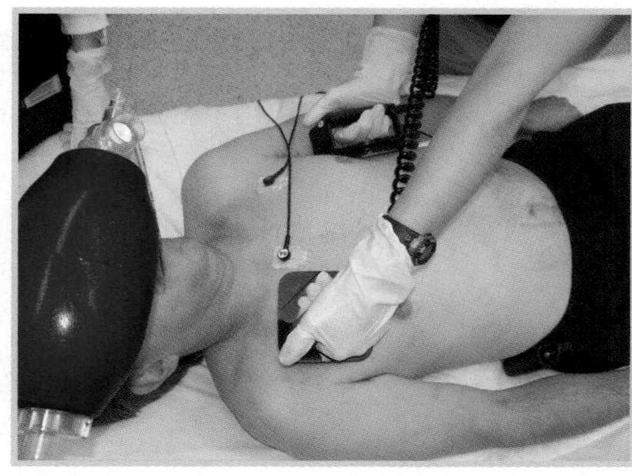

Step 4

Step 5. Cardioversion may need to be repeated at a higher energy level if it is unsuccessful on the first attempt. Ensure that the defibrillator is in synchronization mode before each shock is delivered. The patient should be monitored for several hours after the procedure until the following discharge criteria are met:

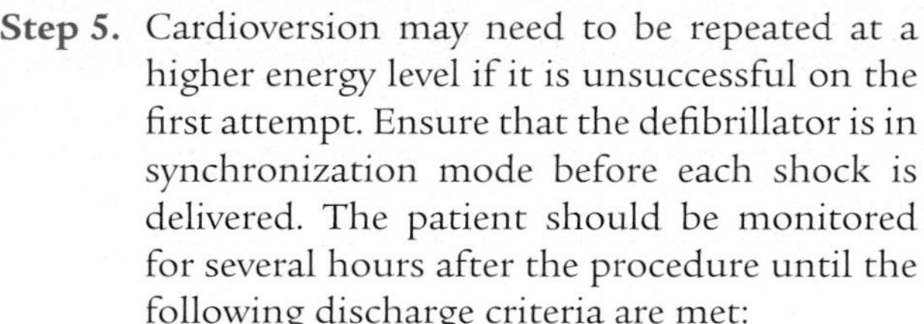

- Return of oxygen saturation to baseline
- Normal vital signs
- Return of level of consiousness to baseline
- Return of baseline ambulatory capacity

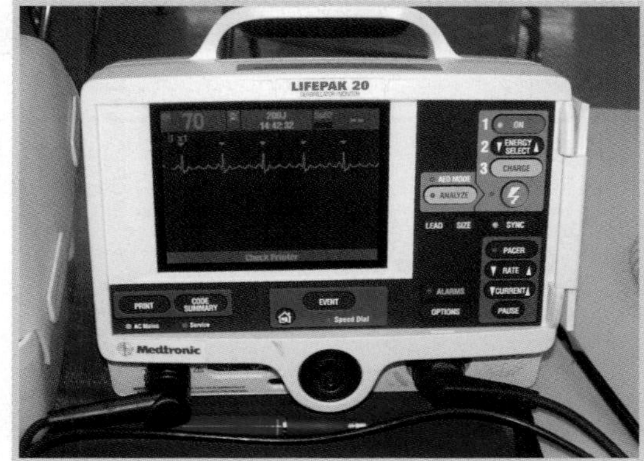

Step 5

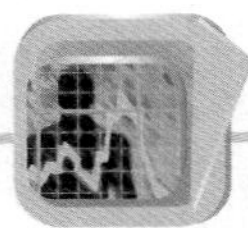

Complications

Bradycardia may be noted in patients with previous inferior myocardial infarction. Patients with digitalis toxicity or electrolyte disturbances such as hyperkalemia may have an increased risk of complications.

Ectopy of the atria or ventricles may be observed in the first 30 minutes after successful cardioversion.

Deterioration to a more unstable rhythm may occur with cardioversion.

Skin burns can occur if adequate gel is not applied to the patient's skin. Commercially available electrode pads have gel incorporated into the pads.

Patients without adequate anticoagulation may experience embolization of an atrial clot with return to sinus rhythm.

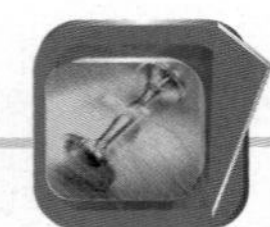

Pediatric Considerations

Supraventricular tachycardia (SVT) can present in children. Infants usually have a heart rate of >220 bpm, whereas children have heart rates of >180 bpm. Sinus tachycardia can be confused with SVT. Children can have a high heart rate due to sinus tachycardia, and this must be differentiated from SVT. (SVT should not have P-waves; sinus tachycardia will have P-waves visible.)

If SVT is unresponsive to adenosine, then synchronized cardioversion may be performed at a dose of 0.5 to 1 J/kg. If initial cardioversion is unsuccessful, the energy dose is increased to 2 J/kg for subsequent attempts. Expert consultation is advised in this situation.

Wide complex tachycardia of ventricular origin can also be seen in children (QRS >0.08 seconds). Energy levels used in cardioversion are the same as in narrow complex tachycardia (0.5 to 1 J/kg initially with repeat dose of 2 J/kg if needed).

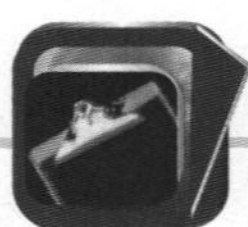

Postprocedure Instructions

The patient should be monitored in a controlled setting capable of resuscitation for several hours postprocedure. If the patient is receiving an antiarrythmic medication, prolonged monitoring may be necessary for dosage adjustment. If anticoagulation therapy is indicated, it will need to be continued for at least 3 months postprocedure and should ideally be delivered 3 weeks prior to cardioversion.

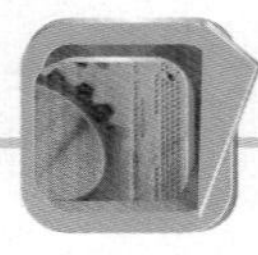

Coding Information and Supply Sources

CPT Code	Description	2008 Average 50th Percentile Fee	Global Period
92960	Cardioversion, elective, external	$485.00	0

ICD-9 Codes

Cardiac arrest	427.5
Atrial fibrillation	427.31
PSVT	427.0

Suppliers

- Emergency Medical Technology, Inc.; 1721 SE Grace, Suite 123, Battle Ground, WA 98604. Phone: 360-667-0368. Web site: http://emergencymedicaltechnology.com/lifepak500aed.html.
- Philips HeartStart Defibrillators; Philips Medical Systems, N.A., 22100 Bothell Everett Highway, P.O. Box 3003, Bothell, WA 98041-3003. Phone: 1-800-722-7900. Web site: http://www.medical.philips.com/main/products/resuscitation/index.html.
- Foremost Equipment, 320 N. Washington Street, Rochester, NY 14625. Phone: 585-586-4880. Web site: http://www.foremostequipment.com/Home/tabid/36/Default.aspx.
- AED Professional, General Medical Devices Company, 411 Colfax Street, Palatine IL 60078. Phone: 1-888-541-2337. Web site: http://www.aedprofessionals.com/.

Patient Education Handout

A patient education handout, "Elective Cardioversion," can be found on the book's companion Web site.

Bibliography

Gurevitz OT, Ammash NM, Malouf JF, et al. Comparative efficacy of monophasic and biphasic waveforms for transthoracic cardioversion of atrial fibrillation and atrial flutter. *Am Heart J.* 2005;149(2):316–321.

Koster RW, Dorian P, Chapman FW, et al. A randomized trial comparing monophasic and biphasic waveform shocks for external cardioversion of atrial fibrillation. *Am Heart J.* 2004:147(5):e1–e7.

Minczac BM, Krim JR. Defibrilation and cardioversion. In: Joberts JR, Hedges JR, eds. *Clinical Procedures in Emergency Medicine.* 4th ed. Philadelphia: Saunders; 2004;226–256.

Siaplaouras S, Buob A, Rötter C, et al. A randomized comparison of anterolateral versus anteroposterior electrode position for biphasic external cardioversion of atrial fibrillation. *Am Heart J.* 2005;150(1):150–152.

2008 MAG Mutual Healthcare Solutions, Inc.'s Physicians' Fee and Coding Guide. Duluth, Georgia. MAG Mutual Healthcare Solutions, Inc. 2007.

CHAPTER 14

Shoulder Reduction

Thomas C. Arnold, MD, FAAEM

Associate Professor and Chairman, Department of Emergency Medicine
Louisiana State University Health Sciences Center, Shreveport, LA

Paul Trisler, MD

Chief Resident, Emergency Medicine Residency
Louisiana State University Health Sciences Center, Shreveport, LA

No other joint in the body is as versatile or complex as the shoulder. Traumatic dislocation of the shoulder joint, if not managed properly, can lead to long-term debility and chronic complications. There are literally hundreds of reduction techniques reported in the literature for shoulder dislocations, and because no single reduction technique is always appropriate for every clinical situation, practitioners who might encounter this injury should be familiar with several different options for shoulder reduction. As with any joint reduction, the keys to successful reduction include knowledge of the anatomy, mastery of the reduction techniques, proper application of adequate procedural sedation, and a calm, gentle manner (see Chapter 4). The skilled practitioner utilizes these tools to entice or coerce the joint back into proper alignment instead of relying on brute-force manipulation. A common pitfall is the underuse of analgesia, thereby making the procedure unnecessarily painful and difficult.

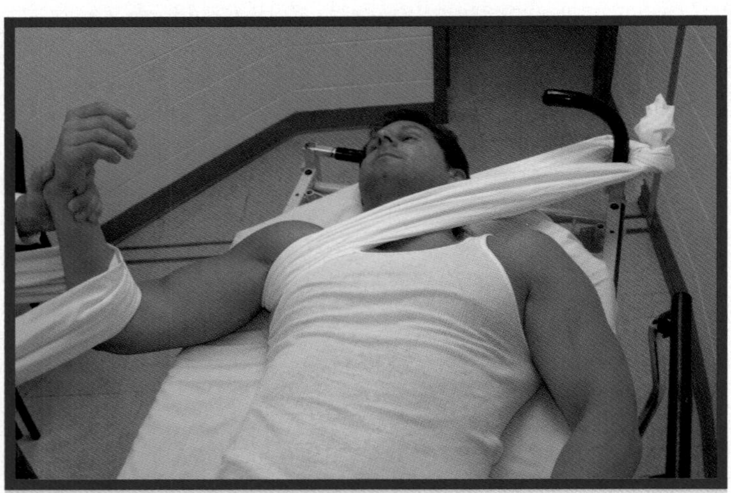

Before any attempts at relocation are begun, it is important to assess and document the neurologic and vascular status of the affected extremity. Serial reassessments after reduction should also be performed and documented. Pre- and postreduction radiographs are prudent to assess for associated fractures unless neurovascular compromise is present, mandating immediate intervention. An understanding the mechanism of injury responsible for the dislocation is important and should alert the practitioner to other commonly associated injuries. One should also keep in mind that inability to reduce the shoulder does not always imply improper technique but may signify a more complicated injury. If unsuccessful after one or two attempts, orthopedic consultation is warranted.

Some patients will present after spontaneously reducing or performing the reduction themselves. It is important to treat these patients no differently than if you performed the reduction. The same evaluation, immobilization, and follow-up referral normally offered all apply. Proper immobilization of the reduced shoulder is just as important as the reduction itself. All patients should have a clear understanding of the complications and possible sequelae of the injured shoulder. Specific follow-up instructions and referral are mandatory.

Dislocations are by convention described in terms of where the distal articulating surface lies in relation to the proximal surface (i.e., the humeral head is anterior to the glenoid fossa in an anterior shoulder dislocation). Three common subclassifications of anterior shoulder dislocations are the subglenoid, subcoracoid, and subclavicular varieties.

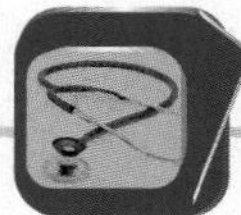

Equipment

- Sheets (2)
- Sufficient personnel (dependant on technique attempted)
- All monitoring equipment and supplies for procedural sedation (see Chapter 4)

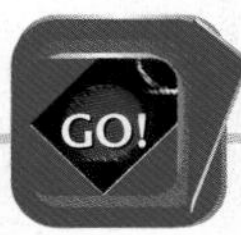

Indications

- Uncomplicated anterior or posterior shoulder dislocations without associated fractures

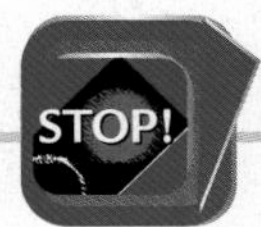

Contraindications

- Practitioners should not attempt reduction more than twice, as this may indicate entrapment of soft tissue or bony fragments in the joint space and not improper technique. Orthopedic consultation is required in these cases.
- If neurovascular status of the extremity is impaired postreduction, other than paresthesia, immediate orthopedic consultation is needed.
- If a fracture is present pre- or postreduction, immediate orthopedic consultation is required.

The Procedure

Anterior Dislocations

Adduction External Rotation Method

Step 1. Place the patient in a supine position with the affected arm adducted to patient's side. The elbow is then flexed to 90 degrees while the arm continues to be held against the lateral chest wall.

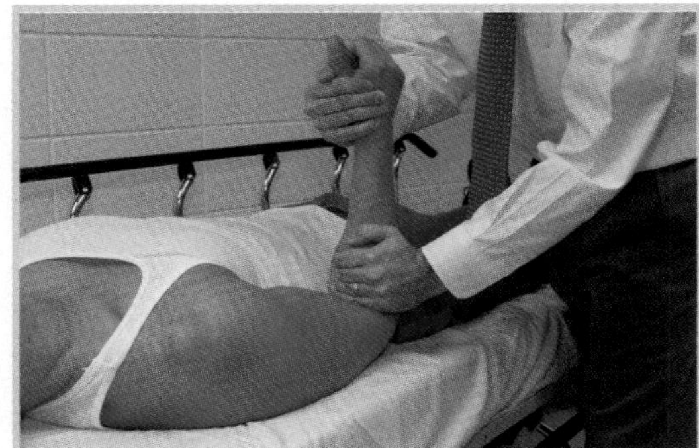

Step 1

Step 2. While gentle traction is maintained in the direction of the patient's feet, the flexed forearm should be slowly rotated 90 degrees in a lateral direction.

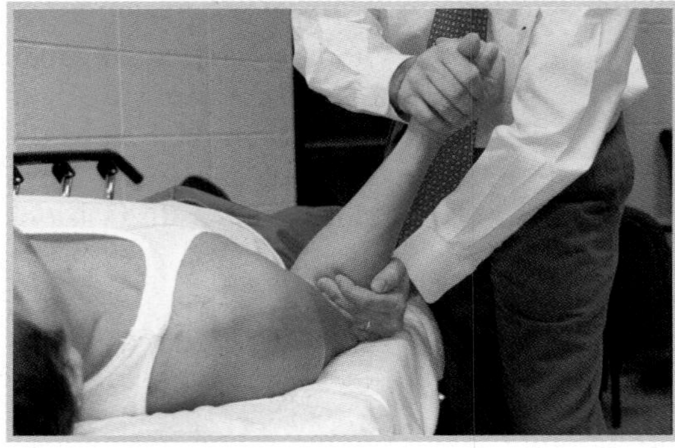

Step 2

Step 3. If reduction has not occurred after 90 degrees of rotation is obtained, slight abduction of the arm away from the chest wall while still in the rotated position may prove successful.

- **PEARL:** Reduction is usually apparent to the patient and the practitioner, as the patient will have improved range of motion and less pain. Commonly, reduction of the joint can be felt by the patient and the practitioner.

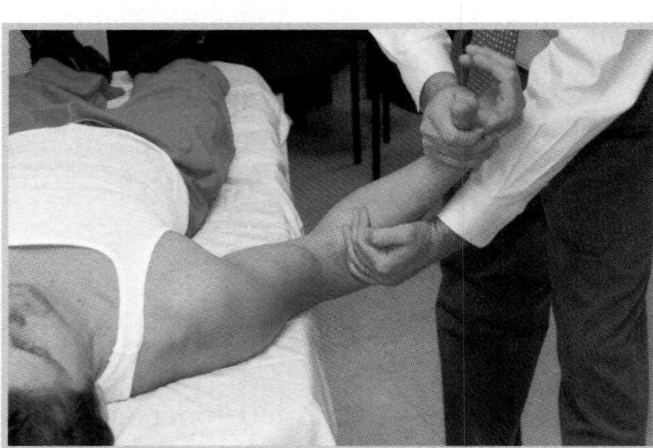

Step 3

STIMSON TECHNIQUE

Step 1. Place the patient in a prone position with the affected arm hanging over the stretcher. Being careful not to obstruct blood flow distally, secure approximately 10 kg of weight to the wrist or forearm of the affected arm creating constant, downward traction of the extremity. Attempt traction for at least 20 to 30 minutes. Reduction will usually occur spontaneously from this position.

- **PEARL:** Reduction is usually apparent to the patient and the practitioner, as the patient will have improved range of motion and less pain. Commonly, reduction of the joint can be felt by the patient and the practitioner.

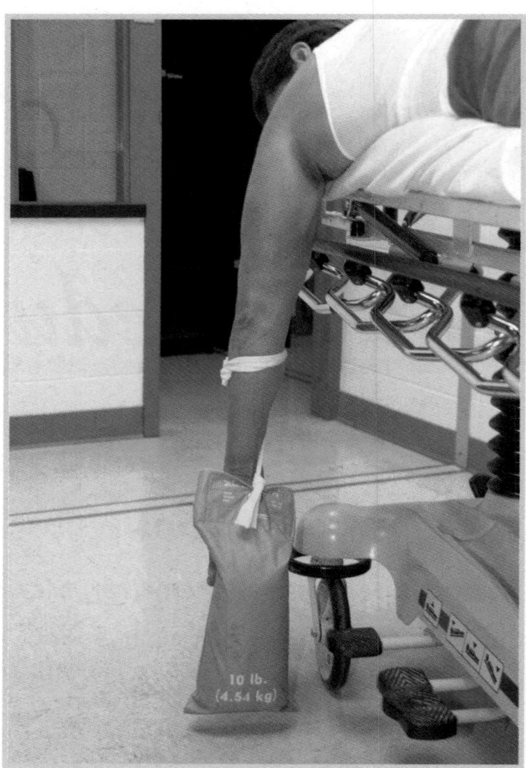

Step 1

Scapular Manipulation

Step 1. Place the patient in a prone position with the affected arm hanging over the stretcher as in the Stimson technique. After adequate sedation, the inferior tip of the scapula is pushed medially while stabilizing the superior aspect of the scapula with the other hand.

- **PEARL:** Reduction is usually apparent to the patient and the practitioner, as the patient will have improved range of motion and less pain. Commonly, reduction of the joint can be felt by the patient and the practitioner.

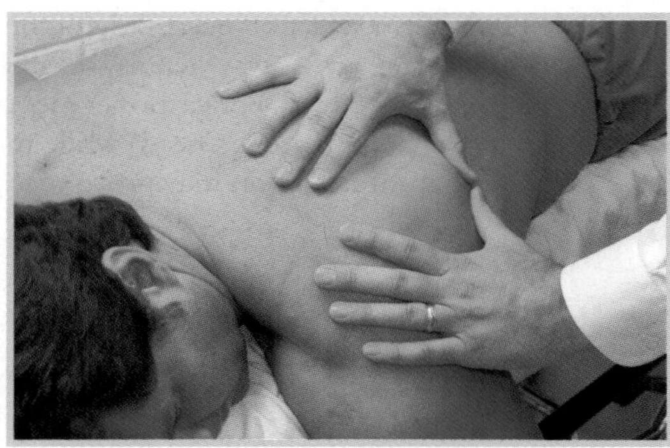

Step 1

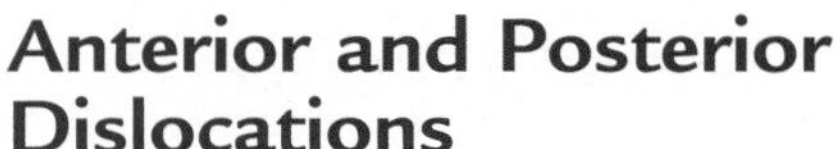

Anterior and Posterior Dislocations

Traction-Countertraction

Step 1. Place the patient in a supine position on a bed or gurney. Place a sheet around the axilla of the affected shoulder and secure it to the stretcher frame above the opposite shoulder.

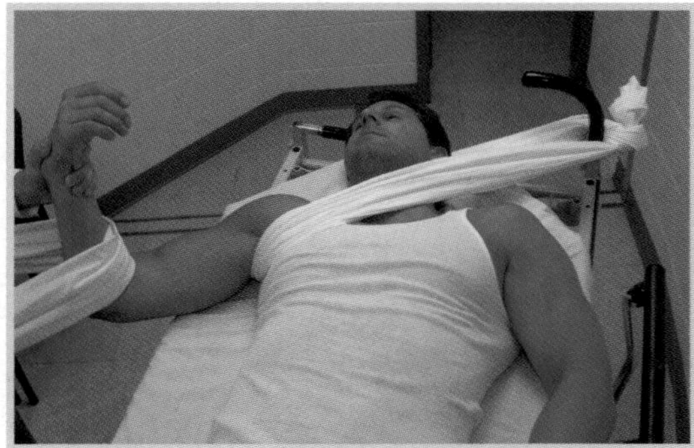

Step 1

Step 2. The practitioner should apply slow, steady traction in a downward direction using a sheet secured around the practitioner's waist and slipped over the forearm flexed at 90 degrees. Traction should be maintained for at least 15 minutes and can be increased simply by leaning backward against the traction sheet.

- **PEARL:** The practitioner should make sure there is ample cleared space provided for the procedure and maintain stable footing at all times.
- **PITFALL:** Care should be taken to let gravity and body weight work to the advantage of the practitioner by leaning backward and avoiding strenuous tugging and risks of back injury.
- **PEARL:** Reduction is usually apparent to the patient and the practitioner, as the patient will have improved range of motion and less pain. Commonly, reduction of the joint can be felt by the patient and the practitioner.

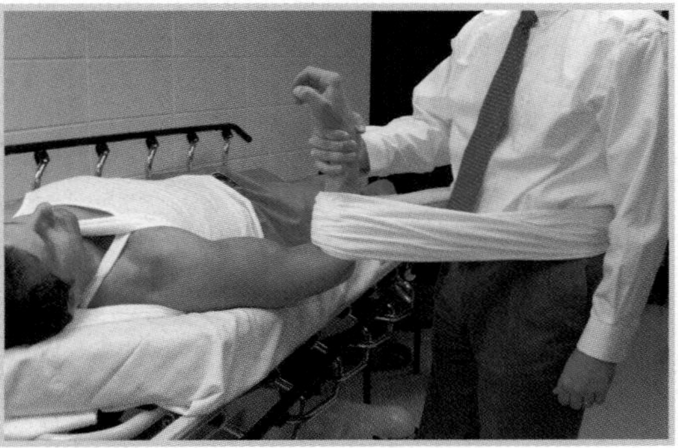

Step 2

Step 3. If reduction has not occurred, slight abduction of the arm away from the chest wall (accomplished by the practitioner moving at an arc toward the patient's head) while maintaining downward traction may prove successful.

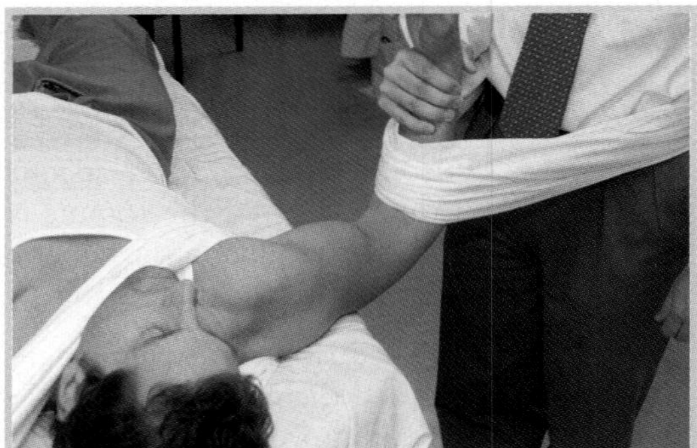

Step 3

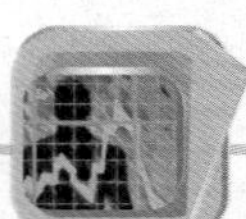

Complications

- Recurrent dislocation
- Vascular and nerve injuries
- Bony injuries
- Rotator cuff injury

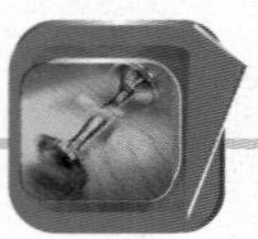

Pediatric Considerations

Immediate referral to an orthopedic surgeon is necessary because of future growth-related considerations.

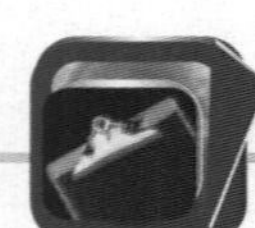

Postprocedure Instructions

- Immobilize the shoulder with an immobilizer or sling and swathe.
- Reassess circulatory status of the extremity and axillary nerve integrity.
- Repeat shoulder x-ray to verify reduction and absence of bony injury.
- Refer patient to an orthopedic surgeon for follow-up within 3 days.

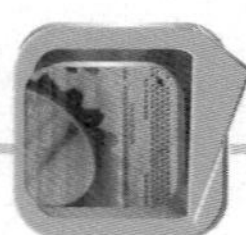

Coding Information and Supply Sources

CPT Code	Description	2008 Average 50th Percentile Fee	Global Period
23650	Closed treatment of shoulder dislocation, with manipulation; without anesthesia	$642.00	90
23655	Requiring anesthesia	$865.00	90

CPT is a registered trademark of the American Medical Association.
2008 average 50th Percentile Fees are provided courtesy of 2008 MMH-SI's copyrighted Physicians' Fees and Coding Guide.

A complete range of shoulder immobilizers and arm slings may be ordered from SupportsUSA, 14275 Midway Rd., Suite 155, Addison, TX 75001. Web site: http://www.supportsusa.com/.

Patient Education Handout

A patient education handout, "Shoulder Dislocation," can be found on the book's Web site.

Bibliography

Doyle WL, Ragar T. Use of the scapular manipulation method to reduce an anterior shoulder dislocation in the supine position. *Ann Emerg Med.* 1996;27(1):92–94.

Lennard F, Martin S. How to immobilise after shoulder dislocation? *Emerg Med J.* 2005;22:814–815.

Mattick A, Wyatt JP. From Hippocrates to the Eskimo—a history of techniques used to reduce anterior dislocation of the shoulder. *JR Coll Surg Edinb.* 2000;45(October);312–316.

Riebal GD, McCabe JB. Anterior shoulder dislocation: a review of reduction techniques. *Am J Emerg Med.* 1991;9(2):180–188.

2008 MAG Mutual Healthcare Solutions, Inc.'s Physicians' Fee and Coding Guide. Duluth, Georgia. MAG Mutual Healthcare Solutions, Inc. 2007.

CHAPTER 15

Exercise Treadmill Testing

Russell D. White, MD

Professor of Medicine, Director, Sports Medicine Fellowship Program
Department of Community and Family Medicine
University of Missouri Kansas City, School of Medicine, Kansas City, MO

George D. Harris, MD, MS

Professor of Medicine, Department of Community and Family Medicine
University of Missouri Kansas City, School of Medicine, Kansas City, MO

Exercise testing is a useful diagnostic procedure performed by appropriately trained primary care physicians. The three major cardiopulmonary reasons for doing exercise testing relate to diagnosis, prognosis, and therapeutic prescription. The predictive value of the exercise test is greatest when test results are combined with family history, current symptoms, and underlying risk factors. This consensus approach of combining clinical information with exercise test data yields 94% sensitivity and 92% specificity. Exercise testing allows the clinician to assess the severity of previously diagnosed disease and to predict the patient's future risk of cardiac events, including death. Following exercise testing a therapeutic exercise program can be prescribed and later assessed for its benefits.

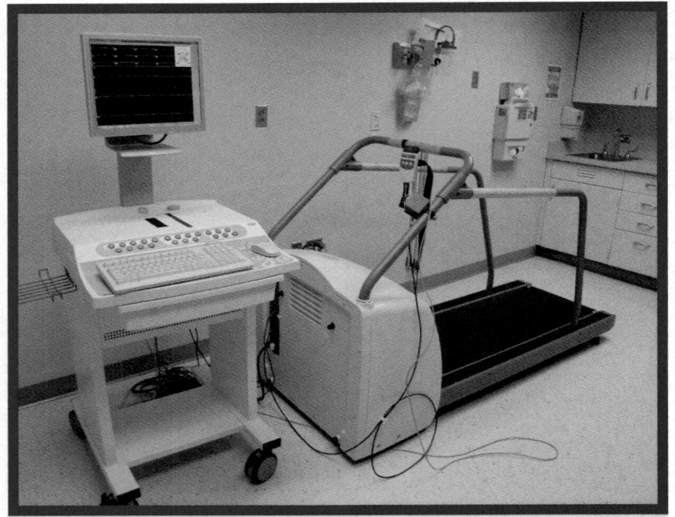

Exercise testing can be utilized in assessing physical fitness, determining functional capacity, diagnosing cardiac disease, defining the prognosis of known cardiac disease, determining an exercise prescription, and guiding cardiac rehabilitation.

To deal with possible complications, one must be trained in advanced cardiac life support (ACLS) protocols. ACLS equipment, including proper medications and a defibrillator, should be available at all times. The most important safety precaution is careful pretest patient evaluation and selection of the proper protocol. The overall risk of a significant cardiac event during an exercise stress test is 0.8 per 10,000 tests. The risk of infarction is 3.5 per 10,000 tests, with a mortality rate of 0.5 to 1.0 in a high-risk population.

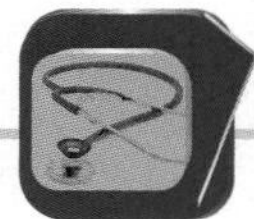

Equipment

- Exercise treadmill device
- Echocardiogram (ECG) machine
- Monitor
- Defibrillator and ACLS equipment (not shown)

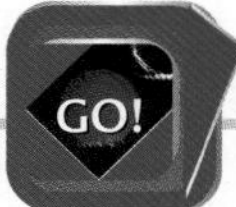

Indications

- Evaluating patients with chest pain
- Screening for latent coronary artery disease
- Determining functional capacity
- Evaluating dysrhythmias
- Early detection of labile hypertension
- Generating an exercise prescription
- Evaluating individual training programs for athletes
- Establishing the severity/prognosis of coronary artery disease
- Evaluating antianginal or antihypertensive therapy
- Evaluating arrhythmias or antiarrhythmia therapy
- Evaluating patients with congestive heart failure
- Evaluating congenital heart disease and valvular dysfunction
- Evaluating the patient after myocardial infarction for risk stratification

Contraindications

Absolute Contraindications

- A recent significant change in the resting ECG, suggesting significant ischemia or other recent cardiac event
- Recent myocardial infarction (within 2 days) or other acute cardiac event
- Unstable angina
- Uncontrolled arrhythmias, causing symptoms or hemodynamic changes
- Severe aortic stenosis
- Uncompensated congestive heart failure
- Acute pulmonary embolus or pulmonary infarction (within 3 months)
- Suspected or confirmed dissecting aneurysm
- Acute infections
- Acute myocarditis or pericarditis
- Uncooperative patients

Relative Contraindications

- Known left main artery stenosis
- Moderately stenotic valvular heart disease
- Electrolyte abnormalities (e.g., hypokalemia, hypomagnesemia)
- Severe systemic hypertension (systolic pressure >200 mm Hg or diastolic pressure >110 mm Hg)
- Uncontrolled tachyarrhythmias or bradyarrhythmias
- Hypertrophic cardiomyopathy or other forms of outflow tract obstruction
- Neuromuscular, musculoskeletal, or rheumatoid disorders that prohibit exercise or are exacerbated by exercise
- Chronic infectious disease (e.g., mononucleosis, hepatitis, AIDS)
- High degree of atrioventricular block (second-degree Mobitz II or third-degree block)
- Ventricular aneurysm
- Uncontrolled metabolic disease (e.g., diabetes mellitus, thyrotoxicosis, or myxedema)

The Procedure

Step 1. Following informed consent, the ECG leads are placed for the exercise test as follows:

- V1—fourth intercostal space right side of the sternum
- V2—fourth intercostal space left side of the sternum
- V3—midway between V2 and V4 (usually overlying the fourth rib)
- V4—fifth intercostal space in the midclavicular line (usually below the left nipple)
- V5—fifth intercostal space in the anterior axillary line
- V6—fifth intercostal space in the midaxillary line
- Right arm lead—right infraclavicular fossa
- Left arm lead—left infraclavicular fossa
- Right lower extremity lead—lower abdomen
- Left lower extremity lead—midback or left lower side

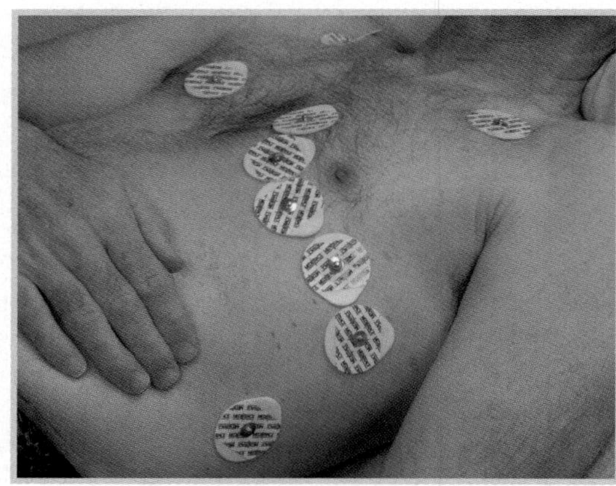

Step 1

- **PITFALL:** Check leads V5 and V6 carefully because often they are not positioned correctly.
- **PEARL:** Reapply brassiere in women to help maintain proper position of leads during the procedure.

Step 2. A baseline ECG is obtained in the supine position and compared with a previous baseline ECG prior to initiating the procedure.

- **PITFALL:** Any change from the previous resting ECG may indicate unstable angina or a recent myocardial event, including infarction, and may be cause to abort the procedure.

Step 3. Initiate the test according to the specified protocol. The modified Bruce protocol allows the patient to become accustomed to the treadmill speed and to smaller increment changes in the inclination or grade prior to starting the more aggressive Bruce protocol. Total exercise time is 8 to 12 minutes for a physiologic response. Each stage is 3 minutes in length. Blood pressure and pulse are recorded with a Borg score (perceived exertion) at the end of each stage (see Table 15-1).

Continue the procedure until the patient reaches peak exercise or develops complications (e.g., arrhythmias, chest pain). If the patient achieves <85% of his maximum predicted heart rate (MPHR) and no abnormalities are found, the results are inconclusive. (MPHR = 220 − age ± 12 beats for 95% confidence limits. This derived value has an extremely wide range and is not specific for the individual patient.)

- **PITFALL:** Observe the monitor for any cardiac abnormalities.
- **PITFALL:** Observe the patient for signs of distress–difficulty maintaining speed and grade, difficulty breathing, or gait abnormalities.
- **PITFALL:** Record any other parameters (e.g., Wright peak flow, pulse oximetry) with each stage of the procedure.

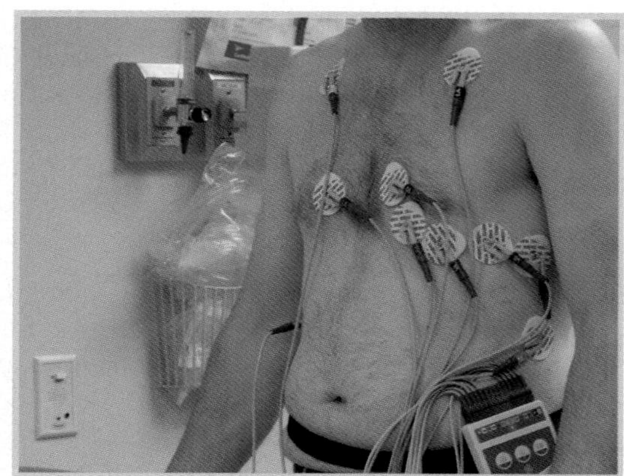

Step 2

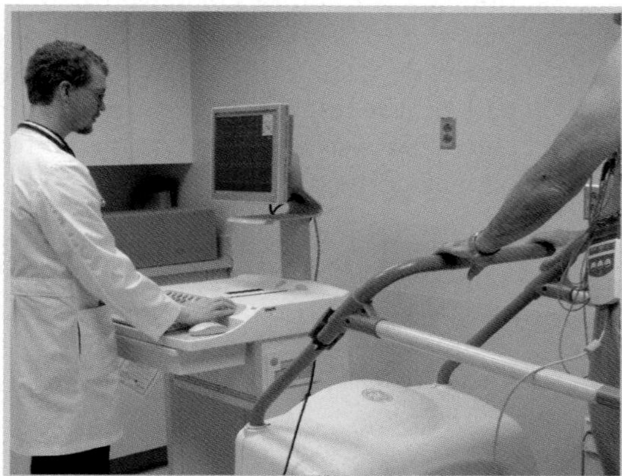

Step 3

TABLE 15-1. Modified Bruce (Gray Cells) and Bruce Protocols

STAGE	SPEED (MPH)	GRADE (%)
0	1.7	0
1/2	1.7	5
1	1.7	10
2	2.5	12
3	3.4	14
4	4.2	16
5	5.0	18
6	5.5	20

- **PITFALL:** Information is valid and more predictable if the patient achieves his personal maximum heart rate determined by high work load (METs), exertional fatigue (Borg scale), and plateau of heart rate (failure of heart rate to increase in response to an increasing workload).

Step 4. The test is terminated, and the patient is put into the recovery (cool-down) period for 1 to 2 minutes. Heart rate and blood pressure are determined at 1 minute. Systolic blood pressure at 3 minutes is divided by the systolic blood pressure at peak exercise. If this ratio is ≥0.91, this parameter a marker for heart disease. Monitoring in the recovery period is continued for 9 minutes or until the patient has returned to baseline blood pressure and heart rate. The leads are then removed from the patient, the test results are carefully reviewed, and a written report is made. Inform the patient of the results.

- **PITFALL:** ECG abnormalities including electrocardiographic wave (ST)-segment changes may occur only in recovery and not during the exercise period. These "recovery-only ST-segment changes" indicate heart disease.

- **PITFALL:** A failure to reduce the heart rate at 1 minute in recovery by at least 12 beats, compared to the maximum exercise heart rate, indicates heart disease.

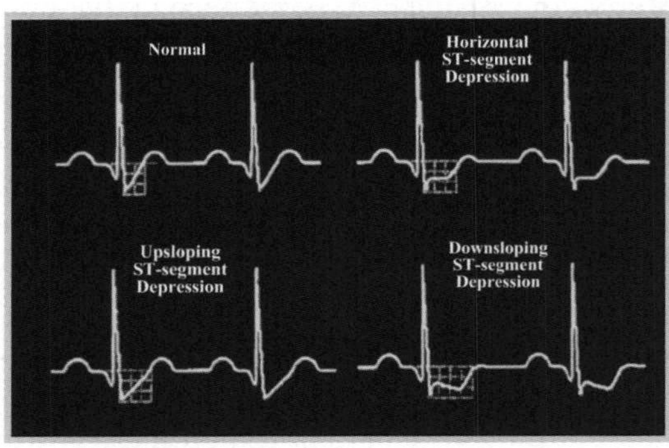

Step 4

Step 5. Interpretation

Myocardial ischemia is defined by ST-segment changes with exercise. The most common findings are a normal response followed by the abnormal responses of upsloping ST-segment depression, horizontal ST-segment depression, and downsloping ST-segment depression.

- Upsloping ST-segment depression: ST-segment depression that is >1.5 mm at 80 msec past the J-point.
- Horizontal ST-segment depression: ST-segment depression that is >1 mm at 60 msec past the J-point.
- Downsloping ST-segment depression: ST-segment depression that is >1 mm at 60 msec past the J-point.

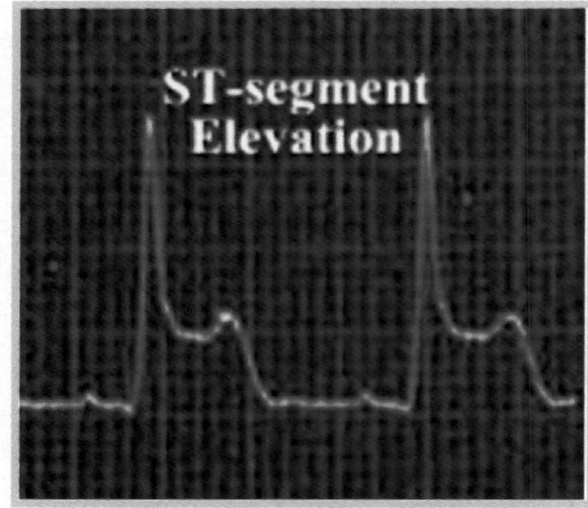

Step 5

- ST-segment elevation (very rare): ST-segment elevation (with J-point elevation) >1 mm at 60 msec past the J-point.
- **PITFALL:** ST-segment depression represents subendocardial ischemia and may not correspond to the anatomic site of pathology (diseased vessel), whereas ST-segment elevation represents transmural ischemia and does correspond with the pathologic anatomic site.

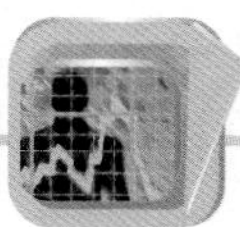

Complications

- Hypotension
- Congestive heart failure
- Accidental physical trauma (e.g., falls)
- Acute central nervous system events (e.g., syncope, stroke)
- Severe cardiac dysrhythmias
- Acute myocardial infarction
- Cardiac arrest
- Death

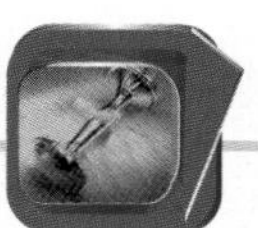

Pediatric Considerations

The clinical reasons for pediatric exercise stress testing include (i) evaluating signs or symptoms induced or accentuated by exercise; (ii) assessing or identifying abnormal responses to exercise in children with known cardiac, pulmonary, or other organ disorders, including myocardial ischemia and arrhythmias; (iii) assessing efficacy of medical or surgical therapies; (iv) assessing functional capacity for recreational, athletic, or vocational activities; (v) establishing baseline data for institution of cardiac, pulmonary, or musculoskeletal rehabilitation; (vi) evaluating prognosis of specific disease states, including serial testing measurements; and (vii) evaluating specific disease states or diagnoses.

These specific disease states or diagnoses include (i) exercise-related symptoms in a child with normal ECG and cardiovascular examination; (ii) exercise-induced bronchospasm studies; (iii) evaluation for long-QTc syndrome; (iv) asymptomatic ventricular ectopy with a normal structural heart; (v) patients with unrepaired or residual congenital cardiac disease who are asymptomatic at rest; (vi) evaluation of patients at risk for myocardial ischemia (e.g., Kawasaki's disease, anomalous left coronary artery circulation, and previous myocardial infarction); (vii) monitoring of heart transplant patients; (viii) patients with hemodynamically stable supraventricular tachycardia (SVT); (ix) patients with stable dilated cardiomyopathy; (x) testing of patients with Marfan's syndrome; and (xi) unexplained syncope with exercise.

Exercise treadmill protocols for pediatric patients are similar to those for adults. Often the Bruce protocol is utilized and then continued into adulthood. This choice permits following the patient on a longitudinal basis over many years with the same protocol. The Balke protocol is also used in pediatric patients, and in some testing centers the cycle ergometer is utilized.

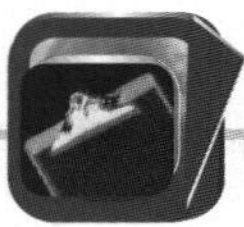

Postprocedure Instructions

The postprocedure written report should include the (i) the heart rate and blood pressure response (include double product); (ii) any dysrhythmias; (iii) the functional aerobic capacity; (iv) ECG changes, especially the ST-segment; (v) results of any other testing parameters (e.g., Wright peak flow measurements, pulse oximetry, glucose determinations); (vi) the presence or absence or myocardial ischemia (probability statement); and (vii) prognosis (based on the Duke treadmill score).

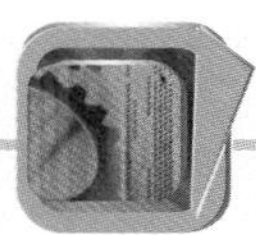

Coding Information and Supply Sources

CPT Code	Description	2008 Average 50th Percentile Fee	Global Period
93000	ECG with interpretation and report	$77.00	XXX
93005	ECG, without interpretation and report	$54.00	XXX
93010	ECG interpretation and report only	$45.00	XXX
93015	CV stress test with supervision, interpretation, and report	$407.00	XXX
93016	CV stress test supervision only	$189.00	XXX
93017	CV stress test supervision only	$110.00	XXX
93018	CV stress test interpretation and report only	$131.00	XXX
94760	Pulse oximetry, single determination	$36.00	XXX
94761	Pulse oximetry, multiple determination	$64.00	XXX
94620	Pulmonary stress testing with pre- and postspirometry and oximetry	$248.00	XXX

XXX, global concept does not apply.

2008 average 50th Percentile Fees are provided courtesy of 2008 MMH-SI's copyrighted Physicians' Fees and Coding Guide.

ICD-9 Codes

401.1 to 429.9	Includes hypertension, coronary artery disease, angina, aneurysm of heart and coronary vessels, cardiomyopathy, atrial fibrillation, and heart failure
780.2	Syncope and collapse
786.05	Shortness of breath
786.06	Tachypnea
786.07	Wheezing
786.50	Chest pain, unspecified
786.51	Precordial pain
786.59	Chest pain, other
V71.7	Observation for suspected cardiovascular disease

Suppliers

- GE Marquette CASE Stress System, Milwaukee, WI. Web site:www.gehealthcare.com.
- Medgraphics Cardio Perfect Stress System, St. Paul, MN. Web site: www.medgraphics.com.
- Quinton Q-Stress Cardiac Stress System, Bothell, WA. Web site: www.quinton.com.
- Spacelabs Burdick Quest Stress Test System, Deerfield, WI. Web site: www.spacelabsburdick.com.
- Welch Allyn PCE PC-Based Exercise ECG System, Skaneateles Falls, NY. Web site:www.welchallyn.com.

Patient Education Handout

A patient education handout, "Exercise Stress Test," can be found on the book's companion Web site.

Bibliography

Ellestad, M. *Stress Testing: Principles and Practices*. 5th ed. New York: Oxford University Press; 2003.

Froelicher VF, Myers J. *Exercise and the Heart*. 5th ed. Philadelphia: Sanders-Elsevier; 2006.

Gibbons RJ, Balady GJ, Bricker JT, et al. ACC/AHA 2002 guideline update for exercise testing: summary article: a report of the American College of Cardiology/American Heart Association Task Force on Practice Guidelines (Committee to Update the 1997 Exercise Testing Guidelines). *Circulation*. 2002;106:1883–1892.

Lane JR, Ben-Schachar G. Myocardial infarction in healthy adolescents. *Pediatrics*. 2007;120:938–943.

Paridon SM, Alpert BS, Boas SR, et al. Clinical stress testing in the pediatric age group: a statement from the American Heart Association Council on Cardiovascular Disease in the Young, Committee on Atherosclerosis, Hypertension, and Obesity in Youth. *Circulation.* 2006;113:1905–1920.

Price DE, Elder K, White RD. Exercise testing. In: O'Connor FG, Sallis R, Wilder R, et al., eds. *Sports Medicine—Just the Facts.* New York: McGraw-Hill; 2004:118–126.

2008 MAG Mutual Healthcare Solutions, Inc.'s Physicians' Fee and Coding Guide. Duluth, Georgia. MAG Mutual Healthcare Solutions, Inc. 2007.

CHAPTER 16

Fishhook Removal

Simon A. Mahler, MD

Assistant Professor, Department of Emergency Medicine
Louisiana State University Health Sciences Center, Shreveport, LA

Fishing is a popular outdoor activity worldwide. In the United States alone, it is estimated that there are more than 34 million anglers. Fishhook injuries are common in both commercial and recreational fishing. Fortunately, most fishhook injuries result in only minor soft tissue trauma. Although patients often have hooks removed in the field, these injuries may be encountered in the office or urgent care setting.

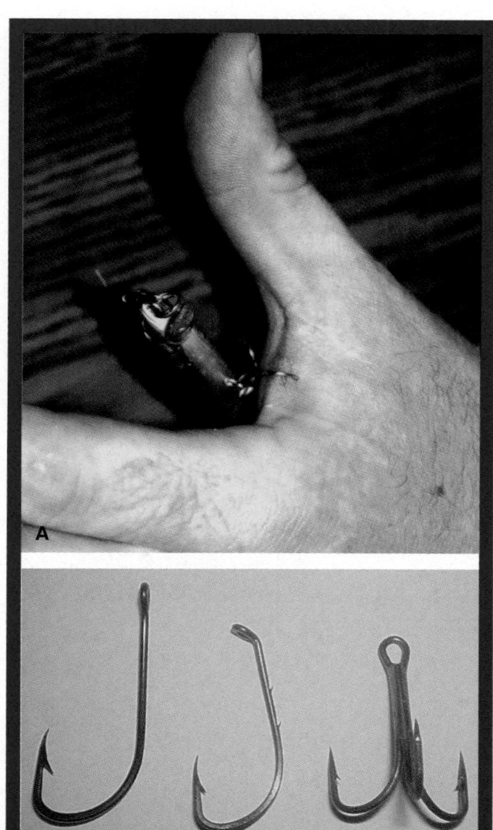

The majority of patients with fishhook injuries present with an embedded hook. The most common locations for these injuries are the hands, face, head, and upper extremities. The special techniques that are required for removal of embedded fishhooks are outlined in this chapter. Although severe injuries are uncommon, ocular involvement could result in a penetrating globe injury and requires emergent ophthalmologic consultation. Hooks with deep tissue penetration in areas that may involve tendons, vessels, nerves, or bone require a thorough evaluation prior to removal. Rarely radiographs or ultrasound may be required to determine the depth of hook penetration and relation to important anatomical structures. Neurovascular status should be assessed in all patients with fishhook injuries.

The optimal fishhook removal technique depends on the type of hook that is embedded. There are many different styles and sizes of fishhooks. However, the most common types are single-barbed straight-shank hooks (A), multibarbed straight-shank hooks (B), and treble hooks (C). Single-barbed straight-shank hooks may be removed using several techniques including the retrograde technique, the string technique, or the needle cover technique. The retrograde technique is the easiest to perform because it does not require special equipment or local anesthesia, but is the least likely to succeed. The string technique can also be used without anesthesia on single-barbed straight-shank hooks. The other hook removal techniques require local anesthesia. The advance and cut techniques are best used for multibarbed and treble hooks.

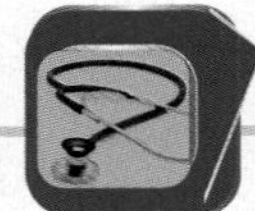

Equipment

- Needle-nosed pliers or needle driver to grasp hook
- Wire cutter or heavy pliers with wire-cutting shear

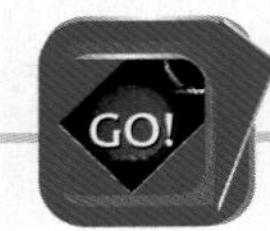

Indications

- Superficially embedded fishhook injuries

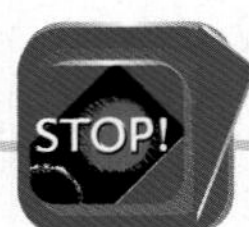

Contraindications

- Ocular involvement
- Deep penetration into tendon, bone, major blood vessel, or nerve

  The string technique should be avoided on mobile structures (earlobes).

The Procedure

Retrograde Technique

Step 1. Downward pressure is applied to the shaft of the hook to disengage the barb. Downward pressure is maintained and the hook is backed out of the skin along the path of entry.

- PITFALL: If resistance is encountered while removing the hook, the procedure should be discontinued and a different technique should be attempted.

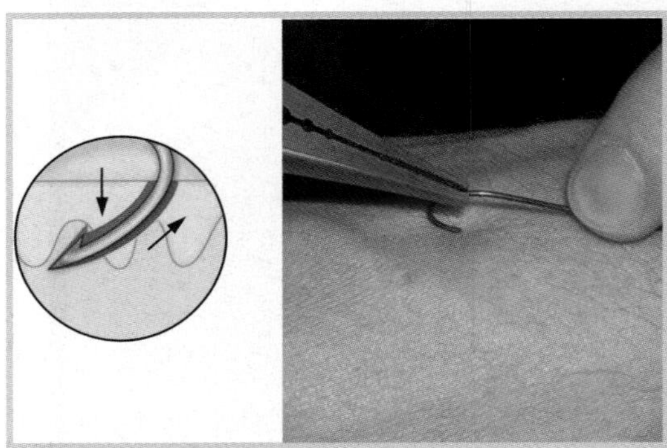

Step 1

String Technique

Step 1. A string is tied to the midpoint of the hook bend and grasped 3 to 4 inches from the hook. Downward pressure is applied to the shaft of the hook to disengage the barb. A firm quick tug on the sting is preformed at a 45-degree angle to the skin while downward pressure on the hook shank is maintained.

- PITFALL: Do not use the string technique on mobile tissue such as earlobes.

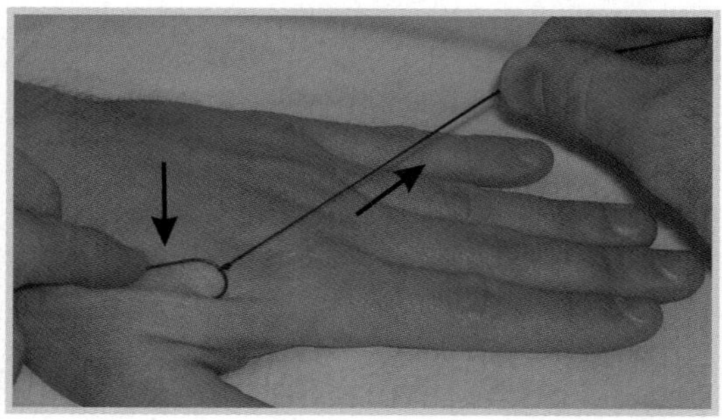

Step 1

Needle Cover Technique

Step 1. Local anesthesia is administered. An 18-gauge needle is advanced along the fishhook until the needle covers the barb of the hook. The hook and needle are backed out of the wound simultaneously.

- PITFALL: Multiple needle stick attempts will increase injury to the surrounding soft tissue and may cause bleeding or hematoma formation.

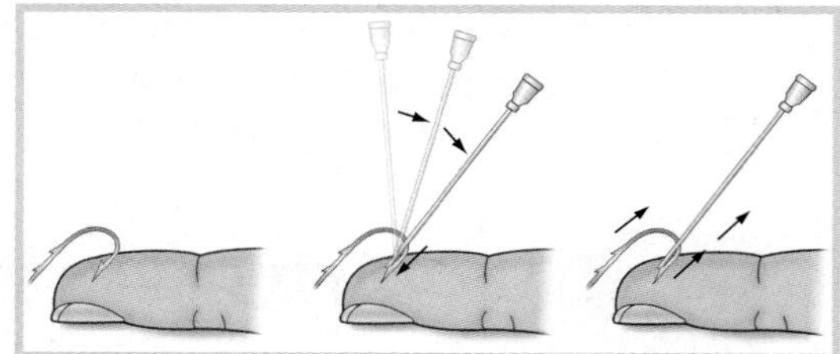

Step 1

Advance and Cut Technique

Step 1. Local anesthesia is administered. Large needle drivers or pliers are used to advance the barb of the hook through the skin. For multibarbed single-shaft hooks, the hook shaft is cut with wire cutters and the hook is pulled forward out of the wound. For single-barbed or treble hooks, the point of the hook including the barb is cut with wire cutters and the hook is backed out of the wound.

- PITFALL: Local anesthesia must be placed where the hook will exit the skin otherwise the procedure will be poorly tolerated.

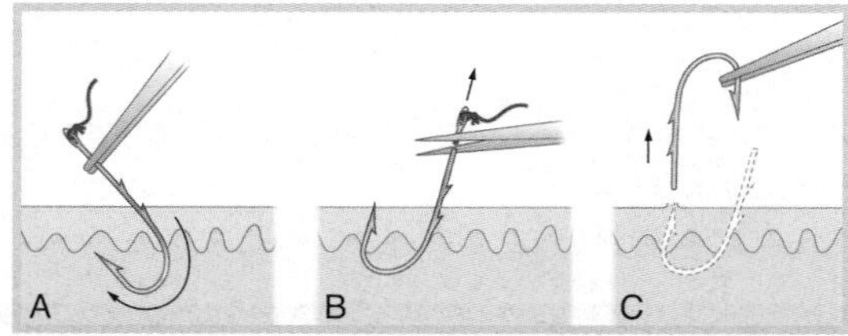

Step 1

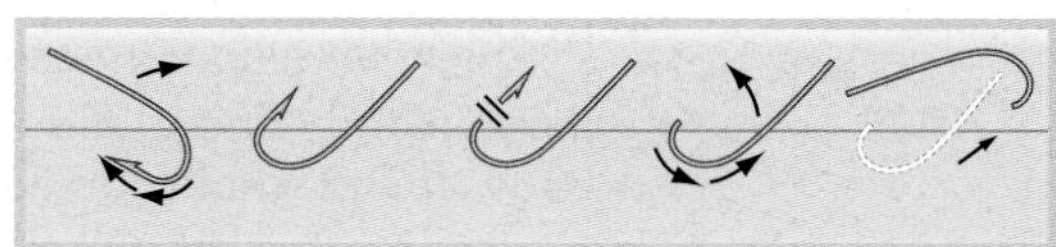

Step 1

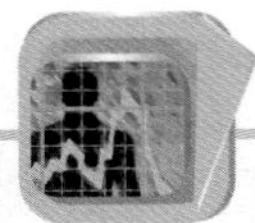

Complications

- Bleeding
- Hematoma
- Infection
- Retained foreign body
- Injury to surrounding structure (tendon, bone, blood vessel, or nerve)

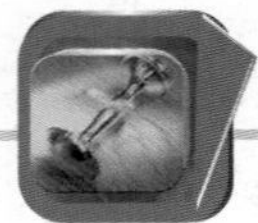

Pediatric Considerations

Although the removal techniques are unchanged, pediatric patients are more likely to be uncooperative because of anxiety. As with any pediatric procedure, it is best to approach the child calmly at his or her level. The child may remain in the parent or caretaker's lap facing toward the clinician. For children younger than 5 years of age, it may be necessary to use a papoose board or conscious sedation.

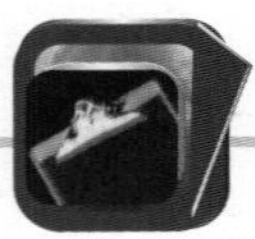

Postprocedure Instructions

After fishhook removal, wounds should be examined carefully for retained foreign bodies. Puncture wounds should generally be left open and covered with a simple dressing. Prophylactic antibiotics are unnecessary for most patients but may be considered in immunocompromised patients such as diabetics. Neurovascular status should be reassessed and tetanus immunization should be confirmed or updated.

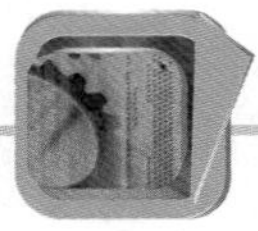

Coding Information and Supply Sources

CPT Code	Description	2008 Average 50th Percentile Fee	Global Period
10120	Incision and removal of foreign body, simple subcutaneous	$165.00	10
10121	Incision and removal of foreign body, complex subcutaneous	$417.00	10
23330	Foreign body removal shoulder subcutaneous	$355.00	10
24200	Foreign body removal upper arm or elbow subcutaneous	$355.00	10

CPT is a registered trademark of the American Medical Association.
2008 average 50th Percentile Fees are provided courtesy of 2008 MMH-SI's copyrighted Physicians' Fees and Coding Guide.

Needle-nosed pliers, wire cutters, and heavy pliers with wire shears are available at any hardware store. A suggested anesthesia tray that can be used for this procedure is listed in Appendix F.

Patient Education Handout

Patient education handouts, "First Aid for Puncture Wounds" and "Fishhook Injuries," can be found on the book's Web site.

Bibliography

Doser C, Cooper WL, Edinger WM, et al. Fishhook injuries: a prospective evaluation. *Am J Emerg Med.* 1991;9:413–415.

Eldad S, Amiram S. Embedded fishhook removal. *Am J Emerg Med.* 2000;18:736–737.

Gammons M, Jackson E. Fishhook removal. *Am Fam Physician.* 2001;63:2231–2236.

Terrill P. Fishhook removal. *Am Fam Physician.* 1993;47:1372.

2008 MAG Mutual Healthcare Solutions, Inc.'s Physicians' Fee and Coding Guide. Duluth, Georgia. MAG Mutual Healthcare Solutions, Inc. 2007.

CHAPTER 17

Endotracheal Intubation

Christopher J. Wolcott, MD
Assistant Clinical Professor of Emergency Medicine, Department of Emergency Medicine
Louisiana State University Health Sciences Center, Shreveport, LA

Endotracheal intubation is a critical, life-saving procedure. To perform the procedure, physicians must rapidly assess the adequacy of the patient's airway and need for ventilatory support. Once the decision to intubate has been made, the procedure should be performed rapidly and skillfully to prevent further deterioration or injury.

The decision to intubate is determined by the patient's failure to (i) oxygenate, (ii) ventilate, or (iii) protect the airway. These problems can occur simultaneously. Failure to oxygenate refers to impairment of gas exchange at the level of the alveoli, resulting in hypoxia and/or hypercarbia. Examples of failure to oxygenate include the patient with pulmonary edema, pneumonia, or pulmonary embolus. Pulmonary fibrosis, asthma, and chronic obstructive pulmonary disease (COPD) are restrictive lung diseases that may lead to a failure to ventilate, or physically move air into and out of the lungs. Ventilatory failure is often the end result of respiratory conditions associated with an increased work of breathing, accessory muscle use, and fatigue. The young and the elderly are particularly susceptible to ventilatory failure from fatigue.

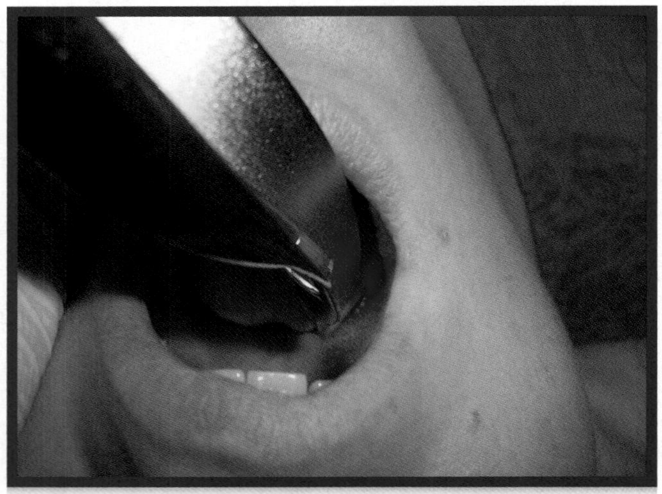

The patient that cannot maintain airway patency or clear secretions requires intubation to protect the airway. Examples of patients who require intubation to prevent aspiration include those with altered mental status from intoxication, closed head injury, central nervous system insult, or severe systemic illness or injury. Patients who require intubation to prevent airway occlusion include those with trauma to neck, upper airway edema, and chemical or thermal burns. The decision to intubate for airway protection is not only based on the patient's current airway status but also on the anticipated clinical course. Intervening early in a relatively stable patient prior to a predicted airway occlusion or compromise allows for a more controlled intubation with fewer complications or risks of failure.

TABLE 17-1. Premedication Drugs

MEDICATION	DOSAGE	DESIRED EFFECT
Atropine	0.01 mg/kg (min 0.1 mg)	Reduces bradycardia and secretions in children
Lidocaine	1.5–2.0 mg/kg	Blunts rise in ICP, reduces cough reflex
Fentanyl	3–5 mcg/kg	Blunts rise in blood pressure and ICP
Defasciculating dose of non-depolarizing paralytic; example, vecuronium	0.01 mg/kg (1/10th normal dose)	Blunts rise in ICP by preventing fasciculations caused by succinylcholine

Rapid Sequence Intubation (RSI) Procedure

A discussion of the technique of endotracheal intubation would not be complete without a discussion of rapid sequence intubation (RSI). RSI is systematic process in which deep sedation and muscle paralysis are used to expedite intubation. Assemble all equipment, check equipment status, select the tube, and confirm cuff integrity. Preoxygenate a spontaneously breathing patient with 100% oxygen. This will saturate the hemoglobin with oxygen and allow more time to place the endotracheal tube before the patient must be reoxygenated by bag-valve mask (BVM). Administer FiO_2 of 100% for 3 minutes by a nonrebreather mask or have the patient take four vital capacity breaths of 100% FiO_2. Note that using positive pressure ventilation with a BVM to preoxygenate or to reoxygenate after a failed intubation attempt can cause gastric distention and increase the risk of vomiting and subsequent aspiration of gastric contents. If the patient is apenic or requires ventilatory support between intubation attempts, the BVM can be used with cricoid pressure. Gentle downward pressure on the cricoid cartilage will compress the esophagus and reduce the chance of gastric insufflation.

Premedication refers to drugs given 3 to 5 minutes prior to sedation and muscle paralysis to blunt the "pressor response" of intubation (Table 17-1). This is the physiologic response caused by manipulation of the larynx, causing an increase in heart rate, blood pressure, intracranial pressure (ICP), and intraocular pressure (IOP).

The induction phase refers to administration of medications to produce deep sedation (Table 17-2). These drugs are given by rapid intravenous push.

TABLE 17-2. Induction Agents

MEDICATION	DOSAGE	COMMENTS
Etomidate	0.3 mg/kg	Protects ICP and maintains blood pressure. Cortisol and aldosterone suppression reported
Thiopental	3–5 mg/kg	Cerebroprotective May cause hypotension and bronchospasm Contraindicated in acute, intermittent, or variegate porphyria
Ketamine	1–2 mg/kg	Potent bronchodilator May cause increased blood pressure and ICP, emergence phenomenon
Propofol	0.5–1.5 mg/kg	Anticonvulsant, antiemetic, lowers ICP Lowers blood pressure

TABLE 17-3. Paralytics

MEDICATION	DOSAGE	TIME TO ONSET	DURATION	COMMENTS
Succinylcholine	1.5 mg/kg	45–60 sec	5–9 min	Depolarizing agent, increases intracranial pressure, increases intraocular pressure, decreases heart rate
Vecuronium	0.08–0.15 mg/kg	2–4 min	25–40 min	Nondepolarizing
Rocuronium	0.6 mg/kg	1–3 min	30–45 min	Nondepolarizing

Finally, give an intravenous paralytic after sedation occurs (Table 17-3). Avoid succinylcholine use in major crush or burn injuries or in any condition with a risk of hyperkalemia. Apply cricoid pressure to reduce the risk of gastric aspiration. Once a neuromuscular blockade is induced, the patient loses protective airway reflexes. Place the endotracheal tube as described in Step 10, confirm its position, and secure it.

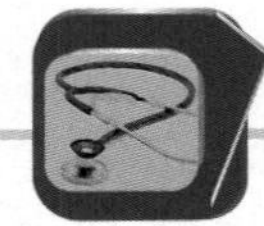

Equipment

All necessary equipment should be kept in an accessible, consistent location. In an emergency department, it is recommended to check the equipment each morning to ensure it is complete and in good working condition.

- Laryngoscope handle (adult and pediatric) with charged batteries
- Laryngoscope blades of various size (shown in Step 1):
  - Miller nos. 3 and 4 for most adults
  - Macintosh nos. 3 and 4 for most adults
  - Miller no. 0 for premature infants and neonates
  - Miller no. 1 for term infants
  - Miller no. 2 for small children
- Endotracheal tubes of various sizes (shown in Step 2):
  - 7.0 to 7.5 mm for most adult females
  - 7.5 to 8.0 mm for most adult males

Although these sizes are the most common, tubes from 2.5 mm to 9 mm should be available.

- BVM attached to high-flow oxygen source
- Suction with tip
- Nasopharyngeal and oropharyngeal airways (shown in Step 1)
- Capnography device (shown in Step 11)
- Stylet
- Spare batteries and light bulbs
- Tracheal tube securing device:
  - Tape and mastic
  - Tracheal cloth ties
  - Commercial devices
- Magill forceps to remove foreign material in posterior oropharynx

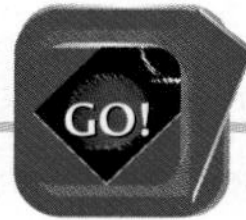

Indications

- Respiratory or cardiopulmonary arrest
- Severe exacerbation of a chronic medical condition, resulting in an unstable patient who cannot oxygenate and/or ventilate, which leads to
  - Hypoxia despite appropriate therapy
  - Hypercarbia, especially with altered mental status
  - Failure to ventilate because of
    - Fatigue
    - Airway obstruction
    - Neuromuscular disease
- Trauma:
  - Central nervous system trauma associated with Glasgow coma scale (CS) ≤8
  - Injury to neck with airway compromise—Listen for stridor or voice changes:
    - Penetrating trauma associated with expanding hematoma
    - Blunt trauma associated with hematoma
  - Severe flail chest
  - Pulmonary injury resulting in poor oxygenation or ventilation
  - Multisystem trauma resulting in an unstable patient
- Loss of airway protection because of altered mental status:
  - GCS ≤8
  - Advanced disease process
  - Intoxication
  - Sepsis
- Anticipated clinical course:
  - Predicted decompensation of medical condition leading to respiratory failure
  - Severely injured patient requiring emergent surgery
  - Inhalation thermal injuries
  - Chemical injuries to the airway
  - Patient with increased work of breathing and fatigue despite therapy
  - Transfer of a patient to another facility with any of the previously mentioned conditions

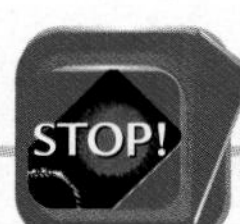

Contraindications (Relative)

- Unstable cervical spine fracture is a relative contraindication but should not prevent intubation when it is required to sustain life. If time permits, a clinician skilled in fiber optic laryngoscopy can intubate with minimal manipulation of the cervical spine.
- Severe facial trauma is a relative contraindication but should not prevent intubation when it is required to sustain life. Debris and blood may prevent visualization of the vocal cords. Cricothyrotomy should be considered in this situation.

The Procedure

Step 1. Prepare the equipment. Confirm the bulb on the laryngoscope is working and properly fits the handle. Inflate the cuff on the endotracheal tube to ensure integrity, and insert the stylet. The equipment should also contain oropharyngeal and nasopharyngeal airways to enable more efficient bag valve mask ventilation should it be needed.

Step 2. Evaluate for a difficult airway. This allows the physician to choose the equipment and method of intubation that will be most successful. If the clinician feels there may be a difficult airway, then another method of intubation should be considered (Table 17-4).

TABLE 17-4. Alternatives to Orotracheal Intubation

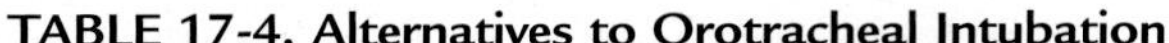

Nasotracheal intubation
Fiberoptic intubation
Intubating laryngeal mask airway
Lighted stylet
Retrograde intubation
Cricothyrotomy

- PITFALL: Factors contributing to difficult intubation include these:
  - An obese patient with a short "bull" neck: This patient will be harder to position and will deoxygenate more quickly. The larynx in a patient with a short neck is often more anterior and higher than normal, leading to difficulty aligning the axes.
  - Large teeth and tongue or the inability to open the mouth more than 3 cm: This leads to less room to place and maneuver equipment in the mouth.
  - Trauma, blood, debris, or vomitus obscure landmarks.
  - Severe ankylosing arthritis or a cervical collar limits movement of cervical spine.

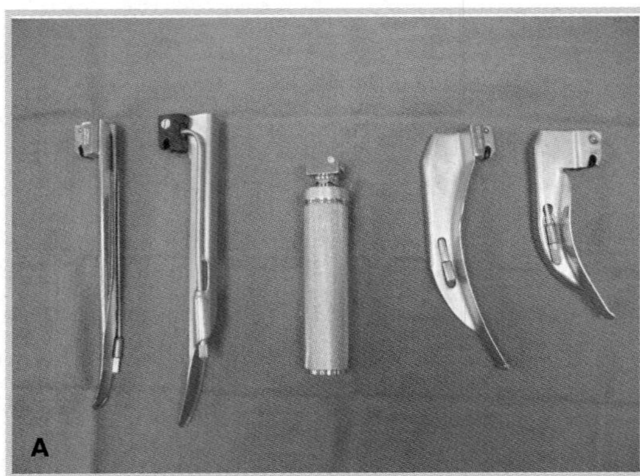

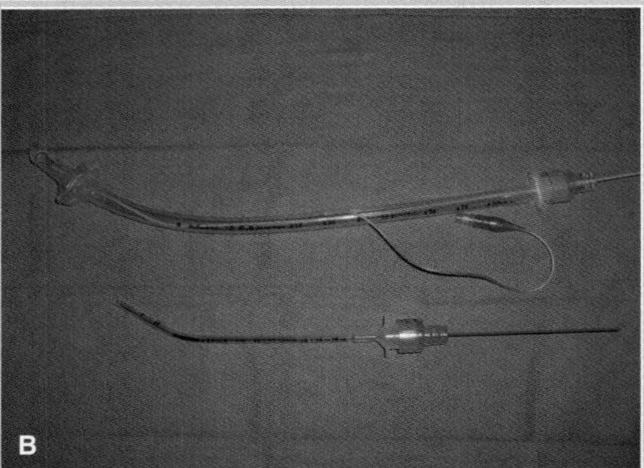

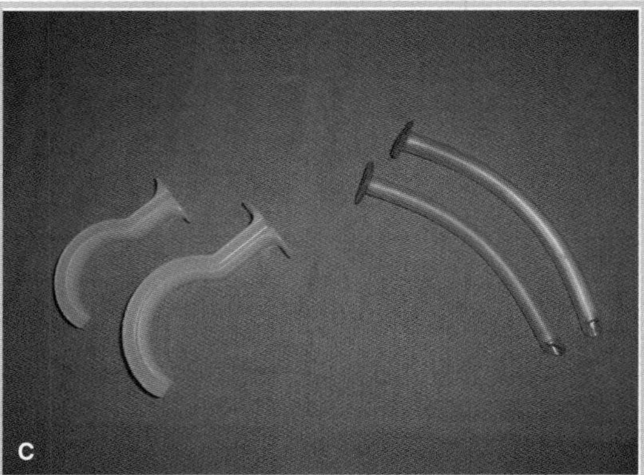

Step 1

Step 3. Position the patient. Place the patient in the "sniffing" position by extending the head on the neck and flexing the neck in relation to the torso. This position better aligns the oral axis with the laryngeal and pharyngeal axes. In the figures, the oral axis is represented by the red line, the laryngeal axis by the blue line, and the pharyngeal axis by the green line. In the neutral position (A), the axes do not line up, making it very difficult to see along the laryngeal axis. Note how the axes are in better alignment when the patient is placed in the sniff position (B).

- **PITFALL:** A patient with a cervical spine injury should not have any movement of the neck and will be more difficult to position.

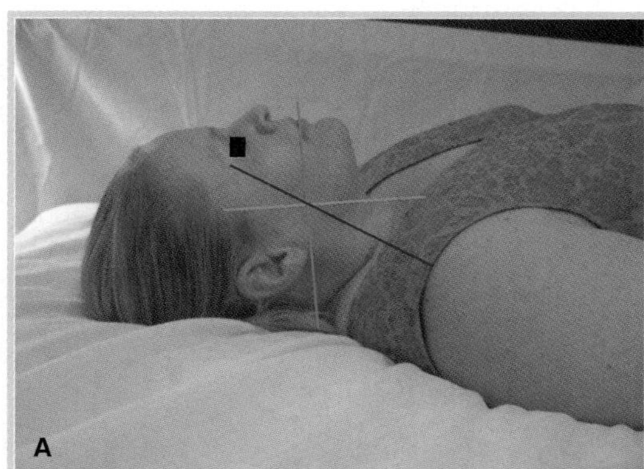

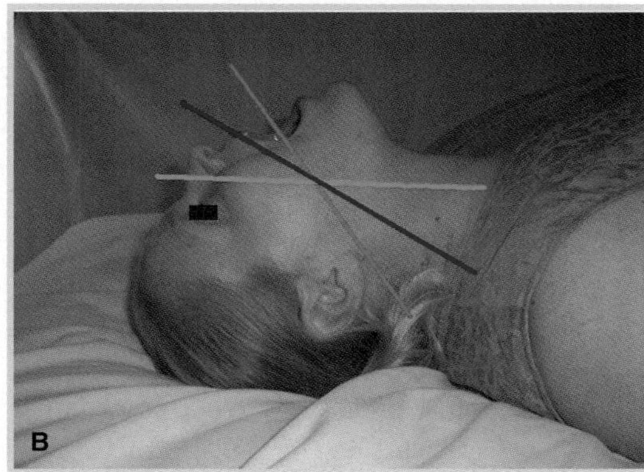

Step 3

Step 4. After adequate sedation and paralysis (see the section on rapid sequence intubation), the physician opens the patient's mouth by placing the right thumb on the lower incisors and right index finger on the upper incisors. Using a scissor-like motion to push the jaw inferiorly with the thumb, the mouth is opened.

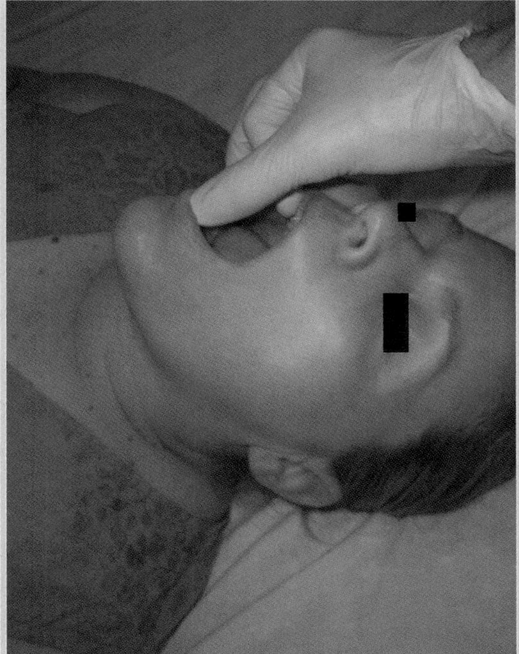

Step 4

Step 5. The operator holds the laryngoscope in the left hand and inserts the tip of the laryngoscope blade between the tongue and the lingual surface of the right mandibular teeth. As the blade is advanced along the lingual surface of the teeth, the tongue is displaced to the left.

- PITFALL: If the blade is started in the center of the mouth, the tongue will not be adequately displaced to the left and will obscure the view.

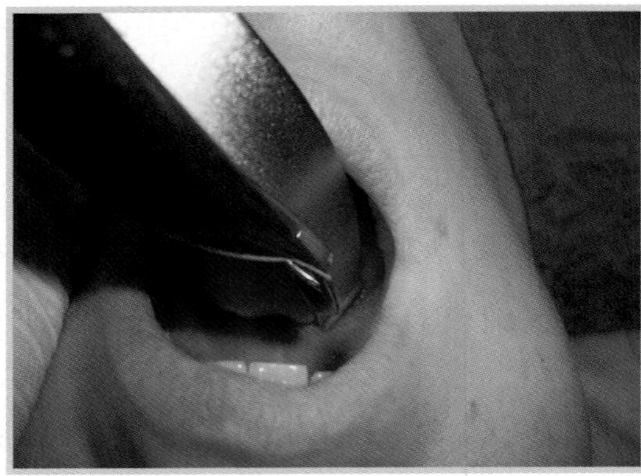

Step 5

Step 6. Advance the blade over the base of the tongue while keeping a gentle "up and out" force on the handle. This force should be directed along the long axis of the handle of the laryngoscope represented by the black arrow. Remember to keep the tongue displaced to the left.

- PITFALL: Rotation of the handle represented by the red arrow in the figure instead of lifting up and out along its axis will lead to the handle or blade pressing against the lips and teeth, causing lacerations or avulsions.

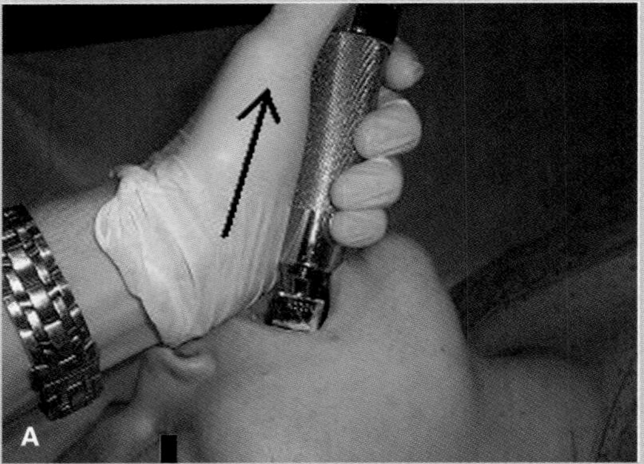

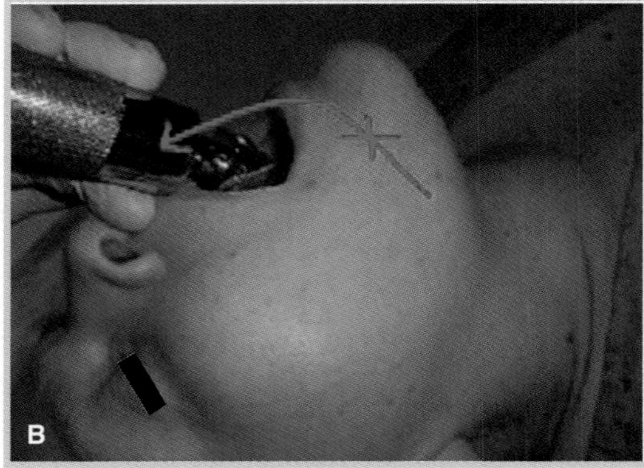

Step 6

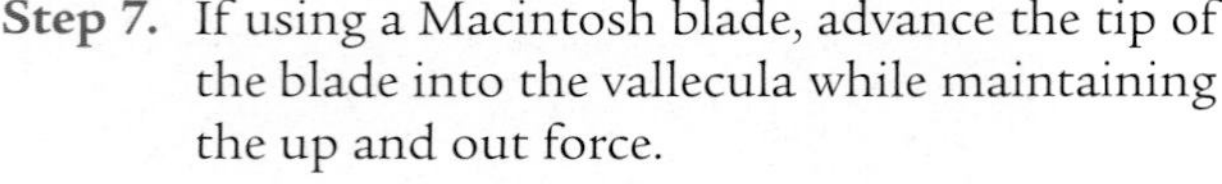

Step 7. If using a Macintosh blade, advance the tip of the blade into the vallecula while maintaining the up and out force.

- PITFALL: Pushing the Macintosh blade too deeply into the vallecula will displace the epiglottis inferiorly, thus obscuring the view of the vocal cords.

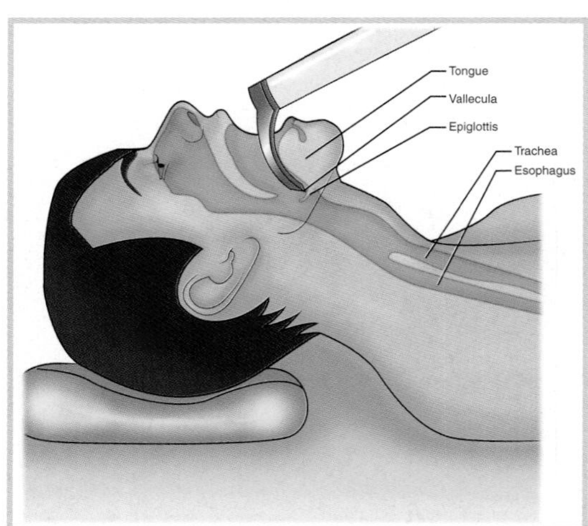

Step 7

Step 8. If using a Miller blade, place the tip just inferior to the epiglottis and lift up and out.

- **PITFALL:** If the Miller blade is passed beyond the epiglottis, the up and out force can lift the larynx and vocal cords out of view.
- **PEARL:** If unable to visualize the vocal cords, the "B.U.R.P." technique may be used. The clinician may apply backward, upward, and rightward pressure to the cricoid cartilage. This will maneuver the larynx into a more favorable position.

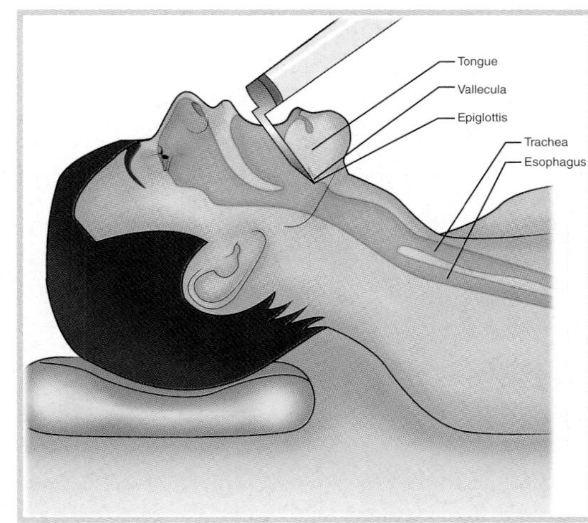

Step 8

Step 9. When the vocal cords are visualized, an assistant should place the endotracheal tube with stylet in the operator's right hand. The operator should never take their eyes off the vocal cords.

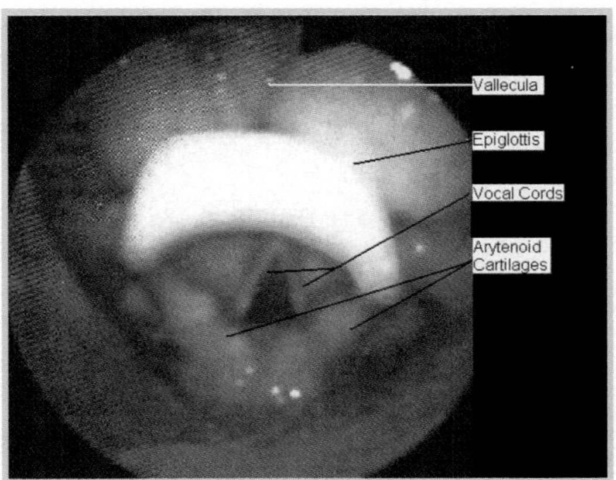

Step 9

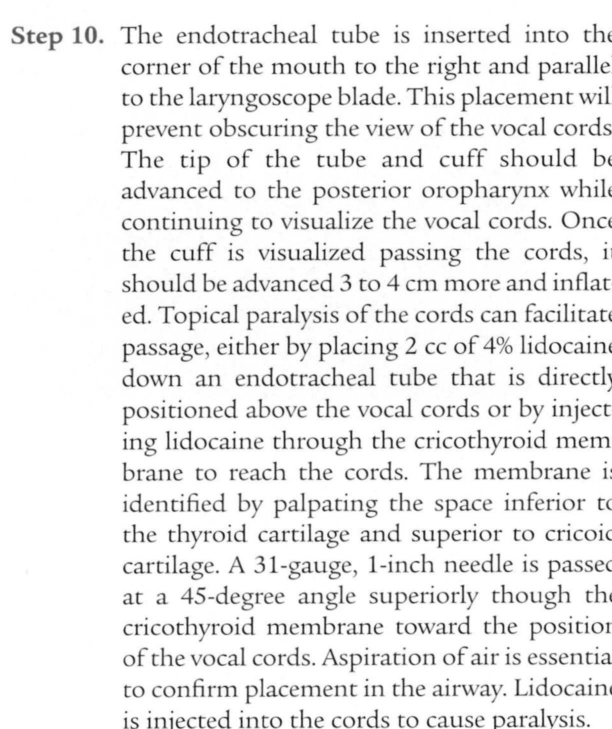

Step 10. The endotracheal tube is inserted into the corner of the mouth to the right and parallel to the laryngoscope blade. This placement will prevent obscuring the view of the vocal cords. The tip of the tube and cuff should be advanced to the posterior oropharynx while continuing to visualize the vocal cords. Once the cuff is visualized passing the cords, it should be advanced 3 to 4 cm more and inflated. Topical paralysis of the cords can facilitate passage, either by placing 2 cc of 4% lidocaine down an endotracheal tube that is directly positioned above the vocal cords or by injecting lidocaine through the cricothyroid membrane to reach the cords. The membrane is identified by palpating the space inferior to the thyroid cartilage and superior to cricoid cartilage. A 31-gauge, 1-inch needle is passed at a 45-degree angle superiorly though the cricothyroid membrane toward the position of the vocal cords. Aspiration of air is essential to confirm placement in the airway. Lidocaine is injected into the cords to cause paralysis.

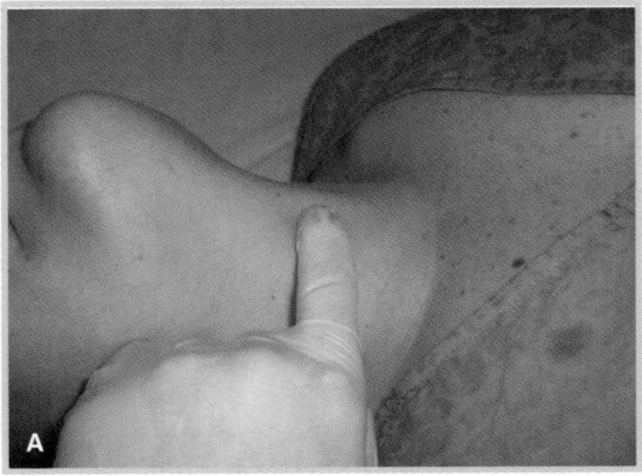

- **PITFALL:** Failure to observe the tube and cuff pass the vocal cords will increase risk of placing the tube into the esophagus.
- **PITFALL:** Forcing the tube between the vocal cords can lead to vocal cord damage. See the section on complications.

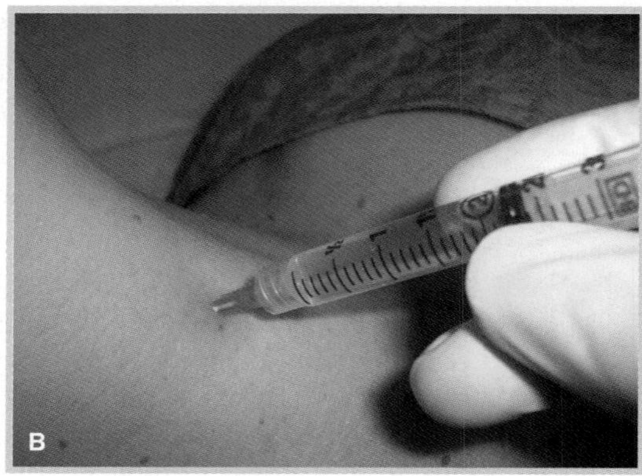

Step 10

Step 11. Confirm placement of endotracheal tube by first auscultating in the bilateral axillae and then epigastrum, followed by observing the chest rise and fall, end tidal CO_2 detection, oxygen saturation, and chest x-ray. An Easy-Cap CO_2 detector will change from purple to yellow when exposed to carbon dioxide.

- **PITFALL:** Failure to auscultate for breath sounds in the axillae may lead to a failure to identify a right mainstem bronchus intubation or esophageal intubation. In a right mainstem bronchus intubation, the clinician may hear breath sounds that have been transmitted from the right lung to the left when listening to the left parasternal area.
- **PEARL:** The desired depth of the tube is 3 to 7 cm above the tracheal carina. This position will prevent damage to the carina by the tube if the patient's head is flexed because flexion of the head can advance the endotracheal tube as much as 2 cm deeper into the trachea.

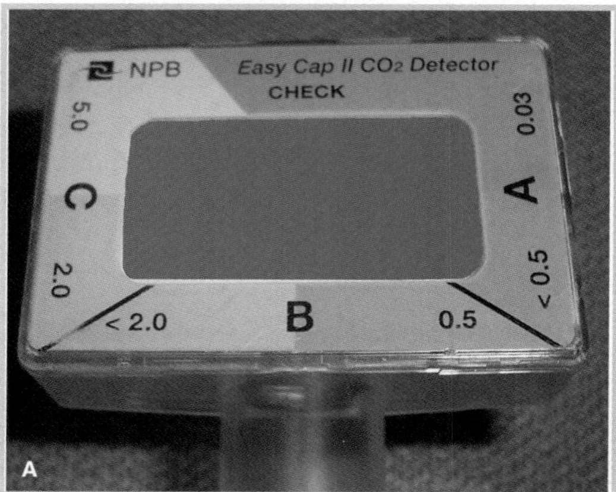

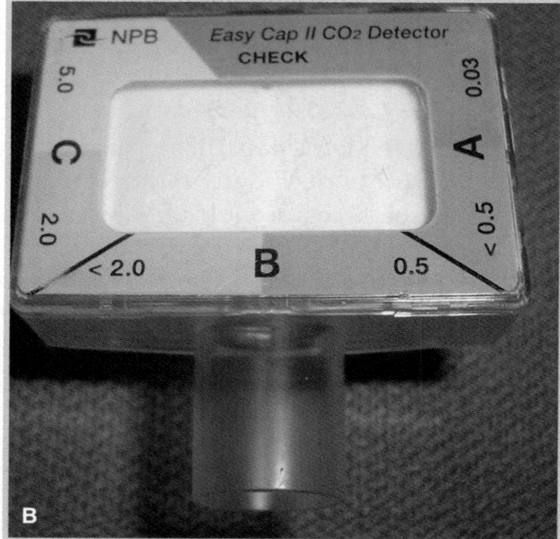

Step 11

Step 12. Secure the endotracheal (ET) tube using tape with mastic, tracheal cloth ties, or a commercial device. The process of using tape to secure ET tube is shown in the figure. Split tape longitudinally as shown. Apply upper segment of tape to face and philtrum and lower segment wraps around tube. Applying mastic to skin will help secure the tape to face.

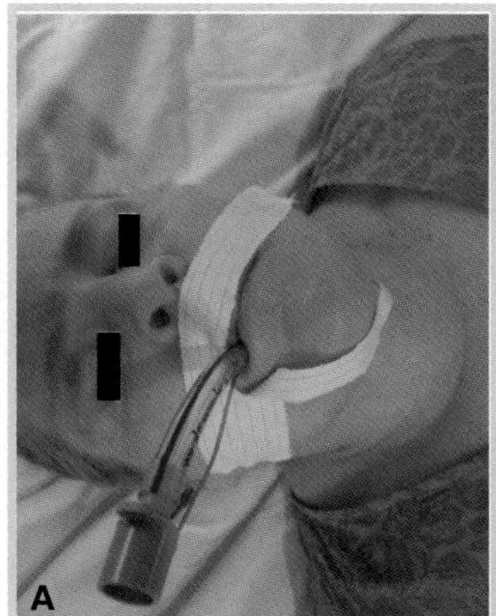

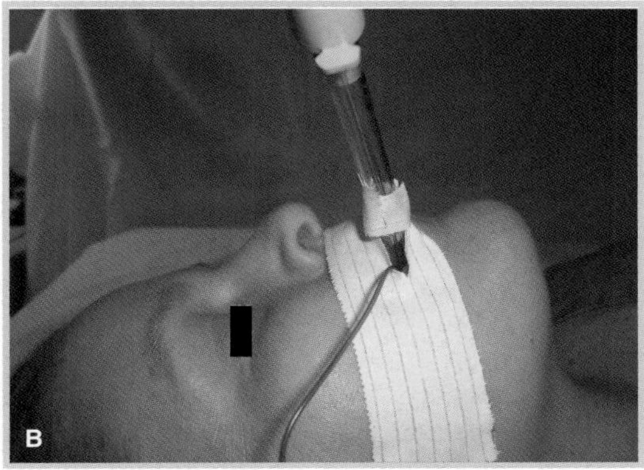

Step 12

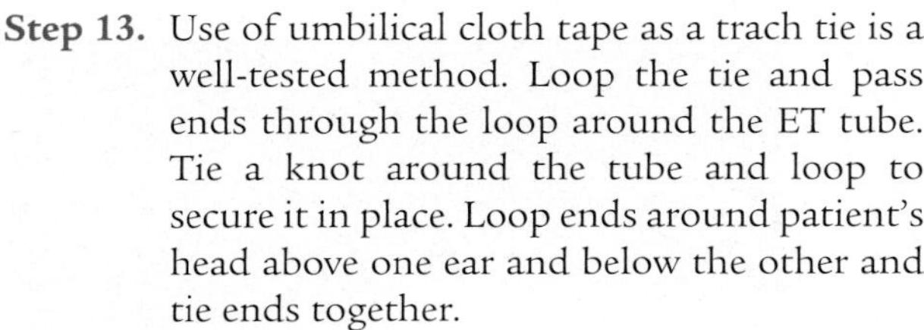

Step 13. Use of umbilical cloth tape as a trach tie is a well-tested method. Loop the tie and pass ends through the loop around the ET tube. Tie a knot around the tube and loop to secure it in place. Loop ends around patient's head above one ear and below the other and tie ends together.

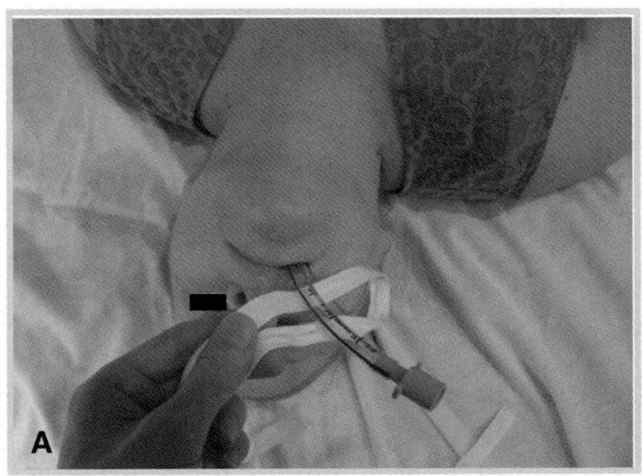

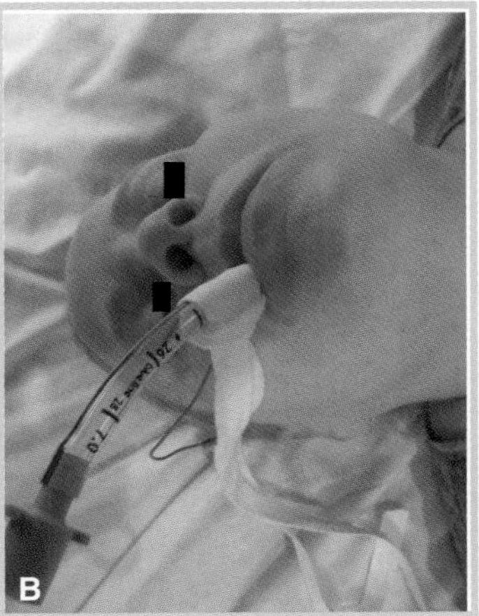

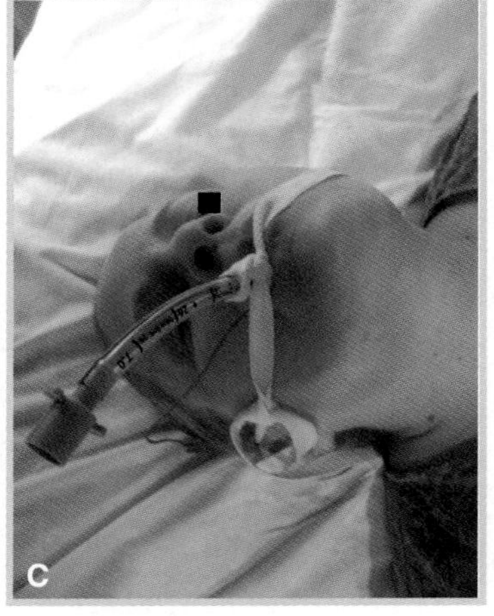

Step 13

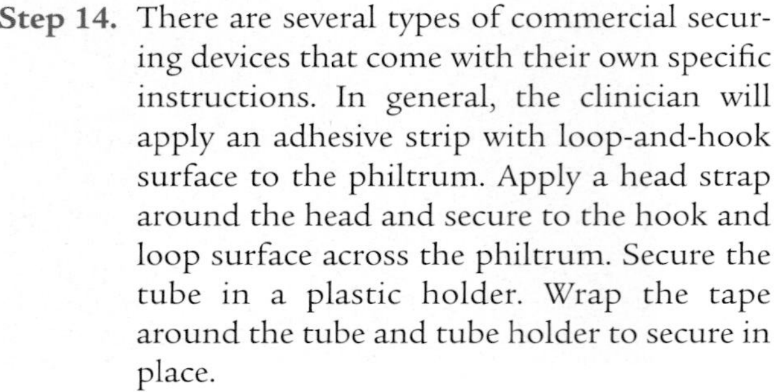

Step 14. There are several types of commercial securing devices that come with their own specific instructions. In general, the clinician will apply an adhesive strip with loop-and-hook surface to the philtrum. Apply a head strap around the head and secure to the hook and loop surface across the philtrum. Secure the tube in a plastic holder. Wrap the tape around the tube and tube holder to secure in place.

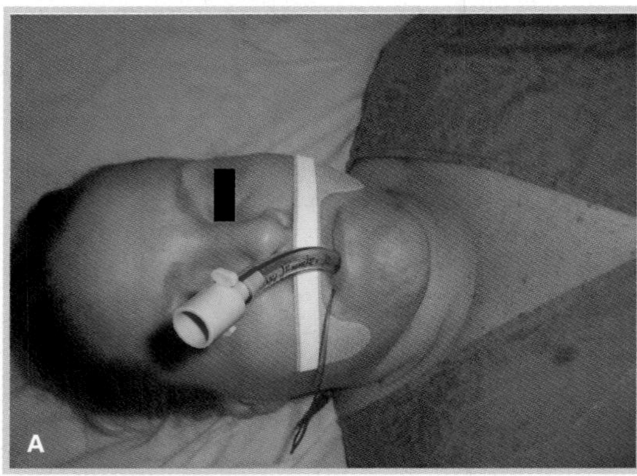

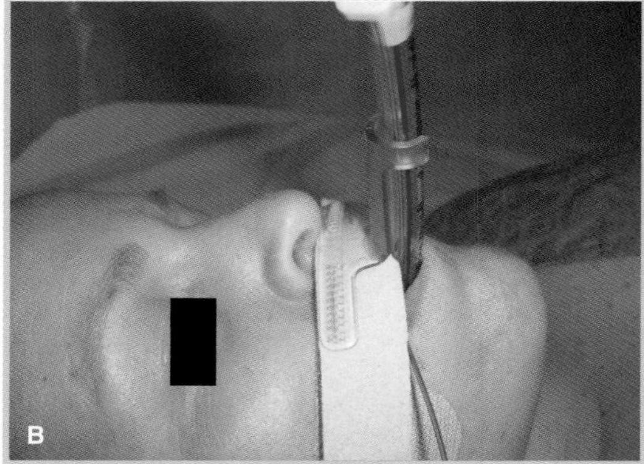

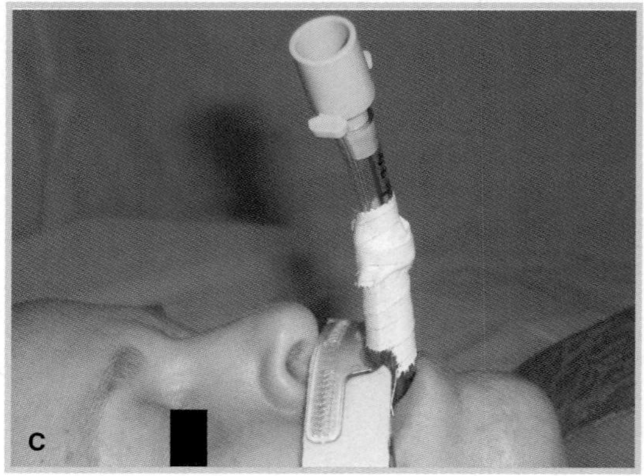

Step 14

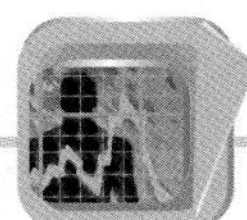

Complications

- Right mainstem bronchus intubation:
  - ET tube is advanced too deeply, and the tip enters the right main stem bronchus.
  - This can cause atelectasis of left lung because of lack of air entering the left lung.
  - Operator should confirm position of the tube through auscultation of equal breath sounds in the axillae and on the chest radiograph.
  - If more intense breath sounds are heard over right side of chest, the tube should be withdrawn while auscultating until equal breath sounds are heard.
- Esophageal intubation:
  - Endotracheal tube is inadvertently placed into the esophagus.
  - Intense air movement is heard over the epigastric area while no breath sounds are heard in lung fields.
  - The patient's vital signs will deteriorate.
  - Some physicians remove the misplaced tube and perform another attempt. Other physicians leave the misplaced tube in place and attempt endotracheal intubation using the misplaced tube to mark the esophagus.
- Vocal cord trauma:
  - Attempting to force an oversized ET tube through narrow vocal cords may cause damage to the cords.
  - Selecting a smaller ET tube will allow easier passage of the tube.
- Oral trauma:
  - Damage to the teeth and lips is common. This usually occurs when the operator attempts to improve visualization by pivoting the laryngoscope in the mouth (shown in Step 6). This will cause the handle to push against the teeth and lips. If all broken teeth and fragments cannot be accounted for, a chest radiograph must be obtained to determine their location.
  - To avoid oral trauma, the laryngoscope handle should be lifted in the "up and out" manner.
- Tracheal perforation by the stylet: The stylet should not extend beyond the tip of the ET tube.
- Aspiration: Positive pressure with the BVM may lead to gastric distention. Cricoid pressure and minimizing BVM use will decrease the amount of gas in the stomach.
- Pneumothorax can occur with positive pressure ventilation especially if the patient has poor lung compliance or if the ET tube was placed in the right mainstem bronchus.
- Arrhythmias may be caused by manipulation of the oropharynx by the laryngoscope. Also, prolonged attempts to place the ET tube may lead to hypoxia, bradycardia, or asystole. Premedication with atropine can blunt the bradycardic response to intubation.

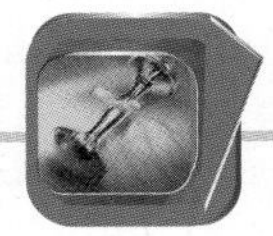

Pediatric Considerations

A child's physiologic response to medical conditions differs from that of an adult. For example, an adult's vital signs may gradually deteriorate with disease progression, allowing the clinician time to respond to an impending cardiovascular or respiratory collapse. In contrast, vital signs in children may remain virtually normal despite progressive deterioration, providing little warning of the need for intervention. Grunting, retractions, nasal flaring, and lethargy are all indicators of poor respiratory status in a pediatric patient.

If the child requires intubation, preoxygenation is critically important. Children cannot tolerate apnea as long as an adult, and shorter attempts to place the tube are warranted. During apnea, a preoxygenated 10-kg child will maintain nearly 100% SaO_2 for approximately 2 to 3 minutes and drop to $<$90% SaO_2 at approximately 4 minutes. The child will then drop from 90% to 0% in $<$45 seconds. A preoxygenated 70-kg adult will maintain oxygen saturation >90% for 8 minutes and then drop from 90% to 0% in 120 seconds.

A child's anatomy is also different from the adult's. The child's head and occiput are proportionally larger and may keep the head in a flexed position. Placing a towel or roll under the shoulders will help extend the neck. Further, the child's tongue is proportionally larger and takes up more of the mouth than in an adult. The tongue must be controlled with the laryngoscope blade to obtain adequate visualization. Finally, the larynx in a child is more proximal than in an adult. This may lead to the placement of the laryngoscope blade too deeply and into the esophagus. Visualization of the entrance of the blade into the posterior oropharynx and advancement into larynx will help identify anatomical structures. A Miller blade is often preferred for infants and children.

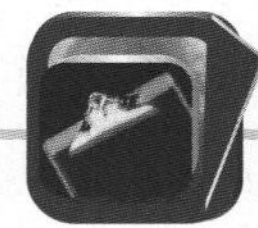

Postprocedure Instructions

After the ET tube is placed and confirmed to be in the correct position, the physician must secure the device using tape and mastic, 0.5-inch cloth umbilical tape, or a commercial device. Ventilator settings must be made. The settings will be based on the patient's weight, medical problem, condition, and desired effect. Settings include but are not limited to ventilator mode, tidal volume, rate, pressure, and oxygen concentration.

- Ventilator modes:
  - Continuous mechanical ventilation (CMV) or assist/control. The ventilator delivers a minimum number of breaths per minute at a set tidal volume (control breath). If the patient takes a breath independently, the ventilator will deliver the preset tidal volume (assist breath). This mode is generally used for patients who are not breathing spontaneously.
  - Synchronized intermittent mandatory ventilation (SIMV). The ventilator delivers a minimum number of ventilations per minute with a set tidal volume as in CMV. However, the patient may breathe spontaneously at rate greater than the ventilator setting and at their own tidal volume. This mode is used when patients are being weaned from the ventilator to allow them to breathe some on their own without risk of respiratory failure due to fatigue.
  - Continuous positive airway pressure (CPAP). The ventilator assists with inhalation by delivering a predetermined pressure in the circuit. This pressure decreases the work of breathing by allowing the patient to overcome airway resistance with less effort. The tidal volume and respiratory rate are determined by the patient's effort. This mode may be used when determining if the patient can be extubated or in various restrictive and obstructive lung diseases.
  - Pressure regulated volume control (PRVC). A form of CMV in which a target volume is set on the ventilator and the ventilator will vary the inspiratory flow of each breath to achieve the set volume at the lowest possible peak pressure. The ventilator adjusts pressure from breath to breath, as the patient's airway resistance and compliance change, in order to deliver a set tidal volume. It also measures the tidal volume of each breath and compares it to the set tidal volume. If the measured volume is less than the set volume, the ventilator will increase the inspiratory pressure to deliver the set tidal volume. If the measured tidal volume is more than the set volume, the ventilator will decrease the pressure. This setting may increase inspiratory time to deliver the set volume without raising pressure above its set upper limit. The PRVC setting is not recommended in asthma or COPD because a longer inspiratory time may cause air trapping and auto-PEEP (positive end-expiratory pressure).
- Tidal volume (VT):
  - VT is the volume of air inspired and expired during each breath.
  - In the past, many experts recommended 10 mL/kg as a good starting point. However, more recent data suggest a lower tidal volume of 6 to 8 mL/kg reduces the risk of barotrauma and ventilator-induced lung injury.

- Respiratory rate:
  - The rate should be adjusted to approach a minute ventilation of 100 mL/kg. This minute ventilation is required to remove carbon dioxide produced by metabolism.
  - The rate should be adjusted with the following considerations:
    - The febrile patient produces 25% more carbon dioxide and requires 25% more breaths.
    - A hypercapneic patient may transiently require an increased respiratory rate to remove excess CO_2. However, providing adequate ventilations through intubation and mechanical ventilation to a previously hypoventilating patient may be sufficient enough to correct hypercapnea without the need for hyperventilation.
  - The rate should be adjusted based on blood gas analysis or end tidal CO_2 monitoring.
- Pressure (PEEP):
  - Pressure is applied to the airway to increase alveolar pressure and keep the small airways open.
  - It may be increased and can improve oxygenation by preventing alveolar collapse.
  - Excess pressure may elicit barotraumas.
  - Most start at 5 to 10 cm H_2O.
- Fraction of inspired oxygen (FiO_2):
  - Concentration of oxygen delivered to the lungs
  - Usually begins with 100% and is titrated down based on arterial blood concentration of oxygen or pulse oximetry

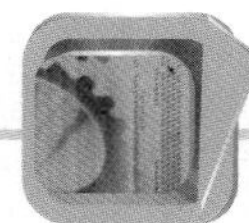

Coding Information and Supply Sources

CPT Code	Description	2008 Average 50th Percentile Fee	Global Period
31500	Intubation, endotracheal, emergency procedure	$415.00	00

CPT is a registered trademark of the American Medical Association.
2008 average 50th Percentile Fees are provided courtesy of 2008 MMH-SI's copyrighted Physicians' Fees and Coding Guide.

The ICD-9 code is used for this procedure is the indication for intubation (symptom/diagnosis).

Supplies for this procedure can be purchased from almost any medical supply house.

Patient Education Handout

A patient education handout, "Endotracheal Intubation," can be found on the book's companion Web site.

Bibliography

Bailey H, Kaplan LJ. Mechanical ventilation. In: Roberts JR, Hedges JR, eds. *Clinical Procedures in Emergency Medicine*. Philadelphia: Saunders; 2004:146–170.

Clinton JE, McGill JW. Basic airway management and decision-making. In: Roberts JR, Hedges JR, eds. *Clinical Procedures in Emergency Medicine*. Philadelphia: Saunders; 2004:53–68.

Clinton JE, McGill JW. Tracheal intubation. In: Roberts JR, Hedges JR, eds. *Clinical Procedures in Emergency Medicine*. Philadelphia: Saunders; 2004:69–99.

Danzl DF, Vissers RJ. Tracheal intubation and mechanical ventilation. In: Tintinalli JE, Kelen GD, Stapczynski JS, eds. *Emergency Medicine: A Comprehensive Study Guide*. New York: McGraw-Hill; 2004:108–119.

Dronen SC, Hopson LR. Pharmacological adjuncts to intubation. In: Roberts JR, Hedges JR, eds. *Clinical Procedures in Emergency Medicine*. Philadelphia: Saunders; 2004:100–114.

Murphy MF, Murphy GW. Mechanical ventilation. In: Walls RM, Murphy MF, eds. *Manual of Emergency Airway Management*. Philadelphia: Lippincott Williams & Wilkins; 2004:320–326.

Schneider RE, Caro DA. Neuromuscular blocking agents. In: Walls RM, Murphy MF, eds. *Manual of Emergency Airway Management*. Philadelphia: Lippincott Williams & Wilkins; 2004:200–211.

Schneider RE, Caro DA. Pretreatment agents. In: Walls RM, Murphy MF, eds. *Manual of Emergency Airway Management*. Philadelphia: Lippincott Williams & Wilkins; 2004:183–188.

Schneider RE, Caro DA. Sedative and induction agents. In: Walls RM, Murphy MF, eds. *Manual of Emergency Airway Management*. Philadelphia: Lippincott Williams & Wilkins; 2004:189–199.

Schneider RE, Murphy MF. Bag/mask ventilation and endotracheal intubation. In: Walls RM, Murphy MF, eds. *Manual of Emergency Airway Management*. Philadelphia: Lippincott Williams & Wilkins; 2004:43–69.

Walls RM. Rapid sequence intubation. In: Walls RM, Murphy MF, eds. *Manual of Emergency Airway Management*. Philadelphia: Lippincott Williams & Wilkins; 2004:22–32.

2008 MAG Mutual Healthcare Solutions, Inc.'s Physicians' Fee and Coding Guide. Duluth, Georgia. MAG Mutual Healthcare Solutions, Inc. 2007.

CHAPTER 18

Mandibular Dislocation Reduction

Christopher J. Wolcott, MD

Assistant Clinical Professor of Emergency Medicine, Department of Emergency Medicine
Louisiana State University Health Sciences Center, Shreveport, LA

The mandible can dislocate anteriorly, posteriorly, laterally, or superiorly. However, mandibular dislocation usually occurs when the mandibular condyle slides anterior to the articular eminence of the temporal bone and becomes trapped secondary to masseter, temporalis, and lateral pterygoid muscle spasm. Dislocation typically occurs when the mouth is opened maximally as during yawning, yelling, or laughing. Further, a direct downward blow to a partially opened mouth can also cause mandibular dislocation.

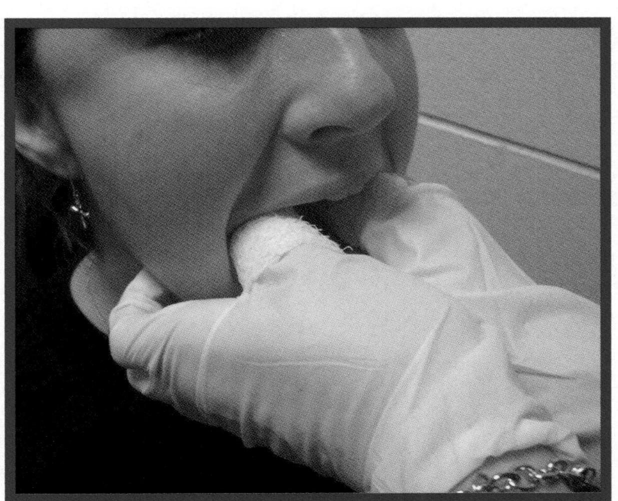

Several factors predispose the patient to mandibular dislocation. For example, laxity of the temporomandibular ligaments in Marfan or Ehlers-Danlos syndromes, prior trauma to the temporomandibular joint, and malformations of the mandibular condyle, fossa, or temporal bone eminence that lead to a shallow joint all predispose a patient to mandibular dislocation.

Patients with mandibular dislocation complain of malocclusion of the teeth and inability to enunciate following an activity that caused maximum opening of the mouth. Inability to fully open or close the mouth and pain due to spasm of muscles of mastication are typically present. Physical findings are dependent on the type of mandibular dislocation. In bilateral mandibular dislocation, the jaw is symmetrically locked open, whereas in unilateral dislocation, the affected side of the mandible is lower than the unaffected side. Finally, the dislocated mandibular condyle may be palpated anterior to the temporal eminence, leaving a depression where the temporomandibular joint is usually felt.

The diagnosis of mandibular dislocation is usually clinical. However, if the diagnosis is in question or in the case of trauma, a panoramic x-ray or computerized tomography (CT) scan of the mandible may be required. Mandibular dislocation is associated with edema and spasm of the masseter muscle. Therefore, reduction of the mandible requires adequate analgesia and muscle relaxation. Intravenous narcotics and benzodiazepines are generally effective for reduction, but conscious sedation may be required.

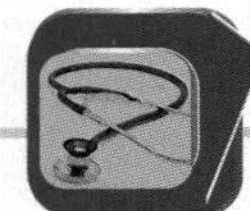

Equipment

- Gauze
- Two tongue depressors
- Intravenous access, oxygen, and monitor if performing conscious sedation (see Chapter 4)

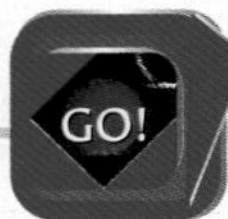

Indications

- Dislocated mandible

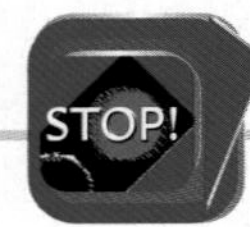

Contraindications

- Fractured mandible
- Open dislocation
- Superior dislocations
- Concurrent trauma or other life-threatening conditions that would preclude an attempt at reduction
- Comorbidities that increase risk with conscious sedation

The Procedure

Step 1. The provider uses gauze to wrap a tongue depressor, which has been cut to size, onto the volar surface of each thumb. The tongue depressor protects the thumbs from being inadvertently bitten. Administer adequate analgesia and provide muscle relaxation.

- **PITFALL:** The provider may not be able to overcome the muscle spasm if the provider fails to administer adequate narcotics and/or benzodiazepines. Moreover, a semi-sedated patient may unknowingly bite down on the provider when reduction attempt is made.

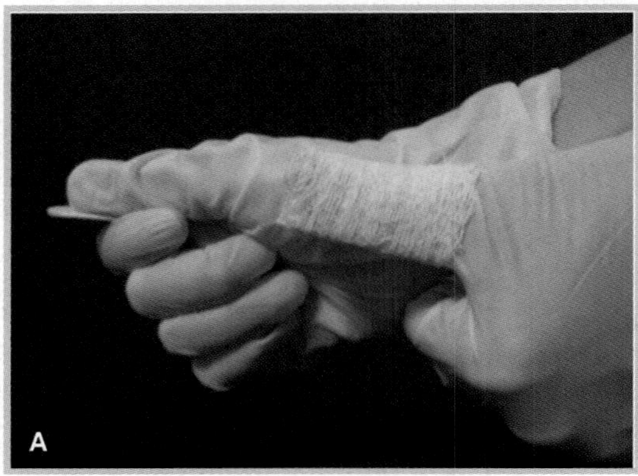
A

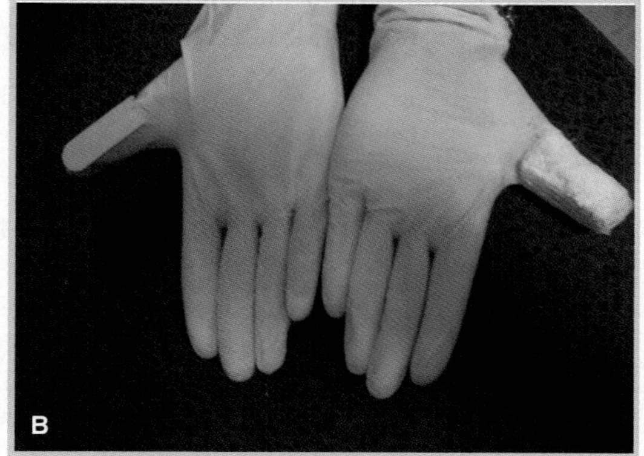

Step 1

Step 2. The provider faces the seated or semirecumbent patient, placing both thumbs on the occlusal surfaces of the lower rear molars. The fingers wrap around the angle and body of the mandible and are placed underneath the medial surface of the jaw. This position allows the provider to firmly grasp the mandible.

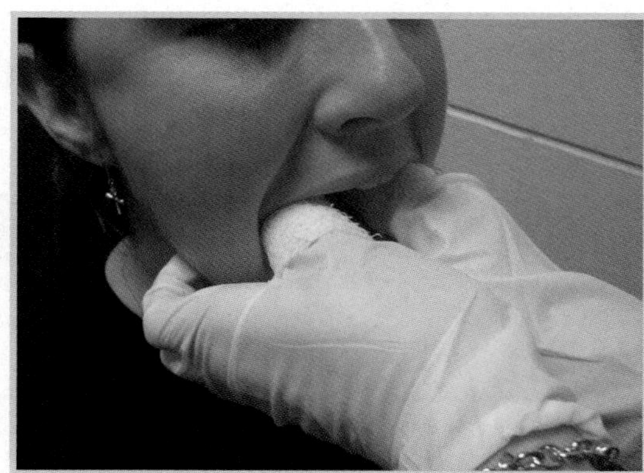

Step 2

Step 3. Apply steady, gentle, downward pressure on the mandible to allow the condyles to clear the articular eminence. Once the anteriorly displaced condyles are inferior to the articular eminence, a posteriorly directed force is applied to slide the condyles back into the mandibular fossa. The patient should be able to immediately close their mouth following successful relocation. Repeat radiographs are generally not necessary.

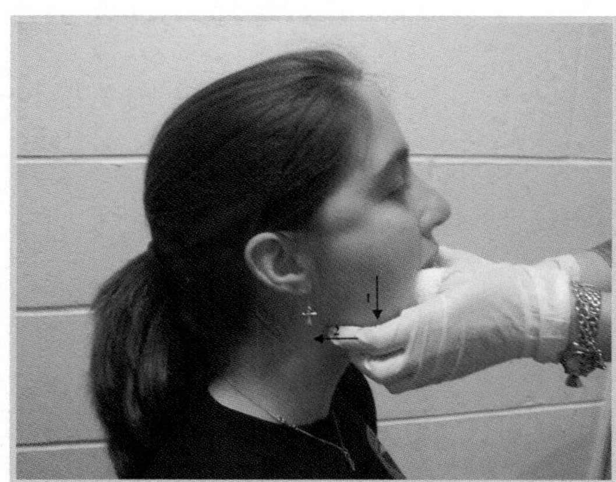

Step 3

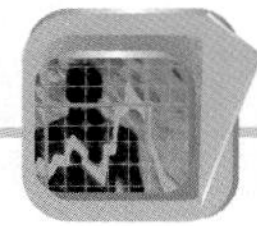

Complications

- Failure to successfully reduce
- Attempt to reduce a fractured mandible

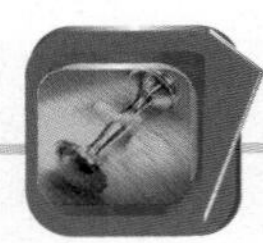

Pediatric Considerations

Although rare in children, the procedure is unchanged.

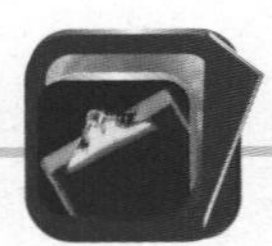

Postprocedure Instructions

Once the mandible is successfully relocated, the patient is placed on a soft mechanical diet for 1 week. The patient should be instructed to avoid activities in which the mouth is opened fully and should be instructed to yawn with a closed mouth. Prescriptions for muscle relaxers, nonsteroidal anti-inflammatory drugs (NSAIDs), and possible narcotic pain medicine should be given to the patient. Finally, the provider should refer the patient to an oral surgeon as an outpatient because they are now at risk for recurrent mandibular dislocation.

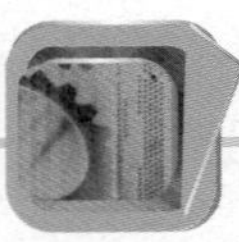

Coding Information and Supply Sources

CPT Code	Description	2008 Average 50th Percentile Fee	Global Period
21480	Reduction of initial mandible dislocation	$349.00	00

CPT is a registered trademark of the American Medical Association.
2008 average 50th Percentile Fees are provided courtesy of 2008 MMH-SI's copyrighted Physicians' Fees and Coding Guide.

Patient Education Handout

A patient education handout, "Mandible (Jaw) Dislocation," can be found on the book's Web site.

Bibliography

Denko K. Emergency dental procedures. In: Roberts JR, Hedges JR, eds. *Clinical Procedures in Emergency Medicine*. Philadelphia: Saunders; 2004:1338–1339.

Haddon R, Peacock WF. Face and jaw emergencies. In: Tintinalli JE, Kelen GD, Stapczynski JS, eds. *Emergency Medicine: A Comprehensive Study Guide*. New York: McGraw-Hill; 2004:1475–1476.

Nelson LS, Needleman HL, Padwa BL. Dental trauma. In: Fleisher GR, Ludwig S, Henretig FM, eds. *Textbook of Pediatric Emergency Medicine*. Philadelphia: Lippincott Williams & Wilkins; 2006:1513–1514.

Upadhye S. Temporomandibular joint dislocation and reduction. In: Reichman EF, Simon RR, eds. *Emergency Medicine Procedures*. New York: McGraw-Hill; 2004:1403–1407.

2008 MAG Mutual Healthcare Solutions, Inc.'s Physicians' Fee and Coding Guide. Duluth, Georgia. MAG Mutual Healthcare Solutions, Inc. 2007.

CHAPTER 19

Office Spirometry

David L. Nelson, MD, LAc
Associate Professor of Clinical Family Medicine
Louisiana State University Health Sciences Center, Shreveport, LA

Dennis R. Wissing, PhD, RRT, CPFT, AE-C
Professor of Cardiopulmonary Science,
Assistant Dean for Academic Affairs, School of Allied Health Professions
Louisiana State University Health Sciences Center, Shreveport, LA

Respiratory disorders such as chronic obstructive pulmonary disease (COPD), emphysema, chronic bronchitis, and asthma are major concerns for the primary care practitioner. Patients often present with a nonspecific cough and shortness of breath, requiring an assessment to determine cause. One simple tool for the practitioner to use to assess the patient's pulmonary status is spirometry. Office or bedside spirometry is a test to determine how much air an individual can blow out and how fast. Spirometry measurements allow the primary care practitioner to determine if the patient has obstructive or restrictive disease or a combination of both during an office visit.

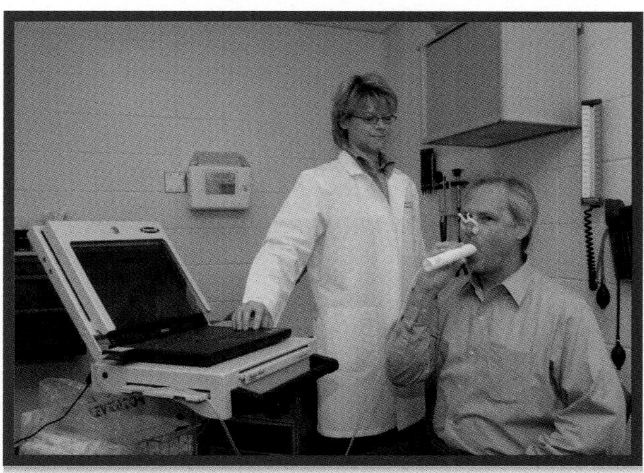

Spirometry measures four numeric values that are useful in assessing the patient:

- Forced vital capacity (FVC) is the total amount of air that can be exhaled following a maximal inspiration. The FVC is reported in liters.
- Forced expired volume in 1 second (FEV 1.0) measures the expired volume during the first second of an FVC maneuver. FEV 1.0 is reported in liters.
- The ratio (FEV 1.0/FVC) is the percentage of the FEV 1.0 compared to the FVC.
- Peak expiratory flow (PEF) is a measurement of how fast a patient can blow out during expiration following a maximal inspiration. The PEF is reported in liters per minute.

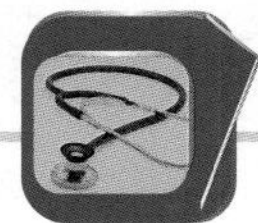

Equipment

- Handheld or desktop portable spirometer
- Disposable pneumotach (mouthpiece)
- Calibration syringe (3 L)
- Printer for hard copy of spirometry results
- Nose clips

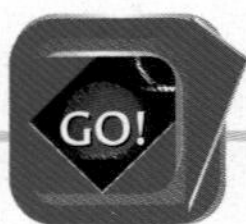

Indications for Spirometry

- Assess severity of COPD.
- Determine existence of lung disease with patients who smoke.
- Diagnose and classify asthma.
- Assess exercise tolerance.
- Diagnose restrictive pulmonary disorders.
- Assess response to bronchodilator.
- Evaluate exposure to inhaled toxins/irritants in the workplace.
- Evaluate for disability benefits.
- Determine preoperative risk for pulmonary complications.
- Monitor disease progression.

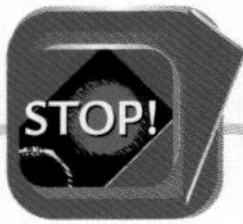

Contraindications

- Inability to cooperate
- Acute respiratory failure
- Moderate to severe persistent asthma

The Procedure

Step 1. The operator should be familiar with the operation of the spirometer. Calibrate the spirometer with a 3-L syringe following the manufacturer's recommendation. Measure and record the patient's height while standing without shoes, and measure and record the patient's weight. Enter the patient's height, weight, age, race, and other data (e.g., smoking history, level of dyspnea) into the spirometer's software program as prompted. Instruct the patient to sit straight in a chair with feet on floor, remove dentures, and loosen any restrictive clothing. Explain why the test is being administered and how the test is to be performed. Demonstrate the procedure using a pneumotach or mouthpiece.

- **PITFALL:** Spirometry should not be performed if the patient has smoked within 4 hours. Smoking can result in acute small airway constriction.

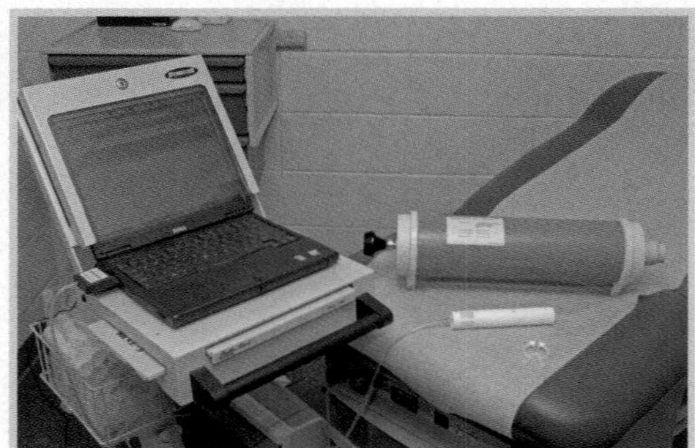

Step 1

Step 2. Apply nose clips. Have the patient place the pneumotach in his or her mouth while maintaining a tight seal with the lips, and assess for leaks. Instruct the patient to breathe normally to acclimate the patient to the procedure and equipment. After several tidal breaths, and at an end-exhalation as noted on the spirometer screen, have the patient take in the deepest breath possible. Immediately following the full deep breath, have the patient blast out air as fast and hard as possible. Continue to have the patient exhale for a minimum of 6 seconds—the volume-time graph should level off.

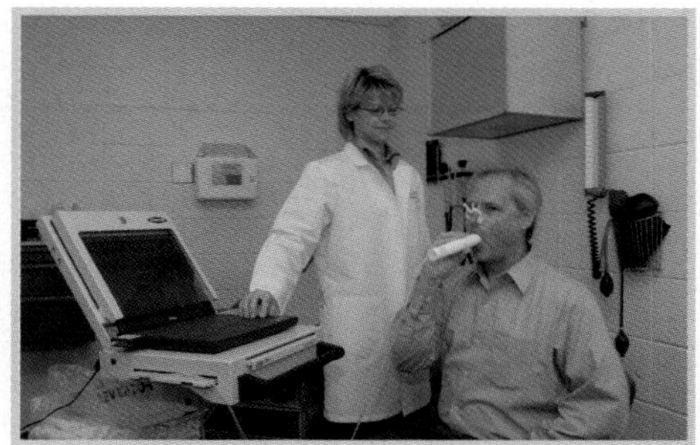

Step 2

Step 3. Encourage longer exhalation if the volume-time graph continues to ascend after 6 seconds. After full expiration, instruct the patient to take in a rapid inspiration to complete the flow-volume loop. Remove the pneumotach and nose clip, and have the patient breathe normally. The procedure is typically repeated two additional times for a total of three acceptable maneuvers.

- **PITFALL:** The accuracy of spirometry depends upon the coaching and correct instructions provided by the practitioner.
- **PITFALL:** The procedure is repeated if the patient performs any of the three maneuvers poorly, so that three tracings with minimal variance in measurements are obtained. Eight attempts is the limit for any given spirometry session.

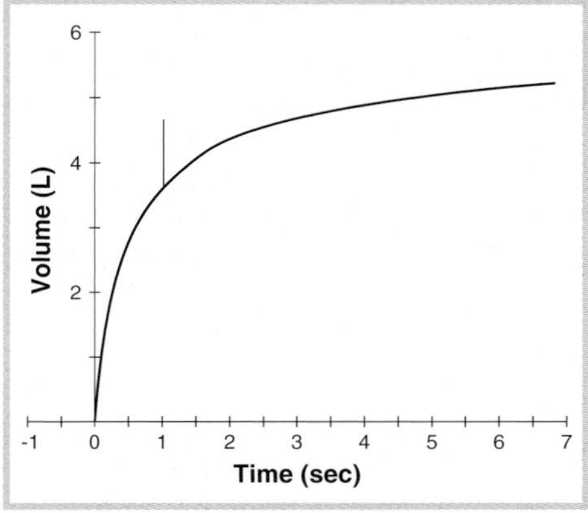

Step 3

Step 4. Review the results and discuss the findings with the patient. If the patient performs <70% of predicted FEV 1.0, the clinician should consider having the patient perform a post-bronchodilator spirogram. Obtain a metered dose inhaler with a beta agonist (e.g., albuterol), and shake the canister to mix the drug and propellant. Attach a holding chamber or spacer to the metered-dose inhaler (MDI), and instruct the patient on proper use of the MDI. Administer four puffs of the beta agonist, wait 15 minutes, and then have the patient perform three spirogram measurements. The patient successfully responds to the inhaled bronchodilator if the FEV 1.0 increases by 12% or more (Table 19-1).

- **PEARL:** It is important that the practitioner records the patient's height, age, gender, and race accurately. These factors affect lung function and are used to determine the patient's predicted spirometry values.

TABLE 19-1. Example of Pre- and Post-bronchodilator Spirometry Measurements from a 56-Year-Old White Female Who is 62 inches Tall and Weighs 133 pounds

Parameter	Predicted	Prebronchodilator	Postbronchodilator
FVC	3.17 L	2.98 L	3.01 L
FEV 1.0	2.47 L	1.25 L	1.88 L[a]
PEF	371 L/min	173 L/min	259 L/min

[a]Represents an increase >12%, showing patient responded to the bronchodilator.

TABLE 19-2. Reasons for Inaccurate Spirometry Measurements

The patient performs a submaximal inspiratory or expiratory effort.
The patient has a leak around the pneumotach.
The patient pauses to forcibly exhale following a maximal inspiration.
The patient coughs during the maneuver.
The patient has poor posture.
The patient inserts their tongue into the pneumotach.
The patient inadvertently closes their glottis.
The patient has an incomplete inspiration or expiration.

The spirometer's software programs will compare the predicted measurements to the patient's actual measured values. From this comparison, a diagnosis can be made.

- **PITFALL:** Even when patient's predicted spirometry values are computed, the normal range of actual spirometer measurements for healthy individuals can vary from 80 to 120%.

Step 5. Determine reliability of spirometry tracings and the repeatability of results. The variance between the largest and second largest force vital capacity should be <150 mL. The variance between the largest and second largest forced expiratory volume in 1 second (FEV 1.0) should be <150 mL. The practitioner should choose the better of the two most similar measurements or allow the spirometer's software program to choose. Table 19-2 shows common reasons for inaccurate spirometry measurements.

- **PEARL:** The patient should have exhaled at least 6 seconds, and longer if the volume-time graph continues to ascend after 6 seconds.

Step 6. Interpretation of the spirometry results. The following figures can assist with the interpretation of spirometry results.

Step 7. Healthy individuals are able to perform a maximal inspiration followed with a maximal expiration. The FVC will be approximately 80% of their predicted values, and their FEV 1.0/FVC ratio will be at least 70%. Obstructive disease is typically diagnosed when these values drop to <80% and 70% of predicted results, respectively. With obstructive disease, there is a decrease in maximal flow rates, and the expiratory curve is scooped out or concave to the x-axis. With restrictive disease, flow rates may be increased while volumes are diminished. Table 19-3 summarizes the changes occurring with spirometry with obstructive and restrictive diseases or when the patient has a combination of both diseases.

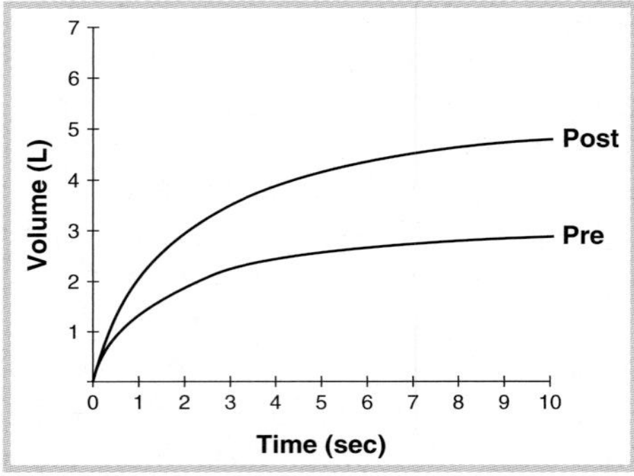

Normal volume-time graph

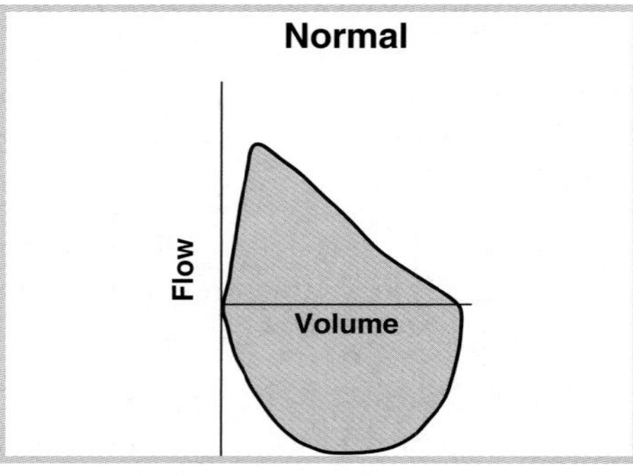

Normal flow-volume loop

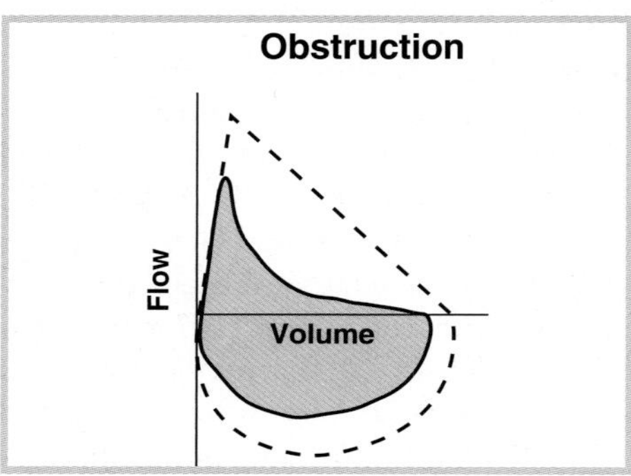

Flow-volume loop pattern with airway obstruction

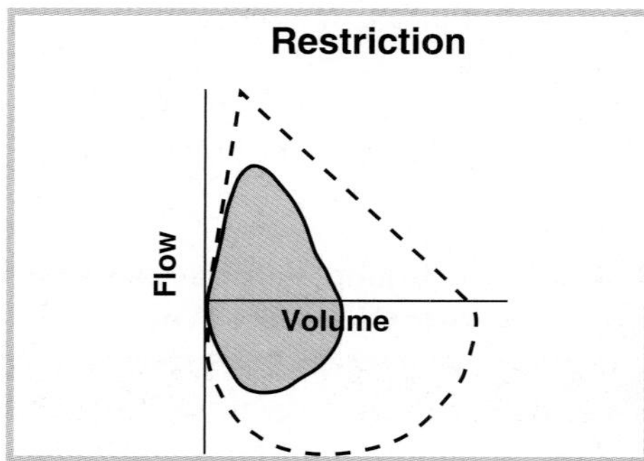

Flow-volume loop pattern with restrictive lung disease

TABLE 19-3. Classification of Pulmonary Abnormalities Based on Spirometry

Parameter	Obstructive	Restrictive	Mixed
FVC	↓ or normal	↓	↓
FEV 1.0	↓	↓ or normal	↓
FEV 1.0/FVC	↓	↑ or normal	↓

■ **PEARL:** There is a good correlation between PEF and FEV 1.0 in asthma, which allows the practitioner to use PEFs to assess the patient with asthma. This correlation decreases with patients with COPD. Airway collapsibility as seen with COPD results in a varying relationship between PEF and FEV 1.0. PEF testing in COPD can be misleading. In addition, PEF does not detect small airway disease, which is common in COPD.

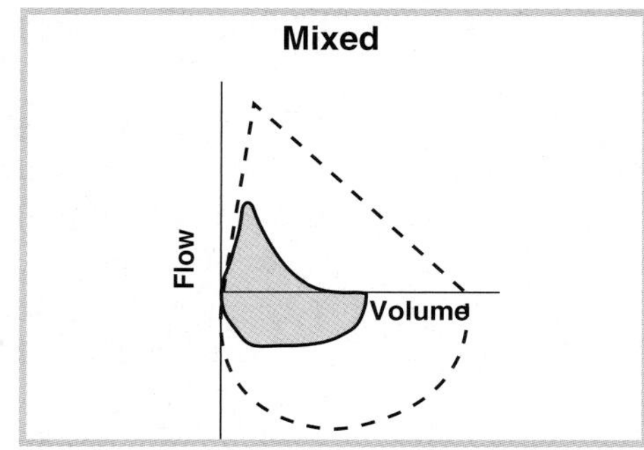

Flow-volume loop pattern with mixed disease pattern

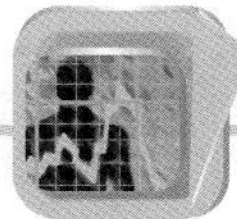

Complications

- Small airway collapse from dynamic airway compression during forced vital capacity can occur in patients with COPD, asthma, emphysema, or chronic bronchitis. This may result in wheezing noted on auscultation.
- Hyperventilation can occur if the patient is not instructed correctly.
- Cross contamination results if the Pneumotach is used by multiple patients.

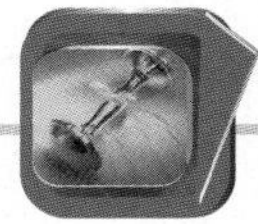

Pediatric Considerations

Children present a challenge to technicians performing spirometry. Careful instruction on correct posture and breathing are essential to performing reproducible test results. Encourage the child to relax as much as possible to prevent undue anxiety.

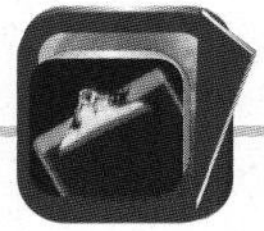

Postprocedure Instructions

- The patient may resume regular activities immediately.
- Although some musculoskeletal pain is common, it should resolve with conservative treatment.
- The patient should follow up with the referring provider.

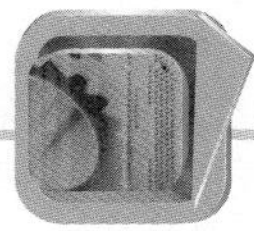

Coding Information and Supply Sources

CPT Code	Description	2008 Average 50th Percentile Fee	Global Period
94010	Spirometry, FVC, and FEV 1.0	$91.00	XXX
94060	Spirometry before and after bronchodilator therapy	$160.00	XXX
94375	Flow-volume loops	$92.00	XXX

XXX, global concept does not apply.

CPT is a registered trademark of the American Medical Association.

2008 average 50th Percentile Fees are provided courtesy of 2008 MMH-SI's copyrighted Physicians' Fees and Coding Guide.

Equipment and supplies can be purchased through several vendors. Pricing varies widely. A brief Internet search for spirometry will yield a host of vendors. Here is a partial list.

- RJ Brindley and Associates, Inc., 337 Bluff RD, Carver, MN 55315-9511. Phone:1-888-448-2834. Web site: http://www.PulmonaryFunction.com.
- Mohawk Medical Mall. Phone: 1-800-962-5660. Web site: http://www.mohawkmedicalmall.com.
- MedFirst Healthcare Supply Inc., 902 JanMar Court, Clermont, FL 34715. Phone: 352-242-0110; fax 352-242-0973. Web site: http://www.medfirstonline.com.
- Medical Solutions Inc., 8633 Jefferson Highway, Osseo, MN 55369. Phone: 888-557-8020. Web site: http://www.medicalsolutionsinc.com.

Patient Education Handout

Patient education handouts, "Spirograms Preprocedure" and "Spirograms Postprocedure," can be found on the book's companion Web site.

Bibliography

Ferguson GT, Enright PL, Buist AS, et al. Office spirometry for lung health assessment in adults: a consensus statement from the National Lung Health Education Program. *Chest.* 2000;117:1146–1161.

Miller MR, Crapo R, Hankinson J, et al. General considerations for lung function testing. *Eur Respir J.* 2005;26:153–161.

Miller MR, Hankinson J, Brusasco V, et al. Standardisation of spirometry. *Eur Resp J.* 2005;26:319–338.

Pauwels RA, Buist AS, Ma P, et al. Global strategy for the diagnosis, management, and prevention of chronic obstructive pulmonary disease: National Heart, Lung, and Blood Institute and World Health Organization global initiative for chronic obstructive lung disease (GOLD) executive summary. *Respir Care.* 2001;46:798–825. http://www.goldcopd.com/. Accessed November 7, 2001.

Pellegrino R, Viegi G, Brusasco V, et al. Interpretive strategies for lung function tests. *Eur Respir J.* 2005;26:948–968.

Wagner J, Clausen JL, Coates A, et al. Standardisation of the measurement of lung volumes. *Eur Respir J.* 2005;26:511–522.

2008 MAG Mutual Healthcare Solutions, Inc.'s Physicians' Fee and Coding Guide. Duluth, Georgia. MAG Mutual Healthcare Solutions, Inc. 2007.

CHAPTER 20

Radial Head Subluxation (Nursemaid's Elbow) Reduction

Simon A. Mahler, MD
Assistant Professor, Department of Emergency Medicine
Louisiana State University Health Sciences Center, Shreveport, LA

Ken Barrick, MD
Senior Resident, Department of Emergency Medicine
Louisiana State University Health Sciences Center, Shreveport, LA

Radial head subluxation is the most common elbow injury in children. It typically occurs in children between the ages of 1 and 4 with a peak incidence between 2 and 3 years of age. However, nursemaid's elbow has been reported in children younger than 6 months old and in those up to 8 years of age. Girls are more likely to be affected than boys, and the left arm is more frequently involved than the right.

Nursemaid's elbow is typically caused by a sudden axial traction on the child's arm. This causes a portion of the annular ligament to slip over the radial head into the radiohumeral joint and become trapped. In most children, the annular ligament strengthens by the age of 5, decreasing the likelihood of the injury in older children.

The classic history suggesting radial head subluxation is that of a "pull injury." Typically the child's arm is pulled while the arm is extended to prevent a fall or the child pulling away. This injury also occurs during playful swinging of a child by the arms. This mechanism accounts for approximately 50% of cases. Other less common mechanisms of injury include falling on the elbow, minor direct trauma, or twisting of the arm. Rarely, there is no history of trauma. Children younger than 6 months of age may present with radial head subluxation as a result of the extremity being trapped under the child's body when rolling over. Nursemaid's elbow may also be the result of child abuse.

Children with nursemaid's elbow present with refusal to move the affected arm. The child typically holds the arm close to the body with the elbow slightly flexed or fully extended and the forearm pronated. The child is usually in no distress until attempts are made to move or examine the arm. With palpation, there may be some tenderness over the anterolateral aspect of the radial head. However, the distal humerus and the ulna are usually not tender. The child will not actively move the involved arm and any attempts to manipulate the extremity will elicit significant discomfort. It is important to examine the entire extremity as well as the clavicle on the affected side to avoid missing other injuries.

Radial head subluxation is a clinical diagnosis. However, this injury should not be confused with a supracondylar fracture, which presents with focal tenderness and swelling. Radiographs are rarely indicated in radial head subluxation but should be obtained if supracondylar fracture is suspected, the mechanism of injury is inconsistent with the classic history for radial head subluxation, or if multiple attempts at reduction are unsuccessful.

There are two methods to reduce a radial head subluxation: the supination/flexion method and the hyperpronation method. Both techniques are effective and can be performed in the office or the emergency department. Although supination/flexion method is traditionally suggested, the hyperpronation technique should also be considered first line. Recent studies suggest that the hyperpronation technique is more likely to be successful on the first attempt and is less painful.

Confirmation of successful reduction occurs when the child voluntarily moves the affected arm. Immediately following reduction, the child may cry and continue to resist arm movement. It may take 5 to 15 minutes before the child moves the affected arm. Following successful reduction, further treatment, immobilization, and activity restriction are not required.

If the patient is not moving the affected arm at 15 minutes, additional attempts may be made to reduce the joint. Hyperpronation is more successful with second attempts than flexion/supination. If multiple attempts are unsuccessful, radiographs of the arm should be obtained. If the radiographs are normal, the child may be placed in a sling and should have a follow-up arranged. Pediatric orthopedic follow-up should be considered, but next-day office follow-up may suffice. Studies suggest that spontaneous movement within 24 hours is common, occurring in 60% of the patients with failed reduction. Unrecognized or unreduced nursemaid's elbows have not been linked to any significant clinical sequelae.

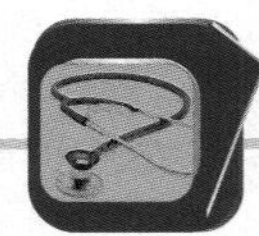

Equipment

- None

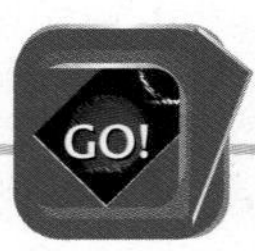

Indications

- Radial head subluxation (nursemaid's elbow)

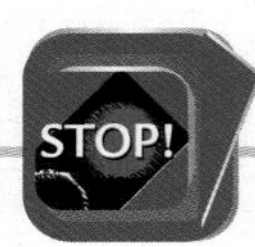

Contraindications

- Suspected fracture

The Procedure

Step 1. For both techniques, approach the child calmly at eye level to reduce anxiety. The child may be more comfortable in the parent or caretaker's lap facing toward the clinician.

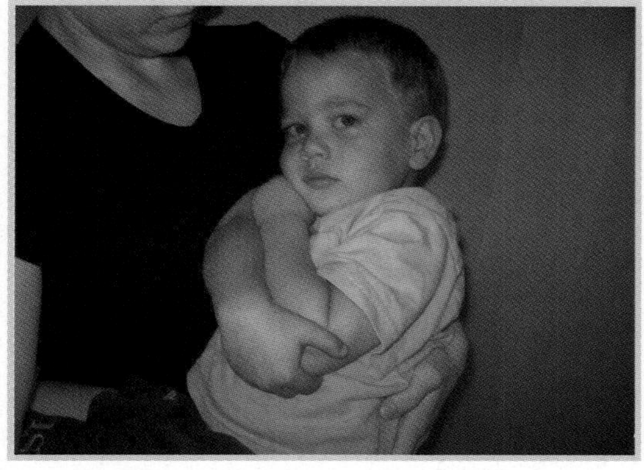

Step 1

Hyperpronation Technique

Step 2. Support the child's affected arm, maintaining the elbow at 90 degrees. Apply moderate pressure to the radial head.

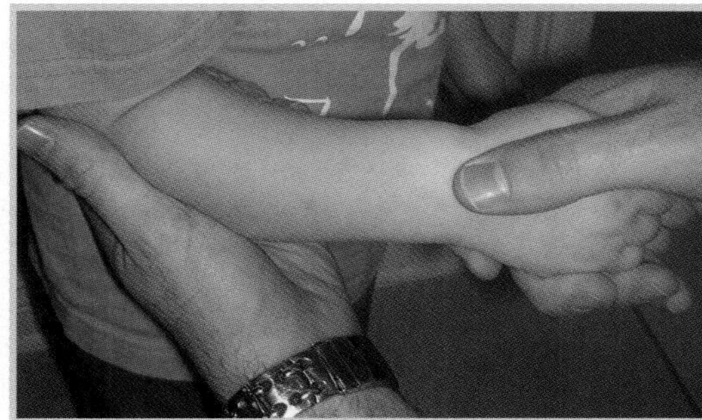

Step 2

Step 3. Grip the forearm with the other hand and pronate the forearm. An audible "click" may be heard, or a "pop" may be felt with successful reduction.

- PITFALL: Crepitus or severe pain suggests an occult fracture and requires discontinuation of the procedure.

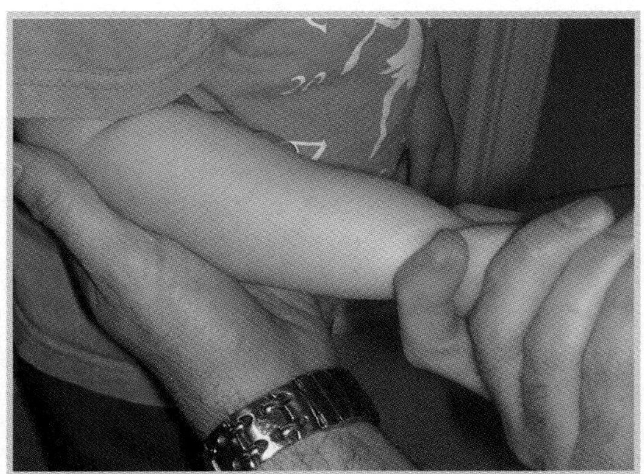

Step 3

Supination/Flexion Technique

Step 2. Support the child's affected arm, keeping the elbow at 90 degrees. Apply moderate pressure to the radial head.

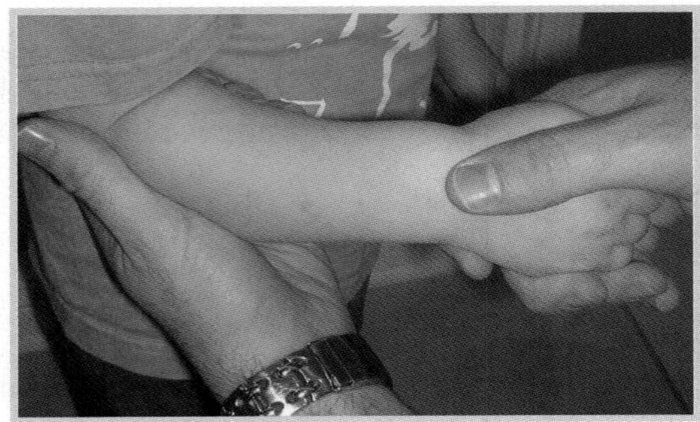

Step 2

Step 3. Grasp the hand or wrist as if shaking hands and apply gentle traction. While maintaining traction, supinate the patient's hand/wrist, then fully flex the affected elbow. An audible "click" may be heard, or a "pop" may be felt with successful reduction.

- PITFALL: Crepitus or severe pain suggests an occult fracture and requires discontinuation of the procedure. The hyperpronation technique should be attempted if the supination/flexion technique fails.

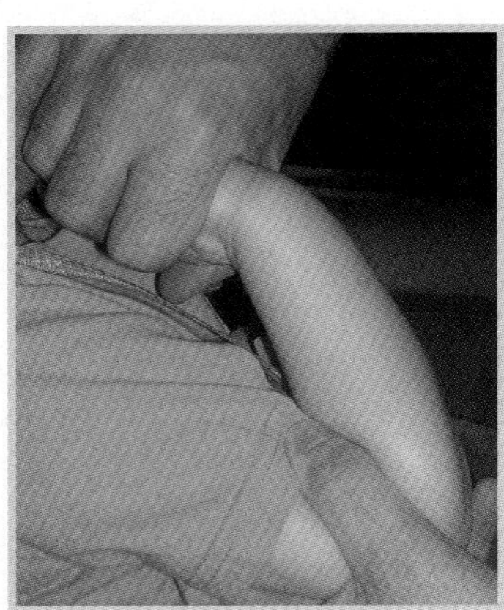

Step 3

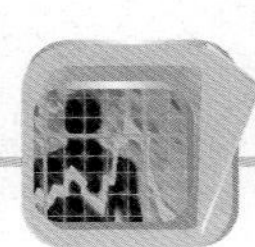

Complications

- Failed reduction

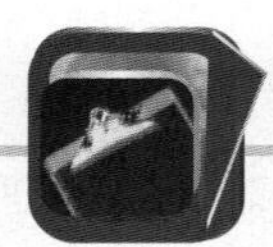

Postprocedure Instructions

It may take 5 to 15 minutes before the child moves the affected arm. Following successful reduction, further treatment, immobilization, and activity restriction are not required. Acetaminophen or ibuprofen can be used for pain as needed. Parents should be informed of reoccurrence risk and avoid pulling their child's arms.

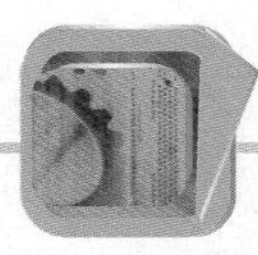

Coding Information and Supply Sources

CPT Code	Description	2008 Average 50th Percentile Fee	Global Period
24640	Treatment of radial head subluxation (nursemaid's elbow), with manipulation	$278.00	10

CPT is a registered trademark of the American Medical Association.
2008 average 50th Percentile Fees are provided courtesy of 2008 MMH-SI's copyrighted Physicians' Fees and Coding Guide.

Patient Education Handout

A patient education handout, “Radial Head Subluxation (Nursemaid’s Elbow),” can be found on the book’s companion Web site.

Bibliography

Green DA, Linares MY, Garcia Pena BM, et al. Randomized comparison of pain perception during radial head subluxation reduction using supination-flexion or forced pronation. *Pediatr Emerg Care.* 2006;22:235–238.

Kaplan RE, Lillis KA. Recurrent nursemaid’s elbow (annular ligament displacement): treatment via telephone. *Pediatrics* 2002;110:171–174.

Macias CG, Bonther J, Wiebe R. A comparison of supination/flexion to hyperpronation in the reduction of radial head subluxations. *Pediatrics.* 1998;102:e10–14.

Quan L, Marcuse EK. The epidemiology and treatment of radial head subluxation. *Am J Dis Child.* 1985;139:1194–1197.

Schunk JE. Radial head subluxation: epidemiology and treatment of 87 episodes. *Ann Emerg Med.* 1990;19:1019–1023.

2008 MAG Mutual Healthcare Solutions, Inc.’s Physicians’ Fee and Coding Guide. Duluth, Georgia. MAG Mutual Healthcare Solutions, Inc. 2007.

CHAPTER 21

Ring Removal

Thomas C. Arnold, MD
Associate Professor and Chairman, Department of Emergency Medicine
Louisiana State University Health Sciences Center, Shreveport, LA

Removal of a tightly lodged ring or ring-like structure from a digit is commonly requested in the clinical or urgent care setting. Reasons for removal range from instant entrapment to gradual constriction after years of wear. Rings should also be removed anytime swelling of the digit is reasonably anticipated such as trauma, envenomation, prolonged illness, skin conditions, surgery, or allergic reaction. As venous outflow is obstructed, the digit becomes increasingly restricted by the ring's tourniquet effects. This digital swelling can leave the digit tightly and painfully trapped at the base of the proximal phalanx. If not promptly treated, complications of nerve damage, ischemia, and digital gangrene are possible. Because many rings have personal significance and value to the patient, when appropriate, several ring-sparing techniques may be attempted to preserve a treasured artifact.

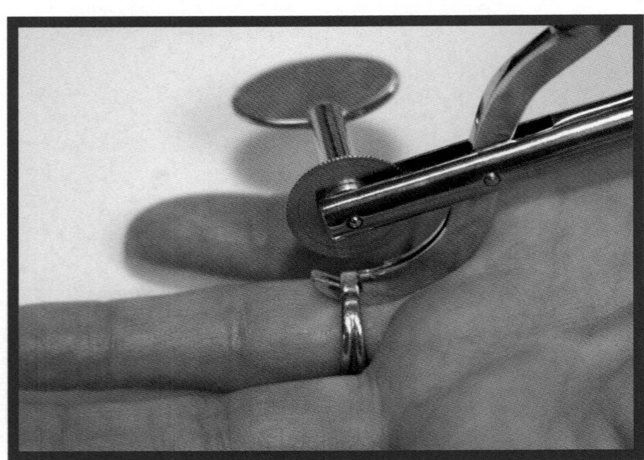

Before attempting ring removal, the digit should be inspected for lacerations, assessed for neurologic compromise by a simple two-point discrimination test, and evaluated for distal digital pulses sought with a Doppler flow meter. If evidence of neurovascular compromise is present (i.e., reduced sensory perception or diminished pulses), ring-sparing techniques should not be attempted and the ring should be promptly removed by cutting. After ring removal, neurovascular integrity of the digit should be re-assessed by tactile sensation and capillary refill. Any deficits suggest that prompt consultation with a hand specialist is warranted.

Initial attempts at ring removal should begin with elevation of the involved extremity to encourage venous and lymphatic drainage. Many times, lubricating the digit with soap, glycerin, or a water-soluble lubricant will allow removal with gentle traction.

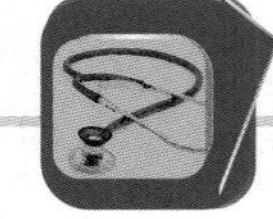

Equipment

- Manual ring cutter
- Pliers
- Curved hemostats
- Umbilical tape (2 to 4 mm wide) or 0-gauge or larger braided suture
- Powder-free, latex surgical glove
- Motorized handheld grinder (such as a Dremel tool)

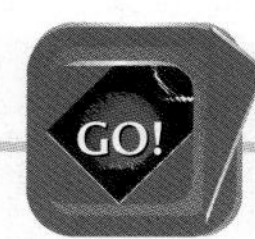

Indications

- Removal of a ring or other constricting object from a swollen digit or one that could potentially become compromised

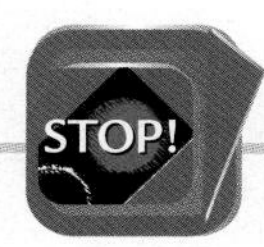

Contraindications

- In the presence of lacerations or neurovascular compromise, the ring-cutting technique should be employed rather than the more time-consuming ring-sparing options.

The Procedure

String Technique

Step 1. After sufficient elevation of the entrapped digit, use the umbilical tape or braided suture to wrap the digit in a spiral fashion from the distal tip toward the ring. Apply the wrap slowly with sufficient tension to allow the interstitial fluid to move gently under the ring, being careful not to apply it tightly enough to obstruct arterial flow.

- PITFALL: Avoid the use of material that is too thin, such as monofilament or thin sutures, because of potential skin damage and decreased effectiveness.

Step 2. Once the wrapping material reaches the ring, the end should be carefully passed beneath the ring. This maneuver may be facilitated by grabbing the umbilical tape end or the suture needle with a small hemostat after passing it under the ring.

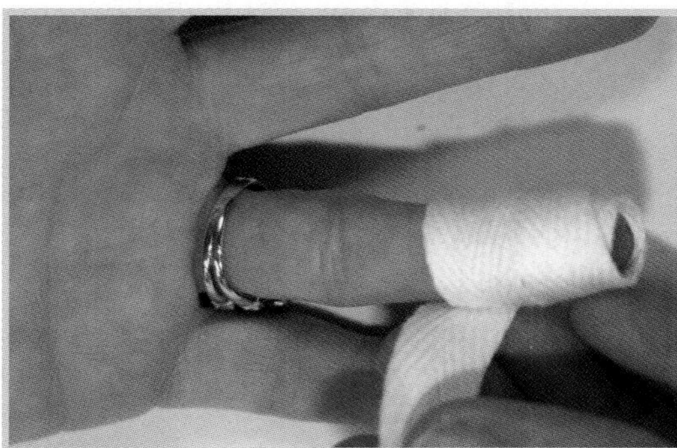

Step 1

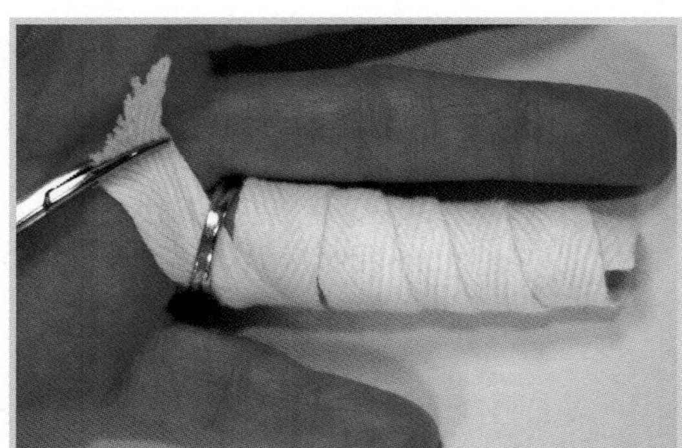

Step 2

Step 3. Generous lubrication of the wrapped digit should be applied after this is accomplished. Then, with gentle traction distalward on the ring, slowly unwind the wrapping material from under the ring, pushing the ring off the digit as it unwraps.

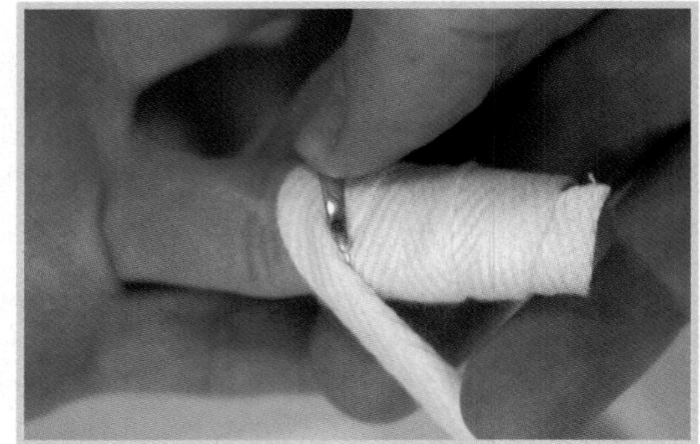

Step 3

Rubber Glove Technique

Step 1. Another method of reducing a markedly swollen digit involves removing a finger from a small, powder-free, latex surgical glove and pulling it onto the swollen digit. (Alternative methods have been described using a penrose drain or rubber/elastic band such as an IV tourniquet in place of the glove finger to reduce the digit edema.) As the edge of the glove finger nears the ring, utilize the small curved hemostats to assist passage of the latex between the ring and the digit.

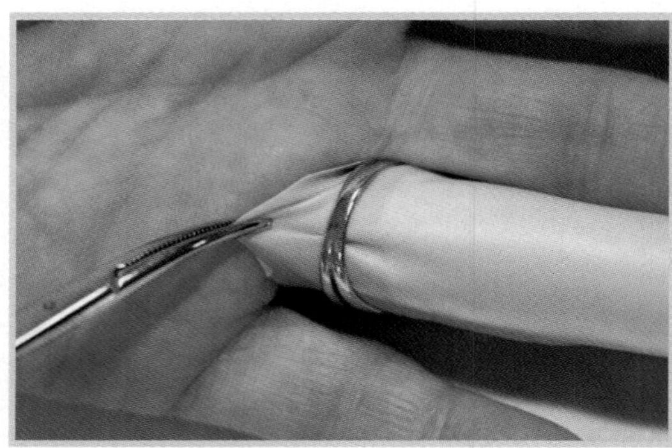

Step 1

- PITFALL: Use latex-free material in anyone with a possible latex allergy because latex could worsen the swelling.

Step 2. Allow the latex to compress the swollen digit uniformly while elevating the digit above the patient's head.

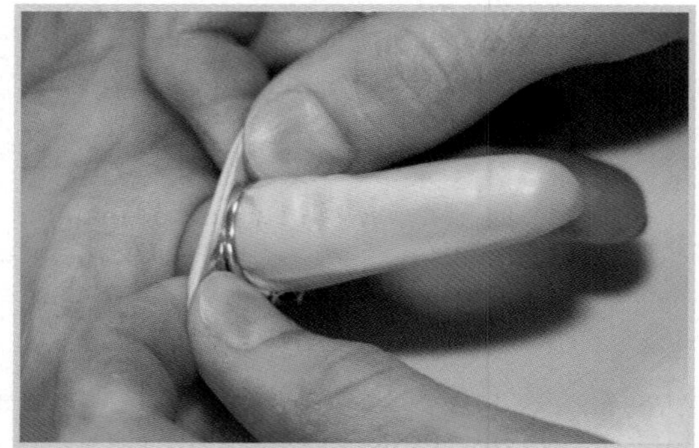

Step 2

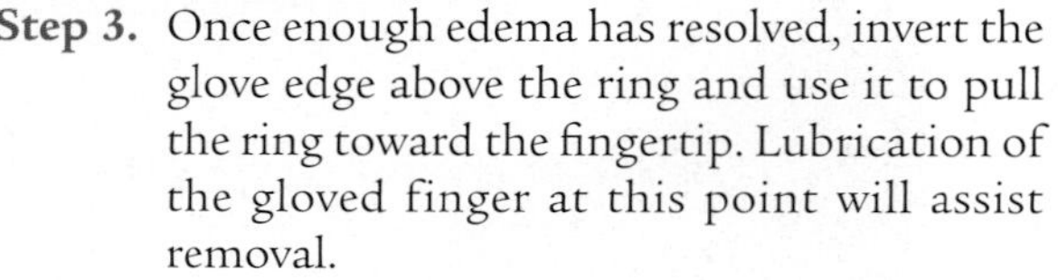

Step 3. Once enough edema has resolved, invert the glove edge above the ring and use it to pull the ring toward the fingertip. Lubrication of the gloved finger at this point will assist removal.

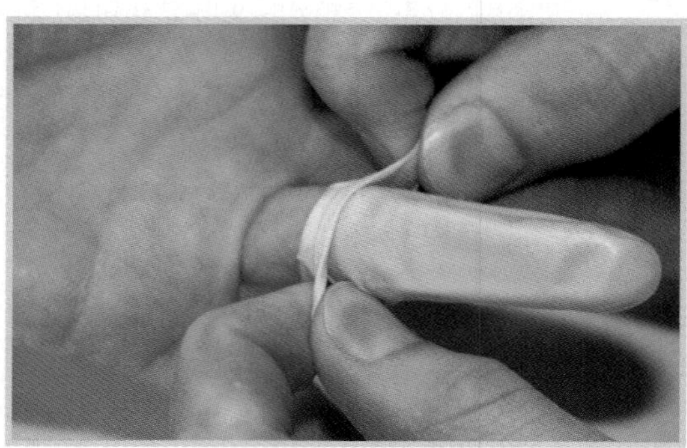

Step 3

Ring Cutting Technique

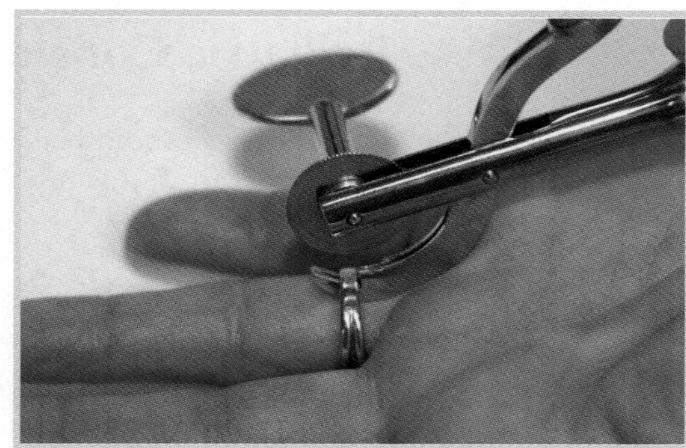

Step 1

Step 1. Select the thinnest or most accessible portion of the ring for the cutting site. The digit guard of the ring cutter should be passed under the ring at the chosen location and serves to protect the digit from injury during the cutting procedure. (If elevation of the cutting site is necessary for placement of the digit guard, the ring may be compressed slightly with pliers. Careful pressure should be applied with the jaws of the pliers placed 90 degrees on either side of the cutting site. This converts the ring shape from circular to elliptical, creating a space between the ring and underlying tissues. This slight lateral compression will displace the neurovascular bundles to the less restricted palmar region and should not compromise their function.)

- PITFALL: Avoid excessive trauma and pressure to the digit. Even with mild pressure, the patient must be warned that some discomfort may be experienced.

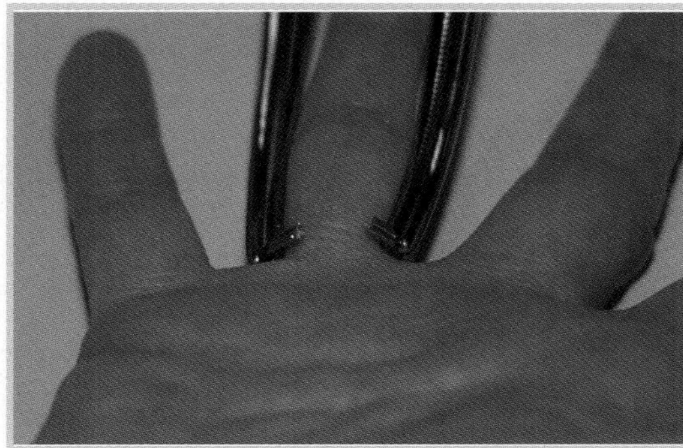

Step 2

Step 2. Once proper positioning of the ring cutter is obtained, rotate the blade lever while maintaining adequate pressure to keep the saw engaged into the metal of the ring. Continue rotation of the saw blade until the ring is completely divided. The two ends of the divided ring are then grasped with pliers or hemostats and pulled apart to open the ring and allow its removal.

- **PEARL:** If the object is too thick or tempered for removal by this method (e.g., steel nuts), consider the use of a motorized, handheld circular cutter/grinder (such as a Dremel tool). A silicone rubber band or other similar material should be placed between the skin and the cutting site to protect the underlying tissue.
- **PEARL:** Two cuts 180 degrees apart are usually necessary for large or hardened objects.

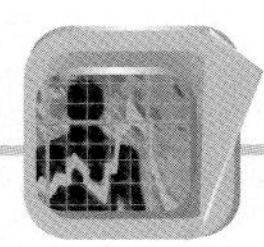

Complications

- Injury to the underlying skin, lymphatics, and neurovascular bundle.
- Fracture of the proximal phalanx or disruption of the finger joint mechanism.
- The benefits, risks, and medical necessity of the ring removal should be considered prior to attempting the procedure.

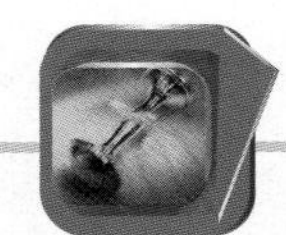

Pediatric Considerations

Consideration should be given to mild sedation and pain control in children experiencing discomfort from this procedure.

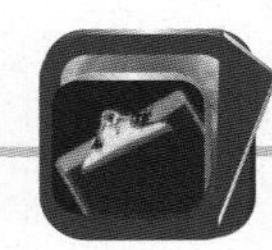

Postprocedure Instructions

A thorough inspection and examination of the finger should be performed after the ring is removed. The chart should document all findings including the presence or absence of two-point discrimination of the digit. Edema of the previously constricted digit should resolve over several hours.

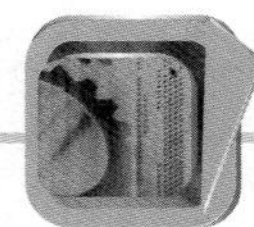

Coding Information and Supply Sources

There is no specific code for ring removal. Use the appropriate evaluation and management (E/M) code for the visit.

Ring cutters may be obtained at Chief Supply Co., 10926 David Taylor Dr., Suite 300, Charlotte, NC 28262. Phone: 888-588-8569. Web site: http://www.chiefsupply.com/home.asp.

Electric and manual versions are available from the Shor International Corporation, 20 Parkway West, Mt. Vernon, NY 10552. Phone: 914-667-1100. Web site: http://shorinternational.com/RingTools.htm.

Patient Education Handout

A patient education handout, "Ring Removal," can be found on the book's companion Web site.

Bibliography

Gallahue FE, Carter WA. Ring tourniquet syndrome. In: Tintinalli JE, Kelen GD, Stapczynski JS, eds. *Emergency Medicine: A Comprehensive Study Guide.* 6th ed. New York: McGraw-Hill; 2004:311–312.

Hiew LY, Juma A. A novel method of ring removal from a swollen finger. *Br J Plastic Surg.* 2000;53:173–174.

Inoue S, Akazawa S, Fukuda H, et al. Another simple method for ring removal. *Am Soc Anesthesiol.* 1995;83(5):1133–1134.

Mizrahi S, Lunski I. A simplified method for ring removal from an edematous finger. *Am J Surg.* 1986;151:412–413.

Paterson P, Khanna A. A novel method of ring removal from a swollen finger. *Br J Plast Surg.* 2001;54:182.

Thilagarajah M. An improved method of ring removal. *J Hand Surg Br.* 1999;24:118–119.

Witz R. Ring removal. *Nurse Pract.* 2002;27(2):54.

2008 MAG Mutual Healthcare Solutions, Inc.'s Physicians' Fee and Coding Guide. Duluth, Georgia. MAG Mutual Healthcare Solutions, Inc. 2007.

CHAPTER 22

Thoracentesis

E. J. Mayeaux Jr., MD, DABFP, FAAFP

Professor of Family Medicine, Professor of Obstetrics and Gynecology
Louisiana State University Health Sciences Center, Shreveport, LA

Thoracentesis is a procedure commonly performed to evaluate or treat fluid collections in the pleural space. Diagnostic thoracentesis is indicated for most newly discovered pleural fluid collection of unknown origin. Approximately 1.5 million individuals in the United States develop a pleural effusion annually, and the cause can be determined in 75% of these cases by performing appropriate cytologic, hematologic, microbiologic, and chemical analyses of the fluid.

Approximately 10 to 20 mL of fluid are normally present in the pleural space. This low-protein fluid acts as a lubricant during respiration. The pleural pressure gradient between the systemic circulation to the parietal surface (chest wall) and the pulmonary circulation to the visceral surface (lung) produces a daily flow of about 10 mL of fluid through the pleural space. Many disease states can produce disruption of hydrostatic pressure, osmotic pressure, capillary permeability, or lymphatic drainage, with the resulting formation of abnormal collections of fluid in the pleural space. Estimates of the volume of pleural fluid can be made from a chest x-ray film. Blunting of the costophrenic angle correlates with 100 to 150 mL of fluid, opacification of one half of a hemithorax is produced by 1.0 to 1.5 L of fluid, and complete opacification of a hemithorax is produced by 2.5 to 3.0 L of fluid.

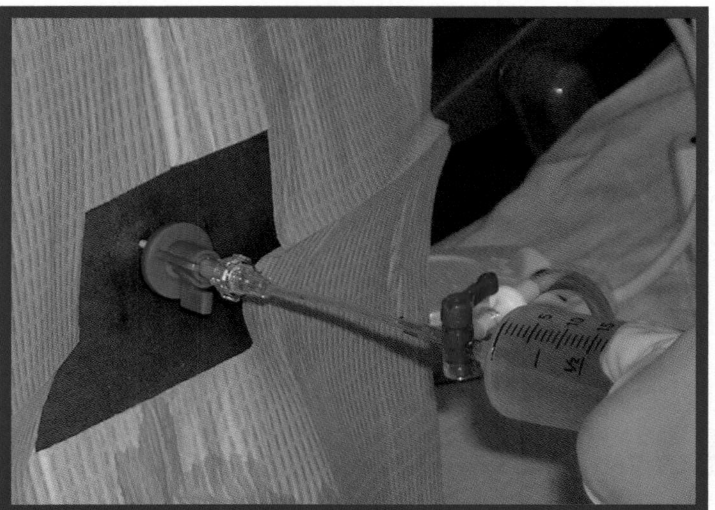

Several laboratory tests help to characterize abnormal pleural fluid collections as transudates or exudates (Table 22-1). Transudates, with a limited number of diagnostic possibilities, are generally associated with imbalances of hydrostatic and oncotic pressures. Transudates are noninflammatory effusions that generally have low numbers of lymphocytes and a predominance of monocytes. Exudates result from a legion of diagnostic possibilities and are caused by pleural inflammation and impaired lymphatic drainage of the pleural space. In acute stages, exudates have high leukocyte counts and a predominance of lymphocytes. The distinction between a transudate and an exudate directs the clinician to the appropriate differential diagnoses and subsequent treatment options (Tables 22-2 and 22-3). Exceptions exist in the classification of effusions, because 20% of effusions associated with pulmonary embolus and 6% associated with malignancy are transudates. Observation of the pleural fluid also can provide clues to its cause (Tables 22-4 and 22-5).

TABLE 22-1. Characteristics of Pleural Exudates[a]

Pleural fluid protein level >3 g/dL[b]
Pleural fluid-to-serum protein ratio >0.5
Pleural fluid lactate dehydrogenase (LDH) level >200 units
Pleural fluid-to-serum LDH ratio >0.6
Pleural fluid pH >7.3
Pleural fluid specific gravity >1.016

[a]Adapted from Erasmus JI, Goodman PC, Patz EF. Management of malignant pleural effusions and pneumothorax. *Radiol Clin North Am.* 2000;38:375–383.
[b]Transudates have the opposite sign (less than the cutoff) for the values listed for exudates (e.g., pleural fluid protein level <3 g/dL).

Medications can produce pleural fluid collections. A number of medications (e.g., procainamide, hydralazine, isoniazid, phenytoin, quinidine) produce drug-induced lupus syndrome and pleural fluid collections that are indistinguishable from those of native lupus erythematosus. Medications that can directly produce effusions include nitrofurantoin, dantrolene, methysergide, methotrexate, bromocriptine, minoxidil, and amiodarone.

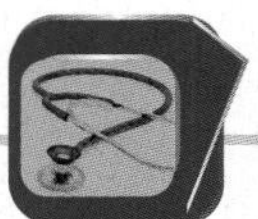

Equipment

Complete trays often include the following items:

- Three-way stopcock and connector tubing
- Luer lock syringe, 60 mL and 5 mL
- Lidocaine hydrochloride (1%), 5 mL
- Anesthesia needles, 25 gauge × 5/8 inch and 22 gauge × 1.5 inches
- Seven-inch Intracath with a 14-gauge needle (some trays do not have a thoracentesis needle)
- Needle guard for the thoracentesis needle
- Drainage tubing
- Fluid collection bag
- Three prelabeled specimen tubes with caps, 10 mL
- Skin prep
- Gauze sponges 3 × 3 inches

TABLE 22-2. Causes and Properties of Transudative Pleural Effusions[a]

Disease[b]	Protein (g/dL)	LDH (Units)
Congestive heart failure	0.6–3.8	10–190
Peritoneal dialysis	<1.0	<100
Urinothorax (urinary obstruction)	<1.0	<175
Nephrotic syndrome	<1.0	<100

[a]Adapted from Sahn SA. The pleura. *Am Rev Respir Dis.* 1998;138:184–234.
[b]Cirrhosis (usually with ascites) and atelectasis usually demonstrate the characteristic pleural fluid-to-serum ratios for protein (<0.5) and lactate dehydrogenase (LDH) <0.6).

TABLE 22-3. Causes and Properties of Exudative Pleural Effusions[a]

Disease[b]	Protein (g/dL)	LDH (Units)
Parapneumonic effusion	1.4–6.1	400–>1,000
Tuberculosis	>4.0	<700
Blastomycosis	4.2–6.6	>225
Histoplasmosis	4.1–5.7	200–425
Coccidiomycosis	3.5–6.5	Ratio >0.6[c]
Cryptococcosis	2.5–5.7	Ratio >0.6[c]
Viral syndrome	3.2–4.9	Ratio >0.6[c]
Mycoplasma infection	1.8–4.9	Ratio >0.6[c]
Carcinoma	1.5–8.0	300
Mesothelioma	3.5–5.5	36–600
Hepatitis	3.0–5.0	Ratio >0.6[c]
Asbestos pleural effusion	4.7–7.5	Ratio >0.6[c]
Rheumatoid pleurisy	Up to 7.3	Frequently >1,000
Injury after myocardial infarction	3.7	202
Uremic effusion	2.1 to 6.7	102 to 770

[a]Adapted from Sahn SA. The pleura. *Am Rev Respir Dis.* 1998;138:184–234.
[b]Exudates associated with pulmonary embolism often have varying levels of protein and lactate dehydrogenase (LDH). Aspergillosis, actinomycosis, nocardiosis, echinococcosis, *Legionella* infection, chylothorax, esophageal perforation, lupus pleuritis, sarcoidosis, pancreatitis, pancreatic pseudocyst, Meigs syndrome, hepatitis, lymphoma, radiation pleuritis, and ruptured upper abdominal abscesses produce the characteristic pleural fluid-to-serum ratios for protein (>0.5) and LDH (>0.6). Pulmonary embolus also produces characteristic ratios in 80% of patients; 20% have transudates.
[c]Ratio refers to the pleural fluid-to-serum ratio of LDH.

TABLE 22-4. Diagnoses Suggested by Examinations of Pleural Fluid[a]

Finding	Suggested Diagnosis
Ammonia odor of the fluid	Urinothorax
Black fluid	*Aspergillus* involvement of the pleura
Bloody fluid	Trauma, traumatic thoracentesis, pulmonary embolism, or malignancy
Brown fluid	Rupture of an amebic liver abscess into the pleural space
Food particles in the fluid	Rupture of the esophagus into the pleural space
Putrid odor of the fluid	Anaerobic infection of the pleura or empyema
Viscous fluid	Malignant mesothelioma due to increased levels of hyaluronic acid
White fluid	Chylothorax, cholesterol in the fluid, or empyema
Yellow-green fluid	Rheumatoid pleuritis

[a]Adapted from Sahn SA. The pleura. *Am Rev Respir Dis.* 1988;38:184–234.

TABLE 22-5. Studies Performed in Complete Pleural Fluid Analysis

Most cost-effective studies: lactate dehydrogenase (LDH), total protein, white blood cell
count and differential count, glucose, and pH[a]
Simultaneously draw serum for protein, LDH, and glucose levels
Consider arterial pH measurement if pleural fluid pH <7.30
Consider serum creatinine (to determine ratio) if uremic pleural effusion is suspected
Determine if the fluid is a transudate or exudate; then consider the following if *exudate:*
■ Infection is suspected: Gram stain, culture and sensitivity, potassium hydroxide (KOH) stain, fungal cultures, acid-fast bacilli smears and culture, specific antigens, titers and cultures depending on clinical presentation
■ Malignancy is suspected: cytology
■ Milky fluid obtained: lipid studies
■ Pancreatitis or esophageal rupture suspected: amylase
■ Rheumatoid or lupus pleuritis suspected: complement levels, rheumatoid factors, LE cells

[a]Studies ordered are based on the clinical presentation; it is not necessary or cost-effective to order the entire battery of tests for every patient.

- Antiseptic prep well
- Towel
- Fenestrated drape
- Puncture site bandage
- Hospital wrap

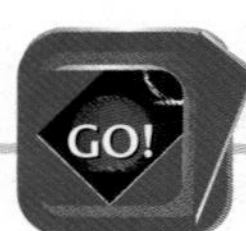

Indications

- Diagnosis of a newly discovered pleural effusion, especially under these circumstances:
  - A unilateral effusion is present, particularly left-sided.
  - Bilateral effusions are present but are of disparate sizes.
  - There is evidence of pleurisy.
  - The patient is febrile.
  - The cardiac silhouette appears normal on a chest radiograph.
  - The alveolar-arterial oxygen gradient is widened out of proportion to the clinical setting.
- Therapeutic removal of fluid for symptomatic improvement (e.g., malignant effusion)

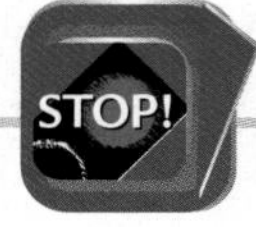

Contraindications (Relative)

- Known cause for the pleural effusion (e.g., congestive heart failure) except when done for symptom relief.
- Bleeding diathesis or anticoagulation
- A small volume of pleural fluid (e.g., in a viral syndrome) if the procedure likely will produce pneumothorax
- Patients on mechanical ventilation
- Active skin infection at the point of needle insertion

The Procedure

Step 1. Secure informed consent as described in Appendix A. The patient is seated, with the arms crossed the body and resting comfortably on a support (e.g., sturdy adjustable table) placed horizontally in front of the body. A footstool can be used to flex the patient's upper legs. The thorax should be as erect as possible. Alternately, for patients who cannot tolerate a seated position, the left lateral decubitus position can be used.

- **PEARL:** Supplemental oxygen is often administered during thoracentesis, both to offset hypoxemia and to facilitate reabsorption of pleural air if pneumothorax complicates the procedure.
- **PITFALL:** Complications can develop if the table supporting the patient suddenly shifts during the procedure. Make sure the table will not shift and that it can support the weight of the patient's torso during the procedure.
- **PITFALL:** Avoid having the patient lean too far forward. Gravitational forces may cause the fluid to shift more anteriorly, increasing the likelihood of a postprocedure pneumothorax.

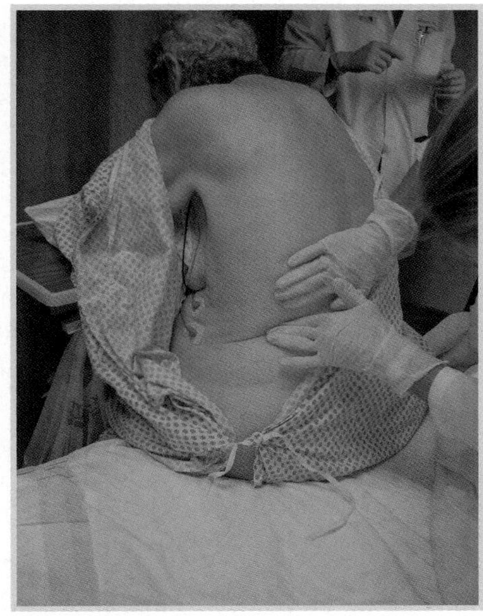

Step 1

Step 2. Determine the level of effusion by percussion or from an x-ray. The level is determined during percussion by the point where the resonant percussion tone of the lungs changes to a dull percussion tone of the fluid from the hollow note of normally expanded lungs.

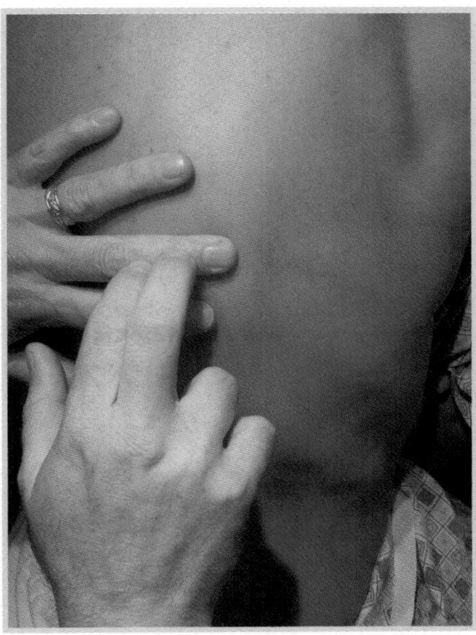

Step 2

Step 3. The needle insertion site should be one intercostal space below the level of effusion, at the upper portion of the rib and midway between the posterior axillary line and the paraspinal muscles. An alternate approach is to insert the needle above the eighth rib, as low in the effusion as possible. Mark the site by indenting the skin firmly with a fingernail or pen cap.

- **PITFALL:** Have the preprocedure chest radiograph immediately available for review. Aspiration of the wrong hemithorax is an embarrassing and dangerous error.
- **PITFALL:** Most experts recommend a lateral decubitus x-ray film to make sure of the fluid layers. Loculated fluid collections can be difficult to tap and are best approached with imaging guidance (i.e., ultrasound or computed tomography scan). Obtain the decubitus films before performing thoracentesis.
- **PITFALL:** Routine approaches that are performed lower in an effusion (to hit the main fluid collection) may have greater risk of liver or splenic perforation.

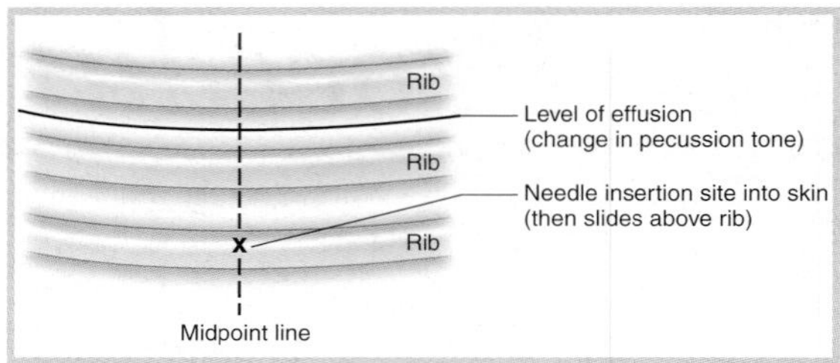

Step 3

Step 4. Apply sterile gloves, and have an assistant open the sterile thoracentesis tray. Swab a large area around the insertion site with povidone-iodine or chlorhexidine (see Appendix E). Alternately, some physicians apply antiseptic solution before application of sterile gloves. Center the fenestration on the drape over the insertion site. Avoid contamination of the sterile gloves during this step.

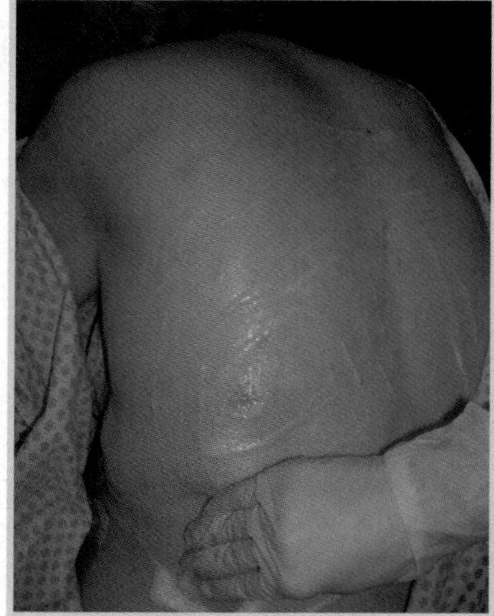

Step 4

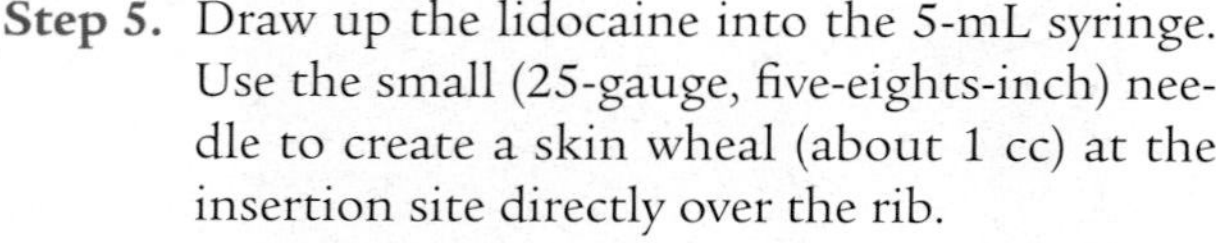

Step 5. Draw up the lidocaine into the 5-mL syringe. Use the small (25-gauge, five-eights-inch) needle to create a skin wheal (about 1 cc) at the insertion site directly over the rib.

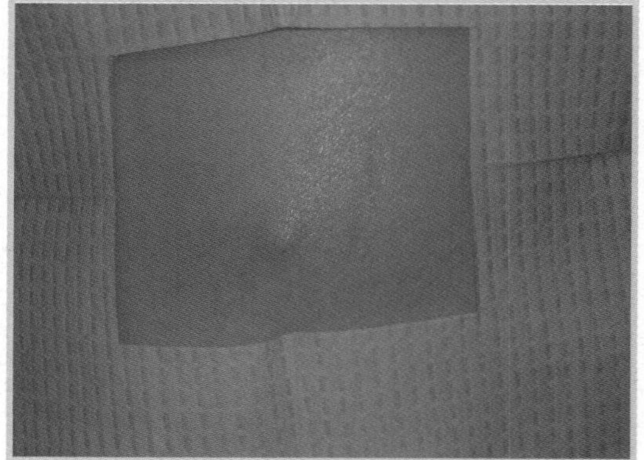

Step 5

Step 6. The larger (22-gauge, 0.5-inch) needle is then placed on the syringe, and the needle tip is inserted to the upper portion of the rib. A small amount (about 1 mL) of anesthetic is administered, and the needle tip is backed up and redirected above the rib until the pleural surface is reached. Some authors advocate administering lidocaine after passing the upper rib every 2 mm of insertion of the needle tip.

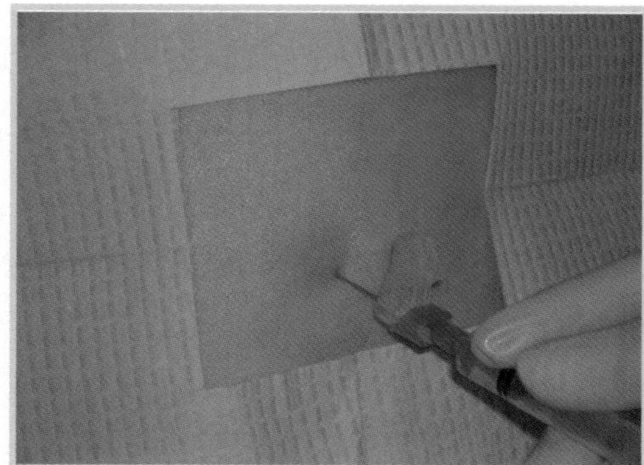

Step 6

Step 7. The path of the needle is a Z-insertion track. On removal of a needle through a Z-track, the natural position of the tissues tends to reduce the chances for leaking fluid.

- **PITFALL:** Extensive bleeding can result from damage to an intercostal artery from the large thoracentesis needle. Always insert the needle just at the upper edge of the rib to avoid the neurovascular bundle that lies beneath each rib.

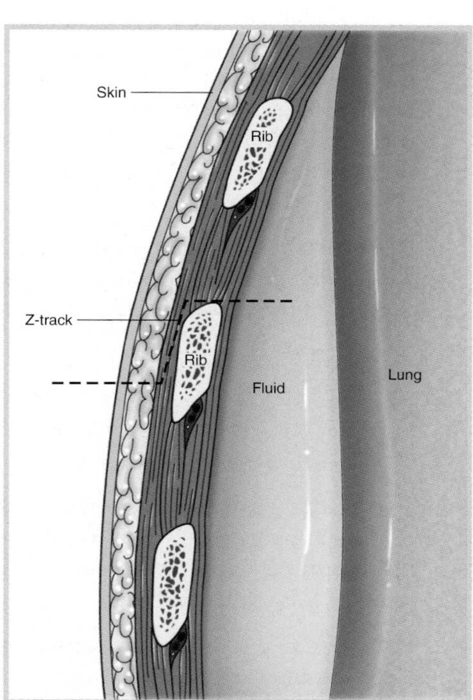

Step 7

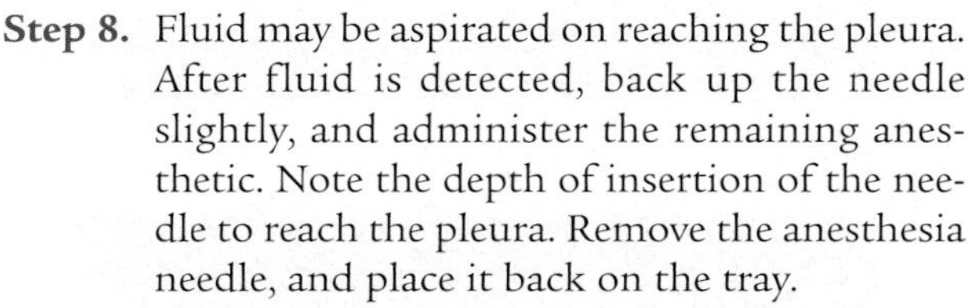

Step 8. Fluid may be aspirated on reaching the pleura. After fluid is detected, back up the needle slightly, and administer the remaining anesthetic. Note the depth of insertion of the needle to reach the pleura. Remove the anesthesia needle, and place it back on the tray.

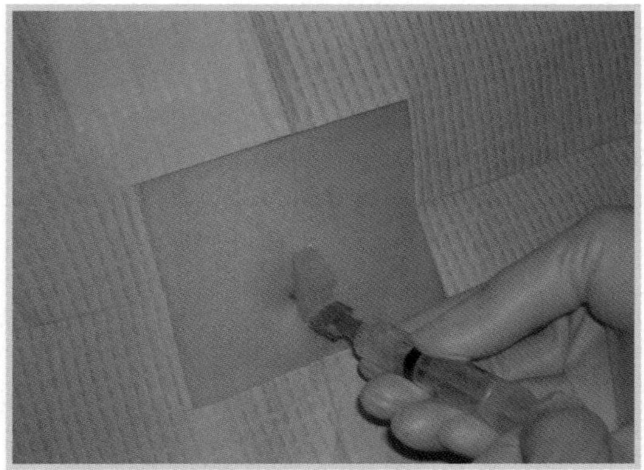

Step 8

Step 9. The thoracentesis needle is attached to the large (60-mL) syringe and inserted through anesthetized skin until the rib is reached. The needle is then redirected above the rib into the pleural space.

- **PEARL:** Some providers recommend adding 1 mL of 1:1,000 heparin to the syringe to prevent clotting of hemorrhagic or highly proteinaceous fluid.

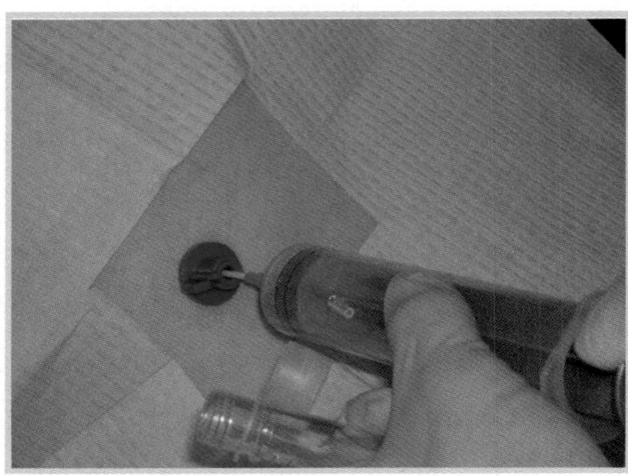

Step 9

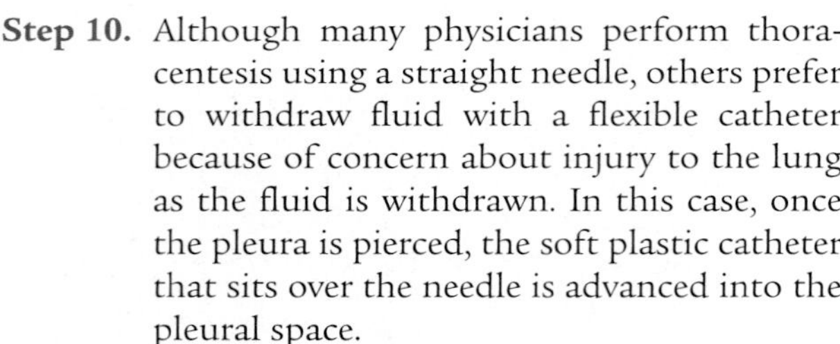

Step 10. Although many physicians perform thoracentesis using a straight needle, others prefer to withdraw fluid with a flexible catheter because of concern about injury to the lung as the fluid is withdrawn. In this case, once the pleura is pierced, the soft plastic catheter that sits over the needle is advanced into the pleural space.

- **PEARL:** The typical needle is a 22-gauge, 1.5-inch needle. A longer needle should be used in the markedly obese patient.

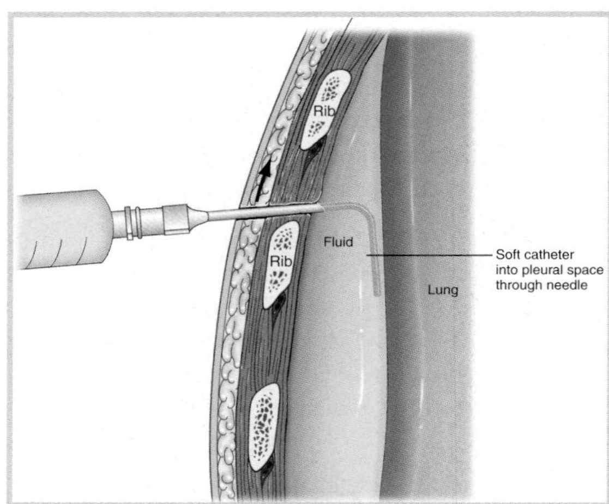

Step 10

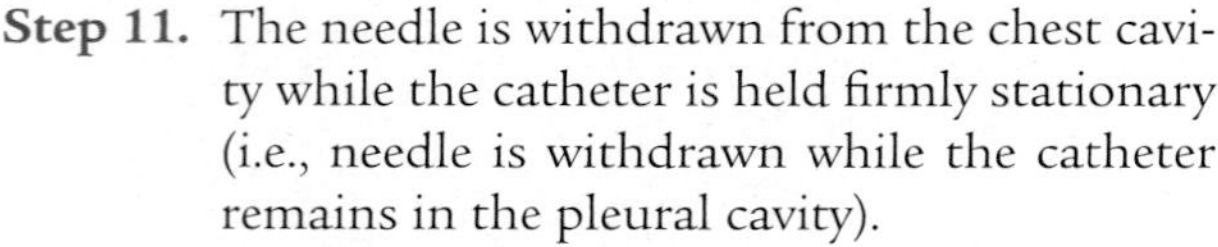

Step 11. The needle is withdrawn from the chest cavity while the catheter is held firmly stationary (i.e., needle is withdrawn while the catheter remains in the pleural cavity).

- **PITFALL:** Make sure an adequate length of catheter is inserted into the pleural space before the needle is withdrawn. It is frustrating if the catheter inadvertently comes out of the pleural space when the needle is withdrawn and before fluid has been obtained.

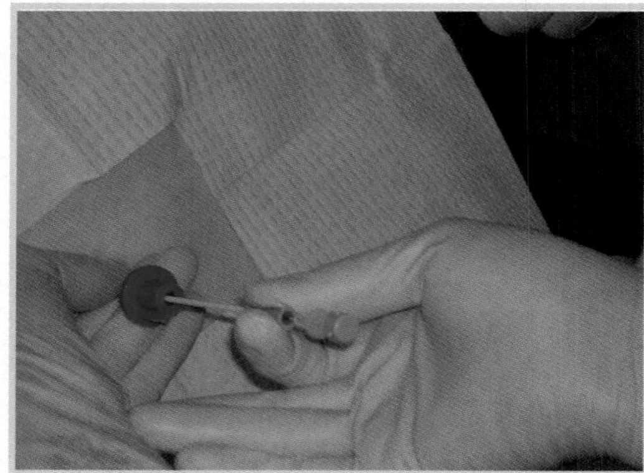

Step 11

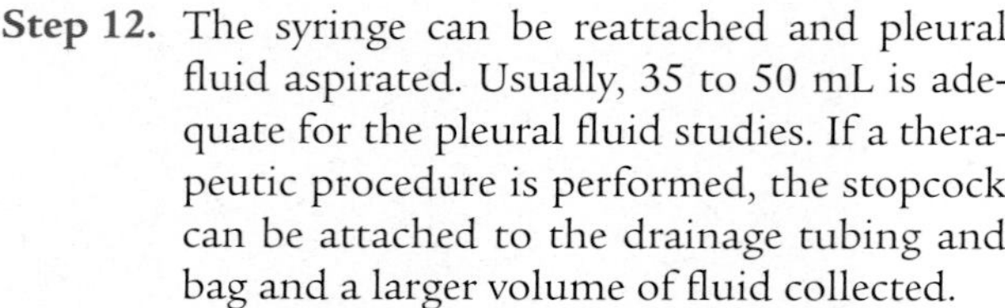

Step 12. The syringe can be reattached and pleural fluid aspirated. Usually, 35 to 50 mL is adequate for the pleural fluid studies. If a therapeutic procedure is performed, the stopcock can be attached to the drainage tubing and bag and a larger volume of fluid collected.

- **PITFALL:** Do not permit air to enter the pleural space during this portion of the procedure.
- **PITFALL:** Do not attempt the removal of more than 1.5 L of fluid in a single setting. Re-expansion pulmonary edema can

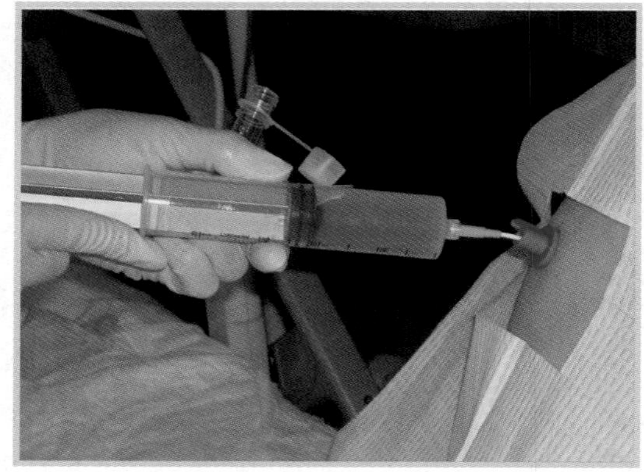

Step 12

result, exacerbating the temporary (and usually minor) hypoxemia that follows thoracentesis. Oxygen should be administered if dyspnea occurs after the procedure. Close clinical monitoring is advocated whenever an individual has more than 1 L of fluid removed.

Step 13. The catheter is removed at the end of the procedure. The insertion site is gently rubbed, and pressure is applied with gauze to the site to ensure the absence of a fluid leak. The skin site is washed clean, and a bandage is applied to the site.

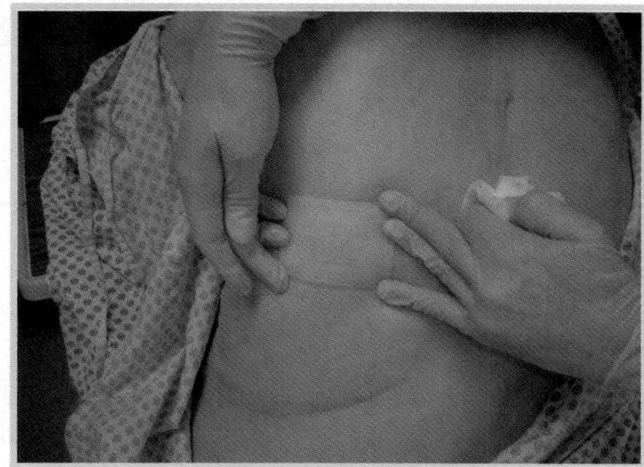

Step 13

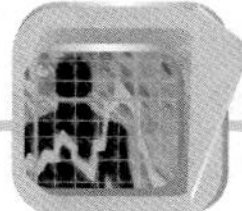

Complications

- The most common complication after thoracentesis is pneumothorax, with an average incidence of 6% to 19%. Uncontrollable coughing during the procedure and the use of a large-bore needle without catheters may increase the likelihood of pneumothorax.
- Re-expansion pulmonary edema can be seen when large effusions are removed or when fluid removal allows atelectatic lung tissue to re-expand, especially if the lung has been collapsed for more than 7 days.
- Hemorrhage develops in <2% of procedures and necessitates thoracic surgery consultation if the bleeding is not controlled in 30 to 60 minutes.
- Pain at the puncture site.
- Empyema or soft tissue infection.
- Spleen or liver puncture.

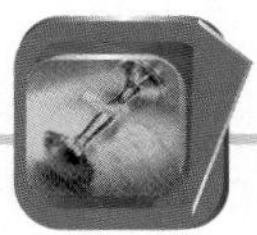

Pediatric Considerations

The procedure is performed similarly in adults and children. However, some children may do better if mildly sedated (see Chapter 122).

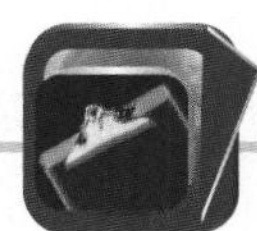

Postprocedure Instructions

Chest radiographs have been routinely performed after thoracentesis. Several studies question the practice and suggest that routine performance of the study in an asymptomatic individual after an uncomplicated procedure adds no management benefit. If multiple needle passes are required before fluid is obtained, if the patient has a history of chest irradiation or a prior sclerosing technique, or if an air leak is detected during the procedure, obtaining a chest radiograph is clearly indicated.

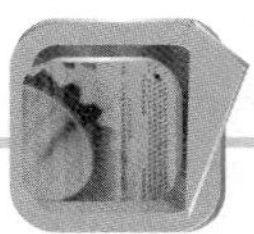

Coding Information and Supply Sources

CPT Code	Description	2008 Average 50th Percentile Fee	Global Period
32421	Thoracentesis, puncture of the pleural cavity for aspiration, initial or subsequent	$358	0
32422	Thoracentesis, with insertion of tube, includes water seal (eg for pneumothorax) when performed (separate procedure)	$508	0

CPT Code	Description	2008 Average 50th Percentile Fee	Global Period
76942-26	Ultrasound guidance for needle placement	$496	XXX
77002-26	Fluoroscopic guidance for needle placement	$396	XXX
77012-26	CT guidance for needle placement	$277	XXX

XXX = Global concept does not apply.
2008 average 50th Percentile Fees are provided courtesy of 2008 MMH-SI's copyrighted Physicians' Fees and Coding Guide.

If imaging is used to guide the needle placement, alternate codes are selected (76003, 76360, or 76942). Code 32002 is used for thoracentesis with insertion of a tube (with or without a water seal) for drainage of a pneumothorax; code 32002 is not used to report chest tube placement for drainage of the pleura of blood or pus (use code 32020).

Thoracentesis trays that include all instruments needed to perform the procedure can be ordered from these suppliers:

- Allegiance Healthcare Corp., McGraw Park, IL 60085. Phone: 847-689-8410. Web site: http://www.cardinal.com/mps/brands/specialprocedures/diagnostictrays.asp.
- AVID Medical, Inc., Toano, VA 23168. Phone: 888-564-7153. Web site: http://www.avidmedical.com.
- WESTNET, Inc., 30 North Street, Canton, MA 02021. Phone: 781-828-7772; fax: 781-828-2011. Web site: http://westnetmed.com/.

Patient Education Handout

A patient education handout, "Thoracentesis," can be found on the book's companion Web site.

Bibliography

Barbers R, Patel P. Thoracentesis made safe and simple. *J Respir Dis.* 1994;15:841–851.

Candeira SR, Blasco LH, Soler MJ, et al. Biochemical and cytologic characteristics of pleural effusions secondary to pulmonary embolism. *Chest.* 2002;121:465–469.

Carlson DW, DiGiulio GA, Gewitz MH, et al. Illustrated techniques of pediatric emergency procedures. In: Fleisher GR, Ludwig S, Henretig FM, et al., eds. *Textbook of Pediatric Emergency Medicine*. New York: Lippincott Williams & Wilkins; 2000:1787–1896.

Colice GL, Curtis A, Deslauriers J, et al. ACCP consensus statement: medical and surgical treatment of parapneumonic effusions: an evidence-based guideline. *Chest.* 2000;118:1158–1171.

Collins TR, Sahn SA. Thoracentesis: clinical value, complications, technical problems, and patient experience. *Chest.* 1987;91:817–822.

Colt HG, Brewer N, Barbur E. Evaluation of patient-related and procedure-related factors contributing to pneumothorax following thoracentesis. *Chest.* 1999;116:134–138.

Erasmus JJ, Goodman PC, Patz EE. Management of malignant pleural effusions and pneumothorax. *Radiol Clin North Am.* 2000;38:375–383.

Fartoukh M, Azoulay E, Galliot R, et al. Clinically documented pleural effusions in medical ICU patients: how useful is routine thoracentesis? *Chest.* 2002;121:178–184.

Heffner JE, Brown LK, Barbieri CA. Diagnostic value of tests that discriminate between exudative and transudative pleural effusions. *Chest.* 1997;111:970–980.

Johnson RL. Thoracentesis. In: Rakel RE, ed. *Saunders Manual of Family Practice*. Philadelphia: WB Saunders; 1996:166–167.

Light RW, MacGregor MI, Luchsinger PC, et al. Pleural effusions: the diagnostic separation of transudates and exudates. *Ann Intern Med.* 1972;77:507–513.

Meeker D. A stepwise approach to diagnostic and therapeutic thoracentesis. *Mod Med.* 1993;61:62–71.

Petersen WG, Zimmerman R. Limited utility of chest radiograph after thoracentesis. *Chest.* 2000;117:1038–1042.

Rubins JB, Colice GL. Evaluating pleural effusions: How should you go about finding the cause? *Postgrad Med.* 1999;105:39–48.

Sahn SA, Good JT. Pleural fluid pH in malignant effusions. *Ann Intern Med.* 1988;108:345–349.

Zuber TJ. *Office Procedures*. Baltimore: Williams & Wilkins; 1999:195–204.

2008 MAG Mutual Healthcare Solutions, Inc.'s Physicians' Fee and Coding Guide. Duluth, Georgia. MAG Mutual Healthcare Solutions, Inc. 2007.

CHAPTER 23

Tick Removal

E. J. Mayeaux Jr., MD, DABFP, FAAFP
Professor of Family Medicine, Professor of Obstetrics and Gynecology
Louisiana State University Health Sciences Center, Shreveport, LA

Many people work and play in nonurban areas where they are exposed to tick bites. The tick bite itself usually is painless and produces harmless effects, such as mild inflammatory reaction or esthetic distaste. However, several medically important illnesses may develop from microorganisms transmitted by the tick, including Rocky Mountain spotted fever, Q fever, typhus, tick fever, tularemia, babesiosis, relapsing fever, and Lyme disease (Figure 1). Tick-borne diseases can be transmitted by through bites and by careless handling of infected ticks. The neurotoxin secreted in the saliva of certain ticks may also result in a progressive ascending paralysis. To limit exposure to potentially pathogenic organisms, expedient and effective tick removal is recommended.

Ticks, like spiders, are arthropods. There are more than 800 species of ticks throughout the world. There are two major families of ticks that bite humans. The Argasidae family (i.e., soft ticks) tends to live around burrows, roots, and nests of birds or reptiles. They attach and feed for minutes to hours and then fall off the prey. The Ixodidae family (i.e., hard ticks) hides in grasses along the sides of animal trails and attach themselves to a passing host. They remain attached until engorged, until they die, or until they are physically removed. In their larval stage, ixodid ticks are known as seed ticks and may infest in great numbers. One anecdotal report demonstrated removal of seed ticks with lindane shampoo.

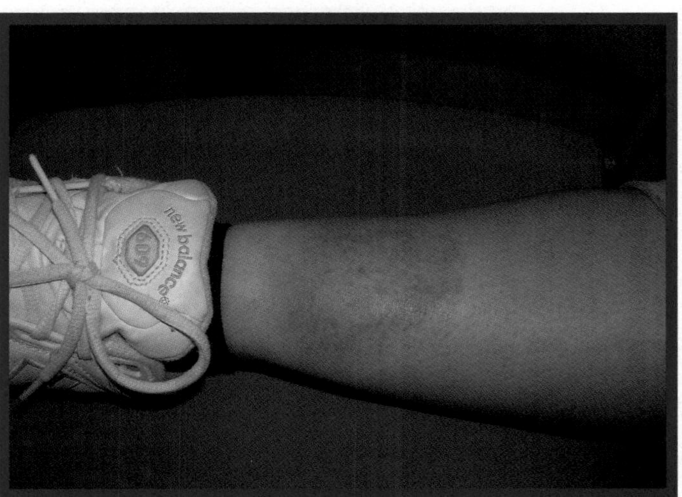

Hard adult ticks are usually best removed mechanically. A tick attaches to its host with mouthparts equipped with specialized structures designed to hold it embedded in the skin. Most species secrete a cement from the salivary glands that toughens into a hard collar around the mouthparts to help hold it in place. After removal, assess whether the tick is intact by inspecting it for the mouthparts. In cases of a particularly tenacious tick or retained mouthparts, a punch biopsy trephine may be used to remove the local skin and any part of the tick that is attached (see Chapter 27, Punch Biopsy of the Skin). If mouthparts are retained in the skin, some providers perform a punch biopsy to remove the remnants of the tick, while others observe for infection.

In the past, the application of petroleum jelly, fingernail polish, 70% isopropyl alcohol, or a hot kitchen match was advocated to induce the detachment of adult ticks. However, ticks are extremely hard to suffocate because their respiratory rate is only 15 breaths per hour, and studies have shown that these methods rarely work. Some of these methods may also increase the likelihood that the tick will regurgitate into the site, promoting disease transmission. These techniques are not recommended. There is one anecdotal report of using a 2% viscous lidocaine, which caused the tick to release after about 5 minutes. It is unknown whether this method increases the risk of disease transmission.

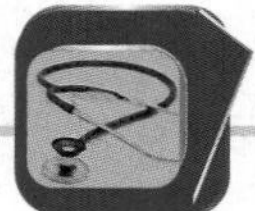

Equipment

- TICKED OFF
- A standard office surgical tray used for simple surgical procedures, found in Appendix G: Instruments and Materials in the Office Surgery Tray.

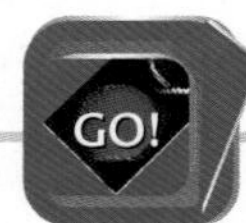

Indications

- Removal of ticks embedded in the skin

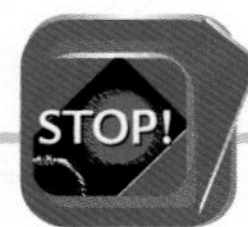

Contraindications

- None

The Procedure

Step 1. Gently paint the surrounding area with chlorhexidine or povidone-iodine. Slide a pair of curved hemostats between the skin and the body of the tick. Straight forceps, tweezers, or gloved fingers also may be used.

- PITFALL: Never squeeze, crush, or puncture the body of the tick, because this may force infectious agents into the wound or onto the examiner.

Step 2. Pull upward and perpendicularly, with steady, even pressure. Place the tick in a container of alcohol, and ask the patient to place the container in a freezer in case subsequent identification is warranted. Disinfect the bite site with povidone-iodine scrub or antibacterial soap.

- PITFALL: Avoid leaving part or all of the arthropod's head or mouthparts. The further from the head traction is applied, the greater the chance parts will be broken off. When using hemostats or other grasping devices, grasp the tick as close to the skin

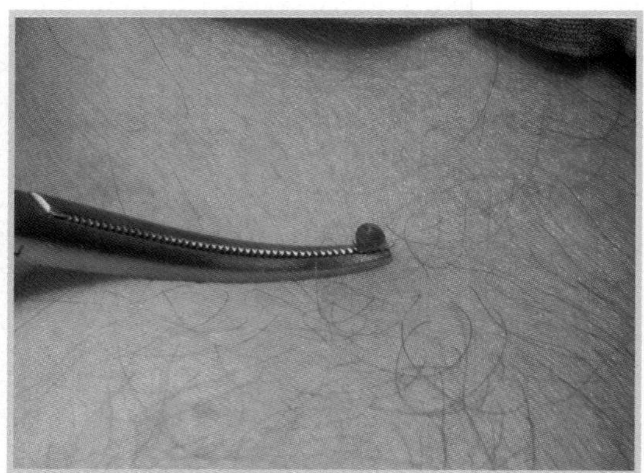

Step 1

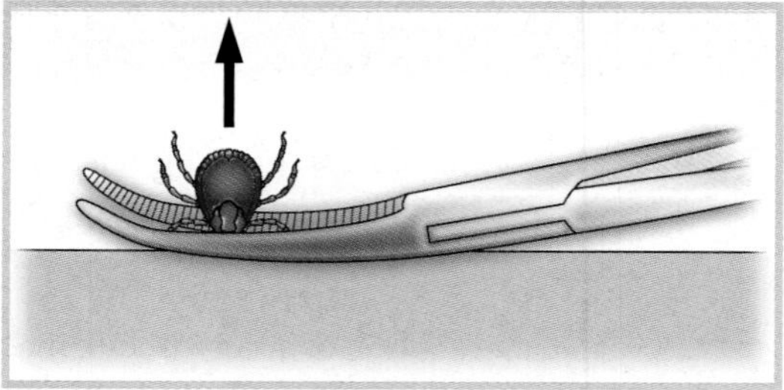

Step 2

surface as possible, and do not twist or jerk the tick.

- **PEARL:** In cases of a particularly tenacious tick or retained mouthparts, a punch biopsy trephine may be used to remove the local skin

Step 3. Alternately, a specific tick removal device, such as the TICKED OFF device, may be used in place of curved hemostats. While holding TICKED OFF vertical to the skin, place the wide part of the notch on the skin near the tick. Applying slight pressure downward on the skin, slide the remover forward so the small part of the notch is up against the tick. Use a slow, continuous, forward-sliding motion of the remover to detach the tick (a motion similar to scooping hard ice cream from a bucket).

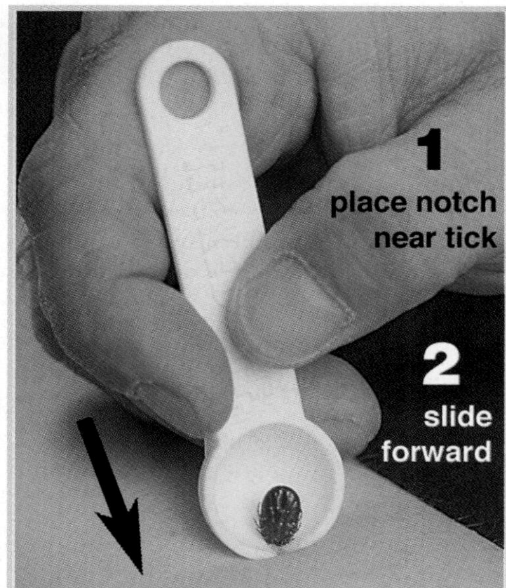

Step 3

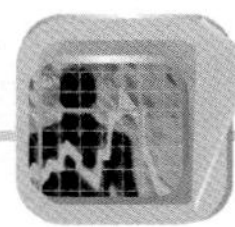

Complications

- Infection
- Bleeding
- Scar formation

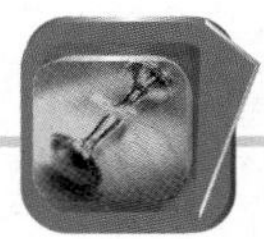

Pediatric Considerations

This procedure is performed in a similar manner for adult and pediatric patients.

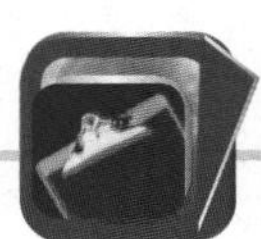

Postprocedure Instructions

Advise patients about the possibility of local or systemic infection, and instruct them to watch for signs of Lyme disease (i.e., erythema marginatum). Excessive bleeding from the removal site is rare and usually is easily controlled with standard measures. Instruct patients on tick infestation prevention methods. When outdoors, protective clothing should be tucked in at the wrists and ankles and sprayed with a tick repellant. Bare skin should have repellant applied every few hours.

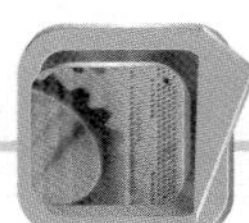

Coding Information and Supply Sources

There is no specific code for tick removal. Code an appropriate office visit, with a punch biopsy code if a Keys punch is used.

TICKED OFF may be purchased at TICKED OFF Inc., 99 Spruce Lane, Dover, NH 03820. Phone: 1-800-642-2485; fax: 603-742-5568; e-mail: tickedoff@ttlc.net. Web site: http://www.tickedoff.com/contact.htm.

CPT Code	Description	2008 Average 50th Percentile Fee	Global Period
11100	Biopsy of skin, subcutaneous	$137	0
11101	Biopsy of each separate or additional lesion (must be reported with 11100)	$81	ZZZ

ZZZ = Code related to another service and is always included in the global period of the other sercive.
2008 average 50th Percentile Fees are provided courtesy of 2008 MMH-SI's copyrighted Physicians' Fees and Coding Guide.

Patient Education Handout

A patient education handout, "Tick Bites," can be found on the book's companion Web site.

Bibliography

Halpern JS. Tick removal. *J Emerg Nurs.* 1988;14:307–309.

Jones BE. Human "seed tick" infestation: *Amblyomma americanum* larvae. *Arch Dermatol.* 1981;117:812–814.

Kammholz LP. Variation on tick removal. *Pediatrics* 1986;78:378–379.

Karras DJ. Tick removal. *Ann Emerg Med.* 1998;32:519.

Munns R. Punch biopsy of the skin. In: Driscoll CE, Rakel RE, eds. *Patient Care: Procedures for Your Practice*. Oradell, NJ: Medical Economics; 1988.

Needham G. Evaluation of five popular methods for tick removal. *Pediatrics* 1985;75:997–1002.

Oteo JA, Casas JM, Martinez de Artola V. Lyme disease in outdoor workers: risk factors, preventive measures, and tick removal methods. *Am J Epidemiol.* 1991;133:754–755.

Patterson J, Fitzwater J, Connell J. Localized tick bite reaction. *Cutis.* 1979;24:168–169, 172.

Pearn J. Neuromuscular paralysis caused by tick envenomation. *J Neurol Sci.* 1977;34:37–42.

Shakman RA. Tick removal. *West J Med.* 1984;140:99.

2008 MAG Mutual Healthcare Solutions, Inc.'s Physicians' Fee and Coding Guide. Duluth, Georgia. MAG Mutual Healthcare Solutions, Inc. 2007.

SECTION TWO

DERMATOLOGY

CHAPTER 24

Cryosurgery of the Skin

E.J. Mayeaux, Jr., MD, DABFP, FAAFP

Professor of Family Medicine, Professor of Obstetrics and Gynecology
Louisiana State University Health Sciences Center, Shreveport, LA

Cryosurgery is a frequently performed ablative procedure used in the treatment of benign, premalignant, and malignant skin growths. Cryosurgery produces controlled destruction of skin lesions by withdrawing heat from the targeted tissue. Historically, physicians have used liquid nitrogen applied with cotton-tipped swabs. Today, most providers generally use a probe tip containing a refrigerant liquid or a device that sprays liquid nitrogen. Human tissue freezes at −2.2°C, with tissue destruction occurring at temperatures at or colder than −10°C. Closed probe systems using nitrous oxide can produce probe tip temperatures in the range of −65°C to −89°C, and liquid nitrogen systems achieve temperatures of −25°C to −50°C. Generally, destruction of benign lesions requires temperatures of −20°C to −30°C. Effective removal of malignant lesions requires temperatures of −40°C to −50°C.

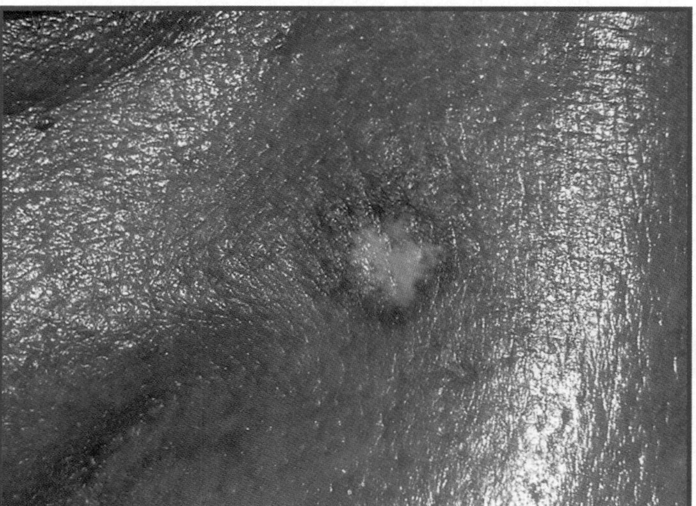

Cryosurgery is best suited for use in patients with light skin and for treatment of lesions in most non-hair-bearing areas of the body. Skin lesions often can be treated in a single session, although some require several treatments.

Cryosurgery produces a ball-shaped sphere of ice in the target tissue. The edge of the ice ball only achieves a temperature of 0°C, and this area usually recovers from the effects of the freeze. Cryosurgery should be performed so that the ice ball extends at least 2 to 5 mm beyond the edge of the lesion being destroyed. Because ice ball formation is symmetric in all directions, the lateral extension of the ice ball from the applicator tip gives a good estimation of the depth of ice penetration into the tissue.

Damage in treated tissue occurs because of intracellular ice formation and electrolyte shifts. The degree of damage depends on the rate of cooling and the minimum temperature achieved. Inflammation develops during the 24 hours after treatment, further contributing to tissue destruction. Keratinocytes need to be frozen to −50°C for optimum destruction. Melanocytes only require a temperature of −5°C for destruction. This is the reason that hypopigmentation is a common side effect following cryotherapy on darker-skinned individuals (Fig. 1).

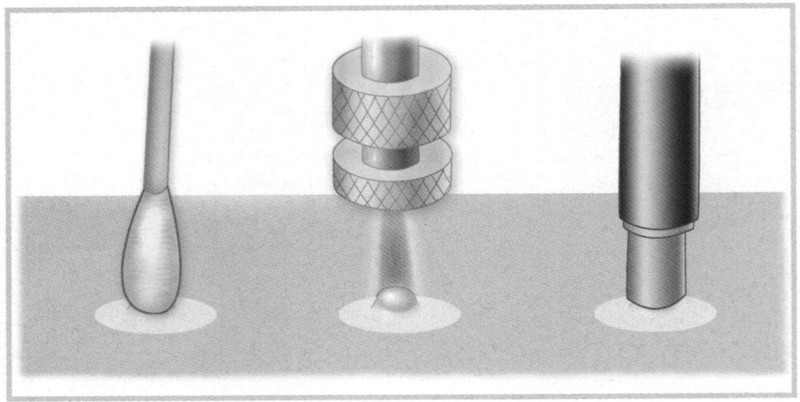

Figure 1

Although there are multiple ways to determine the length of time to freeze, using the timed spot freeze technique may be the safest and most appropriate method for providers who are learning to perform cryosurgery. The standard freezing times are shown in Table 24-1. The freezing time is adjusted according to the skin thickness, vascularity, tissue type, and lesion characteristics.

Many clinicians advocate the performance of double freezes when cryosurgery is performed. The main advantage of the freeze-thaw-freeze technique is that greater cell death is achieved in the zone of tissue that has been previously frozen (but would otherwise recover). This advantage can be significant when treating premalignant or malignant lesions or lesions that resist freezing. Caution should be taken during the thaw phase, because vascular lesions may bleed on thawing. Overfreezing once an adequate freeze ball is achieved can result in disruption of the skin collagen matrix and possible scarring.

Cryosurgery generally produces a burning sensation during the treatment, although the discomfort of injected anesthetic often exceeds the discomfort of the procedure. After the procedure, cryosurgery produces anesthesia in the treated tissues. Frozen tissue reacts with peripheral edema immediately after thawing. Subsequent bulla formation and exudation occur before the area heals in a fine atrophic scar within 4 weeks. The technique produces high cure rates with good cosmetic results.

Certain medical conditions can produce an exaggerated tissue response to the freezing of the skin (listed in the relative contraindications section). Patients with conditions that produce serum cold-induced antibodies (i.e., cryoglobulins) are at greatest risk for marked skin necrosis.

TABLE 24-1. Recommended Cryosurgical Freeze Times for the Standard-Spot Freeze Technique

Time	Technique
5 sec	Actinic keratosis Skin tags Solar lentigo
10 sec	Cherry angioma Common warts Oral mucocele Sebaceous hyperplasia
10–15 sec	Cutaneous horn Pyogenic granuloma
20 sec	Hypertrophic scar Keloid Myxoid cyst
20–30 sec	Dermatofibroma

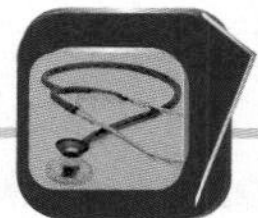

Equipment

- Liquid nitrogen sprayer and liquid nitrogen
- Nitrous oxide tank, regulator, and Cryogun
- Cotton-tipped applicator, forceps (optional), cotton ball, Dewer flask, polystyrene cup, and liquid nitrogen

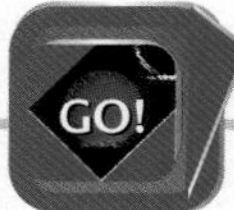

Indications

- Actinic keratosis
- Leukoplakia
- Milia
- Mucocele of the lip
- Pyogenic granuloma
- Seborrheic keratosis
- Sebaceous hyperplasia
- Superficial basal cell carcinoma
- Simple lentigo
- Cherry angioma
- Verrucae vulgaris
- Hypertrophic scars
- Molluscum contagiosum
- Capillary hemangioma of the newborn
- Granuloma annulare
- Solar-induced pigmentation and wrinkling
- Viral warts

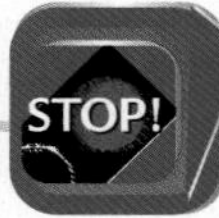

Contraindications

- Lesion for which tissue pathology is required
- Lesion located in an area with compromised circulation
- Melanoma
- Patient unable to accept possibility of pigmentary changes
- Proven sensitivity or adverse reaction to cryosurgery
- Sclerosing basal cell carcinoma or recurrent basal cell or squamous cell carcinoma, particularly when located in a high-risk area (e.g., temple, nasolabial fold)
- Cold intolerance (relative)
- Cold-induced urticaria (relative)
- Collagen disease or autoimmune disease (relative)
- Concurrent treatment with immunosuppressive drugs (relative)
- Cryoglobulinemia (relative)
- Heavily pigmented skin (relative)
- Lesions located in pretibial areas, eyelid margins, nasolabial fold, ala nasi, and hair-bearing areas (relative)
- Multiple myeloma (relative)
- Pyoderma gangrenosum (relative)
- Raynaud disease (especially for procedures on the digits) (relative)
- Active, severe ulcerative colitis

The Procedure

Step 1. Pare down thick, hyperkeratotic lesions that resist cryosurgical treatment. Perform paring with a horizontally held no. 15 scalpel blade using a sawing motion or direct pass through the lesion. Achieve topical hemostasis with an agent such as ferric subsulfate (Monsel solution) before cryotherapy.

- PITFALL: Blood at the surface of the skin acts like an insulator against cryosurgical destruction. Do not perform cryosurgery on an actively bleeding lesion.

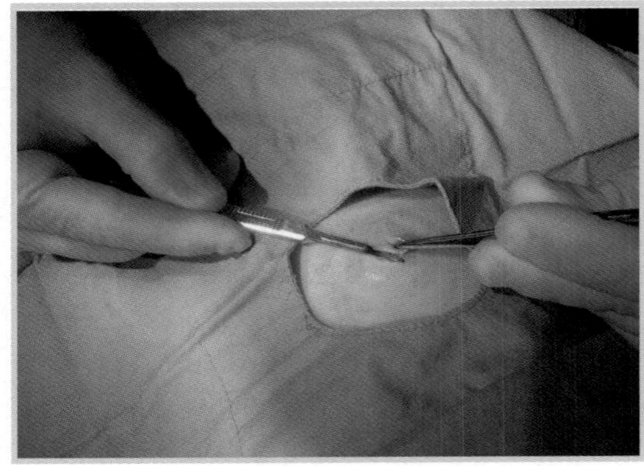

Step 1

Liquid Nitrogen with a Cotton-Tipped Applicator

Step 2. If using a standard long-handled cotton-tipped applicator, expand the head of the applicator by wrapping wisps of cotton pulled from a cotton ball loosely around it.

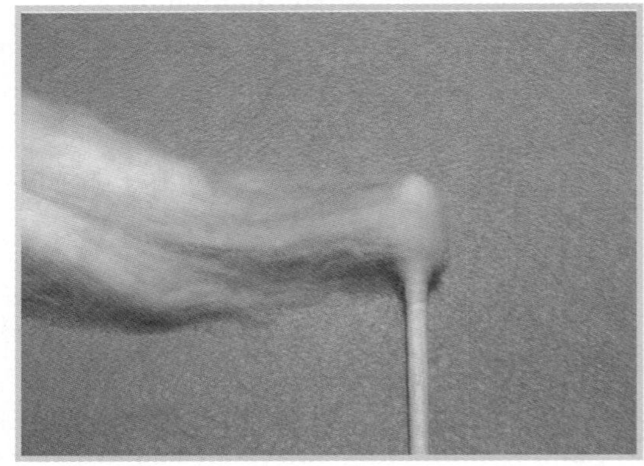

Step 2

Step 3. Place the liquid nitrogen into a disposable polystyrene cup. Dip the cotton-tipped applicator into liquid nitrogen.

- PITFALL: Do not tap the applicator against the lip of the cup (in an attempt to shake off excess liquid nitrogen), because this may remove so much that an adequate freeze will not be possible.
- PITFALL: Adenovirus is capable of survival in liquid nitrogen. The same source of liquid nitrogen should not be used with different patients.

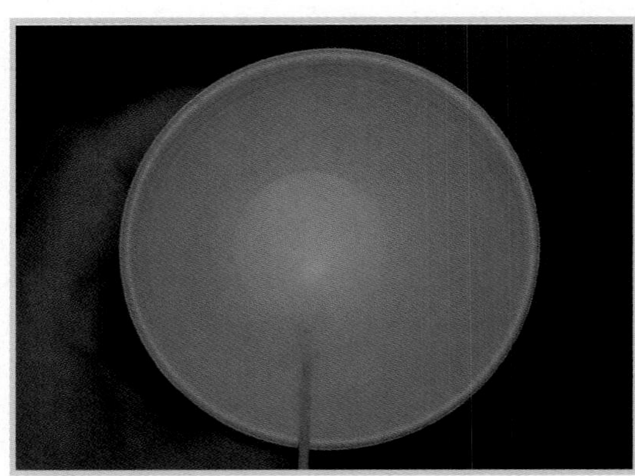

Step 3

Step 4. The applicator is then firmly pressed against the lesion for the desired duration. The dipstick applicator method does not achieve the low temperatures of the spray technique; therefore, this method is suitable only for benign lesions.

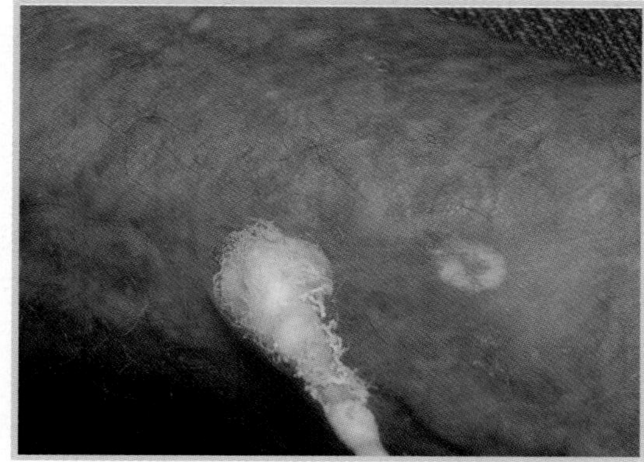

Step 4

Liquid Nitrogen Spray Techniques

Step 2. Position the nozzle of the spray gun 1 to 1.5 cm from the skin surface aimed at the center of the lesion. The spray may be applied directly in a paintbrush fashion or in a rotary pattern.

- **PEARL:** Nozzle sizes B and C are suitable for the treatment of most benign and malignant lesions.
- **PEARL:** Pulsing direct spray is useful to avoid an overexpansion of the treatment site.

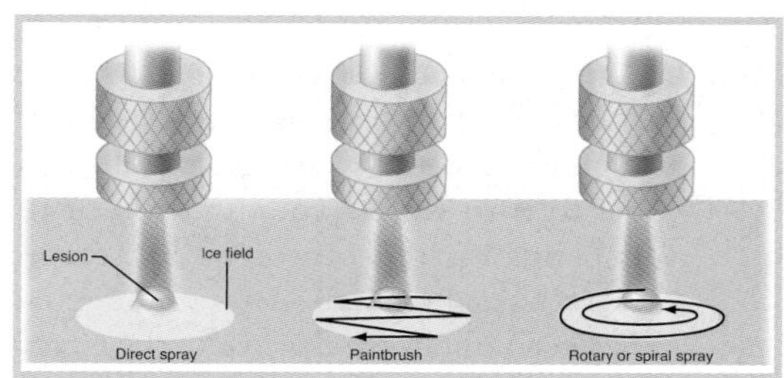

Step 2

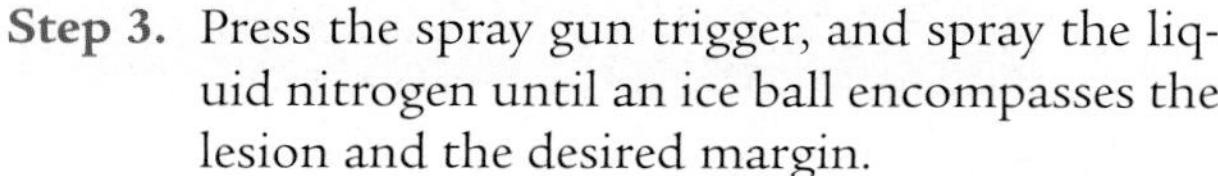

Step 3. Press the spray gun trigger, and spray the liquid nitrogen until an ice ball encompasses the lesion and the desired margin.

- **PEARL:** Ice ball margins for most benign lesions should extend 1 to 2 mm beyond the visible pathologic border. Premalignant lesions need treatment margins of 2 to 3 mm. Malignant lesions require margins of 5 mm of clinically normal skin to ensure adequate depth of treatment.
- **PEARL:** The planned freeze area (with margins) may need to be marked with a skin marker pen before starting the freeze, because freezing may blur the lesion's margin.

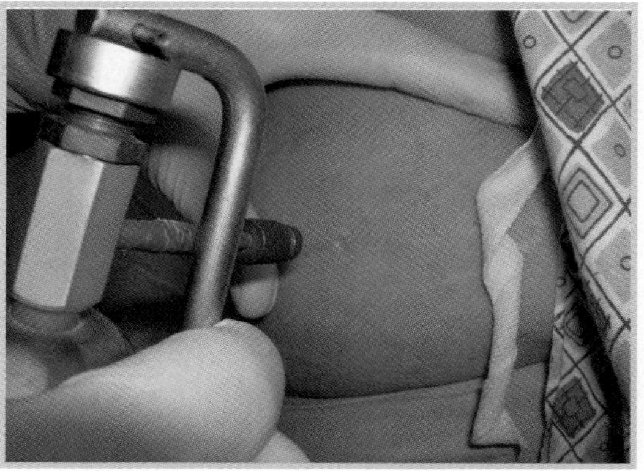

Step 3

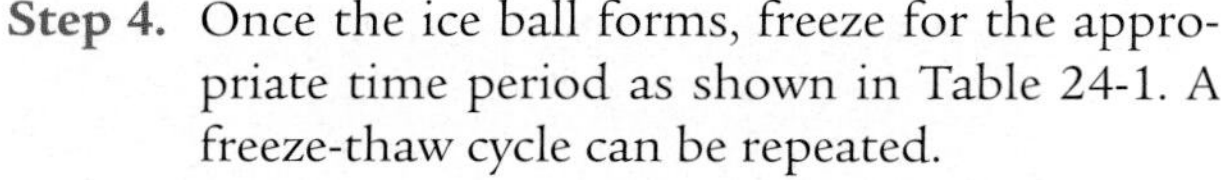

Step 4. Once the ice ball forms, freeze for the appropriate time period as shown in Table 24-1. A freeze-thaw cycle can be repeated.

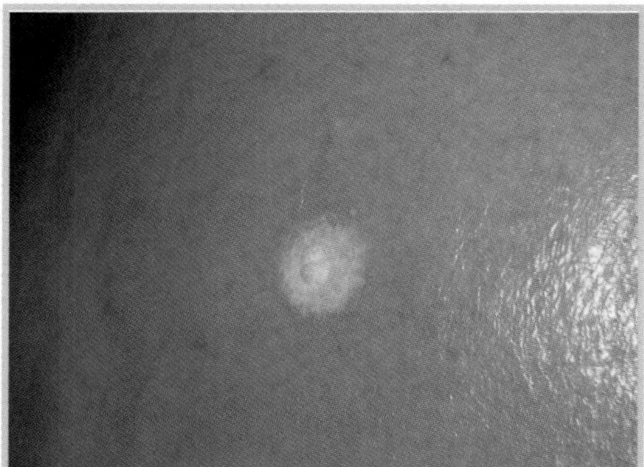

Step 4

Nitrous Oxide or Carbon Dioxide Cryoguns

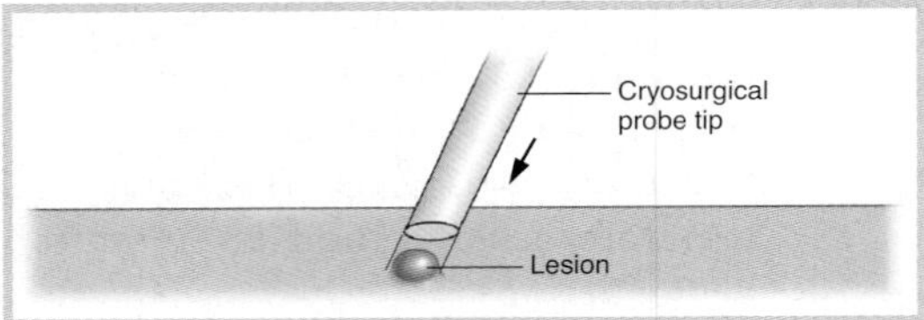

Step 2

Step 2. Select a cryosurgical tip for the procedure that approximates the size of the lesion being treated.

- **PITFALL:** Inadequate treatment of warts using a tip that is too small may result in the formation of a ring wart. Formation of a ring wart does not always imply inadequate treatment, because 5% of properly treated warts result in ring wart formation.
- **PITFALL:** A large, flat tip applied over a small lesion produces excessive tissue destruction and potential scarring.

Step 3. Apply water-soluble gel to the cryotip, and place the tip on the target tissue at ambient (room) temperature. Activate the Cryogun, causing the gel to turn white. The duration of the freeze depends on the time required to produce a proper-sized ice ball. After an adequate freeze has been obtained, deactivate the Cryogun, and allow the probe tip to defrost before disengaging the tip from the target tissue.

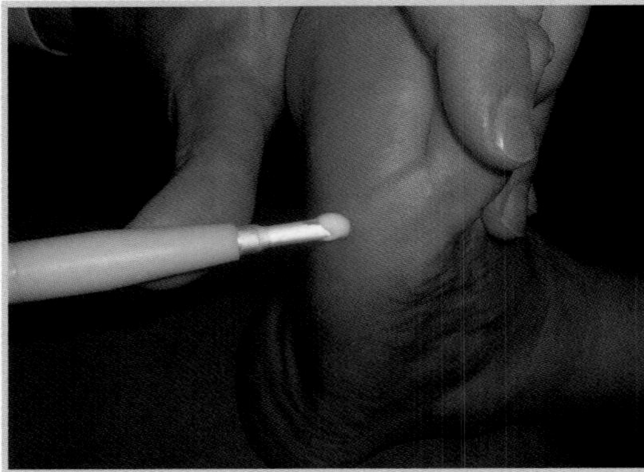

Picture courtesy of Dr. Richard Usatine.

Step 3

- **PITFALL:** Use the size of the ice ball to guide the duration of the procedure. Physicians often use freeze times to guide therapy. Freeze times vary substantially because of factors such as the pressure (amount of refrigerant) in the tank, skin or lesion temperature, and thickness of the lesion.
- **PITFALL:** Do not pull the cryotip off the target tissue before it has defrosted. Withdrawal of applicator tips before defrosting often results in the removal or denuding of the tissue surface.

Forceps Freeze for Small Pedunculated Lesions

Step 2. Pour liquid nitrogen into a disposable polystyrene cup as described previously. Cover the handle of the forceps with a folded 4- × 4-inch gauze to protect the fingers. Then dip the forceps into the liquid nitrogen until it becomes frosted. Pinch the lesion between the tips of the cold forceps until it turns frosty white. Keep the forceps on for an additional 15 seconds and repeat.

- **PEARL:** Lesions will fall off within 1 week and usually heal without problems.
- **PITFALL:** This method is slow and primarily used when few lesions are present.

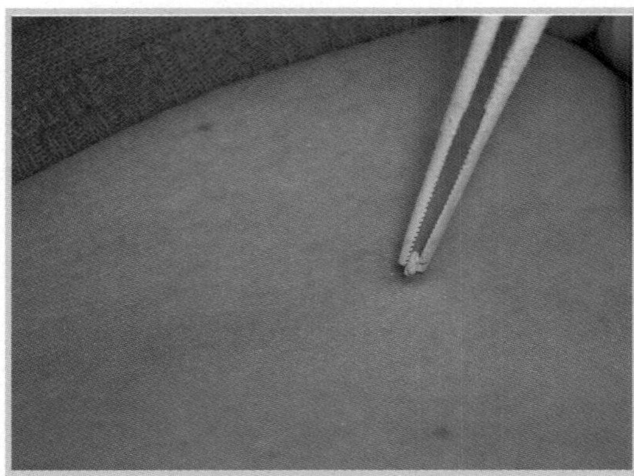

Picture courtesy of Dr. Russell Roberts.

Step 2

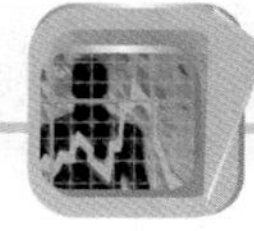

Complications

- Blister formation
- Edema
- Headache (after treatment of facial lesions)
- Pain
- Syncope (vasovagal; rare)
- Bleeding
- Excess granulation tissue formation (rare)
- Infection (rare)
- Atrophy (rare)
- Hypopigmentation
- Hyperpigmentation
- Hypertrophic scarring
- Milia
- Permanent hair loss
- Alteration of sensation
- Temporary, sensory nerve damage (rare)

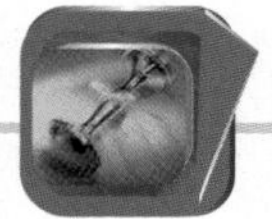

Pediatric Considerations

This treatment is performed in a similar manner in pediatric populations. Consider a topical or injectable anesthetic for younger children, because they are often less tolerant of mild pain.

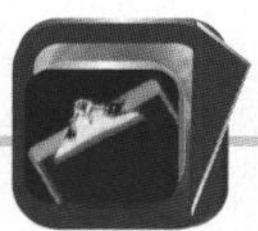

Postprocedure Instructions

Instruct the patient to keep the treated skin clean and to place an antibiotic ointment and bandage on the area after the blister breaks until the wound heals. Because the blister is a sterile bandage that provides moist healing, tell the patient to not open the blister and to allow it to rupture on its own. Have them call your office if the blister becomes painful or drains pus.

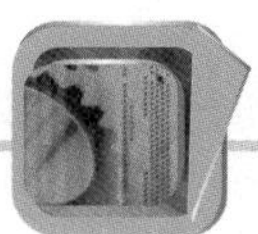

Coding Information and Supply Sources

Specific site treatment codes generally reimburse more than the general codes. Although 17000 and 17003 should be used together when appropriate, 17004 is a stand-alone code for any number beyond 14 lesions and is *not* use with 17000 or 17003.

Note the 17110 to 17111 “destruction of flat warts, molluscum, milia” codes were generalized to “benign lesions.” Destruction performed in certain locations such as penis and vulva can be billed using a specific site destruction code. Malignant lesion destruction (17260 to 17286) provides additional reimbursement when cancerous lesions are ablated.

Office gun applicators, tank units, and hand-held devices can be obtained from these suppliers:

- Wallach Surgical, 235 Edison Road, Orange, CT 06477. Phone: 203-799-2000. Web site: http://www.wallach.com/.
- Brymill Cryogenic Systems, 105 Windermere Avenue, Ellington, CT 06029-3858. Phone: 1-800-777-2796. Web site: http://www.brymill.com/.
- Delasco, 608 13th Avenue, Council Bluffs, IA 51501-6401. Phone: 1-800-831-6273; fax: 1-800-320-9612; e-mail: questions@delasco.com.website: http://www.delasco.com/pcat/1/Cryosurgery/.

CPT Code	Description	2008 Average 50th Percentile Fee	Global Period
11200	Removal (any method) of up to 15 multiple tags, any area	$126.00	10
11201	Removal of each additional 10 lesions (list separately)	$61.00	ZZZ
17000	Destruction benign or premalignant lesion by any method, first lesion (may use *with* 17003)	$102.00	10
17003	Destruction benign or premalignant lesion by any method, 2nd through 14th lesion (list 1 unit for each lesion)	$35.00	ZZZ
17004	Destruction benign or premalignant lesion by any method, ≥15 lesions (do *not* use with 17000 or 17003)	$366.00	10
17110	Destruction (laser, cryo, chemical, surgical) benign lesion other than skin tags or vascular lesions ≤14 lesions	$124.00	10
17111	Destruction benign lesion other than skin tags or vascular lesions by any method, ≥15 lesions	$147.00	10
17260	Destruction malignant lesion by any method TAL ≤0.5 cm	$187.00	10
17261	Destruction malignant lesion by any method TAL 0.6–1 cm	$242.00	10
17262	Destruction malignant lesion by any method TAL 1.1–2 cm	$293.00	10
17263	Destruction malignant lesion by any method TAL 2.1–3 cm	$334.00	10
17264	Destruction malignant lesion by any method TAL 3.1–4 cm	$367.00	10
17266	Destruction malignant lesion by any method TAL >4 cm	$429.00	10
17270	Destruction malignant lesion by any method SNHFG ≤0.5 cm	$236.00	10
17271	Destruction malignant lesion by any method SNHFG 0.6–1 cm	$287.00	10
17272	Destruction malignant lesion by any method SNHFG 1.1–2 cm	$346.00	10
17273	Destruction malignant lesion by any method SNHFG 2.1–3 cm	$396.00	10
17274	Destruction malignant lesion by any method SNHFG 3.1–4 cm	$467.00	10
17276	Destruction malignant lesion by any method SNHFG >4 cm	$550.00	10
17280	Destruction malignant lesion by any method FEENLM ≤0.5 cm	$265.00	10
17281	Destruction malignant lesion by any method FEENLM 0.6–1 cm	$344.00	10
17282	Destruction malignant lesion by any method FEENLM 1.1–2 cm	$403.00	10

CPT Code	Description	2008 Average 50th Percentile Fee	Global Period
17283	Destruction malignant lesion by any method FEENLM 2.1–3 cm	$486.00	10
17284	Destruction malignant lesion by any method FEENLM 3.1–4 cm	$576.00	10
17286	Destruction malignant lesion by any method FEENLM >4 cm	$718.00	10
46916	Destruction of lesion(s), anus (e.g., condyloma, papilloma, molluscum contagiosum, herpetic vesicle), simple; cryosurgery	$424.00	10
46924	Destruction of lesion(s), anus (e.g., condyloma, papilloma, molluscum contagiosum, herpetic vesicle), extensive (e.g., laser surgery, electrosurgery, cryosurgery, chemosurgery)	$1,017.00	10
54050	Destruction of lesion(s), penis (e.g., condyloma, papilloma, molluscum contagiosum, herpetic vesicle), simple; chemical	$245.00	10
54056	Destruction of lesion(s), penis (e.g., condyloma, papilloma, molluscum contagiosum, herpetic vesicle), simple; cryosurgery	$270.00	10
54065	Destruction of lesion(s), penis (e.g., condyloma, papilloma, molluscum contagiosum, herpetic vesicle), extensive (e.g., laser surgery, electrosurgery, cryosurgery, chemosurgery)	$779.00	10
56501	Destruction of lesion(s), vulva; simple (e.g., laser surgery, electrosurgery, cryosurgery, chemosurgery)	$300.00	10
56515	Destruction of lesion(s), vulva; extensive (e.g., laser surgery, electrosurgery, cryosurgery, chemosurgery)	$839.00	10
67850	Destruction of lesion of lid margin (≤1 cm)	$472.00	10

ZZZ, Code related to another service and is always included in the global period of the other service.

CPT is a registered trademark of the American Medical Association.

2008 average 50th Percentile Fees are provided courtesy of 2008 MMH-SI's copyrighted Physicians' Fees and Coding Guide.

TAL, trunk, arms, or legs; SNHFG, scalp, neck, hands, feet, or genitalia; FEENLM, face, ears, eyelids, nose, lips, or mucus membranes.

Patient Education Handout

A patient education handout, "Skin Cryosurgery," can be found on the book's companion Web site.

Bibliography

American Academy of Dermatology Committee on Guidelines of Care. Guidelines of care for cryosurgery. *J Am Acad Dermatol.* 1994;31:648–653.

Andrews MD. Cryosurgery for common skin conditions. *Am Fam Physician*. 2004;69:2365–2372.
Cooper C. Cryotherapy in general practice. *Practitioner.* 2001;245:954–956.
Cryomedics. *Guidelines for Cryosurgery*. Langhorne, PA: Cabot Medical; 1989.
Dawber RP. Cryosurgery: complications and contraindications. *Clin Dermatol.* 1990;8:108–114.
Dinehart SM. Actinic keratoses: scientific evaluation and public health implications. *J Am Acad Dermatol*. 2000;42:S25–S28.
Graham GE. Advances in cryosurgery in the past decade. *Cutis* 1993;52:365–372.
Grealish RJ. Cryosurgery for benign skin lesions. *Fam Pract Recertification J.* 1989;11:21–24.
Hocutt JE. Skin cryosurgery for the family physician. *Am Fam Physician.* 1993;48:445–452.
Kuflik EG: Cryosurgery updated. *J Am Acad Dermatol.* 1994;31(6):925–944; quiz 944–946.
Kuflik EG. Cryosurgery for cutaneous malignancy: an update. *Dermatol Surg.* 1997;23:1081–1087.
Kuwahara RT, Huber JD, Shelley HR. Surgical pearl: forceps method for freezing benign lesion. *J Am Acad Dermatol.* 2000;43:306–307.
Orengo I, Salasche SJ: Surgical pearl: the cotton-tipped applicator—the ever-ready, multipurpose superstar. *J Am Acad Dermatol.* 1994;31(4):658–660.
Torre D. The art of cryosurgery. *Cutis*. 1994;54:354.
Torre D. Cryosurgery of basal cell carcinoma. *J Am Acad Dermatol.* 1986;15:917–929.
Torre D. Cutaneous cryosurgery: current state of the art. *J Dermatol Surg Oncol.* 1985;11:292–293.
Zouboulis CC, Blume U, Buttner P, et al. Outcomes of cryosurgery in keloids and hypertrophic scars: a prospective consecutive trial of case series. *Arch Dermatol.* 1993;129(9):1146–1151.
Zuber TJ. *Office Procedures*. Baltimore: Williams & Wilkins; 1999.
2008 MAG Mutual Healthcare Solutions, Inc.'s Physicians' Fee and Coding Guide. Duluth, Georgia. MAG Mutual Healthcare Solutions, Inc. 2007.

CHAPTER 25

Keloid and Hypertrophic Scar Treatment

E.J. Mayeaux, Jr., MD, DABFP, FAAFP
Professor of Family Medicine, Professor of Obstetrics and Gynecology
Louisiana State University Health Sciences Center, Shreveport, LA

Keloids are benign fibrous scar growths that form because of altered wound healing. These scars are produced with overproduction of extracellular matrix and dermal fibroblasts that have a high mitotic rate. The lesions can be severely disfiguring and painful. *Hypertrophic scars* appear similar to keloids, but they do not extend beyond the margins of the wound. Hypertrophic scars are far less likely to recur once treated.

The precise pathogenesis of keloid formation is unknown, but certain individuals (most commonly of African descent) develop a hyperproliferation of fibroblasts in response to trauma or infection. Any skin damage (including ear piercing, lacerations, and surgery) can cause keloid formation in predisposed individuals. Recurrence after treatment is common.

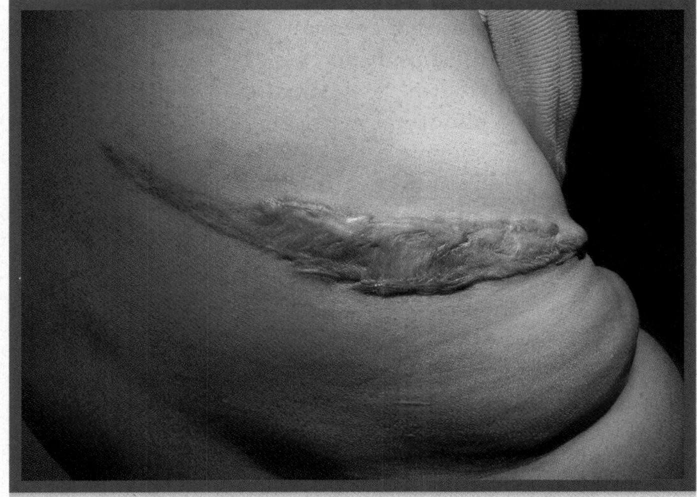

The diagnosis of keloids is based upon the clinical appearance of the lesion. The lesions may be asymptomatic but also may be pruritic, tender to palpation, or occasionally acutely painful. Most commonly, keloids occur on the ears, neck, jaw, presternal chest, shoulders, and upper back. *Acne keloidalis nuchae* refers to a condition resulting in inflamed pustules and papules on the posterior neck that often heal with keloid formation.

The best treatment for keloids is prevention in patients with a known predisposition. This includes preventing unnecessary trauma, such as ear piercing and elective skin surgery, whenever possible. Skin problems that damage the skin in predisposed individuals (e.g., acne, infections) should be treated as early as possible to minimize inflammation. Patients with acne keloidalis nuchae should avoid shaving in the neck region, opting instead for scissors trimming. Multiple medical treatment modalities exist (Table 25-1), and combinations of these therapies are often more effective. The earlier keloids are treated, the more likely it is that they will respond to therapy. However, recurrences are possible despite therapy.

TABLE 25-1. Treatment Options for Keloids and Hypertrophic Scars

Intralesional corticosteroids	Interferon alfa
Excision	Intralesional fluorouracil
Silicone gel sheeting	Intralesional verapamil
Cryosurgery	Laser therapy
Pressure earrings	Imiquimod
Radiation therapy	

Intralesional corticosteroids are the most commonly used therapy for keloids and hypertrophic scars. Seventy percent of patients typically respond to intralesional corticosteroid injection with flattening of keloids, although the recurrence rate may be up to 50% at 5 years. Intralesional therapy has the advantage of delivering the steroid directly into the lesion with minimal systemic effects. The skin also serves as a reservoir, allowing the steroid to act over a period of time. Corticosteroids are diluted prior to injection to minimize patient discomfort and adverse reactions. Saline or lidocaine may be used as a diluent for the corticosteroids. Corticosteroids reduce excessive scarring by reducing collagen synthesis, altering glycosaminoglycan synthesis, reducing production of inflammatory mediators, and reducing fibroblast proliferation. The most commonly used corticosteroid is triamcinolone acetonide (10 to 40 mg/mL) at 4- to 6-week intervals. To dilute a single dose of corticosteroid, it is necessary to gently shake the steroid bottle to resuspend the particles. Normal saline or 1% lidocaine without epinephrine may be used as the diluent. Do not dilute with bupivacaine and other long-acting anesthetics, because the corticosteroid will precipitate in the syringe. Immediately before injecting a lesion, gently shake or roll the syringe to ensure even suspension of the drug in the diluent.

Excision may be used if combined with preoperative, intraoperative, and/or postoperative corticosteroids. Recurrence rates from 45% to 100% have been reported in patients treated with excision alone, but that falls to $<$50% in patients treated with combination therapy. Care should be taken to minimize tension when closing the defect. Postoperative use of imiquimod every other day also may reduce the rate of recurrence.

Silicone gel and sheeting can be used for the management of evolving keloids and the prevention of keloids at the sites of new injuries. It may also be used for the treatment of keloid-related pain and itching. Treatment with silicone gel or sheeting appears to improve elasticity of established abnormal scars, but the evidence is from poor-quality trials. Silicone-gel sheeting and silicone gel are available both by prescription and over the counter. Therapeutic effects appear to be due to a combination of occlusion and hydration, rather than from an effect of the silicone. The sheeting is clear and sticky and should be cut to fit the size of the keloid. It is placed on top of the keloid, taped into place, and left on for 12 to 24 hours per day. The sheet is washed daily and replaced every 10 to 14 days. Effectiveness is judged after a minimum of 2 months of therapy.

Cryosurgery may be used alone or in combination with other treatment modalities. The major side effect is permanent hypopigmentation, which limits its use in darker-skinned patients. Cryosurgery affects the microvasculature and causes cell damage via intracellular crystals, leading to tissue anoxia. Generally, one, two, or three freeze-thaw cycles lasting 10 to 30 seconds each are used. Therapy is repeated once per month until a response occurs. Apply the liquid nitrogen in short application periods because of the possibility of reversible hypopigmentation. Cryotherapy can cause pain and permanent depigmentation in some patients. It combines well as a pretreatment with corticosteroid therapy.

Radiation therapy is highly successful in reducing keloid recurrence, particularly following surgical excision. However, the long-term risk of malignancy from radiation therapy does not justify its use for an essentially benign disorder. It is occasionally used for keloids that are resistant to other therapies and that are unresectable.

Topical imiquimod cream may reduce short-term recurrence postexcision. Mild irritation may be experienced with application of imiquimod, but it otherwise has few side effects. Hyperpigmentation was experienced by more than half of the patients in the study.

Pulsed dye laser treatment can be beneficial for keloids and appears to induce keloid regression through suppression of keloid fibroblast proliferation and induction of apoptosis and enzyme activity. Combination treatment with pulsed dye laser plus intralesional therapy with corticosteroids and/or fluorouracil may be superior to any of the therapies alone. Intralesional fluorouracil (5-FU), interferon alfa, doxorubicin (Adriamycin), or bleomycin may be of benefit for keloids. Some of the drugs can be used in combination with intralesional corticosteroids.

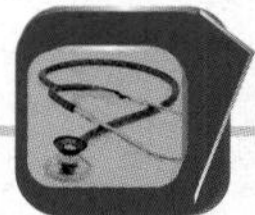

Equipment

- A Luer-Lok (twist-on) syringe (1 cc) with 27- or 30-gauge needle
- Nonsterile gloves
- Alcohol swab
- Gauze, 4 × 4 inches
- Protective eyewear

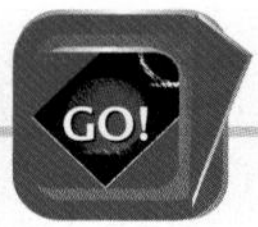

Indications

- Painful or unsightly keloids or hypertrophic scars

Contraindications (Relative)

- Local infection
- Severe bleeding disorders
- Extreme illness that would make wound healing difficult
- Cellulitis in the tissues to be incised
- Conditions that may interfere with wound healing (collagen vascular diseases, smoking, diabetes)
- Concurrent medications that may increase the likelihood of intraoperative bleeding (aspirin, other nonsteroidal anti-inflammatory drugs, warfarin)
- Uncooperative patient

The Procedure

Cryotherapy

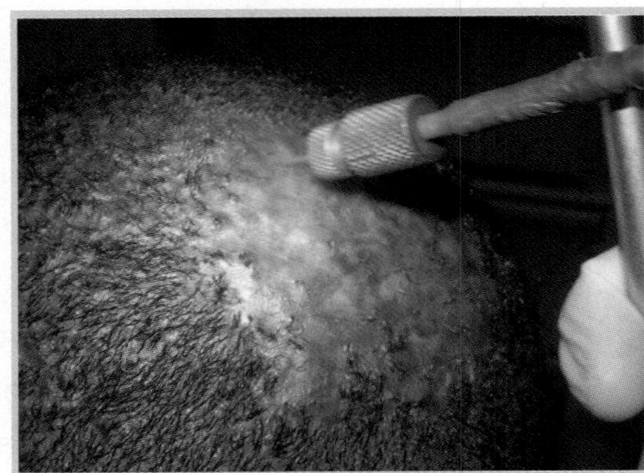

Step 1

Step 1. Apply liquid nitrogen for 10- to 30-second cycles up to three times. Repeat the therapy once per month until response occurs.

- **PITFALL:** Apply the liquid nitrogen in short application periods because of the risk of reversible hypopigmentation or permanent depigmentation in some patients.

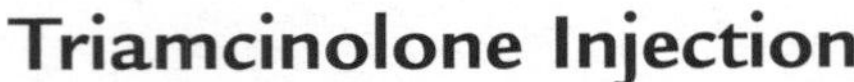

Triamcinolone Injection

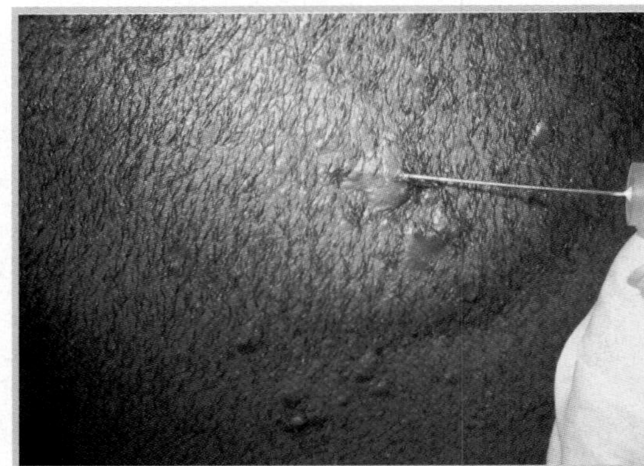

Step 1

Step 1. Consider using eutectic mixture of local anesthetics (EMLA) cream under occlusion for 1.5 hours before injection or pretreatment by applying apply liquid nitrogen for 10 to 30 seconds. Prepare the skin with alcohol. Using a 27- or 30-gauge needle with the bevel directed up toward the skin, inject enough triamcinolone to make the skin rise slightly and the keloid blanch (usually 0.1 to 0.5 mL). Inject into the keloid as the needle is withdrawn from the skin. One-mL syringes are most frequently used because the quantity of medication delivered is usually in the tenths or even hundredths of a milliliter.

- **PITFALL:** Be sure that the injection occurs in the bulk of the lesion and not underneath it, or lipoatrophy may occur. This is easy to recognize because the injected solution flows easily into subcutaneous fat, whereas resistance is felt when it is correctly injected into dermis.
- **PEARL:** Protective eyewear is strongly advised.

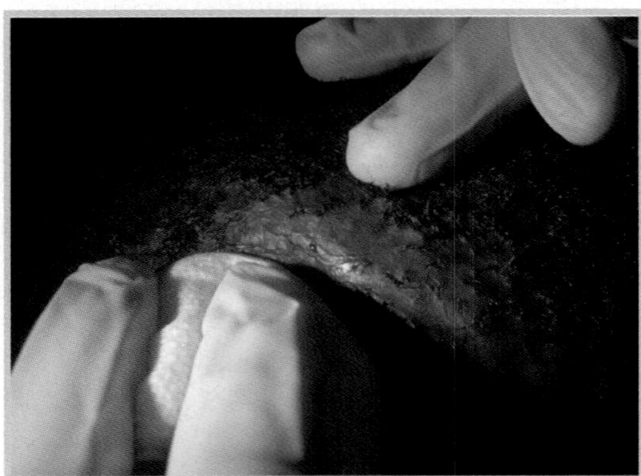

Step 2

Step 2. Be careful not to inject steroid into or immediately underneath the epidermis, because this increases the risk of hypopigmentation. If this occurs, usually resulting from continued pressure on the syringe plunger as the needle exits the skin, gently milk the superficially placed steroid out of the injection hole.

Step 3. For large lesions, the needle should be withdrawn partially and redirected to cover additional areas, or the needle can be removed and reinserted in another site.

- **PITFALL:** Caution is needed to avoid injecting into subcutaneous tissue.
- **PITFALL:** Do not exceed 40 mg of the drug per visit; atrophy and hypopigmentation may occur at higher doses.

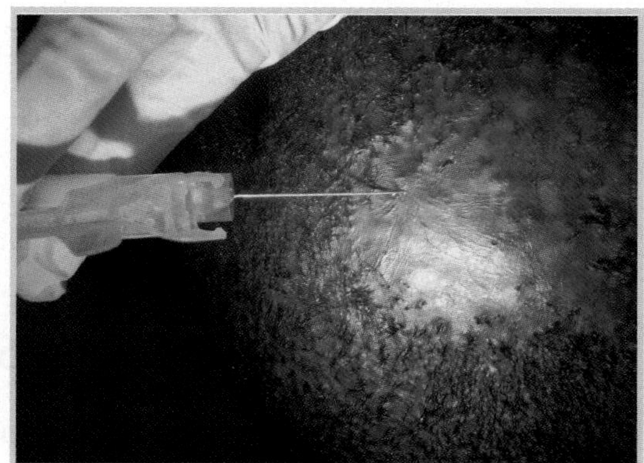

Step 3

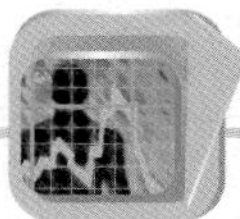

Complications

- Systemic absorption, with potential worsening of control for diabetic patients
- Burning sensation for up to 3 to 5 minutes after injection
- Local skin atrophy
- Hypopigmentation (temporary or permanent)
- Telangiectasia formation
- Sterile abscess formation

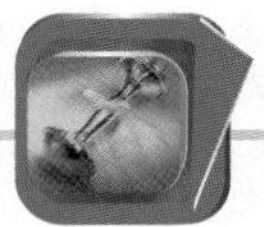

Pediatric Considerations

Keloids are less common in children, but when they occur, the procedure is essentially the same. Consider the use of an occluded topical anesthetic to decrease the pain of injection in children.

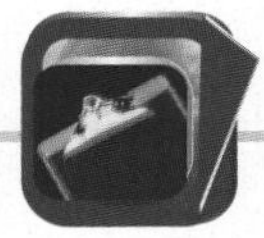

Postprocedure Instructions

Injections can be repeated at monthly intervals. Some providers increase the concentration of triamcinolone by 10 mg/mL each visit on nonfacial lesions until the lesion softens and flattens, then decrease the strength of injections. Keloids often need multiple treatments 3 to 4 weeks apart until there is adequate flattening of the lesion. Surgical excision is recommended if there is no response after four injections.

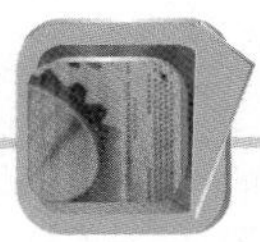

Coding Information and Supply Sources

CPT Code	Description	2008 Average 50th Percentile Fee	Global Period
11900	Injection, intralesional, ≤7 lesions (report once)	$86.00	0
11901	Injection, intralesional, >7 lesions (report once)	$117.00	0

CPT is a registered trademark of the American Medical Association.
2008 average 50th Percentile Fees are provided courtesy of 2008 MMH-SI's copyrighted Physicians' Fees and Coding Guide.

ICD-9 Code

Keloid scar 701.4

Suppliers

Recommended supplies and sources may be found in Appendix I.

Patient Education Handout

A patient education handout, "Keloids," can be found on the book's companion Web site.

Bibliography

Al-Attar A, Mess S, Thomassen JM, et al. Keloid pathogenesis and treatment. *Plast Reconstr Surg.* 2006;117:286–300.

Alster TS. Laser treatment of hypertrophic scars, keloids, and striae. *Dermatol Clin.* 1997;15:419.

Berman B, Bieley HC. Adjunct therapies to surgical management of keloids. *Dermatol Surg.* 1996; 22:126.

Berman B, Flores F. Comparison of a silicone gel-filled cushion and silicon gel sheeting for the treatment of hypertrophic or keloid scars. *Dermatol Surg.* 1999;25:484.

English RS, Shenefelt PD. Keloids and hypertrophic scars. *Dermatol Surg.* 1999;25:631.

Gold MH. Topical silicone gel sheeting in the treatment of hypertrophic scars and keloids: a dermatologic experience. *J Dermatol Surg Oncol.* 1993;19:912.

Hirshowitz B, Lerner D, Moscona AR. Treatment of keloid scars by combined cryosurgery and intralesional corticosteroids. *Aesthetic Plast Surg.* 1982;6:153.

Leventhal D, Furr M, Reiter D. Treatment of keloids and hypertrophic scars: a meta-analysis and review of the literature. *Arch Facial Plast Surg.* 2006;8:362–368.

Nanda S, Reddy BS. Intralesional 5-fluorouracil as a treatment modality of keloids. *Dermatol Surg.* 2004;30:54.

Nemeth AJ. Keloids and hypertrophic scars. *J Dermatol Surg Oncol.* 1993;19:738.

Shaffer JJ, Taylor SC, Cook-Bolden F. Keloidal scars: a review with a critical look at therapeutic options. *J Am Acad Dermatol.* 2002;46:S63.

Slemp AE, Kirschner RE. Keloids and scars: a review of keloids and scars, their pathogenesis, risk factors, and management. *Curr Opin Pediatr.* 2006;18:396–402.

Zouboulis CC, Blume U, Buttner P, et al. Outcomes of cryosurgery in keloids and hypertrophic scars: a prospective consecutive trial of case series. *Arch Dermatol.* 1993;129:1146.

Zurada JM, Kriegel D, Davis IC. Topical treatments for hypertrophic scars. *J Am Acad Dermatol.* 2006;55:1024.

2008 MAG Mutual Healthcare Solutions, Inc.'s Physicians' Fee and Coding Guide. Duluth, Georgia. MAG Mutual Healthcare Solutions, Inc. 2007.

CHAPTER 26

Earlobe Keloid Excision

E.J. Mayeaux, Jr., MD, DABFP, FAAFP

Professor of Family Medicine, Professor of Obstetrics and Gynecology
Louisiana State University Health Sciences Center, Shreveport, LA

Keloids are benign, hard, persistent fibrous proliferations that develop in predisposed persons at sites of cutaneous injury. These deposits of collagen expand beyond the original size and shape of the wound, frequently invading the surrounding skin. Keloids are thought to develop from abnormalities in the synthesis and degradation of collagen.

Earlobe keloids usually appear as shiny, smooth, globular growths on one or both sides of the earlobe. Ear piercing is the most common cause, but other causes include trauma, surgical procedures, and burns. Patients with earlobe keloids usually complain of the cosmetic abnormality, but they may also report pruritus, pain, or paresthesias. Patients may be extremely embarrassed about this condition, and some persons consider keloids to be a major deformity.

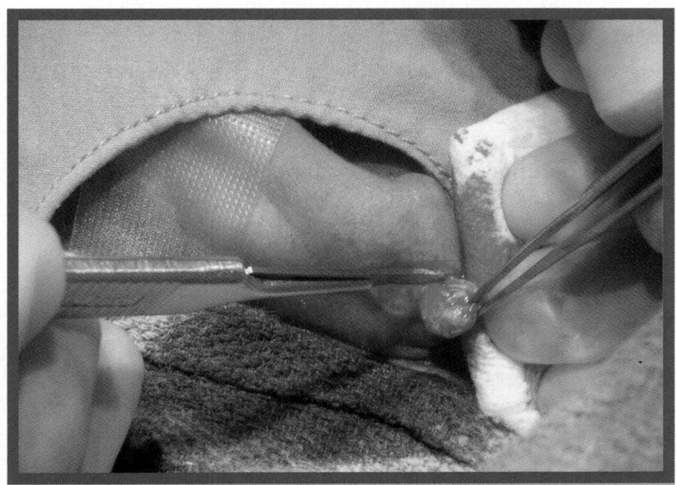

Dumbbell-shaped keloids often distort the pinna. They grow through the pierced ear tract and protrude from both sides of the earlobe. Keloids that are limited to one side of the pinna more commonly appear on the posterior surface of the earlobe. Factors attributable to the piercing technique, allergy to the metal in the earring fastener, or infection behind the ear may explain the increased frequency of posterior growths.

Multiple therapeutic options are available for the treatment of keloids. The location, size, and depth of the keloid, as well as the length of time the keloid has been present, influence the choice of therapy. Combination therapy appears to be the most effective, although there are few comparative studies. Surgical excision, combined with corticosteroid injections and pressure therapy, is the mainstay of therapy for earlobe keloids.

Keloids may be softened and flattened by intralesional corticosteroid therapy. Corticosteroids act on the keloids by producing changes in the ground substance and increasing collagen degradation. Small lesions may be treated using corticosteroid injection as monotherapy. Larger keloids may be softened using corticosteroids, either to relieve pain or as the initial therapy before surgery. Triamcinolone acetonide (10 mg/mL or 40 mg/mL mixed with an equal amount of 1% or 2% lidocaine) is frequently used. A Luer-Lok (twist-on) syringe should be used to administer the injection to prevent separation of the needle when injecting under pressure into a hard keloid. Some providers provide preoperative injections every 3 to 4 weeks for 2 months. Postoperative injections are administered for periods of weeks to months, depending on the patient's clinical progress.

Pressure therapy may be an effective treatment for keloids of the ear following piercing. Pressure earrings, also called Zimmer splints, are splints that are inexpensive and molded to the appropriate size, cosmetically altered to appear as earrings. Simple aluminum finger splints may also be cut, folded, and clamped to the earlobe. The patient may reapply these splints every evening.

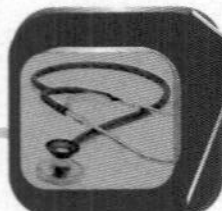

Equipment

- A 1-cc Luer-Lok (twist-on) syringe with 27- or 30-gauge needle
- Nonsterile gloves
- An alcohol swab
- Gauze, 4 × 4 inches
- Protective eyewear

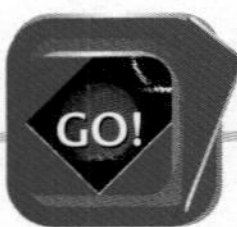

Indications

- Painful or unsightly earlobe keloids

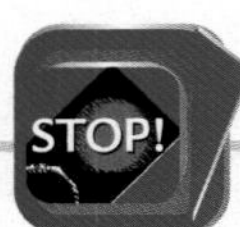

Contraindications (Relative)

- Local infection
- Severe bleeding disorders
- Extreme illness that would make wound healing difficult
- Cellulitis in the tissues to be incised
- Conditions that may interfere with wound healing (collagen vascular diseases, smoking, diabetes)
- Concurrent medications that may increase the likelihood of intraoperative bleeding (aspirin, other nonsteroidal anti-inflammatory drugs, warfarin)
- Uncooperative patient

The Procedure

Core Excision Technique

Step 1. Skin closure is designed to minimize distortion of the earlobe contour and make the lobes look as similar as possible. Inject local anesthetic into the lobe (see Chapter 1), or administer a triamcinolone/lidocaine combination as the local anesthetic. Prep the skin with povidone-iodine or chlorhexidine solution, and allow it to dry (see Appendix E).

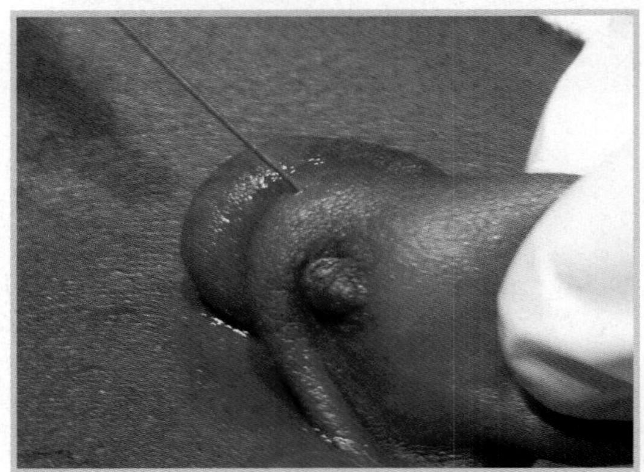

Step 1

- **PEARL:** Prep a wide area so that an undraped area is not inadvertently exposed if the drape slides a little.
- **PEARL:** If the keloid is only in the posterior side, the pinna may be taped over to facilitate removal.

Step 2. Drape the area. Perform a fusiform (elliptical) excision around the base of the keloid. Feel the base of the excision to see if the keloid has formed a "core" or keloid band along the pierced path through the ear. Some providers excise the core, while others leave it in place and inject it with steroids. Other providers will incise the most inferior portion of earlobe creating a V-shape wedge and then close the earlobe.

- **PEARL:** Placing a cotton ball in the external ear canal will prevent blood from draining into the canal.
- **PEARL:** Bleeding is common during earlobe keloid excisions. Although closure and pressure clamping will stop most of the minor bleeding, active bleeders need to be addressed by direct pressure or short-term clamping with hemostats.

Step 3. Using gentle tissue handling, close the defect with fine, simple, interrupted, nonabsorbable, monofilament sutures.

- **PITFALL:** Absorbable sutures should be avoided, because nonabsorbable sutures such as 5-0 nylon may cause less tissue reaction.

Step 4. With both techniques, triamcinolone/lidocaine (without epinephrine) combination can be administered as an injection immediately after surgery if it was not used as the anesthetic solution. Apply ointment to the incision and place a clean gauze over the site.

Step 5. A simple pressure device may be made by taking aluminum finger splints and cutting, folding, and clamping the splint to the earlobe.

- **PEARL:** Leakage of the steroid from the wound can be reduced by applying tape over the incision site.

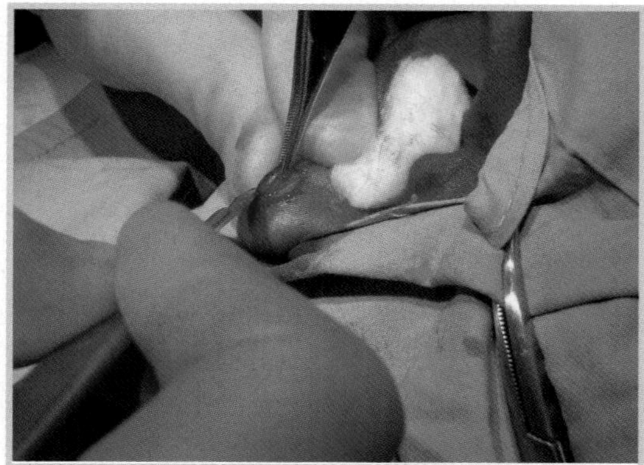

Step 2

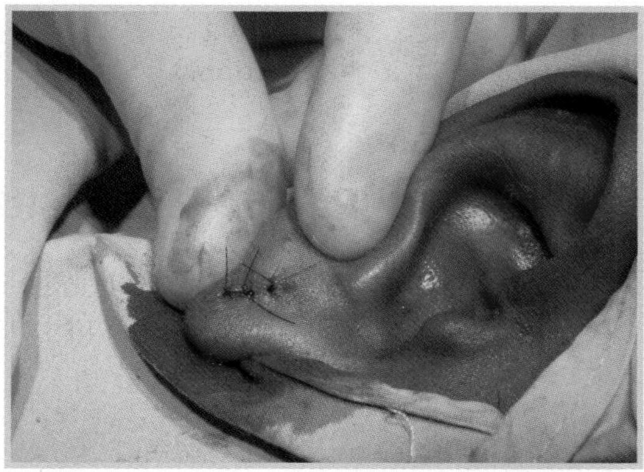

Step 3

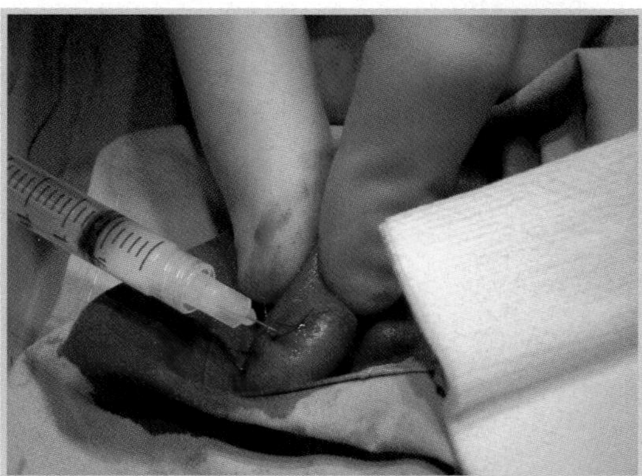

Step 4

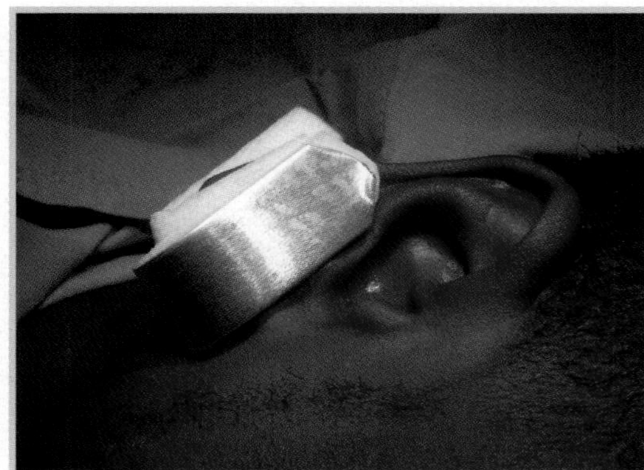

Step 5

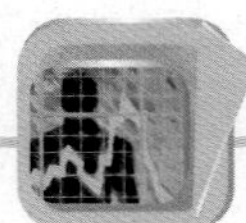

Complications

- Systemic absorption of steroid, with potential worsening of control for diabetic patients
- Burning sensation for up to 3 to 5 minutes after injection
- Local skin atrophy
- Hypopigmentation (temporary or permanent)
- Telangiectasia formation
- Sterile abscess formation
- Reformation of keloid
- Bleeding
- Infection

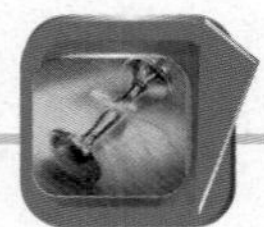

Pediatric Considerations

Keloids are less common in children, but when they occur, the procedure is essentially the same. Consider the use of an occluded topical anesthetic to decrease the pain of injection in children.

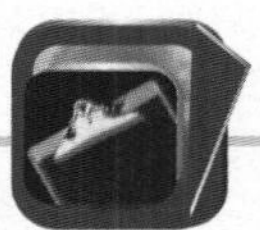

Postprocedure Instructions

Injections can be repeated at monthly intervals. Some providers increase the concentration of triamcinolone by 10 mg/mL each visit on nonfacial lesions until the lesion softens and flattens, then decrease the strength of injections. Keloids often need multiple treatments 3 to 4 weeks apart until there is adequate flattening of the lesion.

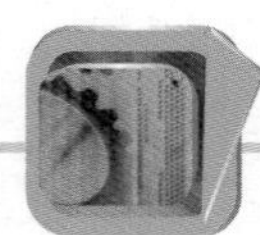

Coding Information and Supply Sources

If a lesion is removed, use the "excision—benign lesion" codes (11400 to 11471).

CPT Code	Description	2008 Average 50th Percentile Fee	Global Period
11900	Injection, intralesional, ≤7 lesions (report once)	$86.00	0
11901	Injection, intralesional, >7 lesions (report once)	$117.00	0
11400	Benign excision TAL <0.6 cm	$178.00	10
11401	Benign excision TAL 0.6–1.0 cm	$226.00	10
11402	Benign excision TAL 1.1–2.0 cm	$289.00	10
11403	Benign excision TAL 2.1–3.0 cm	$347.00	10
11404	Benign excision TAL 3.1–4.0 cm	$441.00	10
11406	Benign excision TAL >4.0 cm	$627.00	10
11420	Benign excision SNHFG <0.6 cm	$179.00	10
11421	Benign excision SNHFG 0.6–1.0 cm	$233.00	10
11422	Benign excision SNHFG 1.1–2.0 cm	$285.00	10
11423	Benign excision SNHFG 2.1–3.0 cm	$385.00	10
11424	Benign excision SNHFG 3.1–4.0 cm	$481.00	10
11426	Benign excision SNHFG >4.0 cm	$683.00	10
11440	Benign excision FEENLMM <0.6 cm	$221.00	10
11441	Benign excision FEENLMM 0.6–1.0 cm	$289.00	10
11442	Benign excision FEENLMM 1.1-2.0 cm	$356.00	10
11443	Benign excision FEENLMM 2.1–3.0 cm	$450.00	10
11444	Benign excision FEENLMM 3.1–4.0 cm	$556.00	10
11446	Benign excision FEENLMM >4.0 cm	$756.00	10

CPT is a registered trademark of the American Medical Association.
2008 average 50th Percentile Fees are provided courtesy of 2008 MMH-SI's copyrighted Physicians' Fees and Coding Guide.
TAL, trunk, arms, or legs; SNHFG, scalp, neck, hands, feet, or genitalia; FEENLMM, face, ears, eyelids, nose, lips, and mucous membranes.

ICD-9 Code

Keloid scar 701.4

Suppliers

Recommended supplies and sources may be found in Appendix I.

Bibliography

Brent B. The role of pressure therapy in management of earlobe keloids: preliminary report of a controlled study. *Ann Plast Surg.* 1978;1:579–581.

Cheng LH. Keloid of the ear lobe. *Laryngoscope.* 1972;82:673–681.

Golladay ES. Treatment of keloids by single intraoperative perilesional injection of repository steroid. *South Med J.* 1988;81:736–738.
Hirshowitz B, Lerner D, Moscona AR. Treatment of keloid scars by combined cryosurgery and intralesional corticosteroids. *Aesthetic Plast Surg.* 1982;6:153–158.
Jackson IT, Bhageshpur R, DiNick V, et al. Investigation of recurrence rates among earlobe keloids utilizing various postoperative therapeutic modalities. *Eur JPlast Surg.* 2001;24:8–95.
Kelly AP. Surgical treatment of keloids secondary to ear piercing. *J Natl Med Assoc.* 1978;70:349–350.
Pollack SV, Goslen JB. The surgical treatment of keloids. *J Dermatol Surg Oncol.* 1982;8:1045–1049.
Rauscher GE, Kolmer WL. Treatment of recurrent earlobe keloids. *Cutis* 1986;37:67–68.
Russell R, Horlock N, Gault D. Zimmer splintage: a simple effective treatment for keloids following ear-piercing. *Br J Plast Surg.* 2001;54:509.
Salasche SJ, Grabski W. Keloids of the earlobes: a surgical technique. *J Dermatol Surg Oncol.* 1983;9:552–956.
Stashower ME. Successful treatment of earlobe keloids with imiquimod after tangential shave excision. *Dermatol Surg.* 2006;32(3):380–386.
Stucker FJ, Shaw GY. An approach to management of keloids. *Arch Otolaryngol Head Neck Surg.* 1992;118:63–67.
Weimar VM, Ceilley RI. Treatment of keloids on earlobes. *J Dermatol Surg Oncol.* 1979;5:591–593.
Zuber TJ, DeWitt DE. Earlobe keloids. *Am Fam Phys.* 1994;49(8):1835–1841.
2008 MAG Mutual Healthcare Solutions, Inc.'s Physicians' Fee and Coding Guide. Duluth, Georgia. MAG Mutual Healthcare Solutions, Inc. 2007.

CHAPTER 27

Punch Biopsy of the Skin

E.J. Mayeaux, Jr., MD, DABFP, FAAFP

Professor of Family Medicine, Professor of Obstetrics and Gynecology
Louisiana State University Health Sciences Center, Shreveport, LA

Punch biopsy is one of the most widely used dermatologic procedures in primary care medicine. This technique obtains a full-thickness skin specimen for histologic assessment. A properly performed punch biopsy frequently yields useful diagnostic information. The technique is simple, rapid, and generally results in an acceptable final cosmetic appearance at the site.

Punch biopsy is performed with a circular blade known as a trephine, which is attached to a pencil-like handle. The instrument is rotated using downward pressure until the blade penetrates into the subcutaneous fat. A cylindrical core of tissue is then cut free and placed in formalin for transfer to the laboratory. Most 3- or 4-mm punch biopsy sites are closed with a single suture. The 2-mm punch biopsy sites frequently do not require suture closure, and Monsel solution can be used for hemostasis if the wound is allowed to granulate.

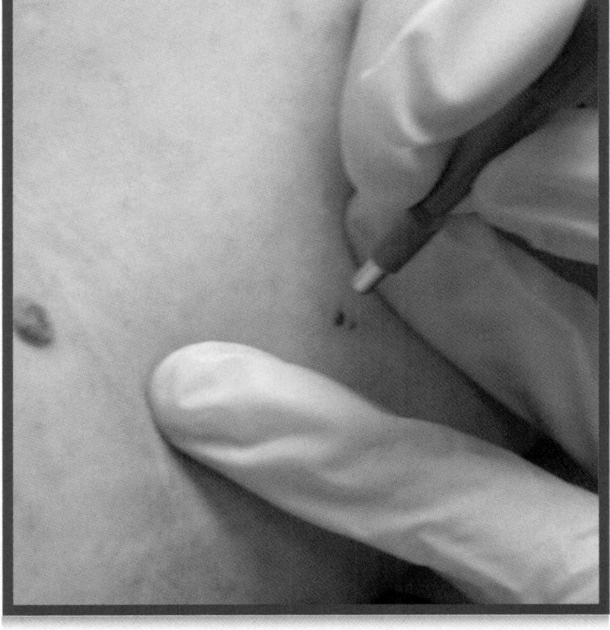

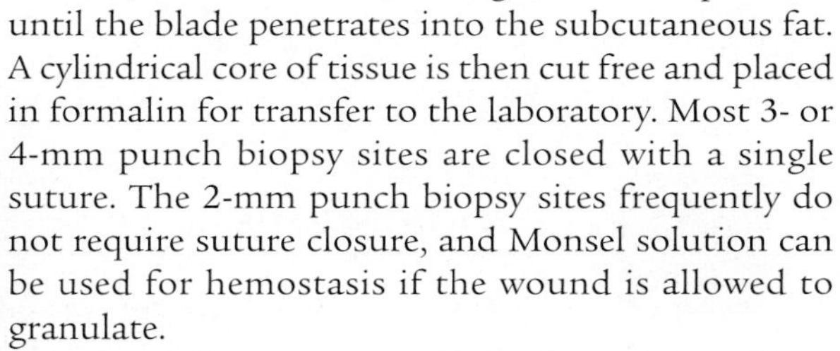

Punch biopsy is generally performed to evaluate lesions of uncertain origin or to confirm or exclude the presence of malignancy. This biopsy technique is considered the method of choice for many flat lesions. Suspected melanomas can be evaluated by this technique, especially when the lesion is too large for easy removal. The yield may be improved if the most suspicious or abnormal-appearing area (darkest, most raised, or most irregular contour) is biopsied. If the suspicion for melanoma is high, some experts feel that it is preferable to perform excisional biopsy to have the entire lesion available for evaluation. Physicians should not fear performing punch biopsy on a melanoma, because the biopsy does not alter the natural course of the disease, and a prompt biopsy expedites definitive treatment.

Punch biopsy used for basal and squamous cell carcinoma has one disadvantage. After these cancers have been diagnosed using the punch technique, the physician is then obligated to perform a definitive full-thickness excisional technique. Superficial techniques that may be employed for these lesions, such as curettage and electrodesiccation, may miss cells that have been driven deeper by the punch instrument.

Providers should be aware of the underlying anatomy when performing a punch biopsy. Certain areas of the body where there is little subcutaneous tissue pose the greatest threat of damaging underlying structures such as arteries, tendons, or nerves. Punch biopsy on the upper cheek can damage the facial or trigeminal nerves, and punch biopsy of the lateral digits or of the thin eyelids should be approached with great caution.

Select the best site for the biopsy. Perform the punch biopsy at the most abnormal appearing site within the most abnormal-appearing solid lesion, except in sclerotic (scarring) lesions which should be biopsied on the leading edge. Tumors of the skin should be biopsied in the center of the lesion, and bullous lesions, ulcers, and sclerotic lesions should be biopsied at the edge. Do not biopsy lesions that have been traumatized, scratched, or significantly modified because biopsy of a traumatized lesion rarely provides useful information. Provide the pathologist with information on the age and sex of the patient, current medications, appearance of the lesion, body location, and suspected diagnosis to increase the chance of gaining useful clinical information from the biopsy.

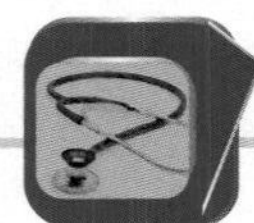

Equipment

- The punch biopsy instrument (trephine) has a plastic, pencil-like handle and a circular scalpel blade. The blade attaches to the handle at the hub of the instrument.
- Basic setup for this procedure includes local anesthesia (1 to 3 mL of anesthetic), the punch biopsy instrument, and sharp iris scissors to cut the specimen free. If the specimen cannot be lifted using the anesthesia needle, Adson pickups without teeth may be used to lift the specimen.
- Suggested suture removal times are listed in Appendix J. A suggested anesthesia tray that can be used for this procedure is listed in Appendix F. Skin preparation recommendations appear in Appendix E.

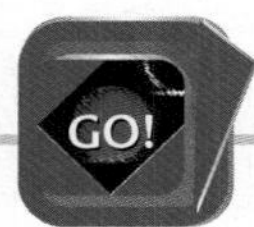

Indications

- Evaluation of skin tumors such as basal cell carcinoma or Kaposi sarcoma
- Diagnosis of bullous skin disorders such as pemphigus vulgaris
- Diagnosis of inflammatory skin disorders such as discoid lupus
- Removal of small skin lesions such as intradermal nevi
- Diagnosis of atypical-appearing lesions such as atypical mycobacterial infection

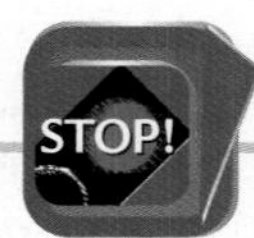

Contraindications

- Lesions overlying anatomic structures likely to be damaged by full-thickness skin biopsy: on the eyelid (globe), on the dorsum of the hand in elderly patients (tendons), on the upper cheek (facial nerve), or on fingers (digital nerves and arteries) (relative contraindication)
- Subcutaneous lesions that cannot be reached with the punch instrument (erythema nodosum)
- Foot and toe lesions in elderly patients or those with peripheral vascular disease

The Procedure

Step 1. Select a punch biopsy instrument of sufficient size (i.e., 3 or 5 mm) to obtain adequate tissue for histologic assessment while minimizing the size of the scar (i.e., 3-mm instrument for biopsy on the face).

- **PEARL:** With small lesions, a punch that is slightly larger than the lesion can remove the entire lesion with the biopsy.

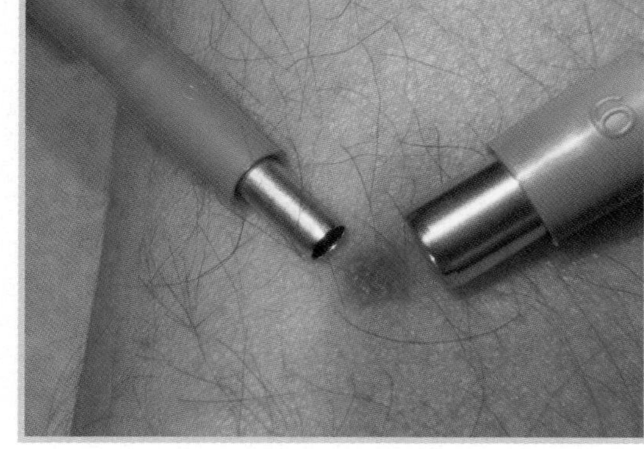

Step 1

Step 2. Perform an intradermal injection of anesthesia (see Chapter 1). Prep the skin with povidone-iodine or chlorhexidine solution, and allow it to dry (see Appendix B: Lines of Lesser Skin Tension (Langer)).

- **PEARL:** Prep a wide area so that an undraped area is not inadvertently exposed if the drape slides a little.

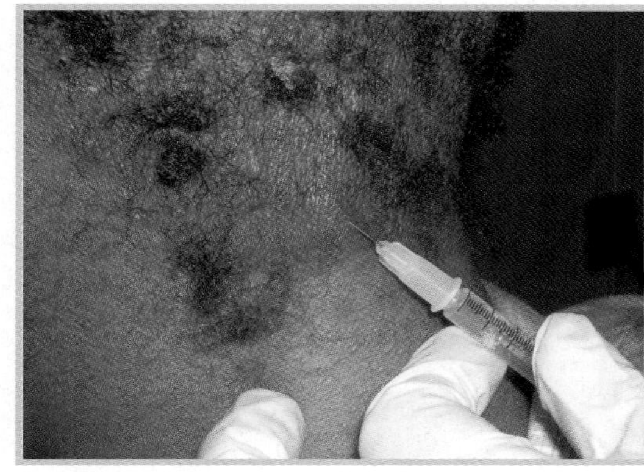

Step 2

Step 3. Prepare for the closure of the punch biopsy site when performing the technique. A circular defect is not easily closed, but an oval or elliptical defect approximates well. After the administration of local anesthesia, stretch the skin *perpendicular* to the lines of least skin tension using the nondominant hand (see Appendix B). After the punch biopsy is performed, relax the nondominant hand, and the circular defect becomes more oval.

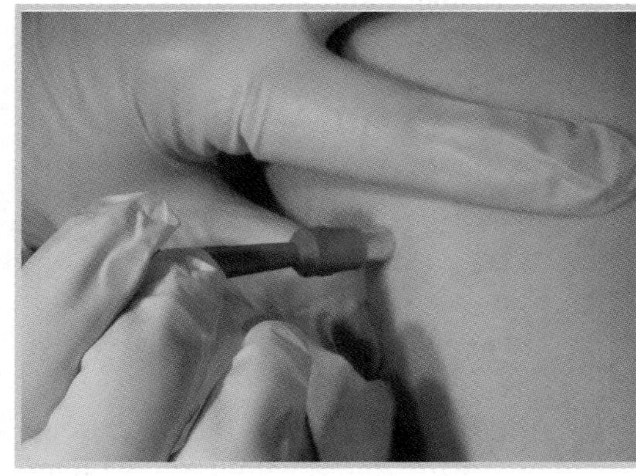

Step 3

Step 4. Rotate the punch biopsy instrument with downward force when performing the biopsy. Turn the blade around its center axis with a back-and-forth motion until the instrument traverses the full thickness of the skin. Be prepared to stop the downward pressure as soon as the instrument penetrates through the skin. When the trephine penetrates the skin into the subcutaneous fat, the operator often notices a "give."

- **PITFALL:** Historically, physicians were instructed to insert the instrument up to the hub. Going to the hub is appropriate where the skin is thick (e.g., upper back) but can damage underlying structures such as nerves or tendons where the skin and subcutaneous tissue is thin. Do not push the instrument to the hub when performing punch biopsy on the upper cheek, nose, or dorsum of the hand.

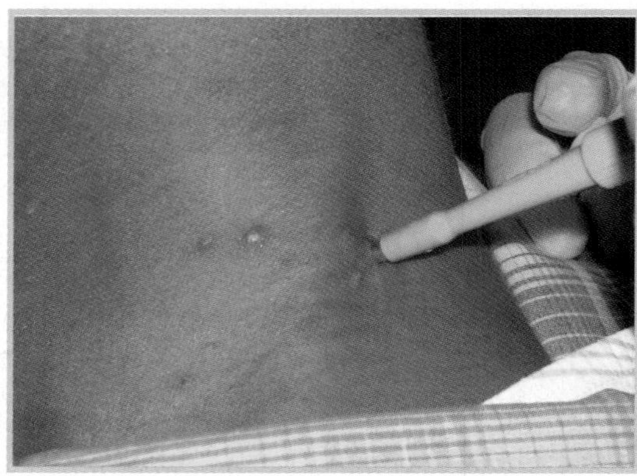

Step 4

Step 5. Lift the specimen with the needle used to anesthetize the skin site, and then cut it free at the base (beneath the dermis) using scissors if necessary.

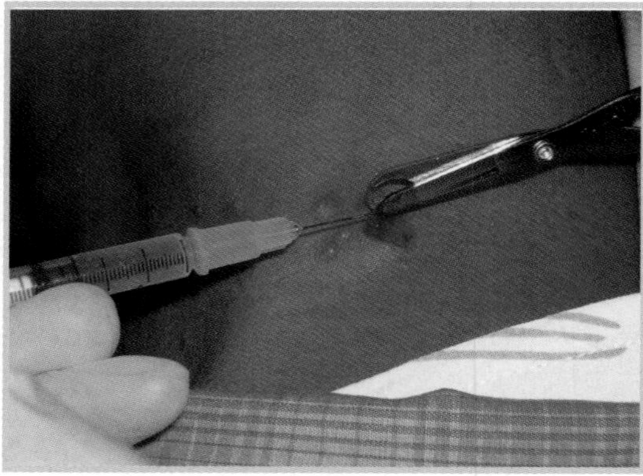

Step 5

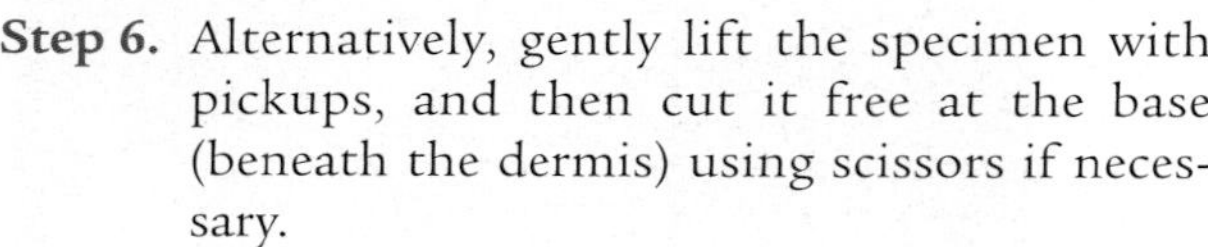

Step 6. Alternatively, gently lift the specimen with pickups, and then cut it free at the base (beneath the dermis) using scissors if necessary.

- **PITFALL:** Many pathologists refuse to examine a skin biopsy specimen that has been crushed. Punch biopsy specimens often are crushed when they are elevated using Adson forceps. Elevate the specimen with the anesthesia needle to avoid crushing the artifact.

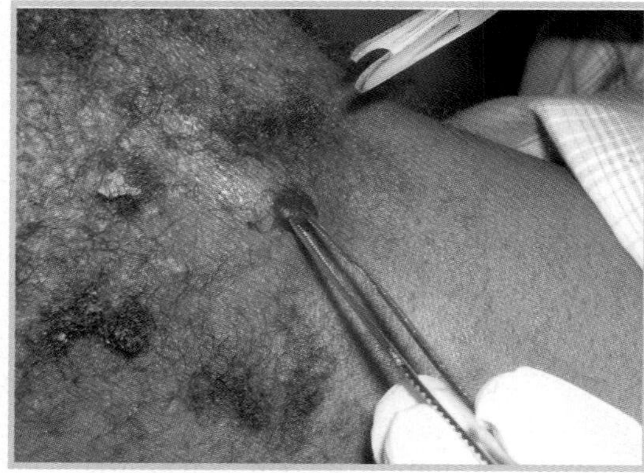

Step 6

Step 7. The defect of small punch biopsies may be left open to heal by second intention, which often produces a small scar. Otherwise, a simple interrupted suture may be placed too close the defect.

- **PEARL:** Make sure the long axis of the final suture line is parallel to the lines of least skin tension.

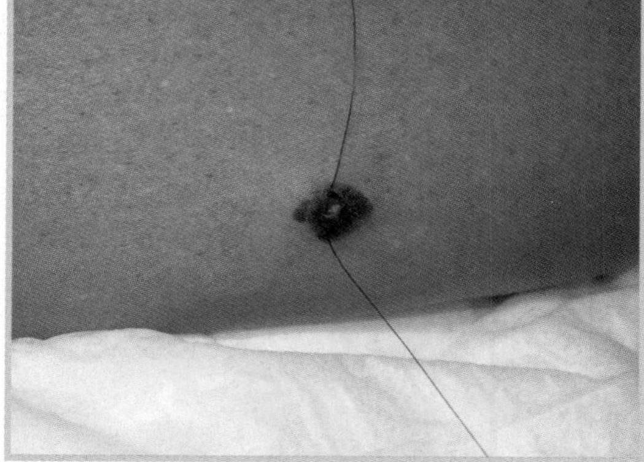

Step 7

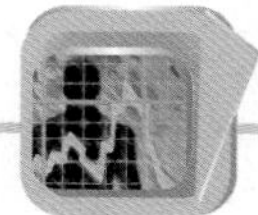

Complications

- Infection
- Bleeding
- Scar formation

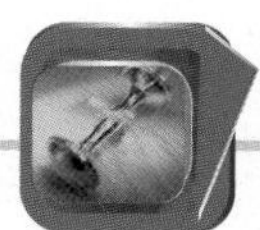

Pediatric Considerations

Generally, pediatric skin has excellent blood flow and heals very well. However, pediatric patients often find it difficult to sit and lie still during lengthy procedures. The patient's maturity and ability to cooperate should be considered before deciding to attempt any outpatient procedure. The maximum recommended dose for lidocaine in children is 3 to 5 mg/kg, and 7 mg/kg when combined with epinephrine. Neonates have an increased volume of distribution, decreased hepatic clearance, and doubled terminal elimination half-life (3.2 hours).

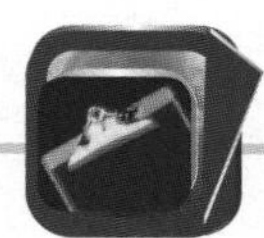

Postprocedure Instructions

Instruct the patient to gently wash an area that has been stitched in 1 day but not to put the wound into standing water for 3 days. Have the patient dry the area well after washing and use a small amount of antibiotic ointment to promote moist healing. Recommend wound elevation to help lessen swelling, reduce pain, and speed healing. Instruct the patient not to pick at, break, or cut the stitches.

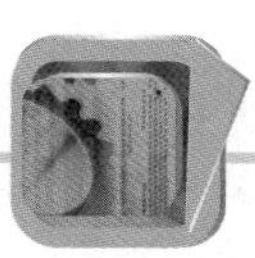

Coding Information and Supply Sources

CPT Code	Description	2008 Average 50th Percentile Fee	Global Period
11100	Biopsy of skin, subcutaneous	$137.00	0
11101	Biopsy of each separate or additional lesion (must be reported with 11100)	$81.00	0

CPT is a registered trademark of the American Medical Association.
2008 average 50th Percentile Fees are provided courtesy of 2008 MMH-SI's copyrighted Physicians' Fees and Coding Guide.

Supplies and ordering information are shown in Appendix G: Instruments and Materials in the Office Surgery Tray.

Patient Education Handout

A patient education handout, "Punch Biopsy of the Skin," can be found on the book's companion Web site.

Bibliography

Fewkes JL. Skin biopsy: the four types and how best to perform them. *Prim Care Cancer.* 1993;13:35–39.

Pariser RJ. Skin biopsy: lesion selection and optimal technique. *Mod Med.* 1989;57:82–90.
Paver RD. Practical procedures in dermatology. *Aust Fam Physician.* 1990;19:699–701.
Phillips PK, Pariser DM, Pariser RJ. Cosmetic procedures we all perform. *Cutis* 1994;53:187–191.
Siegel DM, Usatine RP. The punch biopsy. In: Usatine RP, Moy RL, Tobinick EL, et al., eds. *Skin Surgery: A Practical Guide*. St. Louis: Mosby; 1998:101–119.
Stegman SJ, Tromovitch TA, Glogau RG. Basics of dermatologic surgery. Chicago: Year Book Medical Publishers; 1982.
Swanson NA. *Atlas of Cutaneous Surgery*. Boston: Little, Brown; 1987.
Wheeland RG, ed. *Cutaneous Surgery*. Philadelphia: WB Saunders; 1994.
Zuber TJ. *Office Procedures*. Baltimore: Williams & Wilkins; 1999.
Zuber TJ. Punch biopsy of the skin. *Am Fam Physician.* 2002;65:1155–1158, 1161–1162, 1164, 1167–1168.
Zuber TJ. Skin biopsy techniques: when and how to perform punch biopsy. *Consultant.* 1994; 34:1467–1470.
2008 MAG Mutual Healthcare Solutions, Inc.'s Physicians' Fee and Coding Guide. Duluth, Georgia. MAG Mutual Healthcare Solutions, Inc. 2007.

SECTION THREE

Aesthetic Procedures

CHAPTER 28

Aesthetic Procedures Introduction

Rebecca Small, MD

Assistant Clinical Professor, Director, Medical Aesthetics Training Program, Department of Family and Community Medicine, University of California, San Francisco School of Medicine, Capitola, CA

Minimally invasive procedures have become the primary treatment modalities for facial rejuvenation and enhancement. Traditional treatment options have been limited to surgical interventions, such as facelifts to redrape and lift skin, which give a tighter appearance. However, there has been a shift away from invasive one-time procedures which may radically alter appearance, towards procedures that can enhance appearance in a more natural, subtle way. These procedures are performed in an ongoing capacity to promote and maintain a healthy youthful appearance. Minimally invasive aesthetic treatments today are aimed at reducing the signs of photoaging by relaxing overactive facial muscles with botulinum toxin; filling wrinkles and redefining facial contours with dermal fillers, and improving epidermal hyperpigmentation and vascularities with lasers and intense pulsed light treatments. Statistics published by the American Society for Facial Plastic and Reconstructive Surgery show that of the 11.7 million aesthetic procedures performed in the United States in 2007, 82% were nonsurgical, and the most common procedures performed were botulinum toxin, dermal fillers, laser hair removal, microdermabrasion, and intense pulsed light treatments.

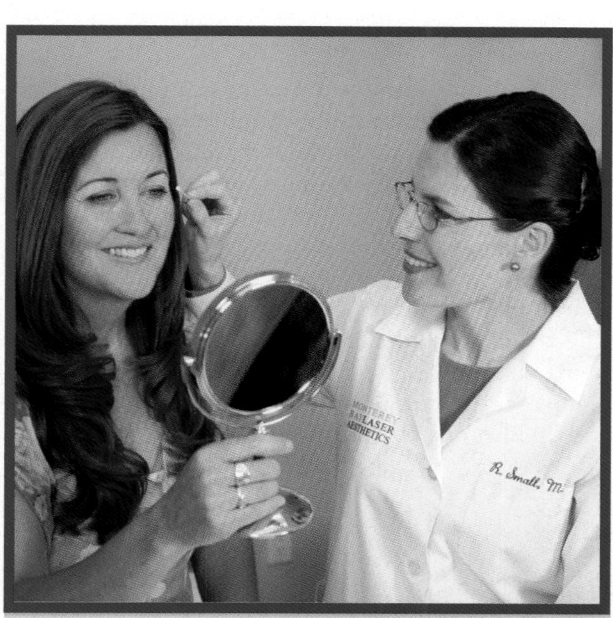

The advances in minimally invasive aesthetic treatments have opened up the aesthetics field to primary care professionals (PCPs), including physicians and nurses in family medicine, obstetrics, internal medicine, and emergency medicine. The skills that these providers have with office procedures and strong doctor-patient relationships make them particularly well suited to provide aesthetic care.

There are several challenges faced by the PCP in performing aesthetic treatments. Obtaining high-quality, evidence-based training has been a barrier; however, with more same-specialty mentors and the emergence of formal training in some primary care residency programs, proper training can be acquired. Selecting aesthetic products and technologies to incorporate into practice can be daunting due to the vast array of therapies available, and treatment options continue to increase as the field of aesthetics grows.

The goal of the following chapters is to provide PCPs with an appreciation for the aesthetic considerations of the aging face and a basic approach to facial rejuvenation utilizing a core group of procedures, the essential medical aesthetic rejuvenation treatments (ARTs). These treatments are highly efficacious, requiring minimal recovery time, have a relatively low risk of side effects, high patient satisfaction, and can be performed safely in the outpatient setting. They form a foundation of aesthetic procedures for PCPs that can be successfully incorporated into primary care practice. In summary, the essential medical ARTs for PCPs include the following:

- Botulinum toxin A (Botox) treatment for
  - Frown lines
  - Crow's feet
  - Horizontal forehead lines
- Dermal filler treatment for
  - Nasolabial folds
  - Oral commissures
  - Lip enhancement
- Laser and intense pulsed light treatment for
  - Permanent hair reduction
  - Photo rejuvenation of benign vascular and pigmented lesions
- Rejuvenation skin care program with
  - Microdermabrasion
  - Chemical peels
  - Topical products
- Sclerotherapy for small varicose veins

Facial Aging

Over time, the skin naturally thins and loses volume as dermal collagen, hyaluronic acid, and elastin diminish. This process of dermal atrophy is accelerated and compounded primarily by sun damage and other extrinsic factors such as smoking. Prematurely photoaged skin exhibits textural changes with wrinkles and roughness; dyschromia with mottled hyperpigmentation and lentigines; vascular ectasias with telangiectasias and cherry angiomas, and undergoes benign and malignant degenerative changes. Hyperdynamic facial musculature contributes to formation of visible lines and wrinkles in the upper one third of the face. Redistribution of facial fat, skin laxity, and biometric changes such as bone resorption, contribute to skin folds and contour changes in the lower two thirds of the face. Specifically, descent of the malar fat pads contributes to deepened nasolabial folds and oral commissures; regression of dentition and resorption of maxillary and mandibular bones accentuates vertical lip lines and the mental crease.

Aesthetic Consultation

Aesthetic consultation is an important part of successfully performing aesthetic treatments. Medical history should be reviewed, including: past medical history, medications, allergies, and past cosmetic history (including results from previous treatments and side effects if any, surgeries, and satisfaction with outcomes). An aesthetic patient intake questionnaire is shown in the figure. Repeated dissatisfaction with past aesthetic treatments is a red flag and can be associated with unrealistic expectations or body dysmorphic disorder, both of which are contraindications to treatment. While discussing the patient's concerns, a mirror should be held between the provider and the patient and the areas of concern simultaneously examined. The areas should be prioritized by the patient and the

AESTHETICS INTAKE FORM

Date:________________

NAME: ________________________________ AGE:______ DOB:__________
Last First

ADDRESS:________________________ CITY:____________ ZIP:__________

HOME PHONE:________________________ ☐ OK TO CONTACT/LEAVE MESSAGE HERE

MOBILE PHONE:________________________ ☐ OK TO CONTACT/LEAVE MESSAGE HERE

WORK PHONE:________________________ ☐ OK TO CONTACT/LEAVE MESSAGE HERE

E-MAIL:________________________ ☐ OK TO CONTACT/LEAVE MESSAGE HERE

OCCUPATION: __________________ REFERRED BY: __________________

INTEREST: ☐ Photo Rejuvenation/IPL ☐ Laser Hair Removal ☐ Botox ☐ Collagen/Restylane/Filler(s)
☐ Medical Skin Care Program (peels, dermaplaning, enzymes) ☐ Skin Tightening Laser ☐ Resurfacing Laser

Medical history	Yes	No
Are you or is it possible that you may be pregnant?		
Are you breastfeeding?		
Do you form thick or raised scars from cuts or burns?		
After injury to the skin (such as cuts/burns) do you have:(circle) Darkening of the skin in that area (hyperpigmentaion) Lightening of the skin in that area (hypopigmentation)		
Hair removal by plucking, waxing, electrolysis in the last 4 weeks?		
Tanning (tanning bed) or sun exposure in last 4 weeks? (circle)		
Tanning products or spray on tan in the last 2 weeks?		
Do you have a tan now in the area to be treated?		
Do you use sunscreen daily with spf 30 or higher?		
History of skin cancer or unusual moles?		
Have you ever had a photosensitive disorder? (E.g. Lupus)		
History of seizures?		
Permanent make-up or tattoos? Where __________		
Have you used Accutane in last 6 months?		
Are you currently taking antibiotics? Which __________		
Are you using Retin-A or Glycolic products? (circle)		
Are you currently under the care of a physician?		
Do you currently smoke?		
Do you have an allergy or sensitivity to lidocaine, latex, sulfa medications, hydroquinone, aloe, bee stings? (circle)		
Life threating allergy to anything?		
Do you have scars on the face?		

Explanation of items marked "Yes":

____

____

Yes	No	Please check all medical conditions past or present
☐	☐	Keloid scarring
☐	☐	Cold Sores
☐	☐	Herpes (genital)
☐	☐	Easy bruising or bleeding
☐	☐	Active skin infection
☐	☐	Moles that changed, itched or bled
☐	☐	Recent increase in amount of hair
☐	☐	Asthma
☐	☐	Seasonal allergies/allergic rhinitis
☐	☐	Eczema
☐	☐	Thyroid imbalance
☐	☐	Poor healing
☐	☐	Diabetes
☐	☐	Heart condition
☐	☐	High blood pressure
☐	☐	Pacemaker
☐	☐	Disease of nerves or muscles
☐	☐	(e.g. ALS, Myasthenia gravis, Lambert-Eaton or other)
☐	☐	Cancer
☐	☐	HIV/AIDS
☐	☐	Autoimmune disease (e.g. rheumatiod arthritis, Scleroderma)
☐	☐	Hepatitis
☐	☐	Shingles
☐	☐	Migaine headaches
☐	☐	Other illness, health problems or medical conditions not listed.

Explanation of items marked "Yes":

____

____

I certify that the medical information I have given is complete and accurate. ______ initials

For Internal Use Only Below This Line

Intake Form120607.sdr

Figure 1 Courtesy of Monterey Bay Laser Aesthetics.

Aesthetics Consultation Form

Name: ______________________________ DOB: ______________

Concerns: ____

____

____

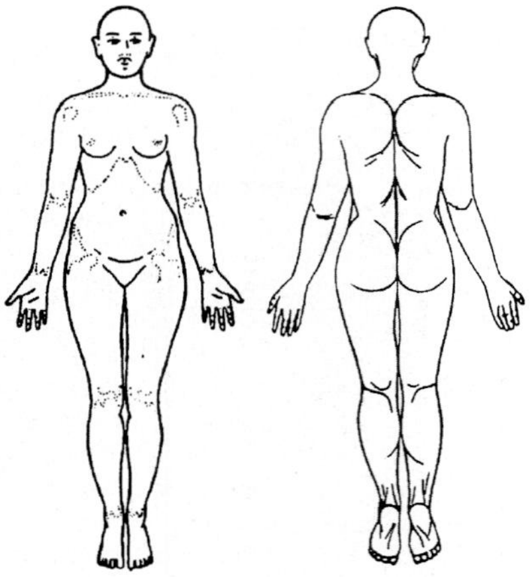

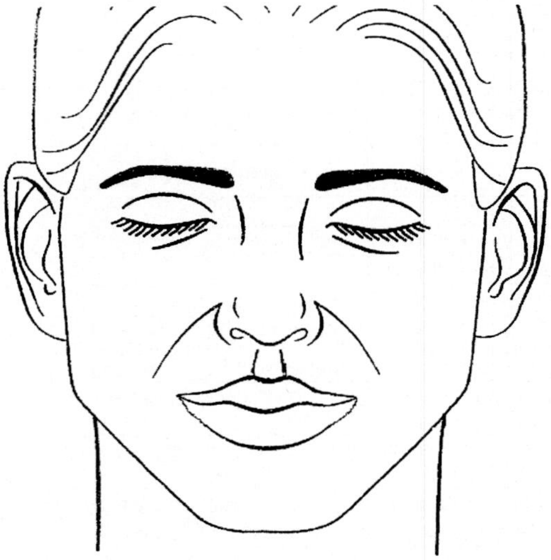

Plan Implementation:

Laser/IPL: ____

____

Botox: ____

____

Filler: ____

____

Other: ____

____

____

Signature Date

Figure 2 Courtesy of Monterey Bay Laser Aesthetics.

treatment options discussed, along with the number of treatments recommended, anticipated results and the cost. Asymmetries, such as uneven eyebrow height, should be pointed out to the patient, noted in the chart and photographed. An aesthetics consultation form is shown in the second figure.

Photographs should be taken prior to treatment, midway through a treatment series, and posttreatment. The patient should be positioned fully upright, looking straight ahead. Photographs are taken of the full face and specific treatment areas in this position, at 90 degrees and 45 degrees. For injectable treatments, photographs should be taken at rest and with active facial movement of the treatment areas. Aesthetic photographic systems, such as Canfield, Profect, and BrighTex, provide standardized angles and lighting, which facilitate consistent photography.

Patients receiving elective aesthetic procedures typically have high expectations of efficacy and low tolerance for side effects. Time should be taken to cover all aspects of the informed consent process, which consists of: (i) discussing the risks, benefits (with emphasis on realistic expectations), alternatives, and complications of the procedure; (ii) providing adequate opportunity for all questions to be asked and answered; (iii) educating the patient about the nature of the aesthetic issue and procedure details (iv) signing the consent form; and (v) documenting the informed consent process in the chart.

CHAPTER 29

Botulinum Toxin Type A for Facial Rejuvenation

Rebecca Small, MD

Assistant Clinical Professor, Director, Medical Aesthetics Training Program, Department of Family and Community Medicine, University of California, San Francisco School of Medicine, Capitola, CA

Treatment of facial lines and wrinkles with botulinum toxin type A has become the most frequently performed cosmetic procedure in the United States today, according to the American Society for Aesthetic Plastic Surgery. It is also one of the most common entry procedures for primary care professionals seeking to incorporate aesthetic procedures into their practice.

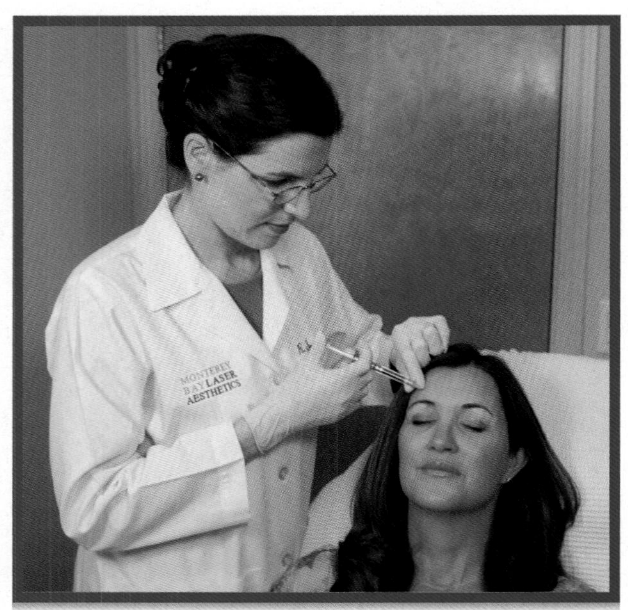

By definition, facial wrinkles formed during muscle contraction are dynamic lines. Over time, dynamic lines may become etched into the skin resulting in permanent or static lines. Botulinum toxin reduces unwanted dynamic and static lines by relaxing overactive facial muscles and smoothing the skin. It is a potent neurotoxin protein derived from the *Clostridium botulinum* bacterium, and exerts its effect at the neuromuscular junction by inhibiting release of acetylcholine. Localized, temporary chemical denervation is achieved through injection of small quantities of botulinum toxin into specific overactive facial muscles.

Botulinum toxin was first noted for its toxic properties, as were atropine and digitalis, but is now routinely used as a medicine to treat clinical conditions such as blepharospasm, strabismus, cervical dystonia, hyperhidrosis, migraines, and muscle spasticity associated with cerebral palsy and strokes. Botulinum toxin was approved by the U.S. Food and Drug Administration (FDA) in 2002 as Botox for cosmetic use to treat the glabella complex muscles, which contribute to frown line formation. All references in this chapter to treatments with botulinum toxin type A refer specifically to Botox, manufactured by Allergan.

Botulinum toxin is used for numerous cosmetic indications; however, treatment to the upper one-third of the face offers the most predictable results, greatest efficacy, and fewest side effects. The three essential medical aesthetic rejuvenation treatments (ARTs) for primary care professionals using botulinum toxin are injections of the: (i) glabella

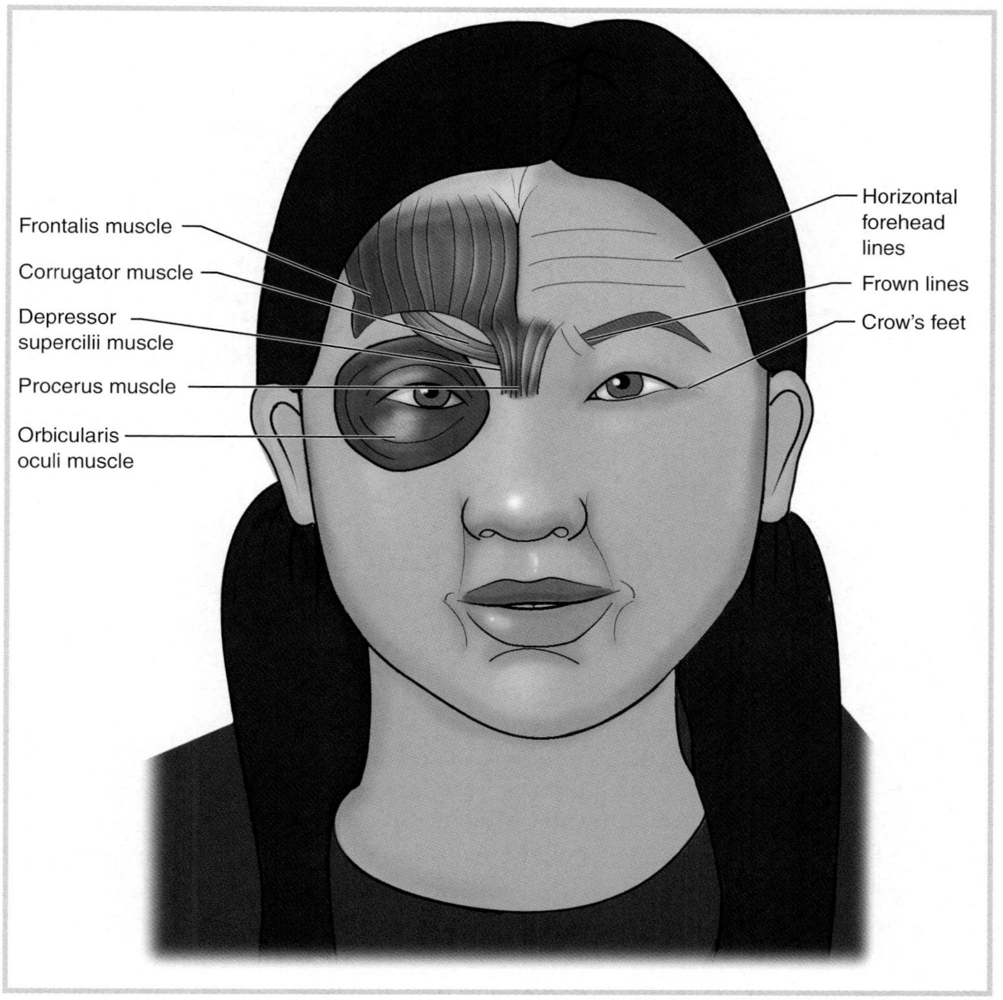

Figure 1

complex muscles, which form frown lines; (ii) frontalis muscle, which forms horizontal forehead lines; and (iii) lateral orbicularis oculi muscles, which form crow's feet (see Figure 1).

Functional Anatomy

A thorough understanding of facial anatomy in the treatment areas is essential prior to performing botulinum toxin procedures. The muscles of facial expression are unique in that they have soft tissue attachments to the skin through the superficial muscular aponeurotic system, unlike most muscles, which have boney attachments. When a muscle contracts, the overlying skin moves with it and wrinkles are formed perpendicular to the direction of the muscle contraction.

Glabella wrinkles, or frown lines, are vertical wrinkles that occur between the medial aspects of the eyebrows. The muscles that contribute to formation of frown lines are the glabellar complex of depressor muscles, which pull the brows medially and inferiorly and include the corrugator supercilii, procerus, depressor supercilii, and medial orbicularis oculi.

Horizontal forehead lines result from contraction of the broad frontalis muscle, which spans the forehead between the temporal fusion lines (see Figure 1). The muscle fibers are vertically oriented, and contraction of this elevator muscle raises the eyebrows, with the lower 2-cm portion having the most marked effect on eyebrow height and shape. The goal of treatment in this area is to partially inhibit activity of the frontalis to reduce horizontal forehead lines while maintaining a desirable eyebrow shape.

Lateral orbital wrinkles commonly known as crow's feet, result from contraction of the lateral portion of the orbicularis oculi, a thin, superficial muscle that encircles the eye. Contraction of the palpebral portion of the orbicularis oculi results in closure of the eyelids. The goal of treatment in this area is to focally inhibit the lateral orbicularis oculi to reduce crow's feet without complete orbicularis oculi inactivation.

Many of the muscles of facial expression interdigitate with one another. While providing treatment with botulinum toxin to one area in isolation will often provide adequate results, in some cases an adjacent area may require concomitant treatment to achieve the desired results. For example, the glabella complex muscles interdigitate to a greater or lesser degree with the frontalis, and treatment of the frontalis in addition to treatment of the glabellar complex may be required to smooth frown lines in some cases.

General Injection Guidelines

- Position the patient comfortably in a reclined position for the procedure, at about 65 degrees.
- Cleanse the treatment areas with alcohol prior to injection and allow alcohol to dry, as alcohol may denature the botulinum toxin.
- Typically no anesthesia is required for botulinum toxin treatments. If necessary, ice may be used prior to injections in all treatment areas except crow's feet, as this makes identification and avoidance of veins more difficult.
- Injections should be made into the "hill" of the contracted muscle.
- Botulinum toxin is injected as the needle is withdrawn and should flow very easily, requiring only a light touch. If resistance is encountered, fully withdraw the needle and reinsert.
- Avoid intravascular injection. Intravascular injection is apparent when the surrounding skin blanches during injection. If this occurs, withdraw the needle partially from the blanched site, reposition, and inject.
- Avoid hitting the periosteum, particularly with frontalis treatments, as this is painful and dulls the needle.
- If bleeding occurs, apply firm pressure directed away from the eye and achieve hemostasis before proceeding to subsequent injection points.

Dosage

The doses and diagrams in this chapter are general treatment recommendations for starting doses and refer exclusively to botulinum toxin type A (Botox) from Allergan. Optimal results are achieved through individualization of treatments based on the patient's observed muscle function and muscle bulk in the treatment areas.

Results and Follow-up

- Some reduction in muscle function is typically seen by the third day after botulinum toxin treatment. Maximal reduction in function of the targeted muscles is visible 1 to 2 weeks after treatment. Botulinum toxin effects are most dramatic for the treatment of dynamic lines. Static lines are slower to respond, usually requiring 2 to 3 consecutive botulinum toxin treatments and deep, static lines may not fully respond even after multiple treatments.

- If muscle activity persists in one or more parts of the treated area, a touch-up procedure may be performed 2 weeks after treatment. The dose is based on the degree of movement remaining in the treated muscle and may range from 2.5 to 10 units. Reassess the treatment area 1 week after the touch-up procedure.
- Return of muscle function in the treatment area is gradual. Patients should follow-up for subsequent treatment when muscle function is regained, prior to facial lines returning to their pretreatment appearance.

Preprocedure Checklist

- Perform an aesthetic consultation and review patient's medical history (see Chapter 28).
- Obtain informed consent (see Chapter 28).
- Take pretreatment photographs with the patient actively contracting the muscles in the intended treatment area and with the muscles at rest.
- Document and discuss any notable asymmetries prior to treatment.
- Minimize bruising by discontinuation of aspirin, vitamin E, St. John's wort and other dietary supplements including ginkgo, evening primrose oil, garlic, feverfew and ginseng for 2 weeks prior to treatment. Discontinue other nonsteroidal anti-inflammatory medications 2 days prior to treatment.

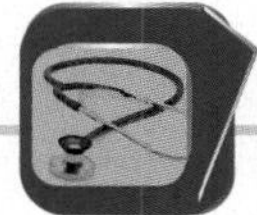

Equipment

Botulinum Toxin Reconstitution

- 5.0-mL syringe
- Botox 100-unit vial
- 10 mL vial 0.9% sterile nonpreserved saline
- 18-gauge, 0.5-inch needle

Botulinum Toxin Treatment

- Reconstituted Botox
- 1.0 mL Luer-Lok syringe
- 30-gauge, 1-inch needle
- 30-gauge, 0.5-inch needle
- 32-gauge, 0.5-inch needle
- Gauze, 3 × 3 inches, nonwoven
- Ice pack

Reconstitution

Using an 18-gauge needle and a 5.0-mL syringe, draw up 4.0 mL of 0.9% nonpreserved sterile saline diluent. Insert the needle at a 45-degree angle into the Botox vial and inject saline slowly, maintaining upward plunger pressure so that the diluent runs down the sides of the vial. Gently swirl the reconstituted Botox vial, and record the date and time of reconstitution on the vial. Note that alcohol can denature Botox and therefore, bottle stoppers must be fully dried.

Concentration

Botox is supplied as a vacuum-dried powder with 100 units per vial. Reconstitution of Botox powder using 4.0 mL of nonpreserved saline results in a concentration of 100 units botulinum toxin per 4.0 mL (100 units/4 mL) or 2.5 units botulinum toxin per 0.1 mL.

Handling

Botox is shipped frozen on dry ice. Prior to and after reconstitution, it should be stored in the refrigerator at a temperature of 2°C to 8°C (35.6°F to 46.4°F). Prior to reconstitution it may be stored for 24 months, per the Botox package insert. After reconstitution, the American Society for Plastic Surgery Botox Consensus Panel recommends using Botox within 6 weeks and notes no loss of potency during that time. The Botox package insert however, recommends using Botox within 4 hours of reconstitution.

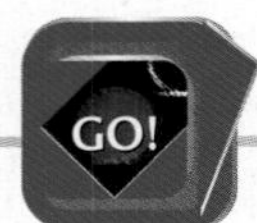

Aesthetic Indications

- Temporary improvement in the appearance of dynamic facial lines and wrinkles.
- FDA approved for treatment of frown lines due to contraction of the glabellar complex muscles. Used off label for all other cosmetic indications, including treatment of lateral orbicularis oculi and frontalis muscles.
- Patients aged 18 to 65 years old. May be used in patients older than age 65, but treatments are less effective if severe static wrinkling is present.

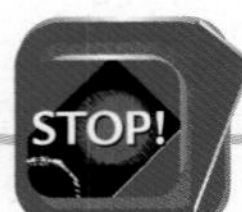

Contraindications

Absolute Contraindications

- Pregnancy (category C)
- Nursing
- Active infection in the treatment area
- Gross motor weakness in the treatment area, for example, due to a history of polio or Bell's palsy
- Neuromuscular disorder or current evaluation for neuromuscular disorder, including but not limited to: amyotrophic lateral sclerosis, myasthenia gravis, or Lambert-Eaton syndrome

Relative Contraindications

- Inability to actively contract muscles in the treatment area prior to the procedure
- Blepharoplasty or laser-assisted in situ keratomileusis (LASIK) surgery within the past 6 months
- Body dysmorphic disorder or unrealistic expectations
- Medications that inhibit neuromuscular signaling which may potentiate botulinum toxin effects, such as: aminoglycosides, penicillamine, quinine, and calcium channel blockers

The Procedure

Frown Lines

Frown lines often convey anger, frustration, and irritation and may be perceived negatively. Improvement of frown lines has therefore become one of the most common aesthetic complaints for which patients seek botulinum toxin treatments. Figure 2A shows a 38-year-old woman with frown lines resulting from active contraction of the glabellar complex muscles. Figure 2B shows the same patient 1 month after her first botulinum toxin treatment attempting to frown. Notice the dramatic posttreatment improvement in frown lines and the elevated medial brow position, due to the lack of depressor muscle function. The duration of botulinum toxin effect in the glabella complex muscles is typically 3 to 4 months.

The glabellar muscles require deep intramuscular injection, and a 30 gauge, 1 inch needle is preferable. Alternatively, a 30 gauge, 0.5 inch needle may be used. Botulinum toxin should be placed within the glabellar complex Safety Zone to minimize the risk of blepharoptosis and eyebrow ptosis. The glabellar complex Safety Zone (shaded gray) is bounded by the vertical lines extending up from the lateral irises (see Figure 3). It is approximately 1–2 cm above the orbital rim and extends inferiorly to a point just below the glabellar prominence.

- **PEARL:** In some patients with broad musculature, the lateral margins of the corrugators may extend outside of the Safety Zone. Avoid injecting the portion of the corrugator that is outside of the Safety Zone.

An overview of botulinum toxin injection points and doses for the treatment of frown lines is shown (Figure 4). The starting dose for women is 20 units botulinum toxin (0.8 mL of reconstituted Botox with 100 units/4 mL) and for men is 25 units botulinum toxin (1.0 mL Botox with 100 units/4 mL).

- **PEARL:** The doses listed in this chapter are recommendations for starting doses and refer exclusively to Botox from Allergan.

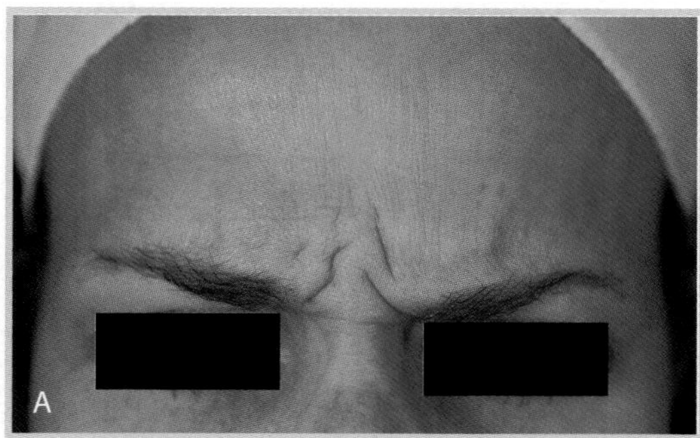

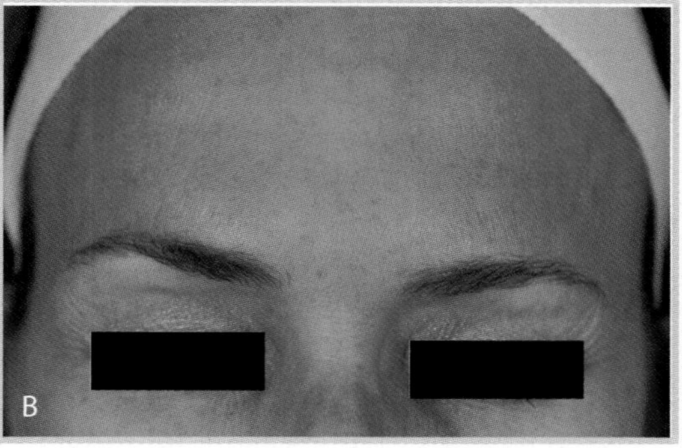

Figure 2

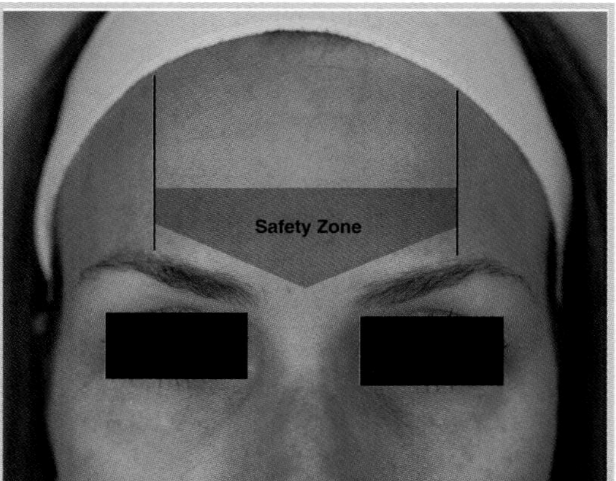

Figure 3

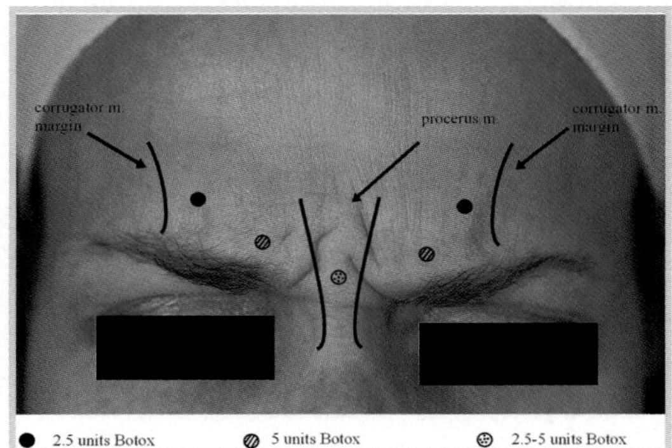

Figure 4

Step 1. The first injection point is at the lateral margin of the corrugator within the Safety Zone. Identify the lateral margin of the corrugator by directing the patient to actively frown. Inject 2.5 units of botulinum toxin 1 to 2 cm above the superior margin of the orbit, at the visible lateral margin of the corrugator. If using the 1-inch needle, insert it part way to about half of its depth.

- **PITFALL:** Do not initiate treatment to the glabella complex if the lateral corrugator margin is not clearly visible.
- **PITFALL:** Inject at least 1 cm above the orbital margin to minimize the risk of blepharoptosis (droopy upper eyelid).

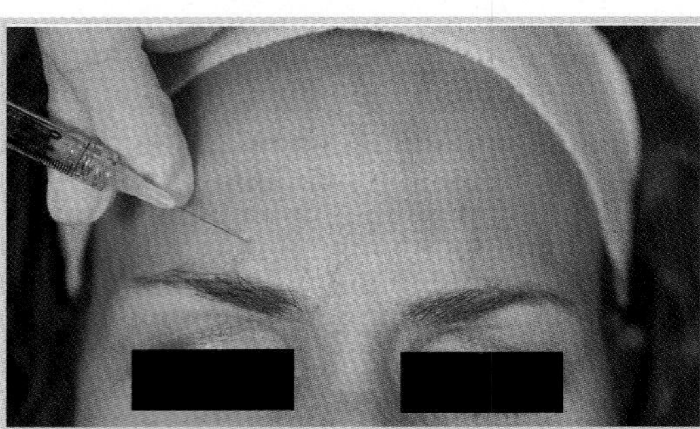

Step 1

Step 2. The second injection site is in the body of the corrugator, approximately 1 cm medial to the first injection site and more inferior, closer to the eyebrow. Direct the needle toward the procerus, inserting the 1-inch needle to the hub, and inject 5 units of botulinum toxin. Repeat Steps 1 and 2 for the contralateral side of the face.

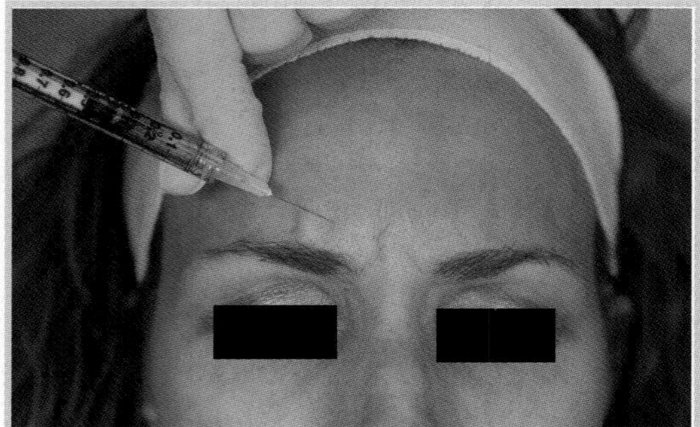

Step 2

Step 3. The third injection site is in the procerus, which is approached inferiorly with the needle directed toward the forehead. With the patient frowning, inject 2.5 to 5 units of botulinum toxin with the 1-inch needle inserted into the procerus to about half its depth.

- **PEARL:** This site tends to bleed, so apply pressure firmly after withdrawing the needle.
- **PEARL:** This third injection site may not be needed if the procerus is adequately injected from the lateral corrugator injection points using the 1 inch needle in the Second Step.

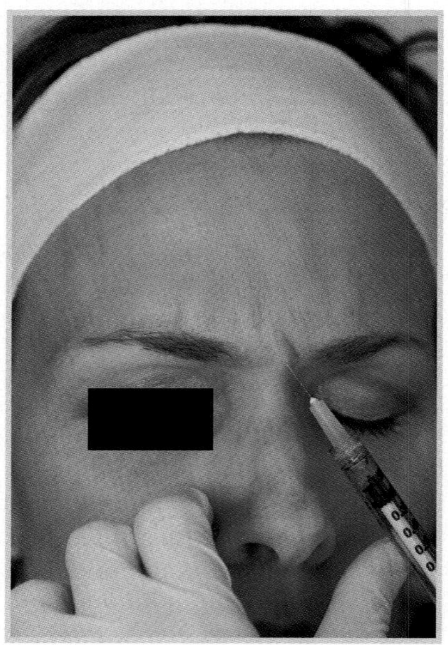

Step 3

Horizontal Forehead Lines

Patients with deep horizontal forehead lines must be assessed for eyebrow ptosis and upper eyelid laxity with the frontalis muscle at rest prior to treatment with botulinum toxin. Avoid treating patients with low-set eyebrows or upper eyelid skin laxity, as frontalis muscle contraction is compensatory to alleviate these issues. The duration of botulinum toxin effect in the frontalis muscle is typically 3 to 4 months. Figure 5A shows a 38-year-old woman with horizontal forehead lines resulting from active contraction of the frontalis muscle. Figure 5B shows the same patient 1 month after botulinum toxin treatment attempting to contract the frontalis muscle.

- **PEARL:** Elicit frontalis muscle contraction by having the patient raise his or her eyebrows as if surprised.

The majority of botulinum toxin is placed within the vertical lines of the frontalis Safety Zone (shaded gray) to minimize the risk of eyebrow ptosis. The frontalis Safety Zone is the area between the vertical lines extending up from the lateral irises, at least 2 cm above the orbital rim, and includes a small area lateral to the vertical lines 2 cm inferior to the hairline (see Figure 6). A 30 gauge, 0.5 inch needle should be used for all injections. The needle tip should be placed in the "hill" of the contracted muscle.

- **PEARL:** As a general rule, do not inject inferior to the lowest horizontal forehead wrinkle.

An overview of botulinum toxin injection points and doses for the treatment of horizontal forehead lines is shown in Figure 7. The starting dose for women is 16 to 22.5 units of botulinum toxin (0.6 to 0.9 mL of reconstituted Botox with 100 units/4 mL) and for men is 20 to 25 units of botulinum toxin (0.8 to 1.0 mL of Botox with 100 units/4 mL).

- **PEARL:** The doses listed in this chapter are recommendations for starting doses and refer exclusively to Botox from Allergan.

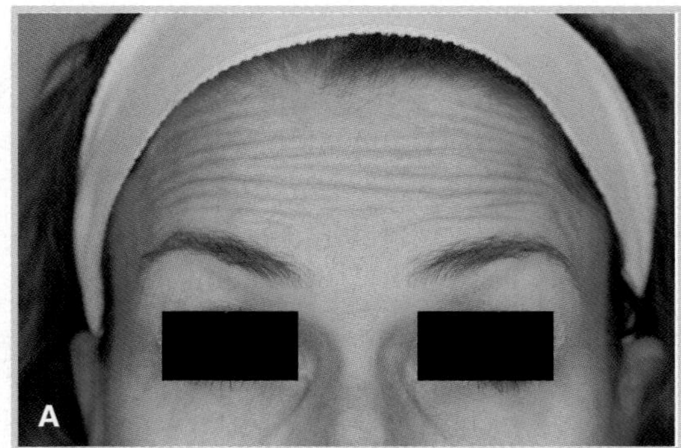

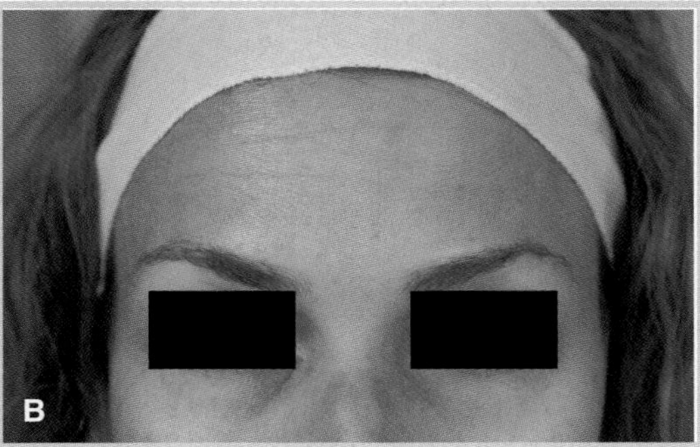

Figure 5

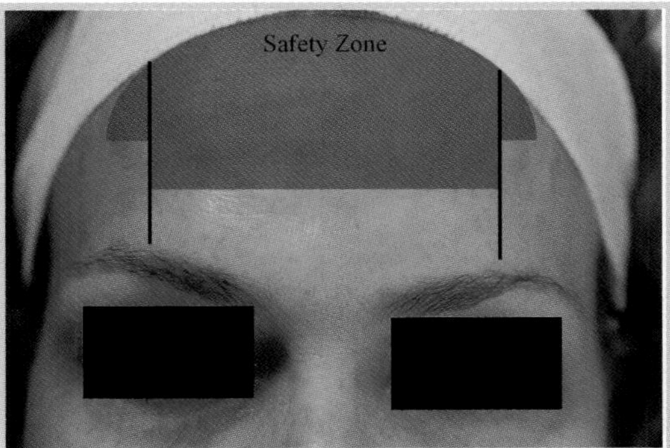

Figure 6

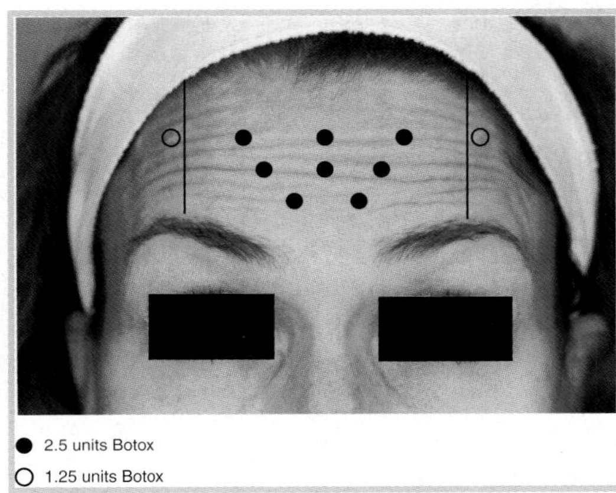

Figure 7

Step 1. While the patient actively raises their eyebrows, inject 2.5 units of botulinum toxin into the "hill" of the frontalis muscle with the needle angled at 30 degrees to raise a wheal. Have the patient relax once the needle is withdrawn.

- **PITFALL:** Avoid injecting too deeply and hitting the periosteum.
- **PEARL:** Change needles after six injections to maintain a sharp needle.

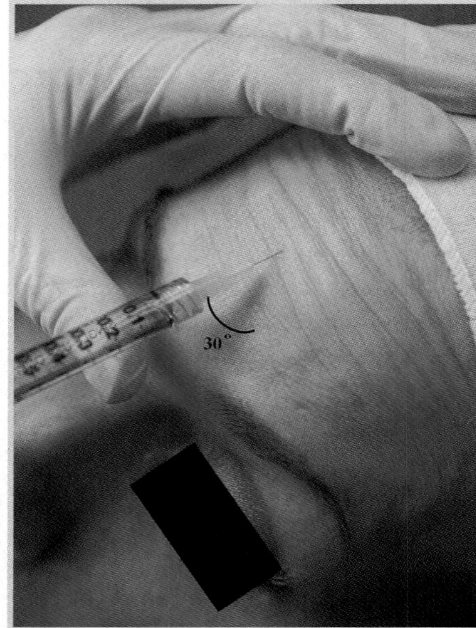

Step 1

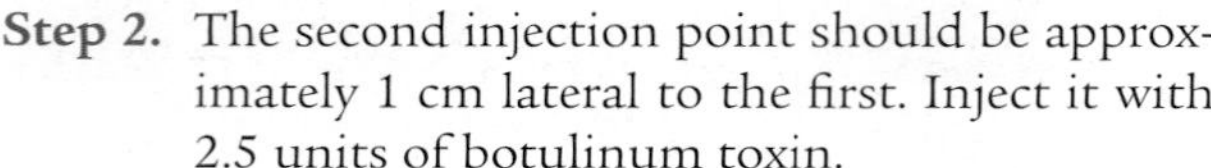

Step 2. The second injection point should be approximately 1 cm lateral to the first. Inject it with 2.5 units of botulinum toxin.

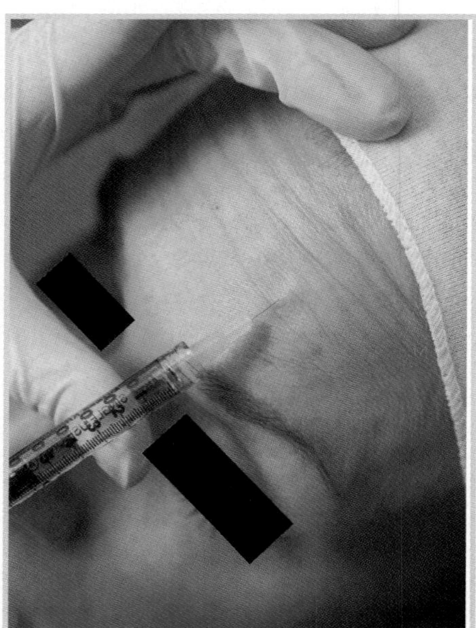

Step 2

Step 3. Continue along each "hill" of the frontalis muscle and proceed superiorly up the forehead. Inject 2.5 units of botulinum toxin at each injection point.

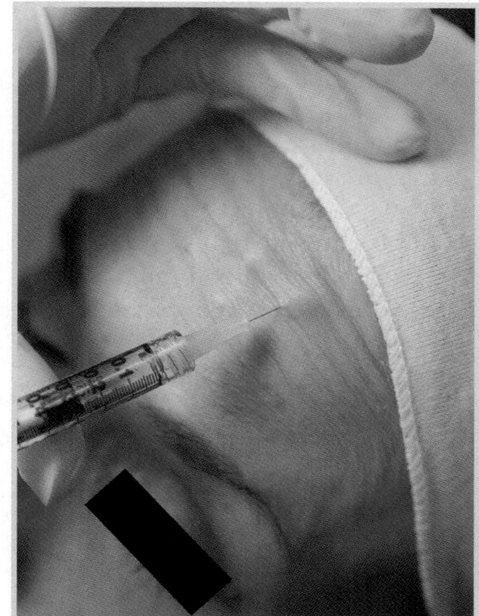

Step 3

Step 4. The last injection should be placed at the maximal point of eyebrow elevation, typically located just lateral to the Safety Zone line, approximately 2 cm inferior to the hair line. Inject 1.25 units of botulinum toxin (0.05 mL of reconstituted Botox, with 100 units/4 mL). Perform botulinum toxin injection symmetrically on the contralateral side of the forehead.

- PITFALL: Omission of this injection may result in a peaked or quizzical eyebrow shape and subsequently require a touch-up.

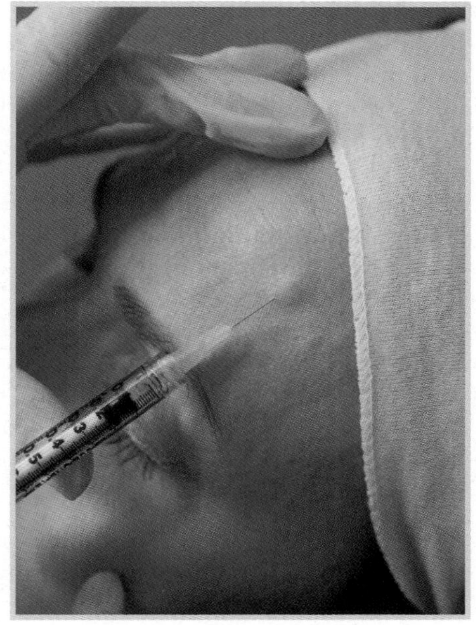

Step 4

Step 5. Patients receiving botulinum toxin treatments for horizontal forehead lines for the first time should be seen 2 weeks after treatment to evaluate eyebrow symmetry and shape. Assess the eyebrow shape at rest and with active elevation. If a peaked eyebrow shape is present with frontalis contraction, inject 1.25 to 2.5 units of botulinum toxin at least 3 cm above the orbital rim, at the most peaked portion of the eyebrow. Reassess in 1 to 2 weeks. Step 5 shows the patient 1 week after receiving 22.5 units of botulinum toxin to the frontalis muscle with mildly peaked eyebrows. She was treated with 1.25 units of botulinum toxin above each peaked eyebrow, and her final result is shown in Figure 5B.

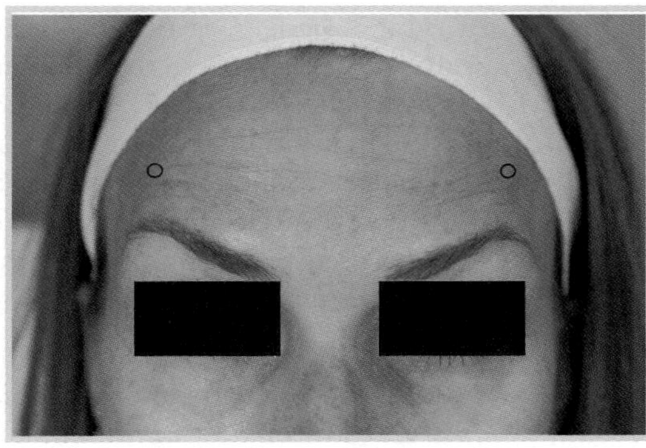

Step 5

Step 6. Eyebrow ptosis can result from botulinum toxin injected laterally, outside of the safety zone or, in the inferior portion of the frontalis, too close to the eyebrows. Eyebrow ptosis can be improved or reversed with injection of botulinum toxin in the orbicularis oculi under the affected eyebrow. Inject 1.25 units of botulinum toxin (0.05 mL of reconstituted Botox with 100 units/4 mL) lateral to the iris in the orbicularis oculi, just beneath the level of the orbital rim as shown in Step 6. Reassess in 1 week.

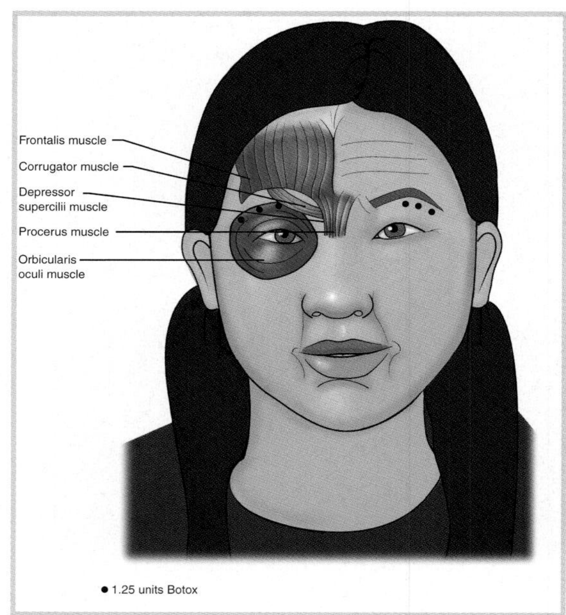

Step 6

Crow's Feet

The pattern of crow's feet resulting from contraction of the lateral orbicularis oculi muscle varies, with some extending superiorly toward the eyebrow and others extending inferiorly toward the cheek. Optimal results with botulinum toxin treatments in the crow's feet area will be achieved by adapting the injection technique outlined here to the individual's pattern of crow's feet.

The duration of botulinum toxin effect in the lateral orbicularis muscle is typically 2.5 to 3 months. Figure 8A shows a 37-year-old woman with crow's feet resulting from active contraction of the lateral orbicularis oculi muscle. Figure 8B shows the same patient 1 month after botulinum toxin treatment attempting to contract the lateral orbicularis oculi muscle.

- **PEARL:** Elicit orbicularis oculi muscle contraction by having the patient smile and squint as if sun is in his or her eyes.

All injection points should be within the crow's feet Safety Zone (shaded gray), the area 1 cm lateral to the orbital rim, above the level of the zygomatic arch, which extends under the eyebrow to the lateral iris. The orbicularis oculi muscle is a thin, superficial muscle, and botulinum toxin should be placed just subdermally using a 30 gauge, 0.5 inch needle to raise a wheal at each injection point. Alternatively, a 32 gauge, 0.5 inch needle may be used to minimize bruising. After each injection, apply firm pressure away from the eye to compress the wheal.

- **PEARL:** Bruising is the most common side effect in the crow's feet area. Look for and avoid veins, which are best seen with oblique lighting.

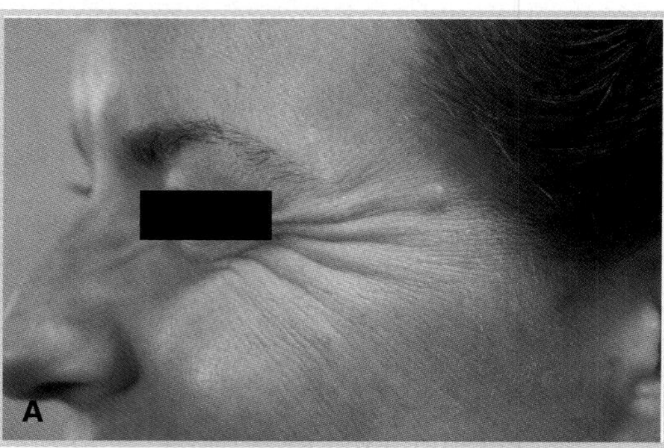

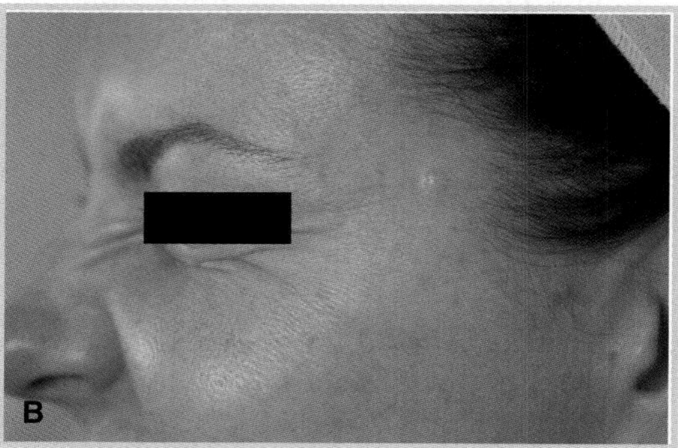

Figure 8

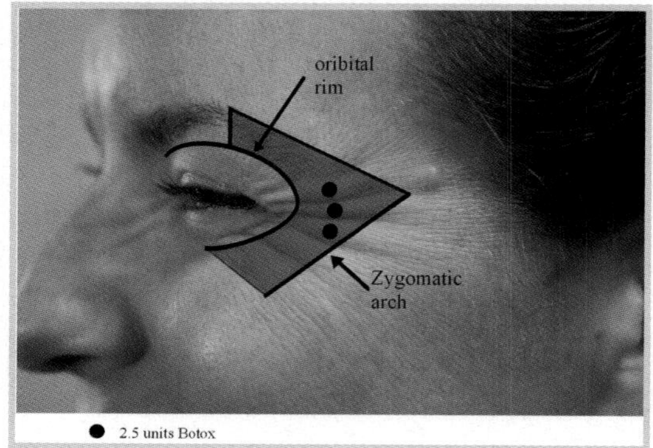

Figure 9

An overview of botulinum toxin injection points and doses for treatment of crow's feet is shown in Figure 10. The starting dose for women is 16 to 20 units of botulinum toxin (0.6 to 0.8 mL of reconstituted Botox with 100 units/4 mL) and for men is 20 to 25 units botulinum toxin (0.8 to 1.0 mL Botox, with 100 units/4 mL).

- **PEARL:** The doses listed in this chapter are recommendations for starting doses and refer exclusively to Botox from Allergan.

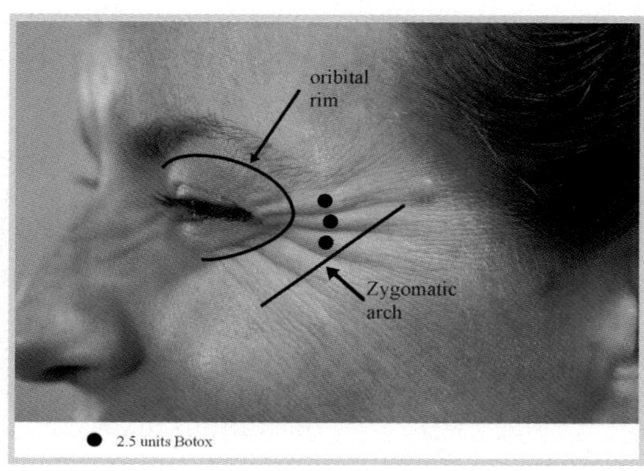

Figure 10

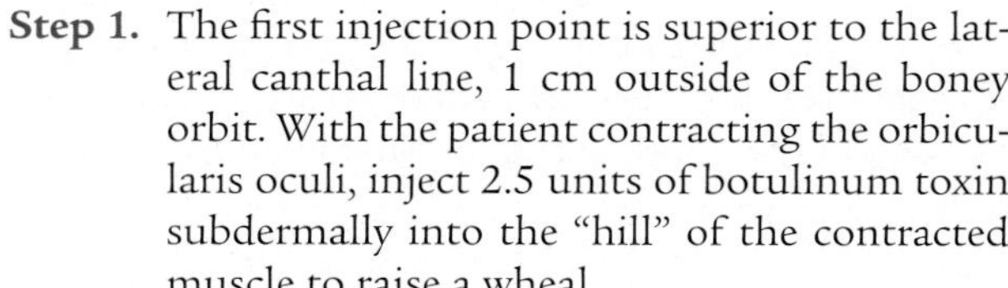

Step 1. The first injection point is superior to the lateral canthal line, 1 cm outside of the boney orbit. With the patient contracting the orbicularis oculi, inject 2.5 units of botulinum toxin subdermally into the "hill" of the contracted muscle to raise a wheal.

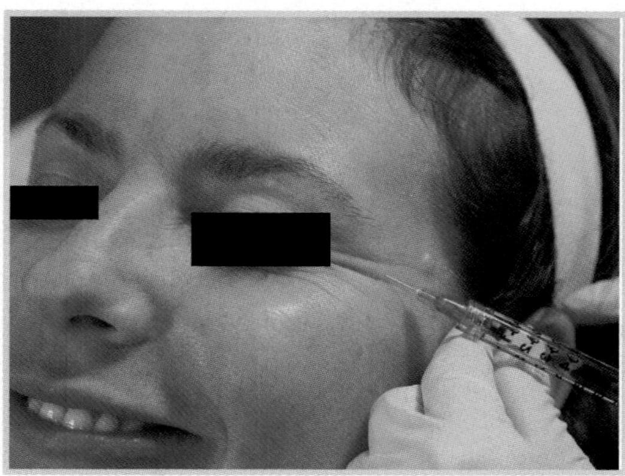
Step 1

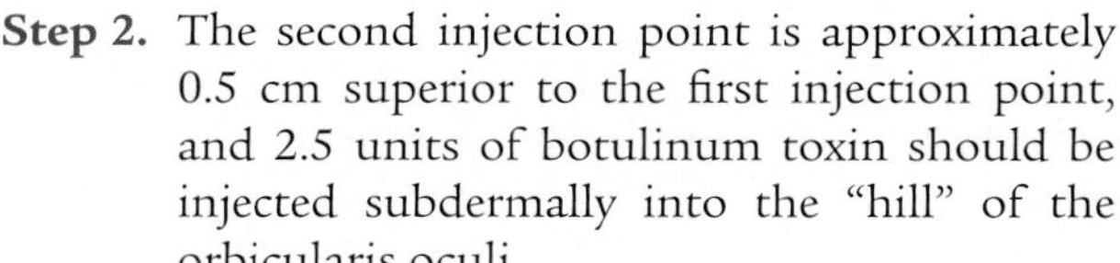

Step 2. The second injection point is approximately 0.5 cm superior to the first injection point, and 2.5 units of botulinum toxin should be injected subdermally into the "hill" of the orbicularis oculi.

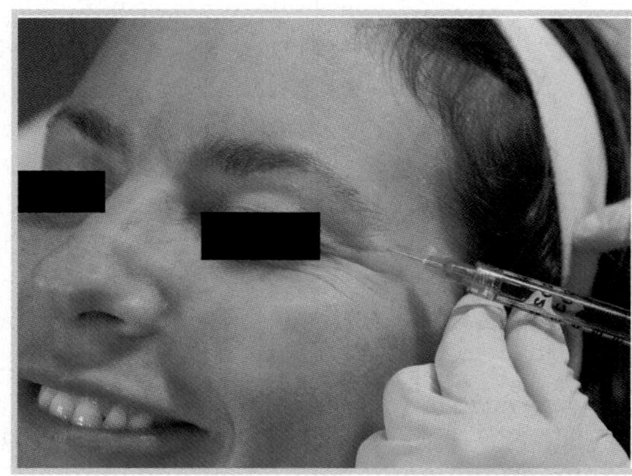
Step 2

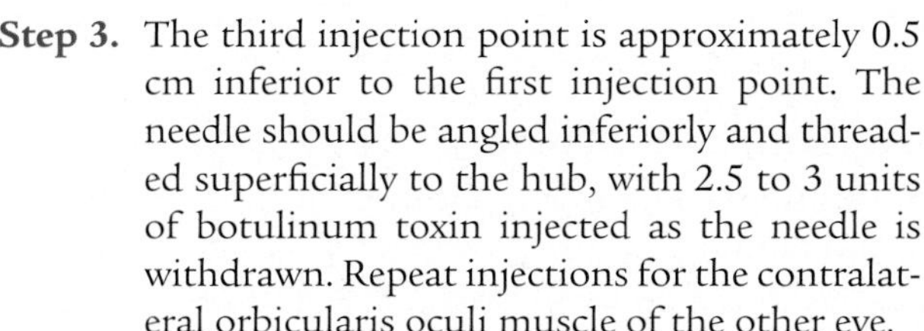

Step 3. The third injection point is approximately 0.5 cm inferior to the first injection point. The needle should be angled inferiorly and threaded superficially to the hub, with 2.5 to 3 units of botulinum toxin injected as the needle is withdrawn. Repeat injections for the contralateral orbicularis oculi muscle of the other eye.

- **PITFALL:** Avoid injecting too deeply and too inferiorly below the level of the zygomatic arch, so as to avoid the zygomatic muscles. Relaxation of the zygomatic muscles can result in cheek ptosis and upper lip ptosis, which may affect oral competence.

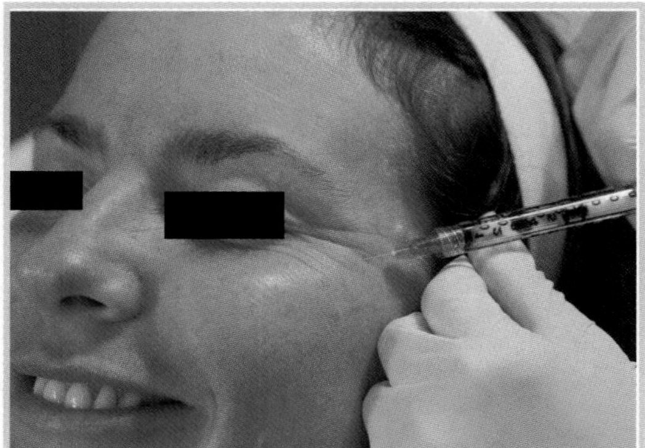
Step 3

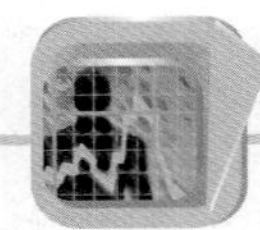

Complications

Common

- Localized burning or stinging pain with injection, bruising, erythema, infection, tenderness, temporary swelling, and mild headache.
- Blepharoptosis (3%) with or without diplopia. Blepharoptosis results from migration of botulinum toxin through the orbital septum, a fascial layer, to the levator palpebrae superioris muscle. Lateral to the Safety Zone line at the boney supraorbital margin, some of the levator palpebrae superioris fibers pass up through the orbital septum, and botulinum toxin can more easily migrate into and relax the levator palpebrae superioris, resulting in blepharoptosis. Blepharoptosis is infrequent and almost always unilateral. It is typically seen as lowering of the affected eyelid 2 to 3 mm, which is most marked at the end of the day with muscle fatigue. It typically resolves spontaneously within 6 weeks. Blepharoptosis may be treated with over-the-counter alpha-adrenergic eyedrops such as Naphcon-A, 1 drop four times per day, or prescription apraclonidine (Iopidine) 0.5% solution, 1 to 2 drops three times per day. These eyedrops cause contraction of an adrenergic levator muscle of the upper eyelid, the Mueller muscle, resulting in elevation of the upper eyelid.
- Eyebrow ptosis.
- Facial asymmetry, including but not limited to smile and eyebrows.
- Oral incompetence with crow's feet treatment.
- Rarely, auto-antibodies against botulinum toxin may be present or develop after treatments, rendering treatments ineffective.

Rare and Idiosyncratic

- Numbness or dysesthesia at the treatment site
- Focal tonic movements
- Periocular swelling
- Extremely rare: immediate hypersensitivity reaction with signs of urticaria, edema, and a remote possibility of anaphylaxis

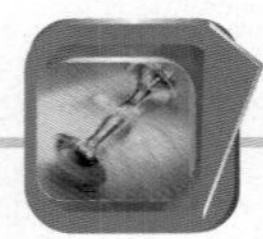

Pediatric Considerations

This treatment is contraindicated for cosmetic uses in pediatric patients.

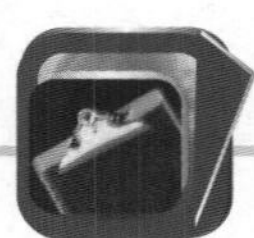

Postprocedure Instructions

On the day of treatment, instruct the patient

- Not to massage the treated areas.
- Avoid lying down for 4 hours immediately after treatment.
- Avoid activities that cause facial flushing, including application of heat to the face, alcohol consumption, exercising, and tanning.
- Ice each site for 10 to 15 minutes every 1 to 2 hours for 1 to 3 days if bruising occurs.

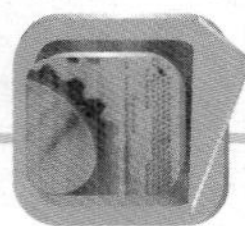

Coding Information and Supply Sources

These procedures are not reimbursable by insurance.

CPT Code	Description	2008 Average 50th Percentile Fee	Global Period
64612	Chemo-denervation of muscles or muscles innervated by the facial nerve.	$482.00	10

CPT is a registered trademark of the American Medical Association.
2008 average 50th Percentile Fees are provided courtesy of 2008 MMH-SI's copyrighted Physicians' Fees and Coding Guide.

Supply Sources

Allergan, Inc., 2525 Dupont Drive, Irvine, CA 92612. Phone: 1-800-377-7790.

Patient Education Handout

A patient education handout, "Botox Treatments," can be found on the book's Web site.

Bibliography

Allergan Inc. Botox cosmetic (botulinum toxin type A) purified neurotoxin complex package insert. Irvine, CA: Allergan, Inc.

Blitzer A, Binder WJ, Brin MF. Botulinum toxin injections for facial lines and wrinkles: technique. In: Blitzer A, ed. *Management of Facial Lines and Wrinkles*. Philadelphia: Lippincott Williams & Wilkins; 2000:303–313.

Carruthers A, Carruthers J. Use of botulinum toxin A for facial enhancement. In: Klein A, ed. *Tissue Augmentation in Clinical Practice*. Taylor & Francis; 2006:117–140.

Carruthers A, Carruthers J, Cohen J. A prospective, double-blind randomized parallel-group, dose-ranging study of botulinum toxin type A in female subjects with horizontal forehead rhytides. *Derm Surg*. 2003;29:461–467.

Carruthers J, Fagien S, Matarasso SL, et al. The Botox consensus group: Consensus recommendations on the use of botulinum toxin type A in facial aesthetics. *Plas Recon Surg*. 2004;114(6)(supp):1–22S.

Carruthers JD, Lowe NS, Menter MA, et al. Botox glabellar lines II study group. Double-blind, placebo-controlled study of the safety and efficacy of botulinum type A for patients with glabellar frown lines. *Plas Recon Surg*. 2003;112:1089.

Hexsel DM, de Almeida AT, Rutowitsch M, et al. Multicenter double-blind study of the efficacy of injections with botulinum toxin type A reconstituted up to 6 weeks before application. *Derm Surg*. 2003;29:523.

Klein, AW. Complications, adverse reactions and insights with the use of botulinum toxin. *Derm Surg*. 2003;29:549–556.

Matarasso SL, Matarasso A. Treatment guidelines for botulinum toxin type A for the periocular region and a report on partial upper lip ptosis following injections to the lateral canthal rhytides. *Plas Reconstr Surg*. 2001;108:208.

Sommer B, et al. Satisfaction of patients after treatment with botulinum toxin for dynamic facial lines. *Derm Surg*. 2003;29:456.

2008 MAG Mutual Healthcare Solutions, Inc.'s Physicians' Fee and Coding Guide. Duluth, Georgia. MAG Mutual Healthcare Solutions, Inc. 2007.

CHAPTER 30

Dermal Fillers for Facial Rejuvenation

Rebecca Small, MD

Assistant Clinical Professor, Director, Medical Aesthetics Training Program, Department of Family and Community Medicine, University of California, San Francisco School of Medicine, Capitola, CA

The use of dermal fillers to correct signs of facial aging such as wrinkles and contour defects is the second most commonly performed cosmetic procedure in the United States today, according to the American Society for Aesthetic Plastic Surgery. This is largely due to increased patient demand for less invasive treatment options and product innovations that have allowed for prolonged duration of treatment effects. Dermal fillers can be used to enhance appearance in a subtle, natural way; require short recovery times; and can be safely performed in the outpatient setting. Consequently, they have become a mainstay of minimally invasive facial rejuvenation procedures.

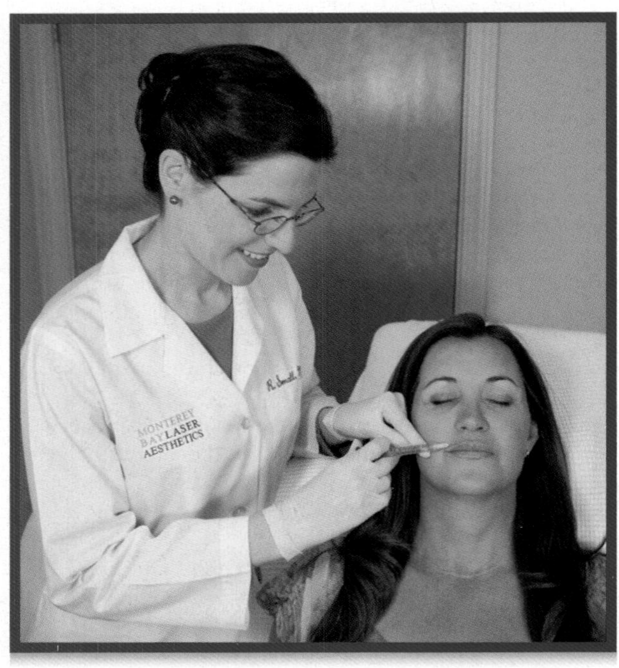

There are numerous injectable products available for facial soft-tissue augmentation. These products, known as dermal fillers, vary by composition, duration of action, palpability, ease of administration, complications, and other factors. It is not within the scope of this chapter to review all dermal filler products but rather to help primary care professionals get started with products and techniques that consistently achieve good outcomes and have low side-effect profiles.

The most versatile dermal fillers currently available are the hyaluronic acid (HA) products. HA is a naturally occurring glycosaminoglycan in the dermal extracellular matrix that provides structural support, nutrients and, through its hydrophilic capacity, adds volume and fullness to the skin. With aging and photo damage, HA is lost from the skin. Injectable HA can temporarily restore dermal volume and correct facial lines and contour defects.

Dermal filler treatments are where art and medicine truly combine. Desirable outcomes depend equally on providers' knowledge of filler products and injection skills, as well as an appreciation for aesthetic facial proportions and symmetry. Dermal fillers have a steeper learning curve than botulinum toxin and require practice to consistently achieve desirable results.

HA fillers are used for many facial aesthetic indications; however, treatment of the lower two thirds of the face yields the most predictable results, with the greatest efficacy and fewest side effects. The three essential dermal filler aesthetic rejuvenation treatments

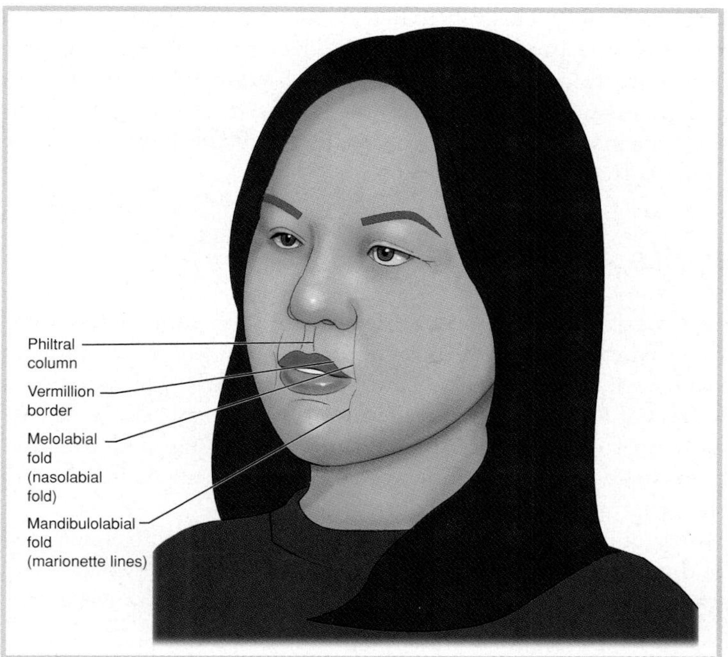

Figure 1

(ARTs) for primary care professionals to treat unwanted facial lines and contour defects are: (i) nasolabial folds (melolabial folds); (ii) oral commissures, marionette lines (mandibulolabial folds); and (iii) lip augmentation as shown in Figure 1.

General Injection Guidelines

Position the patient comfortably, at about a 65 degree reclined position, for the procedure. Prior to injection, prime the needle by depressing the syringe plunger until a small amount of filler extrudes from the needle tip. Ensure that the needle is tightly affixed to the filler syringe because excessive plunger pressure may cause the needle to pop off and filler to be extruded from the syringe.

All injections should be in the dermis. Some plunger resistance during injection should be felt when injecting at the appropriate level in the dermis. When injecting too deeply, in the subcutaneous tissues, there is little to no resistance against injection. When injecting too superficially, the gray needle tip is visible in the skin. The filler should be injected using firm, constant pressure on the syringe plunger as the needle is withdrawn in a linear thread. Visible and palpable bumps of filler seen after treating an area should be compressed between the thumb, placed on the skin, and the first finger, placed intraorally. If bumps do not easily compress, the injector may moisten the bumpy area with water and stretch the area between his or her fingers. The more massage done to a treatment area, the more swelling and bruising will occur.

If blanching occurs while injecting, the blood flow to the treatment site has been compromised either by injecting too much filler into the dermis or injecting intravascularly. Discontinue injecting and massage the area until the tissue appears pink. Injections may be continued in other parts of the treatment area.

Treat one area to injector and patient satisfaction before focusing on another area for treatment.

Dosage and Volume

The volume necessary for treatment must be estimated and discussed with the patient prior to injection. Volumes listed in the chapter are recommendations for starting volumes and refer exclusively to hyaluronic acid fillers formulated without lidocaine, such as Restylane and Juvederm Ultra Plus. The best results are achieved through individualization of treatments based on patients' observed facial anatomy and volume loss in the treatment areas. The maximal volume for Juvederm Ultra Plus is 20 mL/yr. Medicis does not report a maximum annual volume for Restylane; however, the recommended maximal volume per treatment site is 1.5 mL.

Results and Follow-up

Correction of lines and contour defects are seen immediately with filler injections. The treatment area will be swollen for approximately 3 to 5 days postprocedure, and the final appearance of the treatment area will be less full after the swelling resolves. The visible filling effects of Restylane and Juvederm Ultra Plus may persist for 6 to 9 months, and occasionally up to 1 year. Persistence is affected by many factors, including the patient's metabolism, degree of motion in the treatment area, and facial expressivity, and it should not be guaranteed at the time of treatment.

If ongoing treatments are desired, patients should follow-up when the filler appears to be diminishing, at about 6 months. Less volume is typically required for subsequent treatments, provided some volume from the initial treatment is still present.

General Anesthesia Techniques

Providing adequate anesthesia is an essential part of successfully incorporating fillers into practice. Minimizing discomfort improves provider results and offers the patient a better experience. The goal with anesthesia for filler treatments is to achieve maximal anesthesia while minimizing distortion of the treatment area. Four main anesthetic techniques are used prior to filler treatments:

- Regional nerve blocks are ideal for treatment of lips because anesthetic is remote from the treatment area and does not significantly distort lip anatomy (see the Lip Augmentation section).
- Local lidocaine injection is used for treatment of the nasolabial and oral commissure areas. Care should be taken to use the smallest anesthetic volumes possible because infiltration of the anesthetic will result in some distortion of the anatomy. A maxillary nerve block should be used instead of local infiltration in the nasolabial folds when both the upper lip and nasolabial folds are being treated. A mandibular nerve block should be used instead of local infiltration in the oral commissures when both the lower lip and oral commissures are being treated.
- Topical anesthetics may be used in the nasolabial and oral commissure areas. In-office application of a topical anesthetic, such as benzocaine 20%/lidocaine 6%/tetracaine 4% (BLT), with a maximum dose of 1 g applied for 15 minutes, may be used prior to treatment. BLT causes lip edema and is not advised for lip treatments.
- Ice is a good anesthetic and may be used adjunctively with the other methods or alone. Anesthesia is achieved by applying ice immediately before injecting for approximately 5 minutes or until the skin is blanched.

Preprocedure Checklist

- Perform an aesthetic evaluation and review the patient's medical history (see Chapter 28).
- Prophylax with antiviral medication if there is a history of herpes simplex for 2 days prior to procedure and continue for 3 days postprocedure.
- Minimize bruising by discontinuation of aspirin, vitamin E, St. John's wort, and other dietary supplements including ginkgo biloba, evening primrose oil, garlic, feverfew,

and ginseng for 2 weeks prior. Discontinue other nonsteroidal anti-inflammatory medications 2 days prior.

- Take preinjection photographs.
- Document and discuss any notable asymmetries prior to treatment.
- Obtain informed consent.
- Estimate filler volume necessary for treatment and cost.
- Prepare the skin with alcohol.
- Anesthetize the treatment area using the minimal necessary anesthetic volumes so as not to obscure the treatment area.

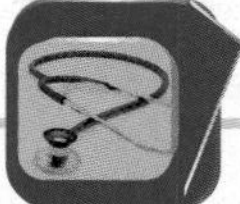

Equipment

Anesthesia

- 5.0-mL syringe
- Lidocaine HCl 2% with epinephrine 1:100,000
- 18-gauge, 1.5-inch needles
- 30-gauge, 0.5-inch needles
- Benzocaine/lidocaine/tetracaine (20:6:4) ointment

Filler Treatment

- Filler syringes of Restylane (20 mg HA/mL) or Juvederm Ultra Plus (24 mg HA/mL)
- 30-gauge, 0.5-inch needles
- Gauze, 3 × 3 inches, nonwoven
- Ice packs

Handling

HA is supplied in individual treatment syringes of 0.8 mL and is a clear colorless gel. Syringes should be stored at room temperature (up to 25°C or 77°F) prior to use.

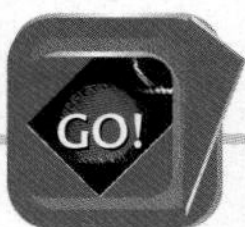

Aesthetic Indications

HA fillers are approved by the U.S. Food and Drug Administration for treatment of moderate to severe facial wrinkles and folds using mid- to deep dermal injections. HA treatment of lips and other cosmetic areas are off-label use.

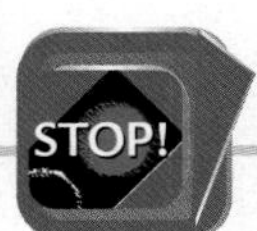

Contraindications

Absolute

- Pregnancy and nursing
- Previous anaphylactic reaction
- Multiple severe allergies
- Keloid formation
- Active infection or inflammation in the treatment area
- Previous allergic response to HA products
- Patient younger than 18 years of age

Relative

- History of easy bruising
- History of poor healing
- Body dysmorphic disorder or unrealistic expectations

The Procedure

Nasolabial Folds

Figure 2A shows a 38-year-old patient with moderate nasolabial folds prior to treatment. Figure 2B shows the same patient 1 week after treatment with an HA filler, Juvederm Ultra Plus, using 0.8 mL (one syringe) in each nasolabial fold for a total volume of 1.6 mL.

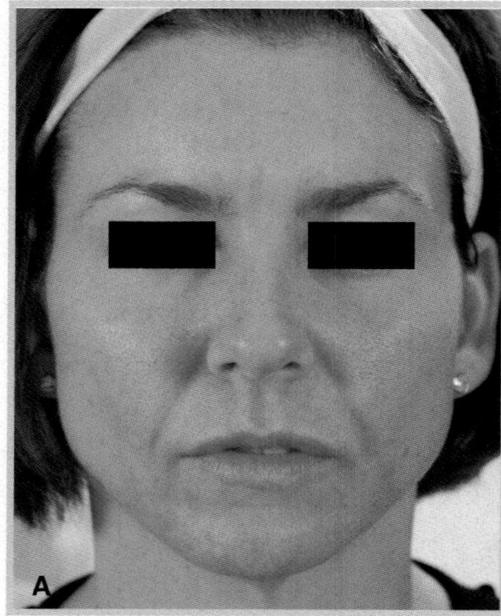
A

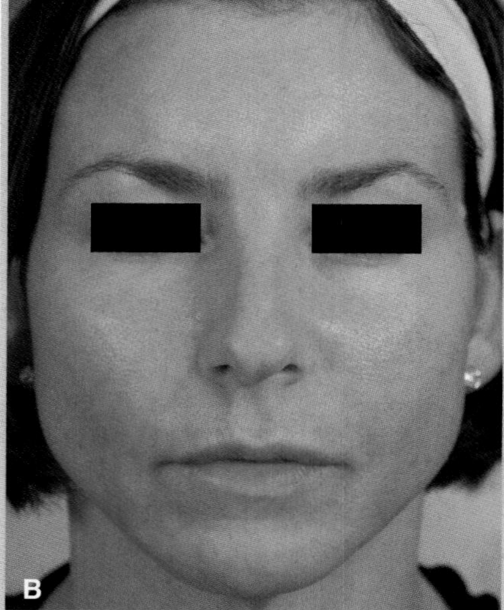
B

Figure 2

There are two methods for providing anesthesia to the nasolabial folds: (i) local infiltration adjacent to the folds (shown in Figure 3) or (ii) an infraorbital nerve block (see the Lip Augmentation section). When treating lips and nasolabial folds in the same visit, an infraorbital nerve block should be used without local infiltration, because this will anesthetize both treatment areas. Topical anesthetic and ice may be used as alternatives to these methods or may be used adjunctively (see Chapter 2). Step 1 shows an overview of injection points and doses for local infiltration of anesthetic for treatment of the nasolabial folds. After preparing the skin with alcohol, lidocaine is injected subcutaneously, superior to the nasolabial fold, with 0.1 mL placed at each injection point. After injecting, compress the injection sites to minimize edema from the anesthetic.

- **PEARL:** Sensitivity increases with proximity to the nose, and injections should start at the inferior injection point first and move superiorly toward the nose.
- **PITFALL:** Placing anesthetic into the nasolabial fold will blunt the fold and make filler treatment volumes more difficult to determine accurately.

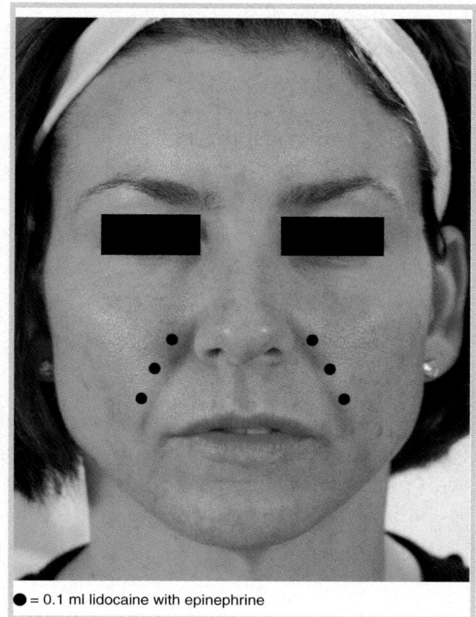

Figure 3

An overview of HA injection points for the treatment of nasolabial folds is shown in Figure 4, where number 1 is the first injection site. The needle is advanced superiorly towards the nose and the filler product is fanned medially at the nasal ala. Mild nasolabial folds typically require 0.4 to 0.8 mL (half to one syringe) of filler per side, and moderate to severe folds require 0.8 to 1.2 mL (one to one and a half syringes) per side. All injections should be placed just medial to the nasolabial fold using a 30-gauge, 0.5-inch needle with the dermal filler syringe.

- **PITFALL:** Care should be taken not to inject lateral to the folds because this can accentuate the folds.
- **PITFALL:** Injections placed too superficially may result in an unsightly visible ridge of filler that can persist in the superficial dermis (see the General Injection Techniques section).
- **PITFALL:** Avoid overfilling the treatment area because the goal of treatment is to blunt, not to eliminate, the nasolabial fold. This is a natural, desired contour of the face.
- **PEARL:** Compress the treated area as described in the General Injection Guidelines section to ensure that the filler is smooth. Threads of filler should not be visible or distinctly palpable after treatment.

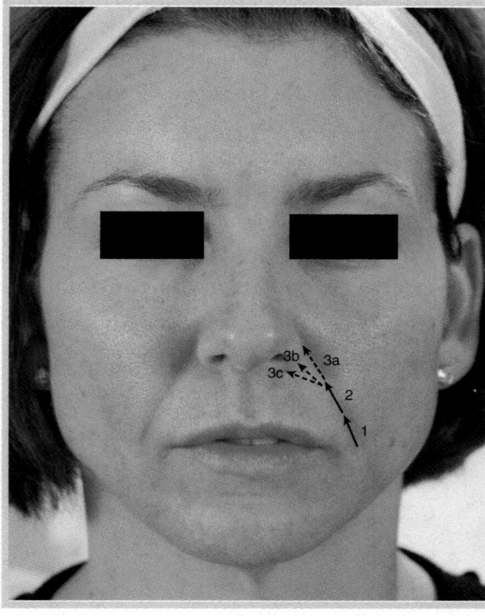

Figure 4

Step 1. The first injection is placed medial and at the inferior point of the fold. The needle should be inserted at a 30 degree angle to the skin and advanced to the hub. Filler should be injected using firm constant pressure on the syringe plunger as the needle is withdrawn.

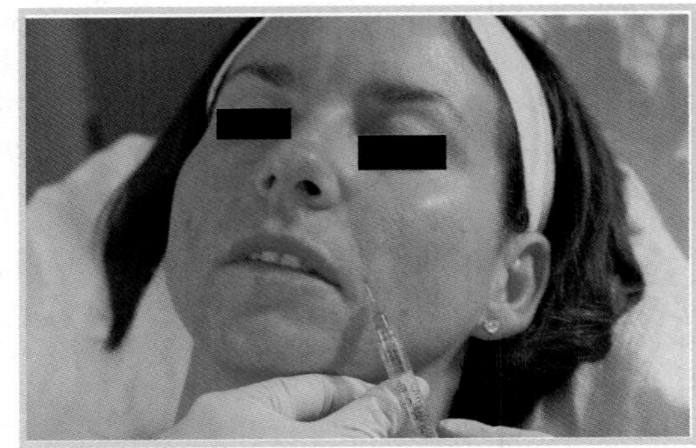

Step 1

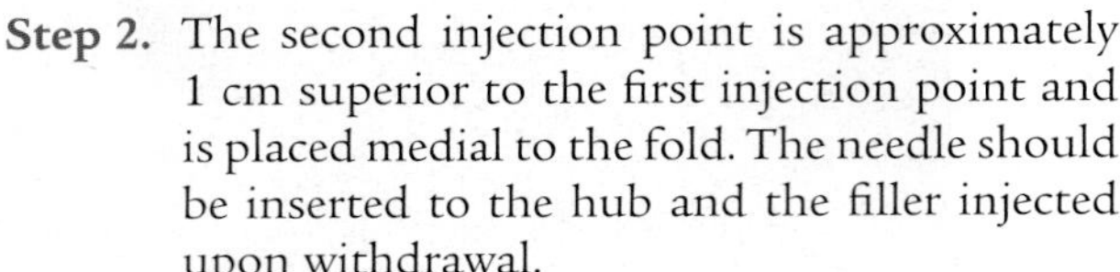

Step 2. The second injection point is approximately 1 cm superior to the first injection point and is placed medial to the fold. The needle should be inserted to the hub and the filler injected upon withdrawal.

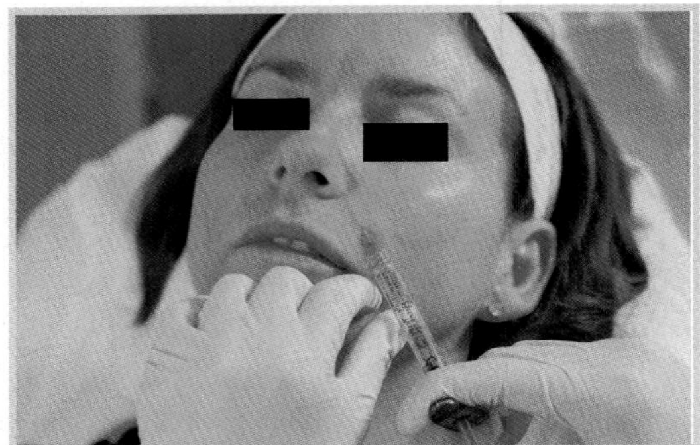

Step 2

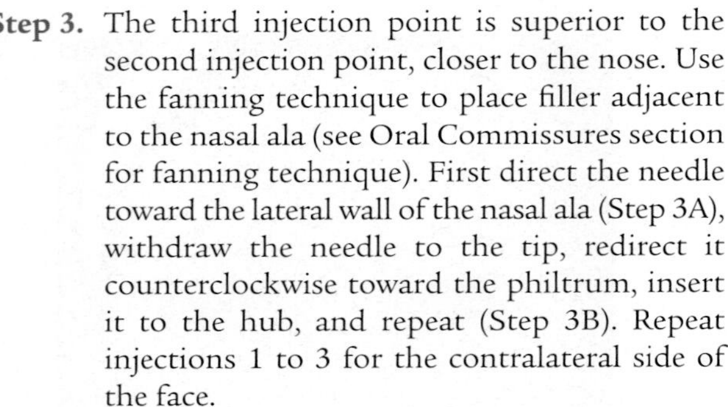

Step 3. The third injection point is superior to the second injection point, closer to the nose. Use the fanning technique to place filler adjacent to the nasal ala (see Oral Commissures section for fanning technique). First direct the needle toward the lateral wall of the nasal ala (Step 3A), withdraw the needle to the tip, redirect it counterclockwise toward the philtrum, insert it to the hub, and repeat (Step 3B). Repeat injections 1 to 3 for the contralateral side of the face.

- **PITFALL:** This is the most sensitive area of the fold, and patients may experience discomfort if not adequately anesthetized.

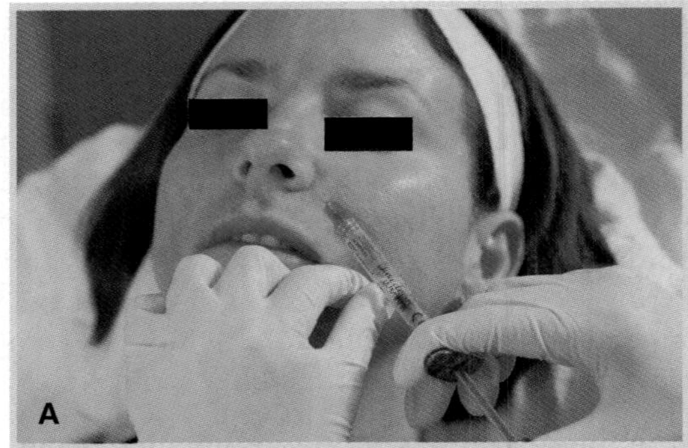

A

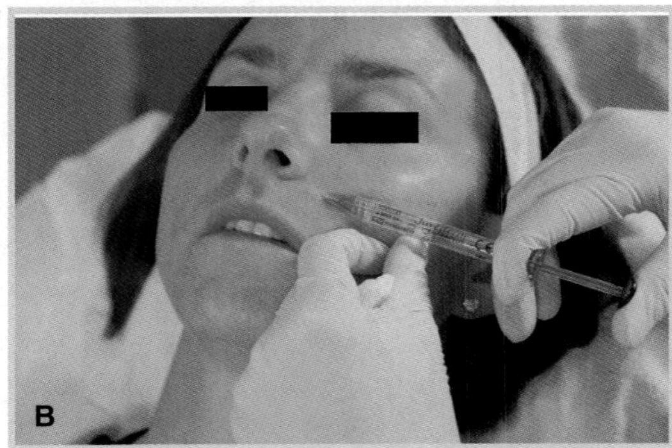

B

Step 3

Figure 5 shows the angular artery which lies at the superior lateral edge of the nasal ala. Tissue ischemia associated with intravascular injection of the angular artery may be seen as a violaceous reticular pattern of the skin along the lateral wall of the nose and/or nasolabial fold. Ischemia can rapidly progress to tissue necrosis, and this complication should be managed urgently. If ischemia occurs, revascularize by massaging the violaceous area and the ala artery, apply heat packs, and give the patient two 325-mg enteric coated aspirins orally. If not improving, apply nitropaste (1-inch dose of Nitro-BID) to the affected area, monitor for hypotension, and contact your local emergency room and/or plastic surgeon.

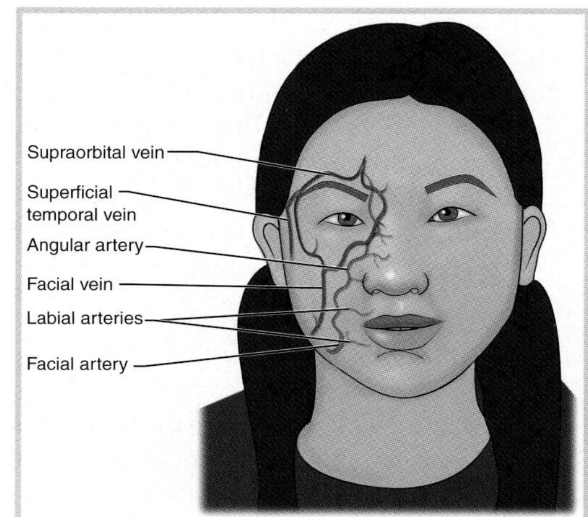

Figure 5

Oral Commissures and Marionette Lines

The corners of the mouth where the upper lips meet the lower lips are called the oral commissures. Volume loss in these areas can lead to depressed oral commissures with downturned corners of the mouth. Skin folds which descend from the oral commissures towards the jaw are known as marionette lines or mandibulolabial folds. Assessment and treatment of the lower facial area should concurrently address both the oral commissures and manionette lines. For the purposes of this chapter, oral commissures and manionette lines will collectively be referred to as the lower face folds (LFF). Figure 1A shows a 70-year-old woman with moderate volume loss in the LFF and downturned corners of the mouth prior to treatment, and Figure 1B shows the same patient 1 week after treatment with a HA filler, Juvederm Ultra Plus, using 0.8 mL (one syringe) per side for a total volume of 1.6 mL. Note the improvement in the downturned corners of the mouth oral commissures, and marionette lines.

There are two methods for providing anesthesia to the LFF: (i) local infiltration in the treatment area and (ii) a mental nerve block (see the Lip Augmentation section). When treating lips and LFF in the same visit, a mental nerve block should be used without local infiltration, because this will anesthetize both treatment areas. Topical anesthetic and ice are alternatives to these methods or may be used adjunctively.

Step 1. Shows an overview of injection points and doses for local infiltration of anesthetic for treatment of the LFF. After preparing the skin with alcohol, 0.1 mL of lidocaine is injected subcutaneously, in the middle of the LFF area, approximately 0.5 cm inferior to the vermillion border and 0.5 cm medial to the marionette line. For patients with moderate and severe LFF that extend inferiorly toward the jaw, a second injection point may be added approximately 1 cm

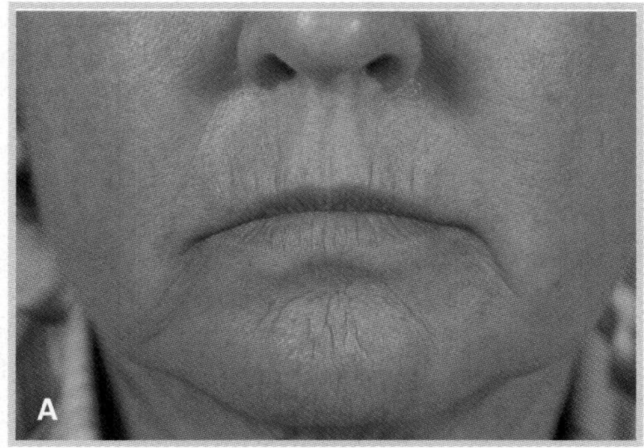

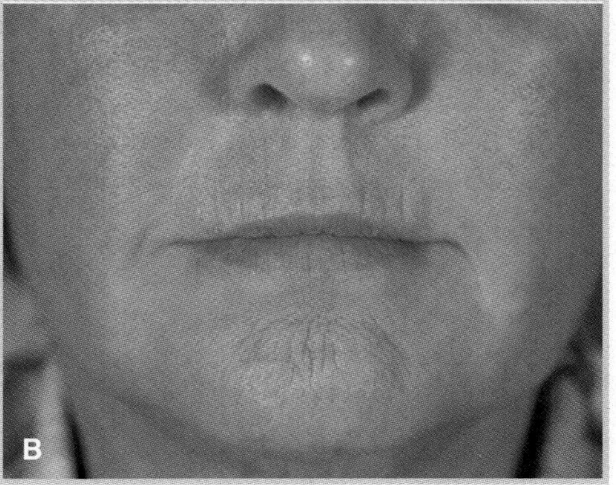

Figure 1

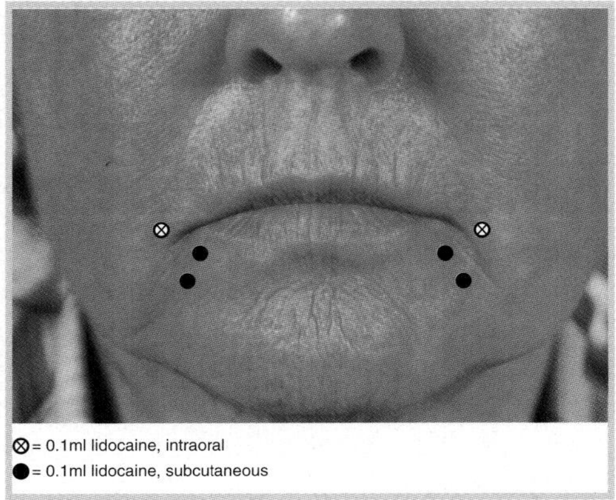

Step 1

inferior to the first point. To anesthetize the corner of lower lip, inject 0.1 mL of lidocaine intraorally in the mucosa at the inferior corner of the mouth (see the Anesthesia section in the Lip Augmentation section). Repeat for the contralateral LFF and corner of the mouth. After injecting, compress the injection sites to minimize edema from the anesthetic.

Step 2. There are two injection techniques for placing filler in the deep dermis that add support to the LFF: fanning and cross hatching. An overview of HA injection points for fanning and cross-hatching techniques for the treatment of the LFF is shown in Step 2.

Fanning utilizes one needle insertion point, whereby a series of adjacent linear threads are injected so that filler is placed in a triangular area in the dermis. From the initial needle insertion point, the needle is advanced to the hub, filler is injected in a linear thread, and the needle is withdrawn to the tip, redirected, and inserted to the hub again.

Cross hatching involves multiple injection points whereby filler is placed in a square area in the dermis. A linear thread of filler is placed, the needle is fully withdrawn and reinserted in an adjacent area, and another linear thread is placed parallel to the first thread. This is repeated at 90 degrees to the first filler threads to form a square area of filler.

Mild LFFs typically require 0.4 mL (half a syringe) of filler per side, and moderate to severe folds require 0.8 mL (one syringe) per side. A 30-gauge, 0.5-inch needle with a dermal filler syringe is used for all injections.

- **PEARL:** Compress the treated area as described in the General Injection Guidelines section to ensure that the filler is smooth. Threads of filler should not be visible or palpable with either technique after treatment.
- **PITFALL:** Avoid overfilling the treatment area because abnormal lip contours, particularly in the lateral upper lip, may result.
- **PITFALL:** Watch for tissue blanching. If this occurs, the area has been overfilled. Manage as described in the General Injection Guidelines section.

Step 3. The first injection point is in the corner of the lower lip (Step 3A). The needle should be inserted at a 30 degree angle to the skin and advanced to the hub (Step 3B). Filler should be injected using firm constant pressure on the syringe plunger as the needle is withdrawn.

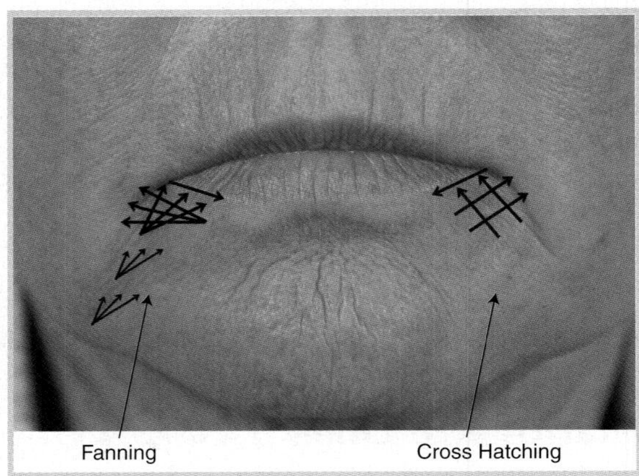

Step 2

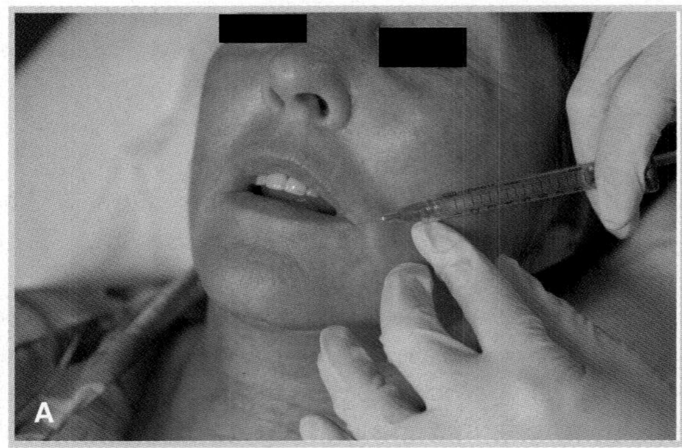

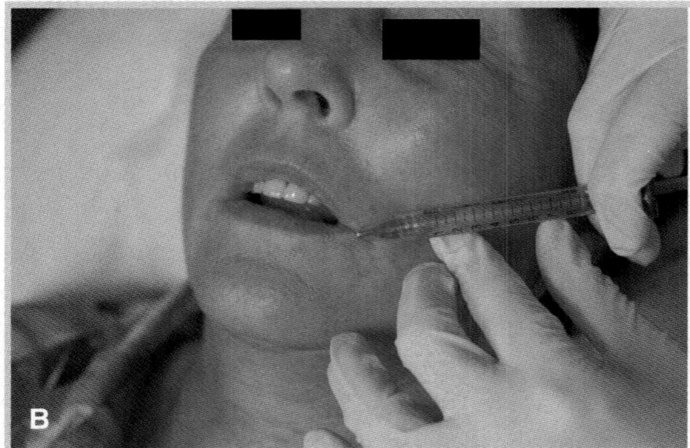

Step 3

Step 4. The second injection point is one needle length below the lower lip vermillion border, just medial to the LFF. The needle is directed toward the vermillion border (Step 4A). Fan the product by withdrawing the needle and redirecting 30 degrees counterclockwise (Step 4B). This is repeated to place a triangular area of filler inferior to and abutting the vermillion border. Note that the blanching seen in Step 4A and 4B is due to the vasoconstrictive epinephrine effect from the local anesthetic.

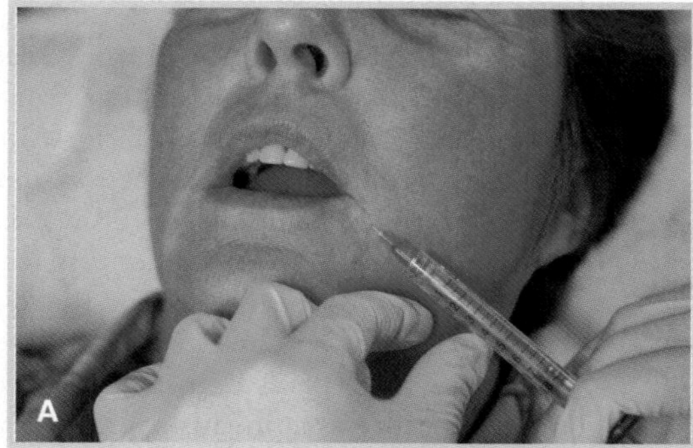

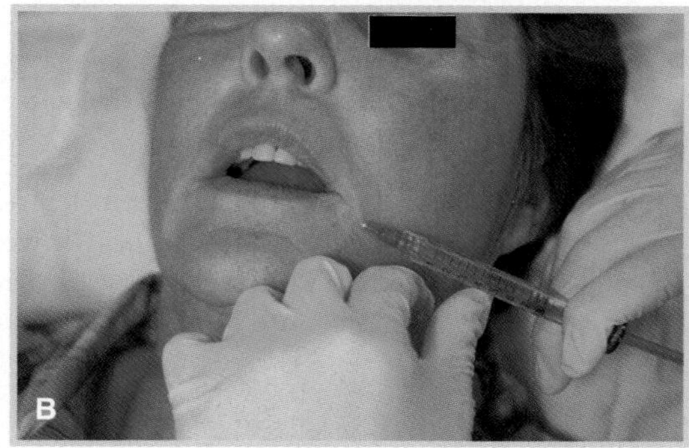

Step 4

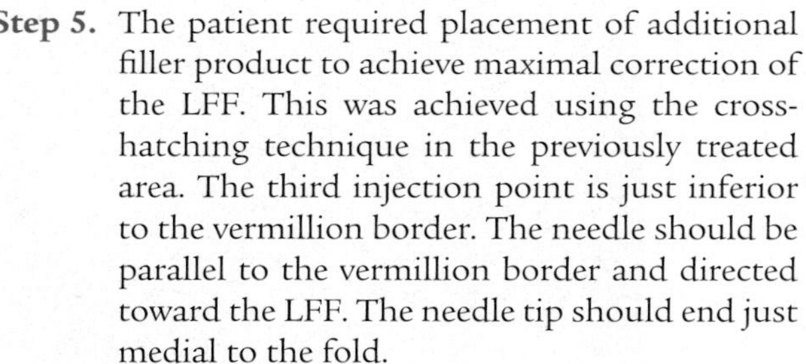

Step 5. The patient required placement of additional filler product to achieve maximal correction of the LFF. This was achieved using the cross-hatching technique in the previously treated area. The third injection point is just inferior to the vermillion border. The needle should be parallel to the vermillion border and directed toward the LFF. The needle tip should end just medial to the fold.

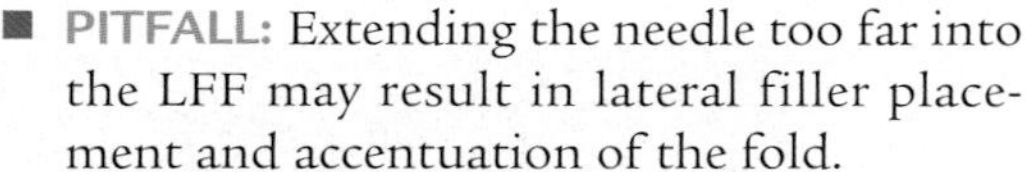

- **PITFALL:** Extending the needle too far into the LFF may result in lateral filler placement and accentuation of the fold.

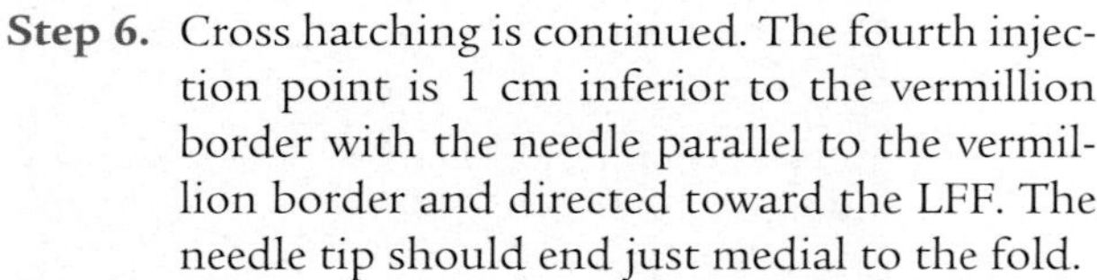

Step 6. Cross hatching is continued. The fourth injection point is 1 cm inferior to the vermillion border with the needle parallel to the vermillion border and directed toward the LFF. The needle tip should end just medial to the fold.

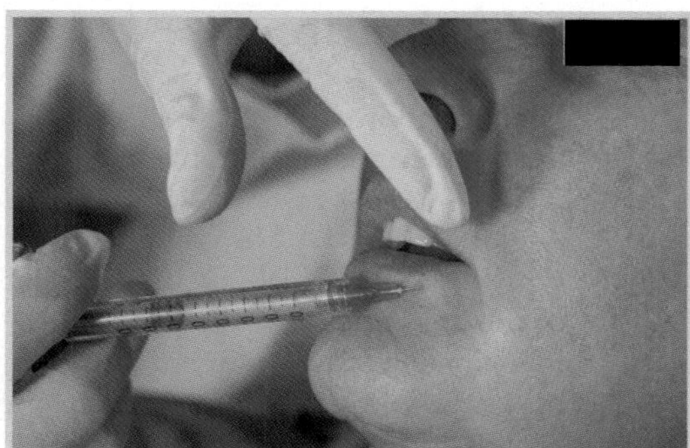

Step 5

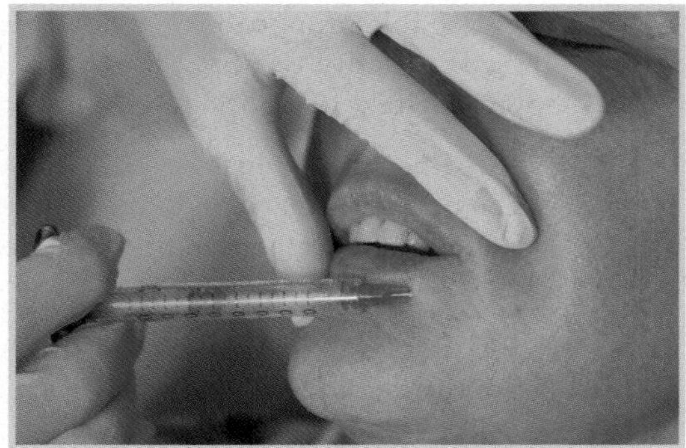

Step 6

Step 7. The remaining inferior portion of the LFF is typically treated using the fanning technique. The fifth injection point is approximately one and a half needle lengths inferior to the vermillion border, with the injection point just medial to the LFF and directed toward the vermillion border (Step 7A). Filler is placed using the fanning technique, where the needle is redirected approximately 30 degrees counter clockwise, and this is repeated, filler is placed in a triangular area in this inferior portion of the LFF (Step 7B).

- **PEARL:** Filler should be placed such that it is continuous with filler already in the dermis and should feel smooth.
- **PEARL:** Successful correction of the LFF is achieved when the lateral lower lip is supported and buttressed by adequate volume and placement of filler as described above.

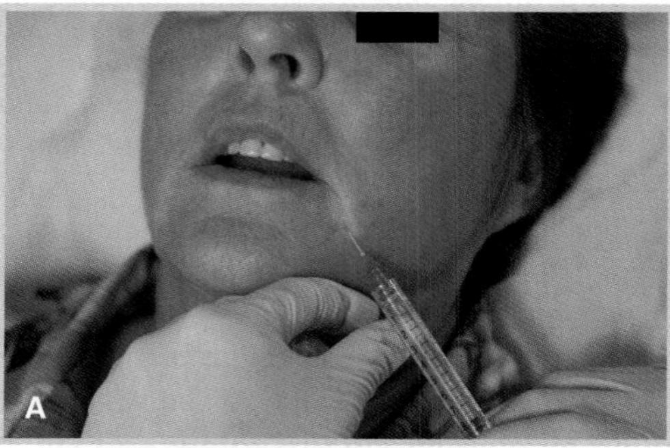

A

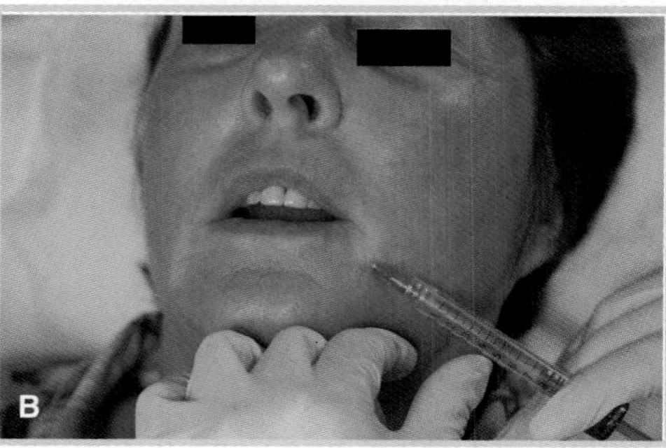

B

Step 7

Lip Augmentation

Figure 1 shows a 38-year-old patient prior to lip augmentation (A), immediately after treatment (B), and 1 week after treatment (C) with a total of 1.6 mL of Juvederm Ultra Plus (two syringes) to the vermillion border and the body of the lips. Note that swelling is most marked immediately after treatment and has resolved by 1 week, leaving only the filler effect. The goal of lip augmentation is to restore a natural fuller appearance to the lip with slight eversion of the vermillion border without overtreating. The desirable proportions for lips are a larger lower lip relative to upper lip with a ratio of approximately 1:2 in lip height.

- **PEARL:** Volume loss is more apparent in the upper lip than the lower lip, and many patients may only need or desire treatment to the upper lip.
- **PEARL:** Track filler volumes closely and administer equal volumes on both sides of a lip unless gross asymmetry is present prior to treating.

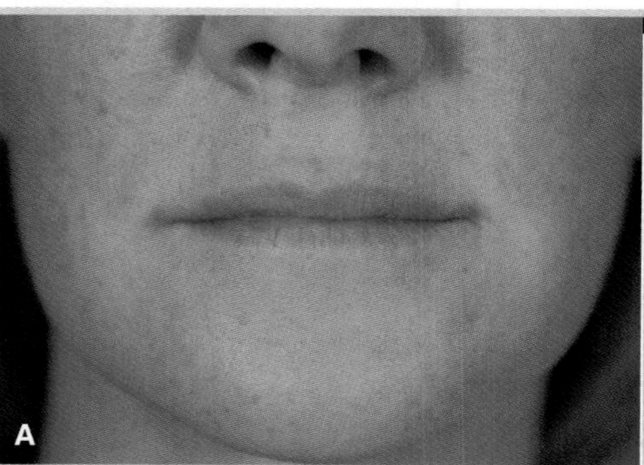

A

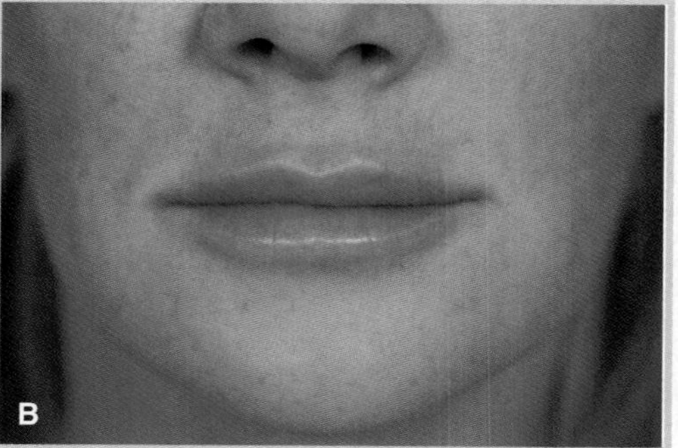

B

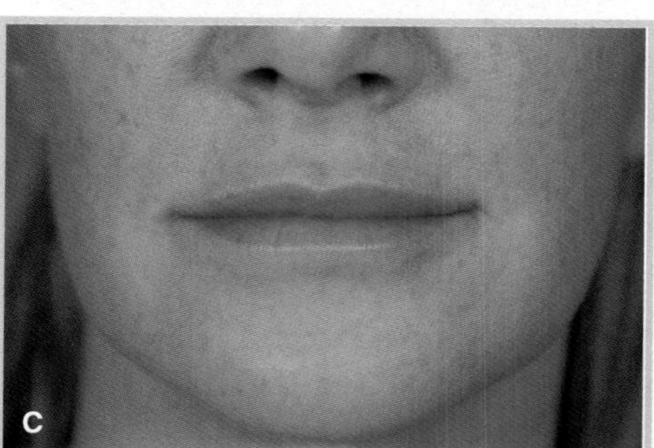

C

Figure 1

On lateral projection, the angle between the upper lip and nose (nasolabial angle) for women should be 95 to 110 degrees and for men 90 to 95 degrees. Figure 2A shows the lateral projection prior to treatment, and Figure 2B shows the nasolabial angle after treatment for the previously mentioned patient.

- **PEARL:** Patients with diminutive upper lips are not good candidates for treatment, and filler injections may result in an unnatural anterior projection of the upper lip or a "duck" lip.

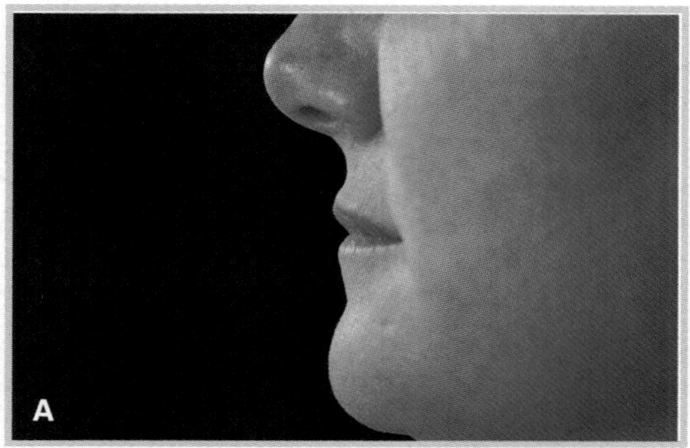

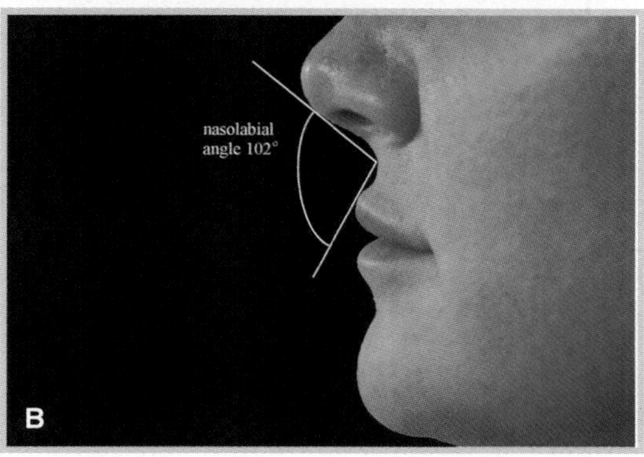

Figure 2

Adequate anesthesia of the lip region prior to filler injection is essential to the success of lip augmentation treatments. Anesthesia for the upper lip requires an infraorbital nerve block and additional mucosal infiltration at the corners of the mouth and at the gingivobuccal junction of the upper lip frenulum. Treatment to the lower lip requires a mental nerve block and additional mucosal infiltration at the corners of the mouth. Figure 3 shows an overview of injection points and doses for fully anesthetizing both the upper and lower lips.

The location of the infraorbital and mental nerves is shown in Figure 4 and can be identified by palpating the nerve foramina. First, palpate the supraorbital notch, which lies along the upper border of the orbit approximately 2.5 cm lateral to the midline of the face, and draw a vertical line down from the supraorbital notch to the mandible. The infraorbital foramen lies on this line and is palpable approximately 1 cm inferior to the infraorbital boney margin. The mental nerve also lies on this line and is palpable just above the margin of the mandible.

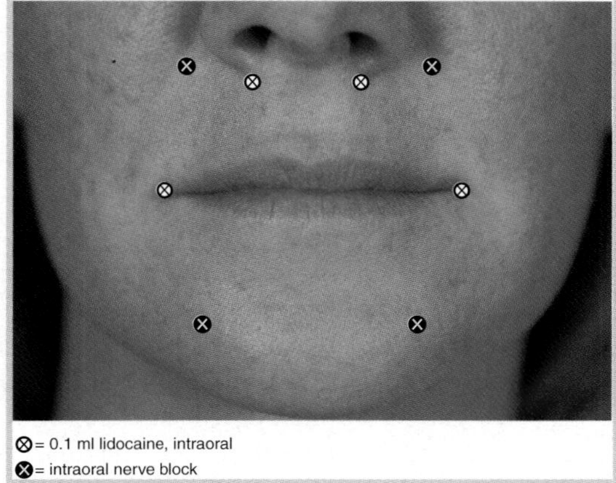

Figure 3

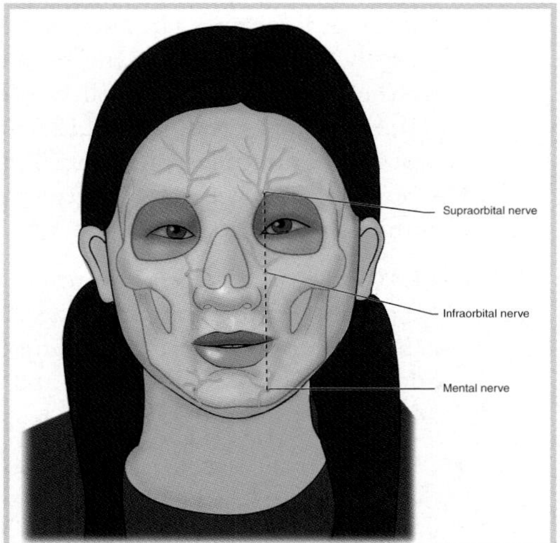

Figure 4

Figure 5 shows the intraoral technique for infraorbital and mental anesthetic nerve blocks to be used prior to lip augmentation.

The infraorbital nerve innervates most of the upper lip, the lower eyelid, lateral portion of the nose, and medial cheek, and an infraorbital nerve block can anesthetize all of these regions (see Figure 6). However, the philtrum and the corners of the mouth are typically poorly anesthetized, because they are at the distal nerve branches, and additional local infiltration is required in these areas.

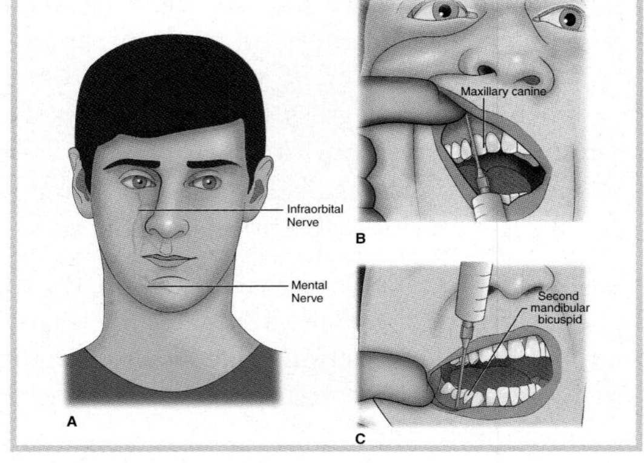

Figure 5

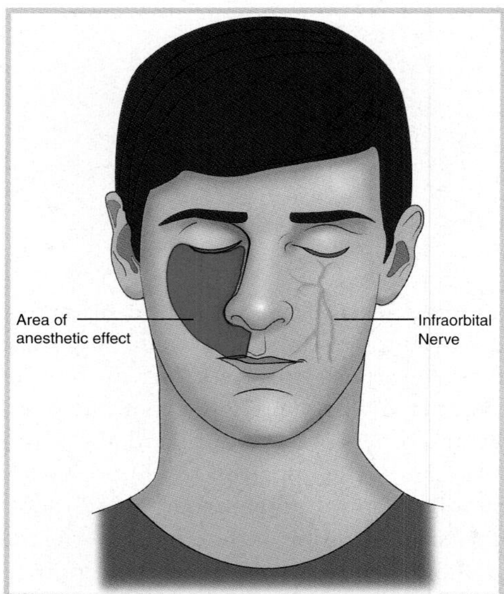

Figure 6

Step 1. Comfortably position the patient upright at about 65 degrees, with their chin tipped upward. Lift the upper lip for good visualization of the gingivobuccal margin, and insert a 30-gauge, 0.5-inch needle at the gingivobuccal margin just lateral to the maxillary canine. Direct the needle superiorly towards the pupil, advance the needle to the hub, and inject 0.5 to 1.0 mL of lidocaine. The anesthetic should flow easily. After removing the needle, compress the deep palpable wheal of lidocaine superiorly towards the infraorbital foramen. Repeat for the contralateral infraorbital nerve. The onset of anesthetic effect is typically 5 to 10 minutes.

- **PEARL:** Test the lip prior to initiating filler treatment. If adequate anesthesia is not achieved, repeat the procedure, injecting an additional 0.5 mL of lidocaine, and wait an additional 10 minutes.
- **PITFALL:** If the needle is angled too anteriorly, lidocaine may be placed in the dermis, and resistance during injection will be encountered.

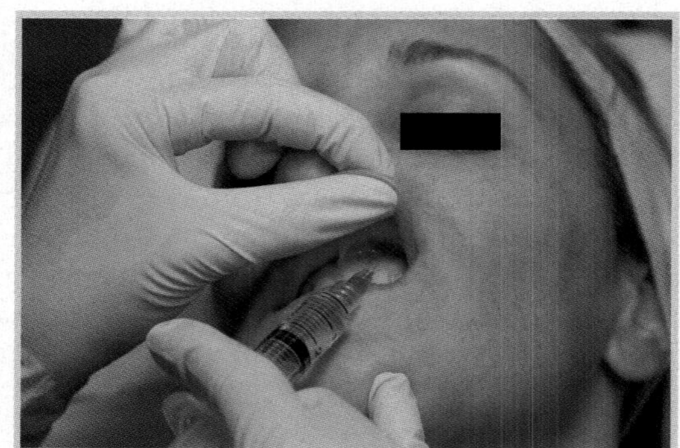

Step 1

The mental nerve innervates most of the lower lip, and a mental nerve block can anesthetize this region (as shown in Figure 7). However, the corner of the mouth is typically poorly anesthetized, and additional local lidocaine infiltration is required.

Step 2. Comfortably position the patient upright at about 65 degrees, with their chin tipped downward. Lift the lower lip for good visualization of the gingivobuccal margin. Insert a 30 gauge, 0.5 inch needle at the gingivobuccal margin just lateral to the first mandibular bicuspid. Direct the needle inferior laterally. Advance the needle halfway to the hub, and inject 0.5 to 1.0 mL of lidocaine. The anesthetic should flow easily. After removing the needle, compress the deep palpable wheal of lidocaine inferiorly towards the mental foramen. Repeat for the contralateral mental nerve. The onset of anesthetic effect is typically within 5 to 10 minutes.

- **PEARL:** Test the lip prior to initiating filler treatment. If adequate anesthesia is not achieved, repeat the procedure, injecting slightly more laterally using an additional 0.5 mL of lidocaine, and wait an additional 10 minutes.

Step 3. The lateral corners of the mouth require additional infiltration of local anesthetic to achieve adequate anesthesia. Inject 0.1 mL of lidocaine intraorally in the mucosa at the corner of the mouth. After the needle is removed, compress the injection site to disburse the lidocaine, and repeat for the contralateral corner of the mouth.

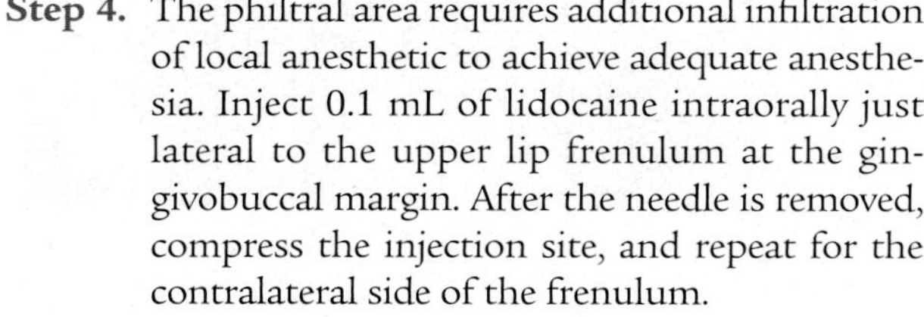

Step 4. The philtral area requires additional infiltration of local anesthetic to achieve adequate anesthesia. Inject 0.1 mL of lidocaine intraorally just lateral to the upper lip frenulum at the gingivobuccal margin. After the needle is removed, compress the injection site, and repeat for the contralateral side of the frenulum.

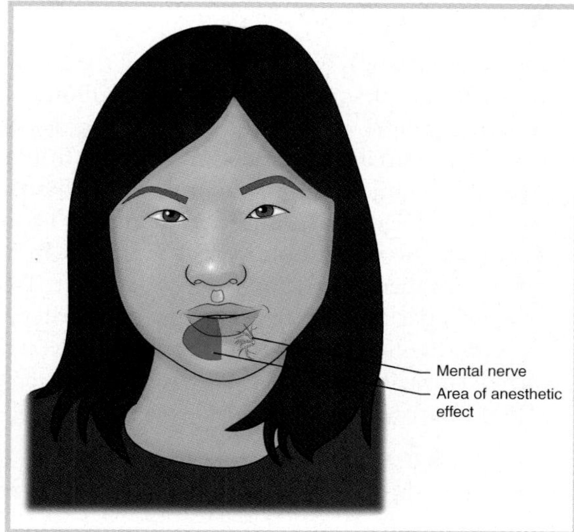

Figure 7

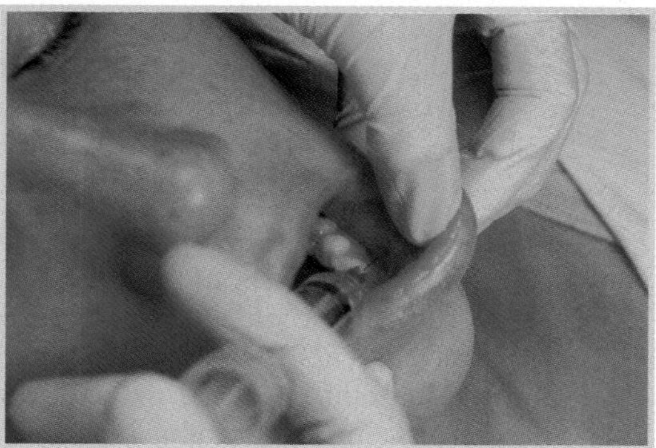

Step 2

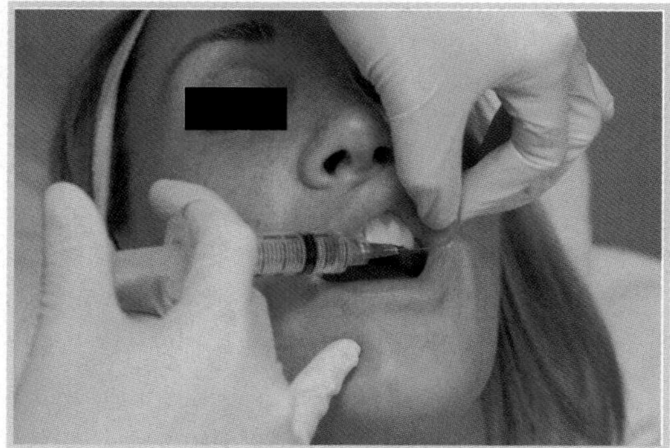

Step 3

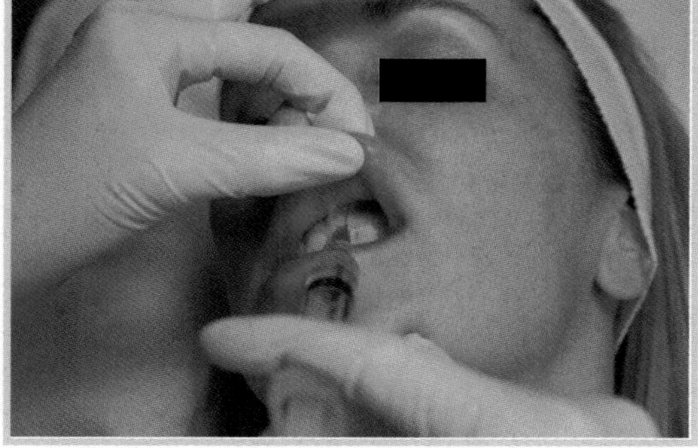

Step 4

Vermillion Border

Lip augmentation involves enhancing the border of the lip with filler injection along the vermillion cutaneous junction, referred to as the vermillion border. Depending on the patient's lip shape and desired fullness, filler may also be injected into the mucosa or "body" of the lip. An overview of HA injection points for lip augmentation of the vermillion border is shown in Figure 8 where number 1 is the first injection point. Treatment of the upper and lower lip vermillion borders require approximately 0.8 mL (one syringe) of Restylane or Juvederm Ultra Plus. A 30-gauge, 0.5-inch needle should be used for injections.

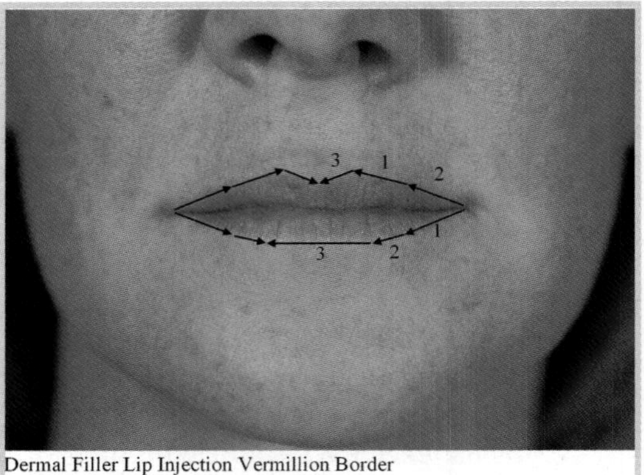

Dermal Filler Lip Injection Vermillion Border

Figure 8

- **PEARL:** The top lip should be injected before the bottom lip.
- **PEARL:** Lip edema can occur fairly rapidly, particularly with Restylane. After completion of treatment to both sides of the lip, the first side that was injected may appear larger. Do not retreat the second side at this time, because this asymmetry likely is due to edema. Re-evaluate the patient 1 week posttreatment.

Step 1. The first injection should be placed such that the tip of the needle ends at the peak of the "M" of the cupids bow. Identify the needle insertion point by measuring with the needle against the lip, as shown in Step 1A. The plane for injection is along the vermillion border in the potential space that exists just below the skin. Insert the needle to the hub, and inject as the needle is withdrawn, as in Step 1B. The filler should flow easily into the potential space of the vermillion border, enhancing the white rolled border of the lip.

- **PEARL:** Vertical lip lines that abut the vermillion border can be effectively treated by augmenting the vermillion border.
- **PITFALL:** Filler should not be visible or palpable as discrete lumps. Compress the treated area as described in the General Injection Guidelines section to ensure that the filler is smooth.
- **PITFALL:** If filler is seen outside of the vermillion border above the lip during injection, stop injecting, compress/massage until no product is visible above the vermillion border, and resume treatment.

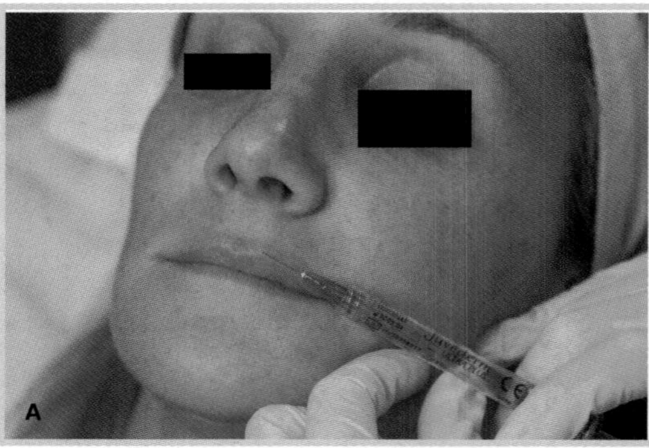

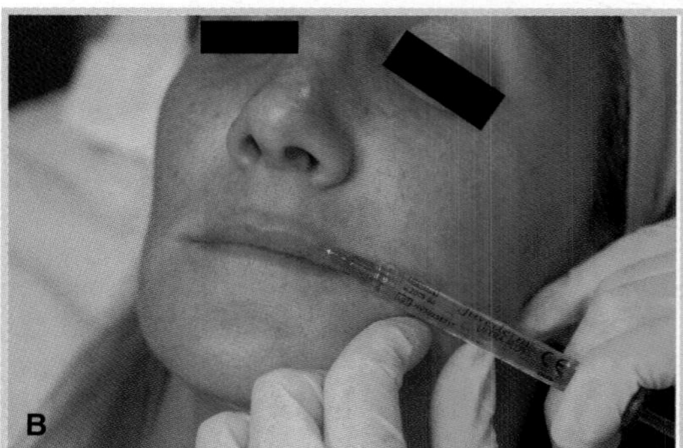

Step 1

Step 2. The second injection point is one needle length lateral to the first injection point. Again, the needle is inserted to the hub, and the filler is smoothly injected as the needle is withdrawn.

- **PEARL:** Do not overfill this lateral-most portion of the lip because this can result in undesired contour changes of the lip.

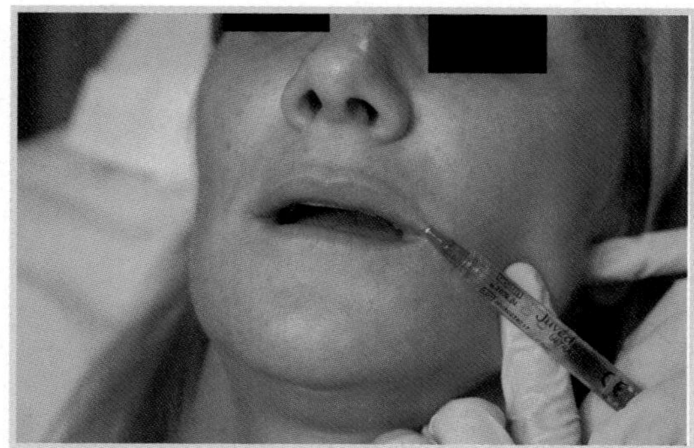

Step 2

Step 3. The third injection point is in the cupid's bow. The needle should be inserted in the peak of the "M" of the cupid's bow and the tip advanced to the nadir of the "M." Smoothly inject filler as the needle is withdrawn. Proceed with filler injections to the lip body if desired; otherwise, complete the vermillion border treatment for the contralateral side of the upper lip.

- **PEARL:** Use small volumes in this area to accentuate the "M" contour.

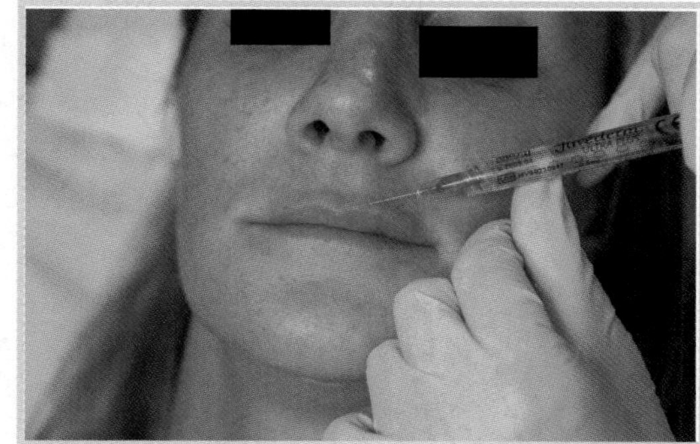

Step 3

Step 4. The first injection in the vermillion border of the lower lip begins at the corner of the lip. The needle is inserted to the hub, and filler is smoothly injected as the needle is withdrawn.

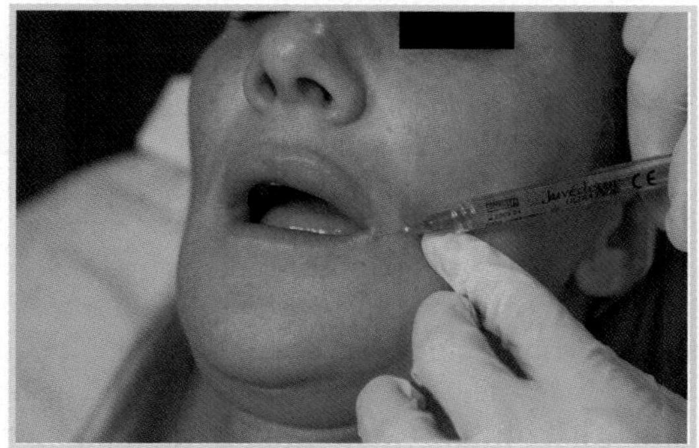

Step 4

Step 5. The second injection point in the vermillion border is placed one needle length medial to the initial injection point, shown in Step 5A. The needle is inserted to the hub, shown in Step 5B, and filler is smoothly injected as the needle is withdrawn.

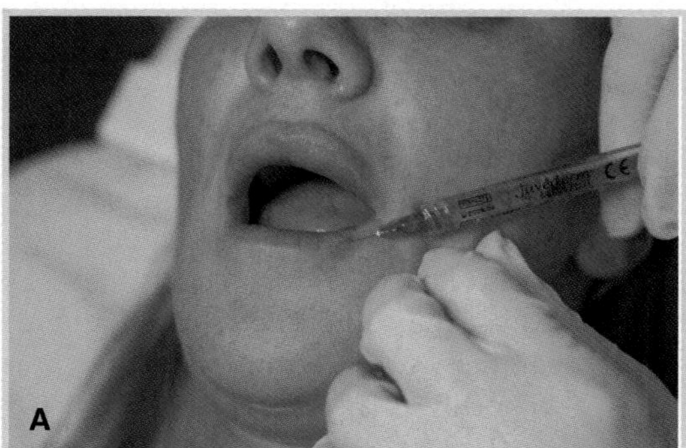

Step 5

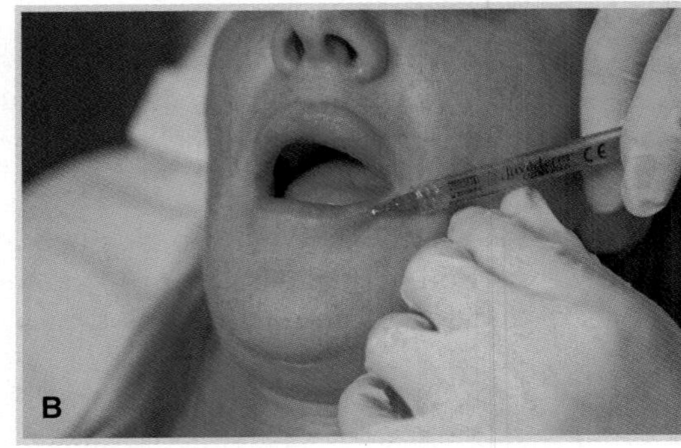

Step 6. The third injection point with filler placement in the middle portion of the lower lip is one needle length medial to the second injection point. Proceed with filler injections to the lip body if desired; otherwise, complete the vermillion border treatment for the contralateral side of the lower lip.

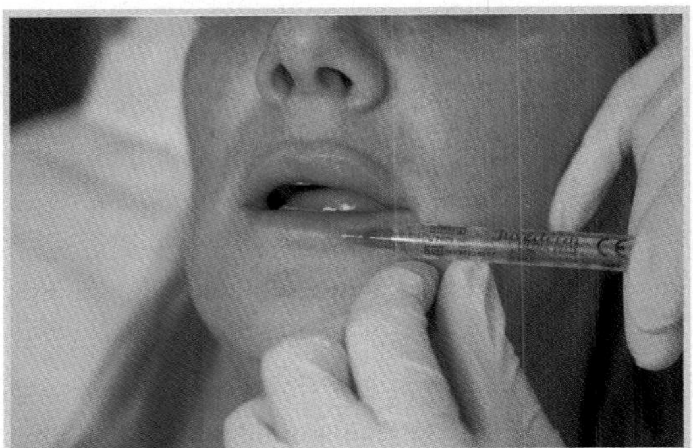

Step 6

Lip Body

After the vermillion border has been treated, additional dermal filler may be placed in the body of the lip. The top lip should be injected before the bottom lip. An overview of HA injection points for lip augmentation to the body of the lip is shown, where number 1 is the first injection point as shown in Figure 9. Treatment of the body of the upper and lower lips requires approximately 0.8 mL (one syringe) of Restylane or Juvederm Ultra Plus. A 30-gauge, 0.5-inch needle should be used for injections.

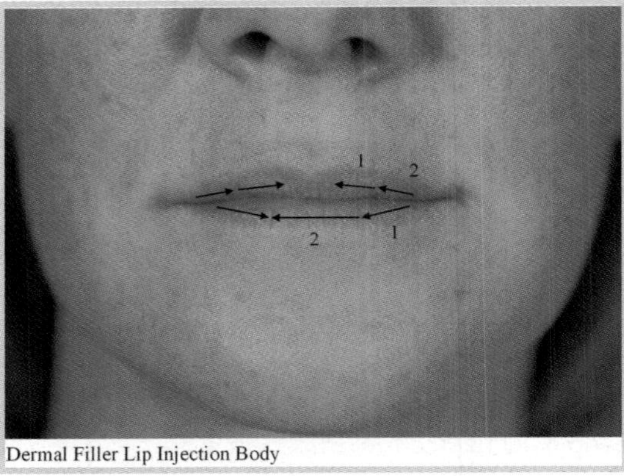

Dermal Filler Lip Injection Body

Figure 9

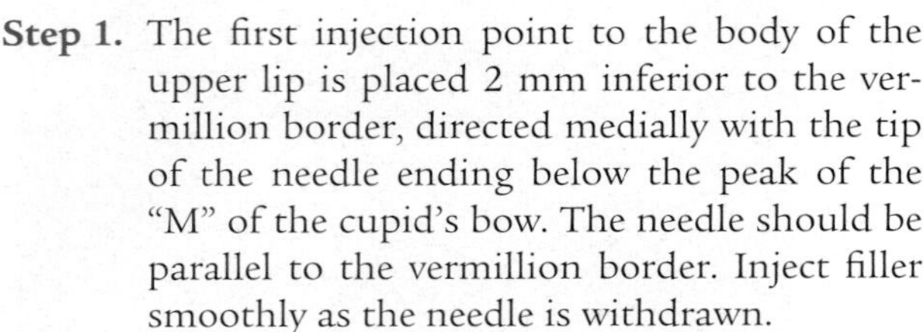

Step 1. The first injection point to the body of the upper lip is placed 2 mm inferior to the vermillion border, directed medially with the tip of the needle ending below the peak of the "M" of the cupid's bow. The needle should be parallel to the vermillion border. Inject filler smoothly as the needle is withdrawn.

- **PITFALL:** Do not inject in the central-most portion of the body of the lip. Filler in the area between the two peaks of the "M" will result in an unnatural protrusion of the upper lip, which is difficult to correct.

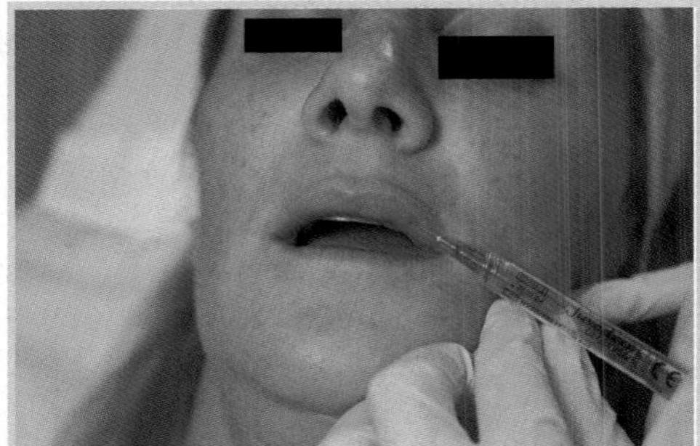

Step 1

Step 2. The second injection point to the body of the upper lip is one needle length lateral to the first injection point.

- **PEARL:** Unlike filler placement in the vermillion border, which typically extends to the corner of the lip, injections in the body of the upper lip do not need to extend to the corner of the lip.

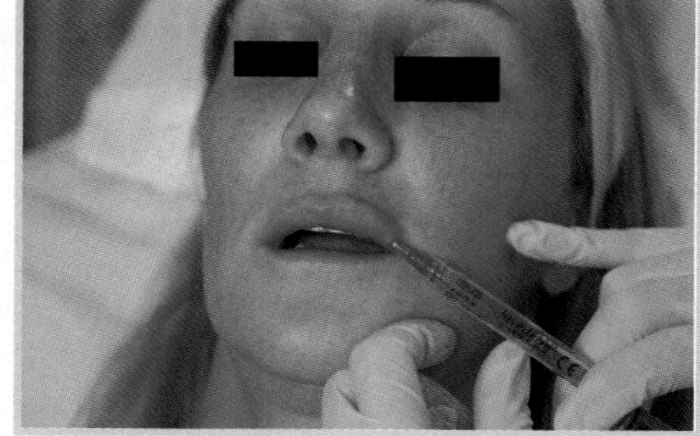

Step 2

Step 3. The first injection point the body of the lower lip is 2 mm medial to the corner of the mouth and 2 mm superior to the vermillion border.

- **PEARL:** Inspect the shape of the lower lip and administer filler volume to match the lip contour as far as possible.

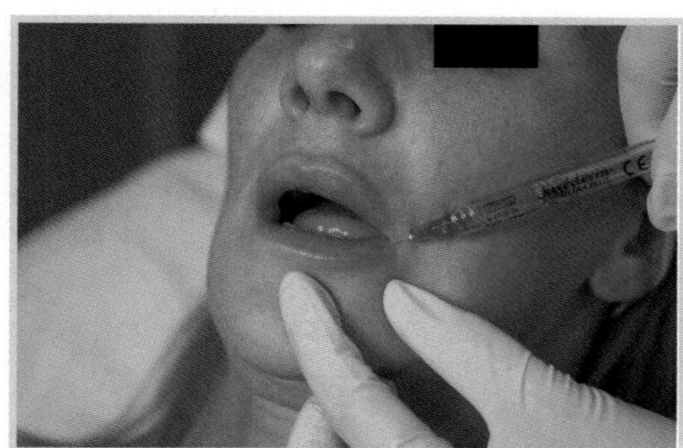

Step 3

Step 4. The second injection point in the body of the lower lip is one needle length medial to the first injection point, shown in Step 4A. Insert the needle to the hub, as shown in Step 4B, and use a more generous amount of filler in this medial portion of the lower lip.

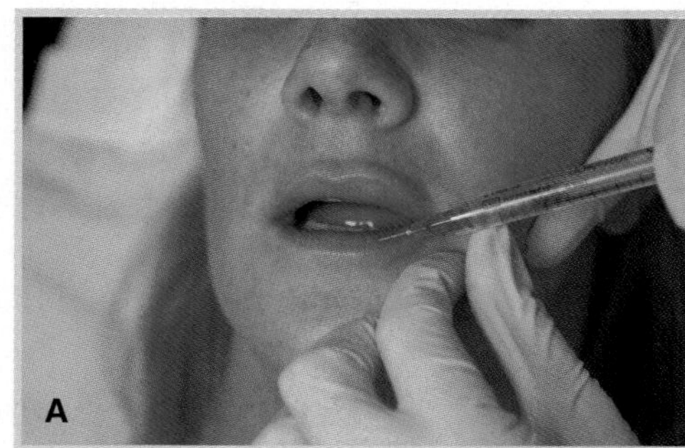

A

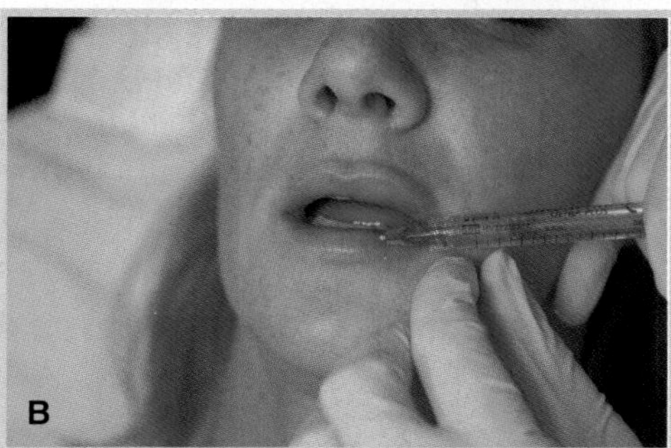

B

Step 4

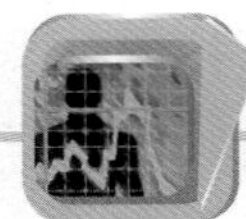

Complications

Common

- Bruising
- Palpable or visible filler
- Asymmetry, overcorrection, or undercorrection
- Prolonged swelling, tenderness, or pain
- Prolonged erythema
- Hyperpigmentation
- Infection
- Allergic reaction
- Migration or extrusion of filler
- Unpredictable persistence of filler, either shorter or longer than anticipated
- Bluish discoloration (Tyndall effect) when filler is placed too superficially in thin skin

Rare and Idiosyncratic

- Hematoma
- Acneic outbreak or milia
- Granulomatous nodules
- Vascular occlusion with skin necrosis
- Extremely rare: immediate hypersensitivity reaction with signs of urticaria, edema, and a remote possibility of anaphylaxis

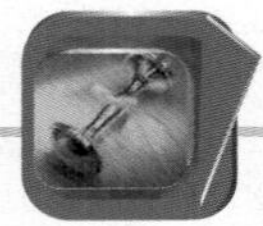

Pediatric Considerations

This procedure is contraindicated for cosmetic uses in pediatric patients.

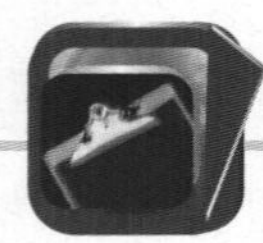

Postprocedure Instructions

Ice each injection site for 10 to 15 minutes every 1 to 2 hours for 1 to 3 days or until the swelling and bruising resolve. Avoid activities that cause facial flushing until the swelling resolves, including application of heat to the face, alcohol consumption, exercising, and tanning. Remind the patient not to massage the filler in the treated areas. Acetaminophen may be used if needed for discomfort.

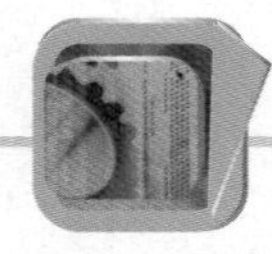

Coding Information and Supply Sources

CPT Code	Description	2008 Average 50th Percentile Fee	Global Period
11950	Subcutaneous injection of filling material; ≤1 mL	$285.00	0
11951	Subcutaneous injection of filling material; 1.1–5.0 mL	$426.00	0

CPT is a registered trademark of the American Medical Association.
2008 average 50th Percentile Fees are provided courtesy of 2008 MMH-SI's copyrighted Physicians' Fees and Coding Guide.

HCPCS Code

Miscellaneous supply A9999

Average fee: $500 per syringe. These procedures are not reimbursable by insurance.

Supply Sources

- Juvederm Ultra Plus: Allergan, Inc., 2525 Dupont Drive, Irvine, CA 92612. Phone: 1-800-377-7790.
- Restylane: Medicis Aesthetics, Inc., 812 N. Hayden Road, Scotsdale, AZ 85258. Phone: 1-866-222-1480.
- Benzocaine/lidocaine/tetracaine (BLT) (20:6:4) ointment: American Health Solutions Pharmacy, 3463 Overland Avenue, Los Angeles, CA 90034. Phone: 310-838-7422.

Patient Education Handout

A patient education handout, "Dermal Filler Treatments," can be found on the book's Web site.

Bibliography

Born T. Hyaluronic acids. *Clin Plas Surg.* 2006;33(4):525–538.

Brandt FS, Boker A. Restylane and perlane. In: Klein A, ed. *Tissue Augmentation in Clinical Practice.* New York: Taylor & Francis; 2006:291–314.

Goldman MP. Optimizing the use of fillers for facial rejuvenation: the right tool for the job. *Cosm Derm.* 2007;20(7)(suppl):S14–25.

Jones J. Patient safety considerations regarding dermal fillers. *Plas Surg Nurs.* 2006;26(3):156–163.

Klein A. The art and architecture of lips and their enhancement with injectable fillers. In: Klein A, ed. *Tissue Augmentation in Clinical Practice.* New York: Taylor & Francis; 2006:337–346.

Klein, A. Temporary dermal fillers—USA experience. In: Lowe NJ, ed. *Textbook of Facial Rejuvenation: The Art of Minimally Invasive Combination Therapy.* United Kingdom: Taylor & Francis; 2002: 189–202.

Murray CA, Zloty D, Warshawski L, et al. The evolution of soft tissue fillers in clinical practice. *Derm Clin.* 2005;23(2): 343–363.

Niamtu J. Facial aging and regional enhancement with injectable fillers. *Cosm Derm.* 2007;20(5)(suppl):S14–20.

Naimtu J. Simple technique for lip and nasolabial fold anesthesia for injectable fillers. *Derm Surg.* 2005;31(10):1330–1332.

Niamtu J. The use of restylane in cosmetic facial surgery. *J Oral Max Surg.* 2006;64(2):317–325.

Sadick, N. Soft tissue augmentation: selection, mode of operation and proper use of injectable agents. *Cosm Derm.* 2007;20(5)(suppl):S8–13.

Salam G, et al. Regional anesthesia for office procedures, part 1: head and neck surgeries. *Am Fam Phys.* 2004;69(3):585–590.

Werschler WP, Kane M. Optimal use of facial filling agents: understanding the products. *Cosm Derm.* 2007;20(5)(suppl):S4–7.

2008 MAG Mutual Healthcare Solutions, Inc.'s Physicians' Fee and Coding Guide. Duluth, Georgia. MAG Mutual Healthcare Solutions, Inc. 2007.

CHAPTER 31

Laser Hair Removal

Rebecca Small, MD

Assistant Clinical Professor, Director, Medical Aesthetics Training Program, Department of Family and Community Medicine, University of California, San Francisco School of Medicine, Capitola, CA

Undesired hair growth is a common aesthetic complaint for which permanent hair reduction treatments are sought by both men and women. Hair density for the body is predetermined by birth; however, the vast majority of hairs are nonvisible because they are either thin, nonpigmented vellus hairs or dormant hairs. Nonvisible hairs may become visible, pigmented terminal hairs through hormonal changes that occur with age. In menopause, these are commonly seen on the chin, upper lip, and anterior neck. For men, new terminal hairs are common on the back and shoulder areas. These changes can be distressing for patients and negatively impact self-image and self-esteem. Increasing patient demand and advances in laser and light-based technologies have made permanent hair reduction treatments widely available, more affordable, and an essential procedure for primary care professionals providing aesthetic care. The purpose of this chapter is to provide primary care professionals with an understanding of laser principles, their application to hair reduction, and a practical approach to treatment techniques.

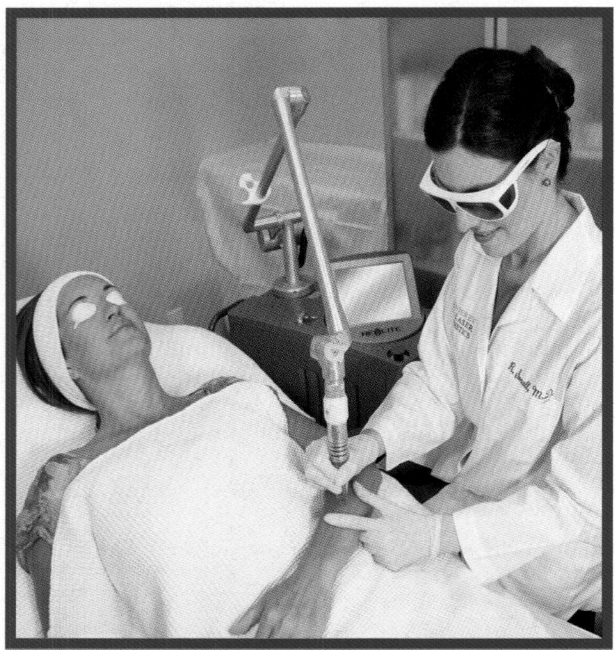

Laser Principles

Hair reduction treatments may be performed with either lasers or intense pulsed light (IPL) devices. Lasers use a lasing medium, such as alexandrite, to produce a single wavelength of light with rays that are highly focused. IPL devices, on the other hand, use a flash lamp such as xenon to produce pulses of light that have of a spectrum of wavelengths, and cut-off filters are used to produce emission peaks at certain desired wavelengths. Both lasers and IPL devices, collectively referred to as *Lasers*, operate under the principle of selective photothermolysis. For the treatment of undesired hair, *Laser* energy is absorbed by melanin, a pigmented chromophore in hair. The melanin in the hair shaft heats up and damages the growth structures of the hair, thereby impairing and reducing hair growth. The surrounding skin, which minimally absorbs energy, is left unaffected.

Melanin can be selectively targeted using particular wavelengths of light. The ideal wavelengths for melanin absorption are those where melanin has greater absorption of energy than other chromophores in the surrounding skin. A chromophore absorption curve (Figure 1A) shows the amount of energy absorbed for various wavelengths by melanin and oxyhemoglobin, the chromophore in red vascular lesions. Notice that

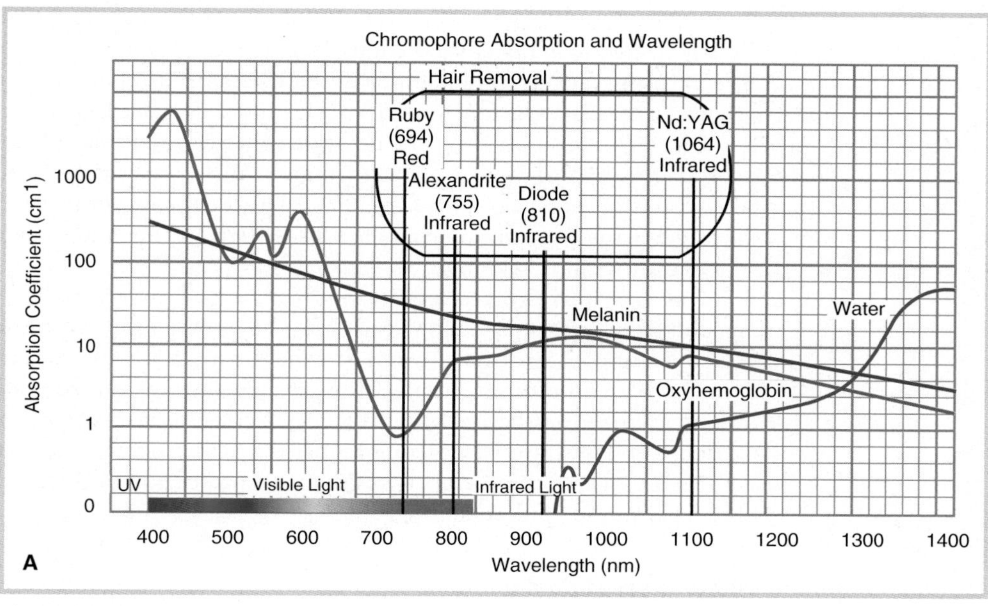

Figure 1A

melanin preferentially absorbs light between 650 and 1,100 nm. These longer wavelengths have a greater depth of penetration to the hair bulb and are the ideal range of wavelengths for treating hair. Hemoglobin preferentially absorbs light at wavelengths between 510 and 600 nm. This range of shorter wavelengths is ideal for treating superficial red vascular lesions, such as facial telangiectasias.

The four main lasers used for hair removal emit wavelengths within this ideal range of melanin absorption ruby (694 nm), alexandrite (755 nm), diode (810 nm) and Nd:YAG (1,064 nm as shown Figure 1A). Figure 1B is an example of an emission spectrum for an IPL device (Palomar StarLux) with the filter for hair reduction (LuxRs handpiece) that shows a peak of wavelengths emitted from 650 to 1,400 nm; this is also the ideal range for melanin absorption.

To achieve efficacious treatments with maximal safety, the provider must have an understanding of basic *Laser* parameters and properties of the targets being treated in the skin. Wavelength selection determines chromophore specificity and the depth of *Laser* energy penetration into tissue. The other main *Laser* parameters include (i) fluence, the amount of energy delivered per unit area (J/cm^2); (ii) pulse width, the duration for which the *Laser* pulse is applied (ms); (iii) spot size, the diameter of the beam emitted (mm); and (iv) repetition rate,

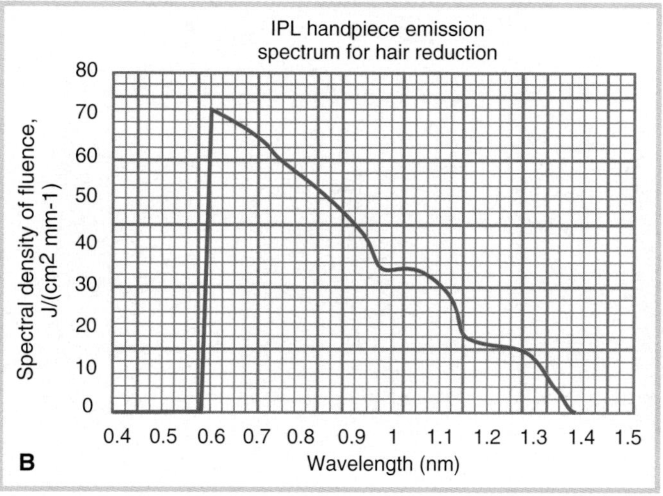

Figure 1B

the number of pulses per second (Hz). The depth of penetration and absorption of energy is directly related to a longer wavelength, larger spot size, longer pulse width, and higher fluence. By using various combinations of these parameters, thermal energy can be specifically supplied to damage the targeted hair while minimizing damage to the surrounding tissue.

Thermal relaxation time (TRT) is the time required for the target tissue exposed to *Laser* energy to cool down by 50% through transfer of heat to surrounding tissues. The pulse duration must be shorter than the TRT of the target to limit thermal damage to the target tissue. For hair follicles, the TRT is 10 to 100 ms, and therefore pulse widths used are typically within this range.

The epidermis is protected during treatments through cooling the skin before, during, and after *Laser* pulses. *Lasers* with built-in cooling mechanisms maintain the *Laser* tip at a constant cool temperature and provide the most reliable contact cooling for the epidermis, which minimizes complications. Systems relying on manually sprayed cryogen or ice water applied to the *Laser* tip provide less consistent epidermal protection. Cooling is particularly important when using higher fluencies, shorter pulse widths, and small spot sizes because these parameters focus the *Laser* more superficially in the skin and are more likely to result in epidermal injury.

Hair Anatomy

Hair follicles are composed of the bulb (which consists of the matrix and dermal papilla) outer root sheath, bulge, and hair shaft (shown in part A of Figure 2). Hair growth occurs in three phases: (1) anagen, the active growth phase during which the hair bulb is most

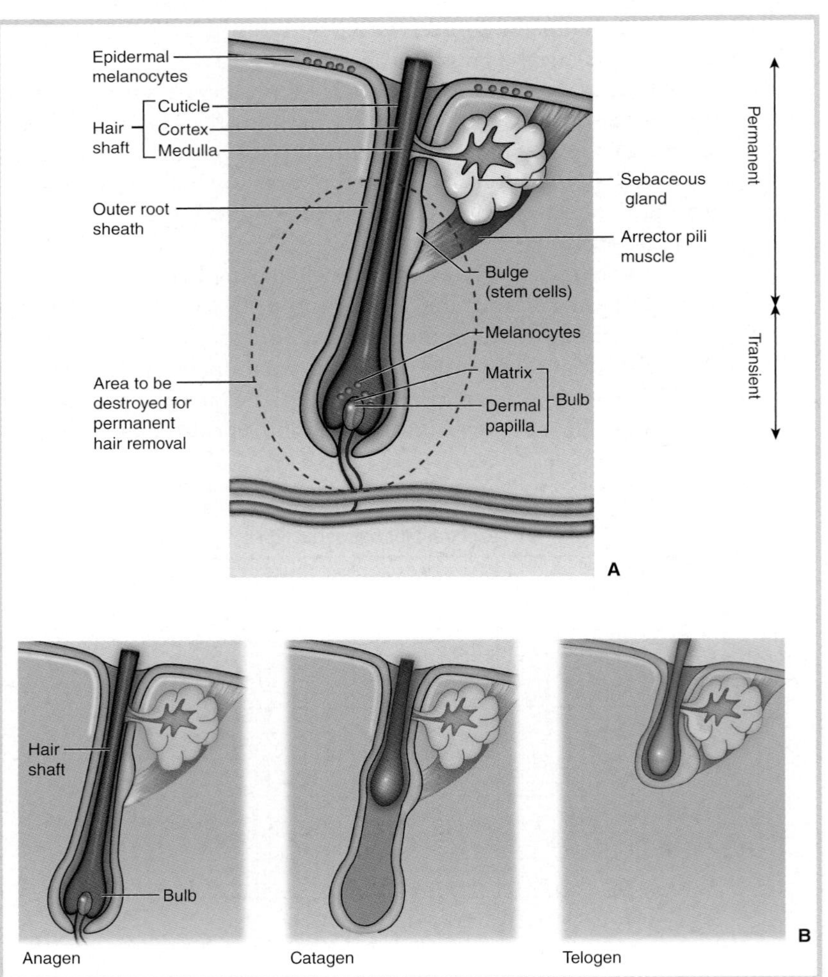

Figure 2

TABLE 31-1. Percentage of Hairs in Anagen Phase and Typical Telogen Duration for Various Areas of the Body

Body Area	Anagen Hair (%)	Telogen Duration (Months)
Scalp	85	3 to 4
Beard	70	2.5
Upper lip	65	1.5
Axillae	30	3
Pubic area	30	3
Arms	20	4.5
Lower legs	20	6

darkly pigmented; (2) catagen, the regression phase when cell division ceases and the follicle begins to involute; and (3) telogen, the resting phase during which the bulb is minimally pigmented (see part B of Figure 2). Hair growth is initiated by epithelial stem cells located in the "bulge," a protrusion near the attachment of the arrector pili muscle. Growth occurs from the rapidly dividing cells of the matrix, which receive their vascular supply from the dermal papilla. Hairs are most susceptible to *Laser* treatment during early anagen phase when the melanin content of the matrix is greatest because *Laser* energy can be most effectively absorbed to heat and damage the hair growth structures. The percentage of hairs in anagen varies for different parts of the body (see Table 31-1), and those areas with the greatest percentage in anagen, such as the scalp, respond most rapidly to *Laser* treatments. The duration of telogen serves as a guideline for the interval between treatments. For example, the lower legs, which have a long telogen phase, require intervals of at least 3 months between treatments, whereas the upper lip, which has a short telogen phase, requires 1 month between treatments (Table 31-1).

Laser Safety

Ocular injury is a risk to both patients and providers, and eyewear specific to the *Laser* in use must be worn. *Lasers* in the visible range of the electromagnetic spectrum, such as the ruby, alexandrite, diode lasers and IPLs, can cause retinal damage, and those in the infrared range, such as the Nd:YAG laser, can cause corneal damage and blindness from severe retinal injury. For treatments in the periocular area, patients must use eye shields, which fit securely over the orbit in place of goggles. Care should always be taken to direct the *Laser* away from the eye. A laser safety officer should be assigned, and a laser safety policy and procedures should be established to ensure that the American National Standards Institute (ANSI) laser safety requirements are met. Some of these laser safety precautions include laser warning signs on doors, coverings on windows and mirrors, and completion of a laser safety checklist prior to performing treatments. The American Society for Laser Medicine and Surgery (ASLMS) has comprehensive training courses in laser safety (see the Suppliers section). ANSI also recommends that all health-care personnel working with *Lasers* have a baseline eye examination prior to employment, immediately after a suspected *Laser* ocular exposure, and upon termination.

Alternative Therapies

Alternatives to *Lasers* for hair reduction include temporary methods such as shaving, chemical depilatories, waxing, and tweezing. Electrolysis is a permanent method of hair reduction by which a high-frequency electric current is applied to the hair bulb through a fine wire electrode. This method is slower and associated with greater discomfort than *Laser* treatments as individual hairs are treated and electric current is applied for seconds, as compared to milliseconds with *Lasers*. Electrolysis is indicated for areas with sparse, fine hairs, such as the upper lip, and for blonde, white, gray, and vellus hairs.

Patient Selection

Appropriate patient selection is fundamental to ensuring the success of treatments. The best candidates for *Laser* hair reduction *(LHR)* are those with fair skin (Fitzpatrick skin types I to III) with dark coarse hair because there is the greatest disparity between the background skin color and the target follicle chromophore. Fitzpatrick skin type classification (see Table 31-2) is used to describe background skin pigmentation and the skin's response to sun exposure. Individuals with more melanin in their skin have darker baseline skin color, are more resistant to sun burning, and are classified as a high Fitzpatrick skin type. In general, Fitzpatrick skin types I to III are Caucasian, IV to V have olive skin tones and are seen in patients with Mediterranean or Latino background, and VI are African American. Darker skin types (IV and V) have a greater risk of epidermal injury and associated hyperpigmentation, hypopigmentation, and burns, because epidermal melanin also serves as a competing target for the *Laser*. Use of a skin-lightening agent, strict sun avoidance, and sun screen prior to treatment can improve outcomes and reduce complications in skin types IV and V. Fitzpatrick skin types VI are at high risk for *Laser* treatments, and providers should consider referral to centers that specialize in treatments for skin type VI.

Patients with grey, white, blonde, and vellus hair are not candidates for LHR treatment because there is inadequate melanin target for the *Laser*. The more fine and light-colored the hair, the less target is present and the poorer the hair reduction results will be.

Addressing patient expectations at the time of consultation is also important for patient satisfaction with *Laser* hair reduction treatments. Terminology must be clarified, and patients must be made aware that treatments result in permanent hair reduction, not permanent hair removal. This can be confusing because the colloquial term for this procedure is *Laser* hair removal. Permanent *Laser* hair reduction is defined by the U.S. Federal Drug Administration as "the long-term, stable reduction in the number of hairs regrowing after a treatment regime." After completing a treatment series, patients will typically experience a 60% to 90% reduction in hair growth; they will not be bald in the treatment area. Hairs that remain are typically finer, lighter, and less problematic.

Patients require a series of treatments regardless of the treatment area, because hairs are in different phases of the growth cycle at any given time. Patients with Fitzpatrick skin types I to III typically require six treatments. Skin types IV and V require eight or more

TABLE 31-2. Fitzpatrick Skin Types

Fitzpatrick Skin Type	Skin Color	Sun Exposure Reaction
I	White	Always burn Never tan
II	White	Usually burn Tan with difficulty
III	White	Sometimes mild burn Tan average
IV	Medium brown	Rarely burn Tan with ease
V	Dark brown	Rarely burn Tan very easily
VI	Black	Never burn Tan very easily

treatments as fluences are started conservatively and increased slowly. The interval between treatments varies by treatment area and is based on the telogen duration. As a general rule, the intervals for treatments to various areas are as follows: the face, 4 to 8 weeks; upper body, 10 to 12 weeks; and lower body, 12 to 14 weeks. Treatments performed at shorter intervals may result in poor outcomes because hairs may be in telogen and thus nonresponsive to the *Laser*.

Results and Follow-up

After the first treatment, patients may experience a prolonged delay in hair regrowth from 1 to 3 months. This is temporary hair reduction, and although patients are usually very pleased with the lack of growth, they should be forewarned that regrowth will occur. Hair regrowth may appear in some parts of the treatment area and not others. This patchy regrowth is normal and indicates that a group of hairs in the anagen phase were effectively treated. After completion of a treatment series, patients may require a touch-up for dormant hairs that have entered the active growth cycle approximately 6 months to 1 year after completion of their series.

Anesthesia

Discomfort associated with *LHR* treatment is usually likened to the snap of a rubber band. Because of the rich sensory nerve supply around hair follicles, *LHR* treatments are rarely free from pain. Anesthesia requirements vary according to the equipment used, patients' tolerance, and treatment area. Most *LHR* devices have built-in cooling in the tip of the *Laser* that contacts the skin for epidermal safety, and this can provide some anesthesia. Some patients may require a topical anesthetic such as EMLA (prilocaine 2½% : lidocaine 2½%), ELA-Max (lidocaine 4%) or BLT (benzocaine 20% : lidocaine 6% : tetracaine 4%) (see Section One). All topical anesthetics should be applied in the office because of safety concerns with lidocaine toxicity. Severe reactions such as hypotension, seizures, and death have been reported where patients self applied excessive doses of lidocaine to large surface areas over a prolonged time. Pretreatment and posttreatment cooling with ice or cold packs at the time of treatment are excellent methods of anesthesia.

Preprocedure Checklist

- Perform an aesthetic consultation and review the patient's medical history (see Chapter 28).
- Determine Fitzpatrick skin type.
- Obtain informed consent (see Chapter 28).
- Take pretreatment photographs.
- Examine the treatment area, and document hair density, coarseness, and color in the treatment area.
- Prophylax with antiviral medication if there is a history of herpes simplex or zoster in or near the treatment area for 2 days prior to the procedure, and continue for 3 days postprocedure.
- Lighten the skin for darker Fitzpatrick skin types (IV to V). Strict sun avoidance for 1 month is requisite with daily use of a full-spectrum sun screen. Use a skin-lightening topical product daily or twice daily for at least 1 month prior to treatment such as hydroquinone or a cosmeceutical such as kojic acid, arbutin, niacinamide, or azelaic acid.
- Perform test spots for skin types III with high-risk ethnic backgrounds (Mediterranean, Latino, and Asian) and skin types IV to V prior to initial treatment. Select appropriate test spot parameters based on the patient's Fitzpatrick skin type and hair characteristics of density, color, and coarseness using the manufacturer's guidelines for spot size, fluence, and pulse width. Test spots should be placed discretely near the desired treatment

area (such as under the chin, behind or inferior to the ear) with 20% overlap of pulses. Test spots should be viewed 3 to 5 days after placement for evidence of hyperpigmentation, burn, or other adverse effect. At each visit, patients requiring test spots should have test spots placed using the fluence and pulse width desired for the subsequent treatment. Inform patients that lack of an adverse reaction with test spots does not ensure that a side effect or complication will not occur with any treatment.

- Patients should shave the treatment area 1 to 2 days prior to treatment. Hair should be barely visible (approximately 1 to 2 mm above the skin) at the time of treatment.
- Patients should avoid direct sun exposure for 1 month prior to treatment and use a full-spectrum sun screen daily in the treatment area; avoid hair removal by waxing, tweezing, or electrolysis 1 month prior to treatment; and avoid bleaching creams, depilatories, or self-tanning products 2 weeks prior to treatment.

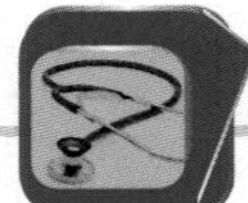

Equipment

- Laser or IPL device appropriate for hair reduction treatments
- Eyewear for the patient and provider that is specific to the laser or IPL used
- Nonalcohol wipes to cleanse treatment area
- Topical anesthetic such as EMLA, ELA-Max, or benzocaine : lidocaine : tetracaine (BLT)
- Clear colorless gel for treatments
- Gauze, 4 × 4 inches
- Ice packs
- Soothing topical product for application after treatment, such as aloe vera gel
- Hydrocortisone cream 1% and 2.5%
- Alcohol wipes for cleaning the *Laser* tip
- Germicidal disposable wipes for sanitizing the *Laser*

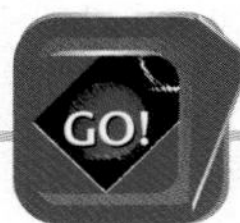

Indications

- Reduction of undesired hair.
- Pseudofolliculitis barbae (PFB) and pseudofolliculitis pubis (PFP). These conditions are due to ingrown hairs and often occur with curly, coarse hair. *LHR* will improve these conditions through hair reduction and formation of finer hairs after a treatment series. However, PFB and PFP may worsen immediately after treatments as hairs may become trapped during the posttreatment extrusion process.
- Hirsutism. This is the development of coarse terminal hairs, sometimes due to increased levels of male androgens. Pathologic conditions associated with hyperandrogenic states include polycystic ovarian syndrome and congenital adrenal hyperplasia. *Laser* hair treatments will not result in permanent hair reduction in patients with untreated hyperandrogenicity. *Hypertrichosis* refers to diffusely increased total body hair, which is typically vellus hair. This condition can be associated with hypothyroidism, anorexia, medications (phenytoin, cyclosporine, phenothiazine), and congenital syndromes and may be unresponsive to *LHR* because of the fine nature of the hair.

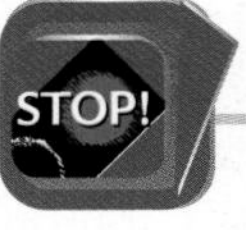

Contraindications

Absolute

- Isotretinoin (Accutane) use in the past 6 months
- Keloid formation or hypertrophic scarring
- Pregnancy and nursing

- Seizures
- Melanoma, or lesions suspected of melanoma, in the treatment area
- Active infection in the treatment area (e.g., herpes or pustular acne)
- Cardiac pacemaker
- Skin type VI
- Recent sun exposure in the last month and/or tanned skin
- Photosensitive disorder (e.g., systemic lupus erythematosus)
- Hair removal by waxing, tweezing, or electrolysis during the previous month
- Use of bleaching creams or depilatories during the past 2 weeks
- Self-tanning product use in the past 2 weeks
- Treatment of eyebrows or any area inside the eye orbit
- History of livido reticularis, a rare autoimmune vascular disease associated with mottled skin discoloration of the legs or arms
- History of erythema ab igne, a rare acquired reticular erythematous rash related to heat exposure with Laser treatments

Relative

- Poor healing
- Recent, undiagnosed increase in hair growth
- Current use of photosensitizing medications (e.g., tetracyclines, St. John's wort, thiazides, etc)
- Use of products containing retinoids, glycolic acids, or hydroxy acids in the treatment area 1 week prior to treatment

The Procedure

The following recommendations are guidelines for hair reduction treatments with IPL devices and are based on the Palomar StarLux using the LuxRs hand piece. There are other IPL systems that are comparable.

Step 1. Results of hair reduction treatment to a patient's axilla are shown before (Figure 3A) and after four IPL hair reduction treatments (Figure 3B) using 100-ms pulse width and 60-J/cm^2 fluence for two treatments and 20-ms pulse width and 40-J/cm^2 for the subsequent two treatments. Initial treatments used a longer pulse width to target the deeper coarser hairs and subsequent treatments used shorter pulse widths for finer, lighter hairs. Notice that some finer lighter hairs are still present posttreatment, as expected.

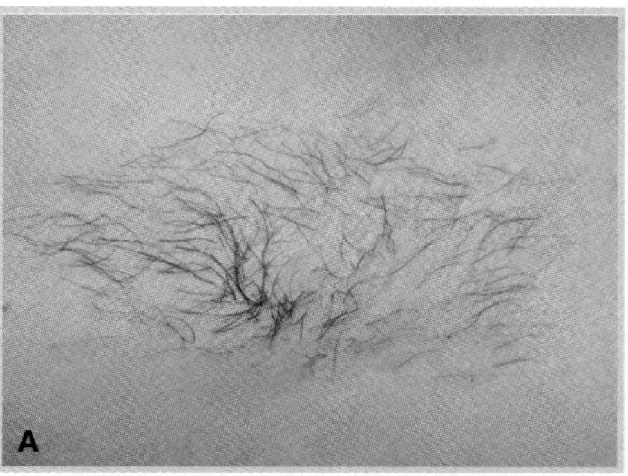

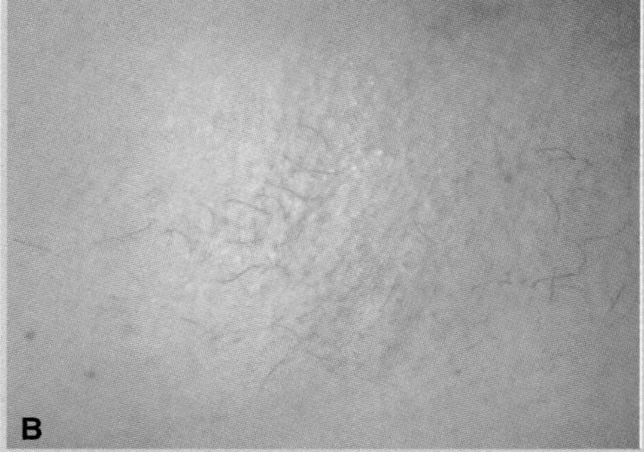

Courtesy of Khalil Khatri, M.D.

Figure 3

Figure 4A shows IPL hair reduction, and Figure 4B shows a significant reduction in hair after six treatments using 20-ms pulse width and increasing fluences over the treatment course from 36 to 40 J/cm^2.

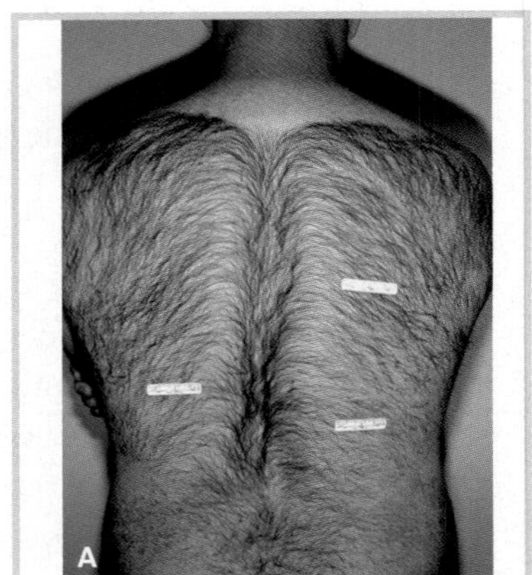

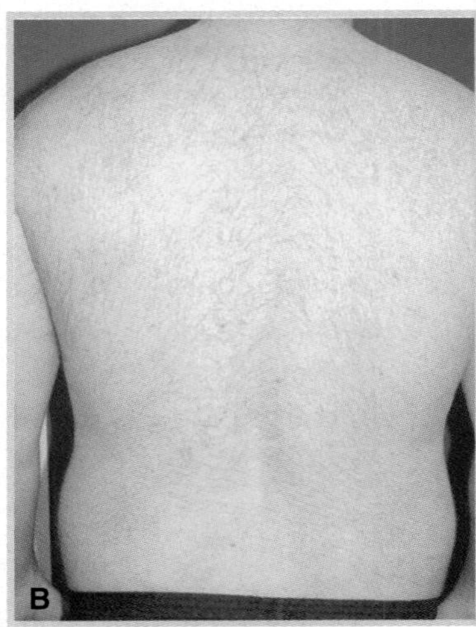

Courtesy of Alan Rockoff, M.D.

Figure 4

Step 1. Comfortably position the patient for treatment, lying flat on the treatment bed. Shave the treatment area if it is unshaven. Step 1 shows the use of a razor for shaving. Cleanse the skin with a non-alcohol wipe. Anesthetize the treatment area if necessary (see Section One). Provide appropriate IPL safety eye protection for the patient and all personnel in the treatment room prior to beginning treatment.

- **PITFALL:** If hair is too long at the time of treatment, singed hair on the skin surface may result in epidermal injury.

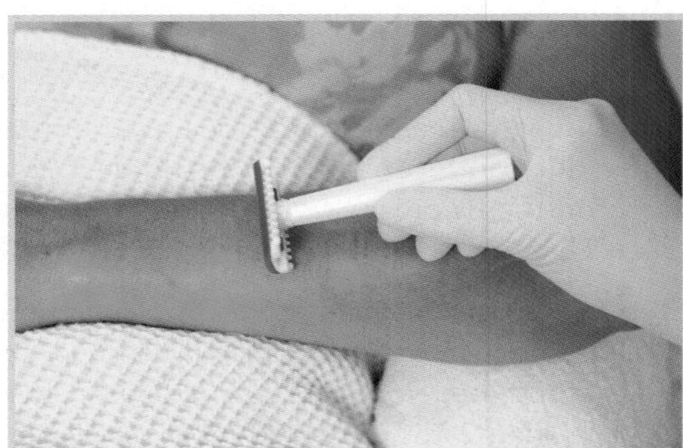

Step 1

Step 2. Operate the IPL device in accordance with your clinic's IPL safety policies and procedures and the manufacturer's guidelines as outlined in the operator's manual. Tattoos and permanent makeup should be covered with wet gauze (see Chapter 32), and treatments must be performed at least 2 inches away from the tattoo.

- **PITFALL:** Full thickness burns may result from treating over tattoos.

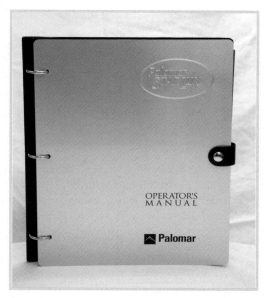

Step 2

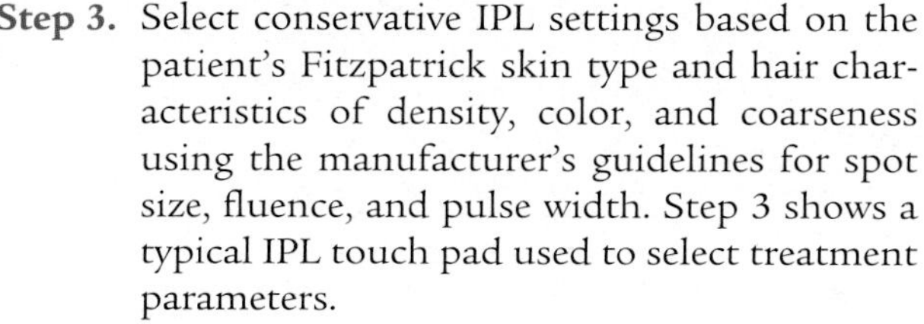

Step 3. Select conservative IPL settings based on the patient's Fitzpatrick skin type and hair characteristics of density, color, and coarseness using the manufacturer's guidelines for spot size, fluence, and pulse width. Step 3 shows a typical IPL touch pad used to select treatment parameters.

- **PEARL:** Darker Fitzpatrick skin types will require longer pulse widths and lower fluences because of their greater risk of epidermal injury.
- **PEARL:** Coarse, dark hairs and areas with higher density of hair, typically seen in the initial treatments, require longer pulse widths and lower fluences.

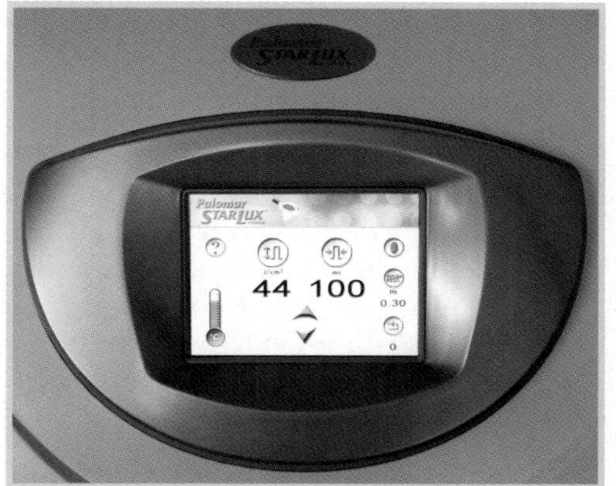

Step 3

Step 4. Perform the procedure. Apply a clear colorless Laser gel to the skin, spreading to a thin 1 to 2 mm layer. Place the IPL tip firmly on the skin, making certain that the entire tip is in contact with the skin and is surrounded by gel. Perform a single pulse in the treatment area and assess for patient tolerance and clinical endpoints (see Figures 5 and 6). In general, there should be subtle endpoints with initial treatments. Adjust IPL settings accordingly until desired clinical end points achieved and then proceed to treat the entire treatment area.

- **PEARL:** Always angle the IPL tip away from the eyes during treatment.

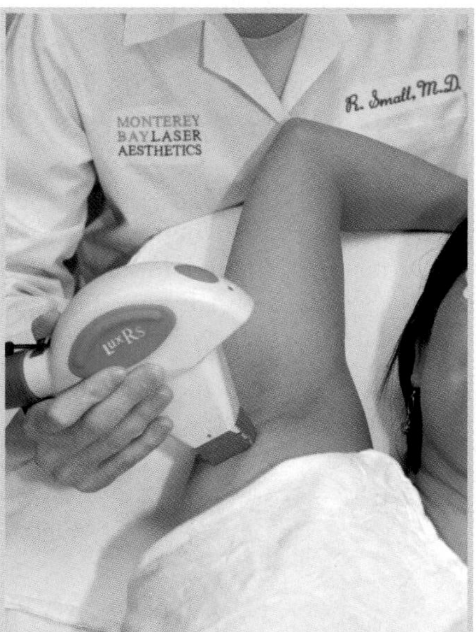

Step 4

- **PEARL:** Ice may be used immediately prior to treatment and after treatment to reduce discomfort. Application of ice after treatment also reduces the incidence of paradoxical hair growth.
- **PEARL:** Continually assess IPL-tissue interaction and clinical endpoints throughout the treatment and adjust the IPL settings accordingly.

Step 5. When performing treatments over large areas such as the upper leg or back, a grid pattern may be drawn using a white pencil to ensure complete coverage of the area as shown in Step 5. The direction of IPL pulses should be toward the provider. The degree of recommended overlap with IPL pulses varies for different devices, but in general, there should be a 20% overlap.

- **PITFALL:** Incomplete coverage of the treatment area will result in noticeable stripes of hair regrowth 1 to 2 weeks after treatment and is associated with patient dissatisfaction.

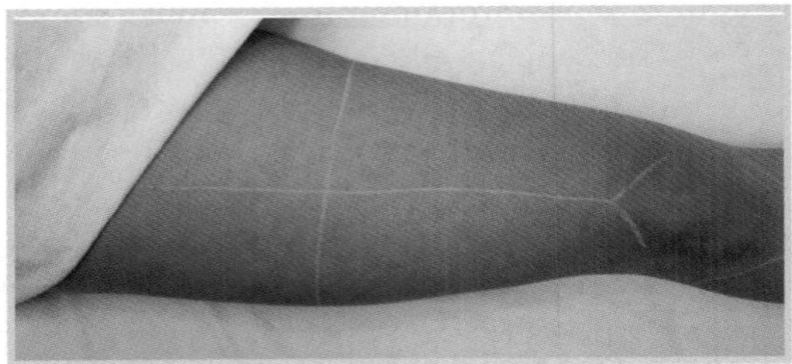

Step 5

Step 6. Decrease the fluence over boney areas and prominences as increased reflection off the bone can intensify treatments and result in overtreatment. Step 6 shows a treatment grid pattern of the lower leg with the tibia outlined as a reminder to reduce the fluence in this boney area.

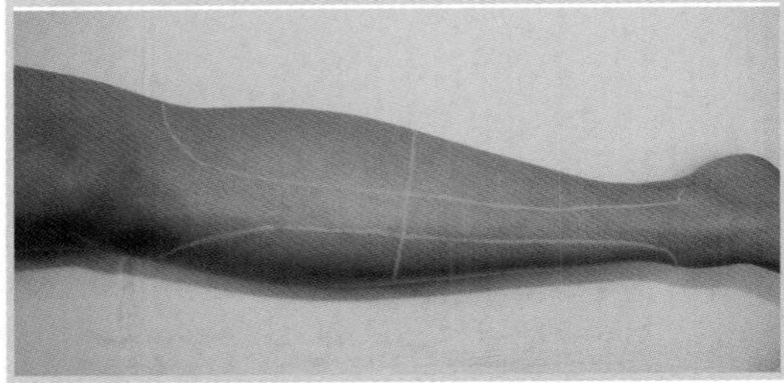

Step 6

Figure 5 shows desired clinical endpoints immediately after an IPL treatment for hair reduction with perifollicular erythema and darkened singed hairs. A burnt sulfur smell may be noticeable immediately after the IPL pulse from singed hairs.

- **PEARL:** Clean the IPL tip between pulses with moist gauze to reduce buildup of singed hair.

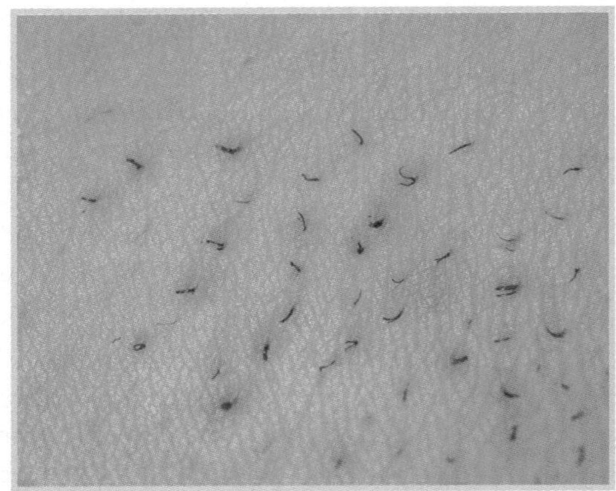

Figure 5

Figure 6 shows the desired clinical endpoint of perifollicular edema (PFE), which typically develops a few minutes after the IPL pulse and indicates that the hair bulb has been effectively treated. PFE is more commonly seen with longer pulse widths.

- **PITFALL:** Confluent PFE or erythema indicates that the IPL settings are too intense and that either the fluence should be decreased or the pulse width increased.

Courtesy of Palomar.

Figure 6

Step 7. For subsequent treatments, fluence should be increased and pulse width decreased according to the manufacturer's guidelines so as to target finer, lighter hairs. In general, only one parameter should be changed to intensify treatments in any given visit. The pulse width should be decreased at subsequent visits to target the finer, lighter hairs. Usually the fluence is increased preferentially for a few treatments to achieve desired clinical endpoints, and pulse width is decreased in the later treatments. These treatment goals are summarized in Step 7.

- **PEARL:** Finer, lighter hairs are the most challenging to treat, and patients must be made aware that once hair becomes too fine, subsequent, more aggressive treatments will not be of therapeutic benefit and may be associated with adverse effects from high fluences.
- **PEARL:** The greatest efficacy with permanent hair reduction is achieved with use of fluencies of at least 30 J/cm^2, a greater number of treatments, and adequately long intervals between treatments that encompass the telogen phase for the treatment area.

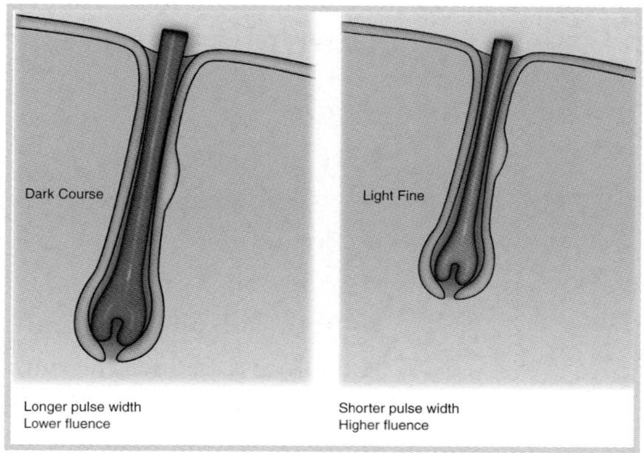

Step 7

Hair regrowth is typically patchy after several hair reduction treatments. Figure 7 shows hair regrowth on a patient's cheek, chin, and anterior neck outlined with a white pencil after five treatments using 100-ms pulse width and 46 to 60 J/cm^2 over three treatments and then 20-ms pulse width and 36 to 40 J/cm^2 for two treatments.

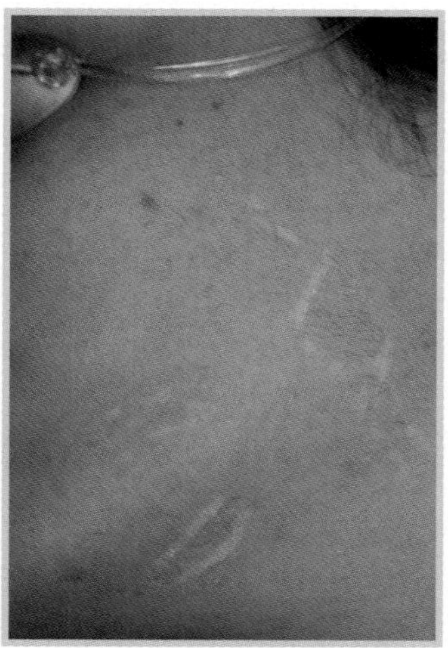

Figure 7

Figure 8A shows an abdomen immediately after IPL treatment for hair reduction that demonstrates excessive erythema and epidermal injury or "branding" from overtreatment. In this case, the device used did not have built-in cooling, and the method of manually spraying cryogen on the IPL tip did not provide adequate cooling. Although it is less common, overtreatment can also be seen with devices that have built-in cooling mechanisms when excessive fluences are used or if a tan is present at the time of treatment. Figure 8B shows the resolution of branding 1 month later.

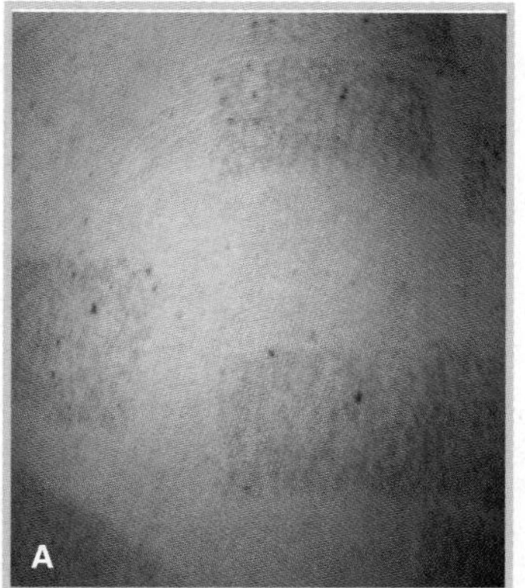

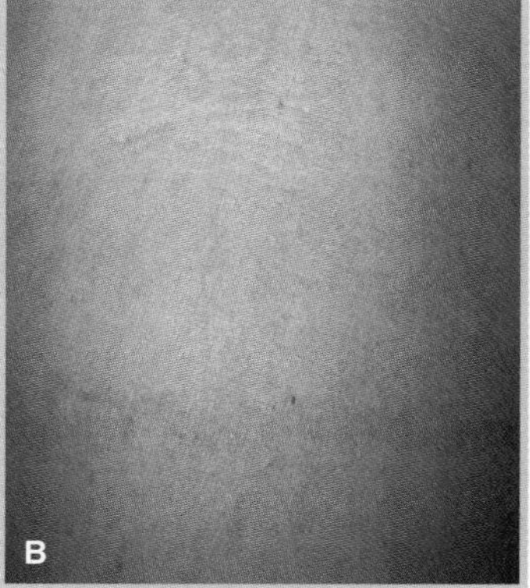

Courtesy of Palomar.

Figure 8

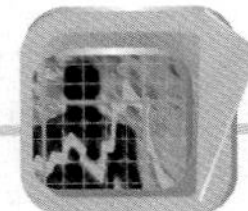

Complications

- Pain
- Hypopigmentation
- Hyperpigmentation
- Eye injury
- Infection
- Burn with blistering and scabbing
- Failure to reduce the number of hairs or hair coarseness
- Damage or alteration to tattoos and permanent makeup
- Reduction in hair adjacent to the treatment area. This can occur because hair follicles may grow at angles to the skin and it is possible to affect hairs adjacent to treatment areas.

Rare and Idiosyncratic

- Scarring.
- Paradoxical hair growth. Stimulation of increased hair growth has been reported in individuals with darker skin types and finer hair, particularly on the cheeks.
- Erythema ab igne (see Chapter 32).

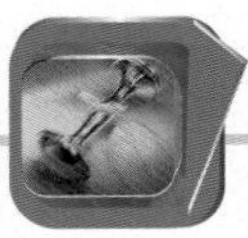

Pediatric Considerations

Hirsute adolescents may be treated with parental consent after hormonal evaluation for hirsutism.

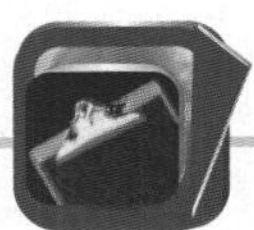

Postprocedure Instructions

Redness and perifollicular edema usually resolve within a few hours to 1 week after treatment and can be managed with application of ice for 15 minutes every 1 to 2 hours and hydrocortisone cream 1% two times per day for 3 to 4 days or until redness resolves. Postinflammatory hyperpigmentation (PIH) can occur with prolonged erythema, and patients should contact their provider if erythema persists for more than 5 days. Pigmentary complications, such as PIH and hypopigmentation, usually resolve in 3 to 6 months but may be permanent. Daily use of a full-spectrum sunscreen (SPF 30 with zinc or titanium) and sun avoidance for 4 weeks after treatment will help minimize the risk of pigmentary changes. Singed hairs may be evident immediately after treatment, and treated hairs may extrude 1 to 2 weeks after treatment. If blistering and/or crusting occur, manage with routine wound care using bacitracin until healed.

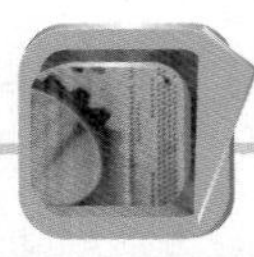

Coding Information and Supply Sources

CPT Code	Description	2008 Average 50th Percentile Fee	Global Period
17380	Epilation (hair reduction) each half-hour	$120.00	0

CPT is a registered trademark of the American Medical Association.
2008 average 50th Percentile Fees are provided courtesy of 2008 MMH-SI's copyrighted Physicians' Fees and Coding Guide.

ICD Codes

704.1 Hirsutism

Insurance

LHR is not reimbursable by insurance. The charges for treatments vary widely and are largely determined by local prices. Patients may pay for individual treatments. However, because *LHR* is only effective with a series of treatments, packages of treatments (usually six) may be offered so that patients achieve the best possible results and have the greatest satisfaction.

Supply Sources

Laser-safe Eyewear

- Glendale, 910 Douglas Pike, Smithfield, RI 02917-1874. Phone: 1-800-500-4739.
- Oculo-plastic, 200 Sauve West, Montreal H3L 1YD, Canada. 1-800-588-2279.

Laser Safety Training Courses

- American Society for Laser Medicine and Surgery (ASLMS), 2100 Stewart Avenue, Suite 240, Wausau, WI 54401. Phone: 1-715-845-9283.

Icing Supplies

- Disposable and reusable ice packs: Cardinal Health, 7000 Cardinal Place, Dublin, OH 43017. Phone: 614-757-5000. Web site: http://www.cardinal.com.

Hair Reduction Lasers and Intense Pulsed Light Suppliers

- Alma Lasers, 485 Half Day Road, Suite 100, Buffalo Grove, IL 60089. 1-866-414-2562 (ALMA). Web site: http://www.almalasers.com/.
- Asclepion Lasers, Im Semmicht 1a, 07751 Jena, Germany. Phone: +49-0-3641-7700-100. Web site: http://www.asclepion.com/.
- Candela, 530 Boston Post Road, Wayland, MA. Phone: 508-358-7400, 1-800-733-8550. Web site: http://www.candelalaser.com/.
- CoolTouch, 9085 Foothills Boulevard, Roseville, CA 95747. Phone: 1-877-858-COOL. Web site: http://www.cooltouch.com/.
- Cutera, 3240 Bayshore Boulevard, Brisbane, CA 94005. Phone: 1-888-4-CUTERA, 415-657-5500. Web site: http://www.cutera.com/.
- Cynosure, Inc./Deka, 5 Carlisle Road, Westford, MA 01886. Phone: 1-978-256-4200, 1-800-886-2966. Web site: http://www.cynosure.com/contact-us/index.php.
- Ellipse, A/S Agern Allé 11, DK-2970 Hørsholm, Denmark. Phone: +45-4576-8808. Web site: http:// www.ellipse.org.
- Energist, 2 Park Pavilions, Clos LLyn Cwm, Off Valley Way, Enterprise Park, Swansea SA6 8QY, UK. Phone: 01792-798768. Web site: http://www.energisint.com/.
- Fotona, 1415 1st Street South, Suite 5, Willmar, MN 56201. Phone: 1-888-550-4113. Web site: http://www.fotonamedicallasers.com.
- General Project, 22 Linnfield Terrace, Phillisburg, NJ 08865. Phone: 908-454-8875. Web site: http://www.generalproject.com.
- HOYA ConBio Europe, 47733 Fremont Blvd., Fremont, CA 94538. Phone: 1-800-532-1064. Web site: http://www.conbio.com.
- IRIDEX, 1212 Terra Bella Avenue, Mountain View, CA 94043. Phone: 650-940-4700. Web site: http://www.iridex.com/.
- Lumenis, 5302 Betsy Ross Drive, Santa Clara, CA 95054. Phone: 408-764-3000. Web site: http://www.lumenis.com/wt/home/home/?flash=true.

- MedArt Corporation, 1479 Glencrest Drive, Suite A, San Marcos, CA 92078. Phone: 760-798-2740. Web site: http://www.medart.dk/.
- Palomar, 82 Cambridge Street, Burlington, MA 01803. Phone: 1-800-725-0627. Web site: http://www.palomarmedical.com/.
- Quantel Medical, 601 Haggerty Lane, Bozeman, MT 59715. Phone: 1-888-660-6726. Web site: http://www.quantelmedical.com.
- Radiancy, 40 Ramland Road South, Suite 10, Orangeburg, NY 10962. Phone: 845-398-1647, 1-888-661-2220. Web site: http://www.radiancy.com/int/press.htm.
- Sciton, 925 Commercial Street, Palo Alto, CA 94303. Phone: 1-888-646-6999. Web site: http://www.sciton.com/.
- SharpLight Technologies, 4-1420 Cornwall Rd., Oakville, Ontario L6J-7W5, Canada. Phone: 905-337-7797. Web site: http://www.sharplightech.com.
- Syneron, 28 Fulton Way, Unit 8, Richmond Hill, Ontario L4B 1L5, Canada. Phone: 905-886-9235, 866-259-6661. Web site: http://www.syneron.com/.

Patient Education Handout

A patient education handout, "Laser Hair Removal," can be found on the book's companion Web site.

Bibliography

Dierickx CC. Hair removal by lasers and other light sources. In: Goldman MP, ed. *Cutaneous and Cosmetic Laser Surgery*. Elsevier; St Louis, Missouri; 2006:135–154.

Levy JL, Ramecourt A. Facial hair removal. In Lowe NJ, ed. *Textbook of Facial Rejuvenation: The Art of Minimally Invasive Combination Therapy*. Taylor and Francis; 2002:245–258.

Rao J, Smalley PJ, Devani A, et al. Laser safety: risks and hazards. In: Goldman MP, ed. *Cutaneous and Cosmetic Laser Surgery*. Mosby Elsevier; London, UK; 2006:293–310.

Sadick NS, Weiss RA, Shea CR, et al. Long-term photoepilation using a broad-spectrum intense pulsed light source. *Arch Dermatol.* 2000;136(11):1336–1340.

Lou WW, Quintana AT, Geronemus RG, et al. Prospective study of hair reduction by diode laser (800 nm) with long-term follow-up. *Derm Surg.* 2000;26:428–432.

Weiss RA, Weiss MA, Marwaha S, et al. Hair removal with a non-coherent filtered flashlamp intense pulsed light source. *Lasers Surg Med.* 1999;24(2):128–132.

Nicolas J. Laser physics for surgical applications. In Keller GS, ed. *Lasers in Aesthetic Surgery.* Thieme, 2001:3–13.

Slatkine M. and Morrow CE. Laser systems and instrumentation for aesthetic surgery. In: Keller GS, ed. *Lasers in Aesthetic Surgery.* Thieme; 2001:14–26.

Cray JE, Laser Safety. In Keller GS, ed. *Lasers in Aesthetic Surgery*. Thieme; 2001:27–33.

Lask G, Eckhouse S, Slatkine M, et al. A comparative study of intense light and laser sources in photoepilation. In: Keller GS, ed. *Lasers in Aesthetic Surgery*. Thieme; 2001: 207–216.

Lacombe V, Thompson I, Keller G. ESC/Sharplan laser hair removal system. In: Keller GS, ed. *Lasers in Aesthetic Surgery*. Thieme; 2001:217–222.

Alster TS and Nanni C. Hair removal with long-pulsed ruby and alexandrite lasers. In: Keller GS, ed. *Lasers in Aesthetic Surgery*. Thieme; 2001:223–229.

Weiss R and Weiss MA. Hair removal with Epilight system. In: Keller GS, ed. *Lasers in Aesthetic Surgery*. Thieme; 2001: 230–237.

2008 MAG Mutual Healthcare Solutions, Inc.'s Physicians' Fee and Coding Guide. Duluth, Georgia. MAG Mutual Healthcare Solutions, Inc. 2007.

CHAPTER 32

Laser Photo Rejuvenation

Rebecca Small, MD

Assistant Clinical Professor, Director, Medical Aesthetics Training Program, Department of Family and Community Medicine, University of California, San Francisco School of Medicine, Capitola, CA

Cumulative sun exposure accelerates the natural intrinsic aging process of the skin and is responsible for many of the skin changes seen with age. Oxidative damage from ultraviolet radiation can cause dysregulation of cellular functions, carcinogenic DNA mutations, and destruction of the skin's extracellular matrix. These cellular insults compound over time and are seen clinically in photoaged skin as benign pigmented lesions with hyperpigmentation and solar lentigines; benign vascular lesions with telangiectasias, poikiloderma of Civatte, rosacea, and cherry angiomas; textural changes with fine lines and laxity; and dysplasia with benign and malignant neoplasia.

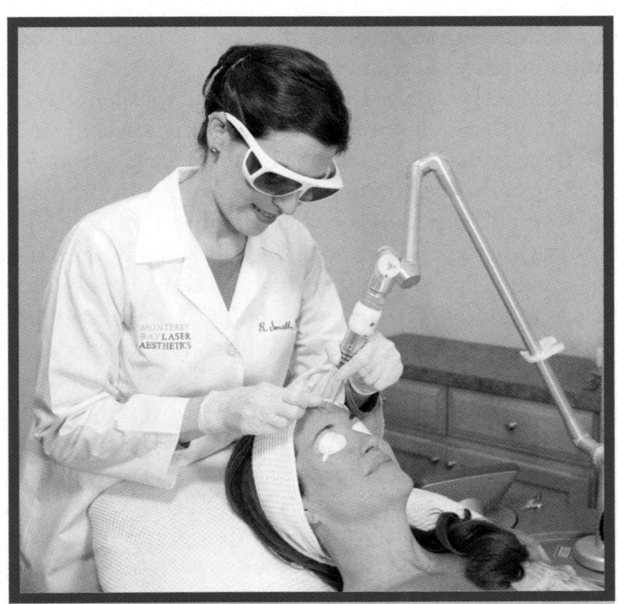

Photo rejuvenation refers to the cosmetic treatment of photoaged skin with laser and light-based technologies. There are many lasers and intense pulsed light (IPL) devices (collectively referred to as *Lasers*) in use today for the treatment of benign pigmented and vascular lesions. These conditions consistently show dramatic improvements with *Laser* treatments, require minimal recovery time, and are associated with high patient satisfaction.

The goals of this chapter are to provide primary care professionals with an understanding of *Laser* principles as they relate to photo rejuvenation and to provide a practical approach to treatment techniques for benign vascular and benign pigmented lesions seen with photoaging. Advances in technology have made *Lasers* widely available, more affordable, and *Laser* photo rejuvenation has become an essential procedure for primary care professionals providing aesthetic care.

Laser Principles

The effects of lasers and IPL devices are both based on the principle of selective photothermolysis. For the treatment of superficial red vascular lesions, *Laser* energy is

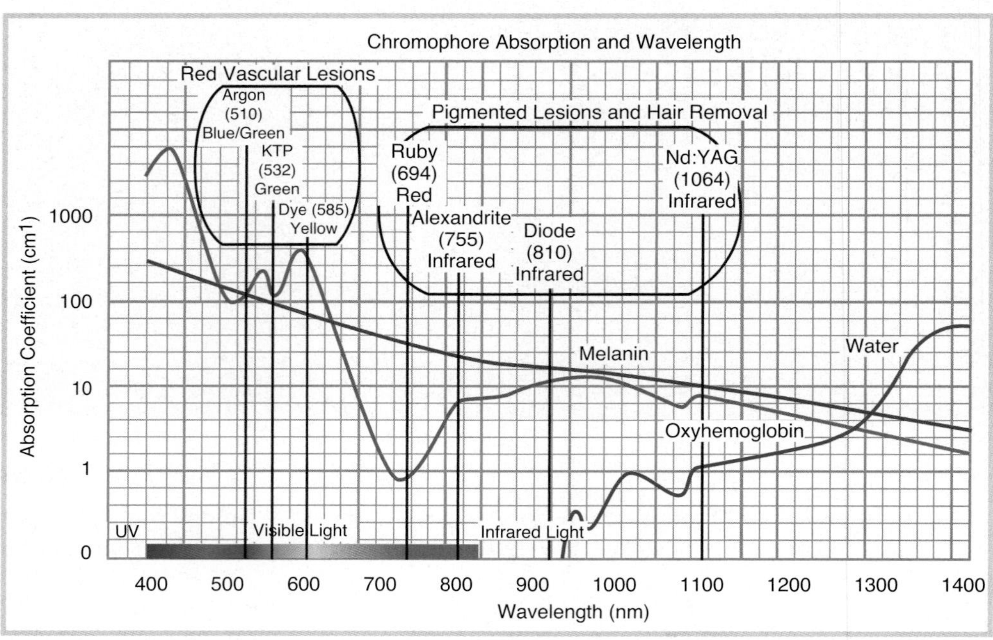

Figure 1A

absorbed by oxyhemoglobin, the target chromophore in red blood vessels. The vessel is heated, causing injury to the vessel wall and perivascular collagen damage, which ultimately results in vessel closure and obliteration with minimal to no thermal damage to the surrounding tissues. For treatment of benign epidermal pigmented lesions, such as lentigines, light energy is absorbed by the target chromophore melanin. Thus, photo rejuvenation treatment of benign pigmented and vascular lesions is achieved through selectively targeting these two main chromophores in the skin, melanin and oxyhemoglobin, while leaving the surrounding skin unaffected.

Particular chromophores can be selectively targeted using different wavelengths of light. For the treatment of superficial red vascular lesions, wavelengths are selected such that light energy is preferentially absorbed by oxyhemoglobin. The absorption spectra in Figure 1A shows the amount of light energy absorbed for various wavelengths by the main chromophores in tissue, oxyhemoglobin and melanin. Oxyhemoglobin preferentially absorbs light between 510 and 600 nm (with peak absorptions at 540 and 580 nm). The main lasers used for treatment of red vascular lesions have emission wavelengths within this ideal oxyhemoglobin absorption range: argon (510 nm), potassium titanyl phosphate or KTP (532 nm), and pulsed dye (585 nm). Melanin preferentially absorbs light between 650 and 1,100 nm. The main lasers used for treatment of epidermal pigmented lesions and hair reduction emit wavelengths within this ideal melanin absorption range: ruby (694 nm), alexandrite (755 nm), diode (810 nm), and Nd:YAG (1,064 nm). The KTP (532 nm) and argon (510 nm) lasers also have high melanin absorption, and these can be used to treat epidermal pigmented lesions as well as vascular lesions.

Selection of the wavelength for *Laser* treatments determines chromophore specificity and the depth of penetration for *Laser* energy. Other laser parameters such as spot size, pulse width, and fluence must also be appropriately selected to effectively target lesions and minimize damage to surrounding tissues. For the treatment of red facial vessels, the size and depth of the vessel determines these laser parameters. Smaller vessels dissipate heat more rapidly, have shorter thermal relaxation times, and therefore require shorter pulse widths to effect vessel damage. Larger red facial vessels are deeper in the dermis and require larger spot sizes, longer pulse widths, and higher fluences for greater depth of penetration into the dermis. The thermal relaxation time for red facial vessels (with luminal diameters of 0.1 to 0.7 mm) is 5 to 50 ms, and therefore pulse widths should be within this range for treatment. When treating epidermal pigmented lesions, short pulse durations (≤50 ms) are effective because most benign pigmented lesions are superficially

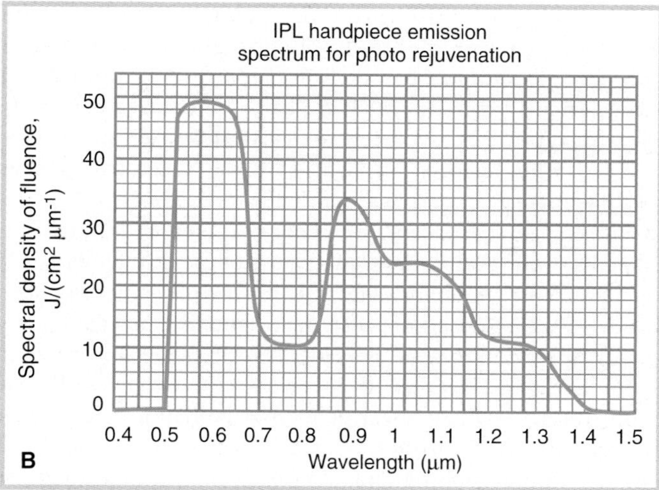

Figure 1B

located in epidermal melanocytes and keratinocytes. Q-Switched lasers, which have very short pulse durations (in the nanosecond range), are effective for reduction of unwanted pigmentation and include 532 nm, ruby (694 nm), alexandrite (755 nm), and Nd:YAG (1,064 nm).

Photo rejuvenation treatments for benign vascular and pigmented lesions using lasers typically require the use of multiple devices because lasers are monochromatic and emit a single wavelength, each of which targets a different chromophore. For example, facial telangiectasias may be treated with a 532-nm laser and lentigines with a 755-nm laser. IPL devices, in contrast, emit a spectrum of wavelengths. Filters are used to produce emission peaks at specified wavelengths corresponding to the chromophores being targeted and the desired depth of penetration for treatment. Figure 1B is an example of an emission spectrum for an IPL device (Palomar StarLux) with a filter for photo rejuvenation (LuxG hand piece) that shows an emission peak from 500 to 670 nm and a second emission peak from 870 to 1,200 nm. Both melanin and oxyhemoglobin are targeted with these wavelengths. More superficial lesions are targeted with the shorter wavelengths, and deeper lesions are targeted with the longer wavelengths. In this way, a single IPL device can be used to target both vascular and pigmented lesions at a variety of depths in the skin. IPLs typically have less versatility in spot size, but other treatment parameters (pulse width and fluence) may be optimized similarly to lasers for delivery of energy to the desired target while sparing the surrounding tissues.

Clinical Considerations

Alternatives to *Lasers* for treatment of benign pigmented and vascular lesions include liquid nitrogen or topical skin-lightening products such as hydroquinone, ablative (fractionated and non-fractionated) such as carbon dioxide and erbium lasers for pigmented lesions, electrocautery for vascular lesions, or no treatment at all. For a discussion of laser safety, see Chapter 31.

Results and Follow-up

Appropriate patient selection is fundamental to ensuring the success of treatments. The best candidates for photo rejuvenation treatment are those with fair skin, which include Fitzpatrick skin types I to III (see Chapter 31 for a review of Fitzpatrick skin types), because they have the greatest disparity between background skin color and target chromophores. Patients with darker skin types have an increased risk of complications such as hyperpigmentation, hypopigmentation, and burns due to competing melanin chromophore in the skin, and treatments should be performed with caution by experienced laser operators. Photo rejuvenation for patients with darker Fitzpatrick skin types IV to V often focuses on reduction of unwanted pigmentation rather than vascular lesions, and the safest devices for treatment are Q-switched Nd:YAG (1,064-nm) lasers.

Photo rejuvenation treatments for benign pigmented lesions may be performed on any sun-exposed area of the body where lentigines are present. However, treatment of lentigines on the face, neck, chest, and hands yield the most consistent results and are associated with the fewest side effects. Results of *Laser* treatments for melasma are variable, and in some cases, hyperpigmentation may be worsened. Noticeable improvements are seen with single treatments for lentigines, but typically a series of three to five IPL treatments is required for dramatic improvements. Fewer treatments may be required with lasers. Patients should be seen at monthly intervals during a treatment series to allow for exfoliation of all flaking microcrusts. An annual maintenance treatment may be required for patients with active outdoor lifestyles despite the regular use of sun screen.

Photo rejuvenation treatments for benign vascular lesions are performed mainly on the face, neck, and chest. The most common lesions are telangiectasias, erythema to telangiectatic rosacea, and poikiloderma of Civatte, which is a pattern of erythema and mottled pigmentation seen most often on the sides of the face, neck, and chest. Larger red facial vessels, which have the most target chromophores, respond more dramatically to treatments than fine lacey red vessels or diffuse erythema. Noticeable improvements are seen with single treatments, but typically a series of three to five IPL treatments is required for improvement. Fewer treatments may be required with lasers. Treatments should be performed at bimonthly intervals to achieve the best results. Vascular lesions may recur, particularly in patients with active lifestyles, and maintenance treatments are recommended annually or biannually. Discrete lesions such as cherry angiomas usually require one or two treatments and do not typically recur.

Anesthesia

Anesthesia is rarely required for photo rejuvenation treatments and is discouraged by the author. Topical anesthetics may contain vasoconstrictive agents that can minimize vascular targets, reducing treatment efficacy. Patient feedback is important in selecting appropriate treatment parameters, and anesthesia obscures this information.

Preprocedure Checklist

- Perform an aesthetic consultation, and review the patient's medical history (see Chapter 28).
- Determine Fitzpatrick skin type (see Chapter 31).
- Obtain informed consent (see Chapter 28).
- Take pretreatment photographs.
- Prophylax with antiviral medication if there is a history of herpes simplex or zoster in or near the treatment area for 2 days prior to procedure, and continue for 3 days after the procedure.
- Lighten skin for darker Fitzpatrick skin types (IV to V). Strict sun avoidance for 1 month is requisite with daily use of a full-spectrum sun screen. Use a topical skin-lightening product daily or twice daily for at least 1 month prior to treatment such as hydroquinone or a cosmeceutical such as kojic acid, arbutin, niacinamide, or azelaic acid.
- Perform test spots prior to the initial treatment for skin type III with high-risk ethnic backgrounds (Mediterranean, Latino, and Asian) and skin type IV and above. Select

appropriate test spot parameters based on the patient's Fitzpatrick skin type and the degree of abnormal pigmentation and/or redness in the treatment area, using the *Laser* manufacturer's guidelines for spot size, fluence, and pulse width. Test spots should be placed discretely near the desired treatment area (under the chin, behind or inferior to the ear) and viewed in 3 to 5 days for evidence of hyperpigmentation, burn, or other adverse effect. At each visit, patients requiring test spots should have test spots placed using the fluence and pulse width desired for the subsequent treatment. Inform patients that lack of an adverse reaction with test spots does not ensure that a side effect or complication will not occur with any treatment.
- All patients should avoid direct sun exposure for 1 month prior to treatments and use a full-spectrum sun screen daily in the treatment area.

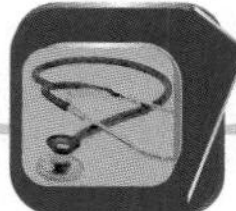

Equipment

- Laser or IPL device appropriate for photorejuvenation treatments
- Eyewear for the patient and provider specific to the laser or IPL being used
- Nonalcohol cleansing facial wipes
- Clear colorless gel for treatments
- Gauze, 4 × 4 inches
- Ice packs
- Soothing topical product for posttreatment application such as aloe gel
- Hydrocortisone cream 1% and 2.5%
- Alcohol wipes for cleaning tip of *Laser*
- Germicidal disposable wipes for sanitizing *Laser*

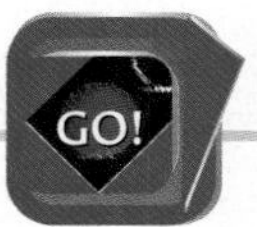

Indications

- Undesired benign pigmentation or benign vascular lesions for cosmesis

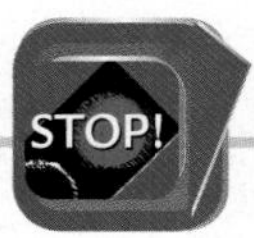

Contraindications

Absolute

- Isotretinoin (Accutane) use in the last 6 months
- Keloid formation or hypertrophic scarring
- Pregnancy and nursing
- Seizures
- Vascular malformations or tumors
- Melanoma or lesions suspected of melanoma in the treatment area
- Active infection in the treatment area (e.g., herpes or pustular acne)
- Cardiac pacemaker
- Skin type VI with lasers and IPL
- Skin type V with IPLs
- Recent sun exposure and/or tanned skin
- Photosensitive disorder (e.g., systemic lupus erythematosus)
- Self-tanning product use 2 weeks prior to treatment

Relative

- Poor healing (due to autoimmune diseases, diabetes, etc.)
- Anticoagulants

- Current use of photosensitizing medications (e.g., tetracyclines, St. John's wort, thiazides, etc.)
- Use of products containing retinoids, glycolic or hydroxy acids in the treatment area 1 week prior to treatment

The Procedure

The following recommendations are guidelines for photo rejuvenation treatments of benign pigmented and vascular lesions with IPL devices and are based on the Palomar StarLux using the LuxG handpiece. There are other IPL systems that are comparable.

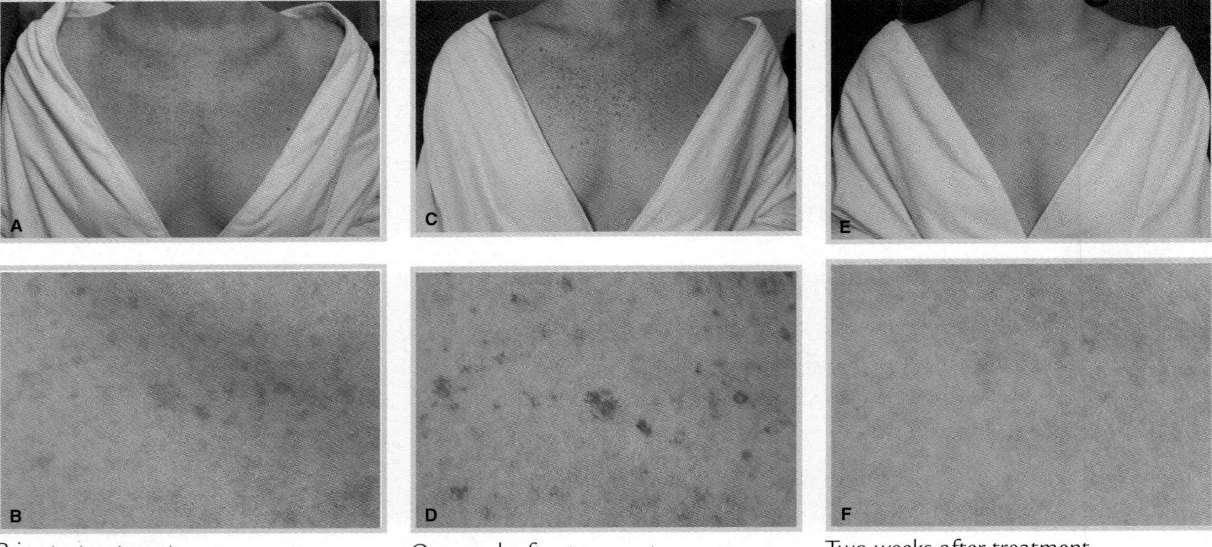

Prior to treatment. One week after treament. Two weeks after treatment.

Figure 2

Results of an initial treatment for lentigines on the chest of a 36-year-old patient are shown in Figure 2. Figures A and B show the patient's chest prior to treatment, C and D show the chest 1 week after treatment, and E and F show the chest 2 weeks after treatment. Note the darkened and flaking appearance of the lentigines 1 week after treatment (C and D) due to micro-crust formation and the significant pigmentation improvement at 2 weeks. Treatment was performed using 20-ms pulse width and 36-J/cm^2 fluence.

IPL photo rejuvenation results for treatment of solar lentigines on the face are shown in Figure 3 using 20-ms pulse width and 38-J/cm^2 fluence.

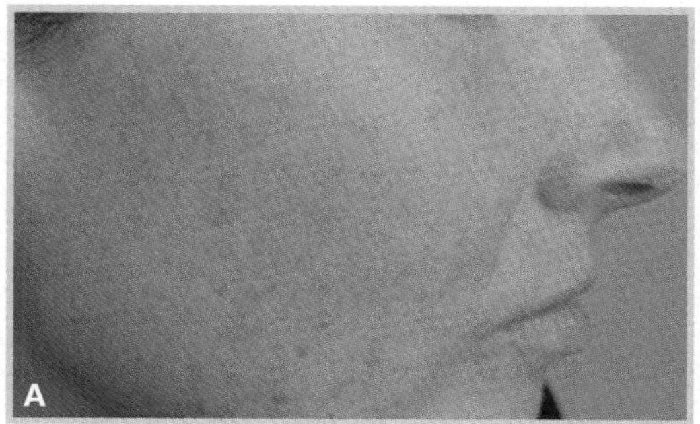

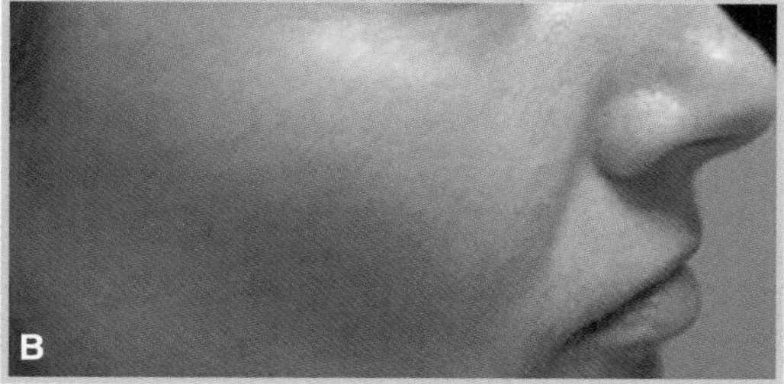

Courtesy of Haneef Alibhai, MD

Figure 3

Figure 4 shows IPL photo rejuvenation results for treatment of solar lentigines on the hands using 40-ms pulse width, 34-J/cm^2 fluence, and two passes.

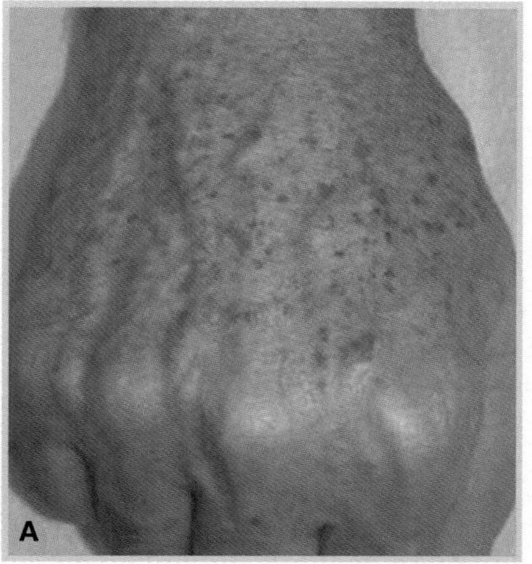

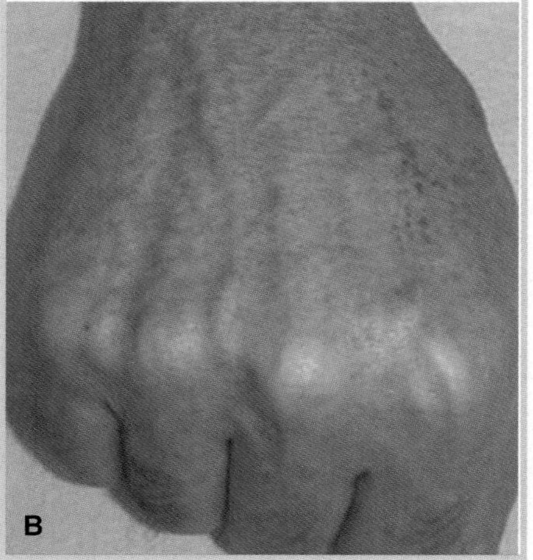

Courtesy of Palomar.

Figure 4

Results of photo rejuvenation treatments for rosacea are shown before (Figure 5A) and after (Figure 5B) a series of five treatments. Note the marked improvement in midface redness and nasal telangiectasias. Treatments were performed using 20-ms pulse width and 40-J/cm^2 fluence.

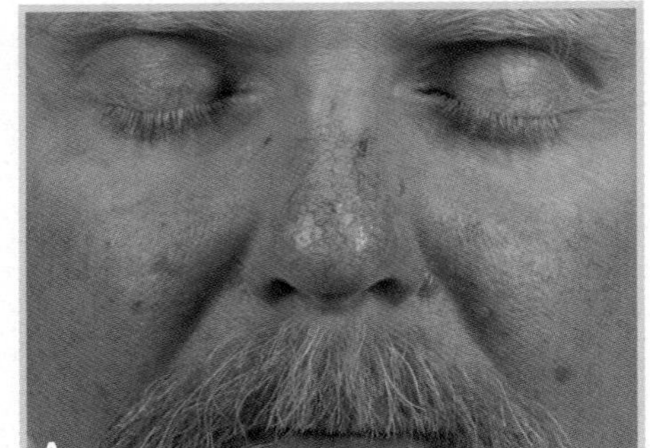

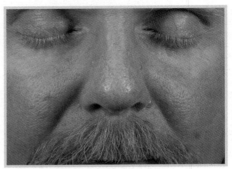

Courtesy of Michael Sinclair, MD

Figure 5

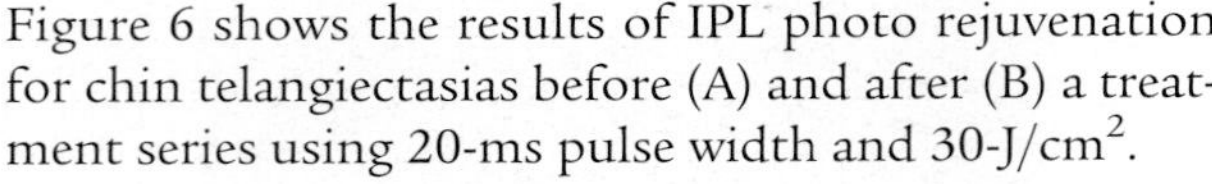

Figure 6 shows the results of IPL photo rejuvenation for chin telangiectasias before (A) and after (B) a treatment series using 20-ms pulse width and 30-J/cm^2.

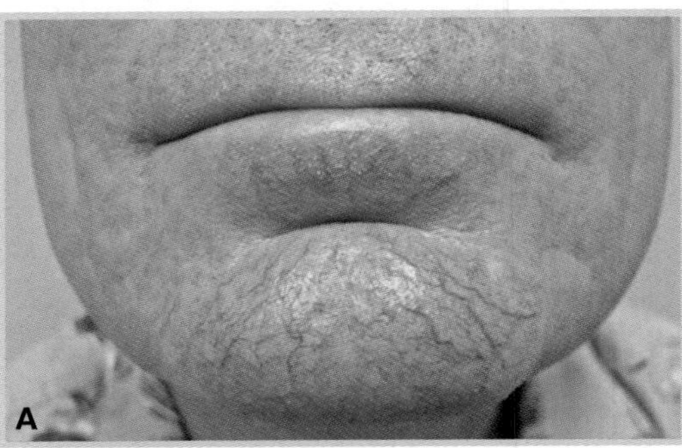

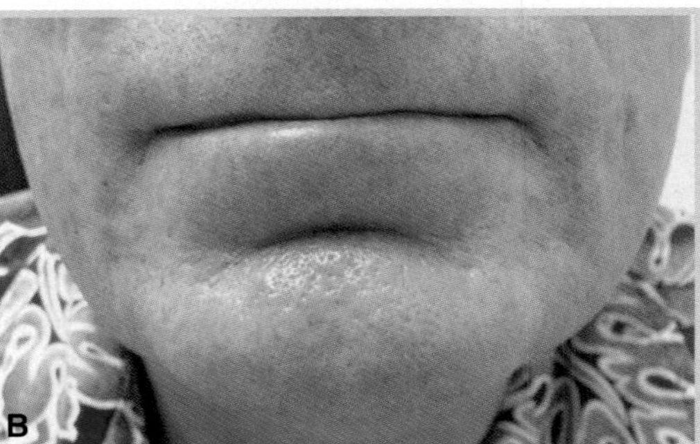

Courtesy of Michael Sinclair, MD

Figure 6

Figure 7 shows the results of IPL photo rejuvenation treatment for a cherry angioma before (A) and after (B) a single treatment using 20-ms pulse width and 40-J/cm^2 fluence.

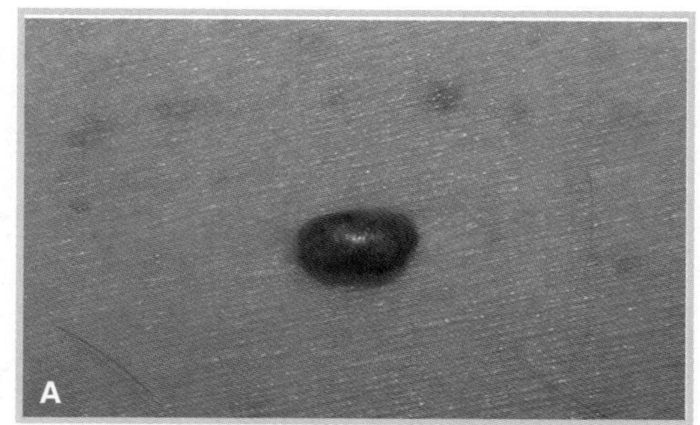

Courtesy of Palomar.

Figure 7

Step 1. Comfortably position the patient for treatment with the treatment bed flat. Cleanse the skin with a non-alcohol wipe. Provide appropriate IPL eye protection for the patient and all personnel in the treatment room prior to beginning treatment. See Supplies section at the end of the chapter for vendor information. Operate the IPL in accordance with your clinic's IPL safety policies and procedures and the manufacturer's guidelines.

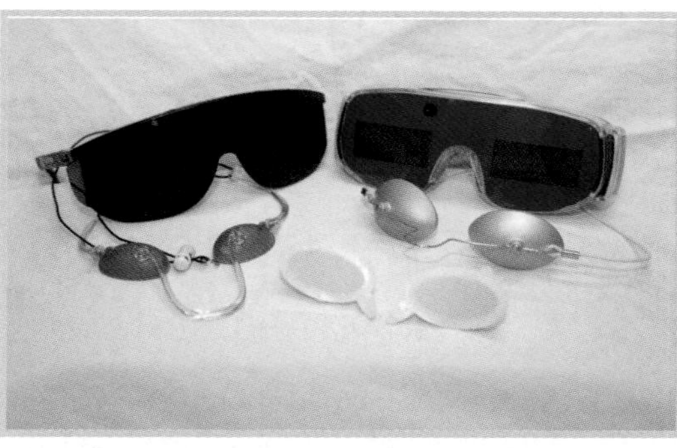

Step 1

Step 2. Tattoos and permanent makeup should be covered with wet gauze, as shown in Step 2, and the IPL tip should be at least 2 inches away from the tattoo during treatment.

- PITFALL: Full thickness burns may result from treating over tattoos.

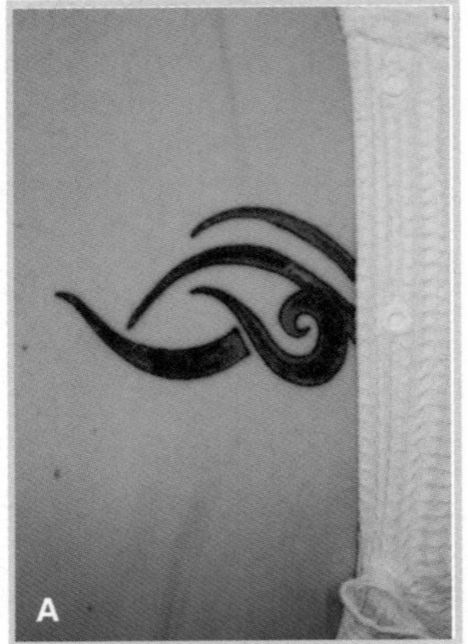

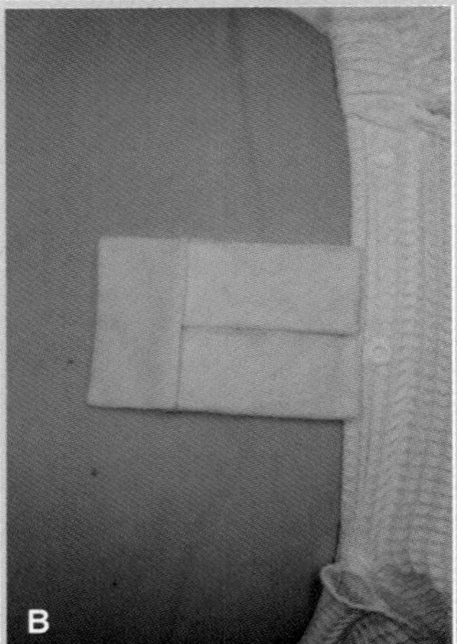

Step 2

Step 3. Select conservative photo rejuvenation settings for the initial treatment based on the patient's Fitzpatrick skin type and the degree of abnormal pigmentation and/or redness in the treatment area, using the IPL manufacturer's guidelines for spot size, fluence, and pulse width. A typical IPL touch pad used to select treatment parameters is shown. The more target present, such as dark lentigines, high density of lentigines or freckles, or intense facial redness, the more conservative the settings should be, with longer pulse widths and lower fluences.

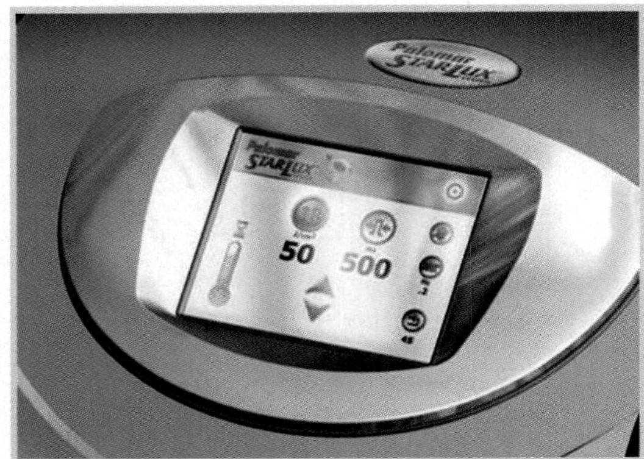

Step 3

Figure 8A shows a patient with moderate to severe photo damage with solar lentigines, requiring more conservative settings. Figure 8B shows a patient with mild photodamage, requiring more aggressive settings of shorter pulse width and higher fluence.

- **PEARL:** The neck and chest are more sensitive to treatments and require more conservative settings than the face.
- **PEARL:** If pigmentation and redness are both present, such as telangiectasias with overlying lentigines, select settings for treatment of pigmentation initially.
- **PEARL:** Type IV skin types will require longer pulse widths and lower fluencies, because there is a greater risk of epidermal injury.
- **PITFALL:** Assess lighter skin types for background actinic bronzing, which is an overall light brown discoloration to the skin. Treatments will also target and reduce this background pigmentation. Excellent coverage must be achieved with 20% overlap of the IPL tip in the treatment area, because untreated areas will be visible as stripes.

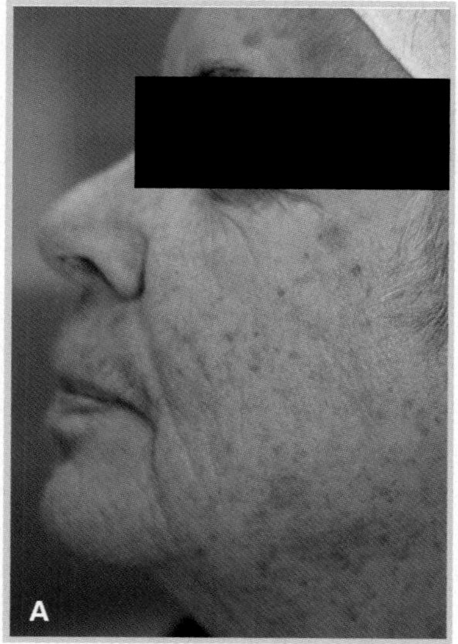

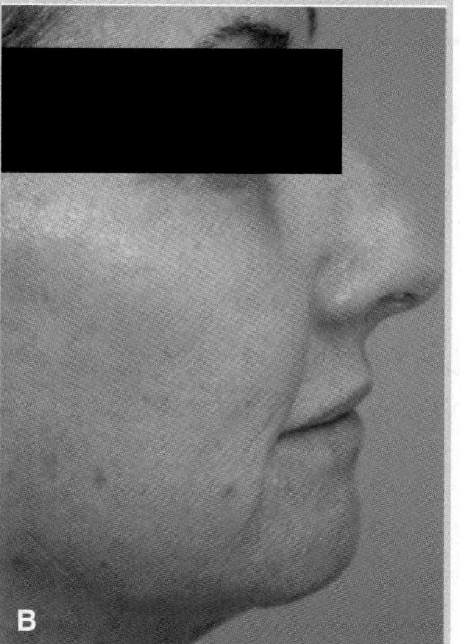

Figure 8

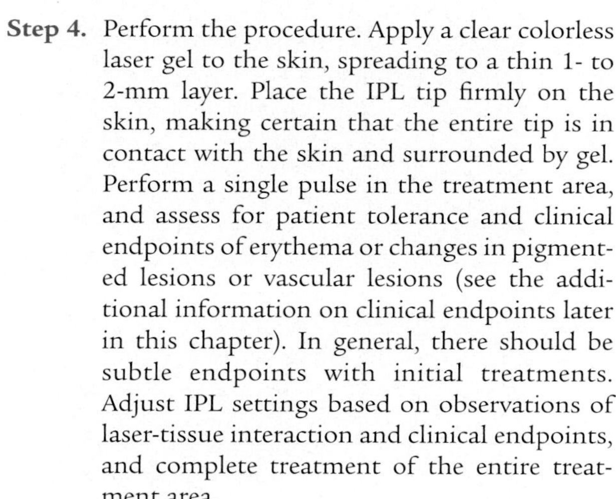

Step 4. Perform the procedure. Apply a clear colorless laser gel to the skin, spreading to a thin 1- to 2-mm layer. Place the IPL tip firmly on the skin, making certain that the entire tip is in contact with the skin and surrounded by gel. Perform a single pulse in the treatment area, and assess for patient tolerance and clinical endpoints of erythema or changes in pigmented lesions or vascular lesions (see the additional information on clinical endpoints later in this chapter). In general, there should be subtle endpoints with initial treatments. Adjust IPL settings based on observations of laser-tissue interaction and clinical endpoints, and complete treatment of the entire treatment area.

- **PEARL:** Always angle the IPL tip away from the eyes during treatment.

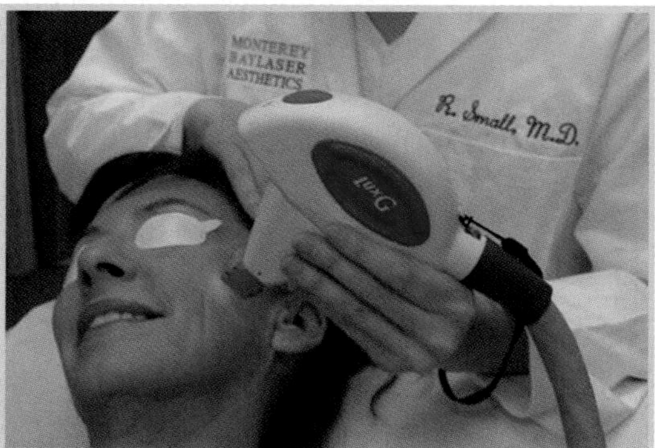

Step 4

Step 5. Step 5 shows a recommended method for IPL treatment of the full face, starting with area 1 and progressing to area 6. The direction of IPL pulses should be toward the provider, with approximately 20% overlap of each pulse.

- **PEARL:** The most sensitive areas are the upper lip (philtrum) and lateral to the nasal ala. When treating the upper lip, have the patient place their tongue over their teeth while keeping their lips closed, to reduce discomfort.
- **PITFALL:** Treating over hair will singe darkly colored hair and may result in overtreatment of the epidermis with blistering, particularly over men's beards, and there is a possibility of permanent hair reduction.

Step 6. After completing treatment of the full face, additional passes may be performed over lesions requiring more intense treatment with slightly higher settings if necessary, based on the presence or absence of clinical endpoints. A template shown in Step 6 may be placed over the lesion to more specifically target the lesion and spare the surrounding skin.

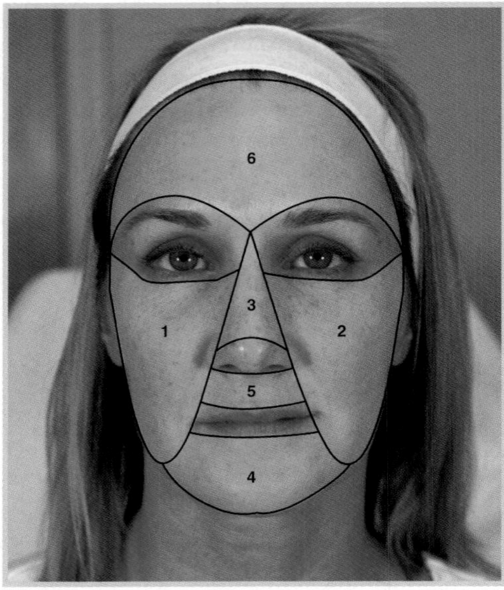

Step 5

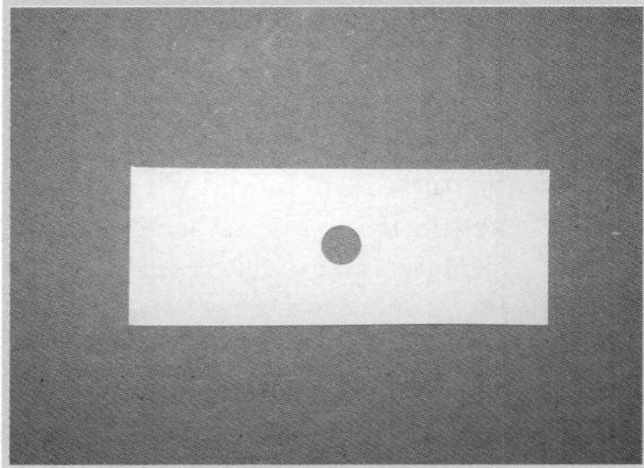

Step 6

Pigmented Lesion Clinical Endpoints

Immediately after treatment, pigmented lesions such as lentigines should darken and appear well demarcated against the background skin, and/or slight erythema around the lesion should be visible. Aggressive treatment will result in a gray or black discoloration of the lentigo. Figure 9A shows a patient's chest immediately after IPL treatment of lentigines on the right half of the chest. Also shown are close-up views of the chest in the treated (Figure 9B) and untreated (Figure 9C).

- **PEARL:** Longer pulse widths are associated with delayed appearance of endpoints, which usually become evident 5 minutes after the IPL pulse.

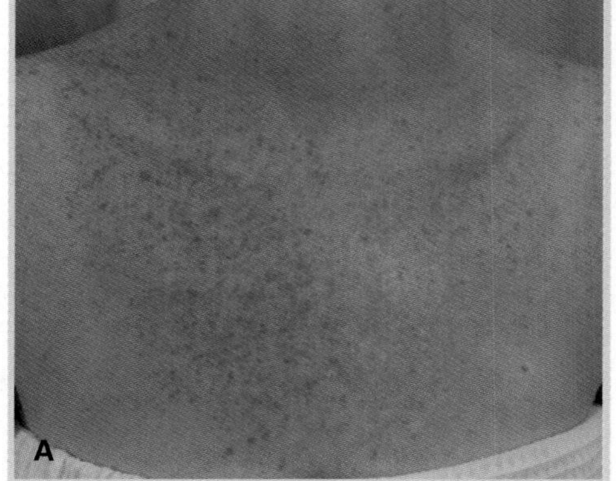

Courtesy of Palomar.

Figure 9

Vascular Lesion Clinical Endpoints

Immediately after treatment, red vascular lesions such as telangiectasias may exhibit blanching or mild surrounding erythema, and larger vessels may appear bluish or dark. Shown in Figure 10A are nasal alar telangiectasias before and immediately after treatment (Figure 10B) using 20-ms pulse width and 38-J/cm^2 fluence. Rarely, a vessel may rupture, and purpura will be seen in patients with thin skin when using short pulse widths and high fluences. Purpura can take 2 weeks to resolve, and patients will require reassurance. Cherry angiomas appear purplish after treatment, gradually regress, and fade in size and color.

- **PEARL:** Some vessels may not appear to change immediately after treatment. Compress the vessel and observe for blanching and refilling. If the vessel does not blanch, it has been adequately treated.

- **PITFALL:** Too much pressure applied with the IPL tip over vascular lesions will reduce the vascular target and render treatments less efficacious.

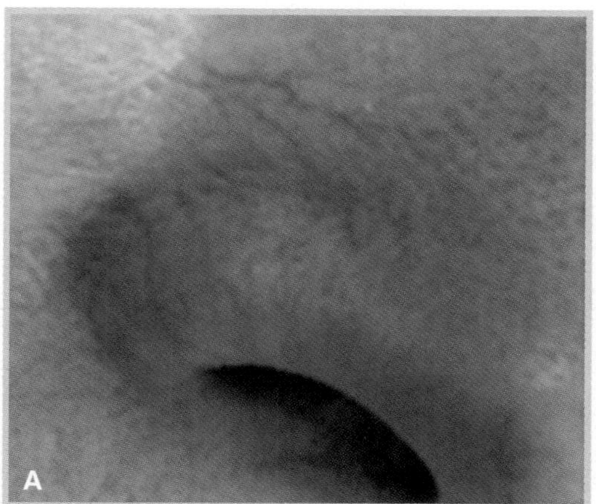

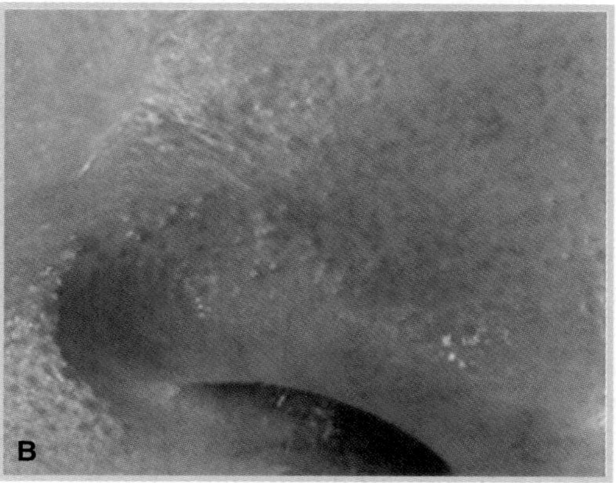

Courtesy of Palomar.

Figure 10

Step 7. For subsequent visits, fluence should be increased and pulse width decreased according to the manufacturer's guidelines so as to target lighter pigmentation and finer vessels. In general, only one parameter should be changed to intensify treatments in any given visit. Usually the fluence is increased for a few treatments to achieve desired clinical endpoints, and pulse width is decreased in the later treatments.

- **PEARL:** Inquire about sun exposure and sun screen use at every visit. If recently sun exposed, wait 1 month before treating to reduce the risk of complications.

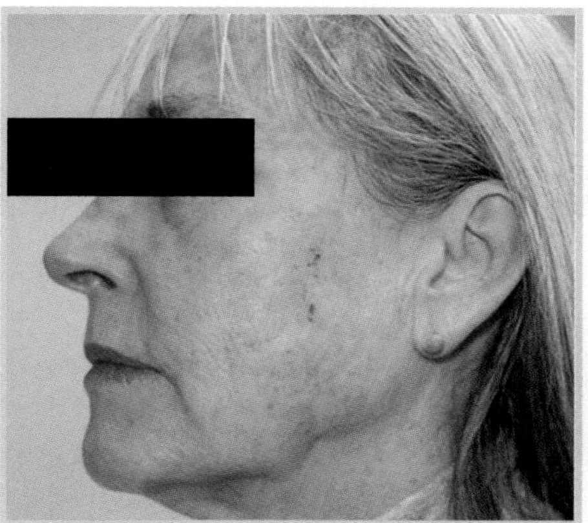

Step 7

- **PEARL:** Do not treat if micro-crusts from the previous treatment are visible. Wait an additional 1 to 2 weeks until all micro-crusts are resolved. Step 7 shows a patient 4 weeks after IPL photo rejuvenation treatment to the face with an area on the left cheek that has persistent micro-crust.

Step 8. After treatment, apply a soothing topical product such as aloe gel. Ice should be applied for 15 minutes to minimize erythema, edema, and reduce discomfort. Step 8 shows ice packs and a cool roller, all of which may be used for icing the treatment area. If the treatment area is significantly erythematous, hydrocortisone cream 1% to 2.5% may also be applied.

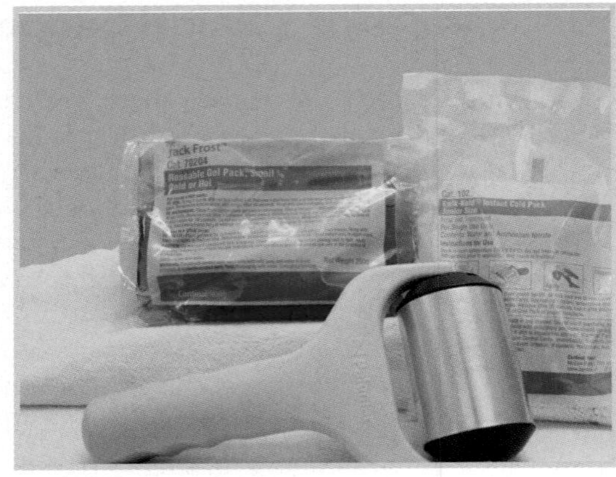

Step 8

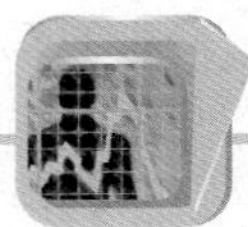

Complications

- Discomfort or pain
- Hypopigmentation
- Hyperpigmentation, including worsening of melasma
- Eye injury
- Infection
- Burn with blistering and scabbing
- Damage or alteration to tattoos and permanent makeup
- Scarring (extremely rare)

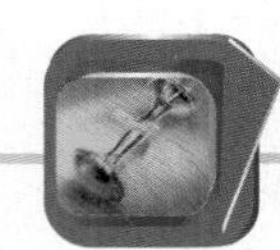

Pediatric Considerations

Pediatric treatments are not contraindicated but are typically performed by physicians specializing in pediatric *Laser* treatments.

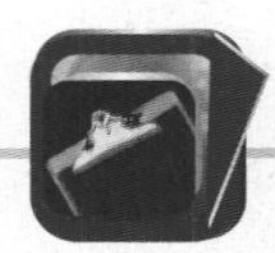

Postprocedure Instructions

Redness and swelling are common, and usually resolve within a few hours to 1 week after treatment. They can be managed with application of ice for 15 minutes every 1 to 2 hours and hydrocortisone cream 1% two times per day for 3 to 4 days or until redness resolves. Pigmented lesions typically continue to darken 1 to 2 days after treatment. The darkened micro-crusts flake off over 1 to 2 weeks, revealing lightened or resolved lesions. Vascular lesions, such as telangiectasias, may gradually recur over 2 to 4 weeks while the patient undergoes a treatment series. Vascular lesions that have turned blue or darkened at the time of treatment will gradually fade over 2 weeks. Postinflammatory hyperpigmentation (PIH) can occur with prolonged erythema, and patients should contact their provider if erythema persists for more than 5 days. Pigmentary complications, such as PIH and hypopigmentation, usually resolve in 3 to 6 months but may be permanent. Daily use of a full-spectrum sun screen (SPF 30 with zinc or titanium) and sun avoidance for 4 weeks after treatment will help minimize the risk of pigmentary changes. If blistering and/or crusting occur, manage with routine wound care using bacitracin until healed.

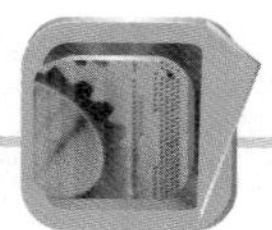

Coding Information and Supply Sources

ICD-9 Codes

Rosacea	695.3
Other dyschromia (solar lentigo, melasma)	709.09
Vascular disorder of the skin (cherry angioma, telangiectasia)	709.1

Laser photo rejuvenation is generally not reimbursable; however, some insurance companies may reimburse for treatment of rosacea. The charges for treatments vary and are largely determined by local prices. Individual treatment prices range from $350 to $500 for a single treatment to a large area such as the face or chest, and $150 to $250 for a small area such as the hands. However, because photo rejuvenation treatments are most effective with a series of treatments, packages of treatments (usually three or five) may be offered so that patients achieve the best possible results.

Supply Sources

Laser-Safe Eyewear

- Glendale, 910 Douglas Pike, Smithfield, RI 02917-1874. Phone: 1-800-500-4739.
- Oculo-plastic, 200 Sauve West, Montreal, H3L 1YD, Canada. Phone: 1-800-588-2279.

Laser Safety Training Courses

- American Society for Laser Medicine and Surgery (ASLMS), 2100 Stewart Avenue, Suite 240, Wausau, WI 54401. Phone: 715-845-9283.

Photo Rejuvenation Lasers and Intense Pulsed Light Suppliers

- American BioCare, 1201 Dove Street, Suite 520, Newport Beach, CA 92660. Phone: 1-800-676-1434. Web site: http://www.medicalbiocare.com/.
- Candela, 530 Boston Post Road, Wayland, MA. Phone: 508-358-7400, 1-800-733-8550. Web site: http://www.candelalaser.com/.
- CoolTouch, 9085 Foothills Boulevard, Roseville, CA 95747. Phone: 877-858-COOL. Web site: http://www.cooltouch.com/.
- Cutera, 3240 Bayshore Boulevard, Brisbane, CA 94005. Phone: 1-888-4-CUTERA, 415-657-5500. Web site: http://www.cutera.com/.
- Cynosure/Deka, 5 Carlisle Road, Westford, MA 01886. Phone: 978-256-4200, 1-800-886-2966. Web site: http://www.cynosure.com/contact-us/index.php.
- DermaMed USA, 394 Parkmount Road, P. O. Box 198, Lenni, PA 19052-0198. Phone: 1-888-789-6342. Web site: http://www.dermamedusa.com/.
- Ellipse A/S, Agern Allé 11, DK-2970 Hørsholm, Denmark. Phone: 45-4576-8808. Web site: http://www.ellipse.org.
- Fotona USA, 1415 1st Street South, Suite 5, Willmar, MN 56201. Phone: 1-888-550-4113. Web site: http://www.fotonamedicallasers.com.
- General Project, 22 Linnfield Terrace, Phillisburg, NJ 08865. Phone: 908-454-8875; fax: 908-454-8938. Web site: http://www.generalproject.com.
- HOYA ConBio Medical and Dental Lasers, 47733 Fremont Blvd.; Fremont, CA 94538. Phone: 1-800-532-1064. Web site: http://www.conbio.com.
- Iridex Corporation, 1212 Terra Bella Avenue, Mountain View, CA 94043. Phone: 1-650-940-4700.
- Lumenis, 5302 Betsy Ross Drive, Santa Clara, CA 95054. Phone: 408-764-3000. Web site: http://www.lumenis.com/.
- Med-Surge, 14850 Quorum Drive, Suite 120, Dallas TX 75254. Phone: 877-354-7845, 972-720-0425. Web site: http://www.medsurgeadvances.com/home.php.

- Quantel Medical, 601 Haggerty Lane, Bozeman, MT 59715. Phone: 1-888-660-6726. Web site: http://www.quantelmedical.com.
- Orion Lasers, 485 Half Day Road, Suite 100, Buffalo Grove, IL 60089. Phone: 1-866-414-ALMA. Web site: http://www.almalasers.com/.
- Palomar, 82 Cambridge Street, Burlington, MA 01803. Phone: 1-800-PALOMAR. Web site: http://www.palomarmedical.com/.
- Sciton, 925 Commercial Street, Palo Alto, CA 94303. Phone: 888-646-6999. Web site: http://www.sciton.com/.
- SharpLight Technologies, 4-1420 Cornwall Rd., Oakville, ON L6J-7W5, Canada. Phone: 905-337-7797. Web site: http://www.sharplightech.com.
- Syneron, 28 Fulton Way, Unit 8, Richmond Hill, ON L4B 1L5, Canada. Phone: 905-886-9235, 866-259-6661. Web site: http://www.syneron.com/.
- WaveLight, Kontichsesteenweg 36, 2630 Aartselaar, Belgium. Phone: 32-3-870-37-63. Web site: http://www.dcmedical.be/FR/dermatologie/lasers/Midon_Vasculair.htm.

Patient Education Handout

A patient education handout, "Photo Rejuvenation," can be found on the book's companion Web site.

Bibliography

Adamic M, Troilius A, Adatto M, et al. Vascular lasers and IPLs: Guidelines for care from the European Society for Laser Dermatology. *J Cosm Laser Therapy*. 2007;9:113–124.

Goldman MP. Laser treatment of cutaneous vascular lesions. In: Goldman MP, ed. *Cutaneous and Cosmetic Laser Surgery*. Mosby Elsevier; 2006:31–91.

Kilmer SL. et al. Diode laser treatment of pigmented lesions. *Lasers Surg Med.* 2000;12(suppl):23.

Lowe JL, Kafaja S. Pigmentation of the ageing face—evaluation and treatment. In: Lowe NJ, ed. *Textbook of Facial Rejuvenation: The Art of Minimally Invasive Combination Therapy*. Taylor & Francis; 2002:73–83.

Railan D, Kilmer S. Treatment of benign pigmented cutaneous lesions. In: Goldman MP, ed. *Cutaneous and Cosmetic Laser Surgery*. Mosby Elsevier; 2006:93–108.

Ross V, et al. Intense pulsed light and laser treatment of facial telangiectasia and dyspigmentation: some theoretical and practical comparisons. *Derm Surg*. 2005;31(9):1188–1198.

Smith KC. Combined erythema and telangiectasia respond quickly to combination treatment with intense pulsed light laser followed immediately by long-pulsed Nd:YAG laser. *Cos Derm*. 2007;20(8):503–505.

Tanghetti EA. The versapulse laser. In: Keller GS, ed. *Lasers in Aesthetic Surgery*. Thieme; 2001:190–194.

Yaghmai D, Garden JM. Treating facial vascular lesions with lasers. In: Lowe NJ, ed. *Textbook of Facial Rejuvenation: The Art of Minimally Invasive Combination Therapy*. Taylor & Francis; 2002: 85–100.

2008 MAG Mutual Healthcare Solutions, Inc.'s Physicians' Fee and Coding Guide. Duluth, Georgia. MAG Mutual Healthcare Solutions, Inc. 2007.

CHAPTER 33

Microdermabrasion

Rebecca Small, MD

Assistant Clinical Professor, Director, Medical Aesthetics Training Program, Department of Family and Community Medicine, University of California, San Francisco School of Medicine, Capitola, CA

Microdermabrasion (MDA) is a minimally invasive mechanical exfoliation procedure for superficial skin resurfacing. Most exfoliation modalities in use today can be broadly classified as chemical exfoliants, which include glycolic and salicylic acid peels and mechanical exfoliants. Mechanical exfoliation treatments range from simple microbead scrubs found over the counter, which partially remove the stratum corneum, to operative procedures such as laser resurfacing and dermabrasion, which can ablate the reticular dermis. The depth of resurfacing achieved with MDA is conservatively in the middle of this spectrum. Although MDA exfoliation can vary from superficial thinning of the stratum corneum to penetration into the upper papillary dermis, the target depth for most MDA procedures is removal of the stratum corneum.

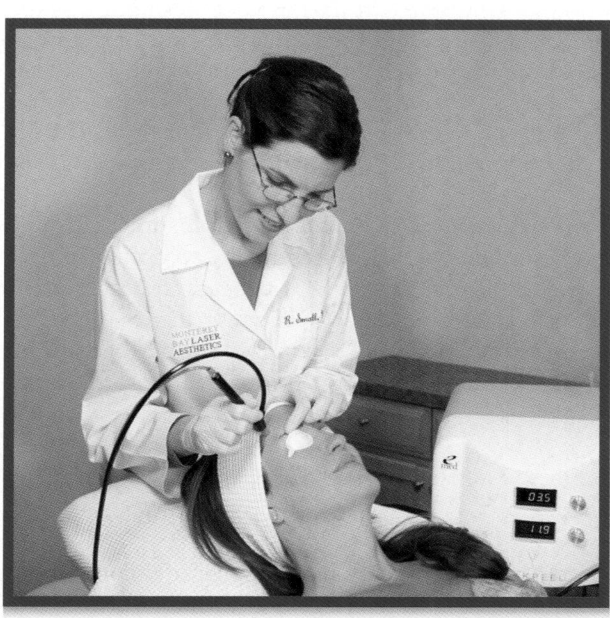

Exfoliation treatments are based on the principles of wound healing. By wounding and removing the uppermost layers of the skin in a controlled manner, cell renewal is stimulated with regeneration of a healthier epidermis and dermis. Histological evaluation of facial skin after repeated MDA treatments demonstrates a reparative wound-healing process with regeneration of a compacted stratum corneum and a smoother epidermis. Skin hydration increases with improved epidermal barrier function, and fibroblast stimulation increases dermal thickness through production of new collagen and elastin.

MDA is commonly used to treat photo-damaged skin and reliably demonstrates improvement in skin texture, coarse pores, comedonal acne, and epidermal hyperpigmentation such as solar lentigines. Treatments may improve fine lines and superficial acne scarring. Certain MDA devices have also shown positive results with rosacea and papulopustular acne.

Traditionally, MDA devices have used crystals as the abrasive element. Negative pressure draws the skin to the hand-piece tip, and crystals superficially abrade the skin's surface as they pass across the epidermis. Used crystals and cellular debris are aspirated and collected separately for disposal after treatment. Each pass of the hand piece removes approximately 15 μm of skin, and two passes of most MDA devices fully remove the stratum corneum. The depth of resurfacing achieved with MDA is comparable to a superficial chemical peel. MDA offers certain advantages over chemical peel treatments such as greater control over the depth of exfoliation, comparatively

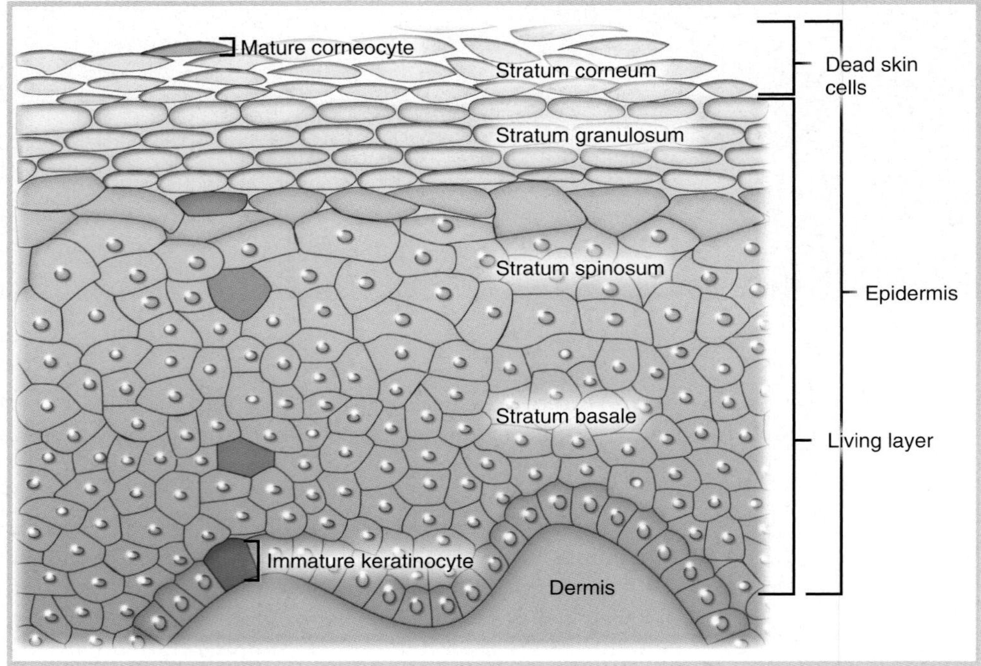

Figure 1

minimal discomfort, and no "downtime" for skin flaking and peeling. Other alternatives to MDA include ablative and nonablative laser resurfacing and dermaplaning, which utilizes a specialized dulled scalpel blade that is passed across the skin.

Recent advances in MDA technology combine exfoliation with dermal infusion. During this process, topical products are delivered into the skin at the time of or immediately after exfoliation. These systems take advantage of the transient disruption to the epidermal barrier that occurs with removal of the stratum corneum to better deliver medications into the deeper dermal layers. Dermal infusion can enhance results for conditions such as dehydration, hyperpigmentation, acne, and rosacea based on the products that are used.

MDA is one of the most commonly performed cosmetic procedures in the United States, with more than a half million treatments performed annually, according to data from the American Society for Aesthetic Plastic Surgery. Treatments are technically straightforward with a low risk of side effects, are associated with a high degree of patient satisfaction, and are well suited to the outpatient office setting. MDA has become an essential medical aesthetic rejuvenation treatment (ART) for primary care professionals who desire to provide aesthetic care.

Anatomy

The outermost layer of the skin, the stratum corneum, is a nonliving layer of corneocytes and lipids, which serves as a barrier against microbial pathogens and environmental irritants and keeps the skin hydrated and protected from injury. Constant renewal is necessary for the epidermis to maintain its integrity and function effectively. In healthy, younger skin, epidermal renewal takes approximately 1 month for keratinocytes to migrate from the living basal layer of the epidermis to the stratum corneum surface, from which they are shed (see keratinocyte migration highlighted in Figure 1). In aged, photo-damaged skin, keratinocyte maturation is slowed, and there is abnormal retention of cells, leading to a thickened, rough stratum corneum. Disruption of the epidermal barrier results in skin dehydration and may cause increased sensitivity. Photo-damaged skin is dull and exhibits dyschromia with solar lentigines and uneven pigmentation. Dermal thinning with loss of collagen and elastin contributes to formation of fine lines. Through stimulating cell renewal in the epidermis and dermis, MDA is able to address many of these changes seen with photo damage and intrinsic aging.

Results and Follow-up

MDA treatments are most commonly performed on the face, neck, chest, and hands. In general, facial skin tolerates more aggressive treatments and tends to show greater improvements than nonfacial areas. Epidermal healing is thought to be related to the density of adnexa (hair follicles and eccrine sweat glands) within a treatment area. The facial epidermis has a greater density of adnexa relative to the nonfacial epidermis, such as the neck and chest, which may account for its greater rejuvenation potential. Other treatment areas include the back and hyperkeratotic areas such as elbows and knees. Treatments may be performed for patients of all Fitzpatrick skin types (see Chapter 31 for Fitzpatrick classifications). However, aggressive treatments should be avoided in darker skin types (IV to VI) because of to their increased risk of postinflammatory hyperpigmentation (PIH). MDA combined with dermal infusion is associated with less posttreatment erythema and reduced risks of PIH.

Results from MDA treatments are cumulative, and typically a series of six treatments is recommended at bimonthly intervals. Results are not usually clinically evident after a single treatment. However, patients who have had little or no skin care previously may report improvements. Maintenance treatments may be performed every 4 to 6 weeks.

The most marked results with MDA are achieved when MDA is used in combination with other rejuvenation treatments such as chemical peels, topical skin care products, laser and intense pulsed light (IPL) photo rejuvenation, and fractional resurfacing. For example, dramatic reduction of benign pigmented epidermal lesions, such as lentigines, can be achieved when MDA is alternated every 2 weeks with laser or IPL photo-rejuvenation treatments. MDA performed prior to fractional resurfacing treatments may also reduce the incidence of posttreatment complications such as milia and acne.

Preprocedure Checklist

- Perform an aesthetic consultation, and review the patient's medical history (see Chapter 28).
- Obtain informed consent (see Chapter 28).
- Take pretreatment photographs (see Chapter 28).
- Prophylax with an oral antiviral medication such as acyclovir or valacyclovir if there is a history of herpes simplex or zoster in or near the treatment area for 2 days prior to procedure, and continue for 3 days postprocedure.
- Prior to MDA, patients should avoid chemical peels, dermal filler injections, waxing, and direct sun exposure for 2 weeks; discontinue use of products containing retinoic acid or alpha-hydroxy acids (e.g., glycolic acid); and avoid botulinum toxin injections for 1 week.

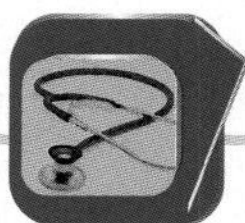

Equipment

- MDA device with abrasive element (e.g., crystals, diamond tips). Aluminum oxide is the most commonly used crystal and is ideal for MDA because it is inert and second only to diamonds in hardness. Other crystals used include sodium chloride, sodium bicarbonate, and magnesium oxide. Crystal-free MDA devices have become popular because of the lack of dust and associated risks of ocular injury. Diamond-tipped devices employ diamond-tipped pads as the abrasive element and can be used with topical solutions for dermal infusion.

- Headband.
- Facial wash and astringent to cleanse and degrease the treatment area.
- Towel to drape the patient.
- Eye protection for the patient with small goggles or moist gauze.
- For crystal MDA devices, the operator should use clear goggles for eye protection and a mask to reduce particle inhalation.
- Gauze, 4 × 4 inches
- Physical sunscreen (with zinc or titanium) and a soothing moisturizer for postprocedure application.
- Saline eyewash.

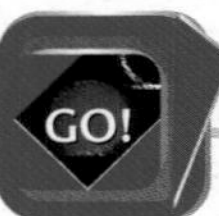

Aesthetic Indications

- Hyperpigmentation
- Rough texture, enlarged pores
- Superficial acne scarring
- Comedonal acne
- Papulopustular acne
- Rosacea and telangiectasias
- Fine wrinkles
- Keratosis pilaris
- Enhanced penetration of topical products

Improvements in papulopustular acne, rosacea, and telangiectasias have been demonstrated with certain MDA devices such as the SilkPeel (diamond-tipped with dermal infusion).

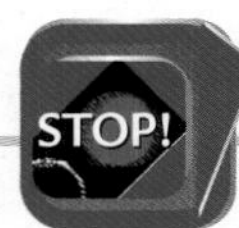

Contraindications

Absolute

- Pregnancy
- Active infection in the treatment area (e.g., herpes simplex and verrucae)
- Melanoma or lesions suspected of malignancy
- Isotretinoin (Accutane) use in the past year
- Dermatoses (e.g., eczema and psoriasis)
- Autoimmune disease
- Sunburn

Relative

- Rosacea and telangiectasias (not recommended with crystal MDA)
- Papulopustular acne (not recommended with crystal MDA)
- Very thin skin or excessive laxity and skin folds
- Anticoagulant therapy
- Unrealistic expectations

The Procedure

The following procedure is for treatments performed with SilkPeel, a crystal-free MDA that uses diamond-tipped pads as the abrasive element and has simultaneous dermal infusion of topical solutions (see Figure 2). Comparisons and recommendations for crystal MDA devices are also included when possible.

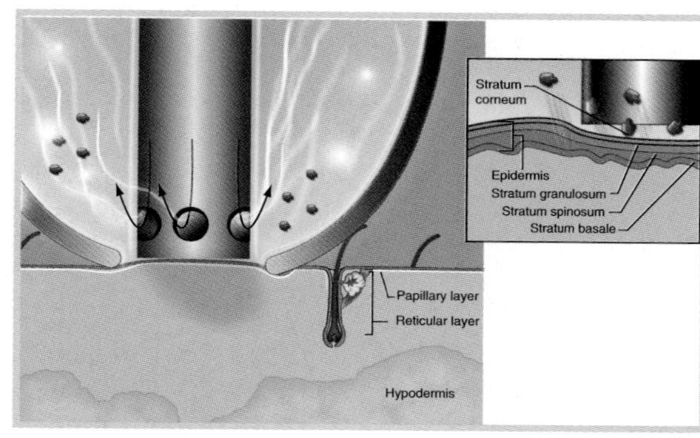

Courtesy of emed.

Figure 2

Results of MDA treatment for papulopustular acne are shown before (Figure 3A) and after 6 treatments (Figure 3B) performed 2 weeks apart. The topical solution used for dermal infusion included 2% salicylic acid.

- PITFALL: Treatment of papulopustular acne and rosacea are contraindicated with crystal MDA devices.

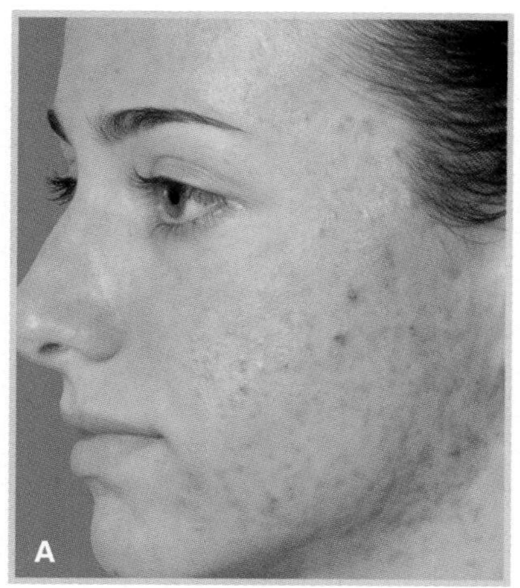

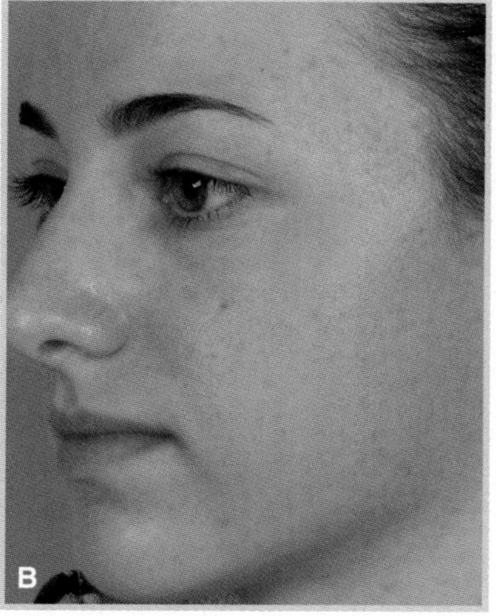

Courtesy of emed.

Figure 3

Results of MDA treatment for hyperpigmentation are shown before (Figure 4A) and after 6 treatments (Figure 4B) performed 2 weeks apart. The topical product used for dermal infusion included hydroquinone, kojic acid, and arbutin.

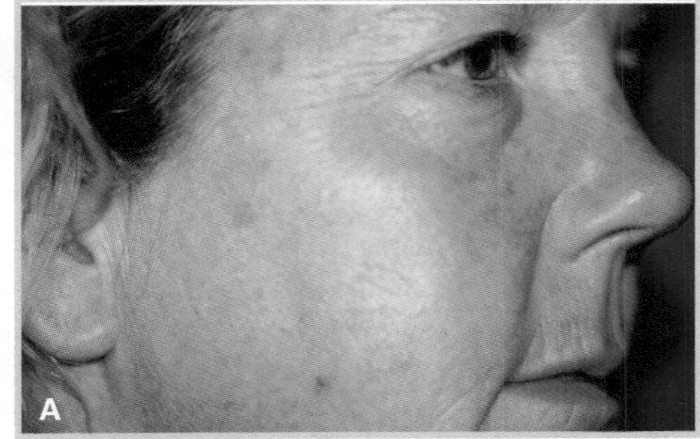

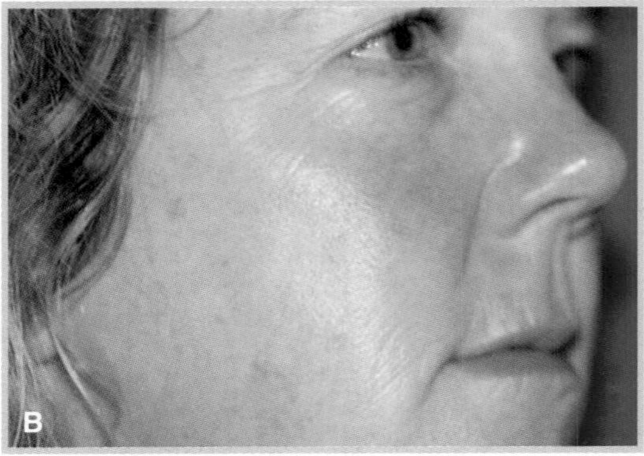

Courtesy of *e*med.

Figure 4

Results of MDA treatment for papulopustular rosacea are shown before (Figure 5A) and after 6 treatments (Figure 5B) performed 2 weeks apart. The topical solution used for dermal infusion was 2% erythromycin and 2% salicylic acid.

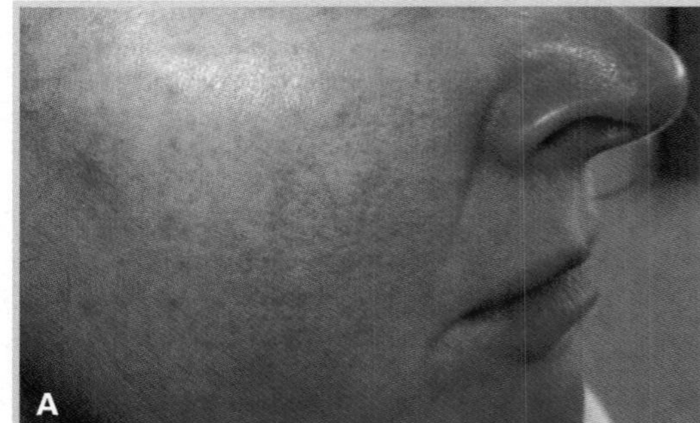

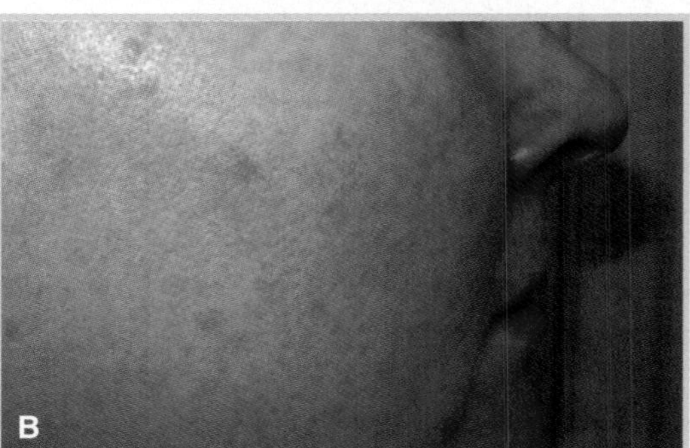

Courtesy of Tejas Desai, MD

Figure 5

Step 1. Perform a detailed skin evaluation prior to initiating treatment (see Skin Analysis Form in Step 1). Fitzpatrick skin type classification is used to describe background skin pigmentation and the skin's response to sun exposure (see Chapter 31 for

SKIN ANALYSIS FORM

Name: ______________________________ DOB: __________________
Last First

Fitzpatrick Skin Type Classification (check one):

_____	Skin Type I	White	Sun exposure reaction always burns, peels, never tans
_____	Skin Type II	White	Usually burns, tans with difficulty
_____	Skin Type III	White	Sometimes mild burn, tans average
_____	Skin Type IV	Moderately brown	Rarely burns, tans easily
_____	Skin Type V	Dark brown	Very rarely burns, tans very easily
_____	Skin Type VI	Black	Never burns, tans very easily

Glogau's Photoaging Classification (check one):

_____	Group I	Mild (28-35 years old)	No keratoses, little wrinkling, no scarring, little or no makeup
_____	Group II	Moderate (35-50 years old)	Early actinic keratoses, slight skin discoloration, early wrinkling, parallel smile lines, mild scarring, little makeup
_____	Group III	Advanced (50-65 years old)	Actinic keratoses, obvious skin discoloration, telangiectasiaa, wrinkling, moderate acne scarring, wears makeup always
_____	Group IV	Severe (65-75 years old)	Actinic keratoses, possible skin cancers, wrinkling, gravitational aging, severe acne scarring, wears makeup thickly

Skin Type

_____ Dry _____ Oily _____ Combination

Pre-Procedure Evalution

Key

LP – Large Pores	D – Dryness	O – Oiliness	M – Milia	C – Comedones
T – Telangectasia	R – Imitation	SC – Scarring	P – Pigmentation	W – Wrinkles

Place abbreviations on facial zones in diagram to note areas of specific conditions and concerns

Zone I _______
Zone II _______
Zone III _______
Zone IV _______
Zone V _______
Zone VI _______
Zone VII _______
Zone Viii _______
Zone IX _______
Zone X _______
Zone XI _______

Other: ____________________

Photo Taken: Yes No

Treatment Plan: ____

Date:__________ Signature:______________________________

Step 1

additional information), which is integral to determining how aggressive treatments may be. The Glogau classification is a baseline measure of a patient's degree of photo damage.

MDA may be performed as a very superficial or superficial skin-resurfacing procedure (see Figure 6 for definitions of skin resurfacing terminology). Depths listed in the figure are from the skin surface down to the layer indicated. The depth of exfoliation with MDA increases with increasing vacuum pressure, number of passes, and a more acute hand piece handle. For diamond-tipped devices, the depth of exfoliation also increases with grit coarseness. Downward pressure on the skin may increase the depth of exfoliation with some diamond-tipped devices. The SilkPeel hand piece has a recessed diamond-tipped pad, and downward pressure on the skin does increase exfoliation depth. For crystal devices, the depth of exfoliation also increases by moving the hand piece more slowly over the skin, using larger particle sizes and higher crystal flow rates.

- **PEARL:** Two passes with the SilkPeel using a 60-grit treatment head and vacuum setting of 5 psi (260 mm Hg) penetrates to 30 to 35 μm and will fully remove the stratum corneum.
- **PEARL:** Two passes with most aluminum-oxide crystal MDAs using a vacuum setting of 4 psi (200 mm Hg) will fully remove the stratum corneum.
- **PITFALL:** Greater depths of penetration have greater potential for improvements but are also associated with greater complication risks. Once the dermis is breached, which is typically evident as bleeding, scarring becomes a consideration.

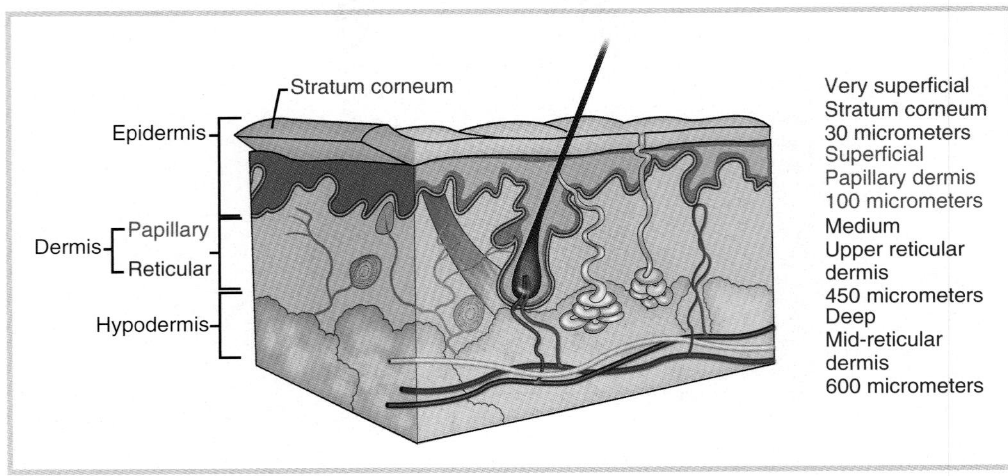

Figure 6

Step 2. Position the patient comfortably, lying supine on the treatment table. Have the patient remove contact lenses, and apply a headband. Cleanse the treatment area with a gentle cleanser and degrease the skin using an alcohol-based astringent. Ensure that the skin is completely dry prior to treatment. Cover the patient's eyes with goggles or moist gauze. For crystal MDA devices, the operator should wear clear eye protection and a mask to reduce particle inhalation.

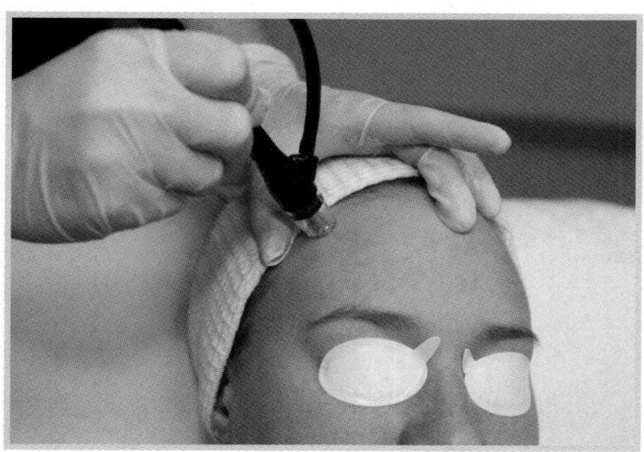

Step 2

Step 3. Select the size and coarseness of the diamond-tipped treatment head (see Step 3). The 6-mm head should be used for the face and the 9-mm head for larger areas, such as the back. Selection of the grit size is based on the aggressiveness of the treatment. The heads range in coarseness from smooth with no diamond chips, fine (120 grit) to coarse (30 grit).

- **PEARL:** With the SilkPeel, most treatments can be performed with the 100-grit head. Hyperkeratotic areas such as elbows and knees respond well to a coarser, 60-grit head. The lips can be treated with the smooth head.
- **PITFALL:** Treatment of the lips is contraindicated with crystal MDA.

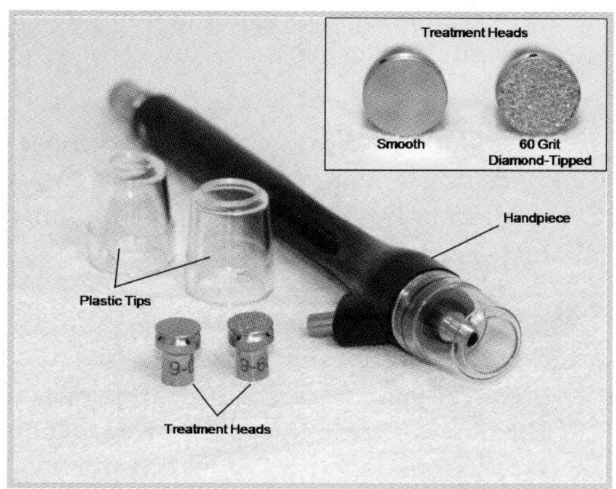

Step 3

Step 4. Set the vacuum flow by occluding the handpiece tip with a gloved finger, as shown in Step 4. The strength of the vacuum affects the depth of resurfacing, and small adjustments in this parameter can fine-tune the intensity of a treatment. Recommended vacuum settings vary by manufacturer. In general, conservative settings should be selected for initial treatments based on the patient's Fitzpatrick skin type, tolerance, and treatment area using the manufacturer's guidelines.

- **PEARL:** The SilkPeel vacuum should be set at 3.5 to 4 psi (180 to 200 mm Hg) for treatment on the face and chest, 2.8 to 3 psi (145 to 155 mm Hg) for the neck, and 5 to 6 psi (260 to 310 mm Hg) for the hands and back. For crystal MDA devices, initial treatment vacuum settings range from 50 to 200 mm Hg and are device dependent.
- **PEARL:** Patients with higher Fitzpatrick skin types are more prone to prolonged postinflammatory erythema PIH, and the lower limits of the range for vacuum settings should be used.
- **PITFALL:** Devices utilizing simultaneous dermal infusion are associated with less discomfort. Patients may experience superficial abrasions without reporting pain

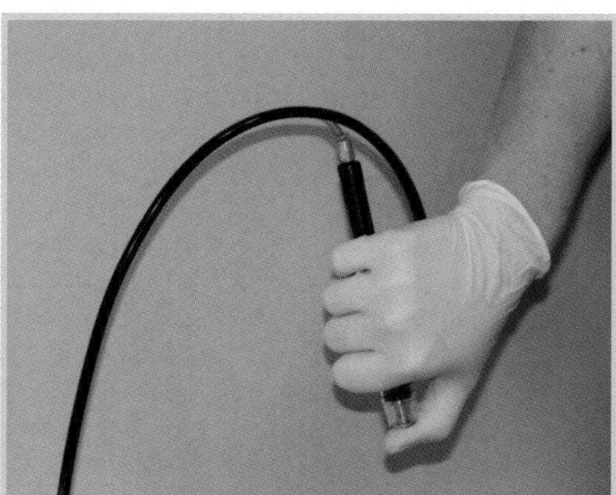

Step 4

during treatment, and patient feedback may be a less reliable indicator of treatment intensity. Observation of tissue response is therefore particularly important in determining vacuum settings with dermal infusion devices.

Step 5. For dermal infusion devices, select a topical solution for dermal infusion based on the presenting condition. Commonly used products include hydroquinone or other botanical lightening agents such as kojic acid and arbutin for treatment of hyperpigmentation; erythromycin and salicylic acid for acne and rosacea; and hyaluronic acid, allantoin, and glycerin for dehydration. Select a solution flow rate for dermal infusion using the manufacturers guidelines.

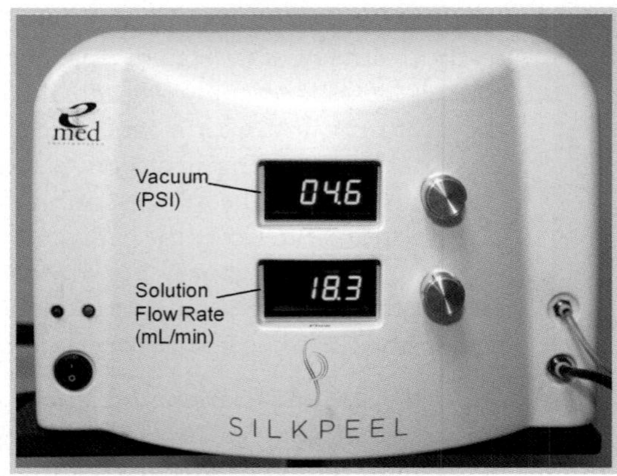

Step 5

- **PEARL:** Two topical solutions may be used during a treatment, for example, to address dehydration and hyperpigmentation.
- **PEARL:** Typical SilkPeel dermal infusion rates range from 15 to 20 mL/min (see Step 5).

Step 6. Move the hand piece smoothly and slowly across the skin as shown in Step 6 for treatment of the face. Exfoliation with the SilkPeel will not occur unless the tip is moving across the skin. For the first pass, strokes should be from the central face to the periphery. The procedure usually starts at the forehead, proceeds down the bridge of the nose, and then covers the cheeks, chin, and mouth. Stretch the skin between the fingers, place the hand piece perpendicular to and in good contact with the skin, and move the hand piece across the skin parallel to the tension line between the fingers. Observe skin for the desired clinical endpoint of mild erythema. Reassess tissue response and patient tolerance throughout the treatment and adjust settings accordingly. After completion of the first pass for the entire face, make a second pass following the same stroke pattern as the first pass. The second pass for crystal MDA is usually perpendicular to the first pass. For treatment of the neck, have the patient lift the chin to extend the neck, use vertical strokes, and perform only one pass. For treatment of the chest, perform two passes with strokes from the midline to the periphery. For treatment of the hands, have the patient make a fist around a towel and perform two passes with strokes parallel and then perpendicular to the axis of the forearm.

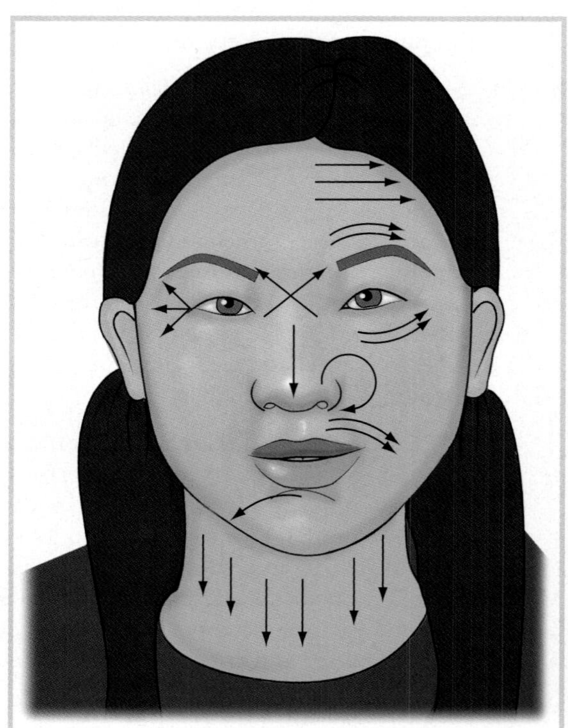

Step 6

- **PITFALL:** Petechiae or pinpoint hemorrhages indicate that the settings are too intense and must be reduced.

TABLE 33-1.

	Thickness (Micrometers)			
Area	**Epidermis**	**Dermis**	**Subcutaneous**	**Total**
Forehead	202	969	1,210	2,381
Upper lip	156	1,061	931	2,143
Chin	149	1,375	1,020	2,544
Cheek	141	909	459	1,509
Eyelids	130	215	248	593
Neck	115	138	544	1,697
Lower lip	113	973	829	1,915
Nose	111	918	735	1,764

- **PEARL:** Reduce treatment intensity near thinned skinned areas such as the periorbital area. With the SilkPeel, reduce the vacuum pressure to 2.8 to 3 psi (145 to 155 mm Hg).
- **PITFALL:** With crystal MDA, do not leave the hand piece in one spot because this will increase abrasion depth and may cause injury to the skin.

Step 7. At subsequent visits, parameters may be increased to intensify treatments. In general, only one parameter should be changed to intensify treatments in any given visit. Typically, the number of passes is increased for a few treatments to achieve the desired clinical endpoints, and vacuum settings are increased in the later treatments. A total of two to four passes may be made on thicker skinned areas (see Table 33.1 for skin thickness in different facial areas) such as the forehead, upper lip, and chin or problematic areas, taking into account tissue response and patient tolerance. Grit coarseness may also be increased at subsequent visits to intensify treatments.

- **PEARL:** Acne scars require more aggressive treatments. With the SilkPeel, a 100-grit head with 6 psi and up to four passes crosshatched over the area may be performed.

Step 8. Apply a soothing topical product and a full-spectrum sunscreen with SPF 30 or greater (containing zinc or titanium).

- **PEARL:** If using a crystal MDA, remove all crystal debris from the face with moist gauze prior to product application, paying close attention to the periorbital area.

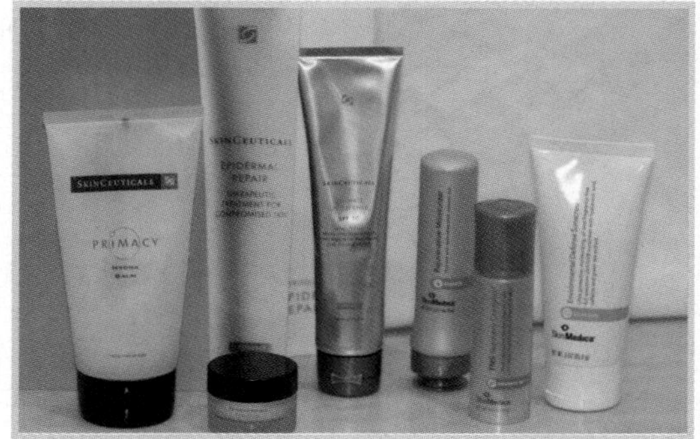

Step 8

Step 9. Sanitize and sterilize reusable equipment parts between patient treatments per the manufacturer guidelines. Step 9 shows the waste container after treatment with skin surface debris and used dermal infusion solution for disposal. After the patient's treatment is completed, the dermal infusion bottle is replaced with a disinfectant solution that is circulated to sanitize the machine prior to the next patient. The diamond-tipped heads are autoclaved after each treatment for sterilization.

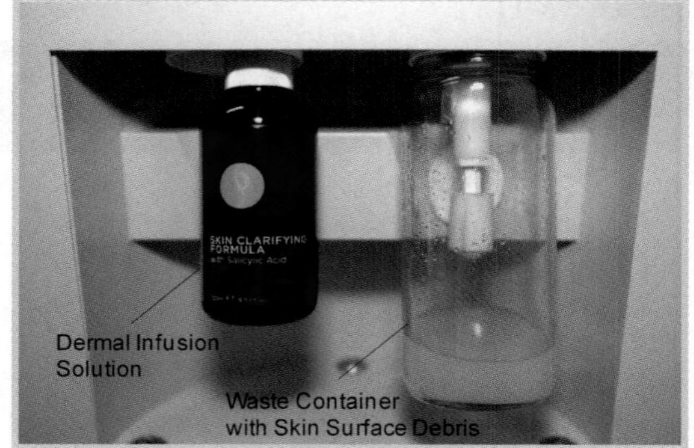

Step 9

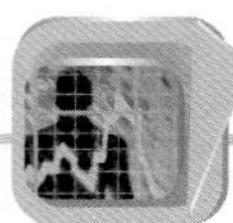

Complications

- Superficial abrasion
- Activation of herpes simplex
- Pain or temporary discomfort
- Prolonged irritation and/or erythema
- Postinflammatory hyperpigmentation (increased risk with high Fitzpatrick skin types)
- Petechiae or purpura
- Ocular injury
- Urticaria (with crystal MDA)
- Remote possibility of scarring

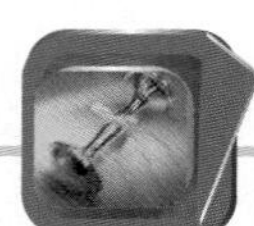

Pediatric Considerations

MDA may be performed for adolescents with parental consent but is otherwise contraindicated for pediatric patients.

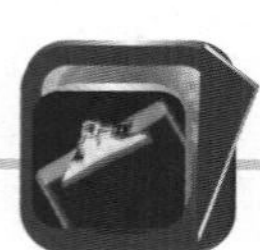

Postprocedure Instructions

Patients typically experience mild erythema and dryness for 1 to 2 days posttreatment with crystal MDA but may not experience these aftereffects with MDA utilizing dermal infusion. A nonocclusive soothing moisturizer may be applied frequently as needed for dryness. The patient should avoid irritating topical products such as retinoids, astringents, glycolic acid, and depilatories and not undergo waxing, dermal filler injections, or laser or IPL treatments for 1 week. The patient should also avoid direct sun exposure for 1 week and use a daily full spectrum sunscreen with SPF 30 or greater (containing zinc or titanium). If scabbing occurs, advise patients to avoid picking, because this may result in scarring, and apply bacitracin daily until healed.

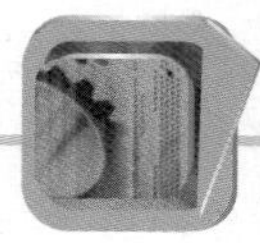

Coding Information and Supply Sources

MDA is not reimbursable by insurance. The charges for treatments vary widely and are largely determined by local prices. Patients may pay for individual treatments, which generally range from $100 to $150. However, because MDA is most effective as a series of treatments, packages of treatments (usually six) may be offered so that patients achieve the best possible results and have the greatest satisfaction.

ICD-9 Codes

Acne vulgaris	706.1
Melasma	709.09
Dyschromia, unspecified	709.0
Wrinkling of skin	701.8
Scarring	709.2

Supply Sources

Microdermabrasion Devices

- Aesthetic Technologies/Parisian Peel (crystal MDA and diamond-tipped MDA), EC-34, Sector I, Salt Lake City, Kolkata 700 064, India. Phone: 408-464-8893. Web site: http://www.mmizone.com/public/web/default.htm.
- Cosmetic R & D (dermal infusion and other abrasives), 4125 Pine Crest Court, Rocklin, CA 95677. Phone: 916-632-9134. Web site: http://dermasweep.com/.
- Edge Systems (crystal MDA and diamond-tipped MDA), 2277 Redondo Avenue, Signal Hill, CA 90755. Phone: 1-800-603-4996. Web site: http://www.edgesystem.net/microdermabrasion.htm.
- *e*med (dermal infusion and diamond-tipped MDA), 31340 Via Colinas, Suite 101, Westlake Village, CA 91362. Phone: 1-888-848-3633. Web site: www.silkpeel.com.
- DermaMed International (crystal MDA), 394 Parkmount Road, P. O. Box 198, Lenni, PA 19052. Phone: 1-888-789-6342. Web site: http://www.megapeel.com/.
- Lumenis (crystal MDA), 5302 Betsy Ross Drive, Santa Clara, CA 95054. Phone: 408-764-3000. Web site: http://www.lumenis.com/wt/home/home/?flash=true.
- Mattioli Engineering (crystal MDA), 7918 Jones Branch Drive, Suite 600, McLean, VA 22102. Phone: 703-312-6000, 877-MATTENG. Web site: http://www.matteng.com/pepita.html.
- Med-Aesthetic Solutions (crystal MDA and ultrasonic MDA), 2033 San Elijo Ave., Suite 200, Cardiff-by-the-Sea, CA 92007. Phone: 760-942-8815. Web site: http://medaestheticsolutions.com/content/view/7/33/.
- RAJA Medical (dermal infusion and other abrasive), 801 South Olive Avenue, Suite 124, West Palm Beach, FL 33401. Phone: 877-880-4184. Web site: http://rajamedical.com/.
- Refine USA (dermal infusion, diamond-tipped MDA, and ultrasonic MDA), 13500 Sutton Park Drive South, Suite 701, Jacksonville, FL 32224. Phone: 866-491-7546. Web site: http://refineusa.com/micro-gem.html.
- Sybaritic (dermal infusion and ultrasonic MDA), 9220 James Avenue South, Bloomington, MN 55431. Phone: 1-800-445-8418. Web site: http://www.sybaritic.com/.
- Syneron (crystal MDA and diamond-tipped MDA), 28 Fulton Way, Unit 8, Richmond Hill, ON L4B 1L5, Canada. Phone: 905-886-9235, 866-259-6661. Web site: http://www.syneron.com/

Patient Education Handout

A patient education handout, "Microdermabrasion Treatments," can be found on the book's companion Web site.

Bibliography

Alam M, Omura N, Dover JS, et al. Glycolic acid peels compared to microdermabrasion: a right-left controlled trial of efficacy and patient satisfaction. *Derm Surg.* 2000;28:475–479.

Bhalla M, Thami GP. Microdermabrasion: reappraisal and brief review of literature. Derm Surg. 2006;32(6):809–814.

Coimbra M, et al. A prospective controlled assessment of microdermabrasion for damaged skin and fine rhytids. *Plast Reconstr Surg.* 2004;113:1438–1443.
Freedman BM, Rueda-Pedraza E, Waddell SP. The epidermal and dermal changes associated with microdermabrasion. *Derm Surg.* 2001;27(12):1031–1034.
Freeman MS. Microdermabrasion. *Facial Plast Surg Clin North Am.* 2001;9(2):257–266.
Grimes P. Microdermabrasion. *Derm Surg.* 2005;31(9):1160–1165.
Hernandez-Perez E, Ibiett EV. Gross and microscopic findings in patients undergoing microdermabrasion for facial rejuvenation. *Derm Surg.* 2001;27(7):637–640.
Karimipour DJ, et al. Microdermabrasion with and without aluminum oxide crystal abrasion: a comparative molecular analysis of dermal remodeling. *J Am Acad Derm.* 2006;54(3):405–410.
Koch RJ, Hanasomo M. Microdermabrasion. *Facial Plast Surg Clin N Am.* 2001;9(3):377–381.
Moy LS, Maley C. Skin management: a practical approach. *Plas Surg Prod.* 2007;Jan:24–28.
Rajan P, Grimes P. Skin barrier changes induced by AL_2O_3 and NaCl microdermabrasion. *Derm Surg.* 2002;28(5):390–393.
Rubin MG, Greenbaum SS. Histologic effects of aluminum oxide microdermabrasion on facial skin. *J Aesth Derm Cosmetic Surg.* 2000;1:237.
Sadick N. A review of microdermabrasion. *Cosm Derm.* 2005;18:351–354.
Spencer JM, Kurtz ES. Approaches to document the efficacy and safety of microdermabrasion procedure. *Derm Surg.* 2006;32(11):1353–1357.
Tejas DD, Moy LS, et al. Evaluation of the SilkPeel system in treating erythematotelangectatic and papulopustular rosacea. *Cosm Derm.* 2006;19(1):51–57.
2008 MAG Mutual Healthcare Solutions, Inc.'s Physicians' Fee and Coding Guide. Duluth, Georgia. MAG Mutual Healthcare Solutions, Inc. 2007.

CHAPTER 34

Radiosurgical Skin Surgery (LEEP)

E. J. Mayeaux Jr., MD, DABFP, FAAFP
Professor of Family Medicine,
Professor of Obstetrics and Gynecology
Louisiana State University Health Sciences Center, Shreveport, LA

Radiosurgery uses high-frequency current in a variety of dermatologic applications. The alternating current output ranges between 100 and 4,000 KHz. At frequencies >100 KHz, cellular membrane depolarization does not occur, so there is no associated shock or muscular contraction. The high-frequency currents operate in the realm of AM radio signals (hence, the name *radiosurgery*). Radiosurgery is used in cosmetic surgery procedures because the high-frequency currents permit smooth cutting through tissue without dissipating heat into surrounding tissues, thereby limiting injury and scarring. Cutting with a high-frequency radiosurgery unit does not involve heat. In fact, the waveforms must be modified to produce heat in the coagulation modes.

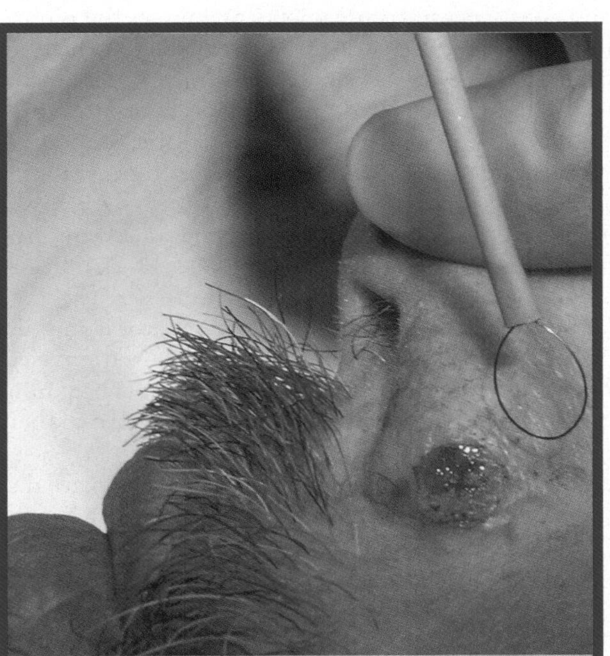

Ablation or thermal tissue destruction also is possible with radiosurgery units. By changing the radiosurgical waveforms, additional heat can be created to increase tissue destruction. Older electrosurgery units were limited to ablative currents because of their lower current frequencies (e.g., Hyfrecator, ConMed Corporation, Utica, NY). Spark-gap or tissue fulgurating procedures are not considered cosmetic, but they are effective in destroying warts or other growths in non-cosmetically important body areas. A small, metal ball electrode can be used for ablation of superficial skin lesions. Flat electrodes are used for matricectomy destruction during surgery for ingrown toenail (see Chapter 63, Ingrown Nail Avulsion and Matrix Ablation). Ablation of unwanted veins and telangiectasias can be performed with fine wires inserted into the veins.

A major application for dermal radiosurgery is the feathering of wound edges after shave excision of lesions (see Chapter 57, Shave Excision). After a lesion has been removed by the shave technique, a scooped-out skin defect usually exists. If this defect is allowed to heal without alteration, a circular, depressed scar may result. The shadow produced by the edges of the depression creates an inferior cosmetic result and draws the attention of an observer's eye. The final cosmetic outcome can be improved by smoothing or feathering the wound edges. Feathering blends the final light color of the scar into the surrounding skin and eliminates any sharp wound edges that can cast shadows on vertical skin surfaces.

Feathering is performed using only a high-frequency cutting current. The technique uses superficial passes of an electrosurgical wire loop over the skin surface. The technique can be used to smooth any irregularity to the skin surface. Because the technique is designed to affect only the skin surface, scarring that results from deeper dermal injury is prevented.

Most generators allow switching between cutting and coagulation modes and can blend a cutting effect with a coagulation effect. These blend modes permit concomitant coagulation hemostasis and surgical excision of tissues. Blend modes represent a greater proportion of coagulation effect that minimizes bleeding but increases thermal damage, and so they are usually not used in skin surgery.

The electrosurgical generator is activated by a foot pedal switch or hand piece with two separate buttons or a bimodal button midshaft. The hand piece handles like a pencil, and the electrodes insert into the distal end. Many, but not all, of the generators can use interchangeable hand pieces and electrodes. Some electrosurgical generators feature a standby mode, which allows for adjustments but does not allow activation until switched to the active mode.

Return (patient) electrodes may be adhesive gel pads or a solid "antenna" and may be either disposable or reusable. They should be applied near the operative site or held in the patient's hands. The wire should be connected to the generator and the circuit tested before the procedure to ensure that the system is functioning correctly. Poor contact between the dispersive pad and the patient may result in a thermal burn at that site.

A smoke evacuator is essential to remove the "plume" produced during the procedure. It filters airborne particles and coexisting microorganisms present in the plume. The operator usually must activate the smoke evacuator prior to turning on the electrosurgical unit. Some manufacturers have combined an electrosurgical unit with a smoke evacuator so that when the generator is activated, the smoke evacuator is automatically activated also. This minimizes plume spillage into the treatment room. A series of microfilters helps remove the carbon, smell, and viral particles generated.

Some radiofrequency units incorporate return electrode monitoring (REM), an excellent safety feature. If the electrical circuit is interrupted during the procedure, unit operation will be inhibited. A warning light and/or an audible tone warns the clinician, for instance, that the patient reference pad has come loose or has not been attached. Isolated circuitry units automatically deactivate the electrosurgical generator if any current that is transmitted to the active electrode is not returned through the patient electrode. Generators with isolated circuitry or return electrode monitoring units help minimize electrical accidents. Most of these special safety features are worth their additional cost.

Electrosurgical units require minimal care. They should be wiped regularly with disinfectants, particularly the dials and switches. Disposable hand pieces, dispersive pads, and tips may be purchased in bulk from various manufacturers, although it is not always possible to use these items on all machines. Disposable hand pieces, dispersive electrode pads, ball electrodes, and loop electrodes minimize the possibility of patient cross contamination. These materials are discarded after each use. Reusable electrodes must be cleaned and disinfected. Debris on ball electrodes may be removed with a scrub pad, followed by a disinfectant soak or gas sterilization. Activation of the electrode for 5 to 10 seconds at a moderate energy level sterilizes the loop but not the insulated baseplate or shaft. Some hand pieces can be sterilized with gas but should not be immersed in a disinfectant solution. The manufacturer's recommendation should always be followed. Smoke evacuation filters should be replaced at intervals in accordance with the manufacturer's recommendations. Grossly contaminated small tubing should be discarded immediately after the procedure.

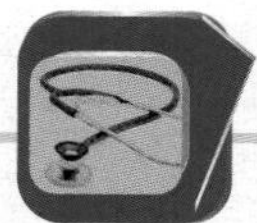

Equipment

- Skin preparation materials are listed in Appendix E: Skin Preparation Recommendations
- Anesthesia supplies may be found in Appendix F: Suggested Anesthesia Tray for Administration of Local Anesthesia and Blocks

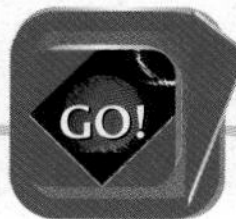

Indications

- Shave or ablation of skin lesions
- Ablation of telangiectasias
- Hemostasis in wounds
- Excision of skin lesions
- Creation of skin flaps to close skin defects
- Rhinophyma planing
- Removal of eyelid lesions
- Matrixectomy for ingrown nails
- Feathering of shave excision sites
- Feathering of skin surface irregularities

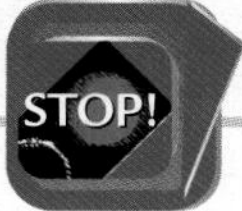

Contraindications

- Application of radiosurgery for treatment of a lesion directly over or near a pacemaker
- Patients in direct contact with metal instruments or metal tables or examination tables
- Ungrounded patients
- Improperly functioning equipment

The Procedure

Step 1. Administer local anesthesia for most excisional, destructive, or feathering radiosurgical procedures. The smoke evacuator tubing should be positioned next to the skin lesion site.

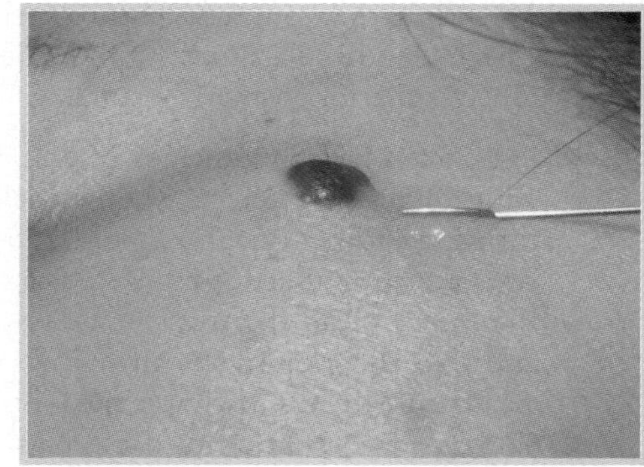

Step 1

Step 2. An electrosurgical shave is similar to cold steel shave excisions (see Chapter 57, Shave Excision) except that the skin lesion may be removed in layers if a pathologic specimen is not needed. When using a dermal loop to remove an elevated or pedunculated lesion, it can be grasped and elevated using Adson forceps. First place the loop over the lesion.

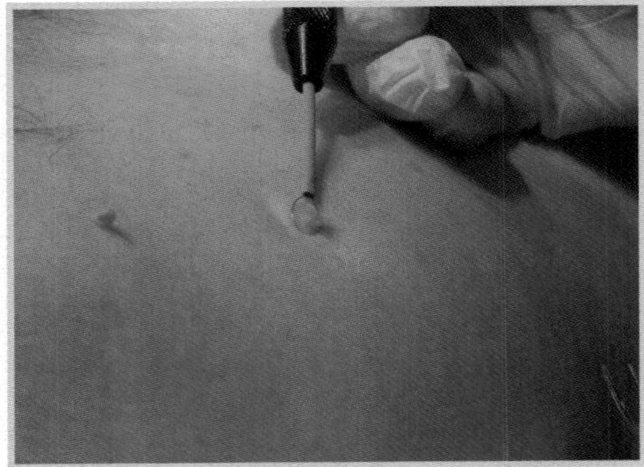

Step 2

Step 3. Elevate the lesion upward through the loop, activate the electrode, and move the electrode horizontally to free the lesion from the underlying tissue. Use a blended (i.e., cutting and coagulation) or pure cutting current for the excision.

- **PITFALL:** With greater upward pull on a lesion, the loop electrode passes deeper in the dermis, and greater scarring results. To avoid excessive upward pull, many physicians shave off lesions without using forceps to elevate the lesion.
- **PITFALL:** Do not use nondermal loop electrodes for excision of skin lesions. Use of larger loop electrodes, such as cervical loops, produces larger defects. Use small, short-shafted dermal loops for better control of the depth of excision and feathering.

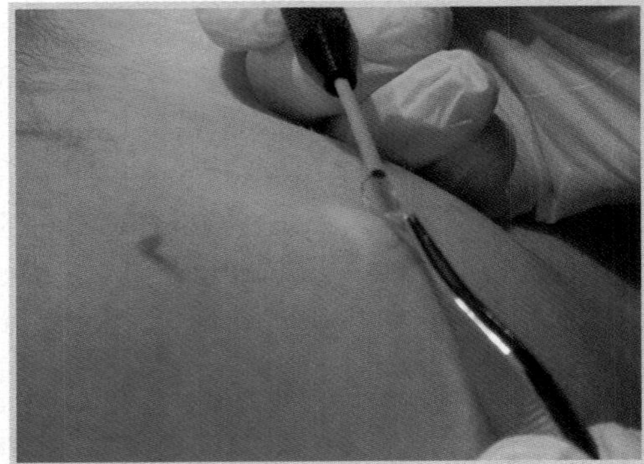

Step 3

Step 4. When shaving flatter lesions, a small loop or slightly bent fine wire can be passed back and forth, slowly shaving down the dermis until the lesion is completely removed and normal dermis exposed.

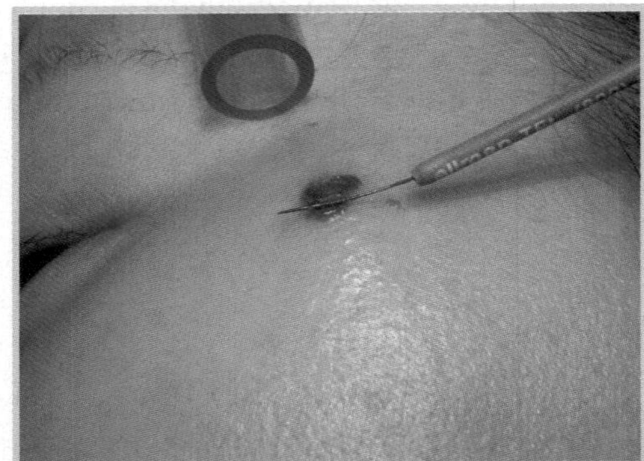

Step 4

Step 5. After a shave excision, a circular, crater-like defect often exists. To perform feathering, the machine setting is set to cutting current only, and the power setting is lowered. Stretch the skin surrounding the treatment site using the fingers on the nondominant hand. Pass the loop over the skin surface with short, back-and-forth motions, eliminating sharp edges and blending the wound edges into surrounding skin. The final wound is smoothed and produces superior cosmetic results.

- **PITFALL:** Novice physicians often produce additional scoop defects when initially performing radiosurgical feathering. To prevent additional scooping defects, stretch the skin around the treatment site tightly, and pass the loop in the air just above the treatment site. Gently lower the loop to the skin surface, and do not drag the loop on the surface during feathering to avoid additional defects and deeper scars.

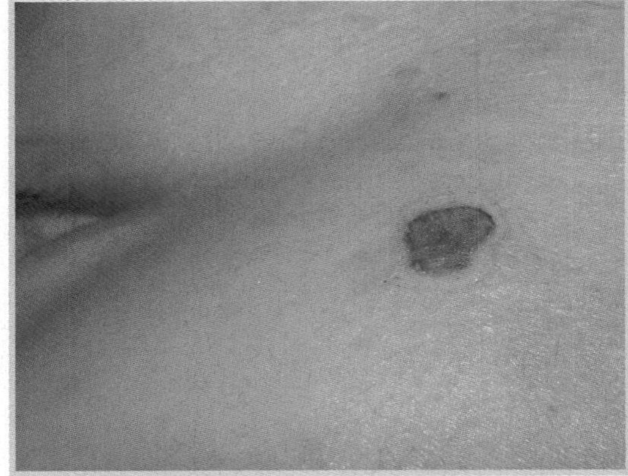

Step 5

Step 6. Perform coagulation (A) ablation of superficial skin lesions or bleeding spots after a shave using coagulation current with a power setting of 3 to 4.5 (30 to 45 W). Hold the ball or needle electrode directly onto the tissue surface to produce a burn (i.e., thermal injury). Fulguration (B) produces an eschar (i.e., dry, burn scab) that limits the depth of thermal injury. To fulgurate, hold the electrode just above the tissue surface, and a spark will travel from the electrode tip to the surface of the skin. The electrode can be gently "bounced" on the skin surface to facilitate this spark-gap or fulguration technique.

- PITFALL: The higher the current setting, the greater the heat applied to the target tissue. Use lower current settings to avoid excessive tissue burns and scarring.

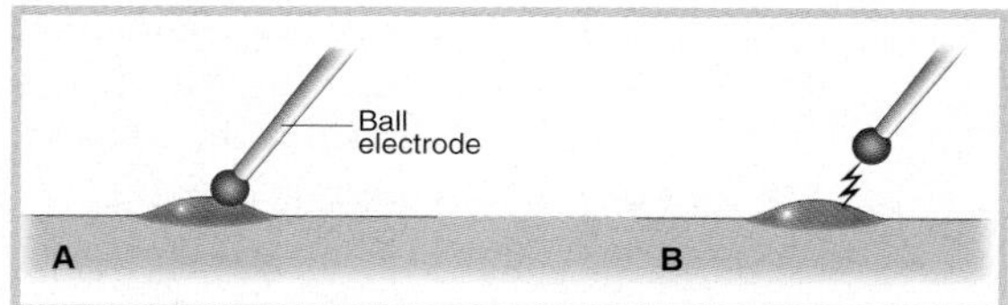

Step 6

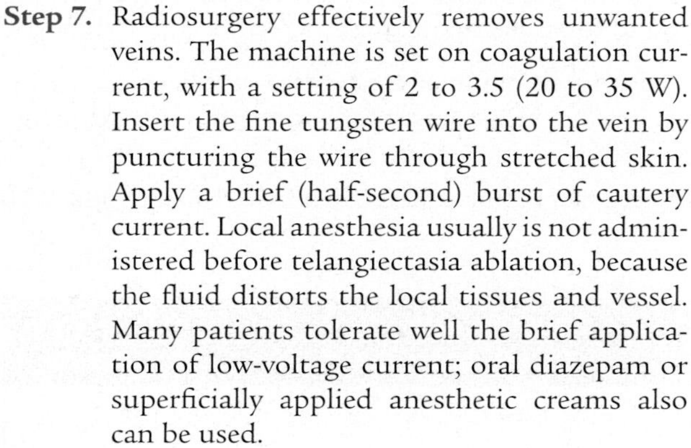

Step 7. Radiosurgery effectively removes unwanted veins. The machine is set on coagulation current, with a setting of 2 to 3.5 (20 to 35 W). Insert the fine tungsten wire into the vein by puncturing the wire through stretched skin. Apply a brief (half-second) burst of cautery current. Local anesthesia usually is not administered before telangiectasia ablation, because the fluid distorts the local tissues and vessel. Many patients tolerate well the brief application of low-voltage current; oral diazepam or superficially applied anesthetic creams also can be used.

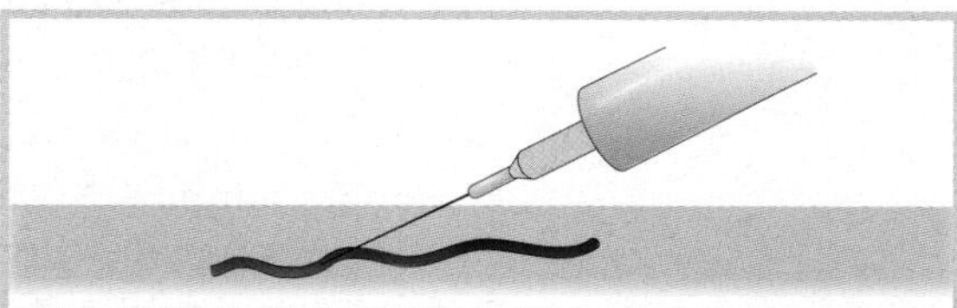

Step 7

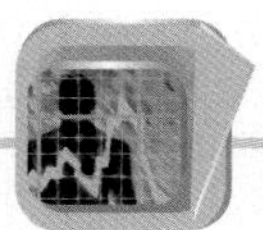

Complications

- Bleeding
- Infection
- Scar formation
- Creating airborne particles and microorganisms
- Unintentional burns

Because radiofrequency treatments have occasionally caused reprogramming of pacemakers, the return electrode should be placed so that the current path does not cross the pacemaker, and pacemaker patients should be monitored after treatment.

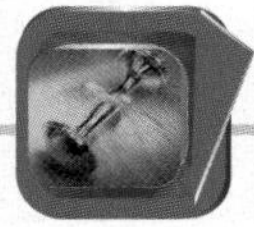

Pediatric Considerations

Generally, pediatric skin has excellent blood flow and heals very well. However, pediatric patients often find it difficult to sit and lie still during lengthy procedures. The patient's maturity and ability to cooperate should be considered before deciding to attempt any outpatient procedure. Sometimes it is necessary to sedate the patient to repair the laceration (see Chapter 122). The maximum recommended dose for lidocaine in children is 3 to 5 mg/kg, and 7 mg/kg when combined with epinephrine. Neonates have an increased volume of distribution, decreased hepatic clearance, and doubled terminal elimination half-life (3.2 hours).

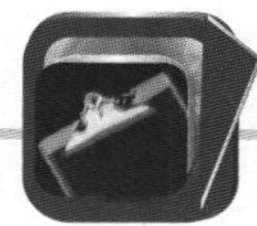

Postprocedure Instructions

Have them use a small amount of antibiotic ointment and cover the wound with a small bandage. Instruct the patient to gently wash an area after 1 day. Have the patient dry the area well after washing and use a small amount of antibiotic ointment to promote moist healing. Instruct the patient not to pick at or scratch the wound.

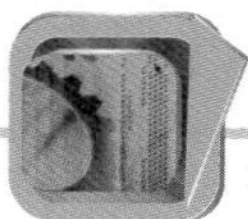

Coding Information and Supply Sources

The CPT codes for shave excision (11300 to 11313) are applied (see Chapter 11). There is no additional reimbursement provided for feathering. The main reasons for performing feathering are the superior cosmetic and functional outcomes.

- LEEP units and associated materials may be obtained from these suppliers:
  - Cooper Surgical, Shelton, CT. Phone: 1-800-645-3760, 203-929-6321. Web site: http://www.coopersurgical.com.
  - Ellman International, Inc., Hewlett, NY. Phone: 1-800-835 5355, 516-569-1482. Web site: http://www.ellman.com.

CPT Code	Description	2008 Average 50th Percentile Fee	Global Period
11300	Trunk, arm, or leg lesion <0.6 cm	$112.00	0
11301	Trunk, arm, or leg lesion 0.6–1.0 cm	$149.00	0
11302	Trunk, arm, or leg lesion 1.1–2.0 cm	$185.00	0
11303	Trunk, arm, or leg lesion >2.0 cm	$224.00	0
11305	Scalp, neck, hands, feet, or genitalia lesion <0.6 cm	$114.00	0
11306	Scalp, neck, hands, feet, or genitalia lesion 0.6–1.0 cm	$161.00	0
11307	Scalp, neck, hands, feet, or genitalia lesion 1.1–2.0 cm	$198.00	0
11308	Scalp, neck, hands, feet, or genitalia lesion >2.0 cm	$228.00	0
11310	Face, ears, eyelids, nose, lips, or MM lesion <0.6 cm	$145.00	0
11311	Face, ears, eyelids, nose, lips, or MM lesion 0.6–1.0 cm	$190.00	0
11312	Face, ears, eyelids, nose, lips, or MM lesion 1.1–2.0 cm	$223.00	0
11313	Face, ears, eyelids, nose, lips, or MM lesion >2.0 cm	$281.00	0

CPT is a registered trademark of the American Medical Association. MM, Mucus membranes.
2008 average 50th Percentile Fees are provided courtesy of 2008 MMH-SI's copyrighted Physicians' Fees and Coding Guide.

- Hemostatic agents such as ferric subsulfate are available from surgical supply houses or the resources listed in Appendix G.
- A suggested anesthesia tray that can be used for this procedure is listed in Appendix F.
- Skin preparation recommendations appear in Appendix E.
- Radiosurgical generators; electrodes for dermatologic, gynecologic, plastic surgery, or ear, nose, and throat uses; smoke evacuators; and other accessories are available from these suppliers:
  - Ellman International, 1135 Railroad Avenue, Hewlett, NY 11557-2316. Phone: 1-800-835-2316. Web site: http://www.ellman.com.
  - Wallach Surgical Devices, 235 Edison Road, Orange, CT 06477. Phone: 203-799-2002. Web site: http://www.wallachsd.com. Cooper Surgical, Shelton, CT. Phone: 1-800-645-3760, 203-929-6321. Web site: http://www.coopersurgical.com
  - Olympus America, Inc., Melville, NY. Phone: 1-800-548-5515, 631-844-5000. Web site: http://www.olympusamerica.com
  - Utah Medical Products, Inc., Medvale, UT. Phone: 1-800-533-4984,801-566-1200. Web site: http://www.utahmed.com

Bibliography

Acland K, Calonje E, Seed PT, et al. A clinical and histologic comparison of electrosurgical and carbon dioxide laser peels. *J Am Acad Dermatol.* 2001;44:492–496.

Bader RS, Scarborough DA. Surgical pearl: intralesional electrodesiccation of sebaceous hyperplasia. *J Am Acad Dermatol.* 2000;42:127–128.

Bridenstine JB. Use of ultra-high-frequency electrosurgery (radiosurgery) for cosmetic surgical procedures [editorial]. *Dermatol Surg.* 1998;24:397–400.

Hainer BL. Electrosurgery for cutaneous lesions. *Am Fam Physician.* 1991;445(suppl):81S–90S.

Hainer BL. Fundamentals of electrosurgery. *J Am Board Fam Pract.* 1991;4:419–426.

Harris DR, Noodleman R. Using a low current radiosurgical unit to obliterate facial telangiectasias. *J Dermatol Surg Oncol.* 1991;17:382–384.

Hettinger DF, Valinsky MS, Nuccio G, et al. Nail matrixectomies using radio wave technique. *J Am Podiatr Med Assoc.* 1991;81:317–321.

Pollack SV. *Electrosurgery of the Skin.* New York: Churchill Livingstone; 1991.

Sebben JE. Electrodes for high-frequency electrosurgery. *J Dermatol Surg Oncol.* 1989;15:805–810.

Wright VC. Contemporary electrosurgery: physics for physicians [editorial]. *J Fam Pract.* 1994;39: 119–122.

Wyre HW, Stolar R. Extirpation of warts by a loop electrode and cutting current. *J Dermatol Surg Oncol.* 1977;3:520–522.

Zuber TJ. Dermal electrosurgical shave excision. *Am Fam Physician.* 2002;65:1883–1886, 1889–1890, 1895, 1899–1900.

Zuber TJ. *Office Procedures.* Baltimore: Williams & Wilkins; 1999.

2008 MAG Mutual Healthcare Solutions, Inc.'s Physicians' Fee and Coding Guide. Duluth, Georgia. MAG Mutual Healthcare Solutions, Inc. 2007.

CHAPTER 35

Sclerotherapy

Michael B. Harper, MD, DABFM
Professor of Clinical Family Medicine
Louisiana State University Health Sciences Center, Shreveport, LA

E. J. Mayeaux Jr., MD, DABFP, FAAFP
Professor of Family Medicine, Professor of Obstetrics and Gynecology
Louisiana State University Health Sciences Center, Shreveport, LA

Sclerotherapy is an inexpensive and generally safe outpatient technique for the removal of unwanted spider (telangiectatic), reticular, and varicose veins. A chemical solution or hypertonic saline is injected into the unwanted vessel using a small (30-gauge) needle. The solution causes an inflammatory reaction at the vessel's endothelial cells, producing obliteration of the vessel and shifting blood into nearby healthy vessels.

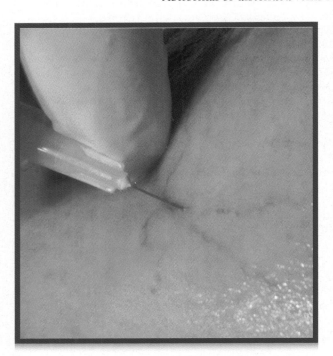

Abnormal or distended veins result from increased vascular pressure transmitted to the superficial vessels. Valves in the deep veins of the lower extremity are thin and fragile, and damage to these valves reduces the unidirectional flow of blood returning to the heart. Many conditions can render the valves nonfunctional, such as the increased blood flow of pregnancy, deep venous thrombosis, venous injury, and increased abdominal pressure (i.e., excessive sitting, leg crossing, or obesity). Other influences, such as hormonal changes in the veins or congenital absence of vein valves, can also produce varicosities.

If hypertonic saline is used as the sclerosing solution, lidocaine usually is mixed with the saline to lessen the discomfort. Two mL of 1% lidocaine hydrochloride (without epinephrine) is added to a 30-mL bottle of 23.4% hypertonic saline, creating a final concentration of 22%. This solution is then placed into 1-cc or 3-cc syringes, and 30-gauge needles are attached to the syringes.

Alternately, physicians may choose to perform sclerotherapy with detergent solutions such as sodium tetradecyl sulfate, which is less painful than hypertonic saline. A 3% solution, made by a compounding pharmacy, is diluted to 0.2% to 0.4%. This is accomplished by drawing up 0.2 cc of solution into a 3-cc syringe and adding 2.8 cc of normal saline, making up 3 cc of 2% sodium tetradecyl sulfate. This strength is used for small veins, 0.4% is used for medium veins, and large veins may require up to 1%.

One to six injections may be needed to effectively treat any vein. When spider veins are injected, interconnections among subcutaneous vessels may permit treatment of a

TABLE 35-1. Initial Consultation Session

- Assess the appropriateness of the candidate. Has the patient undergone prior therapy? A history of dissatisfaction with prior therapy may predict future dissatisfaction. Is there a history of significant vein injury, clots, or predisposing factors? Is the patient taking medications (e.g., hormone therapy) that may exacerbate vein disease? Is the patient willing to wear the support hose after the procedure?
- Educate the patient regarding the major complications of the procedure. Does the patient understand that he or she may experience some discomfort during or after the procedure?
- Assess major pressure influence on the superficial veins from incompetent perforator veins. Perform a cough test (i.e., patient coughs while examiner holds the examining hand over the saphenofemoral junction; if the perforator is incompetent, a pulse is felt). The Brodie-Trendelenburg test uses two examiners. The patient is laid supine, with the legs elevated to a vertical position to drain all the blood from the veins. The examiners hold pressure on the saphenofemoral junction while the patient is stood up; the veins on the posterior lower legs are observed. If there is an incompetent perforator, the veins fill rapidly (<15 to 20 seconds), and then a surge is noted in the filling veins when the pressure over the junction is released.
- To perform photoplethysmography, the patient is seated, and the sensor is placed on the skin 10 cm above the medial malleolus. The ankle is dorsiflexed 10 times by the examiner over 10 to 15 seconds, effectively emptying the blood from the subdermal plexus. In a normal study, refilling occurs in more than 25 seconds; intermediate refilling occurs in 15 to 20 seconds, and severe incompetence of the perforators allows the subdermal veins to refill in <15 seconds.
- Record or chart the presence of abnormal veins. If photographs are obtained, perform them in an area of the office with a dark background (e.g., mounted dark felt).
- Write a prescription for the patient to be fitted for two pairs of 30- to 40-mm Hg, thigh-high support hose. The patient must bring a pair of support hose to the first sclerotherapy session.

large network over a wide area of skin. Wait at least 4 to 6 weeks before reinjecting individual vessels to permit adequate healing and to reduce postinflammatory complications.

Patients desiring sclerotherapy should undergo a pretreatment consultation (Table 35-1). The consultation is used to evaluate potential candidates, map or photograph the extent of their diseased vessels, and educate them regarding the procedure. Education is particularly important, because fewer than 90% of patients of even the most experienced practitioners report full satisfaction with the outcome. Photography can help remind patients of the severity of the disease before therapy.

Sclerotherapy is contraindicated if the procedure is unlikely to produce significant benefit. If a patient has significant pressure extending to superficial veins (e.g., produced by an incompetent perforating vein in the saphenofemoral junction in the groin), abnormal veins will rapidly replace those that are ablated. Competence of the deep venous system can be evaluated with photoplethysmography or a handheld Doppler (similar to the ones used to assess fetal heart tones) with an 8-MHz probe. Functional valves in the deep veins are confirmed with the Doppler by finding unidirectional flow in the veins of the popliteal fossa while squeezing and releasing the calf muscle. Incompetent perforators can also be evaluated by physical examination (e.g., cough test, Brodie-Trendelenburg test).

There are several important principles related to selection of veins for sclerotherapy. Always try to inject proximally into the superficial vein to sclerose it as close to the feeder as possible. Larger veins should be selected and treated before smaller veins and should be emptied whenever possible before injection. Treat an entire vessel, if possible, at a given treatment session, and inject the largest feeding vessel (i.e., tree trunk) when treating a telangiectatic cluster. Large veins (≥4 mm) require larger volumes of sclerosant and are at greater risk of complications. Novice providers may wish to refer these patients to more experienced providers. Patients may need reassurance that large deep veins are normal and should not be treated. The number of injections performed during any one session depends on many factors, including the extent of disease, time available for the procedure, and the patient's tolerance. A typical session may include 10 to 20 injections.

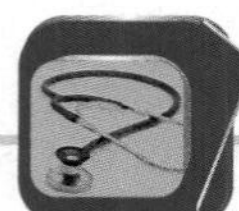

Equipment

- Hypertonic saline 23.4% concentration (use in sclerotherapy is off label): undiluted for midsized vessels (2 to 4 mm), 11.7% (half-strength) for small vessels (1 to 2 mm), and 6% (quarter-strength) for fine vessels (<1 mm).
- Sodium tetradecyl sulfate 3%: 1% for large vessels (4 mm), 0.4% for midsized vessels (2 to 4 mm), and 0.2% for small vessels (<2 mm).
- Polidocanol is commonly used in other countries because it does not cause burning with injection and is less likely to cause skin ulceration or pigmentation changes. The maximum dosage is 2 mg/kg/d. Dilutions are 2% for midsized vessels (2 to 4 mm), 1% for small vessels (1 to 2 mm), and 0.25% to 0.75% for telangiectasias. (No products containing polidocanol are currently approved by the U.S. Federal Drug Administration for marketing in the United States.)
- Syringes (1 or 3 cc) and 30-gauge needles.
- Lidocaine hydrochloride 1% (without epinephrine).
- Normal saline to dilute sodium tetradecyl sulfate or polidocanol.
- A method to assess for incompetent perforating vein.
- Magnifiers or surgical loupes (one to three diopter glasses Isopropyl alcohol).

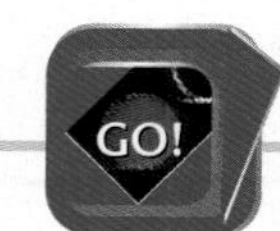

Indications

- Ablation of unwanted spider, reticular, or varicose veins
- Elimination of the symptoms of varicosities such as aching, night cramps, or itching
- Improvement in cosmetic appearance of legs or other affected body sites
- Prevention of complication of leg hypostasis (e.g., dermatitis, ulceration) by diverting blood to healthy vessels

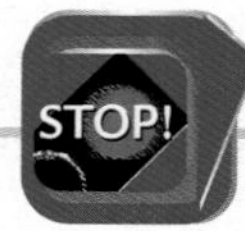

Contraindications

- Uncooperative patient (including refusal to wear support hose after the procedure)
- History of allergic reaction to sclerosing solution (may use alternate solutions)
- Severe peripheral arterial disease that may compromise healing or preclude use of support hose
- Incompetent valves in the deep venous system
- Poorly controlled diabetes
- Pregnancy
- History of thrombophlebitis
- History of pulmonary emboli
- Hypercoagulable states

The Procedure

Step 1. The patient lies flat on the treatment table (prone or supine, depending on the location of the veins being treated). Two lights are positioned from opposite directions to highlight the vessels and limit shadows that can interfere with visualization of the vessels.

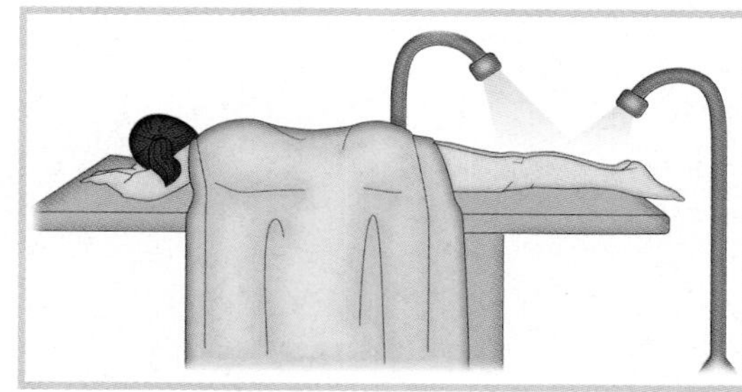

Step 1

Step 2. Check competency of valves in the deep venous system. Use a Doppler with an 8-MHz probe to locate the popliteal artery in the popliteal fossa.

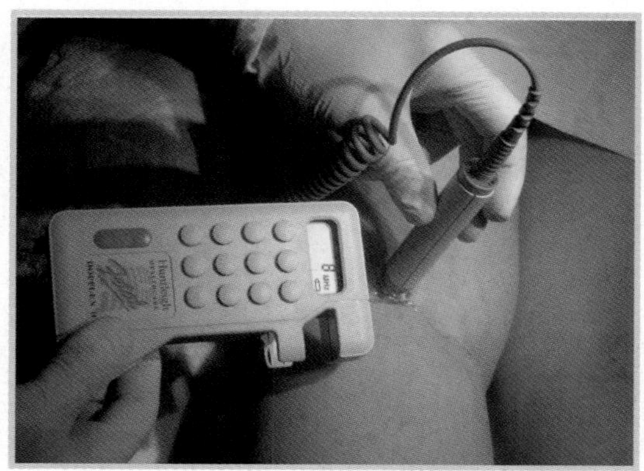

Step 2

Step 3. Move the probe laterally about 1 cm and listen for venous flow while squeezing the calf muscles. The sound is distinctly different from arterial flow and longer in duration. Flow should stop abruptly when the muscle is released unless the valves of the deep venous system allow retrograde flow back into the calf. Functional valves in the deep veins are confirmed by finding only unidirectional flow during the muscle squeeze.

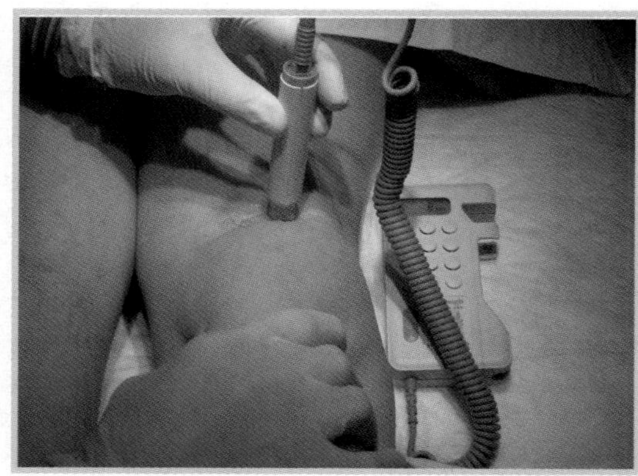

Step 3

Step 4. Pour a colorless antiseptic solution (i.e., isopropyl alcohol or benzalkonium chloride) into a basin containing cotton balls. Apply the solution with the cotton balls to render the skin more transparent and to make the veins easier to visualize.

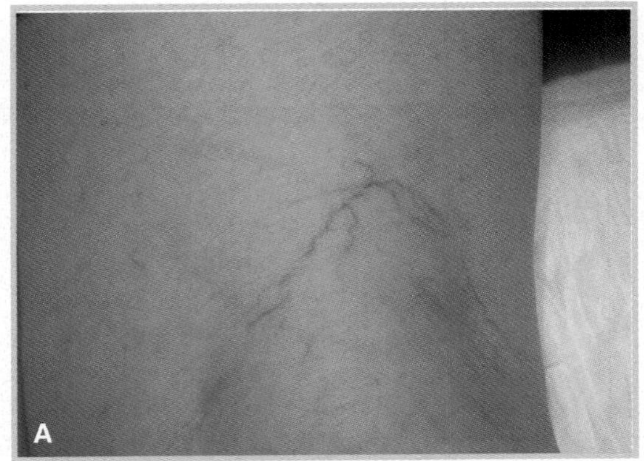

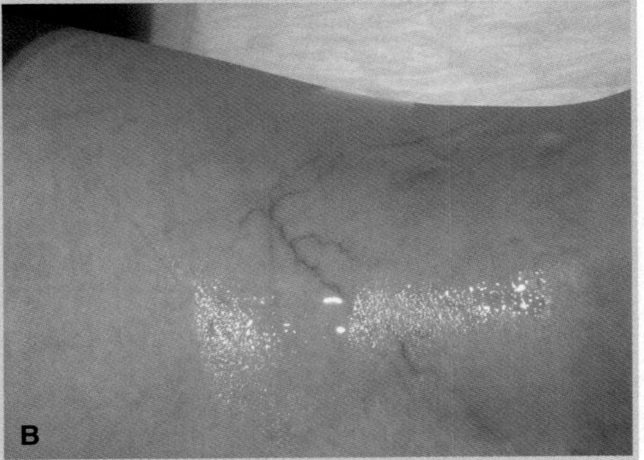

Step 4

Step 5. Use magnifiers or surgical loupes (one to three diopter glasses) to enhance visualization and cannulation of veins.

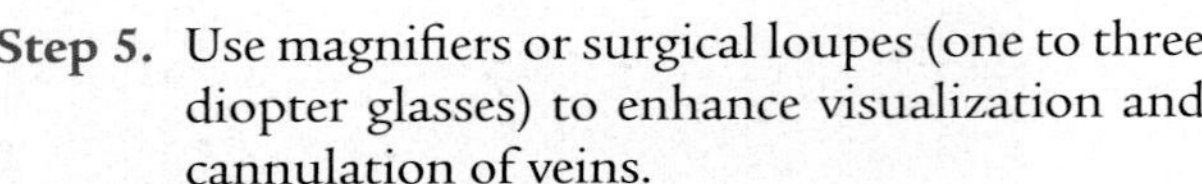

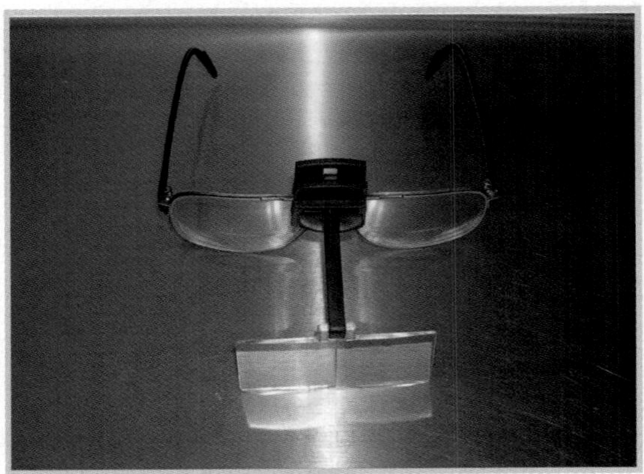

Step 5

Step 6. Bend the needle to a 30- to 45-degree angle with the bevel up. This allows the needle to enter nearly horizontal to the skin surface. Injections should only be performed with the bevel up; this helps to prevent sclerosing fluid from leaking into the tissue. Injections must be intraluminal to prevent complications.

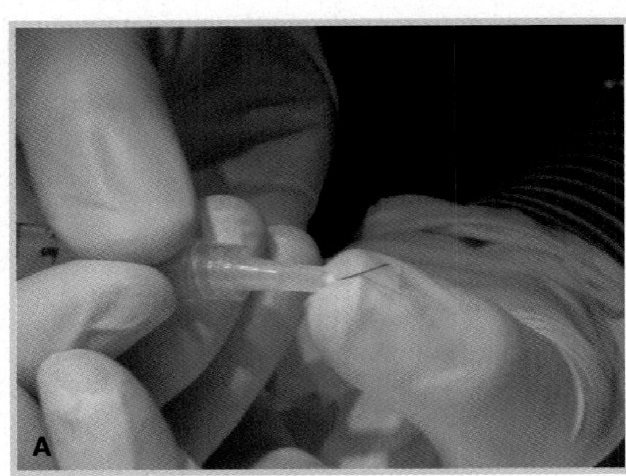

- **PITFALL:** The most common mistake made by novice sclerotherapists is to attempt entry into small vessels with the needle held at too great an angle to the surface of the skin. If the needle is at an angle, the tip frequently passes through a small vessel and deposits the solution in the tissues.

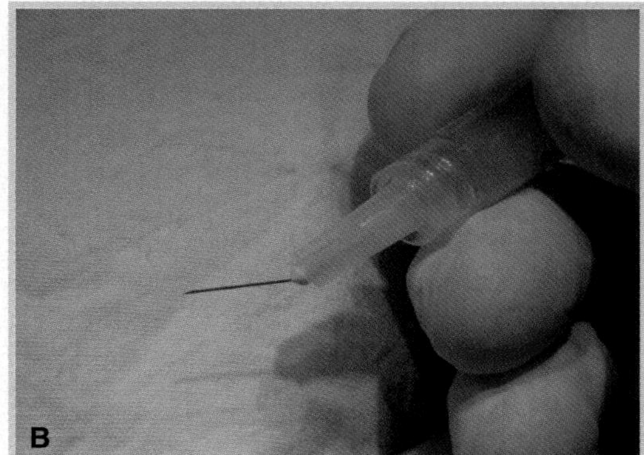

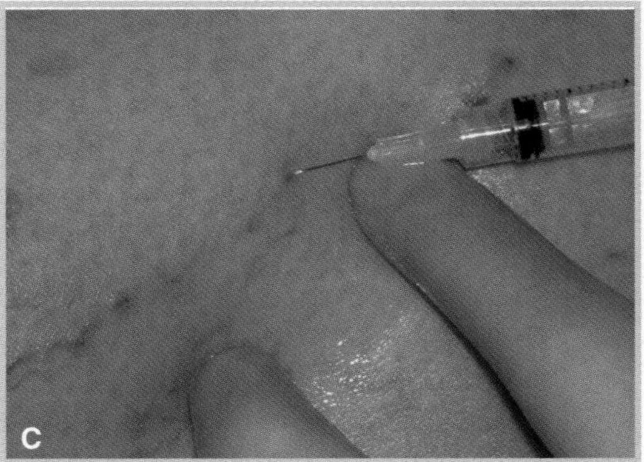

Step 6

Step 7. There are multiple ways of stabilizing the skin for injection. One method is to put the middle finger of the nondominant hand under the needle hub against the skin and the index finger on top of the syringe. The dominate hand can then be used to apply gentle pressure to the syringe plunger.

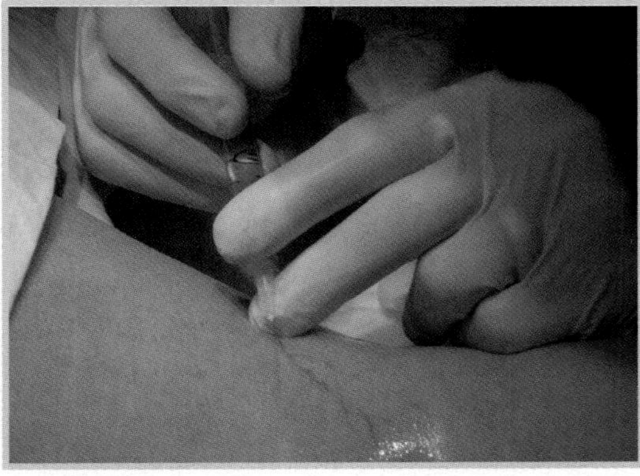

Step 7

Step 8. Alternatively, position the hands to provide three-point traction before injecting a vein. The nondominant hand applies traction using the thumb and index (second) finger. The injecting (dominant) hand's fifth finger is used to provide the third point.

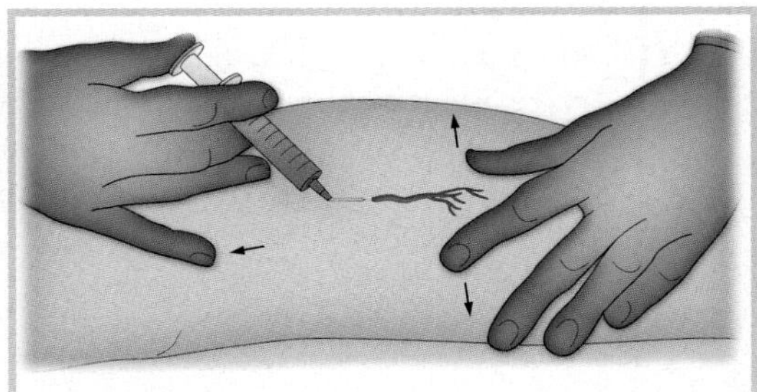

Step 8

Step 9. Injections are administered gently. If the needle tip is intraluminal, the solution will flow easily into the vessel. Observe the needle tip and vessel closely. If a small bleb (or bubble) develops at the injection site, extravasation is likely. The injection should be terminated immediately and the bleb milked into the vein to dissipate the solution. Some physicians advocate infiltrating around extravasation sites with normal saline, but minimal extravasations rarely produce skin necrosis or other complications.

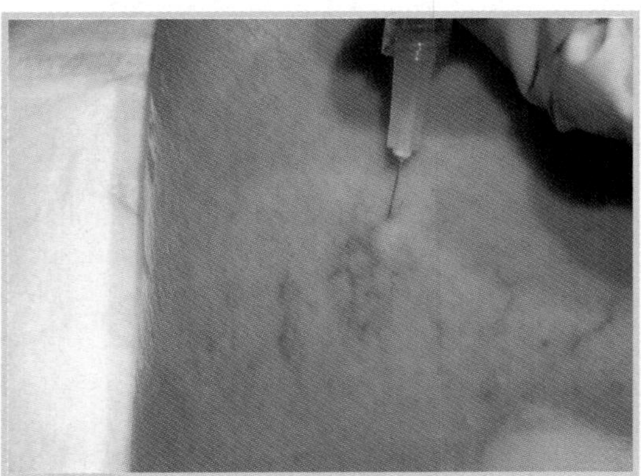

Step 9

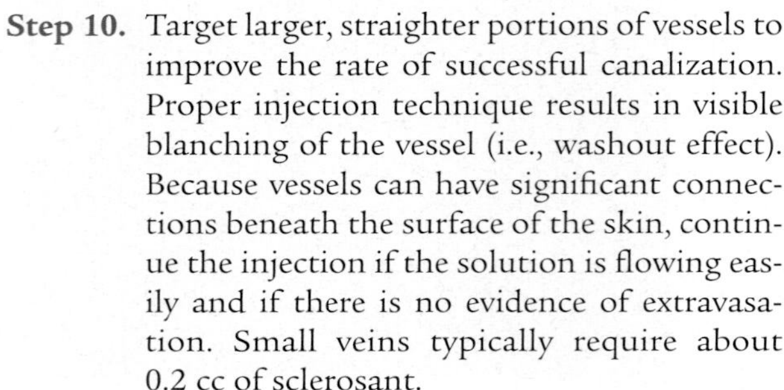

Step 10. Target larger, straighter portions of vessels to improve the rate of successful canalization. Proper injection technique results in visible blanching of the vessel (i.e., washout effect). Because vessels can have significant connections beneath the surface of the skin, continue the injection if the solution is flowing easily and if there is no evidence of extravasation. Small veins typically require about 0.2 cc of sclerosant.

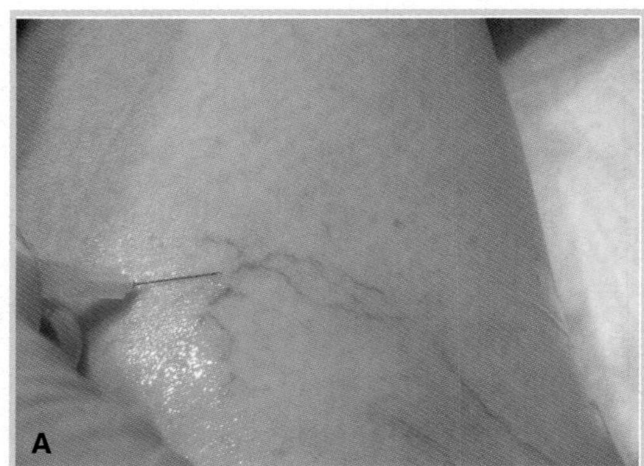

A

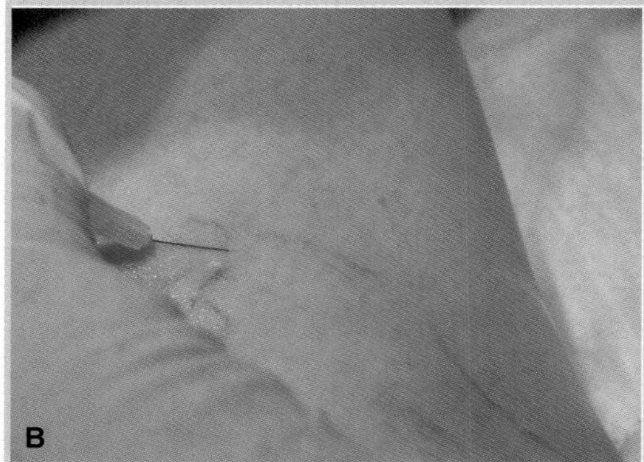

B

Step 10

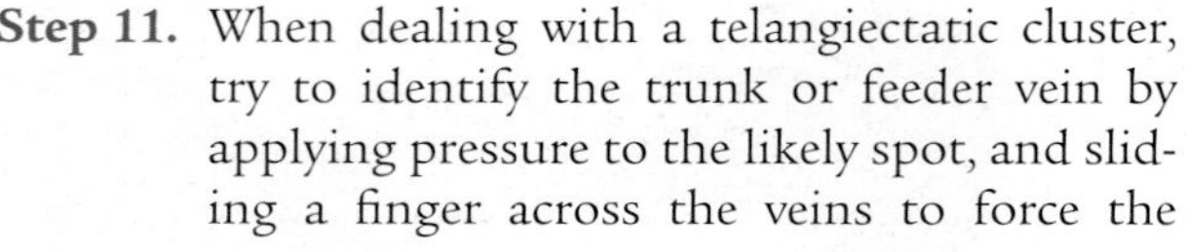

Step 11. When dealing with a telangiectatic cluster, try to identify the trunk or feeder vein by applying pressure to the likely spot, and sliding a finger across the veins to force the

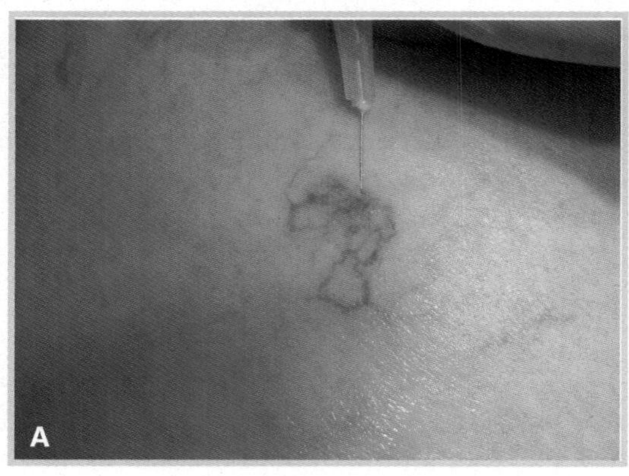

A

blood out of them. If the veins stay blanched longer with pressure applied, you have identified the probable feeder vein. Inject the varicosity near that point until the entire telangiectatic cluster is blanched.

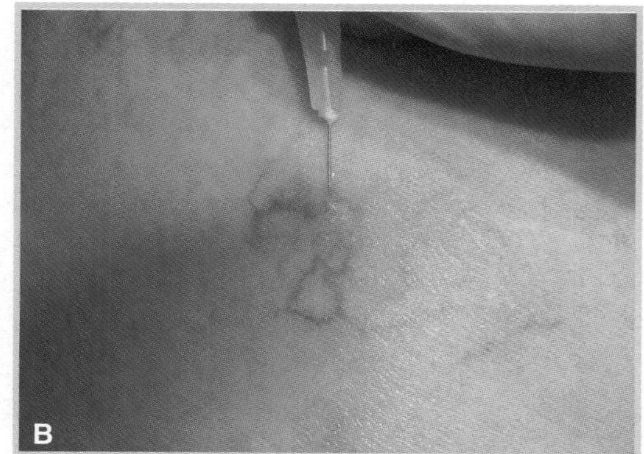

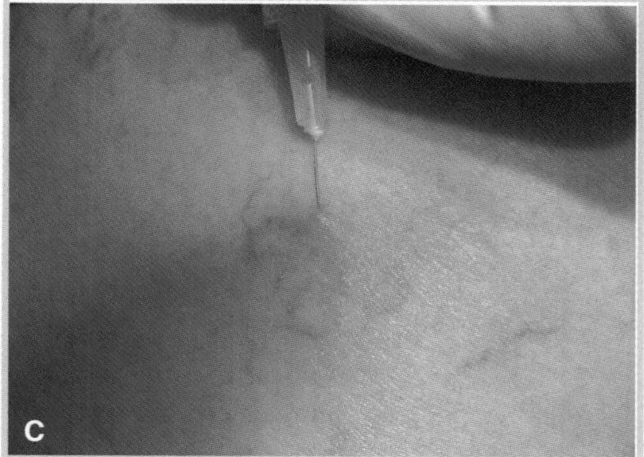

Step 11

Step 12. Immediately after the injection, place pressure on the site with gauze or large cotton balls. The nurse can hold pressure to the site for 30 to 60 seconds while the provider injects another site. Although some providers do not like taping gauze or cotton balls to the skin for fear of tape allergies and tape blistering, others find it a safe and convenient way to keep pressure on the vein from the very beginning.

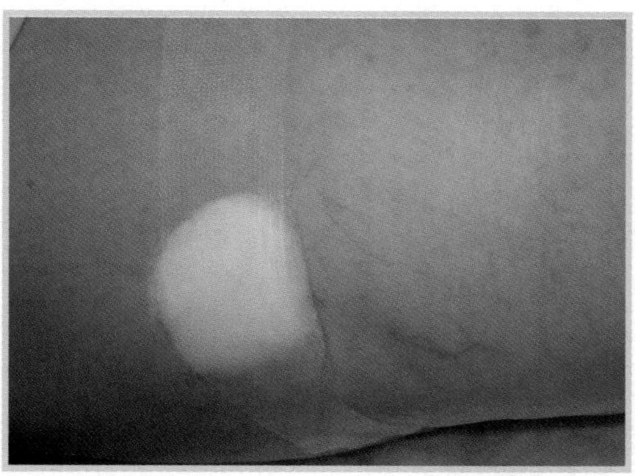

Step 12

Step 13. Fitted support hose are applied while the patient is supine, before standing and refilling the veins. The 2- × 2-inch gauze or cotton ball can be held over the injection sites by hand or with tape as the support hose are rolled up the leg. The patient is instructed to ambulate for 20 minutes after application of the support hose to prevent pooling of sclerosing agents into the deep vein circulation.

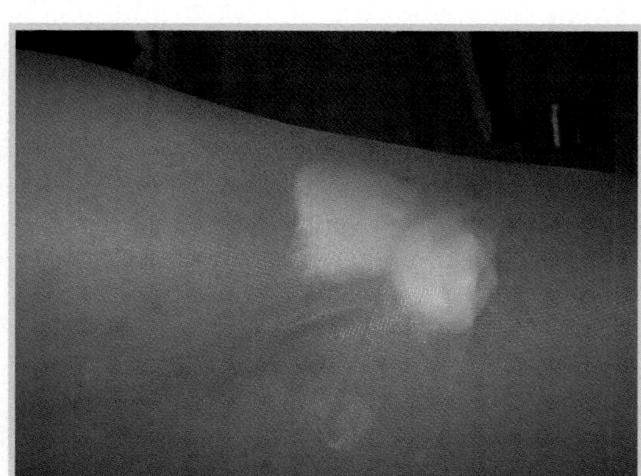

Step 13

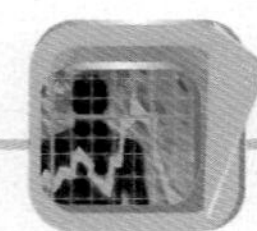

Complications

- Hypertonic saline: Extravasation may cause skin ulceration, and the injection may cause burning.
- Sodium tetradecyl sulfate: The injection may cause burning. Extravasation may cause skin ulceration. Patients may develop an allergy, and anaphylaxis has been reported.
- Polidocanol is less likely than other agents to cause skin ulceration or pigmentation changes. It may cause an allergic reaction.
- Edema.
- Superficial thrombophlebitis: This usually occurs in large vessels and may be treated with aspirin, compression, and nonsteroidal anti-inflammatory drugs (NSAIDs).
- Local tissue necrosis is due to leakage of the sclerosant.
- Cutaneous hyperpigmentation: This occurs in about 30% of patients if hypertonic saline is the sclerosing agent.
- Bruising: This is worsened if larger vessels are injected, when canalization fails, or if there is a lack of compression afterward.
- Temporary swelling: Between 2% and 5% of patients experience pedal and leg edema after the procedure.
- Telangiectatic matting: New appearance of fine (blush) vessels occurs in about 25% of patients.
- Localized urticaria is an allergic local reaction occurring in the first 30 minutes following sclerotherapy.
- Tape compression blister.
- Recurrence of abnormal veins: Most patients develop some new vessels in the next 5 years.
- Anaphylaxis (uncommon).
- Allergic reaction to sclerosing agent.
- Deep venous thrombosis and pulmonary embolus (very rare but serious complication).

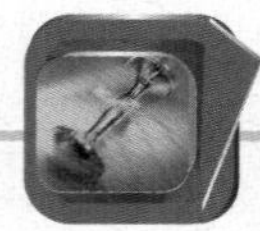

Pediatric Considerations

This procedure is not usually performed in the pediatric population.

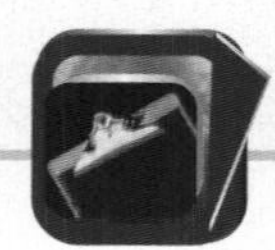

Postprocedure Instructions

After sclerotherapy, patients should wear support hose for the day of and night after the procedure and then daily for at least 10 days (preferably 4 to 6 weeks). The use of support hose limits the refilling of treated vessels and significantly reduces complications after therapy. Patients should be fitted for at least thigh-high, 20- to 30-mmHg support hose after the initial consultation and before the first injection session. Patients with leg hypostasis are encouraged to wear support hose long-term to improve the health of the leg tissues and to reduce recurrences. Patients often prefer lower-pressure (over-the-counter, 10- to 20-mmHg) support hose, but the higher-pressure type of support hose is needed to ensure adeq venous drainage and to prevent stasis complications.

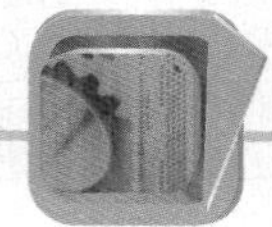

Coding Information and Supply Sources

If bilateral procedures are performed during the session, add the -50 modifier when reporting codes 36468, 36470, and 36471.

CPT Code	Description	2008 Average 50th Percentile Fee	Global Period
36468	Single or multiple injections, spider veins, trunk or limb	$292.00	0
36469	Single or multiple injections, spider veins, face	$318.00	0
36470	Injection of sclerosing solution, single vein	$231.00	10
36471	Injection of sclerosing solution, multiple veins, same leg	$319.00	10
93965	Noninvasive physiologic study, bilateral extremity veins (PPG)	$259.00	XXX
93965	Noninvasive physiologic study, bilateral extremity veins, in hospital (–26)	$130.00	XXX
99002	Handling and fitting of orthotics (office fitting, ordering hose)	$38.00	XXX
99070	Supplies and materials (support hose charge)	Fee determined by cost, markup	XXX

XXX, global concept does not apply.

CPT is a registered trademark of the American Medical Association.

2008 average 50th Percentile Fees are provided courtesy of 2008 MMH-SI's copyrighted Physicians' Fees and Coding Guide.

ICD-9 Codes

Varicose veins of lower extremities	454
Varicose veins with ulcer	454.0
Varicose veins with inflammation	454.1
Varicose veins with ulcer and inflammation	454.2
Varicose veins with other complications	454.8
Asymptomatic varicose veins	454.9

Suppliers

- Hypertonic saline, sodium tetradecyl sulfate, and benzalkonium chloride solution can be obtained from local surgical supply houses or pharmacies.
- Magnifiers and surgical loupes can be obtained from Anthony Products, 7740 Records Street, Indianapolis, IN 46226. Phone: 1-800-428-1610. Web site: http://www.anthonyproducts.com.

Patient Education Handout

A patient education handout, "Sclerotherapy for Varicose Veins," can be found on the book's companion Web site.

Bibliography

Baccaglini U, Spreafico G, Castoro C, et al. Sclerotherapy of varicose veins of the lower limbs. *Dermatol Surg.* 1996;22:883–889.

Goldman MP, Bergan JJ. *Sclerotherapy: Treatment of Varicose and Telangiectatic Leg Veins.* 3rd ed. St. Louis: Mosby-Year Book; 2001.

Goldman MP, Weiss RA, Brody HJ, et al. Treatment of facial telangiectasias with sclerotherapy, laser surgery, and/or electrodesiccation: a review. *J Dermatol Surg Oncol.* 1993;19:899–906.

Green D. Sclerotherapy for varicose and telangiectatic veins. *Am Fam Physician.* 1992;46:827–837.

Hubner K. Is the light reflection rheography (LRR) suitable as a diagnostic method for the phlebology practice? *Phlebol Proctol.* 1986;15:209–212.

Parsons ME. Sclerotherapy basics. *Dermatol Clin.* 2004;22(4):501–508.

Pfeifer JR, Hawtof GD. Injection sclerotherapy and CO_2 laser sclerotherapy in the ablation of cutaneous spider veins of the lower extremity. *Phlebology.* 1989;4:231–240.

Pfeifer JR, Hawtof GD, Minier JA. Saline injection sclerotherapy in the ablation of spider telangiectasia of the lower extremities. *Perspect Plast Surg.* 1990;2:165–170.

Piachaud D, Weddell JM. Cost of treating varicose veins. *Lancet* 1972;11:1191–1192.

Sadick NS. Predisposing factors of varicose and telangiectatic leg veins. *J Dermatol Surg Oncol.* 1992;18:883–886.

Sadick NS, Farber B. A microbiologic study of diluted sclerotherapy solutions. *J Dermatol Surg Oncol.* 1993;19:450–454.

Sadick N, Li C. Small-vessel sclerotherapy. *Dermatol Clin.* 2001;19:475–481.

Tisi PV, Beverley CA. Injection sclerotherapy for varicose veins. *Cochrane Database Syst Rev.* 2002;CD001732.

Weiss MA, Weiss RA, Goldman MP. How minor varicosities cause leg pain. *Contemp Obstet Gynecol.* 1991:113–125.

Weiss RA, Sadick NS, Goldman MP, et al. Post-sclerotherapy compression: controlled comparative study of duration of compression and its effects on clinical outcome. *Dermatol Surg.* 1999;25:105–108.

Weiss RA, Weiss MA, Goldman MP. Physicians' negative perception of sclerotherapy for venous disorders: review of a 7-year experience with modern sclerotherapy. *South Med J.* 1992;85:1101–1106.

Zimmet SE. The prevention of cutaneous necrosis following extravasation of hypertonic saline and sodium tetradecyl sulfate. *J Dermatol Surg Oncol.* 1993;19(7):641–646.

2008 MAG Mutual Healthcare Solutions, Inc.'s Physicians' Fee and Coding Guide. Duluth, Georgia. MAG Mutual Healthcare Solutions, Inc. 2007.

SECTION FOUR

SUTURE TECHNIQUES

CHAPTER 36

Basic Instrument Suture Tie

E. J. Mayeaux, Jr., MD, DABFP, FAAFP

Professor of Family Medicine, Professor of Obstetrics and Gynecology
Louisiana State University Health Sciences Center, Shreveport, LA

Once the suture is satisfactorily placed, it must be secured with a knot. The instrument tie is the most commonly used method of securing sutures in cutaneous surgery. The square knot, or surgeon's knot, is traditionally preferred. The knot should be tightened sufficiently to approximate the wound edges without constricting the tissue and impeding blood flow.

When tying suture knots, properly squaring successive throws is important. That is, each tie must be laid down perfectly parallel to the previous tie by reversing the loops in each successive throw. When tying rope, this is accomplished using the memory aide "left over right and twist, and then right over left and twist." With instrument ties, this is accomplished by alternating sides as the suture is twisted around the needle driver. This procedure is important in preventing the creation of a granny knot, which tends to slip and is inherently weaker than a proper square knot. The first throw in the knotting sequence is often looped or twisted twice, producing the surgeon's knot. When the desired number of throws is completed, the suture material is cut (if interrupted sutures are used) or the next suture may be placed (if running sutures are used). An absolute minimum of three throws are needed for knot security, but some sutures require more throws to remain tied. When in doubt, five throws will hold almost all sutures securely.

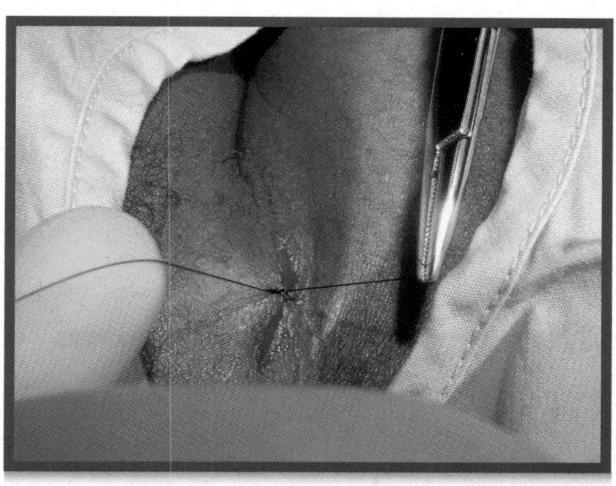

Many varieties of cutaneous suture materials and needles are available. In modern sutures, the suture is swagged (attached) to the needle. Cutting and reverse-cutting needles are most commonly used for skin surgery, although tapered "plastics" needles are also used. Both cutting and reverse-cutting needles have a triangular body. A cutting needle has the point of the triangle on the inner curve of the needle, which is directed toward the wound edge. A reverse-cutting needle has the point of the triangle on the outer curve of the needle, which is directed away from the wound edge and reduces the risk of the suture pulling through the tissue.

A number of various types of sutures are available. They may be monofilaments (Prolene or Ethilon) or multifilamentous (silk). *Tensile strength* is defined as the amount of weight required to break a suture divided by its cross-sectional area. The designation of suture strength is the number of zeros. The higher the number of zeros (1-0 to 10-0), the smaller the size and the lower the strength of the suture. *Memory* is the inherent ability of a material to return to its former shape after being manipulated and is usually related to its stiffness. A suture with a high level of memory is more difficult to handle and more susceptible to becoming untied than a suture with low memory. An absorbable suture is one that will lose most of its tensile strength within 60 days after implantation. Nonabsorbable sutures do not lose tensile strength within 60 days and usually need to be removed.

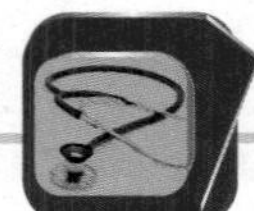

Equipment

- Instruments for skin suture placement are found in Appendix G and can be ordered through local surgical supply houses.
- Suture materials can be ordered from Ethicon, Somerville, NJ. Web site: http://ecatalog.ethicon.com/EC_ECATALOG/ethicon/default.asp.
  - Delasco.com.

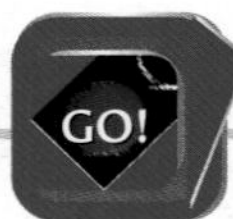

Indications

- Closure of wounds
- Anchoring tubes and devices to the skin

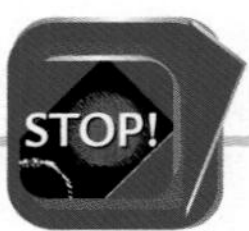

Contraindications (Relative)

- None specifically; see specific suture technique chapters.

The Procedure

Step 1. To prepare the suture for tying, pull it through the skin until a tail of about 2 cm remains. Although there are multiple techniques for an instrument-tying suture, one simple, easy-to-remember method is shown next.

- **PEARL:** A shorter suture tail (about 2 cm) is much easier to work with and better conserves suture than a long tail.

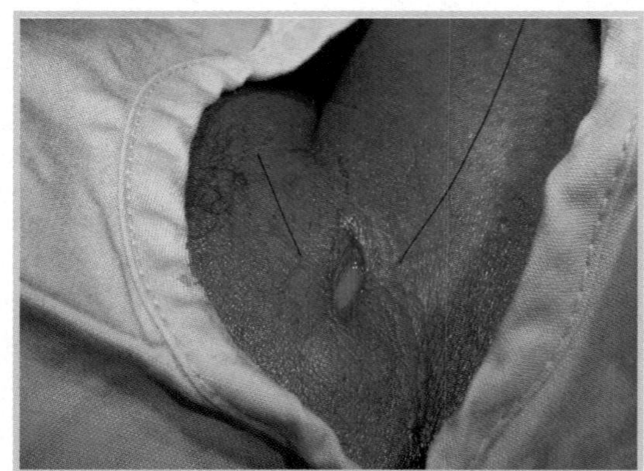

Step 1

Step 2. Be careful not to allow the running end of the suture to accidentally touch nonsterile areas and become contaminated. A simple way to avoid this and keep good control of the needle is to grasp the needle between the thumb and forefinger of the nondominant hand and gently wrap (so as not to pull the tail through the wound) the excess suture around the three middle fingers during the tying procedure.

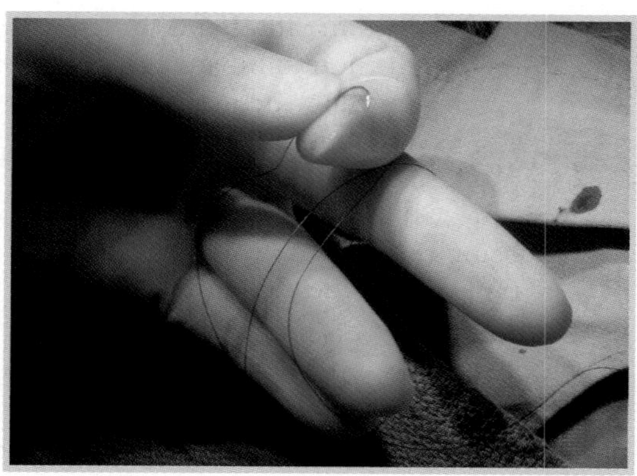

Step 2

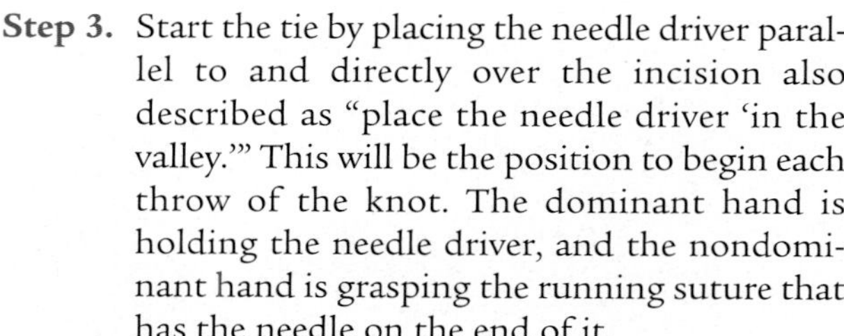

Step 3. Start the tie by placing the needle driver parallel to and directly over the incision also described as "place the needle driver 'in the valley.'" This will be the position to begin each throw of the knot. The dominant hand is holding the needle driver, and the nondominant hand is grasping the running suture that has the needle on the end of it.

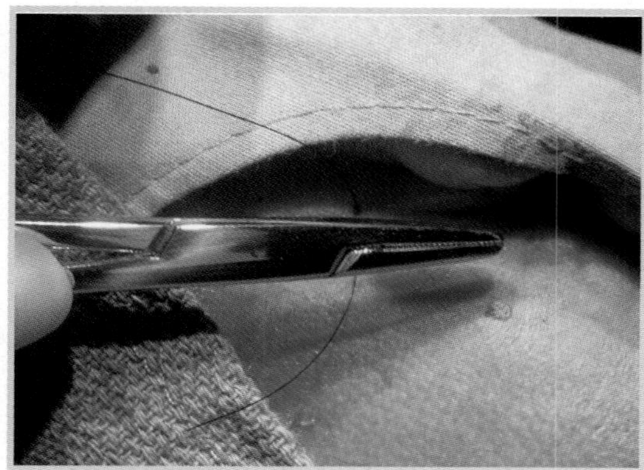

Step 3

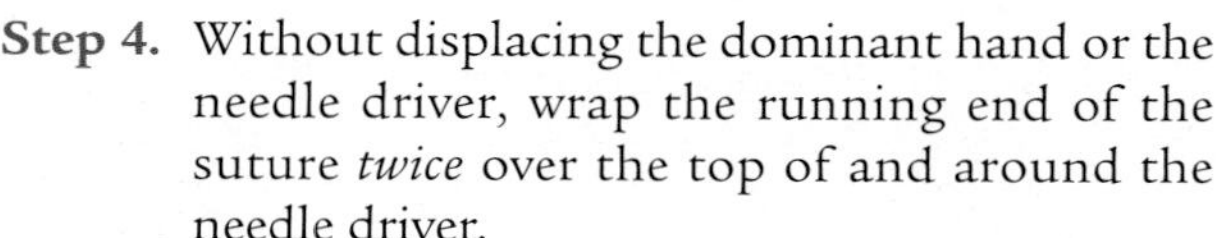

Step 4. Without displacing the dominant hand or the needle driver, wrap the running end of the suture *twice* over the top of and around the needle driver.

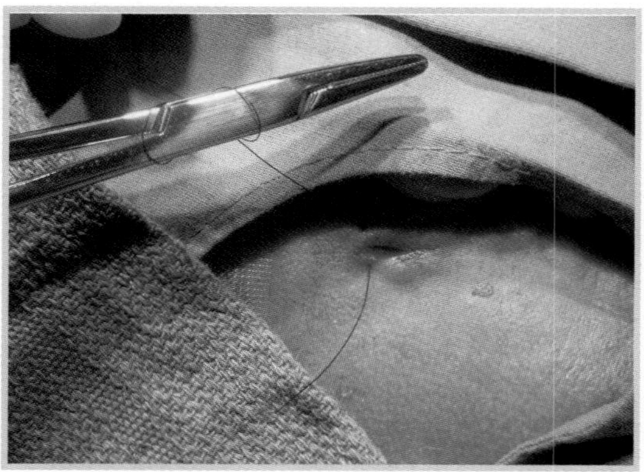

Step 4

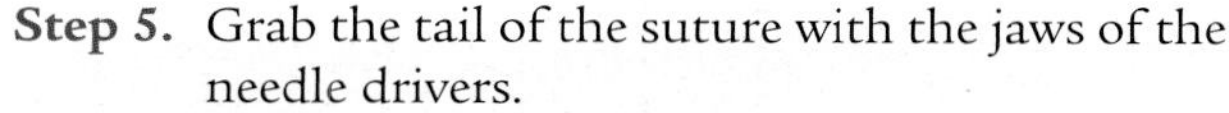

Step 5. Grab the tail of the suture with the jaws of the needle drivers.

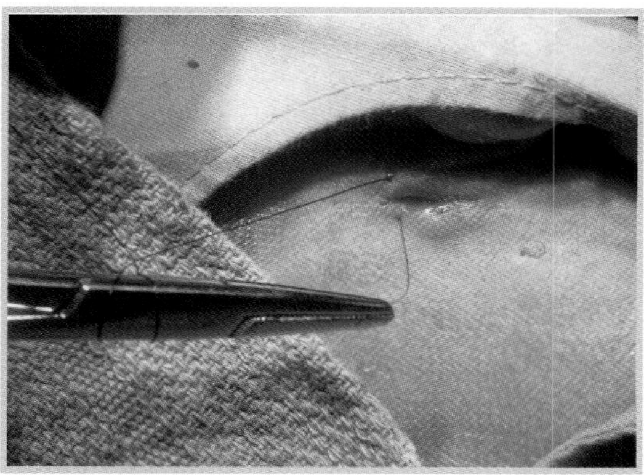

Step 5

Step 6. Pull the dominant hand and needle driver toward the nondominant side, while simultaneously pulling the nondominant hand and running suture toward the dominant side to place the first throw of the surgeon's knot. This will result in the provider's forearms being crossed, and this position will be maintained until the next throw is placed.

- **PITFALL:** Do *not* let go of or reposition the hands, suture, or needle driver until the tie is completed. This method relies on the progressive placement of the hands in each step to correctly tie the knot.

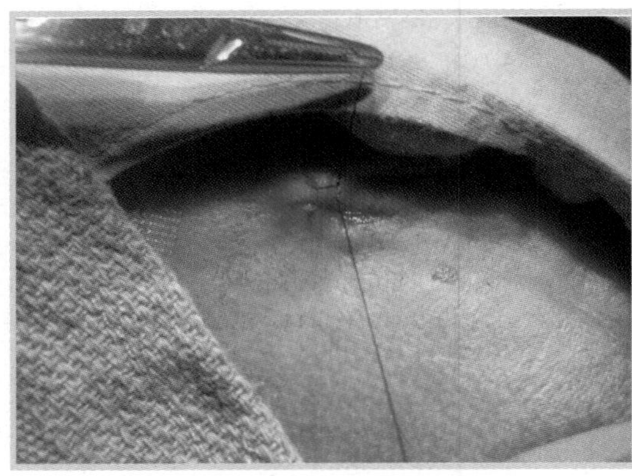

Step 6

Step 7. Now place the needle driver back, parallel to, and directly over the incision in exactly the same position as in Step 2. Wrap the running end of the suture *once* over the top of and around the needle driver.

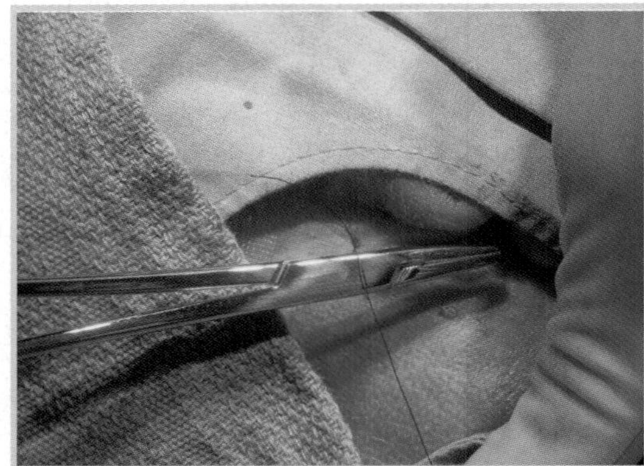

Step 7

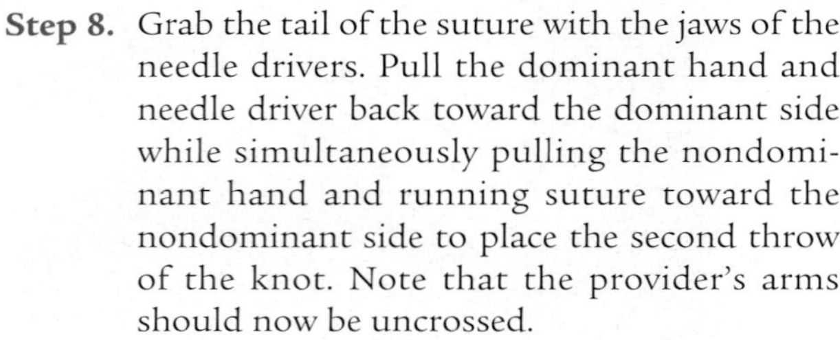

Step 8. Grab the tail of the suture with the jaws of the needle drivers. Pull the dominant hand and needle driver back toward the dominant side while simultaneously pulling the nondominant hand and running suture toward the nondominant side to place the second throw of the knot. Note that the provider's arms should now be uncrossed.

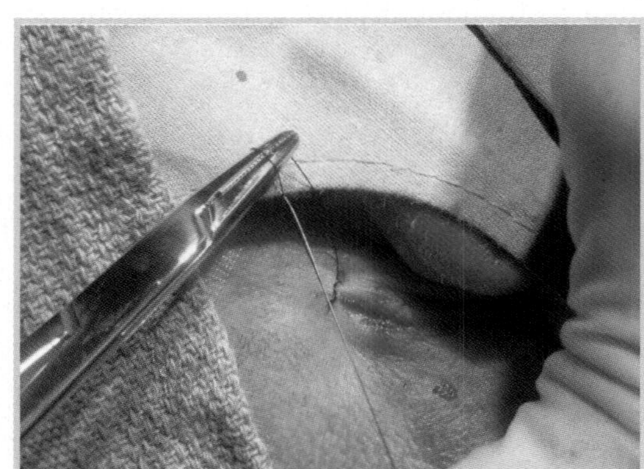

Step 8

Step 9. Steps 2 through 5 are then repeated, with only single wraps for each pass, until the desired number of throws is placed. Cut the suture with suture scissors with approximately 0.5-cm ends.

- **PEARL:** When in doubt about the number of throws to use, remember that five throws will work for most sutures.

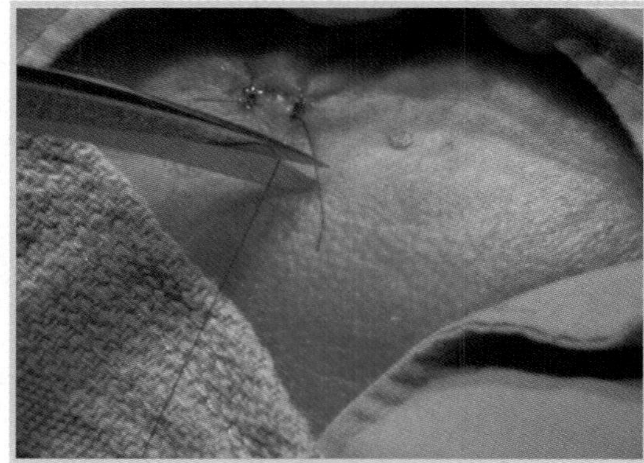

Step 9

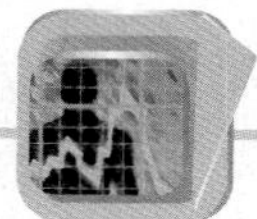

Complications

- Strangulation of skin edges because of excessive tension
- Infection
- Scarring

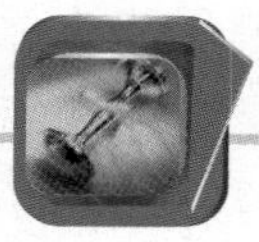

Pediatric Considerations

This technique is the same for patients of all ages.

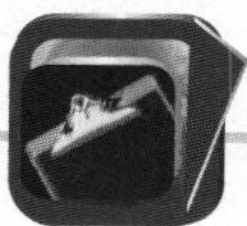

Postprocedure Instructions

Instruct the patient not to pick at, break, or cut the stitches. Have the patient cover the wound with a nonocclusive dressing for 2 to 3 days. A simple adhesive bandage (Band-Aid) will suffice for many small lacerations. Have the patient make an appointment made so the provider can remove any nonabsorbable sutures.

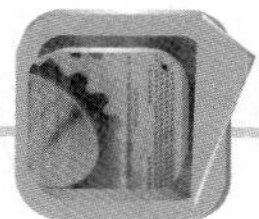

Coding Information and Supply Sources

See the specific suture technique chapters for coding information.

Bibliography

Adams B, Anwar J, Wrone DA, et al. Techniques for cutaneous sutured closures: variants and indications. *Semin Cutan Med Surg.* 2003;22(4):306–316.

Bennett RG. *Fundamentals of Cutaneous Surgery*. St. Louis: CV Mosby; 1988:384–394.

Guyuron B, Vaughan C. A comparison of absorbable and nonabsorbable suture materials for skin repair. *Plast Reconstr Surg.* 1992;89:234.

Hollander JE, Singer AJ. Laceration management. *Ann Emerg Med.* 1999;34:356.

Ivy JJ, Unger JB, Hurt J, et al. The effect of number of throws on knot security with nonidentical sliding knots. *Am J Obstet Gynecol.* 2004;191(5):1618–1620.

Lammers RL, Trott AT. Methods of wound closure. In: Roberts JR, Hedges JR, eds. *Clinical Procedures in Emergency Medicine.* 3rd ed. Philadelphia: WB Saunders; 1998:560–598.

Lober CW, Fenske NA. Suture materials for closing the skin and subcutaneous tissues. *Aesthetic Plast Surg.* 1986;10:245.

McCarthy JG. *Plastic Surgery*. Philadelphia: WB Saunders; 1990:1–68.

Moy RL. Suturing techniques. In: Usatine RP, Moy RL, Tobnick EL, et al., eds. *Skin Surgery: A Practical Guide.* St. Louis: Mosby; 1998:88–100.

Moy RL, Lee A, Zalka A. Commonly used suturing techniques in skin surgery. *Am Fam Physician.* 1991;44:1625–1634.

Moy RL, Waldman B, Hein DW. A review of sutures and suturing technique. *J Dermatol Surg Oncol.* 1992;18:785.

Odland PB, Murakami CS. Simple suturing techniques and knot tying. In: Wheeland RG, ed. *Cutaneous Surgery*. Philadelphia: WB Saunders; 1994:178–188.

Stegman SJ, Tromovitch TA, Glogau RG. *Basics of Dermatologic Surgery*. Chicago: Year Book; 1984:41–42.

Swanson NA. *Atlas of Cutaneous Surgery*. Boston: Little, Brown; 1987:26–28.

Zuber TJ. *Basic Soft-Tissue Surgery*. Kansas City: American Academy of Family Physicians; 1998: 34–38.

2008 MAG Mutual Healthcare Solutions, Inc.'s Physicians' Fee and Coding Guide. Duluth, Georgia. MAG Mutual Healthcare Solutions, Inc. 2007.

CHAPTER 37

Deep Buried Dermal Suture

E. J. Mayeaux Jr., MD, DABFP, FAAFP

Professor of Family Medicine, Professor of Obstetrics and Gynecology
Louisiana State University Health Sciences Center, Shreveport, LA

The deeply buried subcutaneous suture closes dead space, stops subcutaneous bleeding, reduces hematoma and seroma formation, and takes essentially all of the tension off the skin sutures and skin edges. The decreased tension in the healing scar will reduce the final width of a resultant scar. The most common suture materials used in this technique are chromic gut, polyglactin (Vicryl), polyglycolic (Dexon), polydioxanone (PDS), and polyglyconate (Maxon). These sutures are absorbable and do not need to be removed.

Usually, both deep or buried and superficial skin sutures are placed. In multilayered closures, the deep sutures bear virtually all of the tension, and the superficial sutures approximate the epidermal edges for an optimal, cosmetically acceptable result. The eversion obtained with the buried suture carries minimal risk of leaving suture marks. The classic description of the buried suture technique emphasizes that the knot be buried downward. A buried suture allows the physician to remove superficial skin sutures earlier, because wound eversion is maintained longer. The everted wound flattens after wound contraction, providing a good cosmesis.

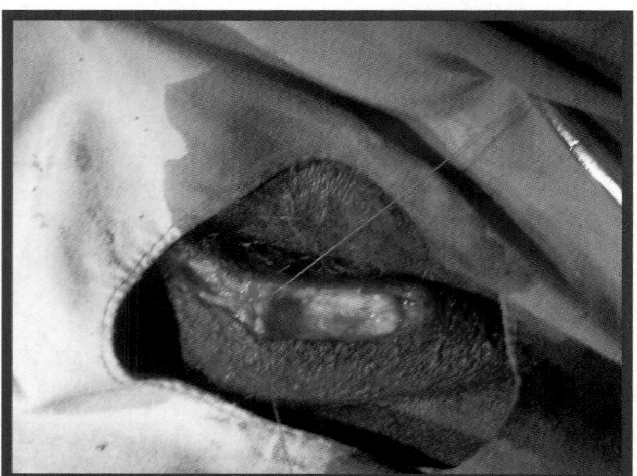

Buried dermal sutures do not increase the risk of infection in clean, uncontaminated lacerations. However, animal studies suggest that deep sutures should be avoided in highly contaminated wounds.

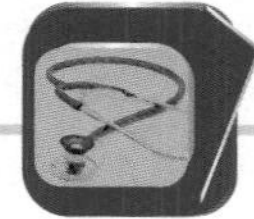

Equipment

- Common skin surgery equipment and the typical skin surgery tray are listed in Appendix G.

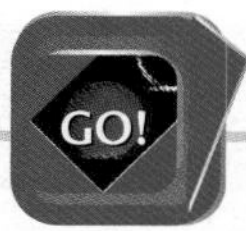

Indications

- Wounds needing tension reduction
- Wounds with deep spaces that may collect blood or fluids
- Large wounds

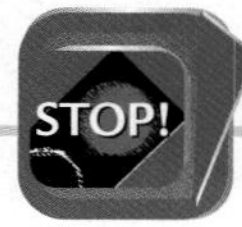

Contraindications

- Inadequate subcutaneous tissue to perform the technique
- Contaminated wounds

Consider vertical mattress sutures if tension reduction is needed.

The Procedure

Step 1. The suture begins in the center of the wound and passes beneath the left wound edge and then back into the center of the wound through the dermis.

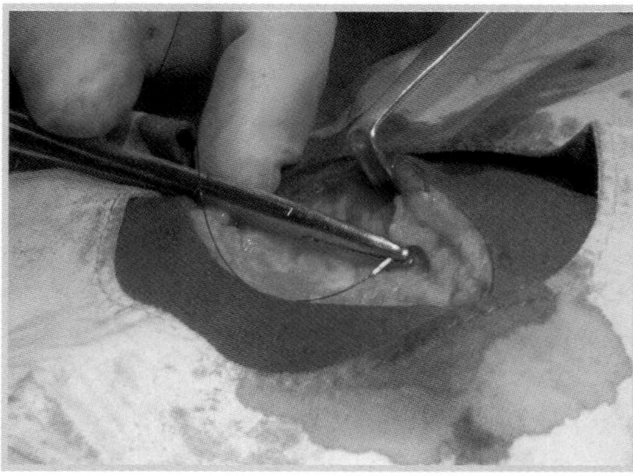

Step 1

Step 2. The needle is placed upside down and backward into the needle holder. It passes through the dermis into the right wound edge and down to the base of the wound. The needle then grabs a small bit of the tissue in the base of the wound.

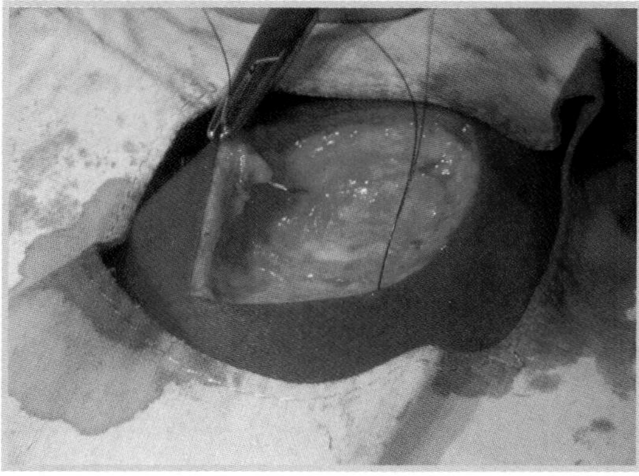

Step 2

Step 3. Both of the suture ends need to be on the same side of the center part of the suture passing across the top of the wound (i.e., toward the operator or away from the operator).

- **PITFALL:** If a suture end is placed on either side of the center part of the suture and tied, the knot will rest on top of the center part of the suture and not be buried in the deep tissue.

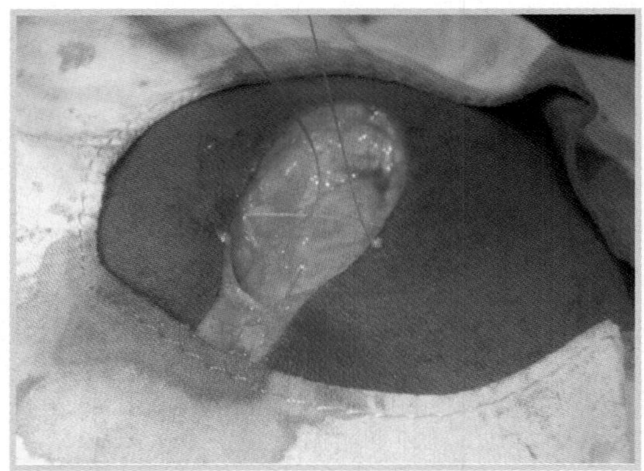

Step 3

Step 4. The knot is tied. Instead of pulling each throw laterally as with most ties, pull the ends of the suture parallel to the wound to deeply bury the knot. Cut the suture tails just above the knot.

- **PEARL:** There should be no more than three to four knots per suture to minimize the risk of the knot migrating through the healing wound through the incision line.

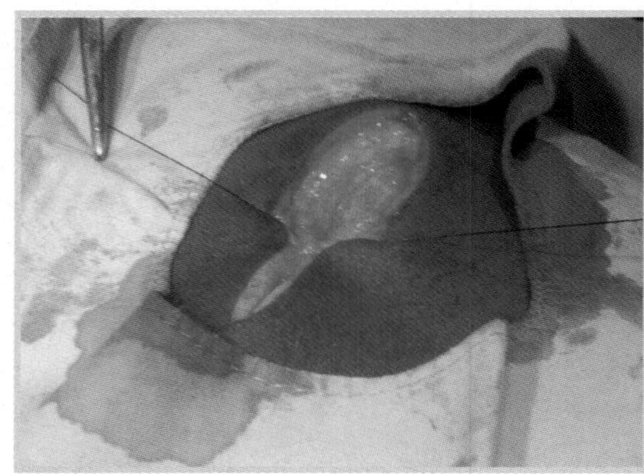

Step 4

Step 5. Usually, a deeply buried suture is placed in the center and/or the ends of the wound.

- **PEARL:** In potentially contaminated wounds, the fewest number of sutures possible should be placed.

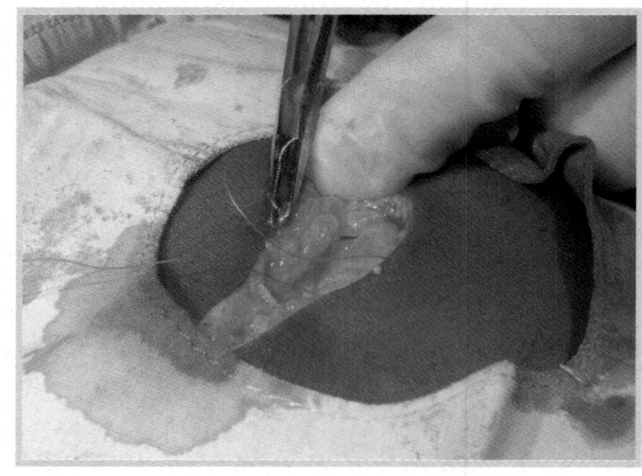

Step 5

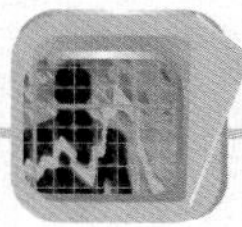

Complications

- Bleeding
- Infection, especially in contaminated wounds
- Scar formation

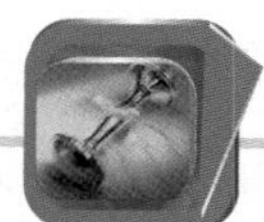

Pediatric Considerations

Deep sutures are particularly useful in children, because they will hold the wound together even if the child picks out the superficial sutures. However, pediatric patients often find it difficult to sit and lie still during lengthy procedures. The maximum recommended dose for lidocaine in children is 3 to 5 mg/kg, and 7 mg/kg when combined with epinephrine. Neonates have an increased volume of distribution, decreased hepatic clearance, and doubled terminal elimination half-life (3.2 hours).

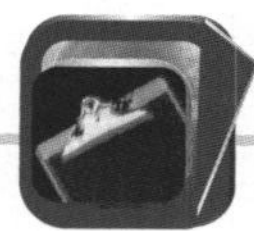

Postprocedure Instructions

Instruct the patient to gently wash the area that has been stitched after 1 day but not to put the wound into standing water for 3 days. Have the patient dry the area well after washing. Have the patient use a small amount of antibiotic ointment to promote moist healing. Recommend wound elevation to help lessen swelling, reduce pain, and speed healing. Instruct the patient not to pick at, break, or cut the stitches.

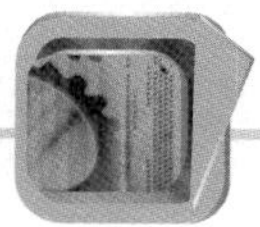

Coding Information and Supply Sources

If a layered closure is required, use intermediate closure codes 12031 to 12057 or complex repair codes 13100 to 13160 in addition to the simple closure codes. Place the intermediate repair code first, then the simple repair code with a -51 modifier.

Simple repair is included in the codes reported for benign and malignant lesion excision (see Chapter 49, Fusiform Excision) and the closure is not reported separately.

CPT Code	Description	2008 Average 50th Percentile Fee	Global Period
12031	Intermediate closure SATAL ≤2.5 cm	$272	10
12032	Intermediate closure SATAL 2.6–7.5 cm	$347	10
12034	Intermediate closure SATAL 7.6–12.5 cm	$438	10
12035	Intermediate closure SATAL 12.6–20.0 cm	$548	10
12036	Intermediate closure SATAL 20.1–30.0 cm	$680	10
12037	Intermediate closure SATAL >30.0 cm	$789	10
12041	Intermediate closure NHFG ≤2.5 cm	$262	10
12042	Intermediate closure NHFG 2.6–7.5 cm	$357	10
12044	Intermediate closure NHFG 7.6–12.5 cm	$462	10
12045	Intermediate closure NHFG 12.6–20.0 cm	$558	10
12046	Intermediate closure NHFG 20.1–30.0 cm	$729	10
12047	Intermediate closure NHFG >30.0 cm	$846	10
12051	Intermediate closure FEENLMM ≤2.5 cm	$341	10
12052	Intermediate closure FEENLMM 2.6–5.0 cm	$426	10
12053	Intermediate closure FEENLMM 5.1–7.5 cm	$527	10
12054	Intermediate closure FEENLMM 7.6–12.5 cm	$645	10
12055	Intermediate closure FEENLMM 12.6–20.0 cm	$822	10
12056	Intermediate closure FEENLMM 20.1–30.0 cm	$1,044	10
12057	Intermediate closure FEENLMM >30.0 cm	$1,211	10

CPT is a registered trademark of the American Medical Association.
2008 average 50th Percentile Fees are provided courtesy of 2008 MMH-SI's copyrighted Physicians' Fees and Coding Guide.

Bibliography

Austin PE, Dunn KA, Eily-Cofield K, et al. Subcuticular sutures and the rate of inflammation in noncontaminated wounds. *Ann Emerg Med.* 1995;25:328.

Borges AF, Alexander JE. Relaxed skin tension lines, Z-plasties on scars, and fusiform excision of lesions. *Br J Plast Surg.* 1962;15:242–254.

Leshin B. Proper planning and execution of surgical excisions. In: Wheeler RG, ed. *Cutaneous Surgery*. Philadelphia: WB Saunders; 1994:171–177.

McGinness JL, Russell M. Surgical pearl: A technique for placement of buried sutures. *J Am Acad Dermatol.* 2006;55(1):123–124.

Mehta PH, Dunn KA, Bradfield JF, et al. Contaminated wounds: infection rates with subcutaneous sutures. *Ann Emerg Med.* 1996;27:43.

Moy RL, Lee A, Zalka A. Commonly used suturing techniques in skin surgery. *Am Fam Physician.* 1991;44:1625–1634.

Stegman SJ, Tromovitch TA, Glogau RG. *Basics of Dermatologic Surgery*. Chicago: Year Book Medical Publishing; 1982:60–68.

Stevenson TR, Jurkiewicz MJ. Plastic and reconstructive surgery. In: Schwartz SI, Shires GT, Spencer FC, et al., eds. *Principles of Surgery*. 5th ed. New York: McGraw-Hill; 1989:2081–2132.

Swanson NA. *Atlas of Cutaneous Surgery*. Boston: Little, Brown; 1987.

Vistnes LM. Basic principles of cutaneous surgery. In: Epstein E, Epstein E Jr, eds. *Skin Surgery*. 6th ed. Philadelphia: WB Saunders; 1987:44–55.

Zalla MJ. Basic cutaneous surgery. *Cutis.* 1994;53:172–186.

Zitelli J. TIPS for a better ellipse. *J Am Acad Dermatol.* 1990;22:101–103.

Zuber TJ, DeWitt DE. The fusiform excision. *Am Fam Physician.* 1994;49:371–376.

2008 MAG Mutual Healthcare Solutions, Inc.'s Physicians' Fee and Coding Guide. Duluth, Georgia. MAG Mutual Healthcare Solutions, Inc. 2007.

CHAPTER 38

Simple Interrupted Suture

E. J. Mayeaux Jr., MD, DABFP, FAAFP
Professor of Family Medicine, Professor of Obstetrics and Gynecology
Louisiana State University Health Sciences Center, Shreveport, LA

The simple interrupted suture has been one of the most commonly employed wound closure techniques in the past century. The goals of suture placement include closing dead space, producing hemostasis, supporting and strengthening the wound until healing increases its tensile strength, approximating skin edges for an aesthetically pleasing and functional result, and minimizing the risk of infection.

The simple suture can be used alone or in conjunction with deep sutures or vertical mattress sutures to provide optimal wound healing and cosmesis. Properly placed interrupted skin sutures incorporate symmetric amounts of tissue from each wound edge, evert the skin edges, and provide wound edge opposition without compromise of tissue blood flow. Interrupted skin sutures allow precise adjustments between stitches. Proper timing for suture removal allows for adequate healing (i.e., strength to the developing scar) and minimizes the development of suture marks (i.e., railroad or Frankenstein marks). Interrupted skin sutures also permit removal of selected stitches (e.g., every other stitch) to individualize the time sutures are present.

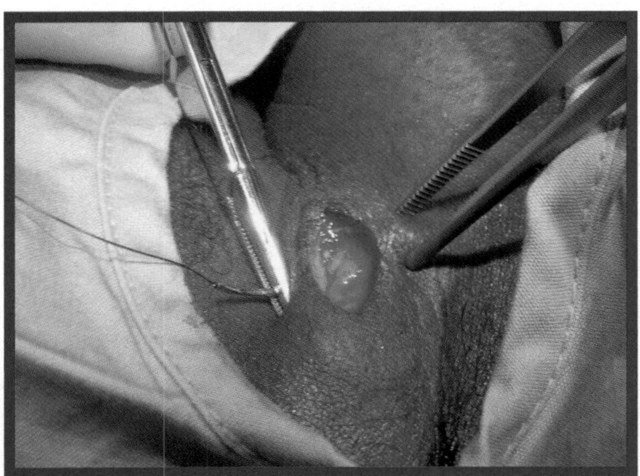

If the wound being closed is traumatic, then irrigation, foreign body removal, and necrotic tissue debridement are the main preventative measures against tissue infection. Otherwise good asepsis during the operative procedure minimizes infections (skin preparation recommendations appear in Appendix E). The skin wound-healing process occurs in several stages. Coagulation involving vasospasm, platelet aggregation, and fibrous clot formation begins immediately following the injury. Proteolytic enzymes released by neutrophils and macrophages break down local damaged tissue. Epithelialization then produces complete bridging of the wound within 48 hours after suturing. New blood vessel growth peaks about 4 days after the injury. Collagen formation is necessary to restore tensile strength to the skin. The collagen-formation process starts within 48 hours of the injury and peaks during the first week. Wound contraction occurs 3 to 4 days following the injury. Collagen production and remodeling continue for up to 12 months.

Wound-edge eversion is an important goal when placing interrupted skin sutures. Healing wounds have a natural tendency to become inverted, with the retraction that occurs over time within scars. Indented or inverted scars can cast a shadow on adjacent surfaces, and the shadow magnifies the appearance of the scar. Everted wounds are created so that the final scar is flat and esthetically pleasing. Eversion is accomplished by incorporating a greater amount of deep tissue in the needle path, which pushes together the deep tissue, causing upward lift to the wound edges.

The simple interrupted skin suture is used in a variety of clinical settings. The technique is used for superficial wounds when single-layer closure is indicated. Suture placement permits functional movement of an area after closure and is especially valuable over the dorsum of the fingers. Although simple sutures can be used to close wide surgical wounds, the distribution of tension to approximate the skin edges may be better handled with vertical or horizontal mattress skin sutures or by placement of deeply buried subcuticular sutures.

Nonabsorbable suture materials such as nylon generally are selected for interrupted suture placement. Smaller-caliber sutures (5-0 and 6-0) tend to produce less skin marking and scarring than larger-caliber sutures (3-0). Placement of tightly clustered sutures close to the wound edge distributes the skin edge tension better than placement of widely spaced sutures set back from the wound edge. Suggested suture removal times are listed in Appendix J.

Wound adhesives (superglues that contain acrylates) are an alternate means for wound closure. Some practitioners believe that wound edge eversion is superior with suture closure, but adhesives can produce good cosmetic results for wounds with closely approximated edges. Wound closure tapes (Steri-Strips) are reinforced microporous surgical adhesive tapes that are used to provide extra support to a suture line, before or after sutures are removed. Wound closure tapes may reduce spreading of the scar if they are kept in place for several weeks after suture removal. They are rarely used for primary wound closure. Stainless steel staples are frequently used in wounds under high tension, including wounds on the scalp and trunk. Advantages of staples include quick placement, minimal tissue reaction, and strong wound closure. Disadvantages include less precise wound edge alignment, cost, and potential for poor cosmetic outcomes.

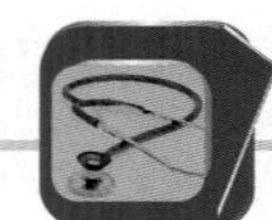

Equipment

- Instruments for simple interrupted skin suture placement are found in Appendix G and can be ordered through local surgical supply houses.
- Suture materials can be ordered from Ethicon, Somerville, NJ (http://ecatalog.ethicon.com/EC_ECATALOG/ethicon/default.asp).
- A suggested anesthesia tray that can be used for this procedure is listed in Appendix F.
- Skin preparation recommendations are shown in Appendix E.

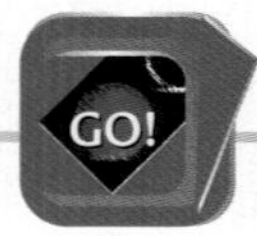

Indications

- Superficial wounds that can be closed in a single layer
- Eversion of wound edges after approximation with mattress or buried sutures
- Marking of skin for correct anatomic approximation (e.g., vermilion border)
- Closure of wounds over areas of movement such as flexor creases or on the dorsum of the fingers

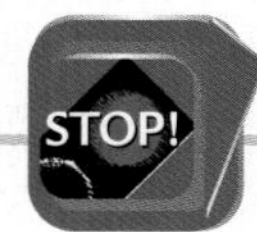

Contraindications (Relative)

- Widely separated wound edges that are better approximated with tension-reducing sutures
- Severe bleeding disorders
- Extreme illness that would make wound healing difficult

- Cellulitis in the tissues to be incised
- Conditions that may interfere with wound healing (collagen vascular diseases, smoking, renal insufficiency, diabetes mellitus, nutritional status, obesity, chemotherapeutic agents, and corticosteroids)
- Disorders of collagen synthesis that affect wound healing, such as Ehlers-Danlos syndrome and Marfan syndrome
- Concurrent medications that may increase the likelihood of intraoperative bleeding (aspirin, other nonsteroidal anti-inflammatory drugs, warfarin)
- Uncooperative patient
- Emergency triage situations that do not allow time for interrupted closure (consider running sutures)

The Procedure

Step 1. A retracted scar on a vertical surface, such as the face, produces a shadow that magnifies the appearance of the scar (A). Wound edges should be everted at closure (B) so that subsequent scar retraction will produce a final scar that is flat (C).

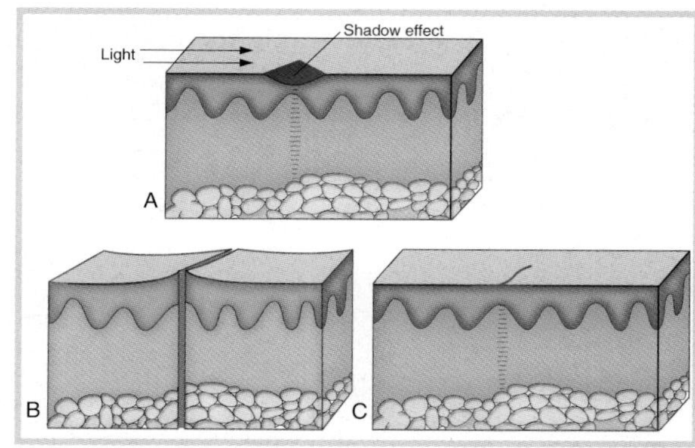

Step 1

Step 2. The poorly performed, "scooped" passage of a suture needle across both wound edges (A) will fail to create proper closure. The stitch should be deeper than it is wide, and similar to the thickness of the dermis. The needle should enter the skin vertically (B) and exit the skin vertically.

- **PEARL:** Gentle handling of the tissue is also important to optimize wound healing. Do not grab or pinch epidermis edges that are expected to heal.

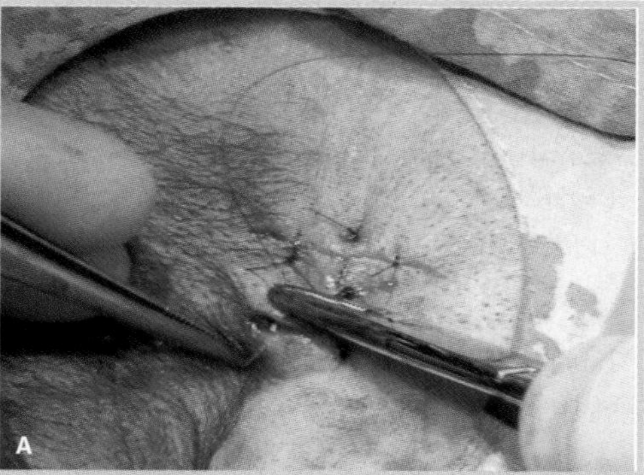

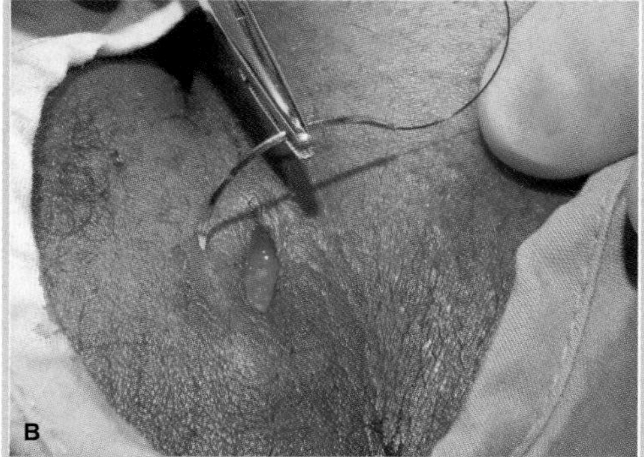

Step 2

Step 3. Symmetric amounts of tissue from each wound edge should be included in the passage of the suture. Uneven bites of tissue in the distance from the edge or the depth of passage (A) produce a closure with uneven edges (B). The resulting scar will cast a shadow and be cosmetically inferior.

- **PITFALL:** Forcefully pushing or twisting the needle when passing it through the tissue will cause the body of the needle to bend or break. Follow the curve of the needle. Do not apply twisting or torquing forces to the needle. Regrasp (remount) the needle in the center of the wound rather than force a small needle through both wound edges. If the needle bends, remove it and open another suture pack. Broken needle tips can result in hours of frustrating searching to find the broken piece.

Step 3

Step 4. The proper needle path to produce wound edge eversion is in the shape of a flask. There are several techniques that will achieve this effect.

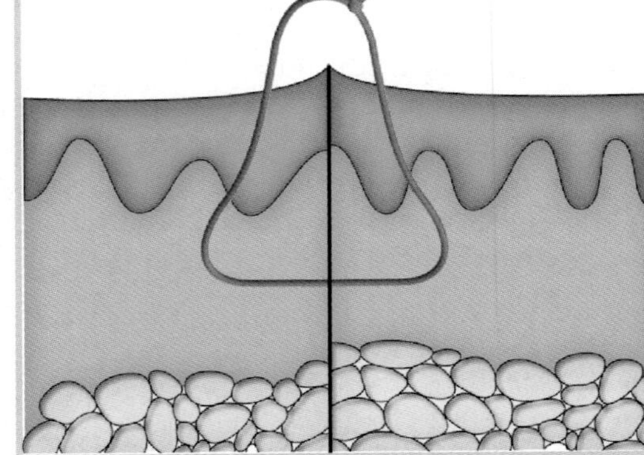

Step 4

Step 4a. The first method involves using the nondominant hand to pinch the skin edges together, causing the tissue to have the appearance of exaggerated eversion. When the nondominant hand relaxes, the tissue returns to its natural position. The suture path is flask shaped, and with tying, the suture produces eversion.

- **PITFALL:** Grasping the wound edges with the fingers increases the risk for an inadvertent needlestick.

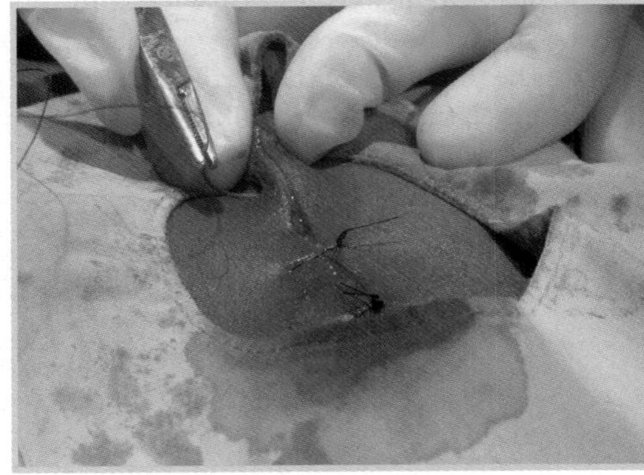

Step 4a

Step 4b. The next method uses the nondominant hand or a forceps to push down on each wound edge, causing the tissue in the deep portion of the wound to move toward the center of the wound. The needle enters the skin vertically and exits the skin vertically. When the nondominant hand relaxes, the tissue returns to its natural position. The suture path is flask shaped, and with tying, the suture produces eversion.

- PITFALL: Pushing down on the wound edges with the fingers increases the risk for an inadvertent needlestick. Instruments can be used to push down on the wound edges to minimize this risk. If the fingers are used, exert added care to minimize the risk of a needle injury.

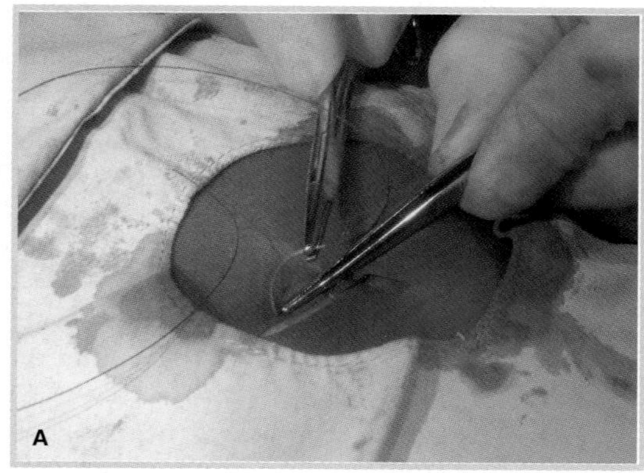

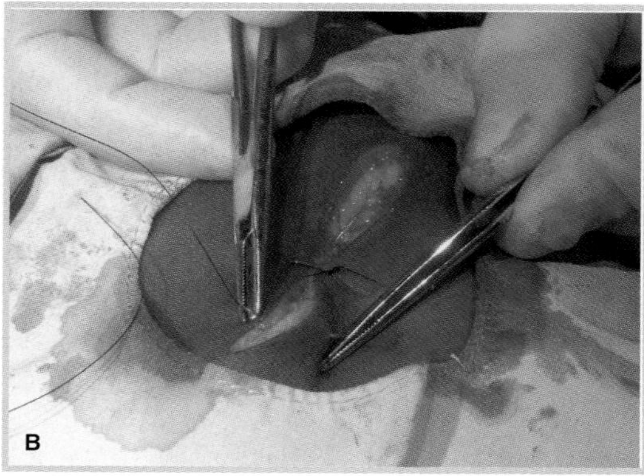

Step 4b

Step 4c. An alternative method to produce a flask-shaped path is technically more difficult. As the needle enters the right wound edge, the nondominant hand grasps tissue beneath the wound edge using forceps and pulls tissue to the center of the wound. Before the needle passes through the opposite wound edge, the deep tissue from that side is pulled to the center of the wound with a backhanded technique.

- PITFALL: Avoid traumatizing the skin or deep tissue with the forceps. Traumatized tissue may necrose, creating excessive time for healing and inferior cosmetic results.

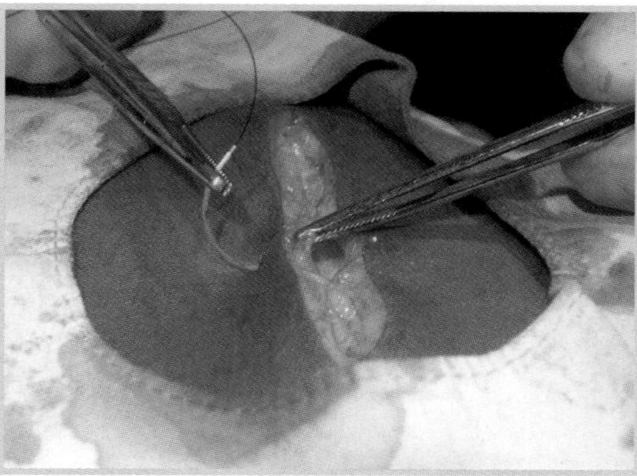

Step 4c

Step 5. Instrument tie the suture (see Chapter 36). Make sure the wound is closed completely without gaps, and add additional interrupted sutures as needed. Antibiotic ointment is placed over the sutured wound, and a dressing is applied.

- **PEARL:** In general, the final sutures should be about as far apart as they are wide.
- PITFALL: Tension in the wound may cause the provider to place sutures with enough tension to strangulate the tissue. Removing tension from a wound with undermining and tension-reducing sutures allows percutaneous sutures to be tied loosely and removed sooner, thereby improving the cosmetic result.
- PITFALL: Make sure to pull the knots off to one side of the incision so that the knot doesn't get buried in the contracting healing wound and causing pain on removal.

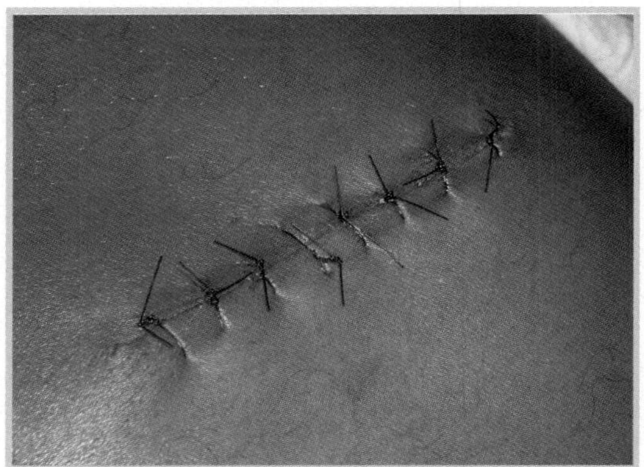

Step 5

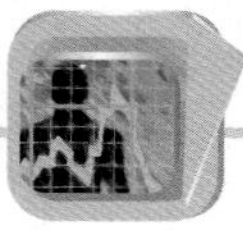

Complications

- Bleeding
- Infection
- Scar formation

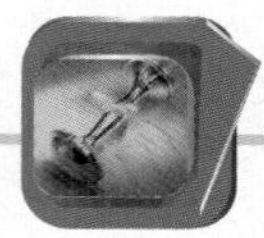

Pediatric Considerations

Generally, pediatric skin has excellent blood flow and heals very well. However, pediatric patients often find it difficult to sit and lie still during lengthy procedures. The patient's maturity and ability to cooperate should be considered before deciding to attempt any outpatient procedure. Sometimes it is necessary to sedate the patient to repair the laceration (see Chapter 122). The maximum recommended dose for lidocaine in children is 3 to 5 mg/kg, and 7 mg/kg when combined with epinephrine. Neonates have an increased volume of distribution, decreased hepatic clearance, and doubled terminal elimination half-life (3.2 hours).

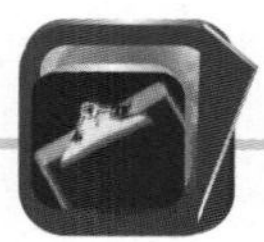

Postprocedure Instructions

Have the patient use a small amount of antibiotic ointment and cover the wound with a small bandage. Instruct the patient to gently wash the area after 1 day. Have the patient dry the area well after washing and use a small amount of antibiotic ointment to promote moist healing. Instruct the patient not to pick at or scratch the wound.

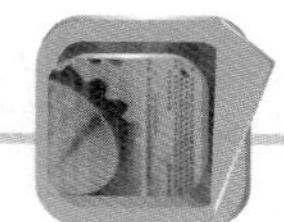

Coding Information and Supply Sources

All codes listed are for superficial wound closure using sutures, staples, or tissue adhesives with or without adhesive strips on the skin surface. If a layered closure is required, use intermediate closure codes 12031 to 12057 or complex repair codes 13100 to 13160.

Add together the lengths of wounds in the same classification and anatomic sites. Use separate codes for repairs from different anatomic sites. Debridement is considered a separate procedure only when gross contamination requires prolonged cleansing or when appreciable amounts of devitalized or contaminated tissue are removed.

CPT Code	Description	2008 Average 50th Percentile Fee	Global Period
12001	Simple repair SNAGTEHF ≤2.5 cm	$220.00	10
12002	Simple repair SNAGTEHF 2.6–7.5 cm	$235.00	10
12004	Simple repair SNAGTEHF 7.6–12.5 cm	$285.00	10
12005	Simple repair SNAGTEHF 12.6–20.0 cm	$408.00	10
12006	Simple repair SNAGTEHF 20.1–30.0 cm	$506.00	10
12007	Simple repair SNAGTEHF >30.0 cm		10
12011	Simple repair FEENLMM ≤2.5 cm	$240.00	10
12013	Simple repair FEENLMM 2.6–5.0 cm	$288.00	10
12014	Simple repair FEENLMM 5.1–7.5 cm	$351.00	10
12015	Simple repair FEENLMM 7.6–12.5 cm	$449.00	10
12016	Simple repair FEENLMM 12.6–20.0 cm	$585.00	10
12017	Simple repair FEENLMM 20.1–30.0 cm	$743.00	10
12018	Simple repair FEENLMM >30.0 cm		10
12020	Treatment of superficial wound dehiscence, simple closure	$397.00	10

CPT is a registered trademark of the American Medical Association.
2008 average 50th Percentile Fees are provided courtesy of 2008 MMH-SI's copyrighted Physicians' Fees and Coding Guide.
SNAGTEHF, scalp, neck, axillae, external genitalia, trunk, extremities, hands, and feet;
FEENLMM, face, ears, eyelids, nose, lips, and mucous membranes.

Patient Education Handout

Patient education handouts, "Stitches" and "Why Get Stitches?," can be found on the book's Web site.

Bibliography

Bennett RG. *Fundamentals of Cutaneous Surgery*. St. Louis: CV Mosby; 1988:384–394.

Brown JS. *Minor Surgery: A Text and Atlas*. 3rd ed. London: Chapman & Hall; 1997:70–96. *Ethicon Wound Closure Manual*. Somerville, NJ: Ethicon; 1994.

Lammers RL, Trott AT. Methods of wound closure. In: Roberts JR, Hedges JR, eds. *Clinical Procedures in Emergency Medicine*. 3rd ed. Philadelphia: WB Saunders; 1998:560–598.

McCarthy JG. *Plastic Surgery*. Philadelphia: WB Saunders; 1990:1–68.

Moy RL, Lee A, Zalka A. Commonly used suturing techniques in skin surgery. *Am Fam Physician*. 1991;44:1625–1634.

Moy RL. Suturing techniques. In: Usatine RP, Moy RL, Tobnick EL, et al., eds. *Skin Surgery*. St. Louis: Mosby; 1998:88–100.

Odland PB, Murakami CS. Simple suturing techniques and knot tying. In: Wheeland RG, ed. *Cutaneous Surgery*. Philadelphia: WB Saunders; 1994:178–188.

Spicer TE. Techniques of facial lesion excision and closure. *J Dermatol Surg Oncol.* 1982;8:551–556.

Stegman SJ, Tromovitch TA, Glogau RG. *Basics of Dermatologic Surgery*. Chicago: Year Book Medical Publishers; 1984:41–42.

Swanson NA. *Atlas of Cutaneous Surgery*. Boston: Little, Brown; 1987:26–28.

Zuber TJ. *Basic Soft-Tissue Surgery*. Kansas City: American Academy of Family Physicians; 1998:34–38.

2008 MAG Mutual Healthcare Solutions, Inc.'s Physicians' Fee and Coding Guide. Duluth, Georgia. MAG Mutual Healthcare Solutions, Inc. 2007.

CHAPTER 39

Corner Suture

E. J. Mayeaux Jr., MD, DABFP, FAAFP

Professor of Family Medicine, Professor of Obstetrics and Gynecology
Louisiana State University Health Sciences Center, Shreveport, LA

The corner suture (also know as the *half-buried horizontal mattress suture* or *tip stitch*) is used to securely suture the tip of a flap of skin into a matching skin defect. If the corner of the flap were to be closed using simple interrupted or running sutures, the two sutures closest to the tip would interfere with the blood supply to the tip, increasing the chance of tip necrosis. Because the corner suture secures the tip without the suture crossing the top of the incision, it does not impede blood flow and may decrease the chance of necrosis of the flap tip.

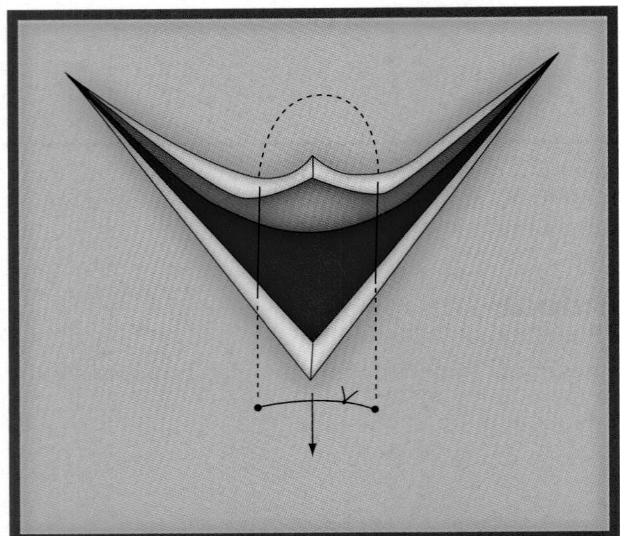

The corner suture is based on the horizontal mattress suture, but the part that passes through the tip is buried in the dermis. It is usually performed using 3-0 to 5-0 nonabsorbable sutures to minimize inflammation in the flap tip. Like most mattress sutures, consider removing the corner sutures earlier than the other sutures in the closure, because the part of the corner suture crossing the surface of the skin may cause damage and scarring if removal is delayed. This is less of a problem with corner sutures than with vertical mattress sutures (see Appendix J).

The main disadvantage of the corner suture is that close approximation of wound edges without trauma to the flap tip can be difficult. Careful control of the tension induced when tying the suture can minimize this problem.

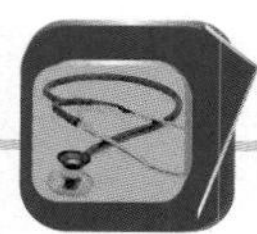

Equipment

Common skin surgery equipment and the typical skin surgery tray are listed in Appendix G.

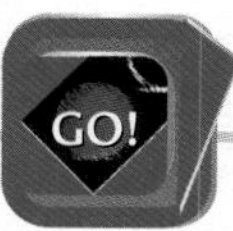

Indications

- Approximating the tip of a skin flap with the corresponding defect
- Approximating corners of skin flaps when performing tissue rearrangements such as T-plasties, V-Y-plasties, and the centers of advancement flaps
- As part of Burow's triangle repairs, especially when suturing unequal length skin edges and when performing tissue rearrangements (such as rotation flaps, O-to-Z-plasties, and the ends of advancement flaps

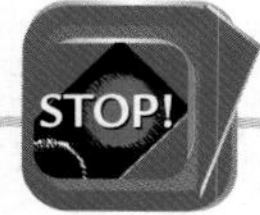

Contraindications (Relative)

- Uncooperative patient
- Wounds best closed by other methods
- Presence of cellulitis, bacteremia, or active infection

The Procedure

Step 1. The corner suture must be laid out correctly to achieve optimal results. It is often helpful to visualize or to draw a baseline that exactly bisects the flap tip and continues through the skin containing the defect into which the tip will be sutured. The entry and exit points of the suture will be parallel to this baseline.

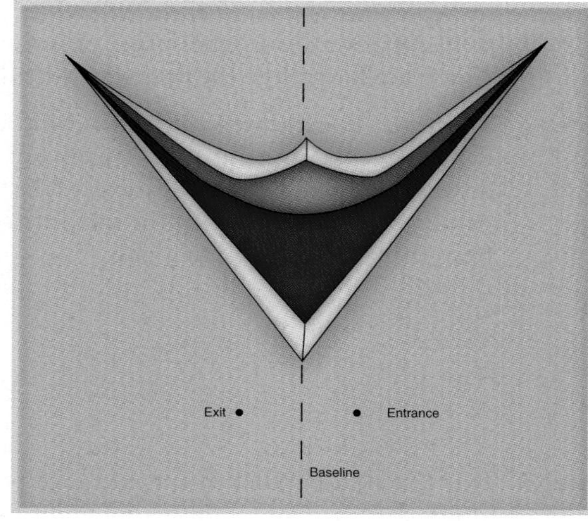

Step 1

Step 2. Begin the suture on the side of the wound containing the defect into which the tip will be sutured. The suture enters through the epidermis about 4 to 8 mm from the skin edge and is passed through the dermis of the wound edge. The path of the needle should be parallel to the baseline.

- **PITFALL:** The needle should *not* go all the way through the skin into the subcuticular tissue, as is the case with most other suturing techniques. The path of the needle is directly into the dermis, at which level it will remain until it exits the skin before tying.

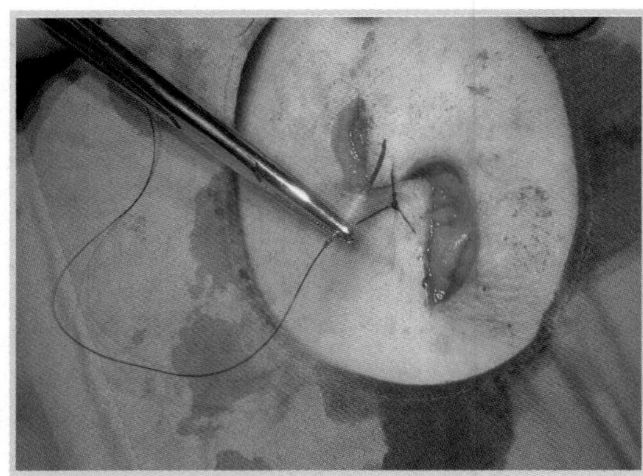

Step 2

Step 3. The needle is then passed horizontally, making a 5-mm loop arcing through the end of tip in the same dermal plane, exiting on the opposite side of the flap tip.

- **PEARL:** This pass may be made with the flap in anatomical position and with the needle drivers in a vertical position. However, many providers find it helpful to *gently* elevate the tip between the sides of pickups (do not actually grab or apply pressure to the flap tip), placing the tip in a vertical position for this pass.
- **PITFALL:** If the flap tip is grasped, the chances of tip necrosis are greatly elevated.
- **PEARL:** Make sure the suture passes symmetrically through the tip for best results.

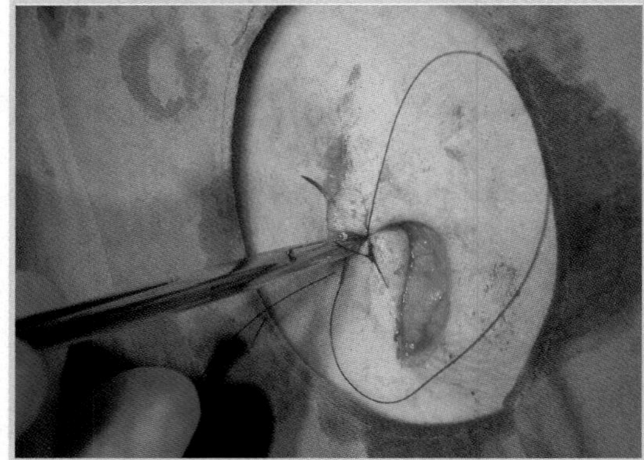

Step 3

Step 4. The needle then reenters the skin to which the flap is being attached at the same level of the dermis. This pass should be parallel to the first pass and the baseline and at the same distance from the baseline as the first pass.

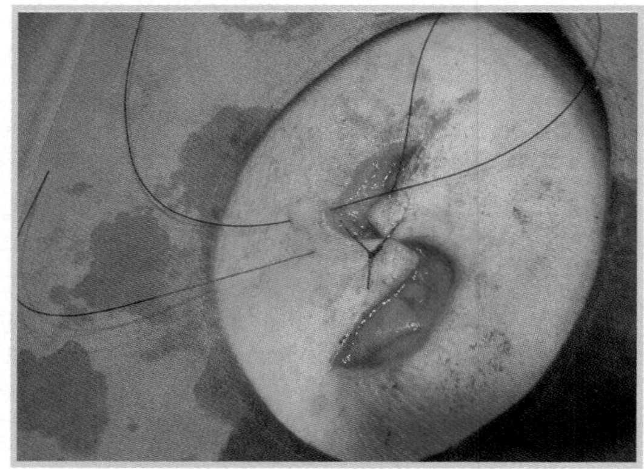

Step 4

Step 5. Exit the skin parallel to the entrance point along the line of pull (baseline) and tie the suture (see Chapter 36, Basic Instrument Suture Tie).

- **PITFALL:** Be careful not to tie the suture too loosely because this will cause poor approximation of the wound edge.
- **PITFALL:** Be careful not to tie the suture too tightly because this can cause bunching of the skin, over- or underriding of the flap tip, or an increased risk of scarring under the knot.

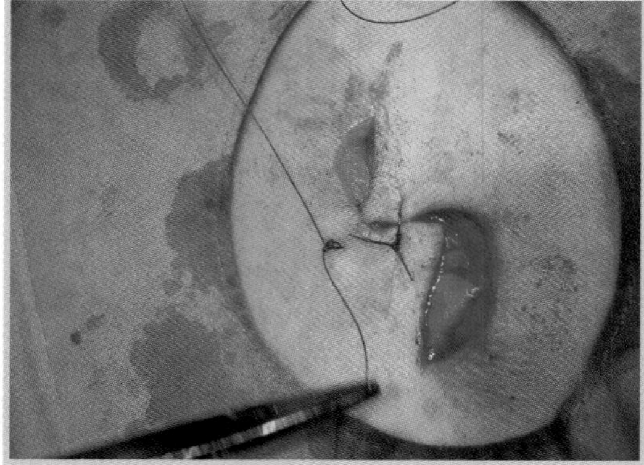

Step 5

Step 6. Multiple corners may be brought together by expanding the arc of the dermal pass to include all of the tips. This is frequently used in advancement and other flaps.

- **PEARL:** Make sure the suture passes symmetrically in a smooth arc through all of the tips for best results.

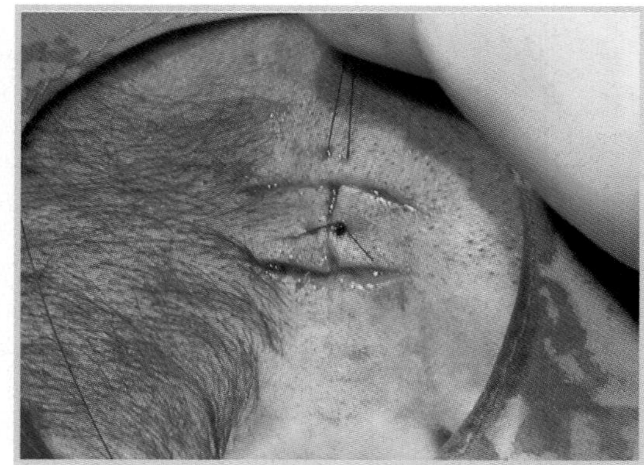

Step 6

Step 7. Similarly, this technique may be used to repair Y-shaped lacerations and stellate lacerations.

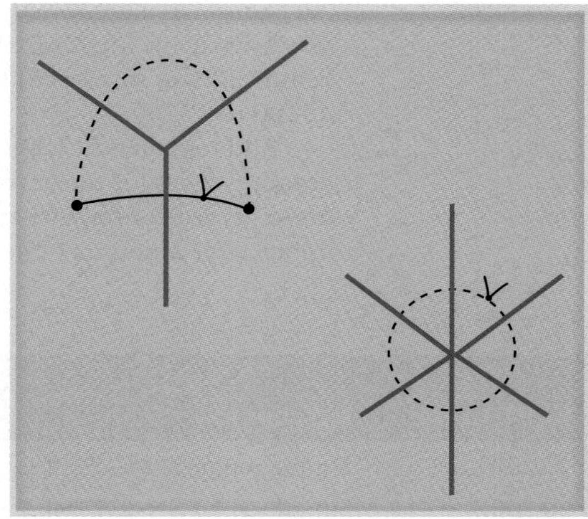

Step 7

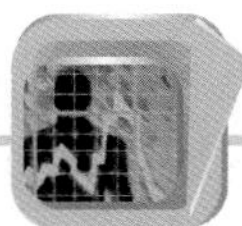

Complications

- Bleeding
- Infection
- Scar formation

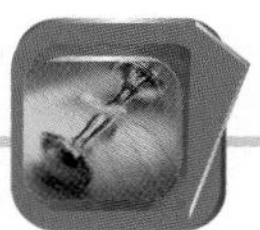

Pediatric Considerations

Generally, pediatric skin has excellent blood flow and heals very well. However, pediatric patients often find it difficult to sit and lie still during lengthy procedures. The patient's maturity and ability to cooperate should be considered before deciding to attempt any outpatient procedure. Sometimes it is necessary to sedate the patient to repair the laceration (see Chapter 122). The maximum recommended dose for lidocaine in children is 3 to 5 mg/kg, and 7 mg/kg when combined with epinephrine. Neonates have an increased volume of distribution, decreased hepatic clearance, and doubled terminal elimination half-life (3.2 hours).

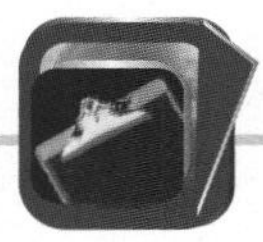

Postprocedure Instructions

Instruct the patient to gently wash an area that has been stitched after 1 day but not to put the wound into standing water for 2 to 3 days. Have the patient dry the area well after washing and use a small amount of antibiotic ointment to promote moist healing. Recommend wound elevation to help lessen swelling, reduce pain, and speed healing. Instruct the patient not to pick at, break, or cut the stitches. Have the patient cover the wound with a nonocclusive dressing for 2 to 3 days. The dressing should be left in place for at least 48 hours, after which time most wounds can be opened to air. Scalp wounds can be left open if small, but large head wounds can be wrapped circumferentially with rolled gauze.

Most uncontaminated wounds do not need to be seen by a provider until suture removal, unless signs of infection develop. Highly contaminated wounds should be seen for follow-up in 2 to 3 days. Give discharge instructions to the patient regarding signs of wound infection.

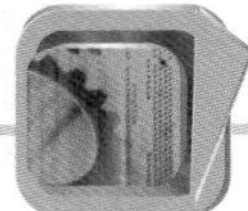

Coding Information and Supply Sources

All codes listed are for superficial wound closure using sutures, staples, or tissue adhesives, with or without adhesive strips on the skin surface. If a layered closure is required, use intermediate closure codes 12031 to 12057 or complex repair codes 13100 to 13160.

Add together the lengths of wounds in the same classification and anatomic sites. Use separate codes for repairs from different anatomic sites. Debridement is considered a separate procedure only when gross contamination requires prolonged cleansing or when appreciable amounts of devitalized or contaminated tissue are removed.

CPT Code	Description	2008 Average 50th Percentile Fee	Global Period
12001	Simple repair SNAGTEHF ≤2.5 cm	$220.00	10
12002	Simple repair SNAGTEHF 2.6–7.5 cm	$235.00	10
12004	Simple repair SNAGTEHF 7.6–12.5 cm	$285.00	10
12005	Simple repair SNAGTEHF 12.6–20.0 cm	$408.00	10
12006	Simple repair SNAGTEHF 20.1 to –30.0 cm	$506.00	10
12007	Simple repair SNAGTEHF >30.0 cm		10
12011	Simple repair FEENLMM ≤2.5 cm	$240.00	10
12013	Simple repair FEENLMM 2.6–5.0 cm	$288.00	10
12014	Simple repair FEENLMM 5.1–7.5 cm	$351.00	10
12015	Simple repair FEENLMM 7.6–12.5 cm	$449.00	10
12016	Simple repair FEENLMM 12.6–20.0 cm	$585.00	10
12017	Simple repair FEENLMM 20.1–30.0 cm	$743.00	10
12018	Simple repair FEENLMM >30.0 cm		10
12020	Treatment of superficial wound dehiscence, simple closure	$397.00	10

CPT is a registered trademark of the American Medical Association.
2008 average 50th Percentile Fees are provided courtesy of 2008 MMH-SI's copyrighted Physicians' Fees and Coding Guide.
SNAGTEHF, scalp, neck, axillae, external genitalia, trunk, extremities, hands, and feet;
FEENLMM, face, ears, eyelids, nose, lips, and mucous membranes.

Bibliography

Adams B, Anwar J, Wrone DA, et al. Techniques for cutaneous sutured closures: variants and indications. *Semin Cutan Med Surg.* 2003;22(4):306–316.

Kandel EF, Bennett RG. The effect of stitch type on flap tip blood flow. *J Am Acad Dermatol.* 2001;44:265–272.

Moy RL, Lee A, Zalka A. Commonly used suturing techniques in skin surgery. *Am Fam Physician.* 1991;44:1625–1634.

Stasko T. Advanced suturing techniques and layered closures. In: Wheeland RG, ed. *Cutaneous Surgery.* Philadelphia: WB Saunders; 1994:304–317.

Stegman SJ. Suturing techniques for dermatologic surgery. *J Dermatol Surg Oncol.* 1978;4:63–68.

Zuber TJ. *Basic Soft-Tissue Surgery*. Kansas City: American Academy of Family Physicians; 1998:34–38.

2008 MAG Mutual Healthcare Solutions, Inc.'s Physicians' Fee and Coding Guide. Duluth, Georgia. MAG Mutual Healthcare Solutions, Inc. 2007.

CHAPTER 40

Horizontal Mattress Suture

E. J. Mayeaux Jr., MD, DABFP, FAAFP

Professor of Family Medicine, Professor of Obstetrics and Gynecology
Louisiana State University Health Sciences Center, Shreveport, LA

The horizontal mattress suture is an everting suture technique that allows separated wound edges to be approximated. The horizontal mattress suture evenly distributes the closure tension along the wound edge by incorporating a large amount of tissue within the passage of the suture thread. The technique is commonly employed for pulling wound edges over a distance or as the initial suture to anchor two wound edges (e.g., holding a skin flap in place).

Thin skin tends to tear with placement of simple, interrupted sutures. The horizontal mattress suture is effective in the closure of fragile, elderly skin or the skin of individuals receiving chronic steroid therapy. The horizontal mattress suture technique also is effective in closing defects of thin skin on the eyelid and in the finger and toe web spaces. Control of bleeding is another advantage of this suture. Hemostasis develops when a large amount of tissue is incorporated within the passage of a suture. The technique can produce effective bleeding control on vascular tissues such as the scalp.

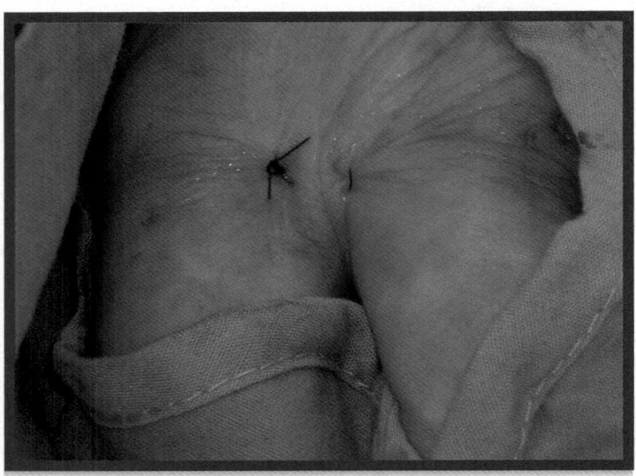

Certain skin defects tend to have skin edges that roll inward. Inversion of the wound edge can retard healing and promote wound complications. The horizontal mattress suture produces strong everting forces on the wound edge and can prevent inversion in susceptible wounds in the intergluteal cleft, groin, or posterior neck. The *running horizontal mattress suture* is also useful for wounds under moderate tension, especially when a more rapid closure is desired.

After placement of horizontal mattress sutures, the loops of suture thread that remain above the skin surface can compress the skin and produce pressure necrosis and scarring. This scarring potential limits the use of the horizontal mattress sutures on the face. Pressure injury commonly develops when the sutures are tied too tightly. Bolsters are compressible cushions placed within the extracutaneous loops of suture to prevent pressure injury to the skin. Some of the commonly used materials in bolsters include plastic tubing, cardboard, and gauze.

Skin compression injury can be reduced by early removal of horizontal mattress sutures. Some authorities recommend removal in 3 to 5 days, with the surrounding interrupted sutures left in place longer. Early suture removal is especially valuable when the horizontal mattress technique is employed in cosmetically important body locations such as the head and neck.

The half-buried horizontal mattress suture combines elements of the horizontal mattress suture with an intradermal closure. It can be used to approximate the corner of a flap (see Chapter 39) or to close normal suture lines, especially along the edges of a flap. This allows for minimum disruption of blood flow to the edge and tip of the newly created flap.

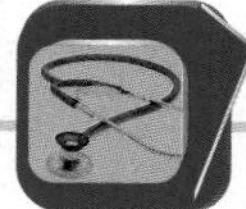

Equipment

- Surgery tray instruments are listed in Appendix G. Consider adding skin hooks to gently handle the skin flaps. Have at least three fine (mosquito) hemostats to assist with hemostasis while developing large skin flaps.
- Suggested suture removal times are listed in Appendix J, and a suggested anesthesia tray that can be used for this procedure is listed in Appendix F. All instruments can be ordered through local surgical supply houses.

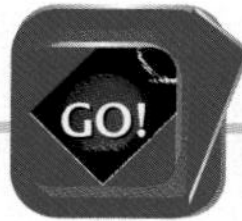

Indications

- Closure of thin or atrophic skin (e.g., elderly skin, eyelids, individuals on chronic steroid therapy)
- Eversion of skin defects prone to inversion (e.g., posterior neck, groin, intergluteal skin defects)
- Closure of bleeding scalp wounds
- Closure of web space skin defects (e.g., finger or toe web spaces)
- Closure of wounds under high tension

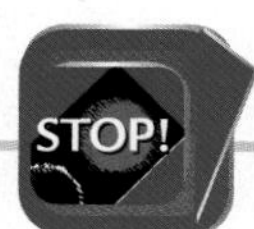

Contraindications (Relative)

- Skin with poor blood flow
- Severe bleeding disorders
- Local infection

The Procedure

Horizontal Mattress Suture

Step 1. The suture needle is passed from the right side of the wound to the left side of the wound, in a manner similar to when starting a simple interrupted suture.

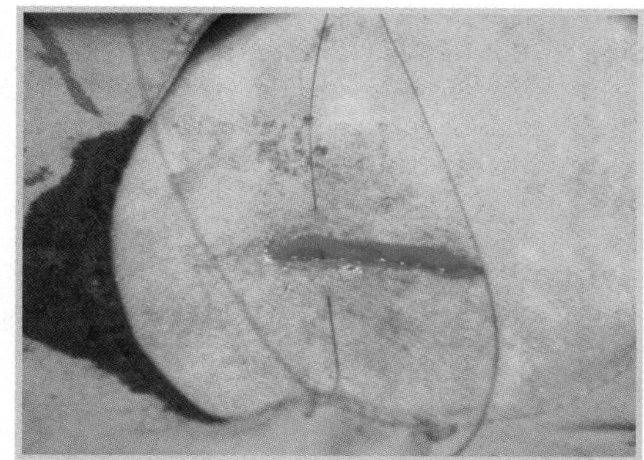

Step 1

Step 2. The entry and exit sites of the wound generally are 4 to 8 mm from the wound edge. Do not tie the suture! The needle is placed backward in the needle driver, and then the suture is passed back from the left side to the right side.

- **PEARL:** The distance down the suture line for the second pass is about one half to two thirds of the suture width across the wound.

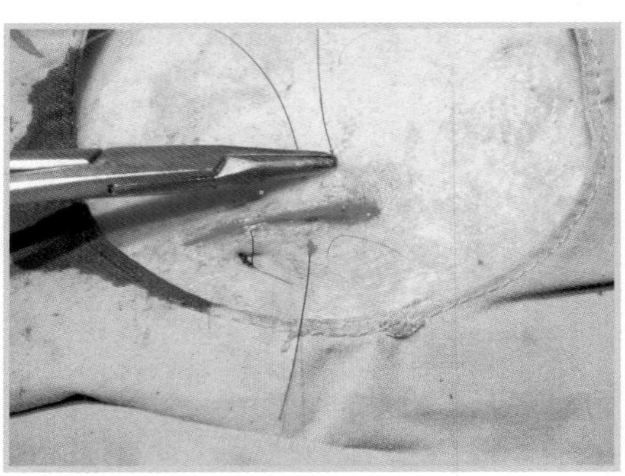

Step 2

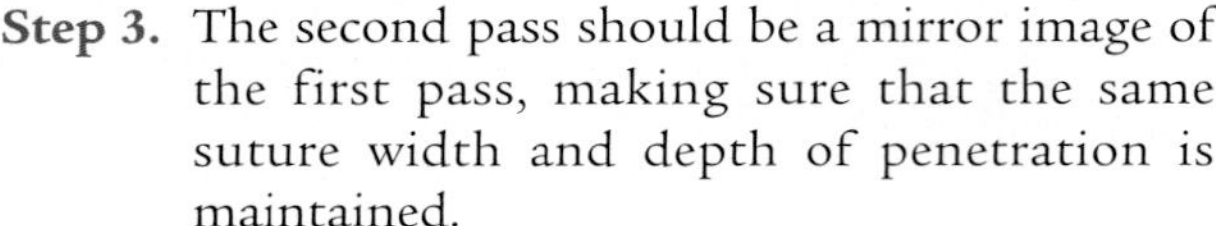

Step 3. The second pass should be a mirror image of the first pass, making sure that the same suture width and depth of penetration is maintained.

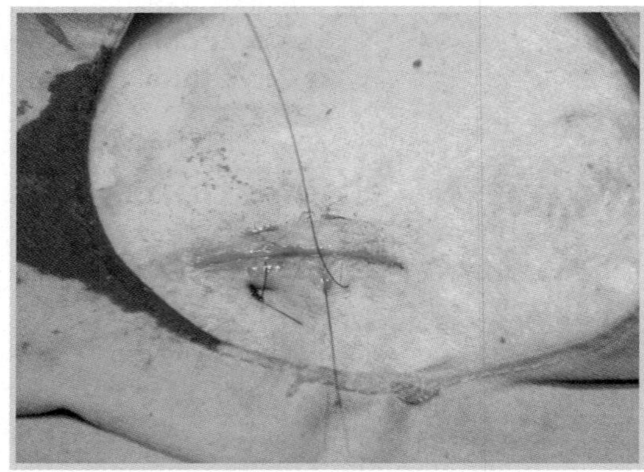

Step 3

Step 4. The horizontal mattress suture is tied, producing skin edge eversion. Tying the suture tightly produces extra eversion.

- **PITFALL:** Although the added eversion may appear beneficial at the time of wound closure, tight knots often produce skin pressure necrosis. Avoid the temptation to tie the horizontal mattress suture tightly.

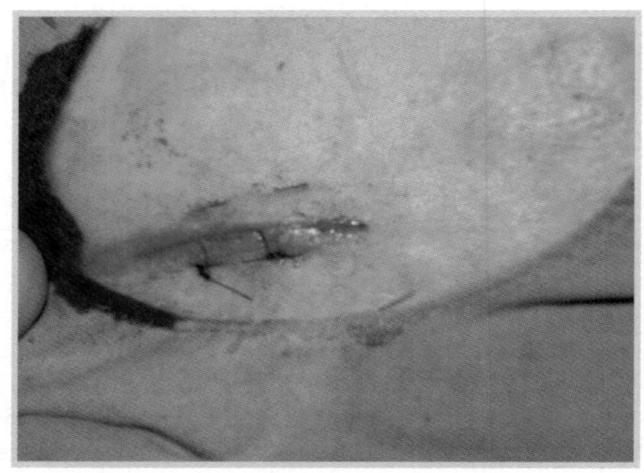

Step 4

Step 5. Bolsters can cushion the skin from the pressure produced by the extracutaneous loops of a horizontal mattress suture. Gauze is used in these bolsters.

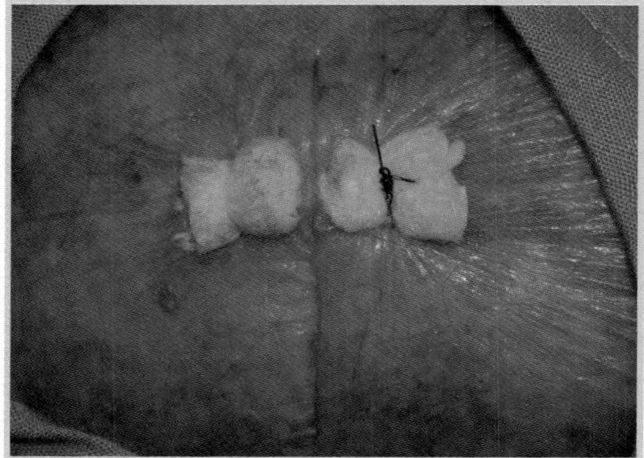

Step 5

Step 6. Horizontal mattress sutures are often used to close a finger web wound.

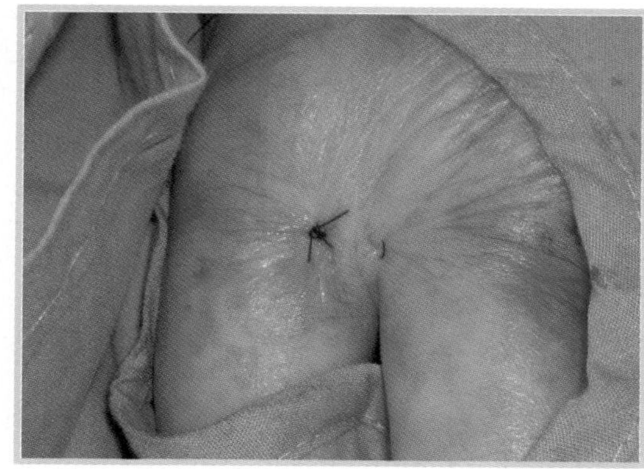

Step 6

Running Mattress Suture

Step 7. The running mattress suture may be used to quickly close a longer laceration. Start by placing a simple interrupted suture but cutting off only the short tail.

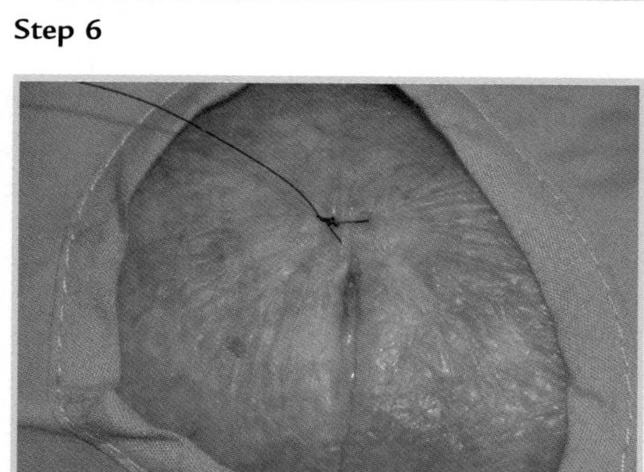

Step 7

Step 8. The needle is then placed backward in the needle driver, and the suture is passed back from the left side to the right side as before.

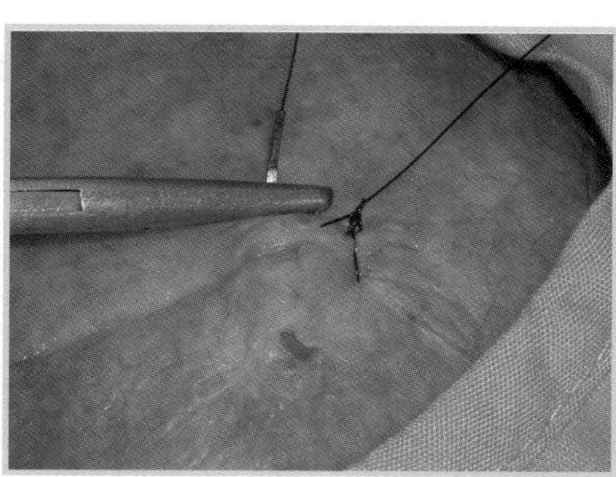

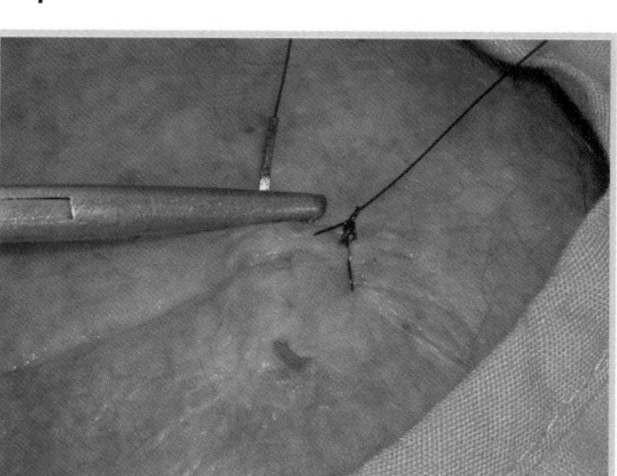

Step 8

Step 9. Rather than securing a completed horizontal mattress stitch, the leading end travels laterally again and then reenters the skin to begin the next horizontal mattress in the series.

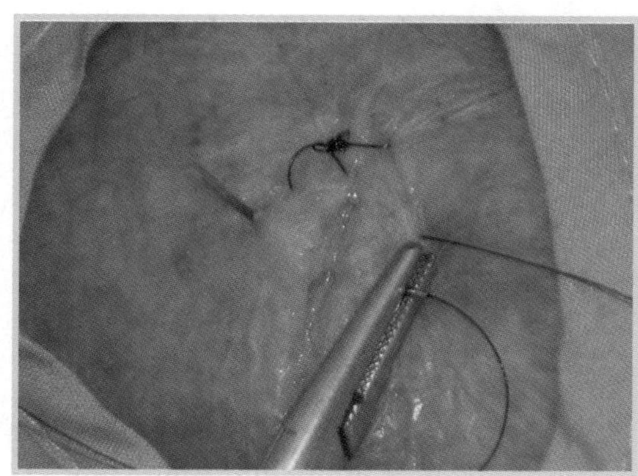

Step 9

Step 10. When the end of the laceration is reached, the last loop of suture is used as the tail to tie off the suture.

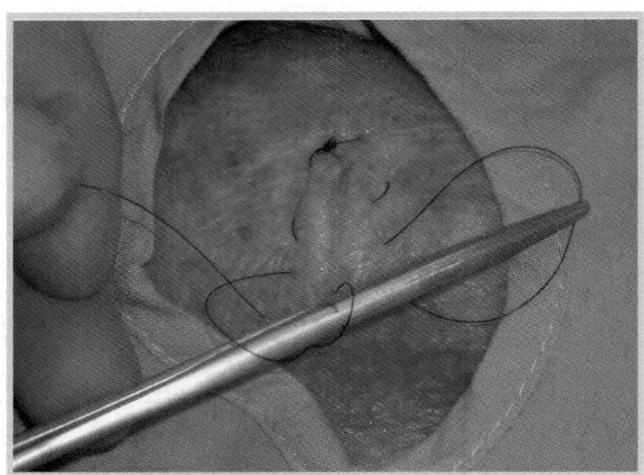

Step 10

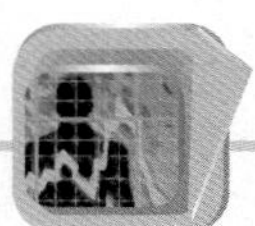

Complications

- Bleeding
- Infection
- Scar formation
- Suture marks, especially if left in place for more than 7 days
- Tissue strangulation and wound edge necrosis if sutures are tied too tightly

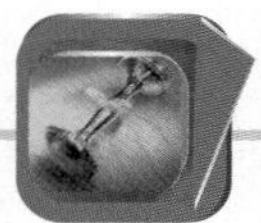

Pediatric Considerations

Generally, pediatric skin has excellent blood flow and heals very well. However, pediatric patients often find it difficult to sit or lie still during lengthy procedures. The patient's maturity and ability to cooperate should be considered before deciding to attempt any outpatient procedure. Sometimes it is necessary to sedate the patient to repair the laceration (see Chapter 122). The maximum recommended dose of lidocaine in children is 3 to 5 mg/kg, and 7 mg/kg when combined with epinephrine. Neonates have an increased volume of distribution, decreased hepatic clearance, and doubled terminal elimination half-life (3.2 hours).

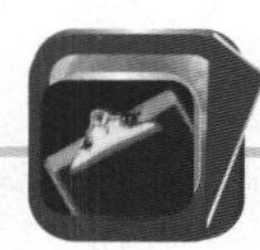

Postprocedure Instructions

Instruct the patient to gently wash an area that has been stitched after 1 day but not to put the wound into standing water for 2 to 3 days. Have the patient use a small amount of antibiotic ointment to promote moist healing. Recommend wound elevation to lessen swelling, reduce pain, and speed healing. Instruct the patient not to pick at, break, or cut the stitches. Have them cover the wound with a nonocclusive dressing for 2 to 3 days. A simple adhesive bandage (Band-Aid) will suffice for many small lacerations. The dressing should be left in place for at least 48 hours, after which time most wounds can be opened to air. Scalp wounds can be left open if small, but large head wounds can be wrapped circumferentially with rolled gauze.

Most uncontaminated wounds do not need to be seen by a provider until suture removal, unless signs of infection develop. Highly contaminated wounds should be seen for follow-up in 2 to 3 days. Give discharge instructions to the patient regarding signs of wound infection.

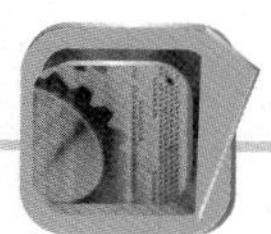

Coding Information and Supply Sources

All codes listed are for superficial wound closure using sutures, staples, or tissue adhesives with or without adhesive strips on the skin surface. The mattress suture closures are considered a variation of single-layered closure, and the codes 12001 to 12021 apply for wound repair.

Add together the lengths of wounds in the same classification and anatomic sites. Use separate codes for repairs from different anatomic sites. Debridement is considered a separate procedure only when gross contamination requires prolonged cleansing or when appreciable amounts of devitalized or contaminated tissue are removed.

CPT Code	Description	2008 Average 50th Percentile Fee	Global Period
12001	Simple repair SNAGTEHF ≤2.5 cm	$220.00	10
12002	Simple repair SNAGTEHF 2.6–7.5 cm	$235.00	10
12004	Simple repair SNAGTEHF 7.6–12.5 cm	$285.00	10
12005	Simple repair SNAGTEHF 12.6–20.0 cm	$408.00	10
12006	Simple repair SNAGTEHF 20.1–30.0 cm	$506.00	10
12007	Simple repair SNAGTEHF >30.0 cm		10
12011	Simple repair FEENLMM ≤2.5 cm	$240.00	10
12013	Simple repair FEENLMM 2.6–5.0 cm	$288.00	10
12014	Simple repair FEENLMM 5.1–7.5 cm	$351.00	10
12015	Simple repair FEENLMM 7.6–12.5 cm	$449.00	10
12016	Simple repair FEENLMM 12.6–20.0 cm	$585.00	10
12017	Simple repair FEENLMM 20.1–30.0 cm	$743.00	10
12018	Simple repair FEENLMM >30.0 cm		10
12020	Treatment of superficial wound dehiscence, simple closure	$397.00	10

CPT is a registered trademark of the American Medical Association.
2008 average 50th Percentile Fees are provided courtesy of 2008 MMH-SI's copyrighted Physicians' Fees and Coding Guide.
SNAGTEHF, scalp, neck, axillae, external genitalia, trunk, extremities, hands, and feet;
FEENLMM, face, ears, eyelids, nose, lips, and mucous membranes.

Bibliography

Adams B, Anwar J, Wrone DA, et al. Techniques for cutaneous sutured closures: variants and indications. *Semin Cutan Med Surg.* 2003;22(4):306–316.

Chernosky ME. Scalpel and scissors surgery as seen by the dermatologist. In: Epstein E, Epstein E Jr, eds. *Skin Surgery.* 6th ed. Philadelphia: WB Saunders; 1987:88–127.

Coldiron BM. Closure of wounds under tension: the horizontal mattress suture. *Arch Dermatol.* 1989;25:1189–1190.

Ethicon Wound Closure Manual. Somerville, NJ: Ethicon; 1994.

Gault DT, Brian A, Sommerlad BC, et al. Loop mattress suture. *Br J Surg.* 1987;74:820–821.

Moy RL, Lee A, Zalka A. Commonly used suturing techniques in skin surgery. *Am Fam Physician.* 1991;44:1625–1634.

Stasko T. Advanced suturing techniques and layered closures. In: Wheeland RG, ed. *Cutaneous Surgery.* Philadelphia: WB Saunders; 1994:304–317.

Stegman SJ, Tromovitch TA, Glogau RG. *Basics of Dermatologic Surgery*. Chicago: Year Book Medical Publishing; 1982.
Swanson NA. *Atlas of Cutaneous Surgery*. Boston: Little, Brown; 1987:30–35.
Zuber TJ. The illustrated manuals and videotapes of soft-tissue surgery techniques. Kansas City: American Academy of Family Physicians; 1998.
Zuber TJ. The mattress sutures: vertical, horizontal, and corner stitch. *Am Fam Physician.* 2002;66:2231–2236.
2008 MAG Mutual Healthcare Solutions, Inc.'s Physicians' Fee and Coding Guide. Duluth, Georgia. MAG Mutual Healthcare Solutions, Inc. 2007.

CHAPTER 41

Running Cutaneous Suture

E. J. Mayeaux Jr., MD, DABFP, FAAFP
Professor of Family Medicine, Professor of Obstetrics and Gynecology
Louisiana State University Health Sciences Center, Shreveport, LA

The running (continuous) cutaneous suture provides a rapid and convenient means of wound closure. This technique is similar to simple interrupted sutures, except that the suture material is not cut and tied with each succeeding suture placement. The suture evenly distributes tension along the length of a wound, thereby preventing damage to the skin edges from excessive tightness of individual sutures. Because suture material is not consumed in creating repetitive knots and cutting ends, this technique can provide cost savings in limiting the use of suture material. This suture method is used primarily in wounds that are well approximated, not under much tension, have a low risk of infection, or require rapid closure.

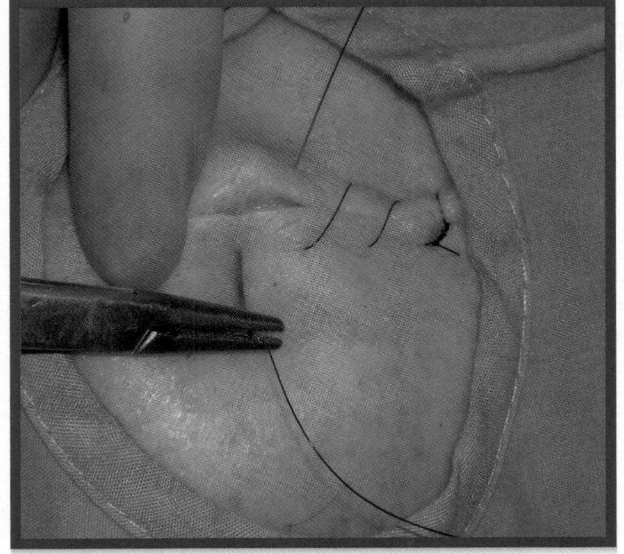

The running cutaneous suture may not provide much skin edge eversion and is generally avoided in cosmetically important areas such as the face. Another disadvantage of a running cutaneous suture is that if the suture thread breaks, the entire wound may dehisce. In addition, this suture may achieve less accurate edge approximation compared with interrupted sutures, final adjustments cannot be made once it is placed, and it can only be removed in its entirety from the skin. A continuous suture does not permit selective removal of sutures in response to healing. Interestingly, the strength of wound closure and the likelihood of dehiscence are equivalent with both interrupted and running sutures. Because the entire suture is removed at one time, slightly longer times before removal are recommended.

The *running locked suture* is a variation of the simple running suture technique. Before beginning each new throw, the needle is looped under the previous external segment of suture crossing the wound. The locked loops counteract some tension on the skin edges, and so this technique may help prevent inversion even in wounds closed under tension. However, the pressure exerted by the external loops may cause focal necrosis. Because this method may produce inferior cosmetic outcomes, it is not commonly used.

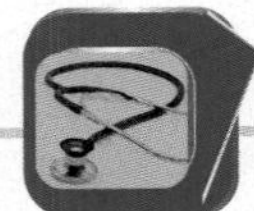

Equipment

- The basic skin-suturing instruments used are listed in Appendix G.
- A suggested anesthesia tray that can be used for this procedure is listed in Appendix F.
- Skin preparation recommendations appear in Appendix E.

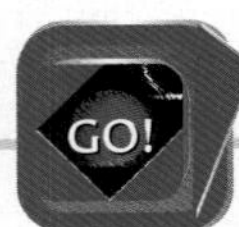

Indications

- Emergency triage situations that do not allow time for interrupted closure
- Closure of long wounds in less cosmetically important (nonfacial) areas
- Shallow wounds with loose skin nearby, such as the scrotum or dorsum of the hand
- To secure a split- or full-thickness skin graft

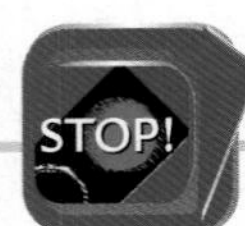

Contraindications (Relative)

- Widely separated wound edges that are better approximated with tension-reducing sutures
- Severe bleeding disorders
- Extreme illness that would make wound healing difficult
- Cellulitis in the tissues to be incised
- Conditions that may interfere with wound healing (collagen vascular diseases, smoking, renal insufficiency, diabetes mellitus, nutritional status, obesity, chemotherapeutic agents, and corticosteroids)
- Disorders of collagen synthesis that affect wound healing such as Ehlers-Danlos syndrome and Marfan syndrome
- Concurrent medications that may increase the likelihood of intraoperative bleeding (aspirin, other nonsteroidal anti-inflammatory drugs, warfarin)
- Uncooperative patient
- Patients with a propensity to pick at wounds or sutures

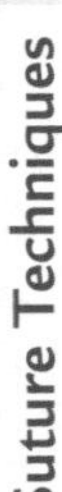

The Procedure

Step 1. The closure begins with placement of a simple interrupted suture at one end of the wound. The free end is cut, but the long end (with the needle attached) is not cut.

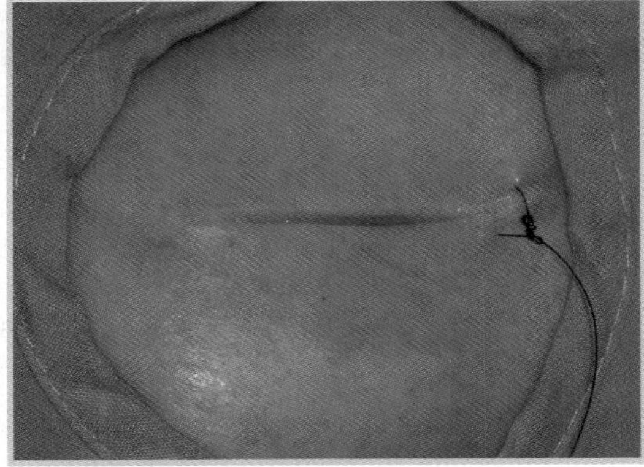

Step 1

Step 2. Reverse the suture needle, move down the incision one suture length, and make another pass across the wound.

- **PITFALL:** Many providers immediately start making diagonal passes across the top of the incision at this point, but this allows the knot to migrate across the incision, loosening the sutures.

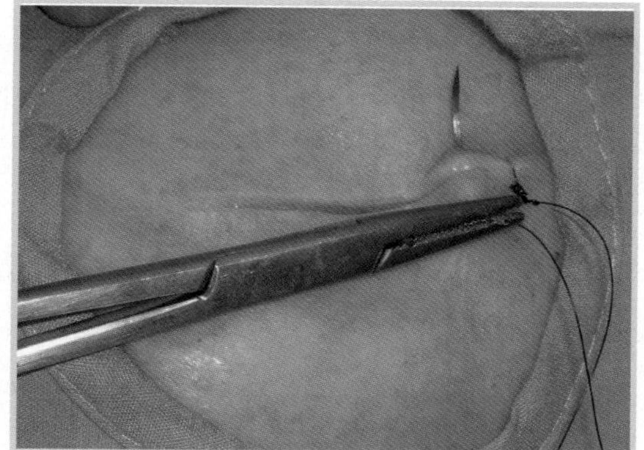

Step 2

Step 3. Multiple passes are made straight across the wound, moving down the wound edge about 4 to 5 mm to initiate each pass, with the suture thread at a 60-degree angle to the wound.

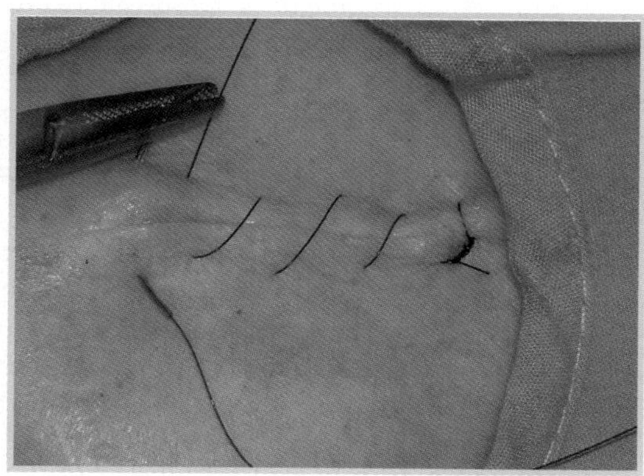

Step 3

Step 4. The suture thread beneath the wound is perpendicular to the long axis of the wound. At the far end of the wound, the suture is tied by looping the suture over the needle driver and reaching back to grasp the final loop across the wound.

- **PEARL:** Make sure the sutures are evenly spaced and the tension is distributed along the suture line.
- **PITFALL:** Do not tie the suture too tightly. The wound edges will bunch up if the final knot is too tight.

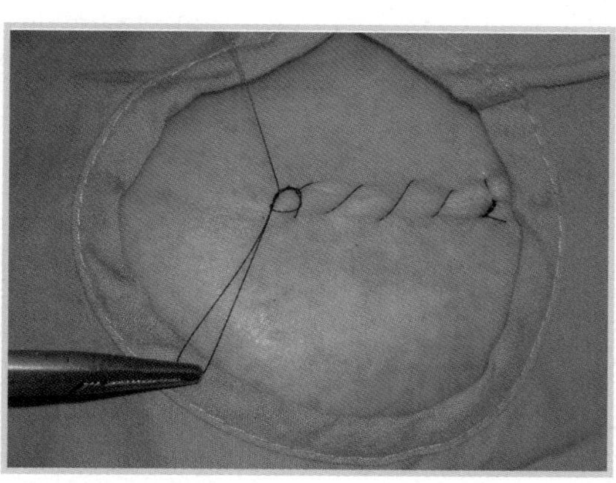

Step 4

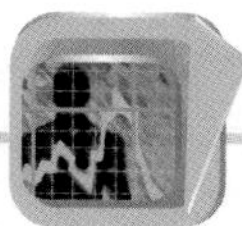

Complications

- Bleeding
- Infection
- Scar formation

- Crosshatch scarring, especially when the suture is pulled too tightly
- Uneven wound edges
- Puckering of the wound
- Wound dehiscence if the suture thread breaks

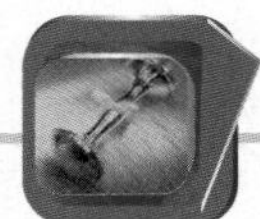

Pediatric Considerations

Generally, pediatric skin has excellent blood flow and heals very well. However, pediatric patients often find it difficult to sit or lie still during lengthy procedures. The patient's maturity and ability to cooperate should be considered before deciding to attempt any outpatient procedure. Sometimes it is necessary to sedate the patient to repair the laceration (see Chapter 122). The maximum recommended dose of lidocaine in children is 3 to 5 mg/kg, and 7 mg/kg when combined with epinephrine. Neonates have an increased volume of distribution, decreased hepatic clearance, and doubled terminal elimination half-life (3.2 hours).

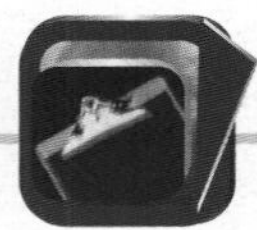

Postprocedure Instructions

Instruct the patient to gently wash an area that has been stitched after 1 day but not to put the wound into standing water for 2 to 3 days. Have the patient dry the area well after washing and use a small amount of antibiotic ointment to promote moist healing. Recommend wound elevation to lessen swelling, reduce pain, and speed healing. Instruct the patient not to pick at, break, or cut the stitches. Have them cover the wound with a nonocclusive dressing for 2 to 3 days. A simple adhesive bandage (Band-Aid) will suffice for many small lacerations. The dressing should be left in place for at least 48 hours, after which time most wounds can be opened to air. Scalp wounds can be left open if small, but large head wounds can be wrapped circumferentially with rolled gauze.

Most uncontaminated wounds do not need to be seen by a provider until suture removal, unless signs of infection develop. Highly contaminated wounds should be seen for follow-up in 2 to 3 days. Give discharge instructions to the patient regarding signs of wound infection.

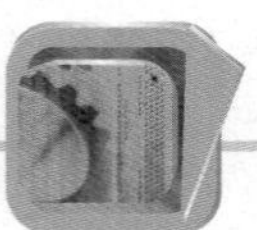

Coding Information and Supply Sources

All codes listed are for superficial wound closure using sutures, staples, or tissue adhesives with or without adhesive strips on the skin surface. If a layered closure is required, use alternate codes: intermediate closure codes 12031 to 12057 or complex repair codes 13100 to 13160.

Add together the lengths of wounds in the same classification and anatomic sites. Use separate codes for repairs from different anatomic sites. Debridement is considered a separate procedure only when gross contamination requires prolonged cleansing or when appreciable amounts of devitalized or contaminated tissue are removed.

CPT Code	Description	2008 Average 50th Percentile Fee	Global Period
12001	Simple repair SNAGTEHF ≤2.5 cm	$220.00	10
12002	Simple repair SNAGTEHF 2.6–7.5 cm	$235.00	10
12004	Simple repair SNAGTEHF 7.6–12.5 cm	$285.00	10
12005	Simple repair SNAGTEHF 12.6–20.0 cm	$408.00	10
12006	Simple repair SNAGTEHF 20.1–30.0 cm	$506.00	10
12007	Simple repair SNAGTEHF >30.0 cm		10
12011	Simple repair FEENLMM ≤2.5 cm	$240.00	10
12013	Simple repair FEENLMM 2.6–5.0 cm	$288.00	10
12014	Simple repair FEENLMM 5.1–7.5 cm	$351.00	10
12015	Simple repair FEENLMM 7.6–12.5 cm	$449.00	10
12016	Simple repair FEENLMM 12.6–20.0 cm	$585.00	10
12017	Simple repair FEENLMM 20.1–30.0 cm	$743.00	10
12018	Simple repair FEENLMM >30.0 cm		10
12020	Treatment of superficial wound dehiscence, simple closure	$397.00	10

CPT is a registered trademark of the American Medical Association.
2008 average 50th Percentile Fees are provided courtesy of 2008 MMH-SI's copyrighted Physicians' Fees and Coding Guide.
SNAGTEHF, scalp, neck, axillae, external genitalia, trunk, extremities, hands, and feet;
FEENLMM, face, ears, eyelids, nose, lips, and mucous membranes.

Bibliography

Adams B, Anwar J, Wrone DA, et al. Techniques for cutaneous sutured closures: variants and indications. *Semin Cutan Med Surg.* 2003;22(4):306–316.

Bennett RG. *Fundamentals of Cutaneous Surgery*. St. Louis: Mosby; 1988:464–465.

Boutros S, Weinfeld AB, Friedman JD. Continuous versus interrupted suturing of traumatic lacerations: a time, cost, and complication rate comparison. *J Trauma*. 2000;48:495–497.

Brown JS. *Minor Surgery: A Text and Atlas*. 3rd ed. London: Chapman & Hall; 1997:70–96.

Lammers RL, Trott AL. Methods of wound closure. In: Roberts JR, Hedges JR, eds. *Clinical Procedures in Emergency Medicine*. 3rd ed. Philadelphia: WB Saunders; 1998:560–598.

Moy RL. Suturing techniques. In: Usatine RP, Moy RL, Tobnick EL, et al., eds. *Skin Surgery: A Practical Guide.* St. Louis: Mosby; 1998:88–100.

Moy RL, Lee A, Zalka A. Commonly used suturing techniques in skin surgery. *Am Fam Physician*. 1991;44:1625–1634.

Stasko T. Advanced suturing techniques and layered closures. In: Wheeland RG, ed. Philadelphia: WB Saunders; 1994:304–317.

Stegman SJ, Tromovitch TA, Glogau RG. *Basics of Dermatologic Surgery*. Chicago: Year Book Medical Publishing; 1984:45–48.

Swanson NA. *Atlas of Cutaneous Surgery*. Boston: Little, Brown; 1987:42–45.

Wong NL. Review of continuous sutures in dermatologic surgery. *J Dermatol Surg Oncol.* 1993;19:923–931.

Zuber TJ. *Basic Soft-Tissue Surgery*. Kansas City: American Academy of Family Physicians; 1998:58–69.

Zukin DD, Simon RR. Emergency wound care: principles and practice. Rockville, MD: Aspen, 1987:51–54.

2008 MAG Mutual Healthcare Solutions, Inc.'s Physicians' Fee and Coding Guide. Duluth, Georgia. MAG Mutual Healthcare Solutions, Inc. 2007.

CHAPTER 42

Running Subcuticular (Intracutaneous) Suture

E. J. Mayeaux Jr., MD, DABFP, FAAFP
Professor of Family Medicine, Professor of Obstetrics and Gynecology
Louisiana State University Health Sciences Center, Shreveport, LA

The running subcuticular (intracutaneous) suture is an elegant but technically demanding and time-consuming technique for wound closure. This suture is commonly used when skin suture marks must be avoided. Certain body locations such as the face, neck, and breast favor the placement of running intracutaneous sutures. This suture also is indicated when closing erythematous forehead skin or facial skin with extensive sebaceous gland activity, which can develop prominent suture marks. This technique is best applied to shallow wounds or to wounds with the edges narrowed by placement of deep buried sutures (see Chapter 37).

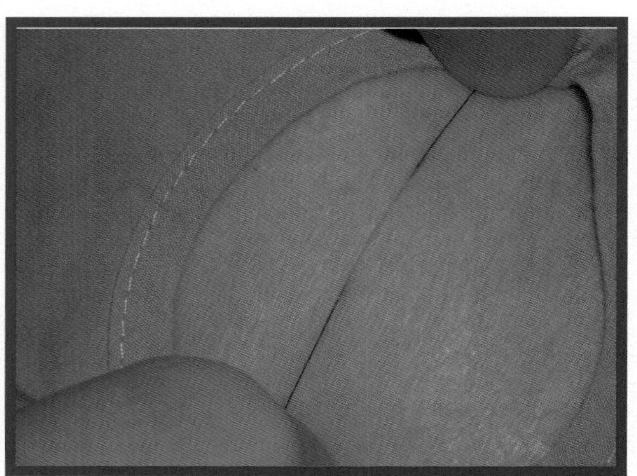

The running intracutaneous suture is placed within the dermis using a horizontal back-and-forth looping action. Although an absorbable suture such as Monocryl or Vicryl is often used, especially for children, some providers prefer a nonabsorbable suture because it produces less tissue reaction. Nonabsorbable intradermal sutures remain in place for 2 to 4 weeks. A slippery suture material such as polypropylene (Prolene) is often selected to facilitate suture removal when nonabsorbable sutures are used. Because long sutures can be difficult to extract after several weeks, placement of extracutaneous loops of suture in the center of a long suture can aid in removal.

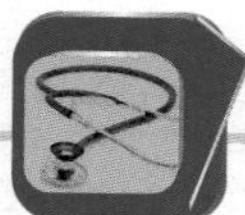

Equipment

- The basic skin-suturing instruments used are listed in Appendix G. A suggested anesthesia tray that can be used for this procedure is listed in Appendix F. Skin preparation recommendations appear in Appendix E.

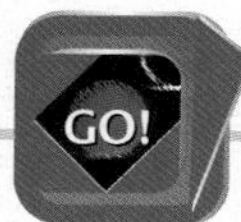

Indications

- Closure of cosmetically sensitive areas where suture marks must be avoided, such as the head and neck
- When closing forehead defects
- When closing facial skin with extensive sebaceous gland activity
- Closure of wounds on highly vascular, ruddy, or plethoric skin
- Closure of wounds on skin subject to increased motion, such as the neck
- Closure of breast wounds or surgical sites that are subject to expansion and suture marks

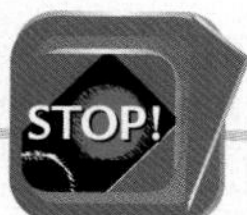

Contraindications (Relative)

- Widely separated wound edges that are better approximated with tension-reducing sutures
- Severe bleeding disorders
- Extreme illness that would make wound healing difficult
- Cellulitis in the tissues to be incised
- Conditions that may interfere with wound healing (collagen vascular diseases, smoking, renal insufficiency, diabetes mellitus, nutritional status, obesity, chemotherapeutic agents, and corticosteroids)
- Disorders of collagen synthesis that affect wound healing such as Ehlers-Danlos syndrome and Marfan syndrome
- Concurrent medications that may increase the likelihood of intraoperative bleeding (aspirin, other nonsteroidal anti-inflammatory drugs, warfarin)
- Uncooperative patient
- Emergency triage situations that do not allow time for interrupted closure (consider running sutures)

The Procedure

Step 1. The running subcuticular suture may be started with a deep buried suture using a slick absorbable suture (See Chapter 37, Deep Buried Dermal Suture).

- **PEARL:** If multiple deep buried sutures are placed to relieve tension in the wound, the knot may be the last deep suture placed at one end.

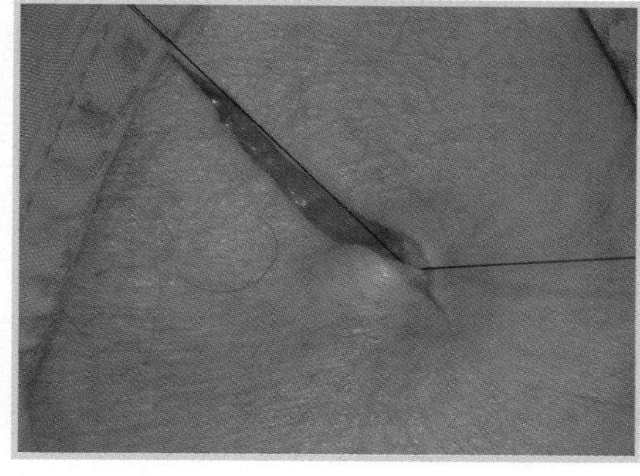

Step 1

Step 2. Pass the needle from the deep space into the midplane of the dermis.

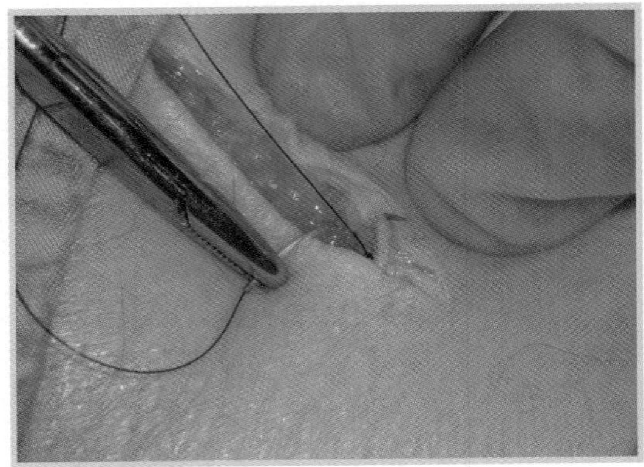

Step 2

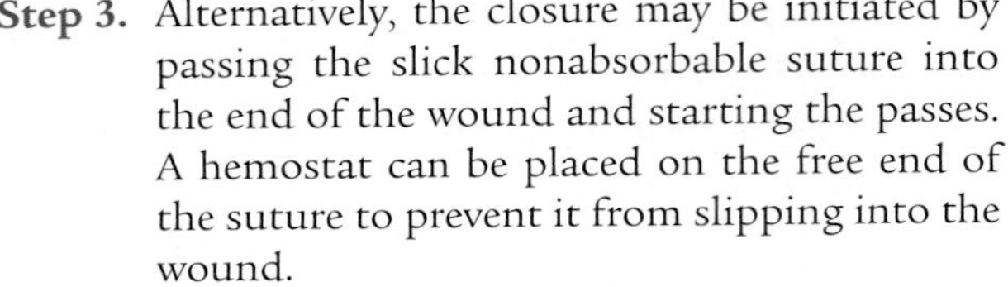

Step 3. Alternatively, the closure may be initiated by passing the slick nonabsorbable suture into the end of the wound and starting the passes. A hemostat can be placed on the free end of the suture to prevent it from slipping into the wound.

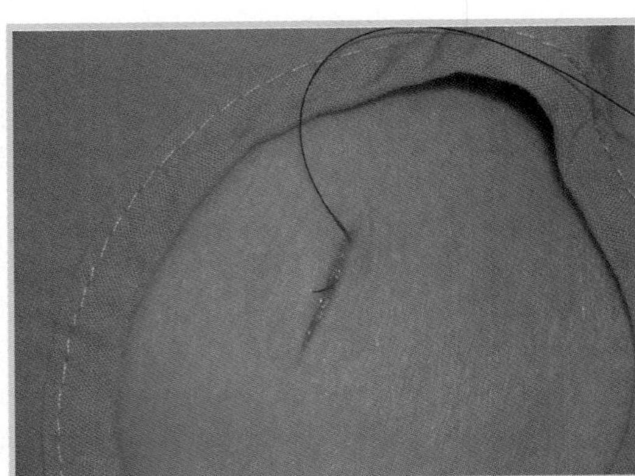

Step 3

Step 4. With either starting method, a horizontal, intracutaneous loop is created back and forth through each side of the wound in the same plane of the dermis. The suture comes straight across the wound with each successive pass.

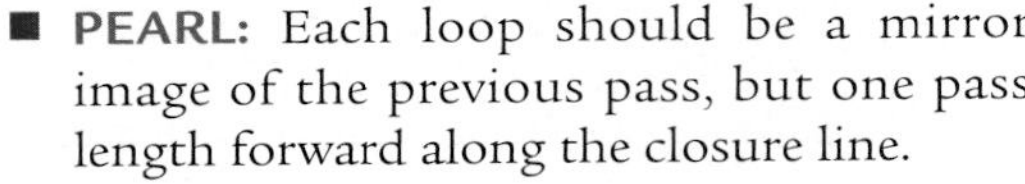

- **PEARL:** Each loop should be a mirror image of the previous pass, but one pass length forward along the closure line.

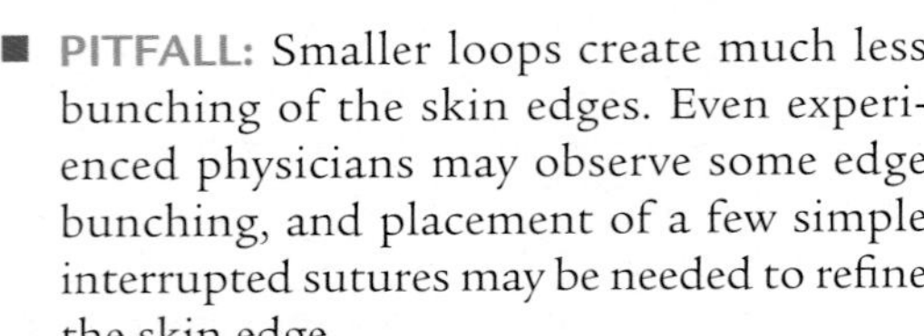

- **PITFALL:** Smaller loops create much less bunching of the skin edges. Even experienced physicians may observe some edge bunching, and placement of a few simple interrupted sutures may be needed to refine the skin edge.

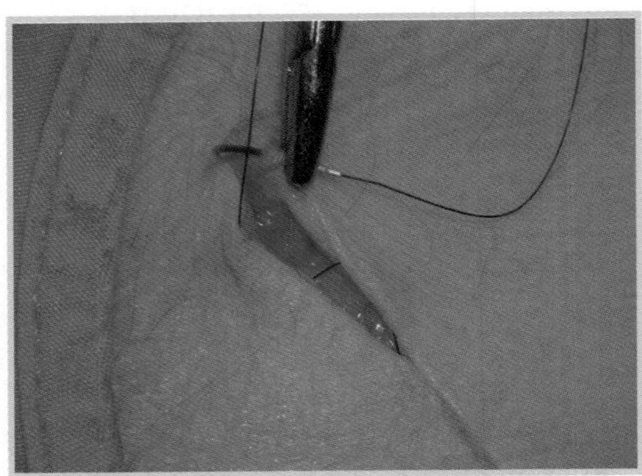

Step 4

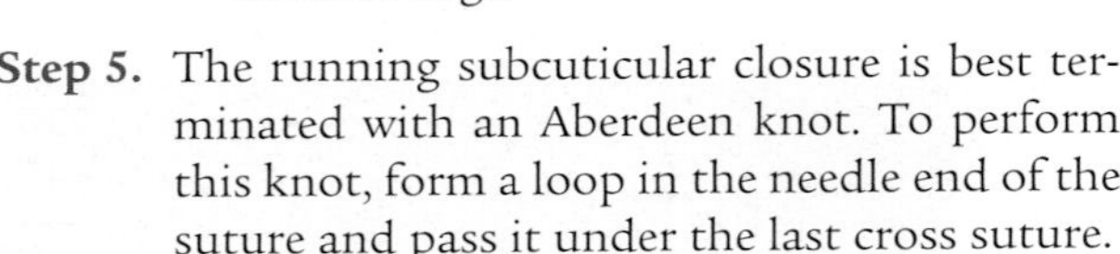

Step 5. The running subcuticular closure is best terminated with an Aberdeen knot. To perform this knot, form a loop in the needle end of the suture and pass it under the last cross suture.

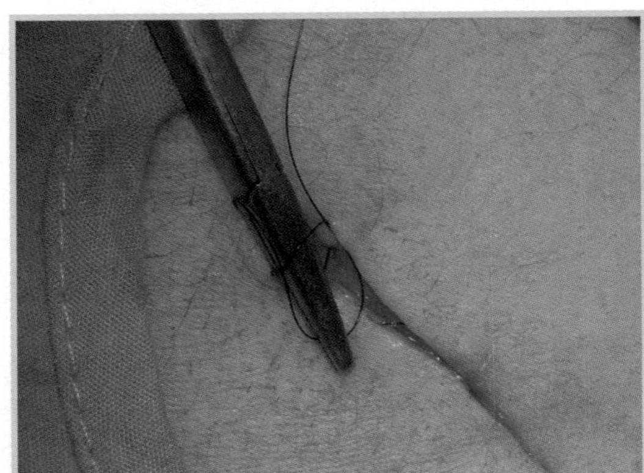

Step 5

Step 6. Pull out all of the slack from the side of the suture exiting the tissue, leaving a well-approximated suture line.

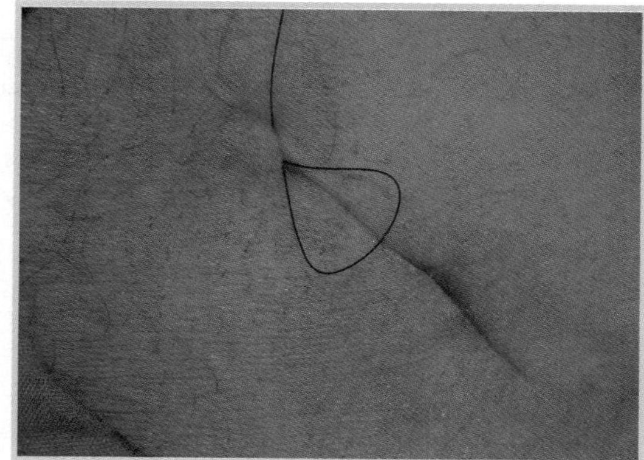
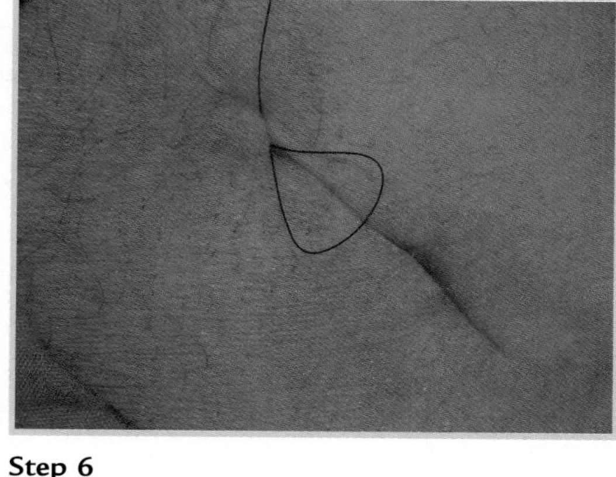

Step 6

Step 7. Again pull a loop of suture from the free end and pass it through the existing loop, pulling the tissue side until it is snug.

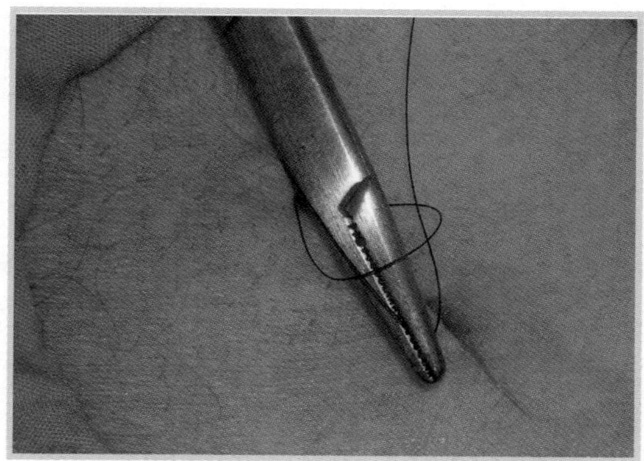

Step 7

Step 8. After pulling four or five loops, pass the needle though the loop and pull it until it is snug.

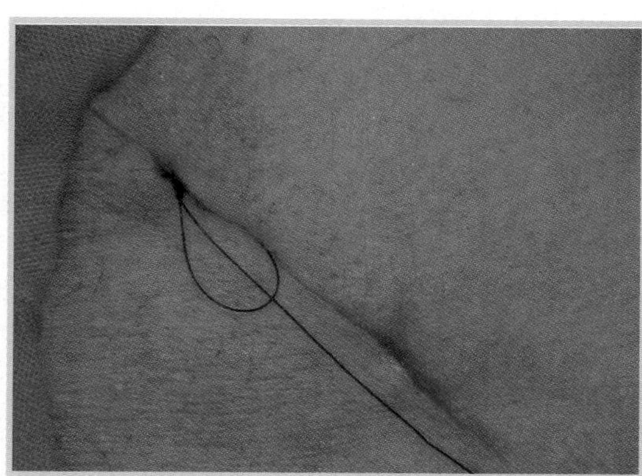
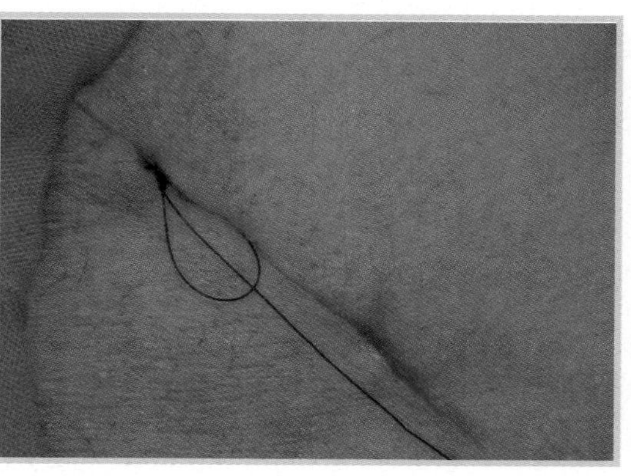

Step 8

Step 9. Cut the suture just above the knot and tuck the free end into the wound.

- **PEARL:** This closure has the distinct advantage of not producing any additional holes in the skin while producing a well-approximated secure suture. There is almost no risk of the suture inadvertently coming loose.

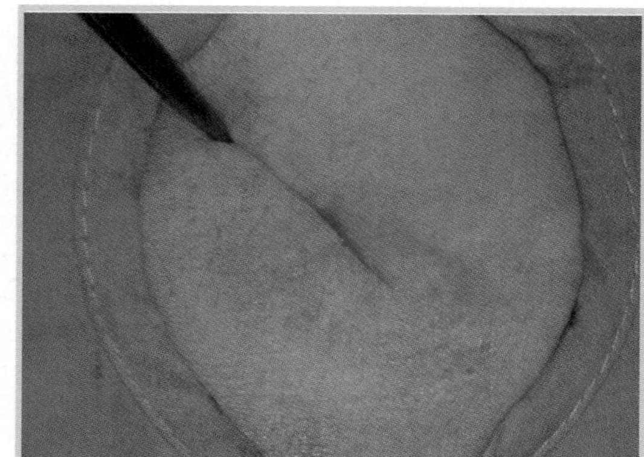

Step 9

Step 10. Alternatively, the suture then exits the wound through the end of the wound. After cutting the needle free, the free ends of suture are secured with tape at the ends of the wound. A knot can be tied on the ends to help the tape hold the suture securely.

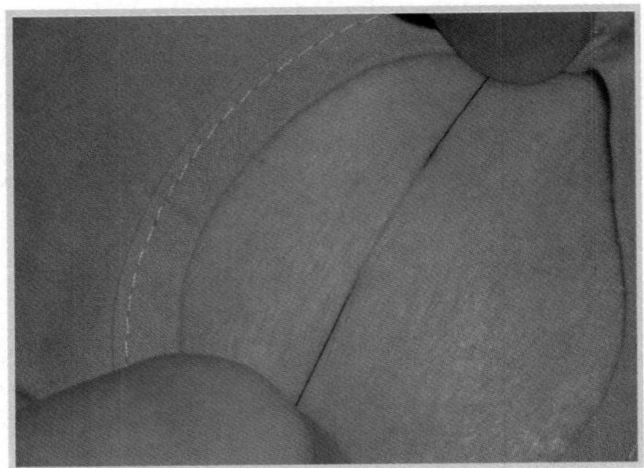

Step 10

Step 11. To facilitate suture removal when using nonabsorbable suture, an extracutaneous loop may be placed in long suture lines. The extracutaneous loop is cut, creating two smaller threads that are easier to extract than one long thread.

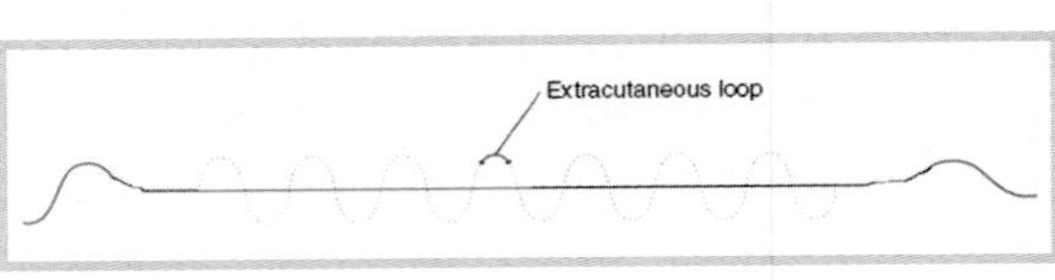

Step 11

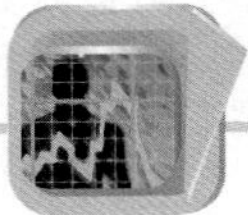

Complications

- Bleeding
- Infection
- Scar formation

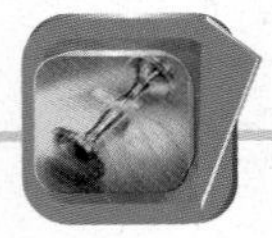

Pediatric Considerations

Generally, pediatric skin has excellent blood flow and heals very well. However, pediatric patients often find it difficult to sit and lie still during lengthy procedures. The patient's maturity and ability to cooperate should be considered before deciding to attempt any outpatient procedure. Sometimes it is necessary to sedate the patient to repair the laceration (see Chapter 122). The maximum recommended dose for lidocaine in children is 3 to 5 mg/kg, and 7 mg/kg when combined with epinephrine. Neonates have an increased volume of distribution, decreased hepatic clearance, and doubled terminal elimination half-life (3.2 hours).

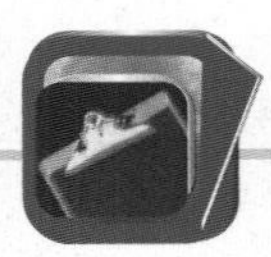

Postprocedure Instructions

Instruct the patient to gently wash an area that has been stitched in 1 day but not to put the wound into standing water for 2 to 3 days. Have the patient dry the area well after washing. Have the patient use a small amount of antibiotic ointment to promote moist healing. Recommend wound elevation to help lessen swelling, reduce pain, and speed healing. Instruct the patient not to pick at, break, or cut the stitches. Have the patient cover the wound with a nonocclusive dressing for 2 to 3 days. A simple adhesive bandage (Band-Aid) will suffice for many small lacerations. The dressing should be left in place for at least 48 hours, after which time most wounds can be opened to air. Scalp wounds can be left open if small, but large head wounds can be wrapped circumferentially with rolled gauze.

Most uncontaminated wounds do not need to be seen by a provider until suture removal, unless signs of infection develop. Highly contaminated wounds should be seen for follow-up in 2 to 3 days. Give discharge instructions to the patient regarding signs of wound infection.

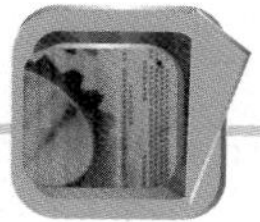

Coding Information and Supply Sources

All codes listed are for superficial wound closure using sutures, staples, or tissue adhesives with or without adhesive strips on the skin surface. If a layered closure is required, use intermediate closure codes 12031 to 12057 or complex repair codes 13100 to 13160.

Add together the lengths of wounds in the same classification and anatomic sites. Use separate codes for repairs from different anatomic sites. Debridement is considered a separate procedure only when gross contamination requires prolonged cleansing or when appreciable amounts of devitalized or contaminated tissue are removed.

CPT Code	Description	2008 Average 50th Percentile Fee	Global Period
12001	Simple repair SNAGTEHF ≤2.5 cm	$220.00	10
12002	Simple repair SNAGTEHF 2.6–7.5 cm	$235.00	10
12004	Simple repair SNAGTEHF 7.6–12.5 cm	$285.00	10
12005	Simple repair SNAGTEHF 12.6–20.0 cm	$408.00	10
12006	Simple repair SNAGTEHF 20.1–30.0 cm	$506.00	10
12007	Simple repair SNAGTEHF >30.0 cm		10
12011	Simple repair FEENLMM ≤2.5 cm	$240.00	10
12013	Simple repair FEENLMM 2.6–5.0 cm	$288.00	10
12014	Simple repair FEENLMM 5.1–7.5 cm	$351.00	10
12015	Simple repair FEENLMM 7.6–12.5 cm	$449.00	10
12016	Simple repair FEENLMM 12.6–20.0 cm	$585.00	10
12017	Simple repair FEENLMM 20.1–30.0 cm	$743.00	10
12018	Simple repair FEENLMM >30.0 cm		10
12020	Treatment of superficial wound dehiscence, simple closure	$397.00	10

CPT is a registered trademark of the American Medical Association.
2008 average 50th Percentile Fees are provided courtesy of 2008 MMH-SI's copyrighted Physicians' Fees and Coding Guide.
SNAGTEHF, scalp, neck, axillae, external genitalia, trunk, extremities, hands, and feet;
FEENLMM, face, ears, eyelids, nose, lips, and mucous membranes.

Bibliography

Bennett RG. *Fundamentals of Cutaneous Surgery*. St. Louis: Mosby; 1988:464–465.

Boutros S, Weinfeld AB, Friedman JD. Continuous versus interrupted suturing of traumatic lacerations: a time, cost, and complication rate comparison. *J Trauma*. 2000;48:495–497.

Brown JS. *Minor Surgery: A Text and Atlas*. 3rd ed. London: Chapman & Hall; 1997:70–96.

Koliyadan SV. Securing subcuticular absorbable suture with buried knots. *Internet J. Surg.* 2005:6(2).

Lammers RL, Trott AL. Methods of wound closure. In: Roberts JR, Hedges JR, eds. *Clinical Procedures in Emergency Medicine*. 3rd ed. Philadelphia: WB Saunders; 1998:560–598.

La Padula A. A new technique to secure an entirely buried subcuticular suture. *Plast Reconstr Surg.* 1995;95:423–424.

Moy RL, Lee A, Zalka A. Commonly used suturing techniques in skin surgery. *Am Fam Physician.* 1991;44:1625–1634.

Moy RL. Suturing techniques. In: Usatine RP, Moy RL, Tobnick EL, et al., eds. *Skin Surgery: A Practical Guide*. St. Louis: Mosby; 1998:88–100.

Smoot EC. Method for securing a subcuticular suture with a minimal buried knot. *Plast Reconstr Surg.* 1998;102:2447–2449.

Stasko T. Advanced suturing techniques and layered closures. In: Wheeland RG, ed. *Cutaneous Surgery:* Philadelphia: WB Saunders; 1994:304–317.

Stegman SJ, Tromovitch TA, Glogau RG. *Basics of Dermatologic Surgery*. Chicago: Year Book Medical Publishing; 1984:45–48.

St John HM. Knot-free subcuticular suture. *Br J Surg.* 1997;84:872.

Swanson NA. *Atlas of Cutaneous Surgery*. Boston: Little, Brown; 1987:42–45.

Wong NL. Review of continuous sutures in dermatologic surgery. *J Dermatol Surg Oncol.* 1993;19:923–931.

Zuber TJ. *Basic Soft-Tissue Surgery*. Kansas City: American Academy of Family Physicians; 1998:58–69.

Zukin DD, Simon RR. *Emergency Wound Care: Principles and Practice*. Rockville, MD: Aspen; 1987:51–54.

2008 MAG Mutual Healthcare Solutions, Inc.'s Physicians' Fee and Coding Guide. Duluth, Georgia. MAG Mutual Healthcare Solutions, Inc. 2007.

CHAPTER 43

Vertical Mattress Suture Placement

E. J. Mayeaux Jr., MD, DABFP, FAAFP

Professor of Family Medicine, Professor of Obstetrics and Gynecology
Louisiana State University Health Sciences Center, Shreveport, LA

The classic vertical mattress suture (also known as the *far-far/near-near* suture) is unsurpassed in its ability to evert skin wound edges. It is commonly employed where wound edges tend to invert, such as on the posterior neck, behind the ear, in the groin, in the inframammary crease, or within concave body surfaces. Because lax skin may also invert, the vertical mattress stitch has been advocated for closure on the dorsum of the hand and over the elbow.

The vertical mattress suture incorporates a large amount of tissue within the passage of the suture loops and provides good tensile strength in closing wound edges over a distance. It is commonly used as the anchoring or tension-reducing stitch when moving a skin flap or at the center of a large wound. The suture also can accomplish deep and superficial closure with a single suture. The vertical mattress suture can provide deeper wound support in situations when buried subcutaneous closure is not advisable (e.g., facial skin flaps). Early removal of vertical mattress sutures is advocated, especially if nearby simple interrupted sutures can remain in place for the normal duration.

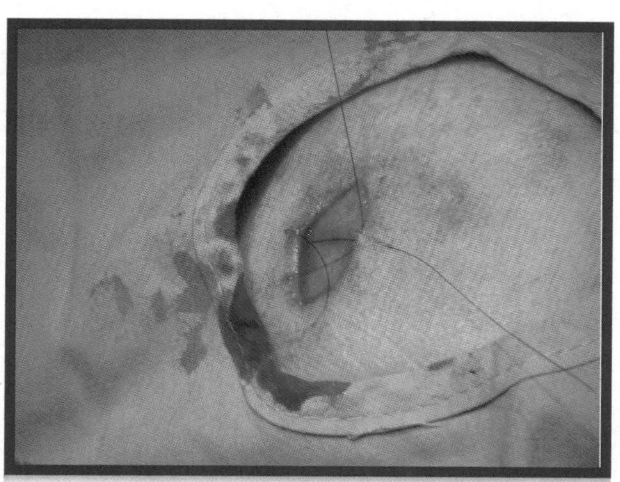

After placement of a vertical mattress suture, the natural process of wound inflammation and scar retraction pulls the externalized loops inward. The potential pressure necrosis and scarring is worsened if the vertical mattress suture is tied too tightly or if a large-caliber suture material is used.

A variation of the vertical mattress suture, known as the *shorthand technique* or *near-near/far-far* technique, has been advocated by some physicians. This variation places the near-near pass of suture first, allowing the clinician to pull up the suture strings to elevate the skin for placement of the far-far loop. The variation is advocated because it can be placed more rapidly than the classic technique. Care must be taken not to tear the skin when lifting the skin after the initial pass.

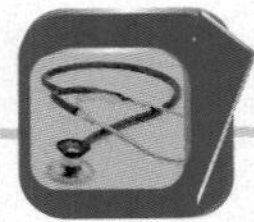

Equipment

- Instruments for simple interrupted skin suture placement are found in Appendix G and can be ordered through local surgical supply houses.
- Suture materials can be ordered from Ethicon, Somerville, NJ (http://ecatalog.ethicon.com/EC_ECATALOG/ethicon/default.asp).
  A suggested anesthesia tray that can be used for this procedure is listed in Appendix F.
- Skin preparation recommendations appear in Appendix E.

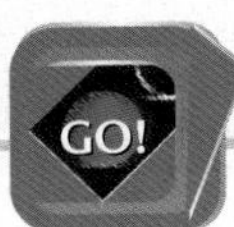

Indications

- Closure of wounds that tend to invert (e.g., back of the neck, groin, inframammary crease, behind the ear)
- Closure of lax skin (e.g., dorsum of the hand, over the elbow)
- Anchoring or tension-reducing stitch when moving a skin flap

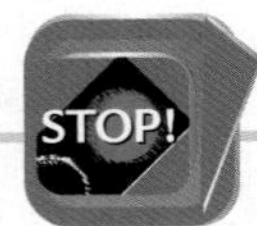

Contraindications

- Skin without enough laxity to close without significant risk of sutures pulling through the skin
- Closure of defects on breast tissue (use a running intracutaneous suture closure)
- Presence of cellulitis, bacteremia, or other active infection
- Uncooperative patient

The Procedure

Classic Vertical Mattress

Step 1. The far-far pass is started with the suture needle entering (and exiting) the anesthetized skin 4 to 8 mm from the wound edge. Pass the suture needle vertically through the skin surface.

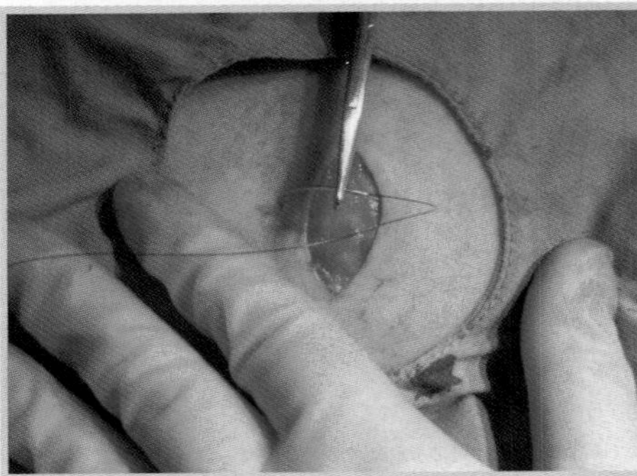

Step 1

Step 2. Place the far-far suture at the same distance and the same depth from the wound edge on both sides.

- PITFALL: Pass the suture needle symmetrically through the tissue. Asymmetric bites through the wound edge can cause one edge to be higher than the other. The creation of a shelf, with one wound edge higher, produces cosmetically inferior scars that are prominent because they cast a shadow.

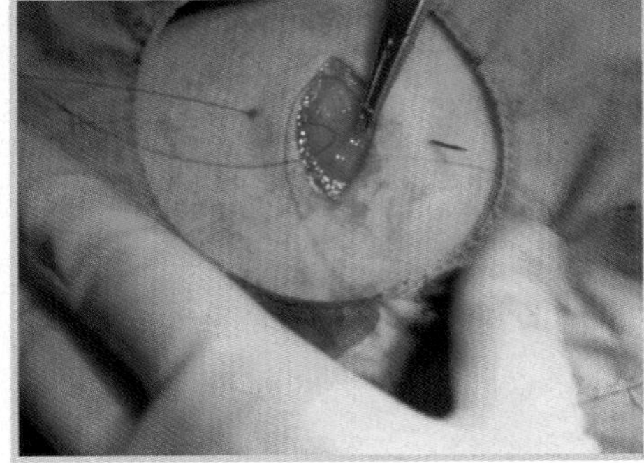

Step 2

Step 3. Place the needle backward in the needle driver. Make the shallower near-near pass within 1 to 2 mm of the wound edge, using a backhand pass. The near-near pass should be mostly within the dermis.

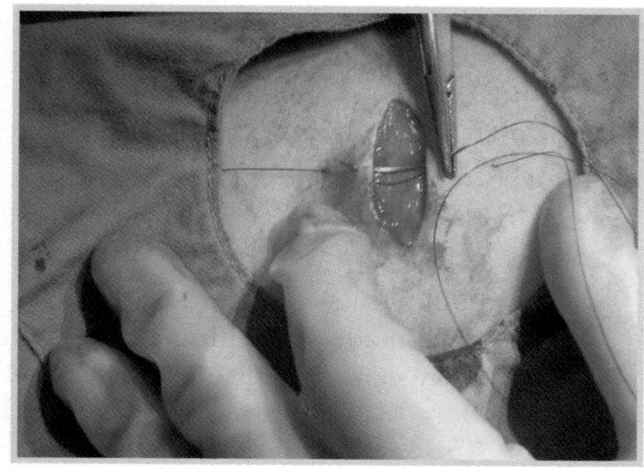

Step 3

Step 4. Tie the suture snugly but gently. Once the wound closure is started and the tension created by the closure is relieved by the vertical mattress suture, the rest of the closure may be accomplished using additional vertical mattress sutures or simple interrupted sutures.

- **PEARL:** If a lot of tension is created by pulling the wound closed, small cloth bolsters made by rolling up the edge of a sponge may be used under the external loops of the suture to spread out the pressure on the skin surface, thereby decreasing the likelihood of necrosis at these points.
- **PITFALL:** Overly tight sutures may produce crosshatch marks.
- **PITFALL:** Novice providers often tie the suture tightly to produce additional eversion. Avoid this temptation, because it results in increased wound scarring.

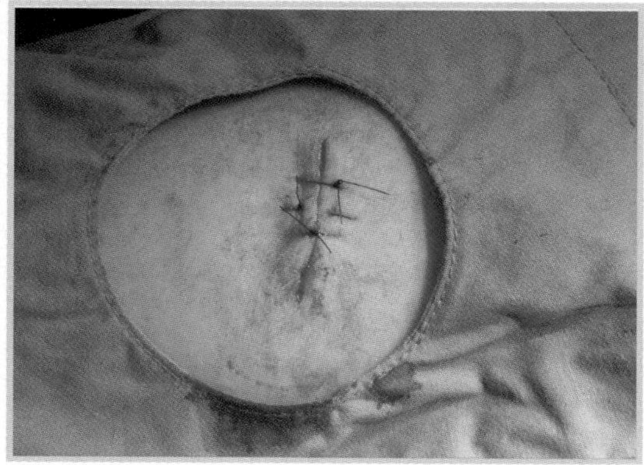

Step 4

Inverted or Shorthand Vertical Mattress

Step 1. The inverted vertical mattress suture is very similar in placement and function to the classic vertical mattress suture, but the placement order is different. First make the shallow near-near pass within 1 to 2 mm of the wound edge, using a backhand pass and with the needle placed backward in the needle driver.

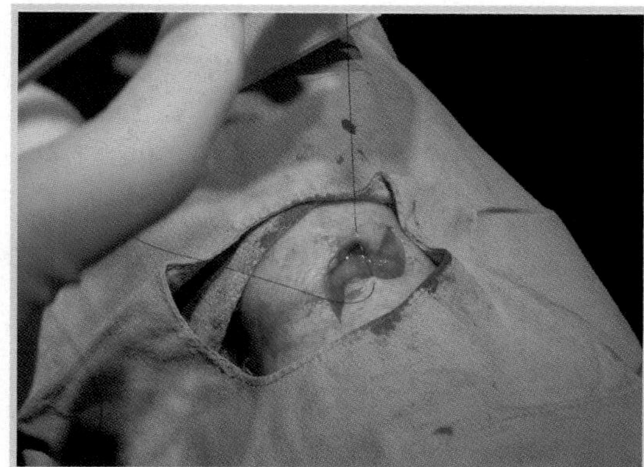

Step 1

Step 2. Then make the far-far pass with the suture needle entering and exiting 4 to 8 mm from the wound edge. Pass the suture needle vertically through the skin.

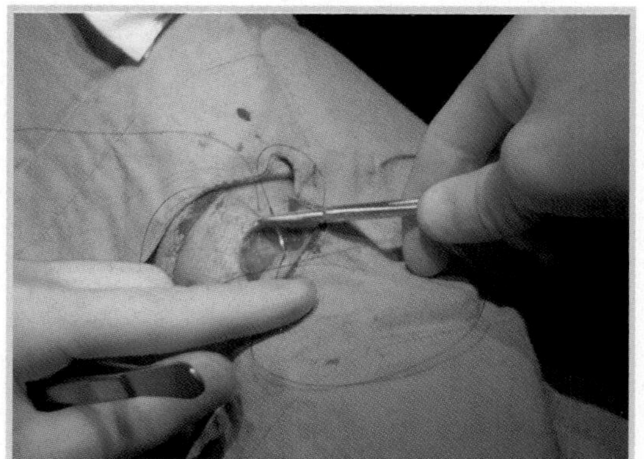

Step 2

Step 3. Tie the suture snugly but gently. Once the wound closure is started and the tension created by the closure is relieved by the vertical mattress suture, the rest of the closure may be accomplished using additional vertical mattress sutures or simple interrupted sutures.

- **PEARL:** If a lot of tension is created by pulling the wound closed, small cloth bolsters made by rolling up the edge of a sponge may be used under the external loops of the suture to spread out the pressure on the skin surface, thereby decreasing the likelihood of necrosis at these points.
- **PITFALL:** Tight sutures may produce crosshatch marks.
- **PITFALL:** Novice providers often tie the suture tightly to produce additional eversion. Avoid this temptation, because it results in increased wound scarring.

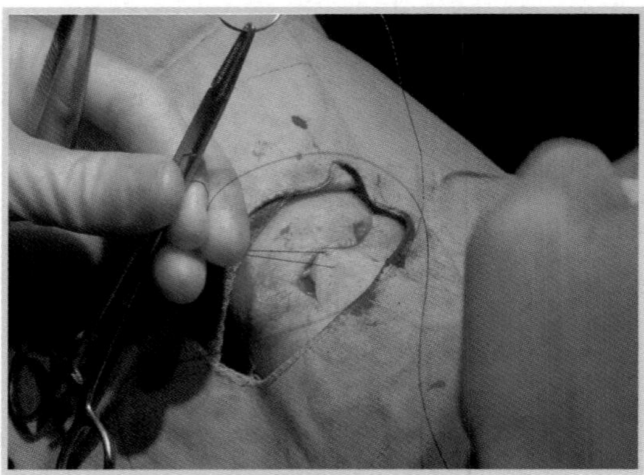

Step 3

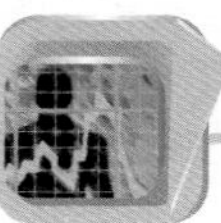

Complications

- Suture marks (i.e., railroad marks or Frankenstein marks) from the suture loops on the skin surface
- Sutures pulling through the skin, especially with closures without enough laxity to close without significant tension
- Bleeding
- Infection
- Scar formation

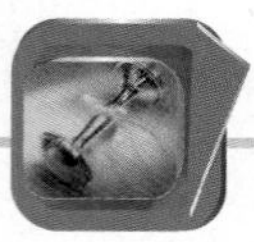

Pediatric Considerations

Generally, pediatric skin has excellent blood flow and heals very well. However, pediatric patients often find it difficult to sit and lie still during lengthy procedures. The patient's maturity and ability to cooperate should be considered before deciding to attempt any outpatient procedure.

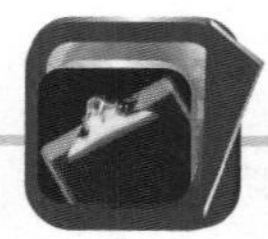

Postprocedure Instructions

Instruct the patient to gently wash an area that has been stitched in 1 day but not to put the wound into standing water for 3 days. Have the patient dry the area well after washing. Have the patient use a small amount of antibiotic ointment to promote moist healing. Recommend wound elevation to help lessen swelling, reduce pain, and speed healing. Instruct the patient not to pick at, break, or cut the stitches. Consider removing the vertical mattress sutures after about half of the time of the removal of adjacent sutures.

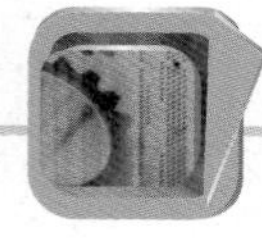

Coding Information

All codes listed are for superficial wound closure using sutures, staples, or tissue adhesives with or without adhesive strips on the skin surface. If a layered closure is required, use intermediate closure codes 12031 to 12057 or complex repair codes 13100 to 13160.

Add together the lengths of wounds in the same classification and anatomic sites. Use separate codes for repairs from different anatomic sites. Debridement is considered a separate procedure only when gross contamination requires prolonged cleansing or when appreciable amounts of devitalized or contaminated tissue are removed.

CPT Code	Description	2008 Average 50th Percentile Fee	Global Period
12001	Simple repair SNAGTEHF ≤2.5 cm	$220.00	10
12002	Simple repair SNAGTEHF 2.6–7.5 cm	$235.00	10
12004	Simple repair SNAGTEHF 7.6–12.5 cm	$285.00	10
12005	Simple repair SNAGTEHF 12.6–20.0 cm	$408.00	10
12006	Simple repair SNAGTEHF 20.1–30.0 cm	$506.00	10
12007	Simple repair SNAGTEHF >30.0 cm		10
12011	Simple repair FEENLMM ≤2.5 cm	$240.00	10
12013	Simple repair FEENLMM 2.6–5.0 cm	$288.00	10
12014	Simple repair FEENLMM 5.1–7.5 cm	$351.00	10
12015	Simple repair FEENLMM 7.6–12.5 cm	$449.00	10
12016	Simple repair FEENLMM 12.6–20.0 cm	$585.00	10
12017	Simple repair FEENLMM 20.1–30.0 cm	$743.00	10
12018	Simple repair FEENLMM >30.0 cm		10
12020	Treatment of superficial wound dehiscence, simple closure	$397.00	10

SNAGTEHF, scalp, neck, axillae, external genitalia, trunk, extremities, hands, and feet;
FEENLMM, face, ears, eyelids, nose, lips, and mucous membranes.

Bibliography

Gault DT, Brain A, Sommerlad BC, et al. Loop mattress suture. *Br J Surg.* 1987;74:820–821.

Jones JS, Gartner M, Drew G, et al. The shorthand vertical mattress stitch: evaluation of a new suture technique. *Am J Emerg Med.* 1993;11:483–485.

Moy RL, Lee A, Zalka A. Commonly used suturing techniques in skin surgery. *Am Fam Physician.* 1991;44:1625–1634.

Snow SN, Goodman MM, Lemke BN. The shorthand vertical mattress stitch—a rapid skin everting suture technique. *J Dermatol Surg Oncol.* 1989;15:379–381.

Stasko T. Advanced suturing techniques and layered closures. In: Wheeland RG, ed. *Cutaneous Surgery*. Philadelphia: WB Saunders; 1994:304–317.

Stegman SJ, Tromovitch TA, Glogau RG. *Basics of Dermatologic Surgery*. Chicago: Year Book Medical Publishing, 1982.

Swanson NA. *Atlas of Cutaneous Surgery*. Boston: Little, Brown; 1987:30–35.

Usatine RP, Moy RL, Tobinick EL, et al. *Skin Surgery: A Practical Guide*. St. Louis: Mosby; 1998.

Zuber TJ. *Basic Soft-Tissue Surgery*. Kansas City: American Academy of Family Physicians; 1998.

Zuber TJ. The mattress sutures: vertical, horizontal, and corner stitch. *Am Fam Physician.* 2002;66:2231–2236.

2008 MAG Mutual Healthcare Solutions, Inc.'s Physicians' Fee and Coding Guide. Duluth, Georgia. MAG Mutual Healthcare Solutions, Inc. 2007.

SECTION FIVE

Skin Surgery

CHAPTER 44

Layout of Skin Procedures

E. J. Mayeaux, Jr., MD, DABFP, FAAFP

Professor of Family Medicine, Professor of Obstetrics and Gynecology
Louisiana State University Health Sciences Center, Shreveport, LA

In determining the best possible layout for closure of a skin excision procedure or wound closure, several factors must be considered. Planning closure of a wound created by an excision procedure should be done before the skin is prepped or cut; it is necessary to understand how different excision procedures and flaps create new lines of tension or pull. Next, defining where the skin has the most laxity from which to pull will help in selecting closure types. Finally, by aligning the inherent stretch properties of the skin and the tension-creating properties of potential closures, adequate closure with the best cosmesis can be obtained.

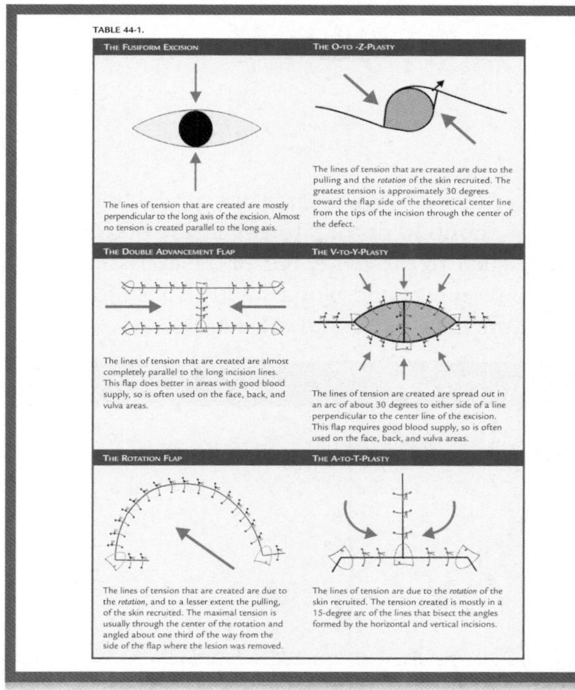

TABLE 44-1.

The Fusiform Excision	The O-to-Z-Plasty
The lines of tension that are created are mostly perpendicular to the long axis of the excision. Almost no tension is created parallel to the long axis.	The lines of tension that are created are due to the pulling and the *rotation* of the skin recruited. The greatest tension is approximately 30 degrees toward the flap side of the theoretical center line from the tips of the incision through the center of the defect.
The Double Advancement Flap	**The V-to-Y-Plasty**
The lines of tension that are created are almost completely parallel to the long incision lines. This flap does better in areas with good blood supply, so is often used on the face, back, and vulva areas.	The lines of tension are created are spread out in an arc of about 30 degrees to either side of a line perpendicular to the center line of the excision. This flap requires good blood supply, so is often used on the face, back, and vulva areas.
The Rotation Flap	**The A-to-T-Plasty**
The lines of tension that are created are due to the *rotation*, and to a lesser extent the pulling, of the skin recruited. The maximal tension is usually through the center of the rotation and angled about one third of the way from the side of the flap where the lesion was removed.	The lines of tension are due to the *rotation* of the skin recruited. The tension created is mostly in a 15-degree arc of the lines that bisect the angles formed by the horizontal and vertical incisions.

How Excision Procedures and Flaps Create New Lines of Tension or Pull

Whenever an opening is created in the skin, some of the remaining skin must be recruited from the area around the defect to primarily close it. As the surrounding skin is pulled, lines of tension are created parallel to the direction of pull. Fusiform (elliptical) excisions and each type of flap or plasty pulls skin from different directions, depending on how skin is recruited to close the skin defect. Generally, the tension is parallel to the direction of pull necessary to close the defect. Table 44-1 lists various closure options. The red arrows in the following figures show the direction of skin tissue generated by the closure.

Determining Where the Skin Has the Most Laxity and Areas of Potential Recruitment

When preparing to do a skin excision procedure or to close an existing skin deficit, the ability of the skin to stretch and move to cover the defect and the cosmetic and

TABLE 44-1.

The Fusiform Excision	The O-to -Z-Plasty
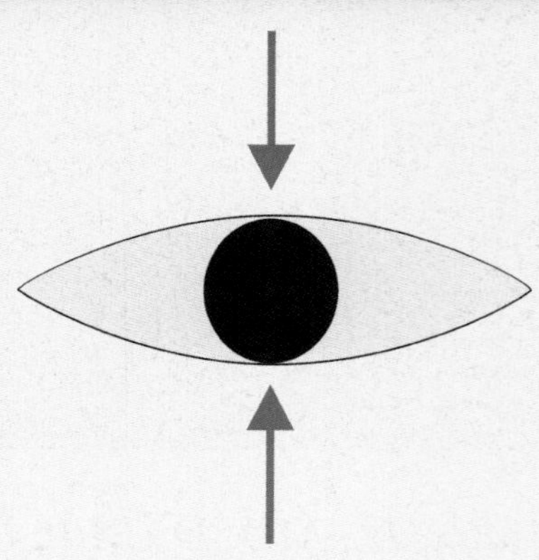 The lines of tension that are created are mostly perpendicular to the long axis of the excision. Almost no tension is created parallel to the long axis.	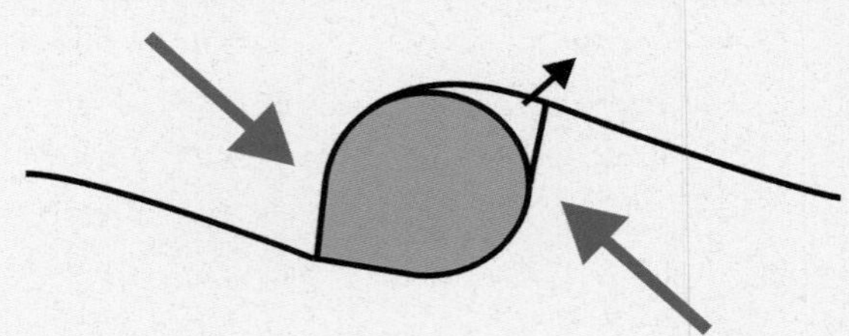 The lines of tension that are created are due to the pulling and the *rotation* of the skin recruited. The greatest tension is approximately 30 degrees toward the flap side of the theoretical center line from the tips of the incision through the center of the defect.
The Double Advancement Flap	**The V-to-Y-Plasty**
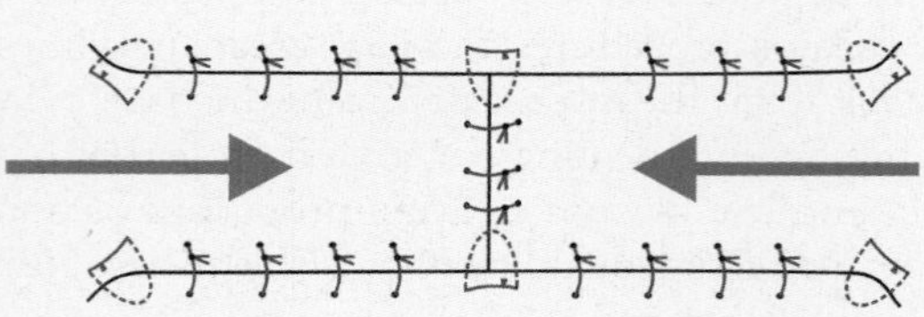 The lines of tension that are created are almost completely parallel to the long incision lines. This flap does better in areas with good blood supply, so is often used on the face, back, and vulva areas.	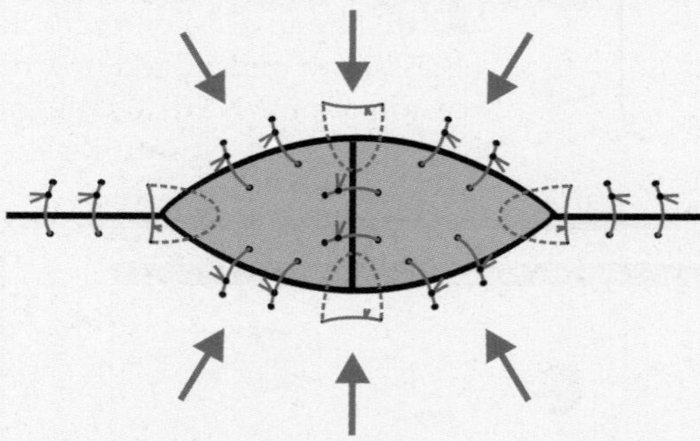 The lines of tension are created are spread out in an arc of about 30 degrees to either side of a line perpendicular to the center line of the excision. This flap requires good blood supply, so is often used on the face, back, and vulva areas.
The Rotation Flap	**The A-to-T-Plasty**
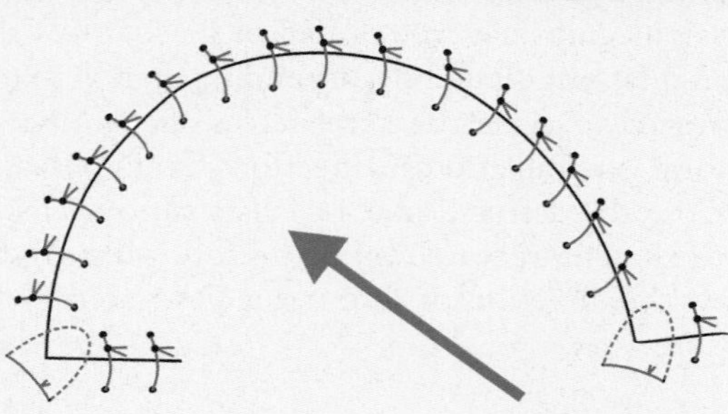 The lines of tension that are created are due to the *rotation*, and to a lesser extent the pulling, of the skin recruited. The maximal tension is usually through the center of the rotation and angled about one third of the way from the side of the flap where the lesion was removed.	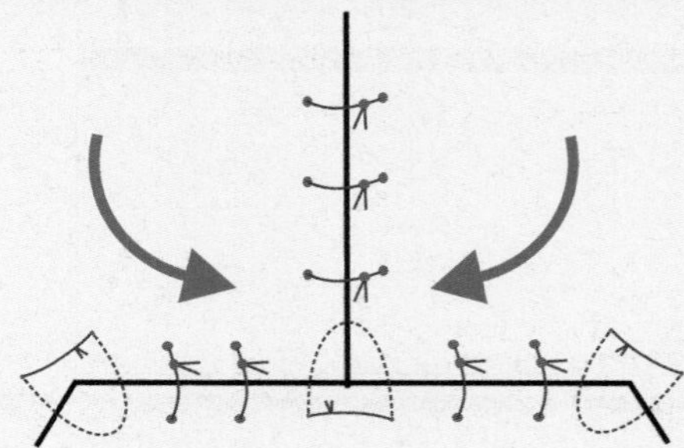 The lines of tension are due to the *rotation* of the skin recruited. The tension created is mostly in a 15-degree arc of the lines that bisect the angles formed by the horizontal and vertical incisions.

functional results of that movement are the primary considerations. The most common problems are encountered in areas where the skin is closely attached or anchored to underlying or protruding structures. Examples include areas over the anterior tibia, around joints, and around protruding modified structures such as the nose, ears, or penis. The cosmetic implications of skin movement are particularly important near mobile, modified skin structures such as eyebrows, sideburns, vulva, and scrotum. Not only are there more limitations to undermining, but changing the shape, angle, or position of these structures can cause serious cosmetic problems. It is also very important around orifices such as the eyes, mouth, and vaginal introitus, because pulling tension in these areas may change their shape, causing cosmetic distress to the patient.

After these problems are identified, the skin can be gently pushed with the surgeon's fingers to determine if there is sufficient laxity to close the defect. The lines of least skin tension are natural lines of laxity in the skin (see Appendix B). Pushing the skin perpendicularly to the lines of least skin tension will reveal the most "give" in the skin.

Aligning Excisions and Potential Closures to Get Adequate Closure and Best Cosmesis

The best cosmetic results are usually achieved when the final closure line (and therefore the scar) lies parallel to the lines of least skin tension. Start choosing possible closures by considering layouts that produce this result. When there is adequate skin to recruit for closure without tension, the fusiform excision is usually the easiest procedure to execute, because the final closure line is straight and easy to plan. Most providers will choose it as the default procedure when starting to lay out a procedure. Eliminate any closures that would pull skin tension from immobile areas or areas that would cause cosmetic problems (such as the eyebrow or mouth, because this would change the contours of these structures).

Next consider where the skin must be recruited to close the defect. Can this area be safely undermined? Also, consider any significant underlying structures, such as arteries, veins, or nerve bundles, that must be avoided during excision or undermining for closure.

Then consider in what directions the skin normally moves and stretches. Because movement stretches the skin, this makes sutures more likely to fail if the closure creates too much tension in the direction of normal skin movement. For example, skin on the back can move in almost any direction, making a V-to-Y-plasty (that pulls some tension from almost all directions) or a rotation flap (that can spread the tension over a wide area, thereby reducing the tension at any particular point) a better choice than a fusiform or advancement flap that pulls all the tension from one direction.

Finally, consider the quality of the blood supply to the skin in the area, because some flaps can be done only in areas of good blood flow.

Examples

For example, when considering a closure on the forehead, the final scar should follow the shape of the eyebrow (line of least skin tension). The skin should not be pulled from the inferior and superior directions, because that could permanently raise some or all of the brow.

This would eliminate the fusiform excision. An O-to-Z-plasty or rotation flap would work, but it would not place most of the closure in line with the lines of least skin tension, would pull the skin at tangential angles, and would make longer scars. A double-V-to-Y-plasty or double advancement flap would put most of the final scar in the lines of least skin tension, not change the shape of the brow, and allow for good closure of the defect. Either of the latter two closures would work well.

Fusiform excisions that line up with the lines of least skin tension will probably cause excessive vertical tension, thereby raising the brow and producing a larger scar. The scar will align with the lines of least skin tension. **Not a good choice.**

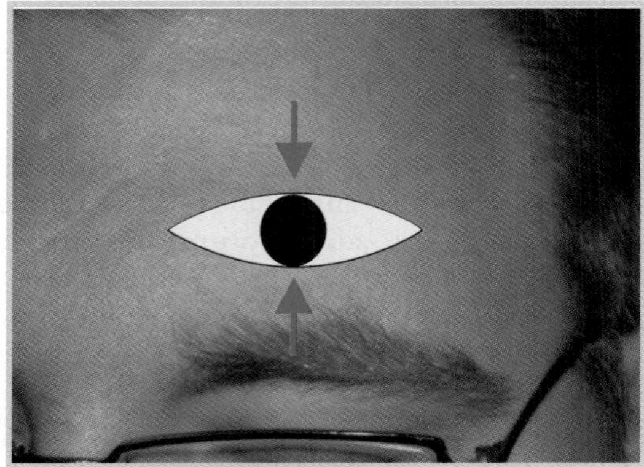

Figure 1

The O-to-Z-plasty will probably raise the lateral part of the brow, and the scar will not align with the least tension skin lines, but will probably close with minimal tension. **Adequate choice.**

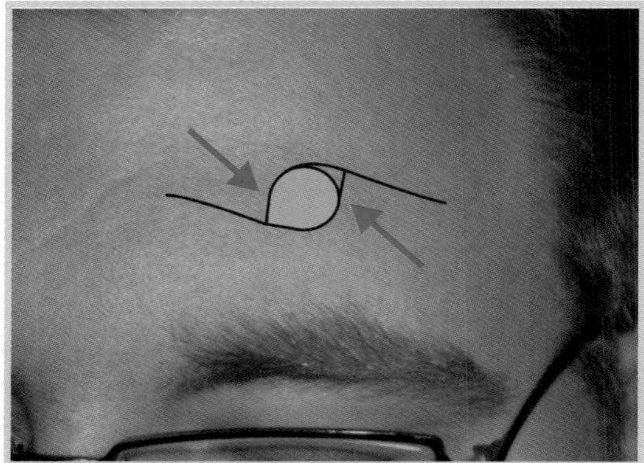

Figure 2

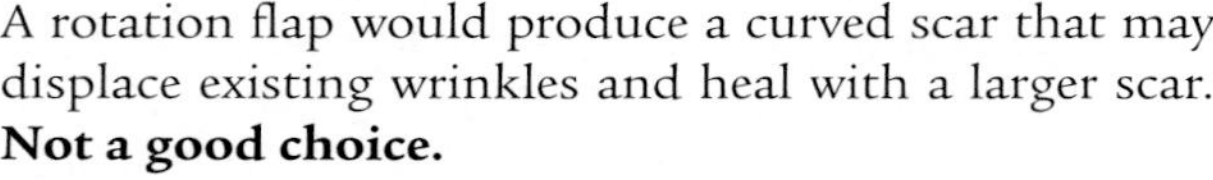

A rotation flap would produce a curved scar that may displace existing wrinkles and heal with a larger scar. **Not a good choice.**

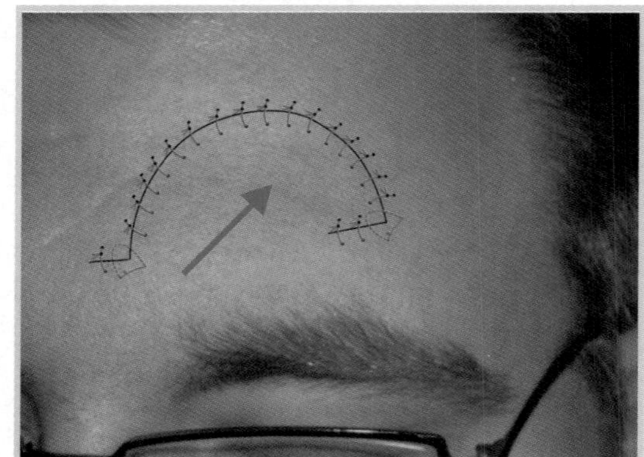

Figure 3

An A-to-T-plasty would produce a large vertical scar that is perpendicular to the lines of least skin tension (and heal with a larger scar). **Not a good choice.**

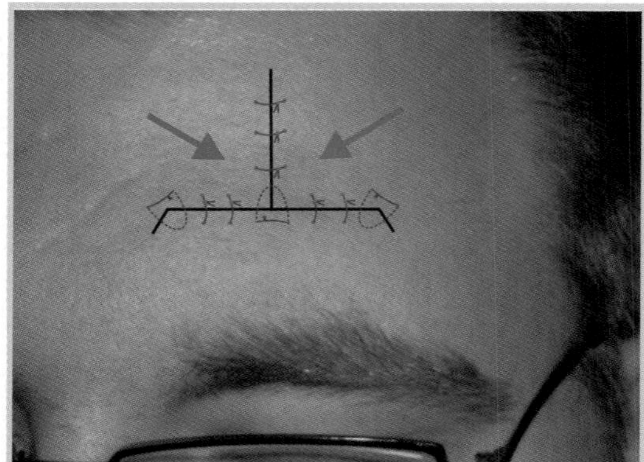

Figure 4

A V-to-Y-plasty pulls minimum tension from any particular direction and aligns well with the lines of least skin tension. It is less likely to alter the shape of the brow. **Good choice.**

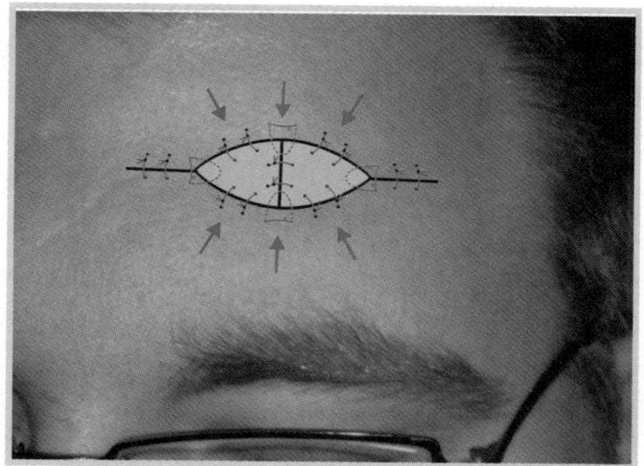

Figure 5

A double advancement flap aligns well with the lines of least skin tension and has essentially no risk of altering the brow. **Good choice.**

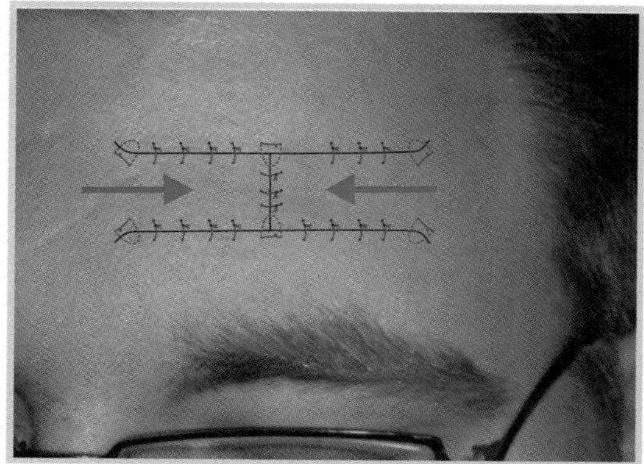

Figure 6

Similarly, in a lesion near an immobile structure or an orifice, a fusiform excision, double V-to-Y-plasty, or rotation flap would put some pull against the structure, increasing the chance of breakdown or cosmetically unappealing scars. The A-to-T-plasty or double advancement flap can close the defect without pulling skin from the direction of the structure. The example shows closures near the mouth but would apply similarly to lesions near the eye, anal edge, or vulva.

A fusiform excision that lines up with the lines of least skin tension will probably cause excessive vertical tension, thereby potentially significantly raising the edge of the lip, pulling down the nasolabial fold (and possible the inferior edge of the nose), and distorting the local anatomy. **Poor choice.**

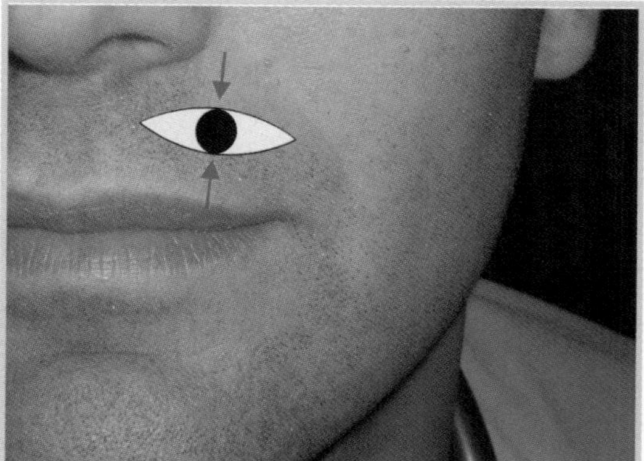

Figure 7

The O-to-Z-plasty would pull from the direction of the nose (limited tissue to pull), possibly distort the nasolabial fold, and may lift the end of the mouth. **Not a good choice.**

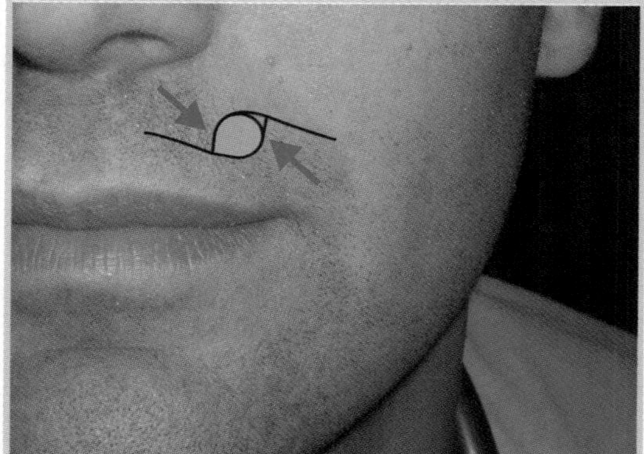

Figure 8

Rotation flap alters the nasolabial fold, alters the local contour, and may alter the hair pattern of the mustache. **Not a good choice.**

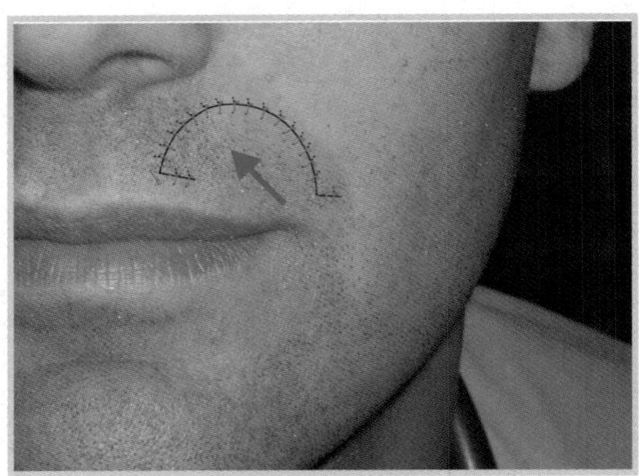

Figure 9

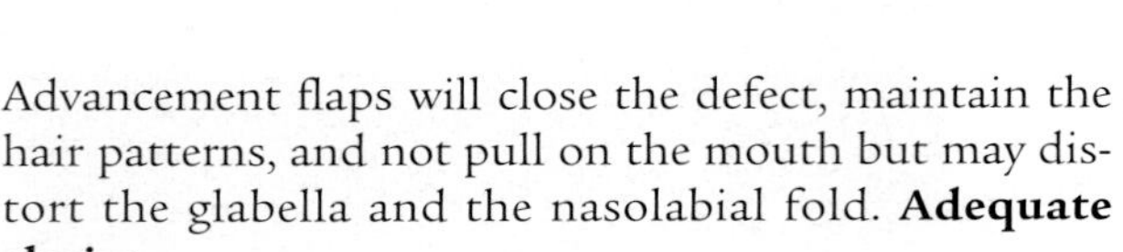

Advancement flaps will close the defect, maintain the hair patterns, and not pull on the mouth but may distort the glabella and the nasolabial fold. **Adequate choice.**

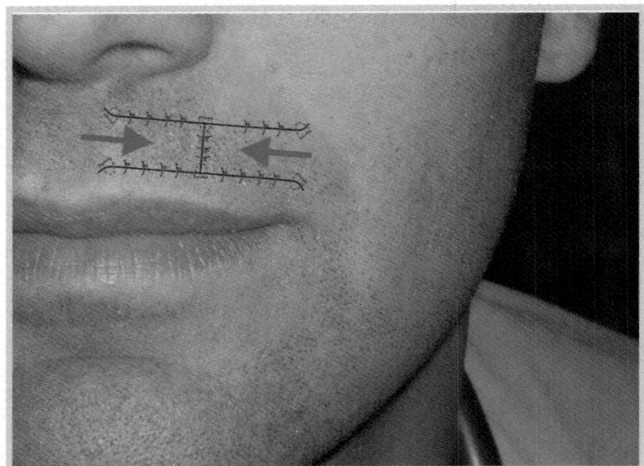

Figure 10

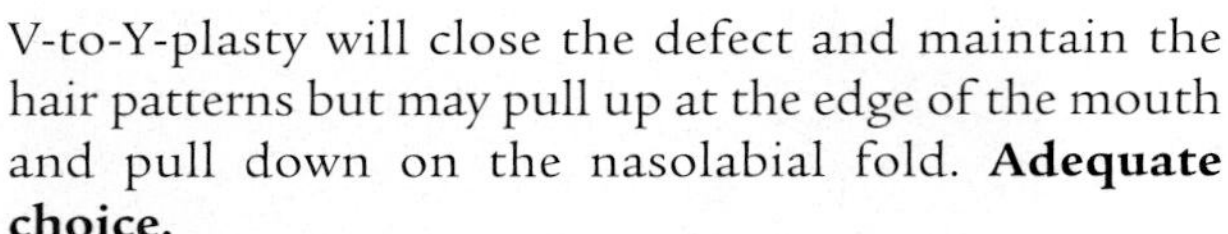

V-to-Y-plasty will close the defect and maintain the hair patterns but may pull up at the edge of the mouth and pull down on the nasolabial fold. **Adequate choice.**

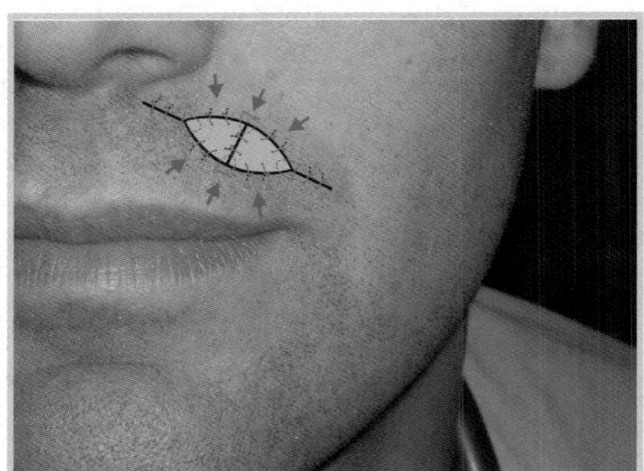

Figure 11

A-to-T-plasty works well because it does not pull tension from the lip, and the skin that is moved matches the skin around it well (the mustache will look normal). **Good choice.**

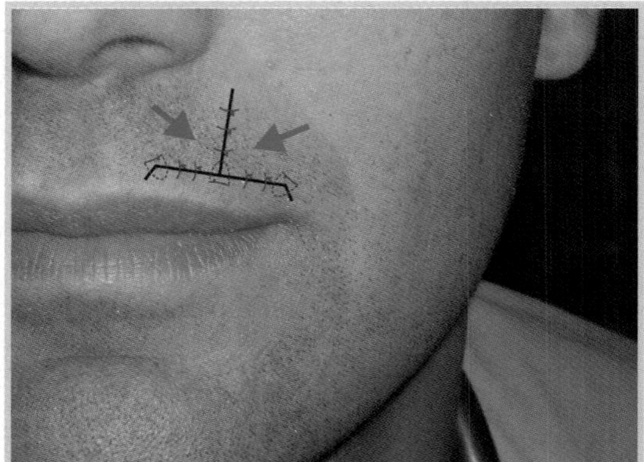

Figure 12

CHAPTER 45

Advancement Flaps

E. J. Mayeaux, Jr., MD, DABFP, FAAFP
Professor of Family Medicine, Professor of Obstetrics and Gynecology
Louisiana State University Health Sciences Center, Shreveport, LA

Local skin flaps provide a sophisticated approach to closing large skin defects produced by trauma or removal of skin lesions. The fusiform (elliptical) excision is the technique most commonly employed for simple lesion removal, but nearby structures (e.g., nose, ear, orifices) can preclude use of this technique by limiting the amount of undermining and loose skin that can be pulled to cover the defect. Nearby skin generally better approximates the needed color and texture to close a defect than skin brought in from a distant site (i.e., skin graft). Local skin flaps can provide excellent functional and cosmetic outcomes.

Advancement flaps represent some of the simplest and most commonly used flap techniques. Advancement flaps move adjacent tissue to close a defect without rotation or lateral movement. The skin may be stretched unidirectionally (i.e., single advancement flap) or bidirectionally (i.e., bilateral advancement flap) to close the defect. Unidirectional pull on tissue can be useful when a certain type of skin is needed for closure. For instance, after removal of a tumor from the outer portion of the eyebrow, the defect should be replaced with hair-bearing skin of the medial eyebrow to prevent a shortened and cosmetically abnormal-appearing eyebrow.

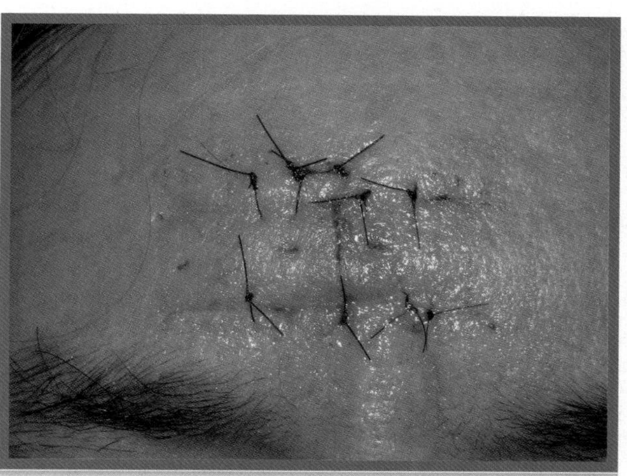

The blood supply for an advancement flap comes from the base of the flap. If a long advancement flap is needed to stretch skin for closure, the blood supply to the flap tip may be compromised. When closing a defect 1 inch in diameter on the face, the single advancement flap should be no longer than 3 inches. Single advancement flaps on less vascular areas of the body do better if limited to a length-to-width ratio of 2.5 to 1. One way to avoid long single advancement flaps is to pull skin from both directions; the bilateral advancement flap generally has less chance of flap tip necrosis.

When removing skin cancer, it is best to ensure clear margins before performance of flap closure. Wide excision around a cancer may provide high rates of cure, but the excessive removal of tissue may limit the cosmetic outcome. Histologic confirmation by Mohs surgery or frozen sections is essential before closure when removing cancers at high risk for recurrence (e.g., morpheaform or sclerosing basal cell carcinomas). Lesions may also be left bandaged for several days pending confirmation of clear margins and closed later.

Preventing complications is an important aspect of performing flap surgery. Strict sterile technique is necessary to avoid wound infections. Excessive stretching of skin should be avoided because necrosis will ensue. Wide undermining of the lateral tissue around a flap aids the closure. Do not pull on the skin edges with forceps because gentle handling prevents excessive scarring. Blood accumulations beneath flaps can interfere with oxygen delivery to the tissue, so excellent hemostasis is required. Bleeding vessels should be clamped or suture-ligated before the flap is sutured, and pressure bandaging is advocated following the procedure.

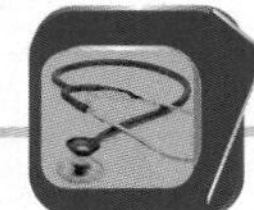

Equipment

- Surgery tray instruments are listed in Appendix G. Consider adding skin hooks to gently handle the skin flaps. Have at least three fine (mosquito) hemostats to assist with hemostasis while developing large skin flaps.
- Suggested suture removal times are listed in Appendix J, and a suggested anesthesia tray that can be used for this procedure is listed in Appendix F. All instruments can be ordered through local surgical supply houses.

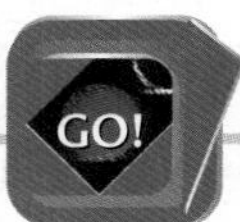

Indications

- Closure of skin defects that require skin pull in line with the long axis of the lesion
- Closure of eyebrow defects
- Repair of defects of the temple area
- Closure of forehead defects
- Closure of cheek defects
- Closure of upper arm defects
- Closure of defects on the tip of the nose
- Closure of defects on the trunk or abdomen
- Closure of forehead skin defects

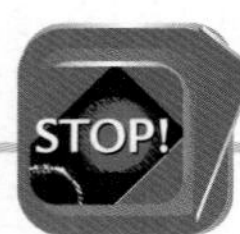

Relative Contraindications

- Practitioner's unfamiliarity or inexperience with techniques
- Cellulitis in the tissues
- Skin unable to be stretched to cover the defect
- Chronic steroid use (and steroid skin effects)

The Procedure

Advancement Flaps

Step 1. Ideally, the long arms for single or bilateral advancement flaps should be placed to align the arms with the lines of least skin tension (see Appendix B, Lines of Lesser Skin Tension [Langer]). The flap placement must also take into account structures that will be distorted if the flap causes tension from this area (e.g., eyes and eyebrows) and structures that anchor the skin (e.g., ears and nose).

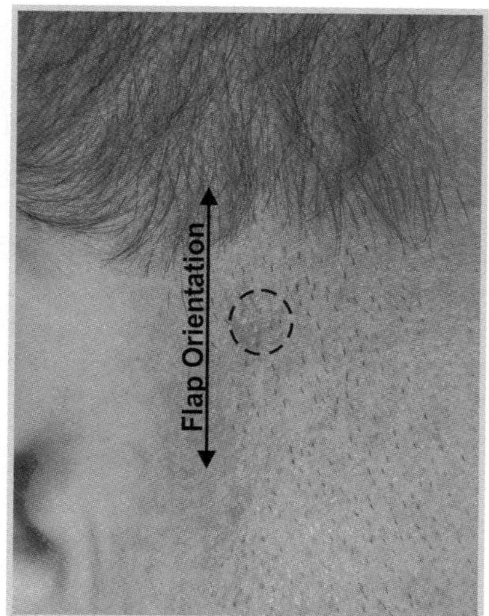

Step 1

Step 2. The advancement flap technique is performed after administration of anesthesia (e.g., field block; see Chapter 2, Field Block Anesthesia). Prep the skin with povidone-iodine or chlorhexidine solution, and allow it to dry (see Appendix E, Skin Preparation Recommendations). The lesion is removed with a rim of normal-appearing skin.

- **PEARL:** Prep a wide area so that an undraped area is not inadvertently exposed if the drape slides a little.

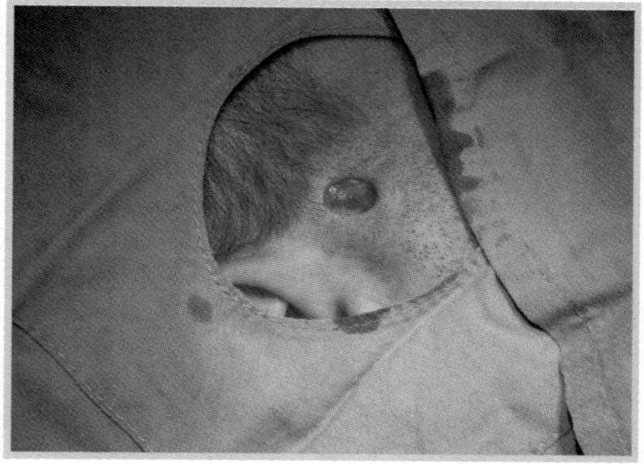

Step 2

Step 3. The defect is squared. The flap arms are incised two to three times the original defect's diameter. The flap and surrounding skin at the base of the flap are undermined with a horizontally held scalpel blade or iris scissors.

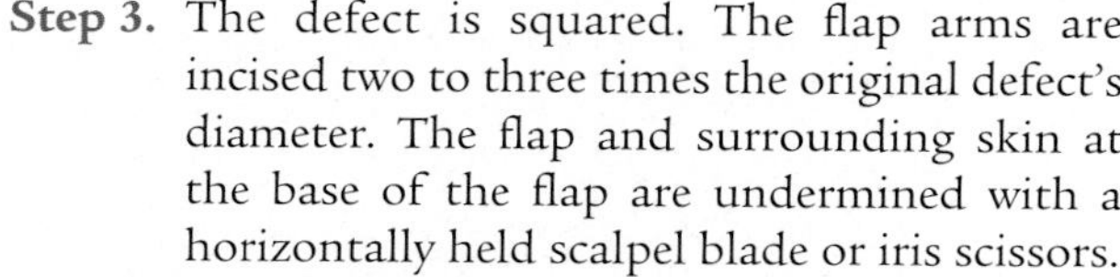

- **PEARL:** Some skin surgeons excise the original lesion in a square, which gives additional tissue in which to get clean margins. This is often easier if the long arms of the H-shape of the flaps are cut first and then the center cuts made connecting the two long arms. This greatly decreases the risk of positive margins.

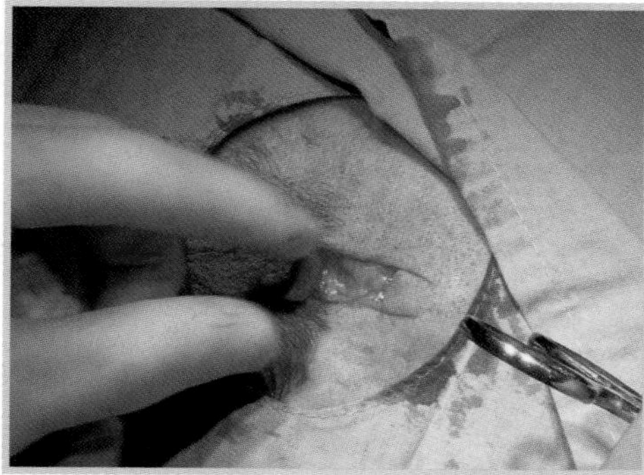

Step 3

Step 4. Attempt to slide the flap to cover the defect using skin hooks or fingertips. If the defect cannot be covered by the flap, the flap can be lengthened. Anchor the flap in place with one or two sutures.

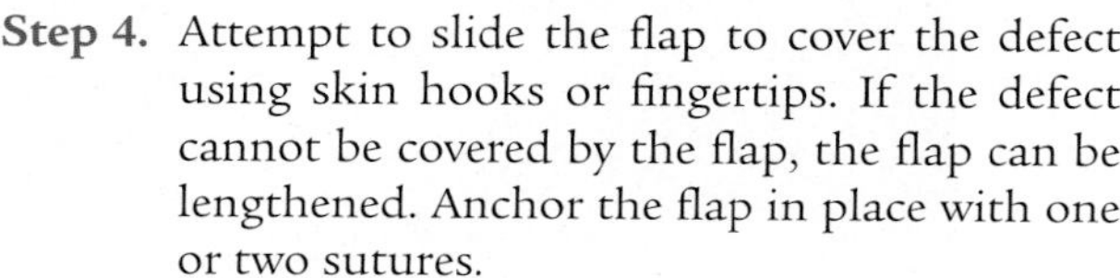

- **PITFALL:** If there is tension on the flap, vertical mattress sutures can be placed instead of simple interrupted sutures to increase blood flow at the suture line (see Chapter 43, Vertical Mattress Suture).

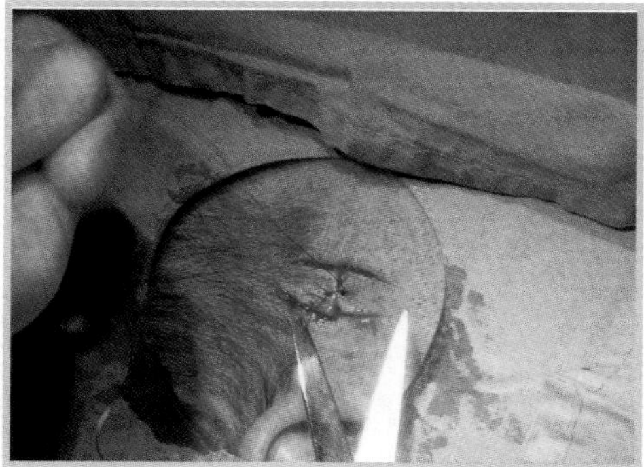

Step 4

- **PITFALL:** The skin often bunches up (i.e., dog ears) near the base of the flap. These dog ears are eliminated by excising triangular pieces of skin (i.e., Burrow triangles) (see Chapter 46, Burrow's Triangle (Dog Ear) Repair).

Step 5. After removal of any redundant tissue, the corners lie flat. Corner sutures (see Chapter 39, Corner Suture) can be placed for the four corners, and interrupted suture is used to complete the flap.

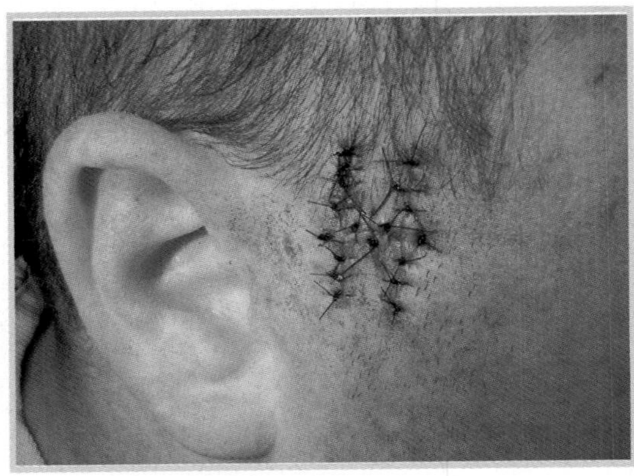

Step 5

Advancement Flaps on the Brow

Step 1. This flap is also is useful in the brow region. After removal of a tumor in the lateral eyebrow, hair-bearing skin is used to close the defect with a single sided advancement flap.

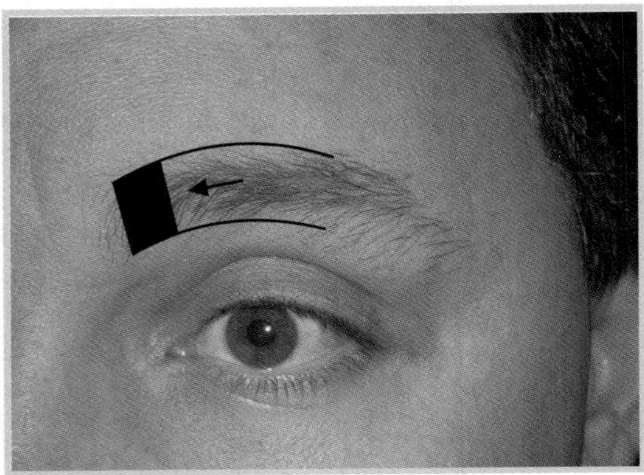

Step 1

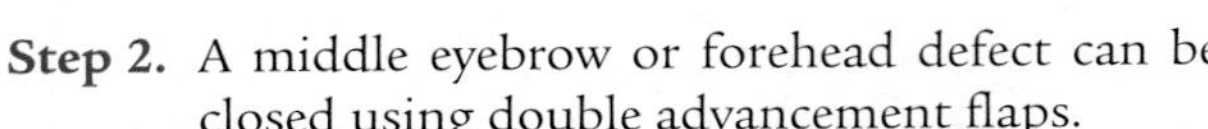

Step 2. A middle eyebrow or forehead defect can be closed using double advancement flaps.

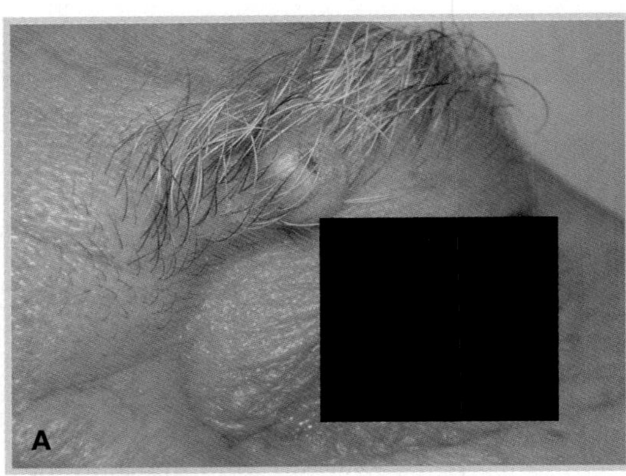

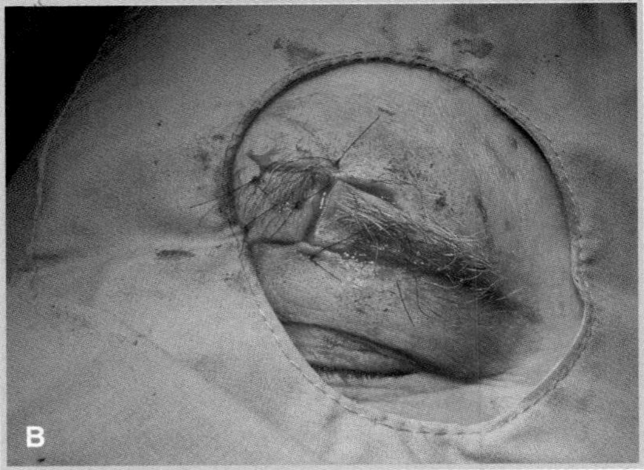

Step 2

Step 3. A square defect is created around the tumor, and the flap arms incised to about 1.5 times the diameter of the defect.

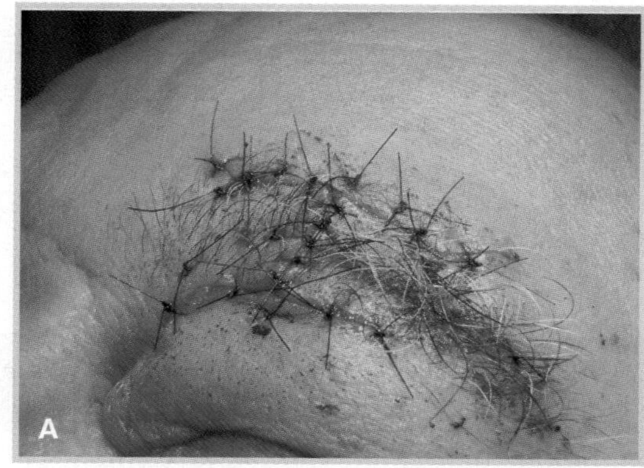

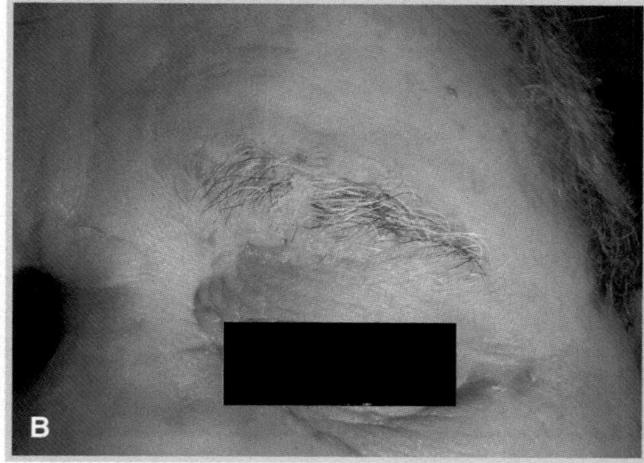

Step 3

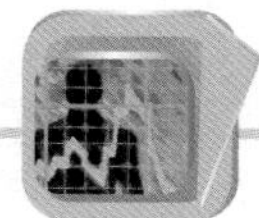

Complications

- Pain, infection, and bleeding
- Nonunion of skin edges
- Scar formation

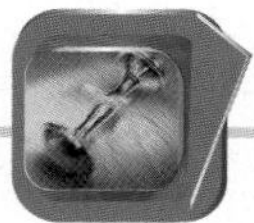

Pediatric Considerations

Generally, pediatric skin has excellent blood flow and heals very well. However, pediatric patients often find it difficult to sit and lie still during lengthy procedures. The patient's maturity and ability to cooperate should be considered before deciding to attempt any outpatient procedure.

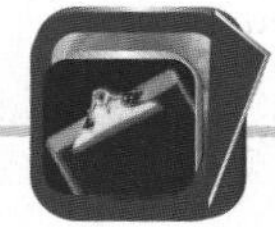

Postprocedure Instructions

Have the patient keep the bandage on and the wound dry for the first 24 hours. After that, it can be cleaned with hydrogen peroxide or gently washed it with soap and water as needed. An antibiotic ointment and bandage should be reapplied until the patient returns or for 2 weeks. Have the patient report signs of infection. Schedule a return appointment for sutures removal (see Appendix J, Recommended Suture Removal Times).

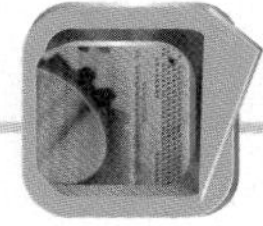

Coding Information

These codes encompass excision or repair, or both, by adjacent transfer or rearrangement, including Z-plasty, W-plasty, V-Y-plasty, rotation flaps, advancement flaps, and double-pedicle flaps. When applied to traumatic wounds, the defect must be developed by the surgeon because the closure requires it, and these codes should not be used for direct closure of a defect that incidentally results in the configuration of one of the flaps or tissue rearrangements. If the configurations result incidentally from the laceration shape, closure should be reported using simple repair codes (see Chapter 38, Simple Interrupted Suture). The excision of benign lesions (CPT 11400–11446) and malignant lesions (CPT 11600–11646) may not be separately reported with codes 14000-14061. All of the following codes are for adjacent tissue transfer or rearrangement, and they refer to defects in the trunk or the following sites: scalp, arms, or legs (SAL); forehead, cheeks, chin, mouth, neck, axillae, genitalia, hands, or feet (FCCMNAGHF); and eyelids, nose, ears, or lips (ENEL).

CPT Code	Description	2008 Average 50th Percentile Fee	Global Period
14000	Trunk ≤10 cm^2	$1,062.00	90
14001	Trunk 10.1–30.0 cm^2	$1,400.00	90
14020	SAL ≤10 cm^2	$1,222.00	90
14021	SAL 10.1–30.0^2	$1,684.00	90
14040	FCCMNAGHF ≤10 cm^2	$1,551.00	90
14041	FCCMNAGHF 10.1–30.0 cm^2	$1,757.00	90
14060	ENEL ≤10 cm^2	$1,841.00	90
14061	ENEL 10.1–30.0 cm^2	$2,254.00	90
14300	Any unusual or complicated area >30 cm^2	$2,749.00	90

CPT is a registered trademark of the American Medical Association.
2008 average 50th Percentile Fees are provided courtesy of 2008 MMH-SI's copyrighted Physicians' Fees and Coding Guide.
SAL, scalp, arms, or legs; FCCMNAGHF, forehead, cheeks, chin, mouth, neck, axillae, genitalia, hands, or feet; ENEL, eyelids, nose, ears, or lips.

Patient Education Handout

Patient education handouts, "Wound and Suture Care for Adults," "Wound and Suture Care for Children," and "Helping Your Child during Medical Procedures" can be found on the book's Web site.

Bibliography

Chernosky ME. Scalpel and scissors surgery as seen by the dermatologist. In: Epstein E, Epstein E Jr, eds. *Skin Surgery*. 6th ed. Philadelphia: WB Saunders; 1987:88–127.

Cook J. Introduction to facial flaps. *Dermatol Clin.* 2001;19:199–212.

Grabb WC. Classification of skin flaps. In: Grabb WC, Myers MB, eds. *Skin Flaps*. Boston: Little, Brown; 1975:145–154.

Grigg R. Forehead and temple reconstruction. *Otolaryngol Clin North Am.* 2001;34:583–600.

Harahap M. The modified bilateral advancement flap. *Dermatol Surg.* 2001;27:463–466.

Shim EK, Greenway HT. Surgical pearl: repair of helical rim defects with the bipedicle advancement flap. *J Am Acad Dermatol.* 2000;43:1109–1111.

Stegman SJ, Tromovitch TA, Glogau RG. *Basics of Dermatologic Surgery*. Chicago: Year Book Medical Publishing; 1982:82–84.

Stegman SJ. Fifteen ways to close surgical wounds. *J Dermatol Surg.* 1975;1:25–31.

Swanson NA. *Atlas of Cutaneous Surgery*. Boston: Little, Brown; 1987:86–91.

Tollefson TT, Murakami CS, Kriet JD. Cheek repair. *Otolaryngol Clin North Am.* 2001;34:627–646.

Vural E, Key JM. Complications, salvage, and enhancement of local flaps in facial reconstruction. *Otolaryngol Clin North Am.* 2001;34:739–751.

Whitaker DC. Random-pattern flaps. In: Wheeland RG, ed. *Cutaneous surgery*. Philadelphia: WB Saunders; 1994:329–352.

Zuber TJ. *Advanced Soft-Tissue Surgery*. Kansas City: American Academy of Family Physicians; 1999:62–72.

2008 MAG Mutual Healthcare Solutions, Inc.'s Physicians' Fee and Coding Guide. Duluth, Georgia. MAG Mutual Healthcare Solutions, Inc. 2007.

CHAPTER 46

Burow Triangle (Dog Ear) Repair

E. J. Mayeaux, Jr., MD, DABFP, FAAFP

Professor of Family Medicine, Professor of Obstetrics and Gynecology
Louisiana State University Health Sciences Center, Shreveport, LA

A *dog ear* (tissue protrusion or tricone) is a protrusion of skin that often results from excessive tissue along one side of the suture line of a flap or plasty. Although the natural elastic properties of the skin allow for primary closure of skin edges with up to 15% difference in lengths, many tissue rearrangement procedures produce greater discrepancies that result in dog ears. In areas of less skin elasticity, tissue protrusions form with less disproportion and tend to be larger. Sometimes excess subcutaneous fat at the apex of a repair may have the appearance of a dog ear. Removal of the excess fat usually alleviates this problem.

Wounds on convex surfaces are more likely to develop dog ears at closure. This is especially pronounced on the extremities, mandible, and chin. As wounds over convex surfaces heal and undergo wound contraction, horizontal scar contraction depresses the central portion of the scar, accentuating dog-ear deformities.

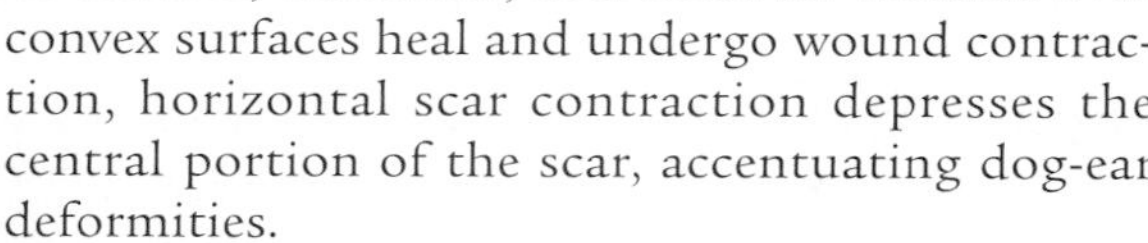

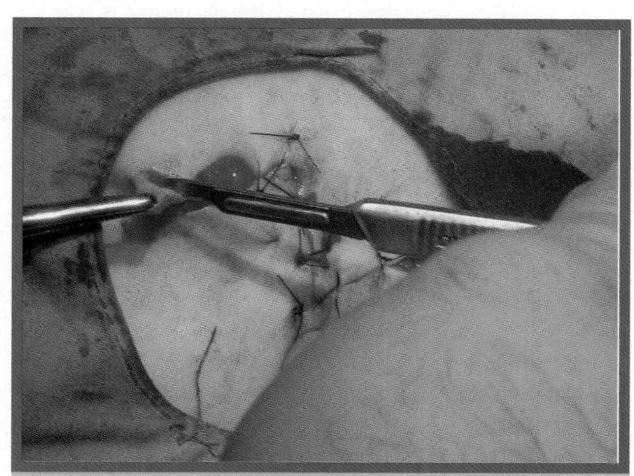

Adherence to basic surgical principles can help limit formation of dog ears. It is very important to maintain the proper 90-degree angle of the scalpel blade with respect to the skin when performing an excision. A beveled edge at the tip of an excision results in excess tissue at the wound apices, producing dog ears that are unlikely to resolve on their own. An undermined wound edge more easily accommodates the horizontal displacement of tissue. If no undermining is performed, the forces of wound closure increase, creating dog ears.

Dog ear correction should be executed with aesthetic concerns. This typically involves positioning the dog ear repair so that it will blend into preexisting wrinkles or anatomic boundaries. Correction of the excessive skin defect is accomplished by removal of a triangular piece of skin known as a *Burow triangle*. Although this technique lengthens the scar, it provides a much-improved cosmetic outcome. Although dog ear repairs can be done anytime during a procedure, it is usually helpful to at least partially close the wound edges before performing the repair. There are many techniques that can be used to correct dog ears. The simplest and most versatile, the Burow triangle repair, is described here.

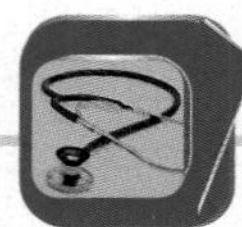

Equipment

Common skin surgery equipment and the typical skin surgery tray are listed in Appendix G.

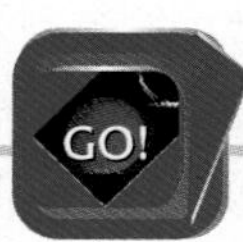

Indications

- Elimination of excess skin when suturing unequal skin length edges, especially when performing tissue rearrangements (such as rotation flaps, O-to-Z-plasties, and the ends of advancement flaps

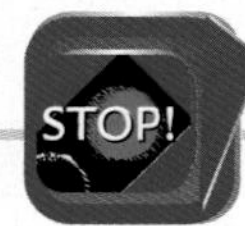

Contraindications

- Uncooperative patient
- Wounds best closed by other methods
- Presence of cellulitis, bacteremia, or active infection

The Procedure

Step 1. Dog ears often result from excess tissue along one side of the suture line of a flap or plasty.

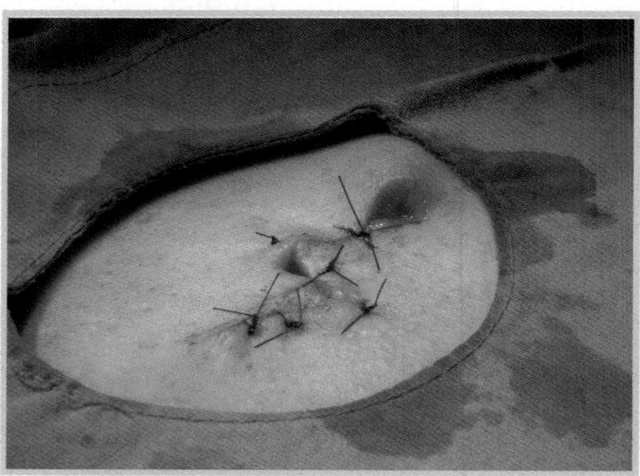

Step 1

Step 2. Start the correction by making an incision at a 120-degree angle to the original incision line.

- **PEARL:** The correct angle produces an incision in the shape of a hockey stick.

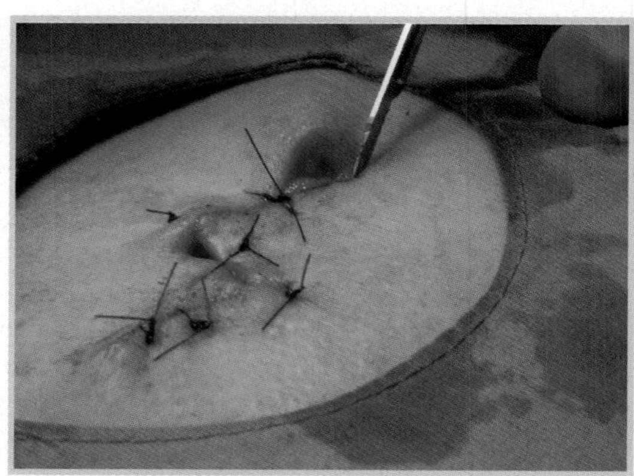

Step 2

Step 3. Undermine the triangular portion of the tissue and lay it flat over the recently made incision.

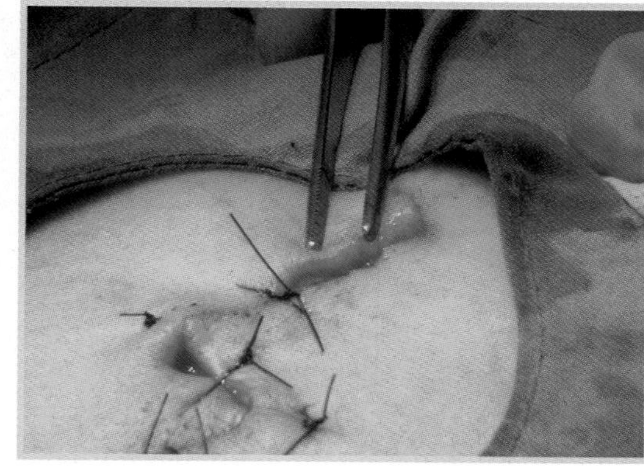

Step 3

Step 4. Using the previous incision as a guide, incise the excess overlying tissue.

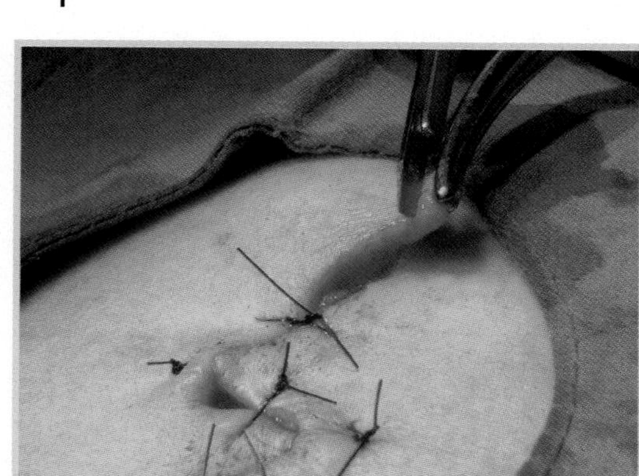

Step 4

Step 5. Lay the newly formed triangular flap into the defect created with the original 120-degree incision and check for fit. If the skin does not lie flat, excise more tissue as necessary to achieve this result.

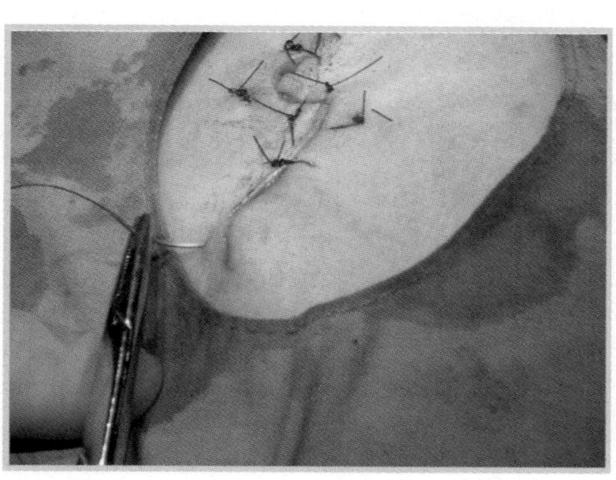

Step 5

Step 6. Place a corner suture to close the corner of the repair (see Chapter 39).

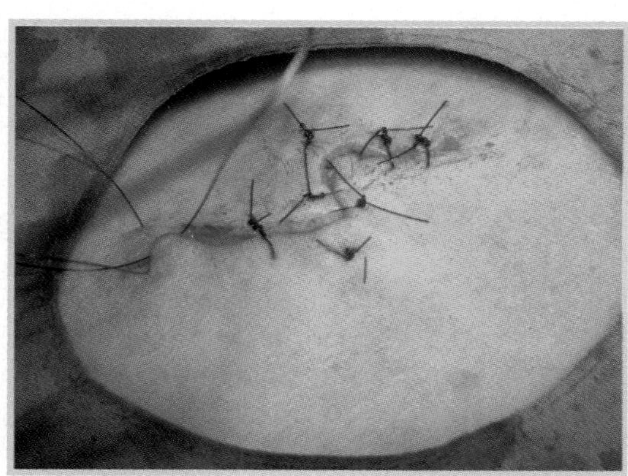

Step 6

Step 7. Use simple interrupted sutures to close any remaining gaps in the suture line.

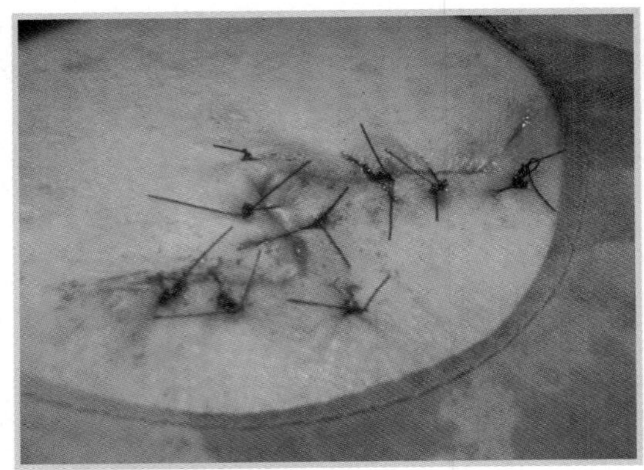

Step 7

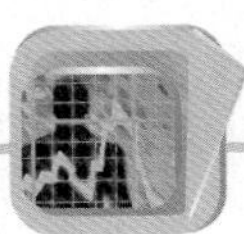

Complications

- Bleeding
- Infection
- Scar formation

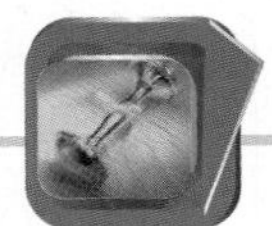

Pediatric Considerations

This technique is the same in pediatric and adult patients.

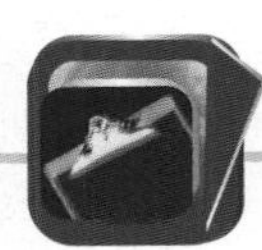

Postprocedure Instructions

Instruct the patient to gently wash an area that has been stitched after 1 day but to not put the wound into standing water for 2 to 3 days. Have the patient dry the area well after washing and use a small amount of antibiotic ointment to promote moist healing. Recommend wound elevation to help lessen swelling, reduce pain, and speed healing. Instruct the patient not to pick at, break, or cut the stitches. Have the patient cover the wound with a nonocclusive dressing for 2 to 3 days. A simple adhesive bandage will suffice for many small lacerations. The dressing should be left in place for at least 48 hours, after which time most wounds can be opened to air. Scalp wounds can be left open if small, but large head wounds can be wrapped circumferentially with rolled gauze.

Most uncontaminated wounds do not need to be seen by a provider until suture removal, unless signs of infection develop. Highly contaminated wounds should be seen for follow-up in 2 to 3 days. Give discharge instructions to the patient regarding signs of wound infection.

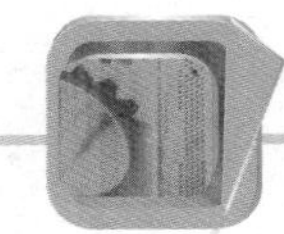

Coding Information and Supply Sources

All codes listed are for superficial wound closure using sutures, staples, or tissue adhesives with or without adhesive strips on the skin surface. If a layered closure is required, use alternate codes: intermediate closure codes 12031 to 12057 or complex repair codes 13100 to 13160.

Add together the lengths of wounds in the same classification and anatomic sites. Use separate codes for repairs from different anatomic sites. Debridement is considered a separate procedure only when gross contamination requires prolonged cleansing or when appreciable amounts of devitalized or contaminated tissue are removed. Simple repair is included in the codes reported for benign and malignant lesion excision.

CPT Code	Description	2008 Average 50th Percentile Fee	Global Period
12001	Simple repair SNAGTEHF ≤2.5 cm	$220.00	10
12002	Simple repair SNAGTEHF 2.6–7.5 cm	$235.00	10
12004	Simple repair SNAGTEHF 7.6–12.5 cm	$285.00	10
12005	Simple repair SNAGTEHF 12.6–20.0 cm	$408.00	10
12006	Simple repair SNAGTEHF 20.1–30.0 cm	$506.00	10
12007	Simple repair SNAGTEHF >30.0 cm		10
12011	Simple repair FEENLMM ≤2.5 cm	$240.00	10
12013	Simple repair FEENLMM 2.6–5.0 cm	$288.00	10
12014	Simple repair FEENLMM 5.1–7.5 cm	$351.00	10
12015	Simple repair FEENLMM 7.6–12.5 cm	$449.00	10
12016	Simple repair FEENLMM 12.6–20.0 cm	$585.00	10
12017	Simple repair FEENLMM 20.1–30.0 cm	$743.00	10
12018	Simple repair FEENLMM >30.0 cm		10
12020	Treatment of superficial wound dehiscence, simple closure	$397.00	10

CPT is a registered trademark of the American Medical Association.
2008 average 50th Percentile Fees are provided courtesy of 2008 MMH-SI's copyrighted Physicians' Fees and Coding Guide.
SNAGTEHF, scalp, neck, axillae, external genitalia, trunk, extremities, hands, and feet;
FEENLMM, face, ears, eyelids, nose, lips, and mucous membranes.

Bibliography

Borges AF. Dog-ear repair. *Plast Reconstr Surg.* 1982;69:707–713.

Dzubow LM. The dynamics of dog-ear formation and correction. *L Dermatol Surg Oncol.* 1985;7:722–778.

Gormley DE. A brief analysis of the Burow's wedge/triangle principle. *J Dermatol Surg Oncol.* 1985;11:121–123.

Gormley DE. The dog-ear: causes, prevention, correction. *J Dermatol Surg Oncol.* 1977;3:194–198.

Metz BJ, Katta R. Burow's advancement flap closure of adjacent defects. *Dermatol Online J.* 2005;11(1):11.

Robertson DB. Dog ear repairs. In: Wheeland RG, ed. *Cutaneous Surgery*. Philadelphia: WB Saunders; 1994:295–303.

Stasko T. Advanced suturing techniques and layered closures. In: Wheeland DG, ed. *Cutaneous Surgery*. Philadelphia: Harcort Brace and Company; 1994:304–317.

Weisberg NK, Nehal KS, Zide BM. Dog-ears: a review. *Dermatol Surg.* 2000;26(4):363–370.

2008 MAG Mutual Healthcare Solutions, Inc.'s Physicians' Fee and Coding Guide. Duluth, Georgia. MAG Mutual Healthcare Solutions, Inc. 2007.

CHAPTER 47

Epidermal Cyst Excision

E. J. Mayeaux, Jr., MD, DABFP, FAAFP

Professor of Family Medicine, Professor of Obstetrics and Gynecology
Louisiana State University Health Sciences Center, Shreveport, LA

Epidermal or sebaceous cysts are frequently encountered in clinical practice. These slowly enlarging lesions commonly appear on the trunk, neck, face, and genitals and behind the ears. The term *epidermal cyst* is preferred over the historically used term *sebaceous cyst*. The cysts usually arise from ruptured pilosebaceous follicles or the lubricating glands associated with hairs or other skin adnexal structures. Within the cyst is a white to yellow, cheese-like substance commonly (but incorrectly) referred to as sebum. The rancid odor associated with some cysts reflects the lipid content of the cyst material and any decomposition of cyst contents by bacteria.

Clinically, the cysts can vary in size from a few millimeters to 5 cm in diameter. Cysts generally have a doughy or firm consistency, and hard, solid-feeling lesions suggest the possibility of alternate diagnoses. The cysts usually are mobile within the skin, unless the cysts have surrounding scar and fibrous tissue from a prior episode of inflammation.

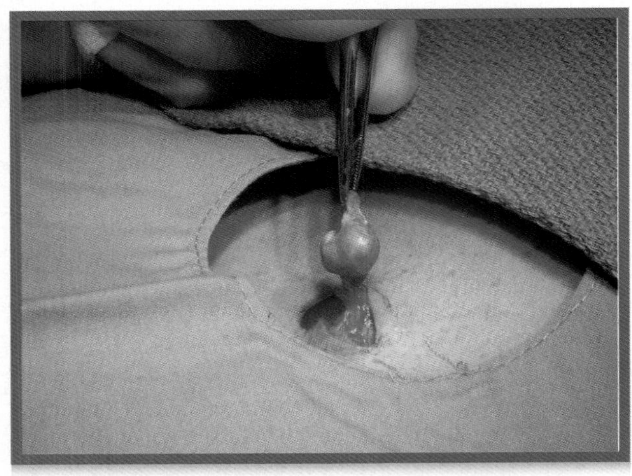

The cyst contents induce a tremendous inflammatory response from the body if they leak out. Epidermal cysts can have a tremendous amount of associated pus when inflamed, but culturing these inflammatory cells often reveals a sterile inflammatory response. Because of the discomfort, redness, and swelling associated with an inflamed cyst, many individuals prefer to have cysts removed before they have the opportunity to leak and become inflamed. Inflamed cysts usually require incision and drainage of the pus and sebaceous material, with removal of the cyst wall at a later date. The inflamed tissues bleed extensively and are unable to hold sutures well for proper closure. After the inflammation resolves, standard incision and removal techniques may be employed to remove the entire cyst. Cyst recurrences are prevented by complete removal of the cyst wall.

Most cysts are simple, solitary lesions. However, some clinical situations warrant added care. Multiple epidermal cysts that are associated with osteomas and multiple skin lipomas or fibromas may represent Gardner syndrome. Gardner syndrome is associated with premalignant colonic and gastric polyps. Dermal cysts of the nose, head, and neck often appear similar to epidermal cysts. However, a dermal cyst can have a thin stalk that connects directly to the subdermal space, and surgery can produce central nervous system infection. Multiple cysts, such as in the fold behind the ear, can be treated alternately with medical therapy (i.e., isotretinoin). When a cyst is removed with any technique, the medical provider should palpate the surgical site to ensure that no tissue or lesions remain. Rarely, the clinician may encounter basal cell carcinoma or squamous cell carcinoma associated with epidermal cysts, and histologic examination of cyst walls is recommended whenever unusual or unexpected clinical findings are encountered.

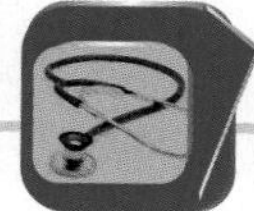

Equipment

- The basic office surgery instruments are used for the standard excision technique (see Appendix G).
- A suggested anesthesia tray that can be used for this procedure is listed in Appendix F.
- Skin preparation recommendations appear in Appendix E.

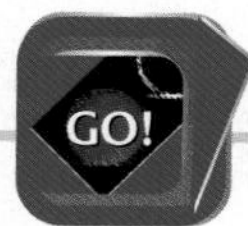

Indications

- Lesions with the clinical findings or appearance of epidermal cysts

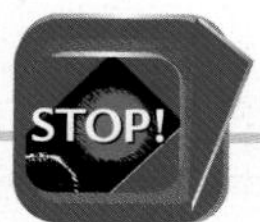

Contraindications (Relative)

- Local cellulitis
- Severe bleeding disorders
- Failed previous minimum excision attempt on the specific lesion

The Procedure

Step 1. Anesthesia is accomplished with a 25-gauge, 1-inch-long needle on the syringe. Insert the needle laterally, angling the needle 45 degrees down to below (behind) the cyst (see Chapter 2). Place an adequate amount of anesthetic (usually 3 to 6 mL) beneath the cyst. Prep the skin with povidone-iodine or chlorhexidine solution, and allow it to dry (see Appendix E).

- **PEARL:** Prep a wide area so that an undraped area is not inadvertently exposed if the drape slides a little.
- **PITFALL:** If the needle tip is placed inadvertently within the cyst, the anesthetic will increase pressure and cause the cyst to explode, often shooting the sebaceous material across the room.

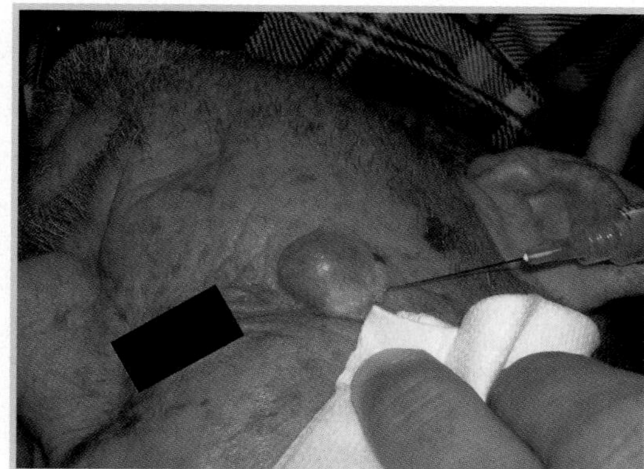

Step 1

Step 2. Make a fusiform excision that is large enough to remove the redundant skin caused by expansion of the cyst. Use care to cut only to the base of the dermis, not into the subcutaneous tissue. Make sure the long axis of the fusiform is parallel to the lines of least skin tension. If the pore is visible, the excision should be designed around it.

- **PITFALL:** Cutting too deeply increases the chances of inadvertent puncture of the cyst, with spillage of the cyst contents and resultant inflammatory response.

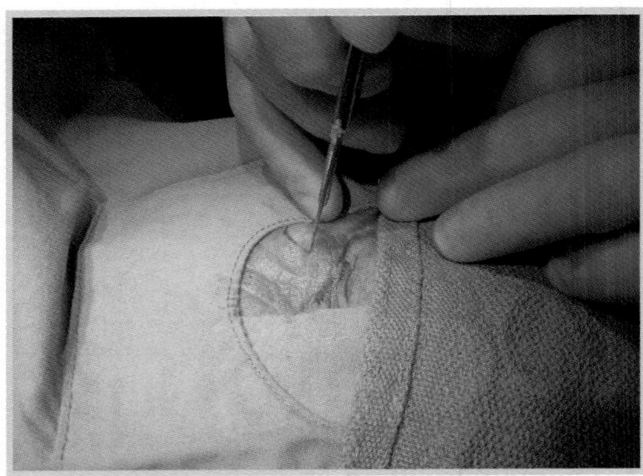

Step 2

Step 3. Carefully open a dissection plane between the skin and the cyst wall. The center of the fusiform incision may be grasped with pick-ups to assist in manipulating the cyst.

- **PEARL:** If the cyst is accidentally entered, use a small hemostat to clamp the hole. It is much easier to excise a full cyst than a deflated one.
- **PITFALL:** The clinician should not be positioned directly over the cyst. Opening a cyst that is under pressure can result in upward spraying of the cyst's contents. Hold some gauze in the nondominant hand to act as a shield when opening the cyst.

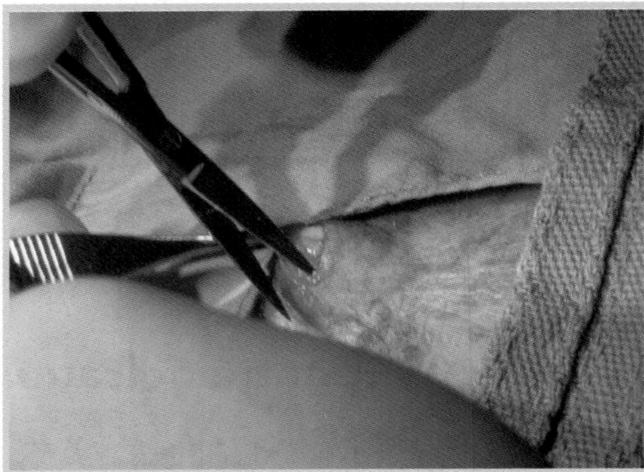

Step 3

Step 4. Dissect around the side of the cyst. Gradually change the angle of the scissors to follow the wall of the cyst. Semisharp dissection usually provides rapid removal with a minimal risk of perforating the cyst.

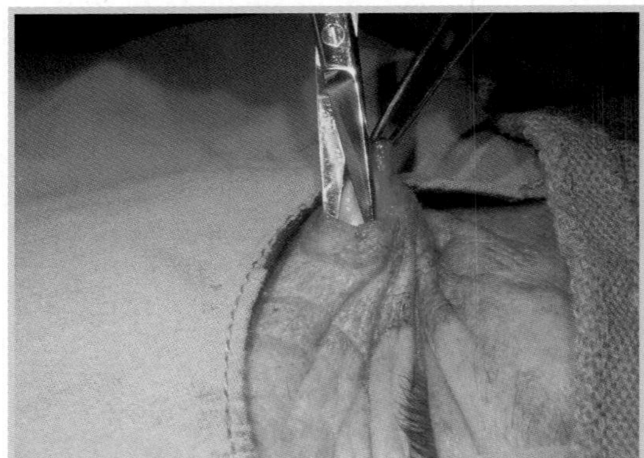

Step 4

Step 5. Continue the removal until the base of the lesion is free.

- **PITFALL:** When attempting to dissect the base of the cyst, be care to not remove excessive normal tissue below the cyst, because this creates a large deep defect that must be closed.

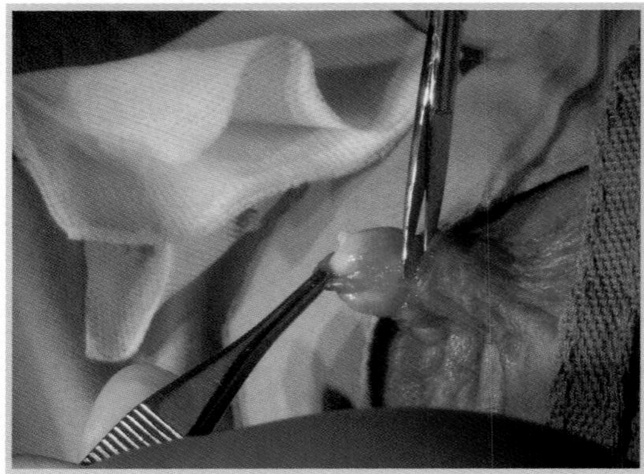

Step 5

Step 6. The wound can be sutured immediately, usually using simple interrupted sutures (see Chapter 38, Simple Interrupted Suture). If a significant defect is present under the skin, place a deep buried suture to close the deep space and approximate the skin edges (see Chapter 37, Deep Buried Dermal Suture).

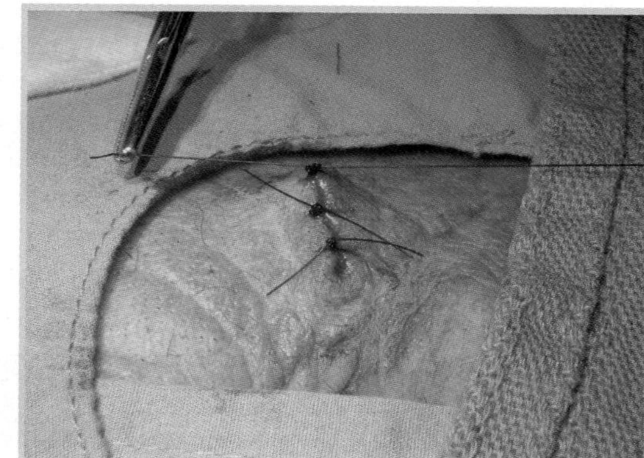

Step 6

Step 7. Incise the cyst and make sure it completely deflates. If there is any thickness or masses in the cyst wall, send it for histologic analysis.

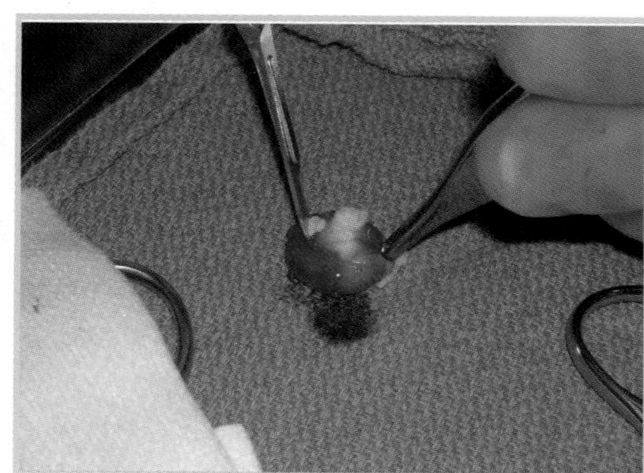

Step 7

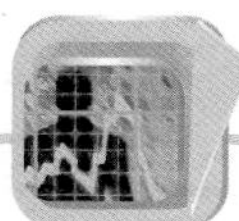

Complications

- Bleeding
- Infection
- Scar formation
- Recurrence

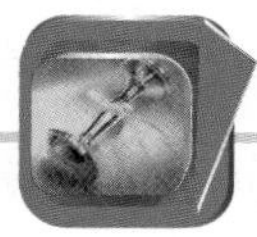

Pediatric Considerations

Although epidermal cysts are rare in the pediatric population, when present, the removal process is the same.

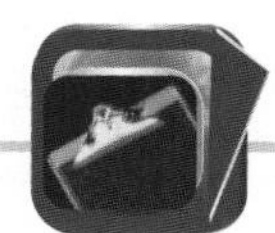

Postprocedure Instructions

Simple epidermal cysts that appear to be completely excised do not generally require follow-up, except for suture removal. If a recurrence is brought to the physician's attention at a later date, standard surgical excision should be attempted.

Instruct the patient to gently wash an area that has been stitched after 1 day but to not put the wound into standing water for 3 days. Have the patient dry the area well after washing and use a small amount of antibiotic ointment to promote moist healing. Recommend wound elevation to help lessen swelling, reduce pain, and speed healing. Instruct the patient not to pick at, break, or cut the stitches.

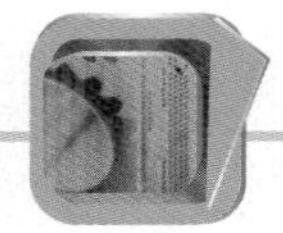

Coding Information and Supply Sources

Use the benign excision codes (11400 to 11446) for removal of these lesions. The code selected is determined by size and location of the lesion. The codes include local anesthesia and simple (one-layer) closure, although the codes can be used if the minimal incision technique is used and no suturing is required. The sites for these codes include the following: trunk, arms, or legs (TAL); scalp, neck, hands, feet, or genitalia (SNHFG); and face, ears, eyelids, nose, lips, or mucous membrane (FEENLMM).

CPT Code	Description	2008 Average 50th Percentile Fee	Global Period
11400	TAL <0.6 cm	$178.00	10
11401	TAL 0.6–1.0 cm	$226.00	10
11402	TAL 1.1–2.0 cm	$289.00	10
11403	TAL 2.1–3.0 cm	$347.00	10
11404	TAL 3.1–4.0 cm	$441.00	10
11406	TAL >4.0 cm	$627.00	10
11420	SNHFG <0.6 cm	$179.00	10
11421	SNHFG 0.6–1.0 cm	$233.00	10
11422	SNHFG 1.1–2.0 cm	$285.00	10
11423	SNHFG 2.1–3.0 cm	$385.00	10
11424	SNHFG 3.1–4.0 cm	$481.00	10
11426	SNHFG >4.0 cm	$683.00	10
11440	FEENLMM <0.6 cm	$221.00	10
11441	FEENLMM 0.6–1.0 cm	$289.00	10
11442	FEENLMM 1.1–2.0 cm	$356.00	10
11443	FEENLMM 2.1–3.0 cm	$450.00	10
11444	FEENLMM 3.1–4.0 cm	$556.00	10
11446	FEENLMM >4.0 cm	$756.00	10

CPT is a registered trademark of the American Medical Association.
2008 average 50th Percentile Fees are provided courtesy of 2008 MMH-SI's copyrighted Physicians' Fees and Coding Guide.
TAL, trunk, arms, or legs; SNHFG, scalp, neck, hands, feet, or genitalia; FEENLMM, face, ears, eyelids, nose, lips, or mucous membrane.

Bibliography

Domonkos AN, Arnold HL, Odom RB. *Andrews' Diseases of the Skin: Clinical Dermatology*. 7th ed. Philadelphia: WB Saunders; 1982.

Farrer AK, Forman WM, Boike AM. Epidermal inclusion cysts following minimal incision surgery. *J Am Podiatr Med Assoc*. 1992;82(10):537–541.

Grocutt M, Fatah MF. Recurrent multiple epidermoid inclusion cysts following rhinoplasty—an unusual complication. *J Laryngol Otol*. 1989;103(12):1214–1216.

Kowand LM, Verhulst LA, Copeland CM, et al. Epidermal cyst of the breast. *Can Med Assoc J*. 1984;131(3):217–219.

Leppard B, Bussey HJ. Epidermoid cysts, polyposis coli and Gardner's syndrome. *Br J Surg*. 1975;62(5):387–393.

Lopez-Rios F. Squamous cell carcinoma arising in a cutaneous epidermal cyst: case report and literature review. *Am J Dermatopathol*. 1999;21:174–177.

Nakamura M. Treating a sebaceous cyst: an incisional technique. *Aesthetic Plast Surg*. 2001;25:52–56.

Suliman MT. Excision of epidermoid (sebaceous) cyst: description of the operative technique. *Plast Reconstr Surg*. 2005;116(7):2042–2043.

Zuber TJ. *Skin Biopsy, Excision and Repair Techniques*. Kansas City: American Academy of Family Physicians; 1998:94–99.

2008 MAG Mutual Healthcare Solutions, Inc.'s Physicians' Fee and Coding Guide. Duluth, Georgia. MAG Mutual Healthcare Solutions, Inc. 2007.

CHAPTER 48

Epidermal Cysts: Minimal Excisional Removal

E. J. Mayeaux, Jr., MD, DABFP, FAAFP

Professor of Family Medicine, Professor of Obstetrics and Gynecology
Louisiana State University Health Sciences Center, Shreveport, LA

Epidermal (sebaceous) cysts are a common complaint in primary care. The cysts arise from the pilosebaceous glands associated with skin adnexal structures. Within the cyst is a white to yellow, cream cheese-like substance commonly (but incorrectly) referred to as *sebum*. Cysts vary in size from a few millimeters to 5 cm in diameter and have a doughy to firm consistency. Some cysts emit a rancid odor, which is due to the lipid content of the cyst and sometimes decomposition of cyst contents by bacteria. The cysts usually are mobile within the skin, unless they have previously ruptured and scarred the surrounding tissue.

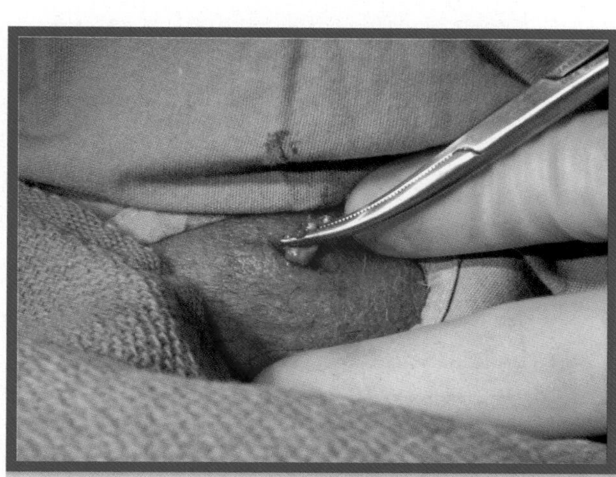

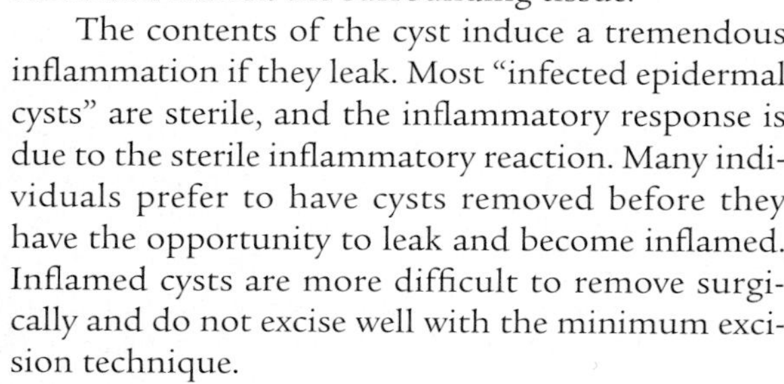

The contents of the cyst induce a tremendous inflammation if they leak. Most "infected epidermal cysts" are sterile, and the inflammatory response is due to the sterile inflammatory reaction. Many individuals prefer to have cysts removed before they have the opportunity to leak and become inflamed. Inflamed cysts are more difficult to remove surgically and do not excise well with the minimum excision technique.

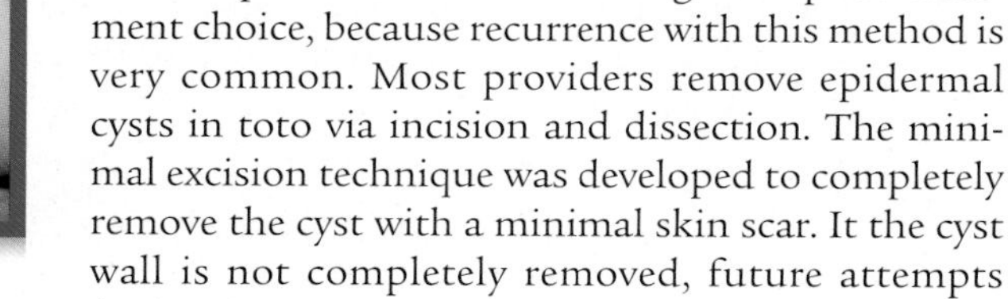

Simple incision and drainage is a poor treatment choice, because recurrence with this method is very common. Most providers remove epidermal cysts in toto via incision and dissection. The minimal excision technique was developed to completely remove the cyst with a minimal skin scar. It the cyst wall is not completely removed, future attempts should be attempted using the standard technique.

Many lesions can be confused with epidermal cysts. If a solid tumor is discovered at the time of the procedure, a biopsy should be obtained. Incisional biopsy can be performed for very large lesions, and excisional biopsy for the smaller lesions. Pilar tumors of the scalp are often confused with epidermoid cysts and may require wide excision because they can erode into the skull.

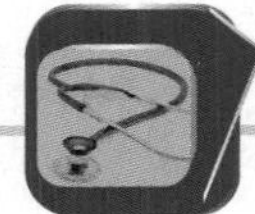

Equipment

- Basic office surgery instruments are used for the standard excision technique (Appendix G). However, the minimal sebaceous cyst removal technique can be performed with a no. 11 scalpel blade, two or three small mosquito hemostats, and sterile gauze.
- A suggested anesthesia tray that can be used for this procedure is listed in Appendix F.
- Skin preparation recommendations appear in Appendix E.

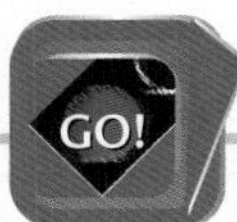

Indications

- Lesions with the clinical findings or appearance of sebaceous cysts, preferably those that have not previously been inflamed or scarred
- Fluctuant or compressible lesions in common areas for sebaceous cysts (e.g., face, neck, scalp, behind the ears, trunk, scrotum)

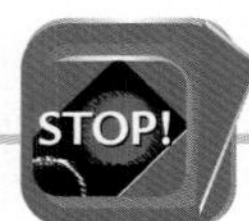

Contraindications (Relative)

- Local cellulitis
- Severe bleeding disorders
- Failed previous minimum excision attempt on the specific lesion. A cyst that has previously ruptured and scarred to the surrounding tissue.

The Procedure

Step 1. Anesthesia is accomplished with a two-step procedure. Begin by placing intradermal anesthesia with a 30-gauge, 0.5-inch-long needle into the skin directly overlying the cyst (see Chapter 1, Local Anesthesia Administration). When the needle tip is correctly placed, there is resistance to injecting the anesthetic within the skin, and a bleb develops in the skin. In the second step, place a field block (see Chapter 2, Field Block Anesthesia).

- PITFALL: If the needle tip is placed inadvertently within the cyst, the anesthetic will increase pressure and cause the cyst to explode, often shooting the sebaceous material across the room.

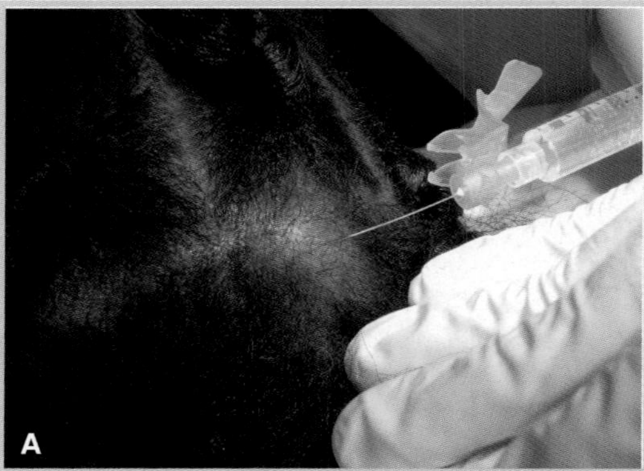
A

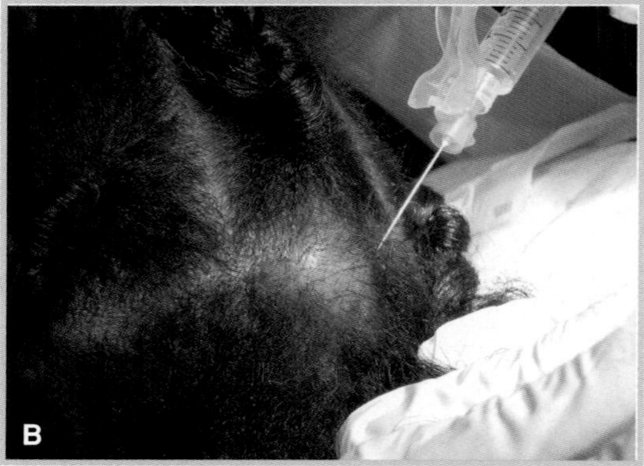
B

Step 1

Step 2. Prep the area. Recommendations for performing skin preps are shown in Appendix E: Skin Preparation Recommendations.

- **PEARL:** When working on the scalp, lightly taping the hair back often facilitates the procedure.

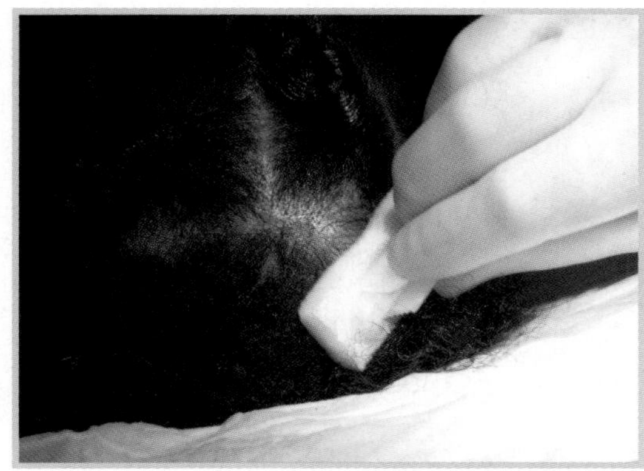

Step 2

Step 3. Create an entry into the cyst by vertically stabbing a no. 11 (sharp-pointed) scalpel blade into the cyst. Usually, a single up-and-down motion is sufficient to create the passage into the cyst. If the cyst is already expressing sebaceous material, use the scalpel to enlarge the opening as necessary.

- **PEARL:** Many operators fail to enter the cyst with the scalpel blade. By directing the blade toward the center of the cyst and inserting until a "give" is felt as the blade tip enters the cyst, the pass of the blade usually will be successful.
- **PITFALL:** The clinician should not be positioned directly over the cyst. Opening a cyst that is under pressure can result in upward spraying of the cyst's contents. Hold some gauze in the nondominant hand to act as a shield when opening the cyst.

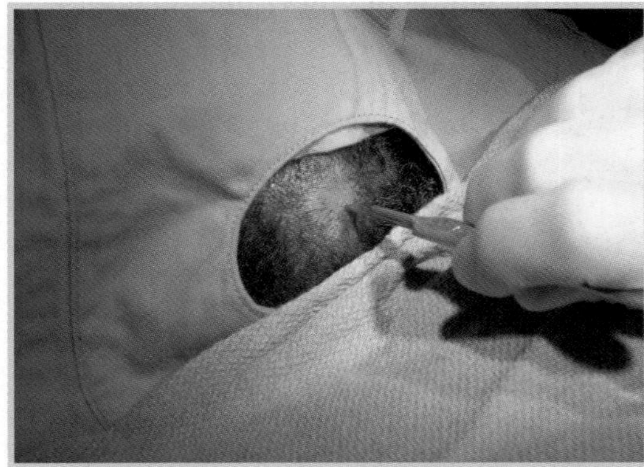

Step 3

Step 4. Alternately, some practitioners prefer the ease afforded by creating a larger opening. A 3- or 4-mm biopsy punch can be inserted directly down into the cyst. The comedone or pore usually is included in the skin that is removed with the biopsy punch. This opening allows much easier emptying of the cyst, but it has the disadvantage of requiring suture closure after the procedure.

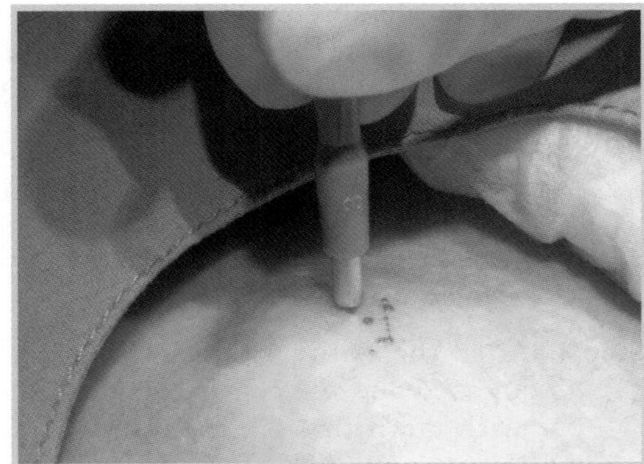

Step 4

Step 5. The cyst contents must be emptied before attempting removal of the cyst wall. Using the thumbs to squeeze the cyst generally provides the greatest possible hand strength. Place the thumbs on opposite sides of the cyst opening. Press straight down with the greatest possible force, and firmly rotate the thumbs toward each other and then up toward the opening.

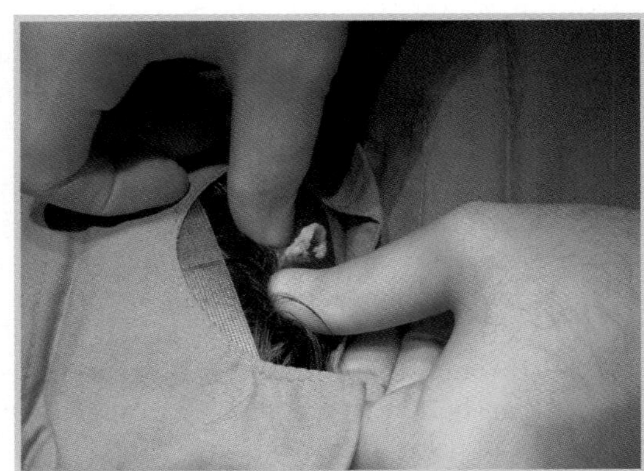

Step 5

Step 6. Squeezing out the cyst's contents can cause the sebaceous material to erupt into the face of the practitioner. A more controlled process involves placing a hemostat into the cyst's opening and squeezing the sebaceous material up into the open hemostat blades. Squeezing is accomplished using fingers on the nondominant hand. After the hemostat fills with material, it is withdrawn with the blades still open, and the sebaceous material is wiped away using gauze. The hemostat is reinserted and the process repeated.

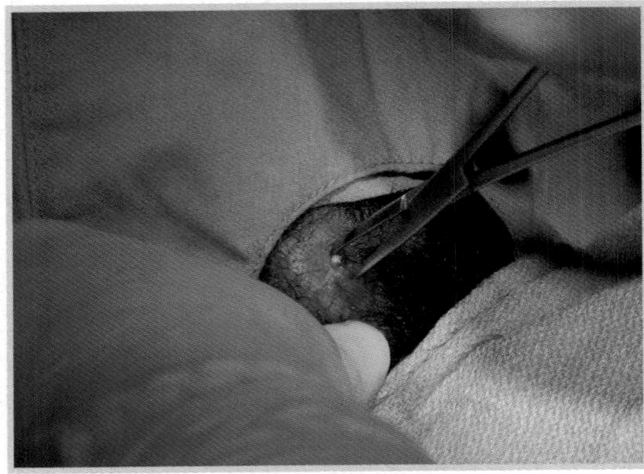

Step 6

Step 7. Use gauze to wipe away sebaceous material on the skin surface. Continue vigorously squeezing until all material is removed. The "kneading" produced from the rocking motion of the thumbs toward the cyst opening helps to loosen the cyst from the surrounding subcutaneous and cutaneous attachments. Move the thumbs around the opening so that the vigorous massaging is performed on all sides of the cyst.

- **PITFALL:** Once the cyst contents have been squeezed out, a mass may be palpated adjacent to the cyst, suggesting that a tumor may be present. It is recommended that the minimal excision technique be abandoned for a formal excision and biopsy. If malignancy is discovered in a cyst wall that is removed at the time of the minimal excision technique, the physician may consider a second excision.

- **PEARL:** Any atypical-appearing lesion or one associated with a palpable irregularity in the cyst wall should be sent for histologic analysis.

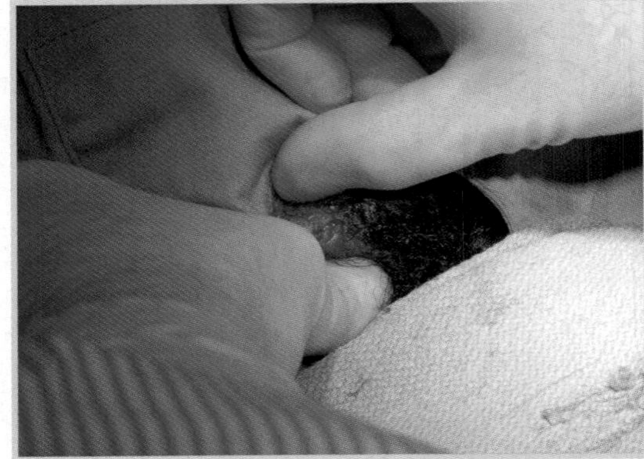

Step 7

Step 8. After the entire site has been vigorously kneaded and the cyst is completely emptied, reach down through the opening and grasp the posterior wall of the cyst. Gently elevate the cyst toward the skin surface. A lateral rocking motion may be helpful.

- **PEARL:** If adhesions are present, they may be reduced by semisharp dissection using Iris scissors.

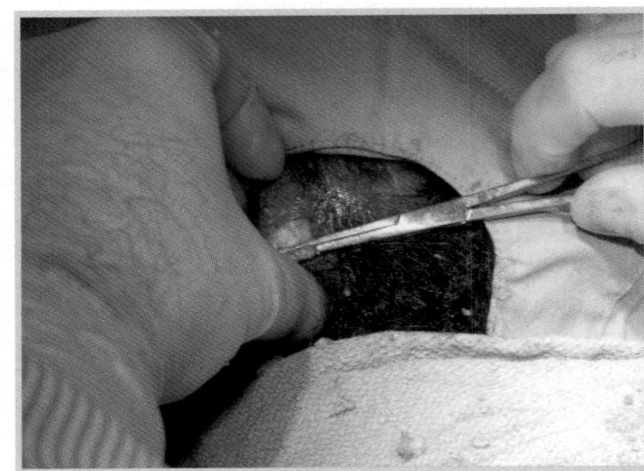

Step 8

Step 9. If resistance is encountered, grasp the cyst wall with a second hemostat just below the initial hemostat application, coming from a horizontal plane. Continue to elevate with both hemostats. If more of the cyst wall slides through the skin opening, the first hemostat can be released and used to regrasp the cyst wall below the second hemostat.

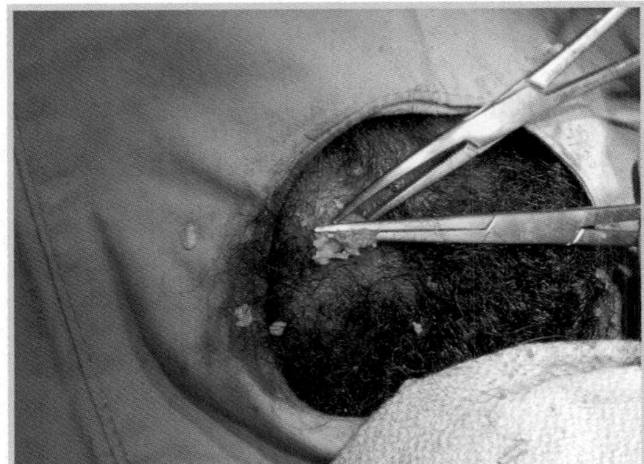

Step 9

Step 10. An attempt is made to remove the entire cyst wall intact. If the cyst wall breaks, enter the skin opening and vigorously grasp in all directions until additional cyst wall is grasped and pulled out. The incision may be closed with simple or hemostatic sutures.

- **PITFALL:** If any cyst wall remains in the wound, the cyst will usually recur. It is critical that the entire cyst wall be removed. Sufficient preprocedure anesthesia should be administered to permit this vigorous tugging within the wound.
- **PITFALL:** Occasionally, previous inflammation of the cyst causes scarring and tethering of the cyst wall to surrounding tissues. This usually prevents removal of the cyst wall by the minimal technique. If the operator is unable to remove the cyst wall using the minimal technique, the operator should convert to a standard removal, making a fusiform excision surrounding the skin opening.

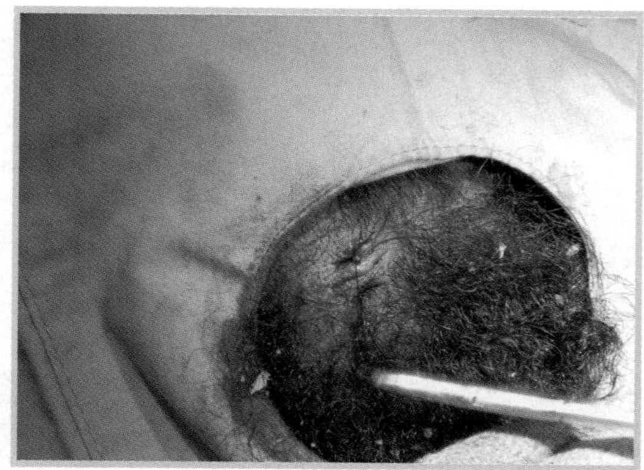

Step 10

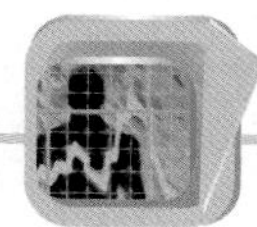

Complications

- Bleeding
- Infection
- Scar formation
- Recurrence

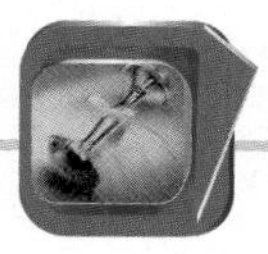

Pediatric Considerations

Although epidermal cysts are rare in the pediatric population, when present, the removal process is the same.

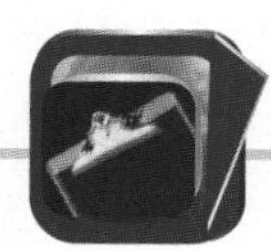

Postprocedure Instructions

Simple epidermal cysts that appear to be completely excised do not generally require follow-up, except for suture removal. If a recurrence is brought to the physician's attention at a later date, standard surgical excision should be attempted.

Instruct the patient to gently wash an area that has been stitched after 1 day but to not put the wound into standing water for 3 days. Have the patient dry the area well after washing and use a small amount of antibiotic ointment to promote moist healing. Recommend wound elevation to lessen swelling, reduce pain, and speed healing. Instruct the patient not to pick at, break, or cut the stitches.

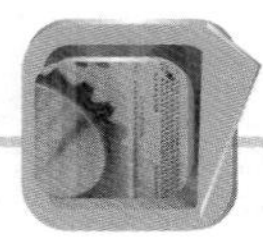

Coding Information and Supply Sources

Use the benign excision codes (11400 to 11446) for removal of these lesions. The code selected is determined by size and location of the lesion. The codes include local anesthesia and simple (one-layer) closure, although the codes can be used if the minimal incision technique is used and no suturing is required.

CPT Code	Description	2008 Average 50th Percentile Fee	Global Period
11400	TAL <0.6 cm	$178.00	10
11401	TAL 0.6–1.0 cm	$226.00	10
11402	TAL 1.1–2.0 cm	$289.00	10
11403	TAL 2.1–3.0 cm	$347.00	10
11404	TAL 3.1–4.0 cm	$441.00	10
11406	TAL >4.0 cm	$627.00	10
11420	SNHFG <0.6 cm	$179.00	10
11421	SNHFG 0.6–1.0 cm	$233.00	10
11422	SNHFG 1.1–2.0 cm	$285.00	10
11423	SNHFG 2.1–3.0 cm	$385.00	10
11424	SNHFG 3.1–4.0 cm	$481.00	10
11426	SNHFG >4.0 cm	$683.00	10
11440	FEENLMM <0.6 cm	$221.00	10
11441	FEENLMM 0.6–1.0 cm	$289.00	10
11442	FEENLMM 1.1–2.0 cm	$356.00	10
11443	FEENLMM 2.1–3.0 cm	$450.00	10
11444	FEENLMM 3.1–4.0 cm	$556.00	10
11446	FEENLMM >4.0 cm	$756.00	10

CPT is a registered trademark of the American Medical Association.
2008 average 50th Percentile Fees are provided courtesy of 2008 MMH-SI's copyrighted Physicians' Fees and Coding Guide.
TAL, trunk, arms, or legs; SNHFG, scalp, neck, hands, feet, or genitalia; FEENLMM, face, ears, eyelids, nose, lips, or mucous membrane.

Patient Education Handout

A patient education handout, "Epidermal (Sebaceous) Cyst," can be found on the book's Web site.

Bibliography

Domonkos AN, Arnold HL, Odom RB. *Andrews' Diseases of the Skin: Clinical Dermatology*. 7th ed. Philadelphia: WB Saunders; 1982.

Johnson RA. Cyst removal: punch, push, pull. *Skin* 1995;1:14–15.

Klin B, Ashkenazi H. Sebaceous cyst excision with minimal surgery. *Am Fam Physician.* 1990;41:1746–1748.

Lieblich LM, Geronemus RG, Gibbs RC. Use of a biopsy punch for removal of epithelial cysts. *J Dermatol Surg Oncol.* 1982;8:1059–1062.

Lopez-Rios F. Squamous cell carcinoma arising in a cutaneous epidermal cyst: case report and literature review. *Am J Dermatopathol.* 1999;21:174–177.

Nakamura M. Treating a sebaceous cyst: an incisional technique. *Aesthetic Plast Surg.* 2001;25:52–56.

Richards MA. Trephining large sebaceous cysts. *J Plast Surg.* 1985;38:583–585.

Vivakananthan C. Minimal incision for removing sebaceous cysts. *Br J Plast Surg.* 1972;25(1):60–62.

Vogt HB, Nelson RE. Excision of sebaceous cysts: a nontraditional method. *Postgrad Med.* 1986;80:128–334.

Zuber TJ. Minimal excision technique for epidermoid (sebaceous) cysts. *Am Fam Physician.* 2002;65:1409–1412, 1417–1418, 1420, 1423–1424.

Zuber TJ. *Office Procedures.* Baltimore: Williams & Wilkins; 1999:97–105.

Zuber TJ. *Skin Biopsy, Excision and Repair Techniques.* Kansas City: American Academy of Family Physicians; 1998:94–99.

2008 MAG Mutual Healthcare Solutions, Inc.'s Physicians' Fee and Coding Guide. Duluth, Georgia. MAG Mutual Healthcare Solutions, Inc. 2007.

CHAPTER 49

Fusiform Excision

E. J. Mayeaux, Jr., MD, DABFP, FAAFP

Professor of Family Medicine, Professor of Obstetrics and Gynecology
Louisiana State University Health Sciences Center, Shreveport, LA

The fusiform excision technique is one of the most versatile and frequently used office surgery procedures. The technique is used to remove benign and malignant lesions on or below the skin surface. The technique can be used to remove lesions entirely (i.e., excisional biopsy) or to remove a portion of a large lesion (i.e., incisional biopsy) for histologic assessment. The major advantage is that the procedure often affords a one-stage diagnostic and therapeutic intervention.

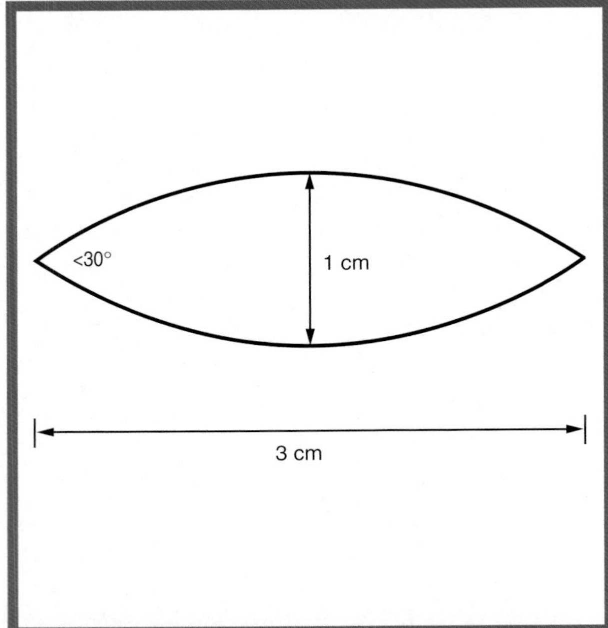

The fusiform technique historically has been misnamed the *elliptical excision*. Properly designed fusiform excisions resemble a biconcave lens rather than an oval ellipse. The corners of the fusiform excision should have angles ≤30 degrees, and the length of a proper fusiform excision is three times the width.

The fusiform excision incorporates several important dermatologic techniques (Table 49-1). The techniques are combined to reduce subcutaneous hematoma formation, prevent development of seromas beneath the wounds, and produce good cosmetic outcomes. These various techniques are illustrated in this and subsequent chapters.

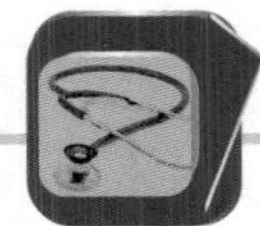

Equipment

- The recommended surgical tray for office surgery is listed in Appendix G. Suggested suture removal times are listed in Appendix J.
- A suggested anesthesia tray that can be used for this procedure is listed in Appendix F.
- Skin preparation accommodations appear in Appendix E.

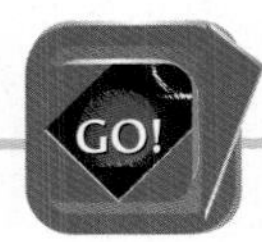

Indications

- Removal of pigmented melanocytic nevi to identify melanoma and ascertain the depth of the lesion
- Small tumors or skin cancers that can be removed with fusiform excision

- Incisional biopsy of a large lesion when excision is not feasible
- Flat lesions not readily amenable to shave excision
- Lesions on convex surfaces that are not amenable to shave excision
- Removal of subcutaneous tumors

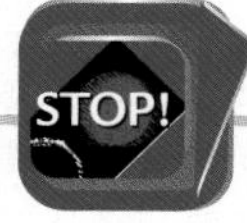

Contraindications (Relative)

- Severe bleeding disorders
- Extreme illness that would make wound healing difficult
- Cellulitis in the tissues to be incised
- Conditions that may interfere with wound healing (collagen vascular diseases, smoking, diabetes)
- Concurrent medications that may increase the likelihood of intraoperative bleeding (aspirin, other nonsteroidal anti-inflammatory drugs, warfarin)
- Uncooperative patient

TABLE 49-1. Techniques Incorporated into the Fusiform Excision

Excision aligned with the lines of least skin tension; See Appendix B
Local or field block anesthesia
Application of appropriate skin margins; Appendix D
Sterile draping of the surgical site; Appendix E
Smooth, continuous incisions with the scalpel
Lifting skin edges using skin hooks
Undermining of skin edges
Placement of interrupted, deep buried, subcutaneous sutures; Chapters 36–18
Simple, interrupted skin sutures; Chapter 38
Placement of sutures using the halving technique
Eversion of wound edges
Moist wound healing using antibiotic or other ointment

The Procedure

Step 1. The fusiform excision should be designed so that the long axis of the fusiform parallels the lines of least skin tension (Appendix B) and with an adequate margin (Appendix D). Draw the fusiform excision on the skin using a skin marking pen before initiating the procedure. A properly designed fusiform excision is three times as long as it is wide.

- **PITFALL:** Many experienced physicians perform fusiform excision without drawing out the skin incision lines. After the sterile drapes are placed on the skin, the nearby landmarks may be covered, causing the physician to incorrectly orient the excision.
- **PITFALL:** Some providers want to save as much tissue as possible and draw the fusiform excision with kthe length only two times the width. These so-called football excisions create elevations of tissue at the ends (i.e., dog ears). The attempt to excise less tissue often produces inferior cosmetic results.

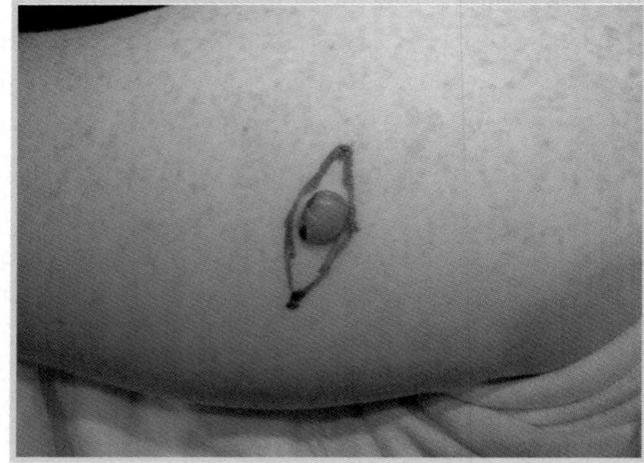

Step 1

Step 2. Perform field block anesthesia (see Chapter 2). Insert the needle within the fusiform island of skin to be excised. The operator should not create needle tracks in surrounding skin that will not be excised. Plan the anesthesia injections to create a large enough numb area to allow for undermining parallel to the long axis. Prep the skin with povidone-iodine or chlorhexidine solution, and allow it to dry (see Appendix E).

- **PEARL:** Prep a wide area so that an undraped area is not inadvertently exposed if the drape slides a little.

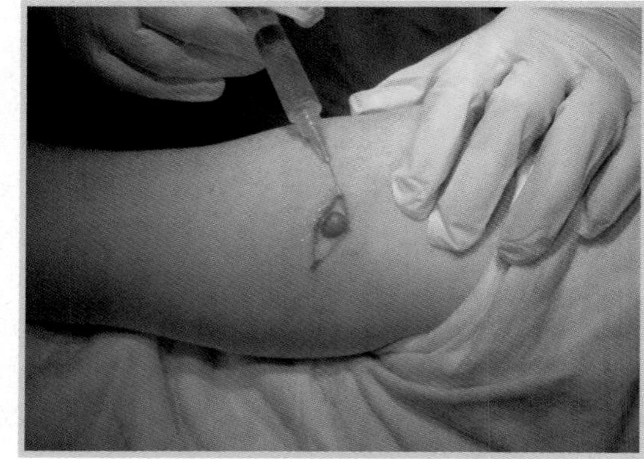

Step 2

Step 3. Create smooth, vertical skin incisions using a no. 15 scalpel. The scalpel blade is held vertically at the corner of the wound and punctures the skin using the point of the blade. The blade handle is then dropped down, and a smooth, continuous stroke is used to create the wound edge. The blade should be passed firmly enough to penetrate the dermis.

- **PITFALL:** Many inexperienced operators make a short pass with the scalpel, stop to inspect the incision, and then make an additional short pass. This creates crosshatch

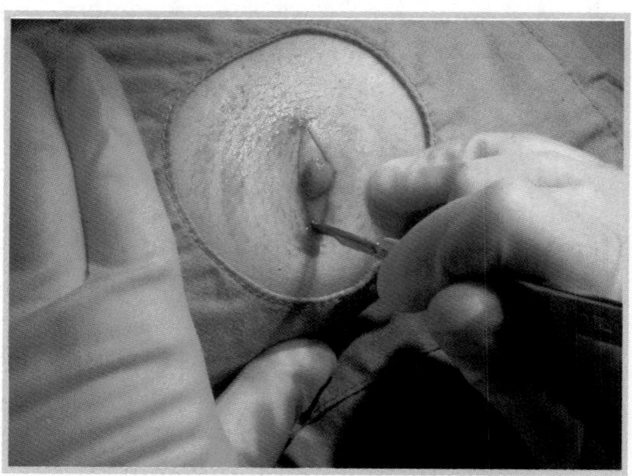

Step 3

marks and an irregular skin edge. Smooth, confident passes with the scalpel avoid jagged edges.

- **PITFALL:** Create the incision with the blade vertical to the skin surface. Novice surgeons often angle the blade under the lesion, creating a wedge excision. Angled edges will not evert well.

Step 4. Grasp the corner of the central fusiform island of skin with Adson forceps, and elevate the island. Use a scalpel or scissors to horizontally excise the island from the subcutaneous fat. After the lesion is cut free, immediately place the specimen in a container of formalin for histologic assessment in the laboratory.

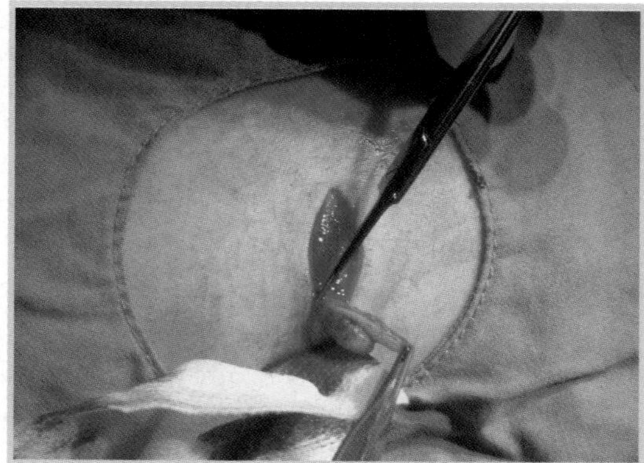

Step 4

Step 5. Undermining can be performed with a scalpel blade, with scissors, or bluntly using a hemostat. Elevate the skin edges using skin hooks, not forceps. If pickups are used, use them only to lift and not to grasp tissue. The safest level of undermining is in the fat, just below the dermal-fat junction, to avoid damaging nerves that traverse the deeper levels of the fat. To create 1 cm of wound edge relaxation, 3 cm of undermining is required. Undermine the wound corners to release any tethering at these locations.

- **PITFALL:** Elevating skin edges using skin hooks prevents the damage and subsequent scarring that often result from handling the edges with forceps.
- **PEARL:** A cheap, disposable skin hook can be created by bending the tip of a 1-inch, 20-gauge needle with the needle driver.
- **PEARL:** Using retractors, or using pickups as a retractor, eliminates damage to the skin edge.

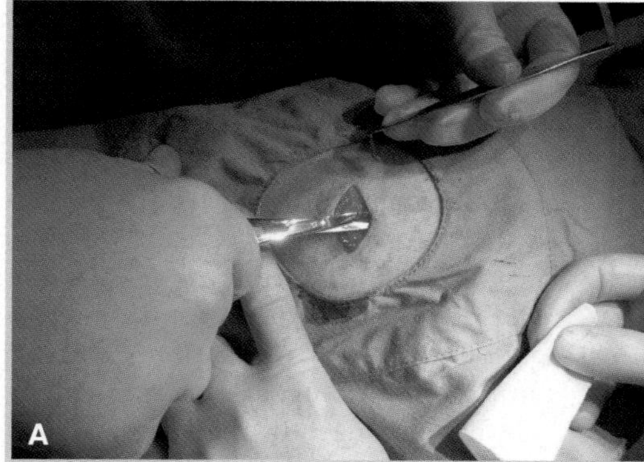

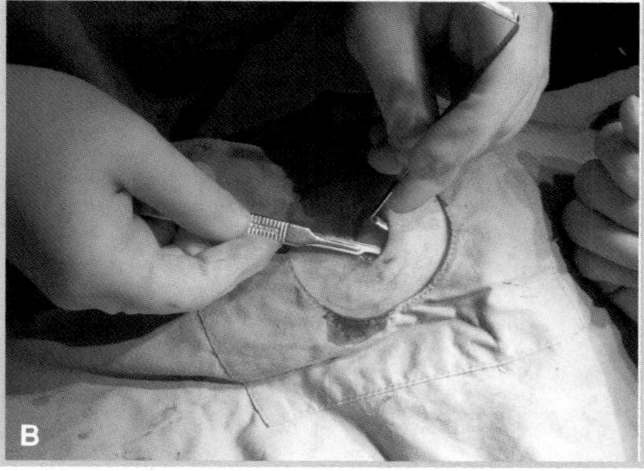

Step 5

Step 6. Lightly press the edges of the wound together with your fingertips. If it closes with light pressure, it is ready to suture. If it does not close with light pressure, more undermining or a tension reducing suture technique may be required.

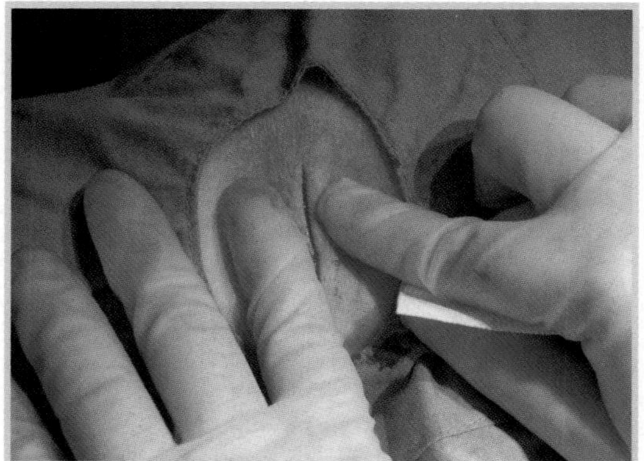

Step 6

Step 7. Place a deeply buried subcutaneous stitch or a vertical mattress stitch to close dead space and decrease local tension if necessary. Remember that the deeply buried sutures do not evert the skin edges. Eversion can be achieved by proper placement of simple interrupted sutures or vertical mattress sutures.

- PITFALL: Inexperienced providers frequently are distracted by the minor bleeding (especially from facial wounds) produced by undermining. The closure of the deeper tissues using deep, buried sutures almost always stops the bleeding. Physicians should move quickly to perform the deep buried closure, rather than waste time applying gauze to the wound.

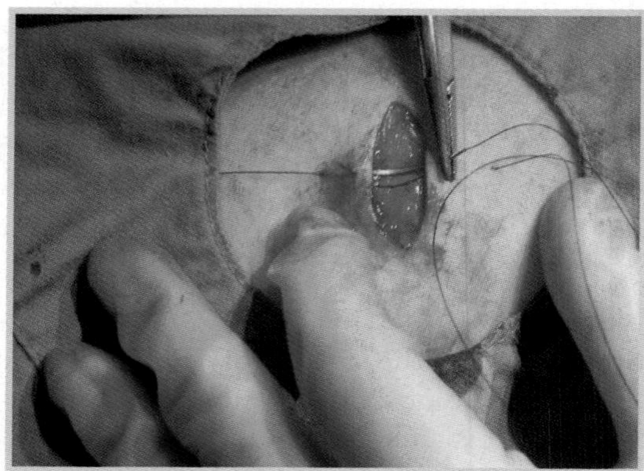

Step 7

Step 8. To close the wound using the halving principle, place a suture in the center of a wound first. The next sutures are placed in the center of the remaining wound defects. This prevents uneven edges (i.e., dog ears), which can be produced when suturing from one end of the wound to the other. Clean the wound with normal saline. Antibiotic or other ointments applied to the wound immediately after the procedure help to promote more rapid and improved healing at the site. Then apply a sterile bandage. If the excision was on an extremity, gauze may be wrapped around the extremity to apply mild pressure and avoid the pain of tape removal.

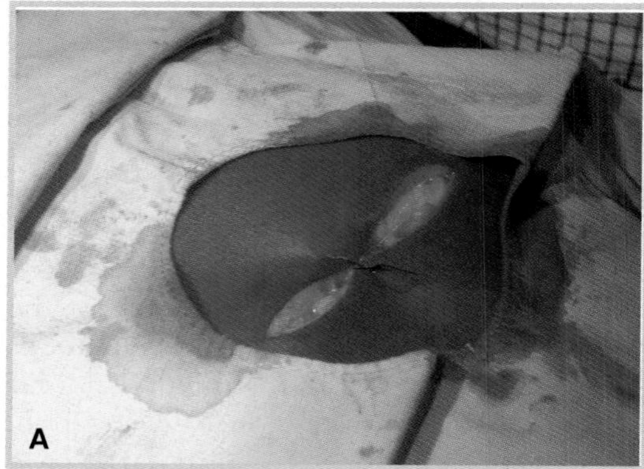

A

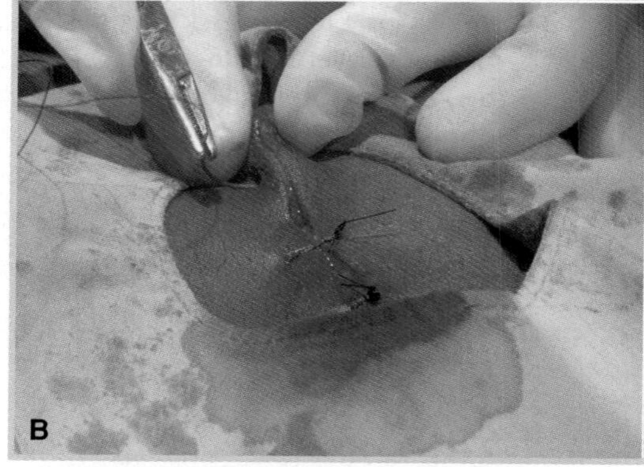

B

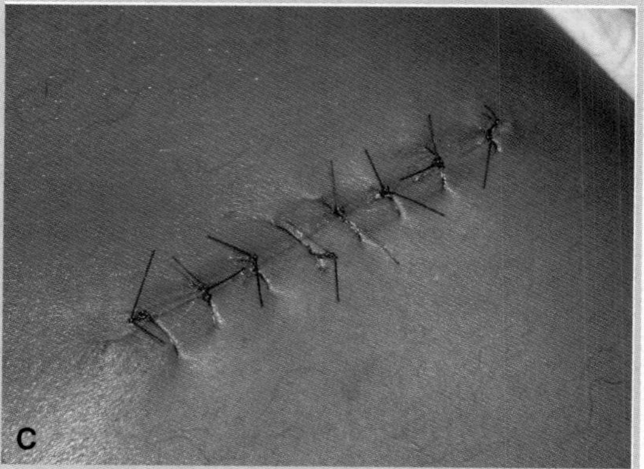

C

Step 8

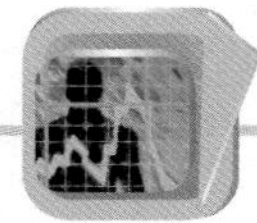

Complications

- Pain, infection, and bleeding
- Nonunion of skin edges
- Scar formation
- Incomplete excision of lesion

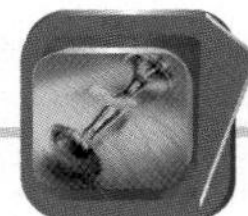

Pediatric Considerations

Generally, pediatric skin has excellent blood flow and heals very well. However, pediatric patients often find it difficult to sit and lie still during lengthy procedures. The patient's maturity and ability to cooperate should be considered before deciding to attempt any outpatient procedure. The maximum recommended dose for lidocaine in children is 3 to 5 mg/kg, and 7 mg/kg when combined with epinephrine. Neonates have an increased volume of distribution, decreased hepatic clearance, and doubled terminal elimination half-life (3.2 hours).

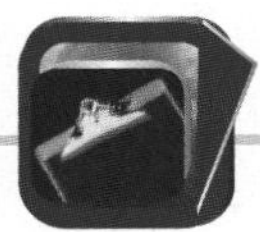

Postprocedure Instructions

Instruct the patient to gently wash an area that has been stitched after 1 day but not to put the wound into standing water for 3 days. Have the patient pat dry the area thoroughly after washing, and use a small amount of antibiotic ointment to promote moist healing. Recommend wound elevation to help lessen swelling, reduce pain and speed healing. Instruct the patient not to pick at, break, or cut the stitches.

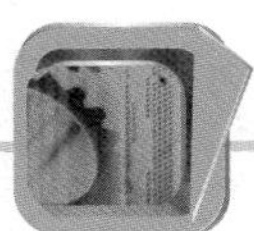

Coding Information and Supply Sources

All codes listed are for superficial wound closure using sutures, staples, or tissue adhesives with or without adhesive strips on the skin surface. If a layered closure is required, use alternate codes: intermediate closure codes 12031 to 12057 or complex repair codes 13100 to 13160.

Add together the lengths of wounds in the same classification and anatomic sites. Use separate codes for repairs from different anatomic sites. Debridement is considered a separate procedure only when gross contamination requires prolonged cleansing or when appreciable amounts of devitalized or contaminated tissue are removed.

If a lesion is removed, use either "Excision—benign lesion" codes (11400 to 11471) or "Excision—malignant lesion" codes (11600 to 11646).

CPT Code	Description	2008 Average 50th Percentile Fee	Global Period
11400	Benign excision TAL <0.6 cm	$178.00	10
11401	Benign excision TAL 0.6–1.0 cm	$226.00	10
11402	Benign excision TAL 1.1–2.0 cm	$289.00	10
11403	Benign excision TAL 2.1–3.0 cm	$347.00	10
11404	Benign excision TAL 3.1–4.0 cm	$441.00	10
11406	Benign excision TAL >4.0 cm	$627.00	10
11420	Benign excision SNHFG <0.6 cm	$179.00	10
11421	Benign excision SNHFG 0.6–1.0 cm	$233.00	10

11422	Benign excision SNHFG 1.1–2.0 cm	$285.00	10
11423	Benign excision SNHFG 2.1–3.0 cm	$385.00	10
11424	Benign excision SNHFG 3.1–4.0 cm	$481.00	10
11426	Benign excision SNHFG >4.0 cm	$683.00	10
11440	Benign excision FEENLMM <0.6 cm	$221.00	10
11441	Benign excision FEENLMM 0.6–1.0 cm	$289.00	10
11442	Benign excision FEENLMM 1.1–2.0 cm	$356.00	10
11443	Benign excision FEENLMM 2.1–3.0 cm	$450.00	10
11444	Benign excision FEENLMM 3.1–4.0 cm	$556.00	10
11446	Benign excision FEENLMM >4.0 cm	$756.00	10
11600	Malignant excision TAL <0.6 cm	$268.00	10
11601	Malignant excision TAL 0.6–1.0 cm	$316.00	10
11602	Malignant excision TAL 1.1–2.0 cm	$369.00	10
11603	Malignant excision TAL 2.1–3.0 cm	$455.00	10
11604	Malignant excision TAL 3.1–4.0 cm	$535.00	10
11606	Malignant excision TAL >4.0 cm	$761.00	10
11620	Malignant excision SNHFG <0.6 cm	$309.00	10
11621	Malignant excision SNHFG 0.6–1.0 cm	$389.00	10
11622	Malignant excision SNHFG 1.1–2.0 cm	$448.00	10
11623	Malignant excision SNHFG 2.1–3.0 cm	$544.00	10
11624	Malignant excision SNHFG 3.1–4.0 cm	$717.00	10
11626	Malignant excision SNHFG >4.0 cm	$922.00	10
11640	Malignant excision FEENLMM <0.6 cm	$364.00	10
11641	Malignant excision FEENLMM 0.6–1.0 cm	$465.00	10
11642	Malignant excision FEENLMM 1.1–2.0 cm	$550.00	10
11643	Malignant excision FEENLMM 2.1–3.0 cm	$724.00	10
11644	Malignant excision FEENLMM 3.1–4.0 cm	$888.00	10
11646	Malignant excision FEENLMM >4.0 cm	$1,175.00	10

CPT is a registered trademark of the American Medical Association.
2008 average 50th Percentile Fees are provided courtesy of 2008 MMH-SI's copyrighted Physicians' Fees and Coding Guide.
TAL, trunk, arms, or legs; SNHFG, scalp, neck, hands, feet, or genitalia;
FEENLMM, face, ears, eyelids, nose, lips, and mucous membranes.

Patient Education Handout

Patient education handouts, "Fusiform Excision Procedure," "After the Fusiform Excision," and "Scars," can be found on the book's Web site, .

Bibliography

Borges AF, Alexander JE. Relaxed skin tension lines, Z-plasties on scars, and fusiform excision of lesions. *Br J Plast Surg.* 1962;15:242–254.

Jobe R. When an "ellipse" is not an ellipse [Letter]. *Plast Reconstr Surg.* 1970;46:295.

Leshin B. Proper planning and execution of surgical excisions. In: Wheeler RG, ed. *Cutaneous Surgery*. Philadelphia: WB Saunders; 1994:171–177.

Moy RL, Lee A, Zalka A. Commonly used suturing techniques in skin surgery. *Am Fam Physician.* 1991;44:1625–1634.

Stegman SJ, Tromovitch TA, Glogau RG. *Basics of Dermatologic Surgery*. Chicago: Year Book Medical Publishing; 1982:60–68.
Stevenson TR, Jurkiewicz MJ. Plastic and reconstructive surgery. In: Schwartz SI, Shires GT, Spencer FC, et al., eds. *Principles of Surgery*. 5th ed. New York: McGraw-Hill; 1989:2081–2132.
Vistnes LM. Basic principles of cutaneous surgery. In: Epstein E, Epstein E Jr, eds. *Skin Surgery*. 6th ed. Philadelphia: WB Saunders; 1987:44–55.
Zalla MJ. Basic cutaneous surgery. *Cutis*. 1994;53:172–186.
Zitelli J. TIPS for a better ellipse. *J Am Acad Dermatol*. 1990;22:101–103.
Zuber TJ. *Office Procedures*. Baltimore: Williams & Wilkins; 1999.
Zuber TJ, DeWitt DE. The fusiform excision. *Am Fam Physician*. 1994;49:371–376.
2008 MAG Mutual Healthcare Solutions, Inc.'s Physicians' Fee and Coding Guide. Duluth, Georgia. MAG Mutual Healthcare Solutions, Inc. 2007.

CHAPTER 50

Lipoma Excision

E. J. Mayeaux, Jr., MD, DABFP, FAAFP

Professor of Family Medicine, Professor of Obstetrics and Gynecology
Louisiana State University Health Sciences Center, Shreveport, LA

Lipomas are benign, adipose-issue tumors that can arise anywhere on the body. Lipomas frequently are encountered on the upper half of the body, with common sites including the head, neck, shoulders, and back. Most lesions are confined to the subcutaneous tissues, but lesions occasionally penetrate between fascial planes and even into muscle. Subfascial lipomas are most commonly found in the neck.

Lipomas can vary from the size of a pea to that of a soccer ball. The tumors are composed of lobules of fat encased in a thick, fibrous capsule. The adipose tissue within lipomas is often indistinguishable from normal fat. Delineation of a lipoma may be achieved by searching for the limits of the capsule. Lobules are connected by a thinner stroma or fibrous bands that can extend to deep fascia of the skin and produce dimpling. These bands may prevent easy enucleation of an encapsulated lipoma.

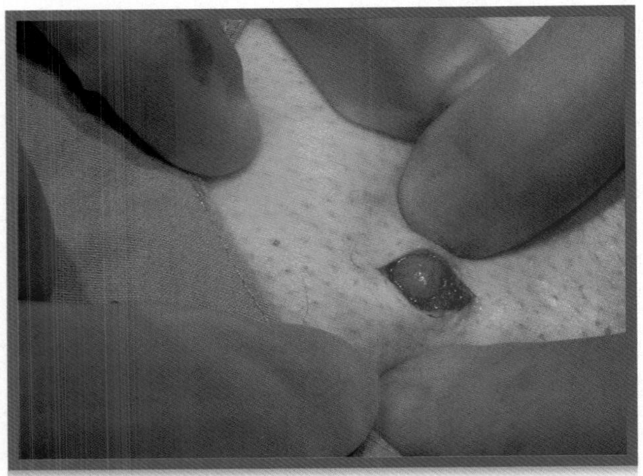

Lipomas often produce a rounded mass that protrudes above surrounding skin. On palpation, the lesions usually feel smooth, lobulated, compressible, and dough-like. Lipomas are generally not tender, although adiposis dolorosa (Dercum disease) is a condition with painful or tender truncal or extremity lipomas. Dercum disease is most commonly encountered in women in the later reproductive years. Lipomas often grow slowly and can increase in size if the patient gains weight. During times of weight loss or starvation, lipomas do not decrease in size.

The presence of multiple lipomas is known as lipomatosis, and the condition is more common in men. Hereditary multiple lipomatosis is an autosomal dominant condition that produces widespread lipomas over the extremities and trunk. Madelung disease refers to benign symmetric lipomatosis of the head, neck, shoulders, and proximal upper extremities. It is uncommon to find malignancy in a lipoma (i.e., liposarcoma) when a patient displays multiple lipomas. Liposarcoma is found in 1% of lipomas and is most commonly encountered in lesions on the lower extremities, shoulders, and retroperitoneal areas. Other risk factors for liposarcoma include large size (>5 cm), associated calcification, rapid growth, or invasion into nearby structures or down through fascia and into muscle.

Nonexcisional techniques for lipoma removal include steroid injection and liposuction. Steroid injections produce fat atrophy and are best performed on smaller lesions (<1 inch in diameter). A one-to-one mixture of 1% lidocaine and triamcinolone acetonide in a dosage of 10 mg/mL is injected into the center of the lesion. Often, multiple injections given over 1 to 3 months are required for an adequate response. Liposuction can be performed in the office using large-gauge needles attached to 20-mL or larger syringes (after field block anesthesia using diluted lidocaine) or in the operating room using standard suction curettes. Complete eradication of the lipoma cells can be difficult to achieve with liposuction, and rapid regrowth of the lesion may result. Liposuction is an attractive option for lipomas located in areas where large scars should be avoided (e.g., face).

Small lipomas are often surrounded by a well-developed and easily identified capsule. After the creation of a small incision, these lesions can be extruded through the wound with the application of pressure to surrounding skin. Enucleation can also be achieved by combining the use of a dermal curette with pressure. Larger lipomas often do not display such a well-defined capsule, and distinguishing normal from lipomatous fat can be a challenge.

Large lipomas can be removed by leaving the top of the tumor attached to a small island of overlying skin. This skin can be grasped and retracted when dissecting around the lipoma. The deeper yellow color (due to increased density) often seen in lipomas can help visually identify the tumor. Skin markings made before the procedure also aid in identifying the extent of the tumor. Care must be exerted when dissecting the base of the wound to avoid creating trauma to deep structures such as arteries, nerves, or muscle. After the tumor is removed, inspect the base of the wound carefully to identify any lobules of tumor that may have been left.

Small bleeding vessels at the base of the wound can be clamped with hemostats or tied off with absorbable sutures in a figure-eight pattern. The wound bed should be dry (i.e., bleeding controlled) before closure is attempted. Deep wounds often require the use of larger-gauge absorbable sutures, because significant tension may be required to close the dead space created by removal of a large tumor. Historically, Penrose drains were used to facilitate blood and fluid drainage from these deep wounds. Drains increase bacterial counts in wounds and often are not needed if meticulous hemostasis and suture closure of the deep wound are properly performed.

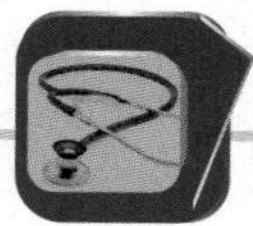

Equipment

- A standard surgery tray can be used for removal of lipomas (see Appendix G). Consider adding two or three larger hemostats (e.g., Kelly clamps) to the surgery tray to allow easier grasping of the lipoma.
- Suggested suture removal times are listed in Appendix J.
- A suggested anesthesia tray that can be used for this procedure is listed in Appendix F.
- Skin preparation recommendations appear in Appendix E.

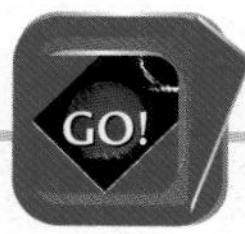

Indications

- Removal of tumors that are symptomatic (i.e., producing pain or discomfort)
- Removal to improve body contour and appearance
- Removal to relieve anxiety regarding the diagnosis

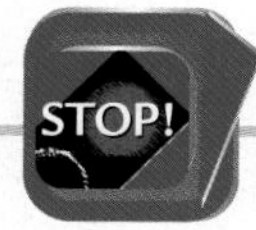

Contraindications

- Uncooperative individual
- Tumors at increased risk for malignancy (i.e., >5 cm in diameter, displaying associated calcification, invading nearby structures, growing rapidly, invading deeper structures such as fascia, or in high-risk sites such as the lower legs or shoulders) without a prior biopsy result to document the benign nature of the lesion (relative contraindication)

The Procedure

Step 1. Palpate the tumor to determine its extent. Consider drawing an outline of the tumor on the skin with a skin marking pen. Small lesions can be removed through a straight incision. For a large lesion, outline a fusiform excision that overlies the center of the tumor and whose long axis coincides with the nearby lines of least skin tension. The fusiform incision should be designed to be about two thirds of the diameter of the underlying lipoma.

- **PITFALL:** Do not draw on the skin using ballpoint pens. Ballpoint pens can traumatize skin, and the ink tends to wash off when the skin preparation is performed. Using a surgical skin marking pen is likely to provide an outline of the tumor that will guide the excision and last throughout the surgery.

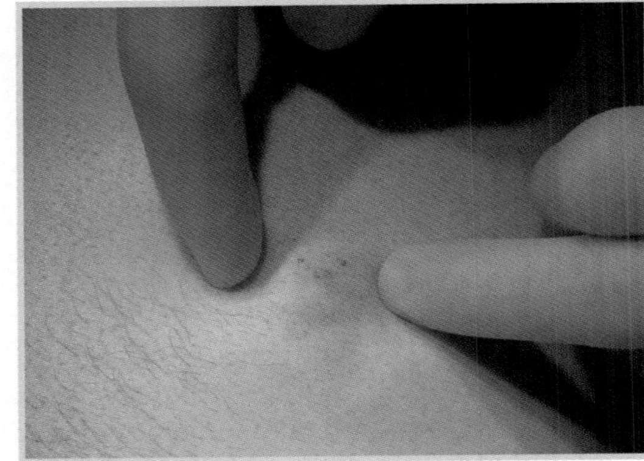

Step 1

Step 2. Field block anesthesia can be achieved by injecting beneath and lateral to the outlined lesion using long (1.25- or 1.5-inch) needles. A sufficient volume of lidocaine should be administered around the periphery of the lesion to surround the tumor (see Appendix F). Cleanse the skin with povidone-iodine or chlorhexidine solution, making sure to avoid wiping away the skin markings (see Appendix E). The area is draped with sterile towels.

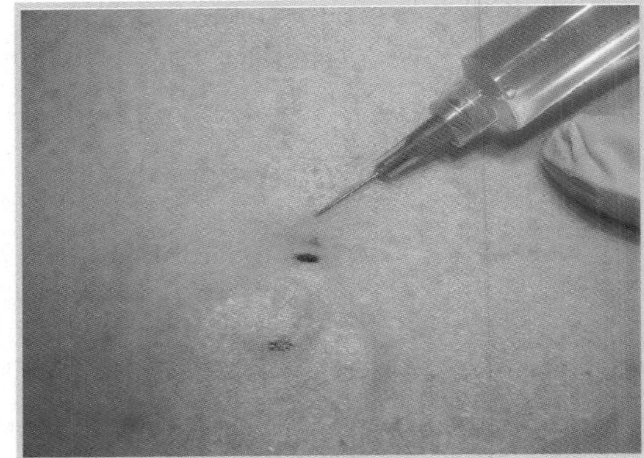

Step 2

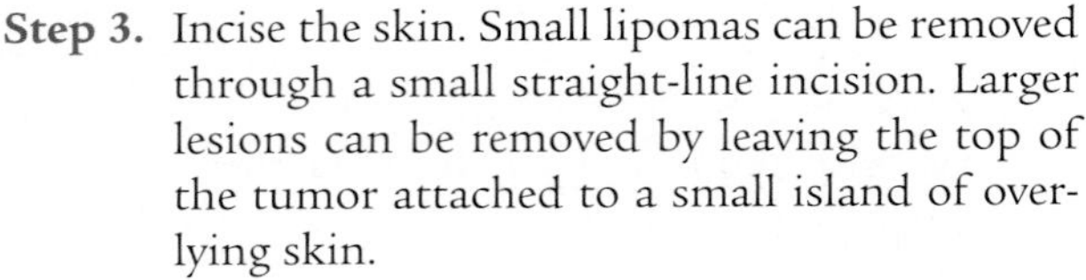

Step 3. Incise the skin. Small lipomas can be removed through a small straight-line incision. Larger lesions can be removed by leaving the top of the tumor attached to a small island of overlying skin.

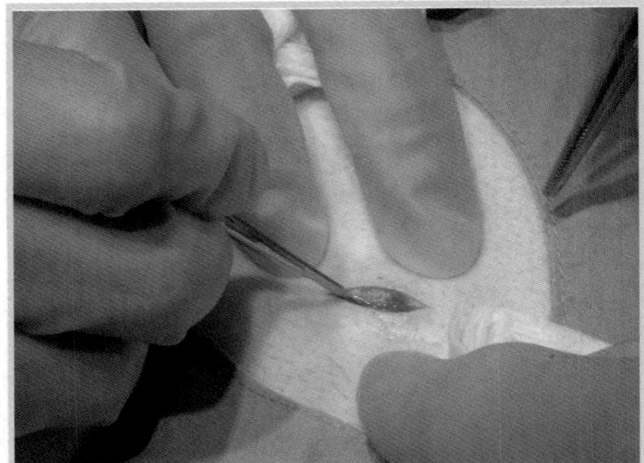

Step 3

Step 4. Dissect down to and around the top of the lipoma.

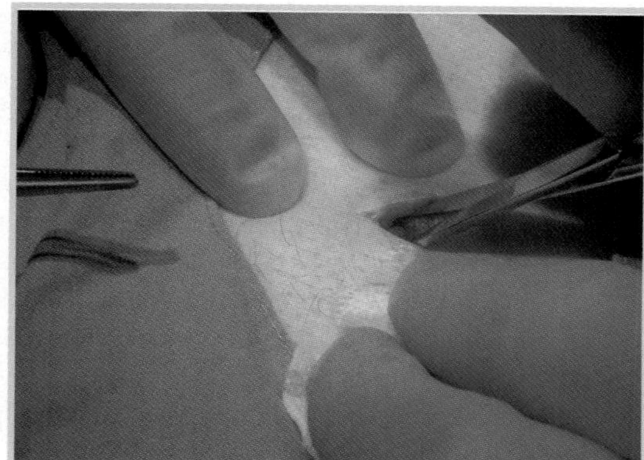

Step 4

Step 5. Small lipomas may often be enucleated by applying pressure around the lesion and upward.

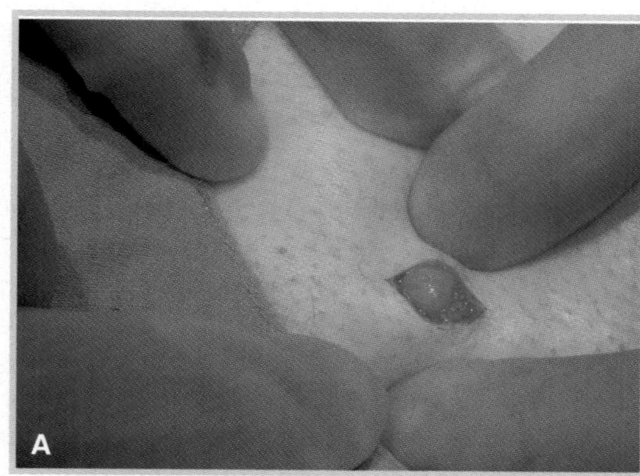

Step 5

Step 6. If using a fusiform excision, do not undermine the central fusiform island of skin. Carry the incision down to the level of the fat or to the lipoma capsule. Use an Allis clamp or large Kelly clamp to grasp the center of the island of skin, which remains attached to the underlying lipoma. Use the clamp to provide traction to undermine lateral skin and to dissect around the lipoma.

- PITFALL: Some physicians prefer to make a simple incision through skin rather than create a fusiform island of skin. Traction applied directly on the lipoma produces tearing through the tissue, and closure after large lipoma removal leaves redundant skin unless a fusiform section of skin is removed.

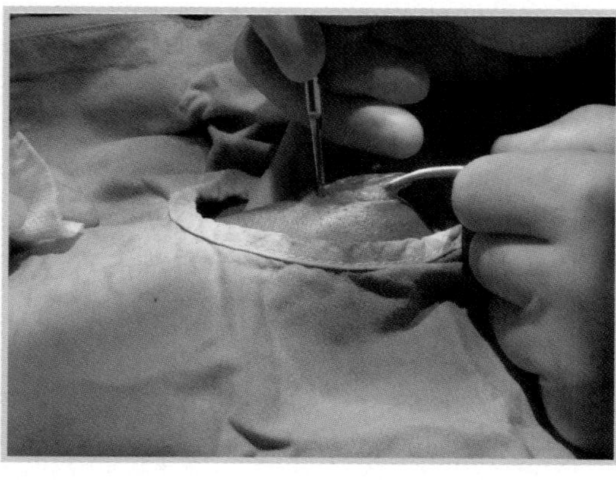

Step 6

Step 7. Use a gloved finger, iris scissors, or scalpel blade to carefully dissect around the entire lesion. The entire lipoma can often be delivered through the smaller fusiform skin incision.

- PITFALL: Care must be taken to avoid damaging structures beneath the lipoma, such as nerves, arteries, or muscle. Because visualization may be poor beneath the lesion, blunt dissection is often advocated for freeing the underside of the lipoma. A finger is often a sensitive and effective tool for this part of the operation.
- PITFALL: Bleeding may occur during dissection and delivery of the tumor. Bleeding vessels can be briefly clamped with small hemostats to provide adequate hemostasis before wound closure.

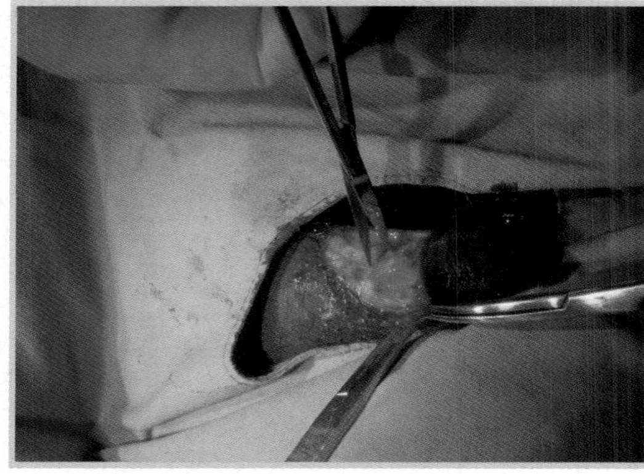

Step 7

Step 8. Deeply buried sutures are placed to close a large defect after removal of the lipoma (see Chapter 37). Large-caliber absorbable sutures (e.g., 3-0 or 4-0 polyglycan) are used and should grasp a significant portion of lateral tissue so that it will not tear when closing the deep space. Significant tension may be placed on these sutures when closing large spaces.

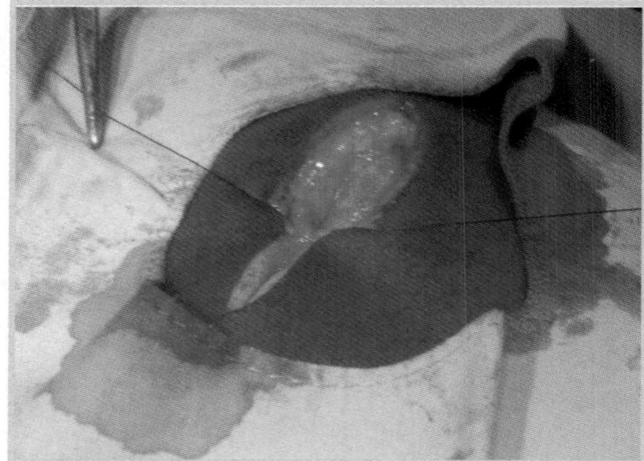

Step 8

Step 9. Alternatively, a smaller excision may be closed with vertical mattress sutures.

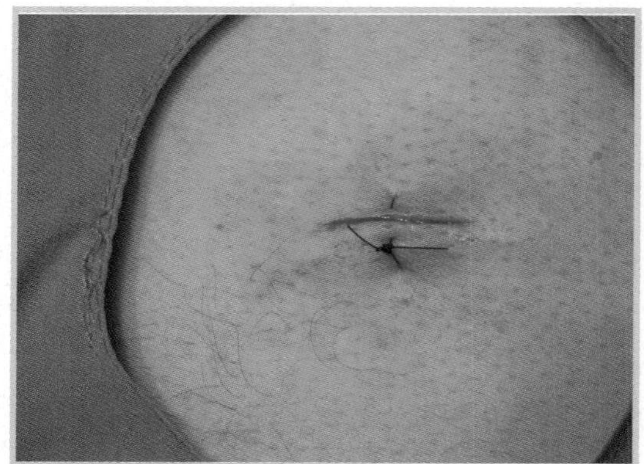

Step 9

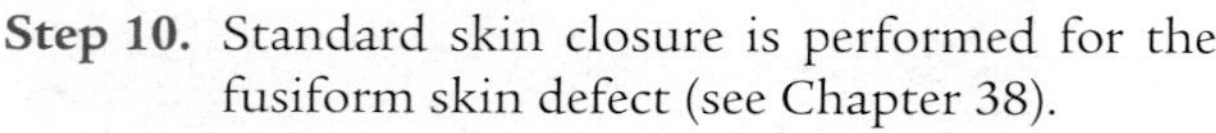

Step 10. Standard skin closure is performed for the fusiform skin defect (see Chapter 38).

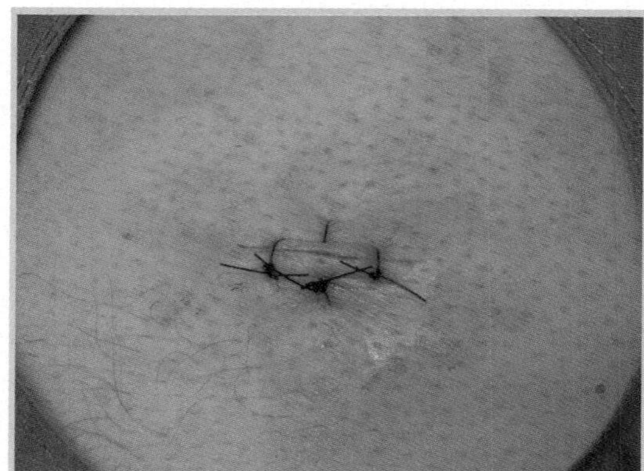

Step 10

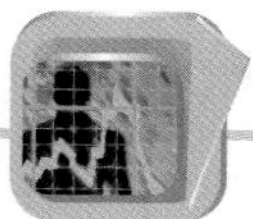

Complications

- Recurrence
- Surgical infection/cellulitis/fasciitis
- Ecchymosis
- Hematoma/seroma formation
- Injury to nearby nerves with permanent paresthesia/anesthesia (rare)
- Injury to nearby vessels/vascular compromise (rare)
- Permanent deformity secondary to removal of a large lesion (rare)
- Excessive scarring with cosmetic deformity or contracture (rare)
- Muscle injury/irritation (rare)
- Fat embolus (rare)
- Periostitis/osteomyelitis (rare)

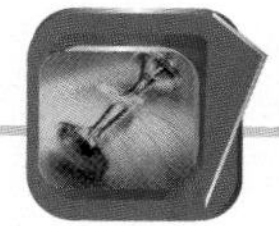

Pediatric Considerations

Although lipomas are rare in the pediatric population, when present, the removal process is the same.

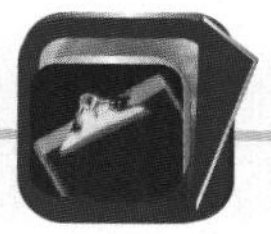

Postprocedure Instructions

Simple epidermal cysts that appear to be completely excised do not generally require follow-up, except for suture removal. If a recurrence is brought to the physician's attention at a later date, standard surgical excision should be attempted.

Instruct the patient to gently wash an area that has been stitched after 1 day but to not put the wound into standing water for 3 days. Have the patient dry the area well after washing and use a small amount of antibiotic ointment to promote moist healing. Recommend wound elevation to help lessen swelling, reduce pain, and speed healing. Instruct the patient not to pick at, break, or cut the stitches.

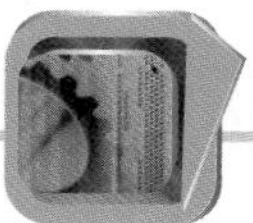

Coding Information and Supply Sources

Lipoma removal can be reported using the benign excision codes. The benign excision codes include removal of the benign subcutaneous lesion with simple skin closure. Enucleation is usually reported with these codes. Intralesional injection is reported using the 11900 code.

CPT Code	Description	2008 Average 50th Percentile Fee	Global Period
11400	Benign excision TAL <0.6 cm	$178.00	10
11401	Benign excision TAL 0.6–1.0 cm	$226.00	10
11402	Benign excision TAL 1.1–2.0 cm	$289.00	10
11403	Benign excision TAL 2.1–3.0 cm	$347.00	10
11404	Benign excision TAL 3.1–4.0 cm	$441.00	10
11406	Benign excision TAL >4.0 cm	$627.00	10
11420	Benign excision SNHFG <0.6 cm	$179.00	10

11421	Benign excision SNHFG 0.6–1.0 cm	$233.00	10
11422	Benign excision SNHFG 1.1–2.0 cm	$285.00	10
11423	Benign excision SNHFG 2.1–3.0 cm	$385.00	10
11424	Benign excision SNHFG 3.1–4.0 cm	$481.00	10
11426	Benign excision SNHFG >4.0 cm	$683.00	10
11440	Benign excision FEENLMM <0.6 cm	$221.00	10
11441	Benign excision FEENLMM 0.6–1.0 cm	$289.00	10
11442	Benign excision FEENLMM 1.1–2.0 cm	$356.00	10
11443	Benign excision FEENLMM 2.1–3.0 cm	$450.00	10
11444	Benign excision FEENLMM 3.1–4.0 cm	$556.00	10
11446	Benign excision FEENLMM >4.0 cm	$756.00	10

CPT is a registered trademark of the American Medical Association.
2008 average 50th Percentile Fees are provided courtesy of 2008 MMH-SI's copyrighted Physicians' Fees and Coding Guide.
TAL, trunk, arms, or legs; SNHFG, scalp, neck, hands, feet, or genitalia; FEENLMM, face, ears, eyelids, nose, lips, and mucous membranes.

Intermediate closure codes can be added to an excision code if deeply buried subcutaneous sutures are placed.

CPT Code	Description	2007 Average 50th Percentile Fee	Global Period
12031	SATAL ≤2.5 cm	$272.00	10
12032	SATAL 2.6–7.5 cm	$347.00	10
12034	SATAL 7.6–12.5 cm	$438.00	10
12035	SATAL 12.6–20.0 cm	$548.00	10
12036	SATAL 20.1–30.0 cm	$680.00	10
12037	SATAL >30.0 cm	$789.00	10
12041	NHFG ≤2.5 cm	$262.00	10
12042	NHFG 2.6–7.5 cm	$357.00	10
12044	NHFG 7.6–12.5 cm	$462.00	10
12045	NHFG 12.6–20.0 cm	$558.00	10
12046	NHFG 20.1–30.0 cm	$729.00	10
12047	NHFG >30.0 cm	$846.00	10
12051	FEENLMM ≤2.5 cm	$341.00	10
12052	FEENLMM 2.6–5.0 cm	$426.00	10
12053	FEENLMM 5.1–7.5 cm	$527.00	10
12054	FEENLMM 7.6–12.5 cm	$645.00	10
12055	FEENLMM 12.6–20.0 cm	$822.00	10
12056	FEENLMM 20.1–30.0 cm	$1,044.00	10
12057	FEENLMM >30.0 cm	$1,211.00	10

CPT is a registered trademark of the American Medical Association.
2008 average 50th Percentile Fees are provided courtesy of 2008 MMH-SI's copyrighted Physicians' Fees and Coding Guide.
SATAL, scalp, axilla, trunk, arms, or legs (excluding hands and feet); NHFG, neck, hands, feet, or external genitalia; FEENLMM, face, ears, eyelids, nose, lips, or mucous membranes.

ICD-9 Codes

Lipoma	214.9
Lipoma skin	214.1
Lipoma face	214.0

Supplies

A standard surgery tray can be used for removal of lipomas (see Appendix G).

Patient Education Handout

A patient education handout, "Lipomas," can be found on the book's companion Web site,.

Bibliography

Benjamin RB. *Atlas of Outpatient and Office Surgery*. 2nd ed. Philadelphia: Lea & Febiger; 1994:385–392.

Bennett RG. *Fundamentals of Cutaneous Surgery*. St. Louis: Mosby; 1988:726–731.

Brown JS. *Minor Surgery: A Text and Atlas*. 3rd ed. London: Chapman & Hall Medical; 1997:222–223.

Campen R, Mankin H, Louis DN, et al. Familial occurrence of adiposis dolorosa. *J Am Acad Dermatol*. 2001;44:132–136.

Christenson L, Patterson J, Davis D. Surgical pearl: use of the cutaneous punch for the removal of lipomas. *J Am Acad Dermatol*. 2000;42:675–676.

Digregorio F, Barr RJ, Fretzin DF. Pleomorphic lipoma: case reports and review of the literature. *J Dermatol Surg Oncol*. 1992;18:197–202.

Eskey CJ, Robson CD, Weber AL. Imaging of benign and malignant soft tissue tumors of the neck. *Radiol Clin North Am*. 2000;38:1091–1104.

Humeniuk HM, Lask GP. Treatment of benign cutaneous lesions. In: Parish LC, Lask GP, eds. *Aesthetic Dermatology*. New York: McGraw-Hill; 1991:39–49.

Makley JT. Benign soft tissue lesions. In: Evarts CM, ed. *Surgery of the Musculoskeletal System*. 2nd ed. New York: Churchill Livingstone; 1990:4795–4818.

Moraru RA. Lipomas. Emedicine Web site. http://www.emedicine.com/DERM/topic242.htm. Accessed November 7, 2001.

Salam GA. Lipoma excision. *Am Fam Physician*. 2002;65:901–905.

Sanchez MR, Golomb FM, Moy JA, et al. Giant lipoma: case report and review of the literature. *J Am Acad Dermatol*. 1993;28:266–268.

Zuber TJ. *Skin Biopsy, Excision, and Repair Techniques*. Kansas City: American Academy of Family Physicians, 1999:100–106.

2008 MAG Mutual Healthcare Solutions, Inc.'s Physicians' Fee and Coding Guide. Duluth, Georgia. MAG Mutual Healthcare Solutions, Inc. 2007.

CHAPTER 51

O-to-Z-plasty

E. J. Mayeaux, Jr., MD, DABFP, FAAFP
Professor of Family Medicine, Professor of Obstetrics and Gynecology
Louisiana State University Health Sciences Center, Shreveport, LA

The O-to-Z-plasty is a versatile closure technique used for large defects that are not appropriately closed with a fusiform (elliptical) excision technique. Because of the multiple clinical indications, the O-to-Z-plasty can be readily learned by generalist physicians and used frequently in practice. Advantages of the technique include the sparing of tissue, closure mostly aligning with the lines of least skin tension, and production of a broken line (Z-shaped) final scar. The O-to-Z flap technique generally produces excellent cosmetic results.

The O-to-Z-plasty combines advancement and rotation techniques, and some authors characterize it as a transposition flap. The O-to-Z flap can be envisioned as a large fusiform excision, with only the central circular area around the lesion excised. On each side of the central circular area, only one of the arms of the fusiform excision is incised. A flap is created on each side, and these two flaps are joined centrally to create a final Z-shaped scar.

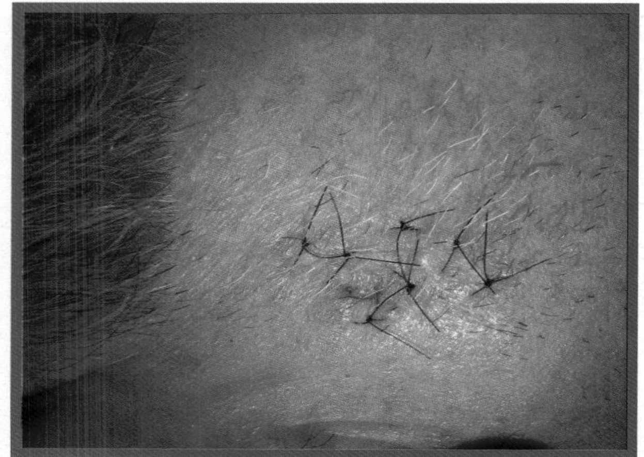

Large fusiform excisions can result in the removal of a large amount of tissue and subsequent pull on surrounding structures with closure of the wound. For instance, a large fusiform excision just above the eyebrow can produce permanent elevation of the eyebrow. Fusiform excisions on the upper lip can elevate the vermilion border. Because less total tissue is removed, the O-to-Z-plasty can obviate the difficulty of lateral pull on surrounding structures when closing the wound.

Skin flaps are most commonly performed where the blood supply is extensive. The O-to-Z-plasty receives its blood supply through large pedicle bases (i.e., portion of the fusiform incisions that are not incised) and can sometimes work well even on sites with less vigorous blood flow. As with all skin flap techniques, meticulous attention to hemostasis is required.

When the O-to-Z-plasty is performed after skin cancer removal, it is preferable to ensure clear margins using frozen sections or Mohs surgery before performing wound closure. Because these options may not be available to an office physician, a sufficient margin of normal-appearing skin must be removed around and beneath a cancer (see Appendix D) before closure is attempted. Postprocedure pressure dressings are recommended to reduce hematoma formation beneath the flaps and the development of complications.

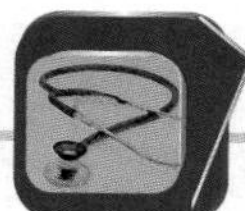

Equipment

- Appendix G lists the instruments included in a standard skin surgery tray.
- Suggested suture removal times are listed in Appendix J.
- A suggested anesthesia tray that can be used for this procedure is listed in Appendix F.

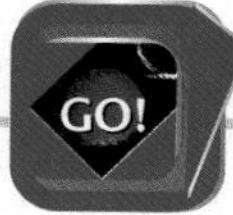

Indications

- Lesion removal next to linear structures that should not be pulled
- Lesion removal on the upper lip
- Closure of defects on the chin or beneath the chin
- Closure of large forehead defects (especially if just above the eyebrows or near the hairline)
- Repair of scalp defects
- Closure of defects in temple region, lateral face beneath the ear, or along the mandible

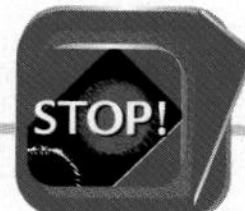

Contraindications (Relative)

- Closure of defects on breast tissue (use a running intracutaneous suture closure)
- Widely separated wound edges that are better approximated with deeply buried sutures
- Severe bleeding disorders
- Extreme illness that would make wound healing difficult
- Cellulitis in the tissues to be incised
- Conditions that may interfere with wound healing (collagen vascular diseases, smoking, diabetes)
- Concurrent medications that may increase the likelihood of intraoperative bleeding (aspirin, other nonsteroidal anti-inflammatory drugs, warfarin)
- Uncooperative patient

The Procedure

The O-to-Z-plasty is based on the fusiform excision, with the overall length of the excision being three times the width. The long axis is aligned so that it is parallel to the lines of least skin tension (Appendix B) and has an adequate margin (Appendix D). However, in the O-to-Z-plasty, only one incision line (i.e., arm) is performed on each side of the central circular excision. The incision lines are drawn to slope toward a theoretical central line. One incision arm is above the central line, and one incision arm is below the central line.

- **PITFALL:** Make sure the incision arms are on opposite sides of the central line! Many

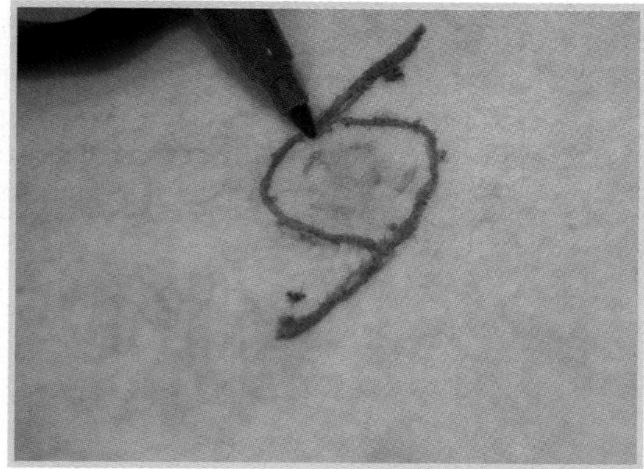

Figure 1

novice practitioners unintentionally incise both arms on the same side of the central line, necessitating performance of a fusiform excision or an advancement flap technique.

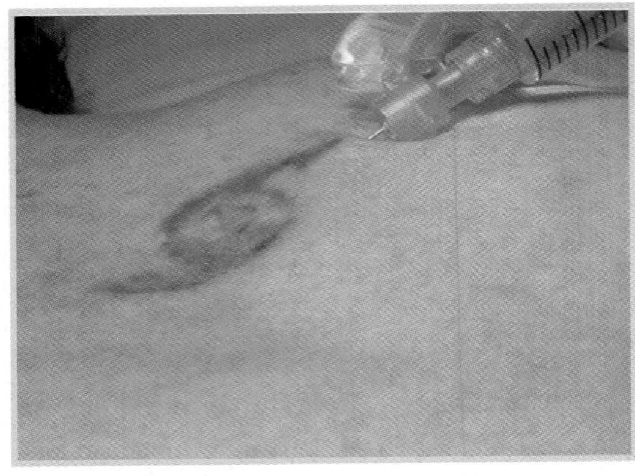

Step 1

Step 1. Perform field block anesthesia (see Chapter 2). Plan the anesthesia injections to create a large enough numb area to allow for undermining parallel to the long axis, as in a fusiform excision. Prep the skin with povidone-iodine or chlorhexidine solution, and allow it to dry (see Appendix E).

- **PEARL:** Prep a wide area so that an undraped area is not inadvertently exposed if the drape slides a little.

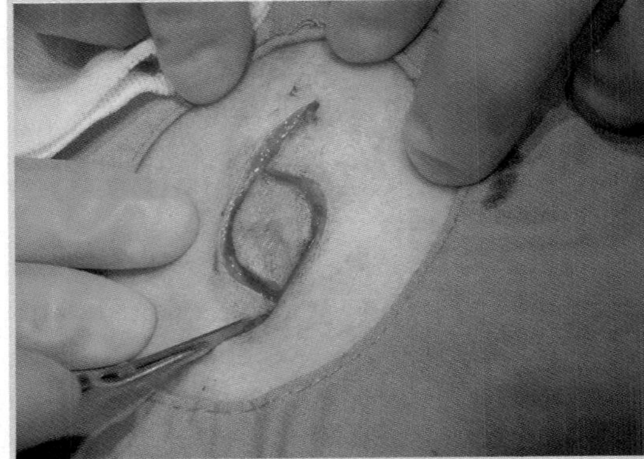

Step 2

Step 2. Incise gentle sloping lines that end at the theoretical central line. The arms should be approximately 1.5 to 2 times the diameter of the central circular excision.

- **PEARL:** The center island containing the lesion may be excised first, although smoother excision lines occur when all of the excision is made at once. The corners of the central island are squared (if the island is removed first) to facilitate approximation of the flaps.

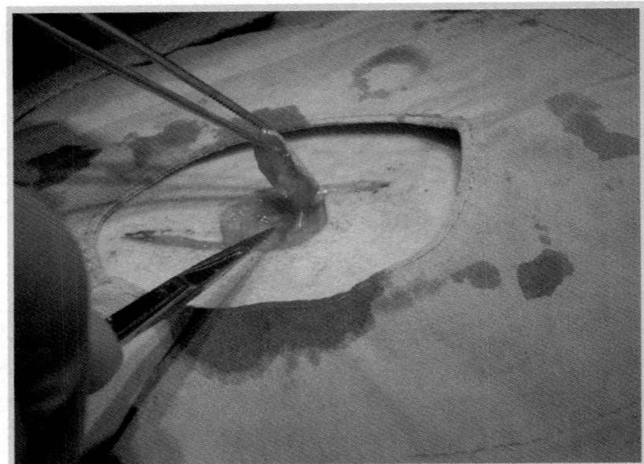

Step 3

Step 3. The central island of skin containing the lesion is undermined, removed, and sent for histologic analysis.

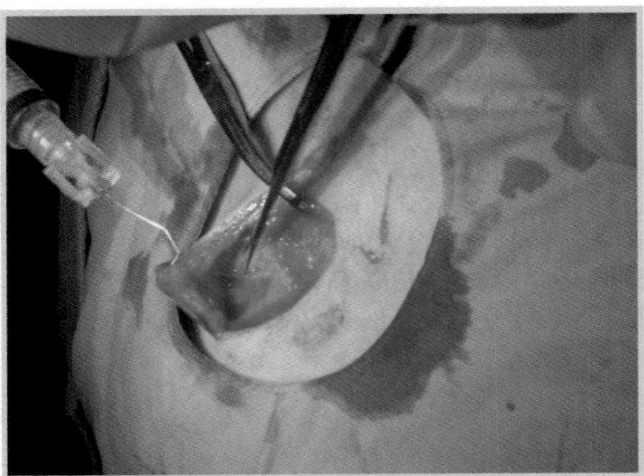

Step 4

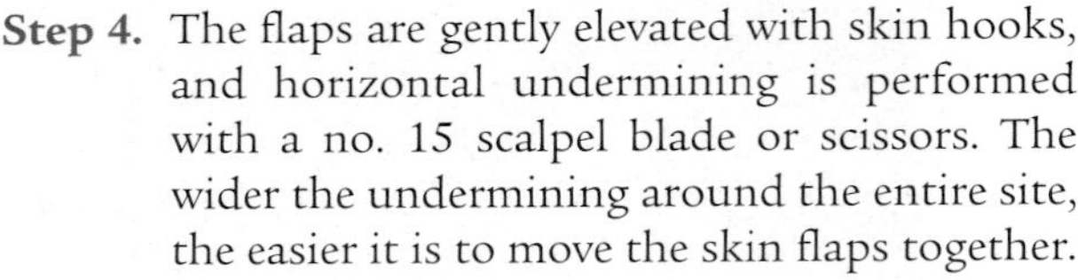

Step 4. The flaps are gently elevated with skin hooks, and horizontal undermining is performed with a no. 15 scalpel blade or scissors. The wider the undermining around the entire site, the easier it is to move the skin flaps together.

Step 5. Test to see if the flaps are lax enough to come together without significant tension. If there is too much tension to close the flaps with minimal finger pressure, then more undermining of the flaps may be necessary.

- **PITFALL:** If the flaps are well undermined and still do not close with minimal pressure, check the overall length of the flaps. If the length-to-width ratio is <3:1, it is difficult to close the flaps, and there will be a greater risk of necrosis of all or part of the flaps due to lack of blood flow.

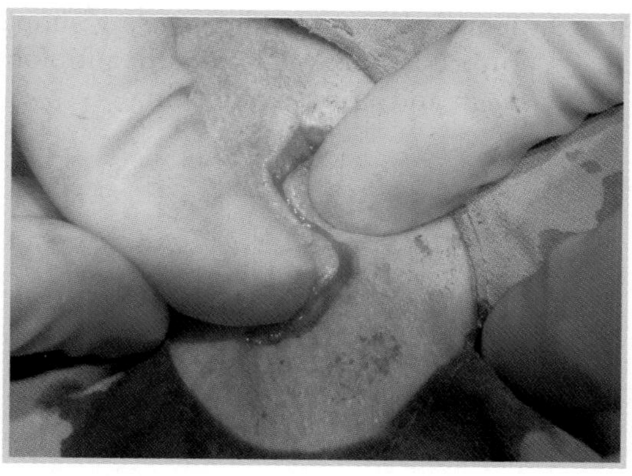

Step 5

Step 6. The two flaps are brought together and anchored with one or two vertical mattress sutures. Place the anchoring stitch in the center of both flaps.

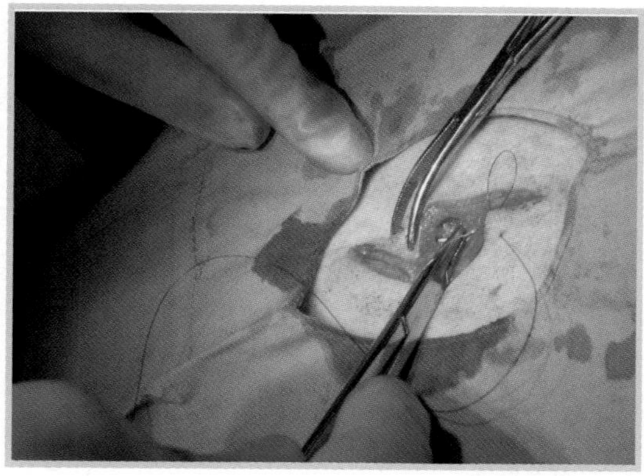

Step 6

Step 7. Corner stitches are placed in the flap tip corners. See Chapter 39, Corner Suture. Elevated tissue formations at the ends of the arms (dog ears) may develop and are dealt with in the next step.

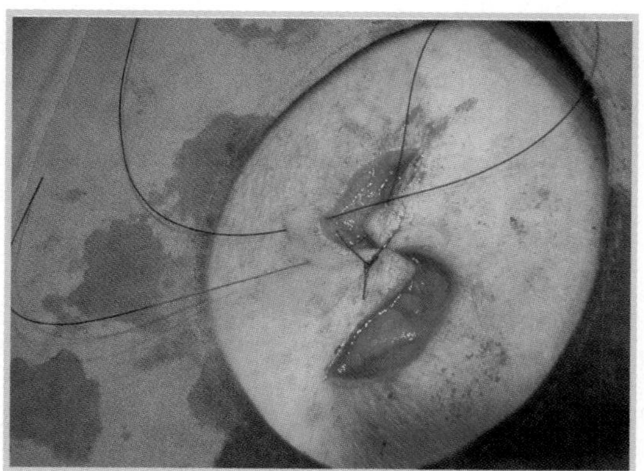

Step 7

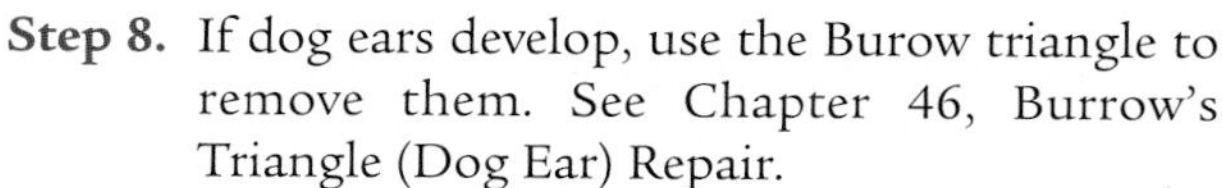

Step 8. If dog ears develop, use the Burow triangle to remove them. See Chapter 46, Burrow's Triangle (Dog Ear) Repair.

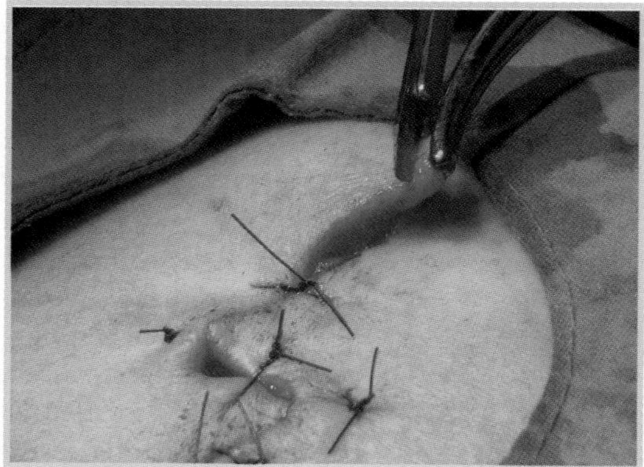

Step 8

Step 9. Finish closing the defect using simple interrupted sutures. Dress with antibiotic ointment and a pressure dressing.

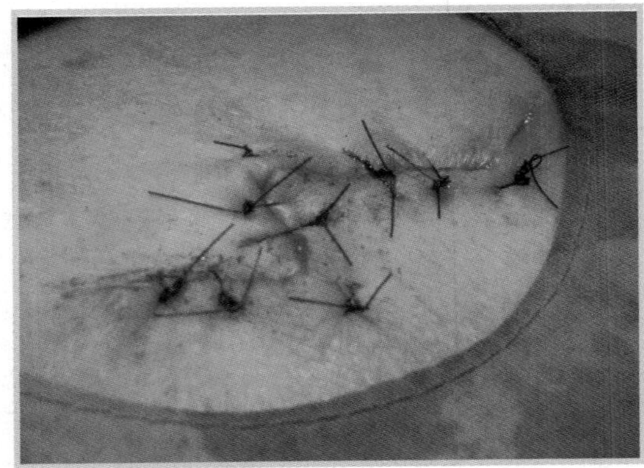

Step 9

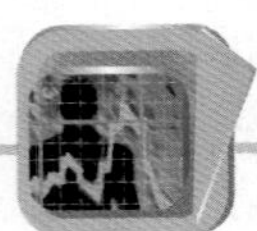

Complications

- Pain, infection, and bleeding
- Nonunion of skin edges
- Scar formation
- Incomplete excision of lesion

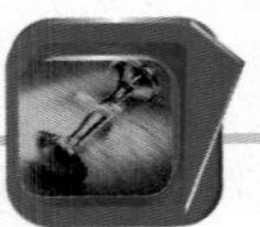

Pediatric Considerations

Generally, pediatric skin has excellent blood flow and heals very well. However, pediatric patients often find it difficult to sit and lie still during lengthy procedures. The patient's maturity and ability to cooperate should be considered before deciding to attempt any outpatient procedure. The maximum recommended dose for lidocaine in children is 3 to 5 mg/kg, and 7 mg/kg when combined with epinephrine. Neonates have an increased volume of distribution, decreased hepatic clearance, and doubled terminal elimination half-life (3.2 hours).

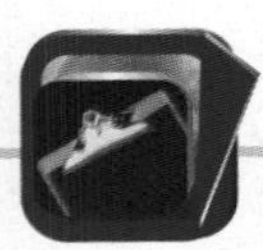

Postprocedure Instructions

Instruct the patient to keep the pressure bandage on the rest of the day, then gently wash the area that has been stitched the next day. The patient should not put the wound into standing water for 3 days. Have the patient cleanse dry the area well after washing and use a small amount of antibiotic ointment to promote moist healing. Recommend wound elevation to help lessen swelling, reduce pain, and speed healing. Instruct the patient not to pick at, break, or cut the stitches.

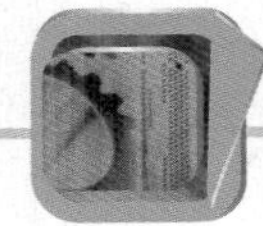

Coding Information and Supply Sources

These codes encompass excision or repair, or both, by adjacent transfer or rearrangement, including Z-plasty, W-plasty, V-Y-plasty, rotation flaps, advancement flaps, and double-pedicle flaps. When applied to traumatic wounds, the defect must be developed by the surgeon because the closure requires it, and these codes should not be used for direct closure of a defect that incidentally results in the configuration of one of the flaps or plasties. If the configurations result incidentally from the laceration shape, closure should be reported using simple repair codes.

CPT Code	Description	2008 Average 50th Percentile Fee	Global Period
14000	Trunk ≤10 cm^2	$1,062.00	90
14001	Trunk 10.1–30.0 cm^2	$1,400.00	90
14020	SAL ≤10 cm^2	$1,222.00	90
14021	SAL 10.1–30.0^2	$1,684.00	90
14040	FCCMNAGHF ≤10 cm^2	$1,551.00	90
14041	FCCMNAGHF 10.1–30.0 cm^2	$1,757.00	90
14060	ENEL ≤10 cm^2	$1,841.00	90
14061	ENEL 10.1–30.0 cm^2	$2,254.00	90
14300	Any unusual or complicated area >30 cm^2	$2,749.00	90

CPT is a registered trademark of the American Medical Association.
2008 average 50th Percentile Fees are provided courtesy of 2008 MMH-SI's copyrighted Physicians' Fees and Coding Guide.
SAL, scalp, arms, or legs; FCCMNAGHF, forehead, cheeks, chin, mouth, neck, axillae, genitalia, hands, or feet; ENEL, eyelids, nose, ears, or lips.

Bibliography

Chernosky ME. Scalpel and scissors surgery as seen by the dermatologist. In: Epstein E, Epstein E Jr, eds. *Skin Surgery*. 6th ed. Philadelphia: WB Saunders; 1987:88–127.

Hammond RE. Uses of the O-to-Z-plasty repair in dermatologic surgery. *J Dermatol Surg Oncol.* 1979;5:205–211.

Stegman SJ. Fifteen ways to close surgical wounds. *J Dermatol Surg.* 1975;1:25–31.

Stegman SJ, Tromovitch TA, Glogau RG. *Basics of Dermatologic Surgery*. Chicago: Year Book Medical Publishing; 1982:77–78.

Swanson NA. *Atlas of Cutaneous Surgery*. Boston: Little, Brown; 1987:102–104.

Vural E, Key JM. Complications, salvage, and enhancement of local flaps in facial reconstruction. *Otolaryngol Clin North Am*. 2001;34:739–751.

Whitaker DC. Random-pattern flaps. In: Wheeland RG, ed. *Cutaneous Surgery*. Philadelphia: WB Saunders; 1994:329–352.

Zuber TJ. *Advanced Soft-Tissue Surgery*. Kansas City: American Academy of Family Physicians; 1998:92–97.

2008 MAG Mutual Healthcare Solutions, Inc.'s Physicians' Fee and Coding Guide. Duluth, Georgia. MAG Mutual Healthcare Solutions, Inc. 2007.

CHAPTER 52

Purse-String Suture Closure

E. J. Mayeaux, Jr., MD, DABFP, FAAFP

Professor of Family Medicine, Professor of Obstetrics and Gynecology
Louisiana State University Health Sciences Center, Shreveport, LA

The purse-string suture can be used to provide complete or partial closure of round skin defects. This running suture is placed horizontally in the dermis. Skin from the entire periphery of the defect is uniformly advanced by the tension placed on the purse-string suture. Large circular defects may be closed or made smaller by utilizing a running purse-string suture.

The purse-string suture eliminates the excision of healthy skin adjacent to the wound. It can function as the primary closure for small skin defects. It can also serve as a partial closure for larger defects by reducing the wound surface area, and allowing the remainder of the wound to granulate. Alternatively, the residual defect can be closed using either a skin graft or a transfer of adjacent tissue.

Standing wedges may be cut in advance of the closure. This converts the round defect into a stellate defect that may be closed with a purse-string or classic multiple corner sutures. This technique obviates the need for placement of secondary sutures in a side-to-side fashion, which could interfere with the healing in the central portion of the repair. These side-to-side buried sutures produce tension that could cut through the central graft. The wound can be further supported temporarily during the initial postoperative period by placing overlying mattress sutures.

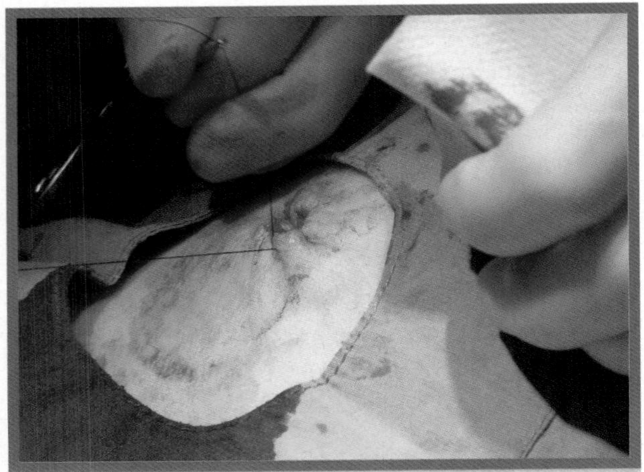

Skin has extensive viscoelastic properties that allow it to stretch and expand when placed under constant tension. When the tension in a skin closure is constant, stress relaxation occurs that causes the tension to gradually decrease. Using the purse-string suture, the wound margin length can be considerably reduced, with no long-term distortions of the surrounding skin and a satisfactory scar. During the time necessary for healing, skin remodeling occurs, eliminating concentric skin folds and tissue distortions.

In the immediate postoperative period, the suture is usually surrounded by a large number of concentric redundant skin folds, and there may be some distortion of the nearby structures. Both of these problems typically improve spontaneously over a period of a month, as the skin naturally stretches under the constant tension, and often completely disappear by the time the suture is removed in 4 to 6 weeks. The scars also tend to orient themselves along the lines of least skin tension line over the ensuing month. Some scar widening may occur over time, especially when larger sutures (0-1 or more) are used or are left in place longer than 6 weeks. The final scar is always shorter than the original defect. Patients need to be carefully prepared for the initial skin distortion and the extended period that the suture remains in the skin.

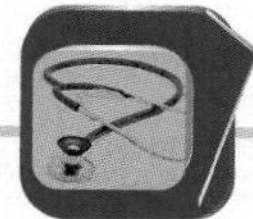

Equipment

- Surgery tray instruments are listed in Appendix G. Consider adding skin hooks to gently handle the skin flaps. Have at least three fine (mosquito) hemostats to assist with hemostasis while developing large skin flaps.
- Suggested suture removal times are listed in Appendix J, and a suggested anesthesia tray that can be used for this procedure is listed in Appendix F. All instruments can be ordered through local surgical supply houses.

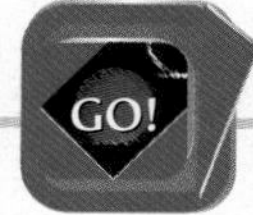

Indications

- Closure of round skin defects that are not amenable to other low-tension closures
- Temporary reduction of skin defects during malignancy excision procedures
- Reconstruction of postsurgical wounds in elderly patients with loose or thin, sun-damaged skin
- Operative defects on the distal legs and feet where there is limited skin laxity
- Closures in patients who are unable or unwilling to appropriately limit their level of activity following surgery

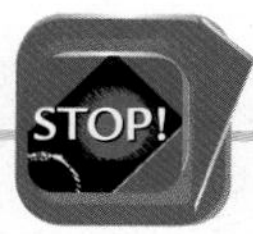

Contraindications

- Poor skin vascular supply
- Diseases causing poor vascular supply to the skin (e.g., atherosclerotic heart disease, diabetes, smoking, collagen vascular disease, prior irradiation, severe anemia, anticoagulation)
- History of poor wound healing, hypertrophic scarring, or keloid formation
- Uncooperative patient
- Presence of cellulitis, bacteremia, or active infection

The Procedure

Standard Purse-String Closure

Step 1. After removal of the skin lesion with an adequate margin, a round or ovoid defect is left.

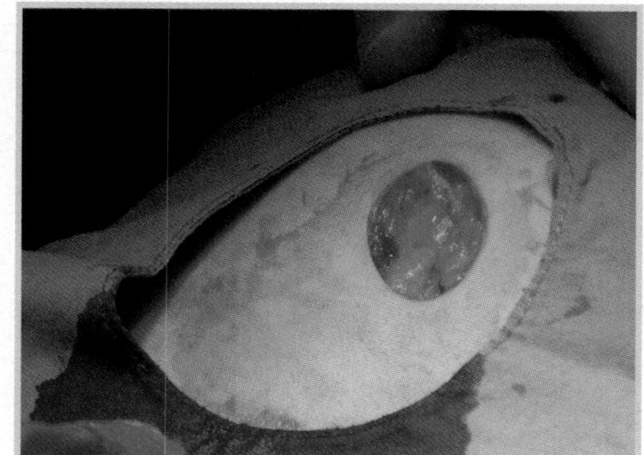

Step 1

Step 2. A 2-0 or larger nylon or Prolene suture is passed into the middermis.

- **PITFALL:** Using a suture smaller than 2-0 may result in suture breakage with tying or the suture pulling through the dermis before it is time for removal.

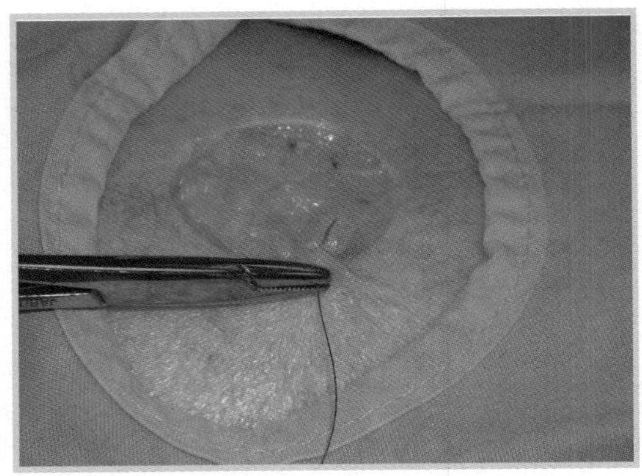

Step 2

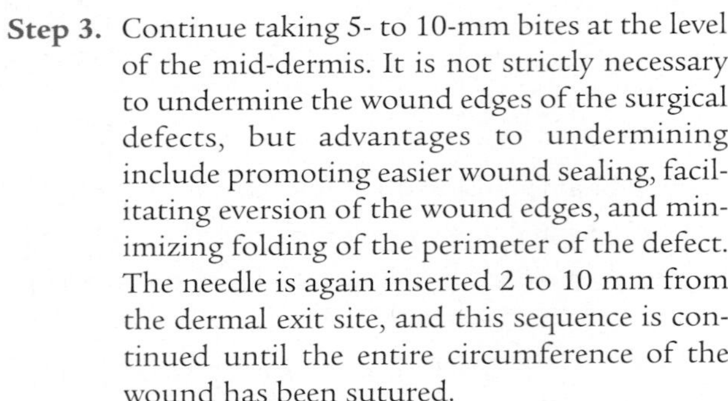

Step 3. Continue taking 5- to 10-mm bites at the level of the mid-dermis. It is not strictly necessary to undermine the wound edges of the surgical defects, but advantages to undermining include promoting easier wound sealing, facilitating eversion of the wound edges, and minimizing folding of the perimeter of the defect. The needle is again inserted 2 to 10 mm from the dermal exit site, and this sequence is continued until the entire circumference of the wound has been sutured.

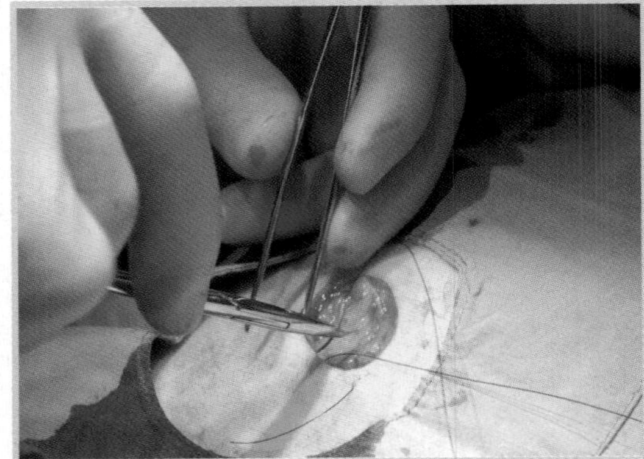

Step 3

Step 4. If the final purse string is going to be long, it may be difficult to extract the suture at the time of removal. Consider placing an external loop, which can be cut to facilitate removal.

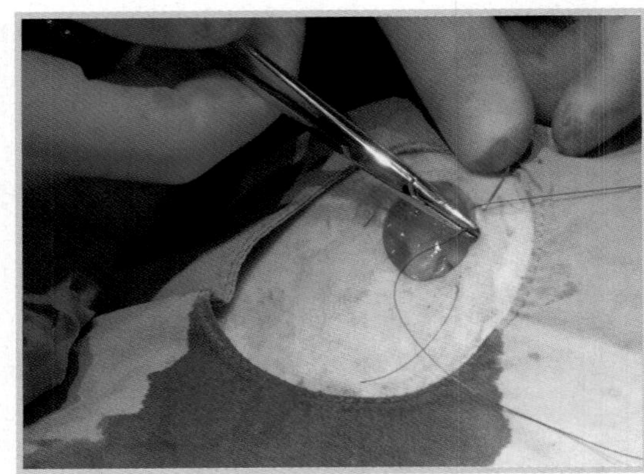

Step 4

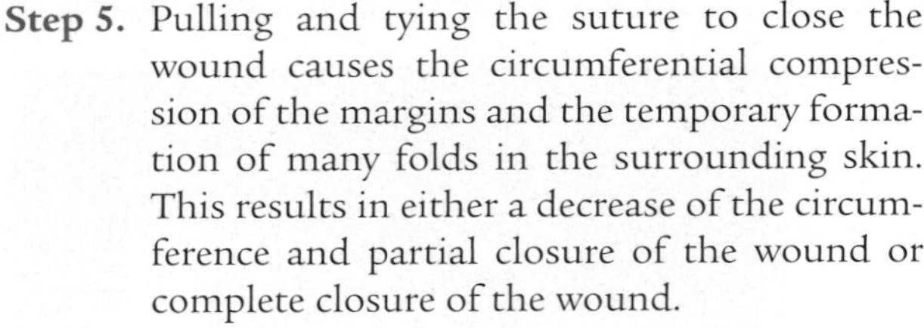

Step 5. Pulling and tying the suture to close the wound causes the circumferential compression of the margins and the temporary formation of many folds in the surrounding skin. This results in either a decrease of the circumference and partial closure of the wound or complete closure of the wound.

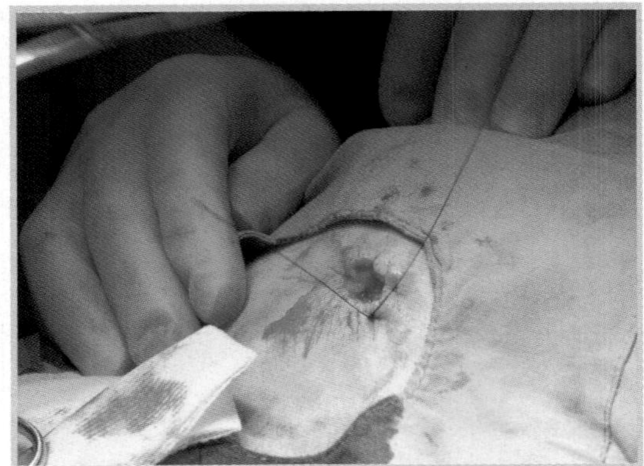

Step 5

Step 6. Partially closed wounds can then be packed with an absorbable gelatin sponge (i.e., Gelfoam). Alternatively, a final closure may be completed using a few external interrupted or vertical mattress sutures. Apply an antibiotic ointment and then a nonadherent pad, followed by a pressure dressing.

- **PEARL:** Minimal undermining of the wound margins is necessary, which may help maximize skin vascularity.

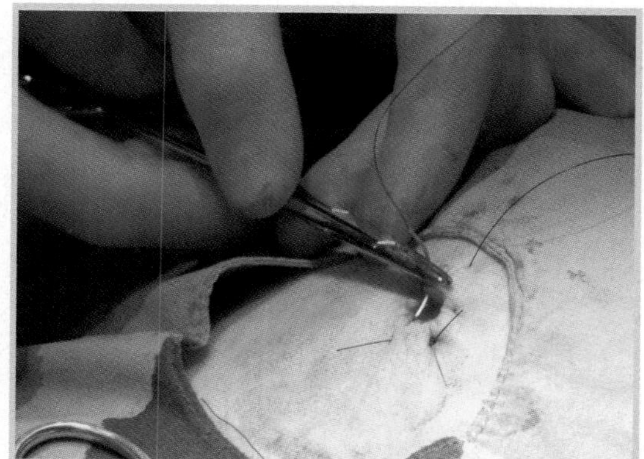

Step 6

Stellate Purse-String Closure

Step 1. After the round defect is created by removal of the skin lesion with an adequate margin, draw and excise four wedges equidistant from each other around the defect.

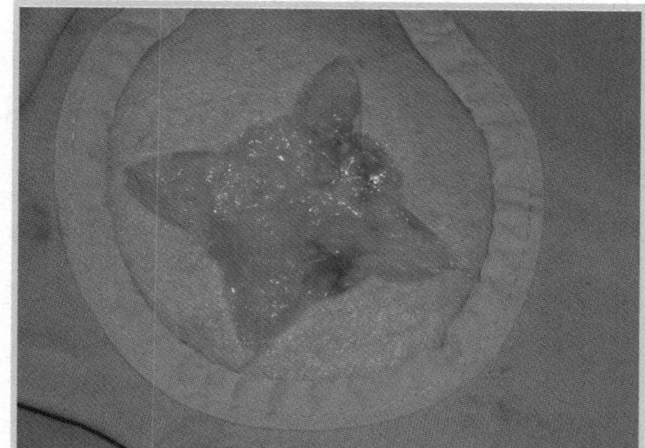

Step 1

Step 2. Then the suture can be placed as described previously with a deep pass crossing the opening of each wedge defect. Alternatively, the suture can be passed only through the base of the defect in a circular pattern in a manner similar to that used to close stellate wounds (see Chapter 39, Corner Suture).

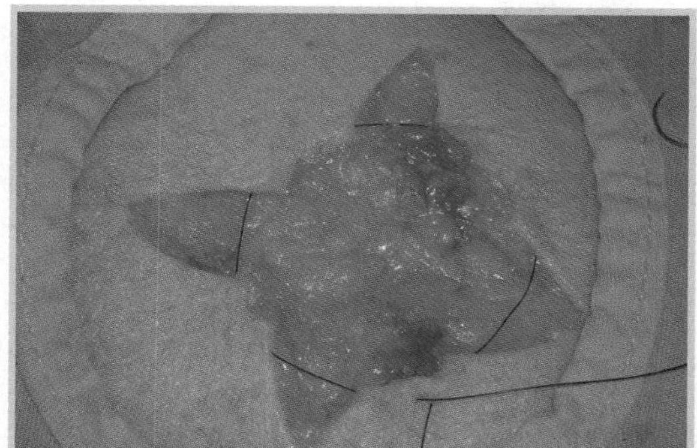

Step 2

Step 3. Pulling and tying the suture to close the wound causes complete closure of the defect without the folds in the surrounding skin found in the traditional method.

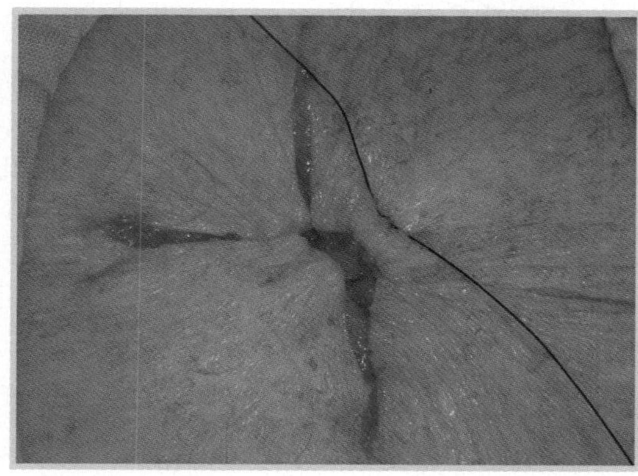

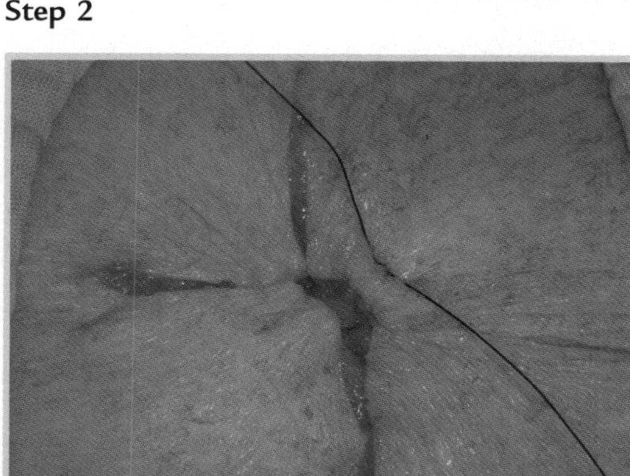

Step 3

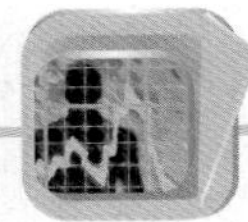

Complications

- Pain, infection, and bleeding
- Nonunion of skin edges
- Sensory changes (often subside with time)
- Skin necrosis
- Dehiscence
- Hypertrophic scarring (often resolves spontaneously within 12 months)
- Suture marks
- Alopecia
- Widening of the scar (especially on the scalp)
- Exuberant granulation tissue
- Postoperative pain

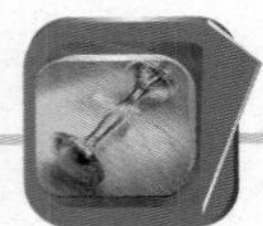

Pediatric Considerations

Generally, pediatric skin has excellent blood flow and heals very well. However, pediatric patients often find it difficult to sit or lie still during lengthy procedures. The patient's maturity and ability to cooperate should be considered before deciding to attempt any outpatient procedure. It is rare to have to do such wide excisions on pediatric patients, which is fortunate because parents are often less accepting of scars for their children than they are for themselves.

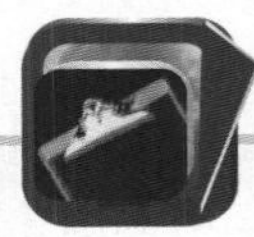

Postprocedure Instructions

Apply topical antibiotics and a dressing after the procedure. Have the patient keep the bandage on and the wound dry for the first 24 hours. After that, it can be gently washed with soap and water as needed. An antibiotic ointment and bandage should be reapplied after each washing until the patient returns.

Any external sutures should be removed in 5 to 8 days to avoid any suture marks. The purse-string suture should be left in place for a minimum of 4 weeks, although waiting 6 to 8 weeks produces better results. Educate the patient that suture removal too early (<4 weeks) often results in a worse cosmetic outcome. Have the patient report signs of infection.

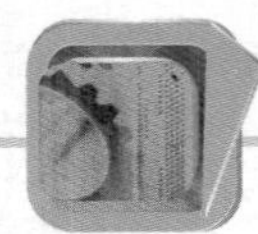

Coding Information

These codes encompass excision or repair, or both, by adjacent transfer or rearrangement, including Z-plasty, W-plasty, V-Y-plasty, rotation flaps, advancement flaps, and double-pedicle flaps. When applied to traumatic wounds, the defect must be developed by the surgeon because the closure requires it, and these codes should not be used for direct closure of a defect that incidentally results in the configuration of one of the flaps or plasties. If the configurations result incidentally from the laceration shape, closure should be reported using simple repair codes.

CPT Code	Description	2008 Average 50th Percentile Fee	Global Period
14000	Trunk ≤10 cm^2	$1,062.00	90
14001	Trunk 10.1–30.0 cm^2	$1,400.00	90
14020	SAL ≤10 cm^2	$1,222.00	90
14021	SAL 10.1–30.0^2	$1,684.00	90
14040	FCCMNAGHF ≤10 cm^2	$1,551.00	90
14041	FCCMNAGHF 10.1–30.0 cm^2	$1,757.00	90
14060	ENEL ≤10 cm^2	$1,841.00	90
14061	ENEL 10.1–30.0 cm^2	$2,254.00	90
14300	Any unusual or complicated area >30 cm^2	$2,749.00	90

CPT is a registered trademark of the American Medical Association.
2008 average 50th Percentile Fees are provided courtesy of 2008 MMH-SI's copyrighted Physicians' Fees and Coding Guide.
SAL, scalp, arms, or legs; FCCMNAGHF, forehead, cheeks, chin, mouth, neck, axillae, genitalia, hands, or feet; ENEL, eyelids, nose, ears, or lips.

Bibliography

Benelli, L. A new periareolar mammaplasty: the "round block" technique. *Aesthetic Plast Surg.* 1990;14:93.

Berschadsky M. Periareolar subcuticular pursestring suture. *Plast Reconstr Surg.* 1999;104:1203.

Ciatti S, Greenbaum SS. Modified purse-string closure for reconstruction of moderate/large surgical defects of the face. *Dermatol Surg.* 1999;25:215–219.

Cohen PR, Martinelli PT, Schulze KE, et al. Closure of round cutaneous postoperative wounds with the purse string suture. *South Med J.* 2006;99(12):1401–1402.

Cohen PR, Martinelli PT, Schulze KE, et al. The cuticular purse string suture: a modified purse string suture for the partial closure of round postoperative wounds. *Int J Dermatol.* 2007;46(7):746–753.

Cohen PR, Martinelli PT, Schulze KE, et al. The purse-string suture revisited: a useful technique for the closure of cutaneous surgical wounds. *Int J Dermatol.* 2007:46;341–347.

Dang M, Greenbuam SS. Stellate purse-string closure. *Dermatol Surg.* 2000;26:495–496.

Dinner MI, Artz JS, Foglietti MA. Application and modification of the circular skin excision and pursestring procedures. *Aesthetic Plast Surg.* 1993;17(4):301–309.

Marconi F. The dermal purse-string suture: A new technique for a short inframammary scar in reduction mammoplasty and dermal mastopexy. *Ann Plast Surg.* 1989;22:484.

Peled IJ, Zagher U, Wexler MR. Purse-string suture for reduction and closure of skin defects. *Ann Plast Surg.* 1985;14(5):465–469.

Shelton RM. Repair of large and difficult-to-close wounds. *Dermatol Clin.* 2001;19:535–553.

Tremolada C, Blandini D, Beretta M, et al. The "round block" purse-string suture: a simple method to close skin defects with minimal scarring. *Plast Reconstr Surg.* 1997;100(1):126–131.

2008 MAG Mutual Healthcare Solutions, Inc.'s Physicians' Fee and Coding Guide. Duluth, Georgia. MAG Mutual Healthcare Solutions, Inc. 2007.

CHAPTER 53

Rhomboid Flap

E. J. Mayeaux, Jr., MD, DABFP, FAAFP

Professor of Family Medicine, Professor of Obstetrics and Gynecology
Louisiana State University Health Sciences Center, Shreveport, LA

Local skin flaps provide a superior approach to closing skin defects with like-appearing skin from nearby areas. The common fusiform (elliptical) excision (Chapter 49) is the technique most commonly employed for simple lesion removal, but nearby structures (e.g., nose, ear, orifices) can limit its use. The long straight scar line produced by the fusiform also tends to draw the eye more and thus be less cosmetically appealing than procedures that produce a less noticeable, broken line.

Nearby skin generally better approximates the needed color, hair pattern, and texture to close a defect than skin brought in from a distant site (i.e., skin graft). Local transposition skin flaps, such as the rhomboid flap (Limberg flap), can provide both excellent functional and cosmetic outcomes. They also allow closure of skin defects near orifices and fixed structures that limit the amount of skin that can pulled from those areas.

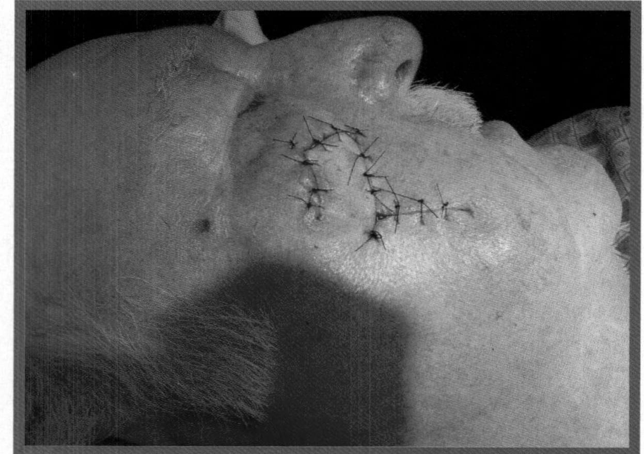

Preventing complications is an important aspect of performing flap surgery. Proper skin prep (see Appendix E) and strict sterile technique is necessary to avoid wound infections. Excessive handling of skin should be avoided because necrosis may ensue. Wide undermining of the tissue around a flap aids the closure without flap-necrosing tension. Do not pull on the skin edges with forceps or roughly handle the skin edges; gentle handling promotes healing. Excellent hemostasis is required for proper healing, so bleeding vessels should be clamped or suture-ligated before the flap is sutured. Pressure bandaging is advocated following the procedure.

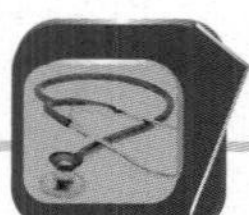

Equipment

- Surgery tray instruments are listed in Appendix G. Consider adding skin hooks to gently handle the skin flaps. Have at least three fine (mosquito) hemostats to assist with hemostasis while developing large skin flaps.
- Suggested suture removal times are listed in Appendix J, and a suggested anesthesia tray that can be used for this procedure is listed in Appendix F. All instruments can be ordered through local surgical supply houses.
- Also see Appendix E: Skin Preparation Recommendations.

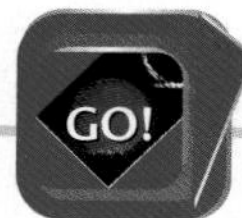

Indications

- Closure of skin defects that have limited skin that matches the area to be removed
- Closure of defects around eyes/eyebrows
- Closure of defects on the lips
- Closure of a defect over the glabella
- Closure of a large hand defect
- Closure of cheek defects

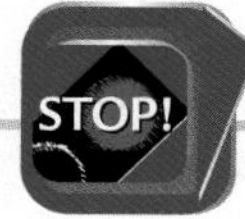

Contraindications (Relative)

- Practitioner's unfamiliarity or inexperience with the techniques
- Cellulitis in the tissues
- Skin unable to be stretched to cover the defect
- Chronic steroid use (and steroid skin effects)

The Procedure

Step 1. The rhomboid flap has several potential uses, especially around the eyes, lips, and glabella. Lay out the flap to minimize pull applied to structures that may be distorted by the added tension.

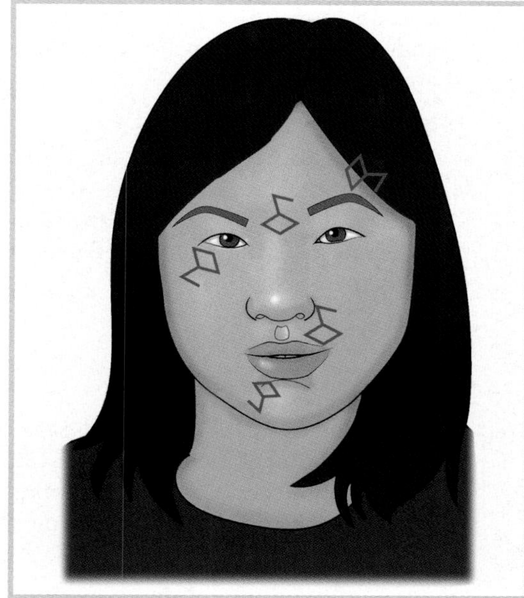

Step 1

Step 2. The rhomboid flap is based on geometry of the rhomboid or diamond. When planned and executed correctly, it is an equilateral parallelogram with the oblique angles equaling 120 degrees and the acute angles equaling 60 degrees. The length of all of the lines (labeled "L") will vary, but each line will be exactly the same length. The horizontal line that extends to the side (labeled "C") is the same length as the all of the other lines, and if it were extended into the diamond, it would bisect both 120 degree angles.

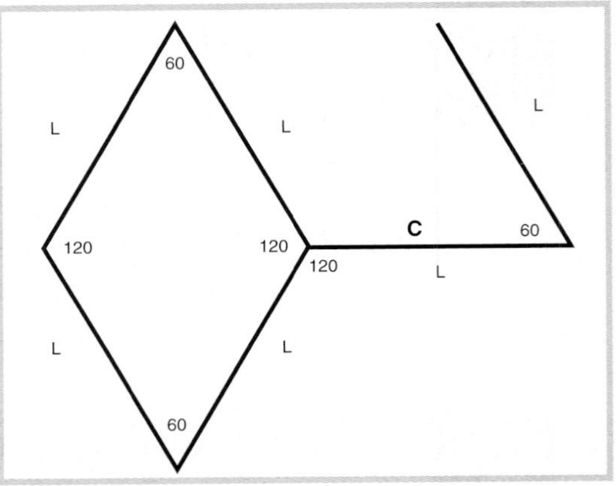

Step 2

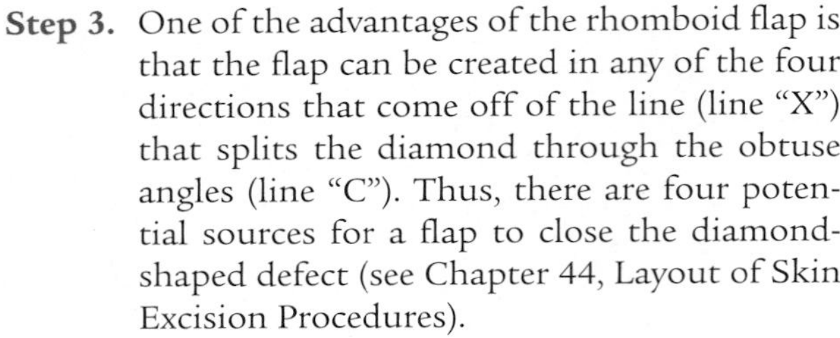

Step 3. One of the advantages of the rhomboid flap is that the flap can be created in any of the four directions that come off of the line (line "X") that splits the diamond through the obtuse angles (line "C"). Thus, there are four potential sources for a flap to close the diamond-shaped defect (see Chapter 44, Layout of Skin Excision Procedures).

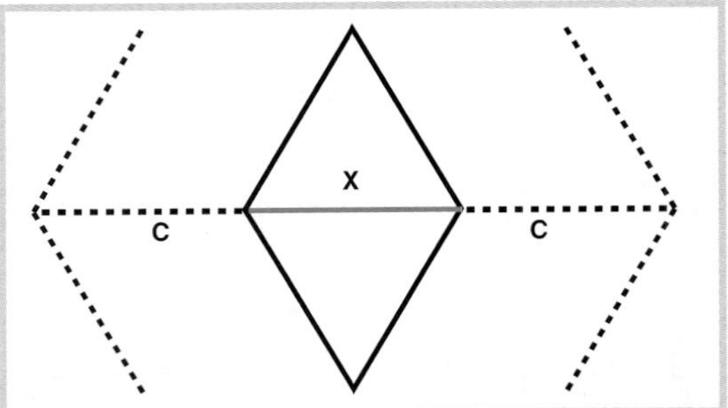

Step 3

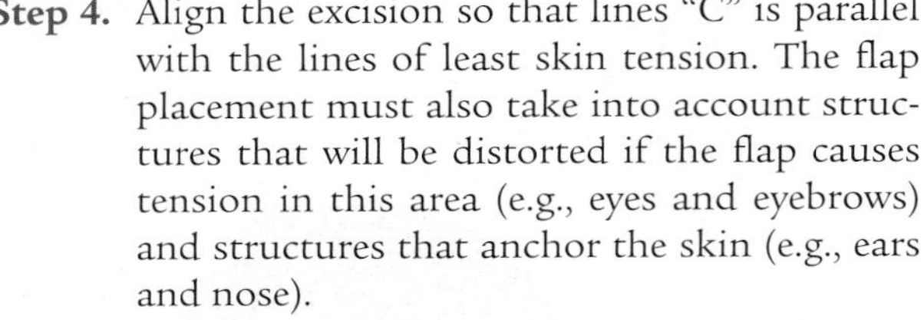

Step 4. Align the excision so that lines "C" is parallel with the lines of least skin tension. The flap placement must also take into account structures that will be distorted if the flap causes tension in this area (e.g., eyes and eyebrows) and structures that anchor the skin (e.g., ears and nose).

- **PEARL:** Consider using a permanent skin marker to mark the cut lines for the flap before the procedure, even if you do not normally need to mark flaps. The correct geometry of the rhomboid flap is critical to its success.

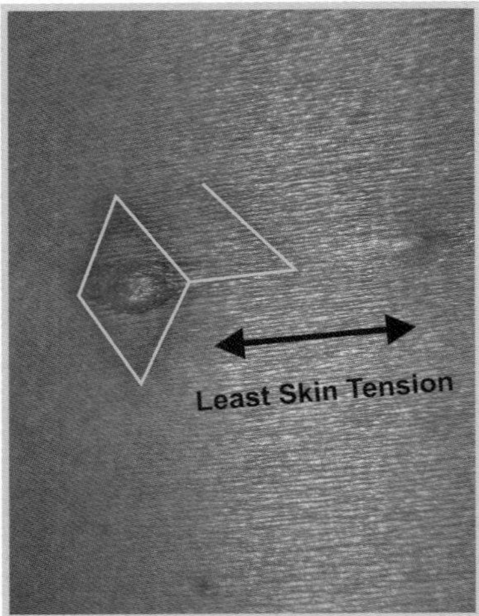

Step 4

Step 5. The rhomboid flap technique is started after administration of a field block (see Chapter 2). The lesion is removed in a diamond shape, with a margin of normal-appearing skin (see Appendix D).

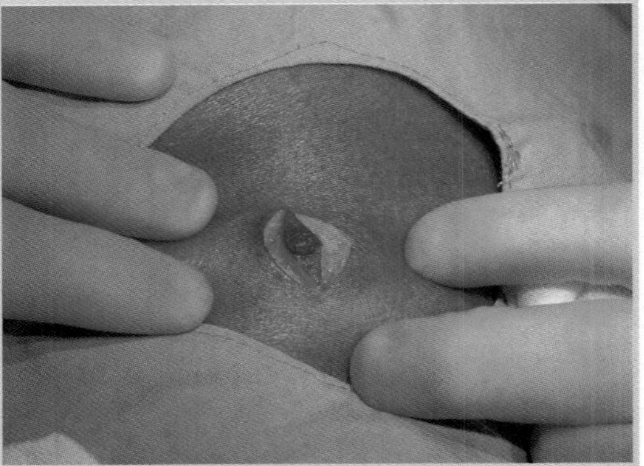

Step 5

Step 6. Prep the skin with povidone-iodine or chlorhexidine solution, and allow it to dry (see Appendix E). The flap is incised, making sure the correct geometry is maintained.

- **PEARL:** When checking the geometry of the cuts, always release any tension being held on the skin, because it can distort the geometry.
- **PEARL:** Prep a wide area so that an undraped area is not inadvertently exposed if the drape slides a little.

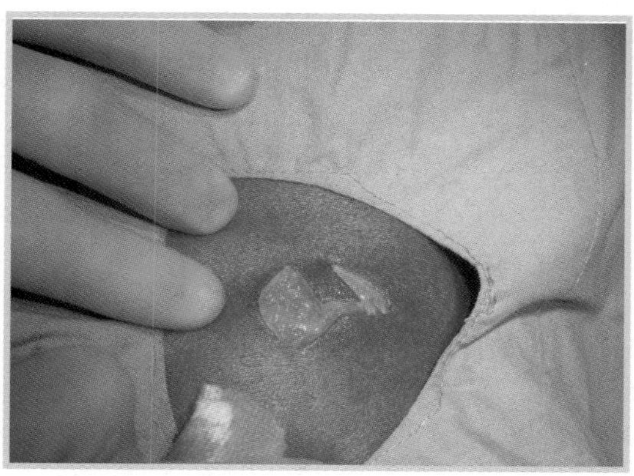

Step 6

Step 7. The flap is undermined with a horizontally held scalpel blade or iris scissors.

- **PITFALL:** Do not excessively undermine the flap base, because this can compromise blood flow to the flap.

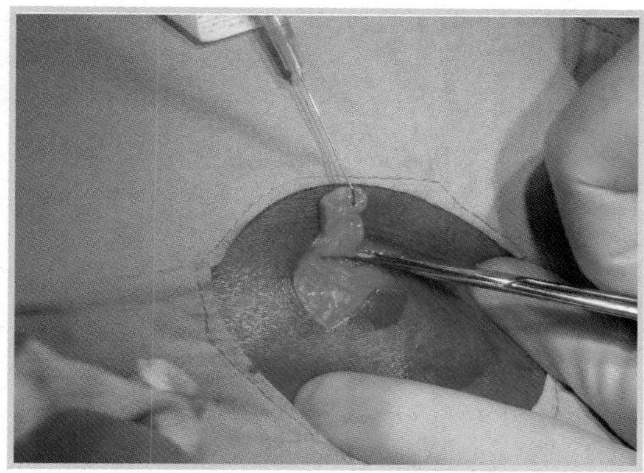

Step 7

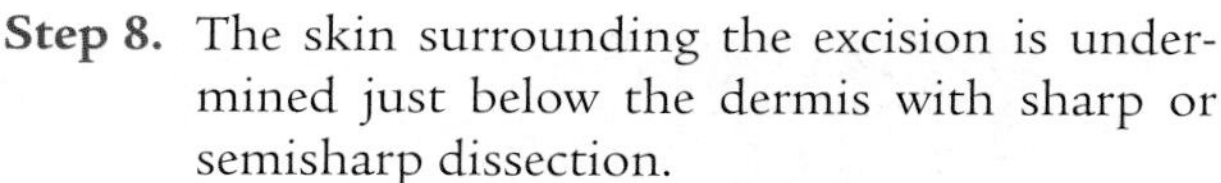

Step 8. The skin surrounding the excision is undermined just below the dermis with sharp or semisharp dissection.

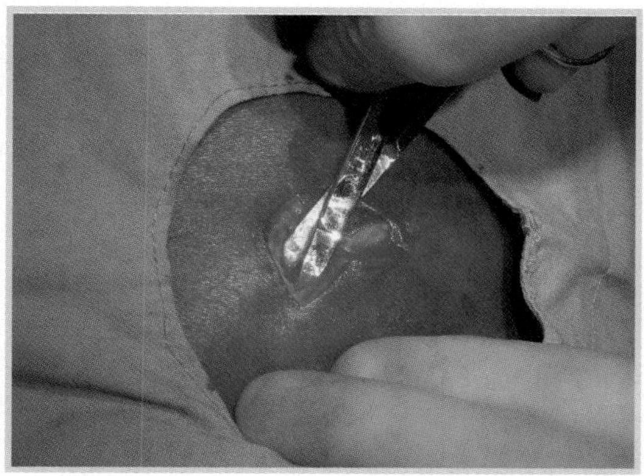

Step 8

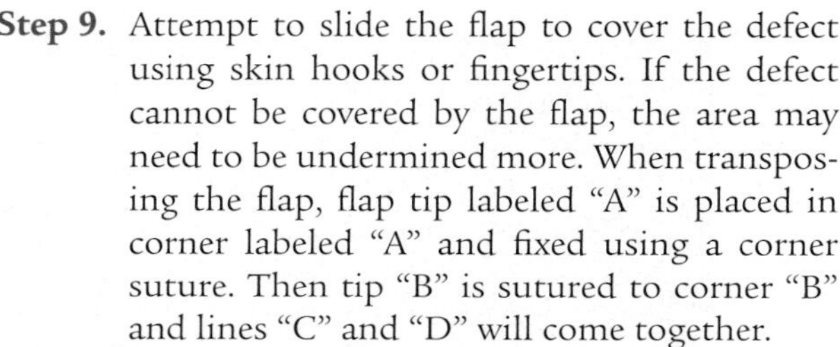

Step 9. Attempt to slide the flap to cover the defect using skin hooks or fingertips. If the defect cannot be covered by the flap, the area may need to be undermined more. When transposing the flap, flap tip labeled "A" is placed in corner labeled "A" and fixed using a corner suture. Then tip "B" is sutured to corner "B" and lines "C" and "D" will come together.

- **PITFALL:** The skin may bunch up (i.e., make a dog ear) near the base of the flap. If it is significant, it is eliminated by excising triangular pieces of skin at a 120-degree angle (i.e., Burrow triangles).

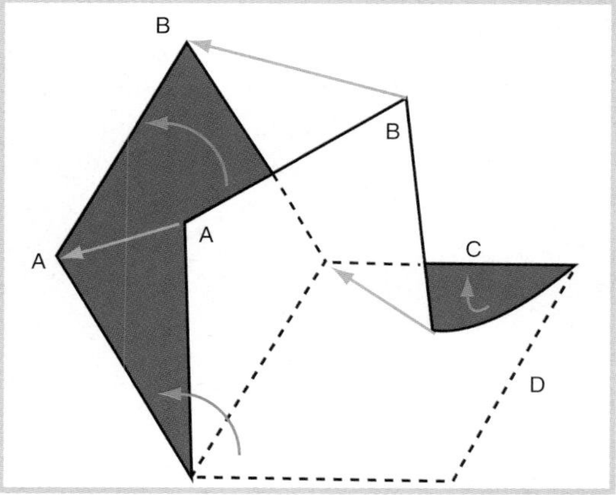

Step 9

Step 10. Transpose the flap by using a corner suture (see Chapter 39) to anchor the first corner (both labeled "A").

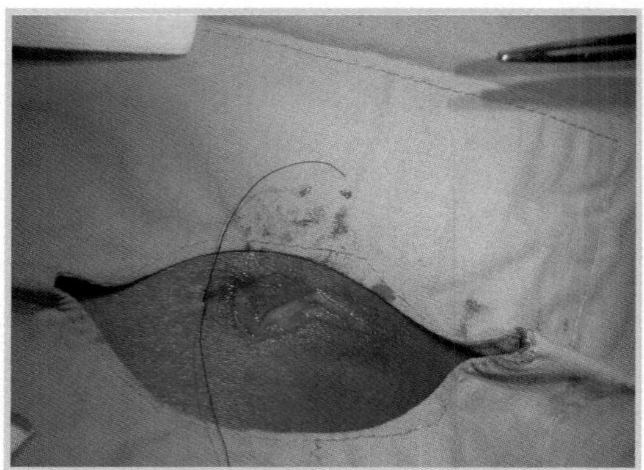
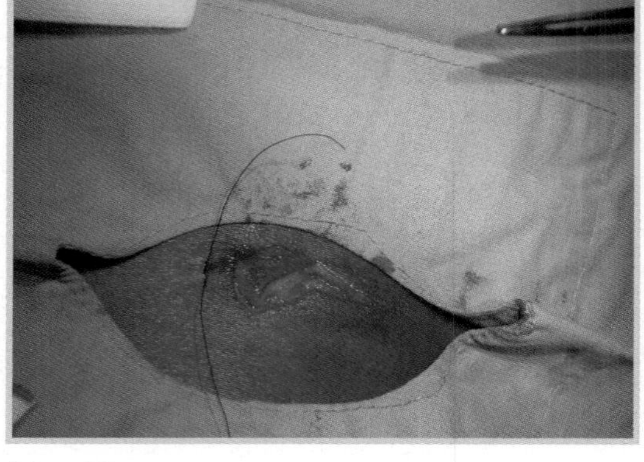

Step 10

Step 11. Then place a corner suture to anchor the tip of the flap into its corner (both labeled "B"). Note: The rest of the flap comes together and the closure appears more obvious.

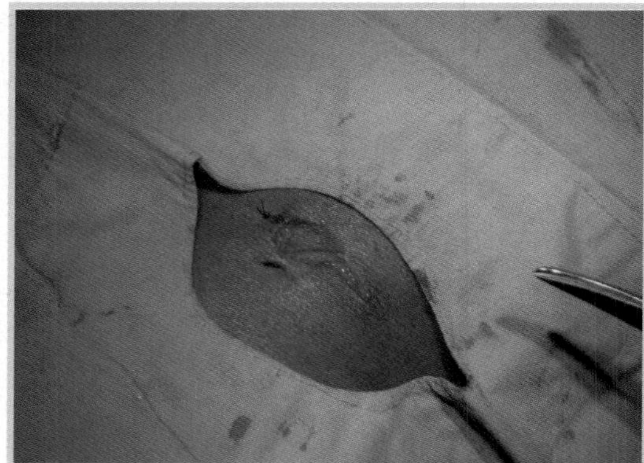

Step 11

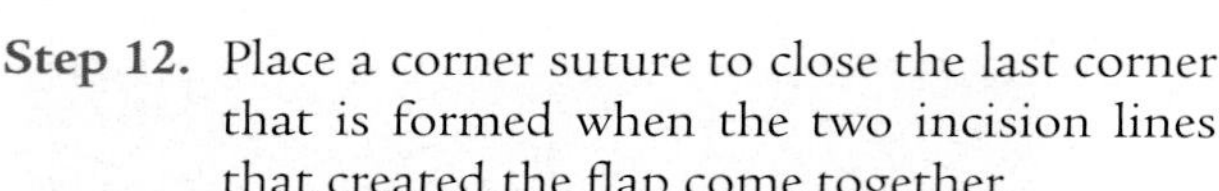

Step 12. Place a corner suture to close the last corner that is formed when the two incision lines that created the flap come together.

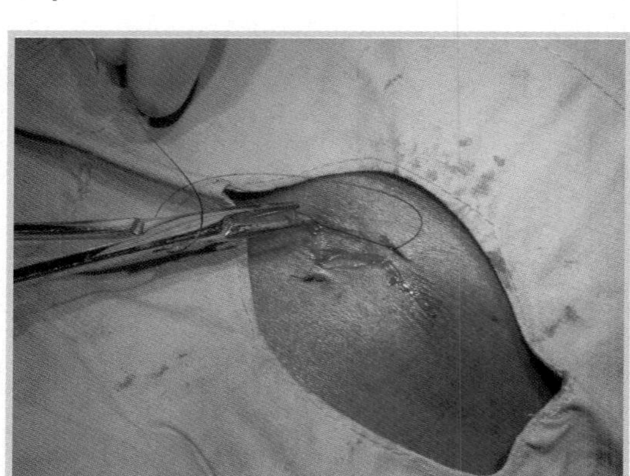

Step 12

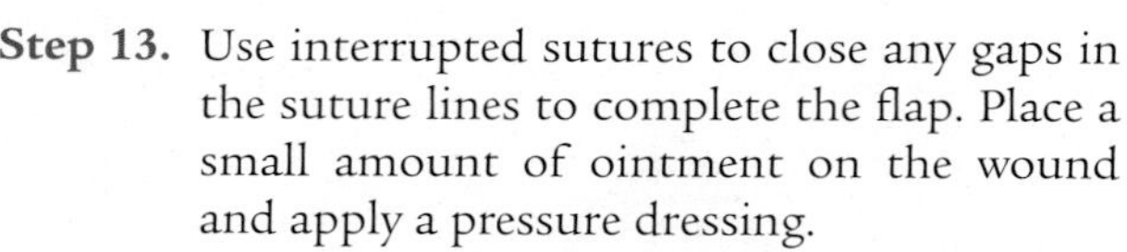

Step 13. Use interrupted sutures to close any gaps in the suture lines to complete the flap. Place a small amount of ointment on the wound and apply a pressure dressing.

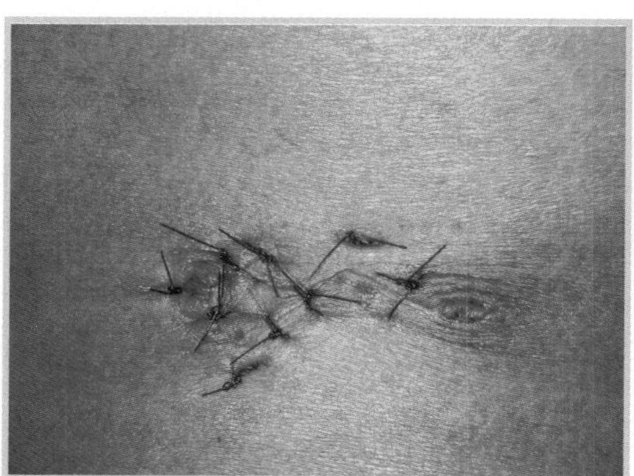

Step 13

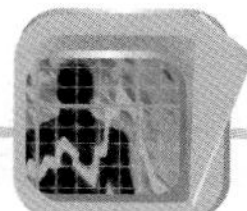

Complications

- Pain, infection, and bleeding
- Nonunion of skin edges
- Scar formation

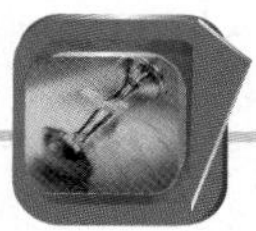

Pediatric Considerations

Generally, pediatric skin has excellent blood flow and heals very well. However, pediatric patients often find it difficult to sit and lie still during lengthy procedures. The patient's maturity and ability to cooperate should be considered before deciding to attempt any outpatient procedure.

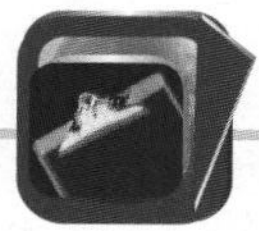

Postprocedure Instructions

Have the patient keep the bandage on and the wound dry for the first 24 hours. After that, it can be cleaned with hydrogen peroxide or gently washed with soap and water as needed. An antibiotic ointment and bandage should be reapplied after each washing until the patient returns or for 2 weeks. Have the patient report signs of infection. Schedule a return appointment for suture removal (see Appendix J).

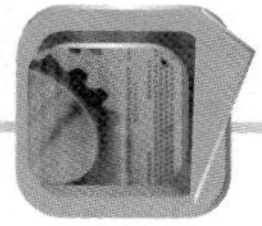

Coding Information

These codes encompass excision or repair, or both, by adjacent transfer or rearrangement, including Z-plasty, W-plasty, V-Y-plasty, rotation flaps, advancement flaps, and double-pedicle flaps. When applied to traumatic wounds, the defect must be developed by the surgeon because the closure requires it, and these codes should not be used for direct closure of a defect that incidentally results in the configuration of one of the flaps or plasties. If the configurations result incidentally from the laceration shape, closure should be reported using simple repair codes.

CPT Code	Description	2008 Average 50th Percentile Fee	Global Period
14000	Trunk $\leq$10 cm^2	\$1,062.00	90
14001	Trunk 10.1–30.0 cm^2	\$1,400.00	90
14020	SAL $\leq$10 cm^2	\$1,222.00	90
14021	SAL 10.1–30.0^2	\$1,684.00	90
14040	FCCMNAGHF $\leq$10 cm^2	\$1,551.00	90
14041	FCCMNAGHF 10.1–30.0 cm^2	\$1,757.00	90
14060	ENEL $\leq$10 cm^2	\$1,841.00	90
14061	ENEL 10.1–30.0 cm^2	\$2,254.00	90
14300	Any unusual or complicated area >30 cm^2	\$2,749.00	90

CPT is a registered trademark of the American Medical Association.
2008 average 50th Percentile Fees are provided courtesy of 2008 MMH-SI's copyrighted Physicians' Fees and Coding Guide.
SAL, scalp, arms, or legs; FCCMNAGHF, forehead, cheeks, chin, mouth, neck, axillae, genitalia, hands, or feet; ENEL, eyelids, nose, ears, or lips.

Patient Education Handout

A patient education handout, "Skin Flap Closures," can be found on the book's Web site.

Bibliography

Becker FF. Rhomboid flap in facial reconstruction: new concept of tension lines. *Arch Otolaryngol.* 1979;105(10):569–573.

Calhoun KH, Seikaly H, Quinn FB. Teaching paradigm for decision making in facial skin defect reconstructions. *Arch Otolaryngol Head Neck Surg.* 1998;124(1):60–66.

Chernosky ME. Scalpel and scissors surgery as seen by the dermatologist. In: Epstein E, Epstein E Jr, eds. *Skin Surgery*. 6th ed. Philadelphia: WB Saunders; 1987:88–127.

Connor CD, Fosko SW. Anatomy and physiology of local skin flaps. *Facial Plast Surg Clin North Am.* 1996;4:447–454.

Cook J. Introduction to facial flaps. *Dermatol Clin.* 2001;19:199–212.

Larrabee WF, Trachy R, Sutton D, et al. Rhomboid flap dynamics. *Arch Otolaryngol.* 1981;107(12):755–757.

Ling EH, Wang TD. Local flaps in forehead and temporal reconstruction. *Facial Plast Surg Clin North Am.* 1996;4:469.

Lober CW, Mendelsohn HE, Fenske NA. Rhomboid transposition flaps. *Aesthetic Plast Surg.* 1985;9(2):121–124.

Lister GD, Gibson T. Closure of rhomboid skin defects: the flaps of Limberg and Dufourmentel. *Br J Plast Surg.* 1972;25:300–314.

Stegman SJ. Fifteen ways to close surgical wounds. *J Dermatol Surg.* 1975;1:25–31.

Tollefson TT, Murakami CS, Kriet JD. Cheek repair. *Otolaryngol Clin North Am.* 2001;34:627–646.

Whitaker DC. Random-pattern flaps. In: Wheeland RG, ed. *Cutaneous Surgery*. Philadelphia: WB Saunders; 1994:329–352.

2008 MAG Mutual Healthcare Solutions, Inc.'s Physicians' Fee and Coding Guide. Duluth, Georgia. MAG Mutual Healthcare Solutions, Inc. 2007.

CHAPTER 54

Rotation Flap

E. J. Mayeaux, Jr., MD, DABFP, FAAFP

Professor of Family Medicine, Professor of Obstetrics and Gynecology
Louisiana State University Health Sciences Center, Shreveport, LA

Rotation flaps are local flaps that use adjacent tissue rotated in an arc to close skin defects. They are composed of skin and associated subcutaneous tissue devoid of segmental vessels. They ultimately rely on arterial perforators that course superficially to supply blood via the dermal and subdermal plexuses. Rotation flaps should be designed to place closure lines parallel to the lines of least skin tension (see Appendix B) and take advantage of adjacent areas of skin laxity or redundancy.

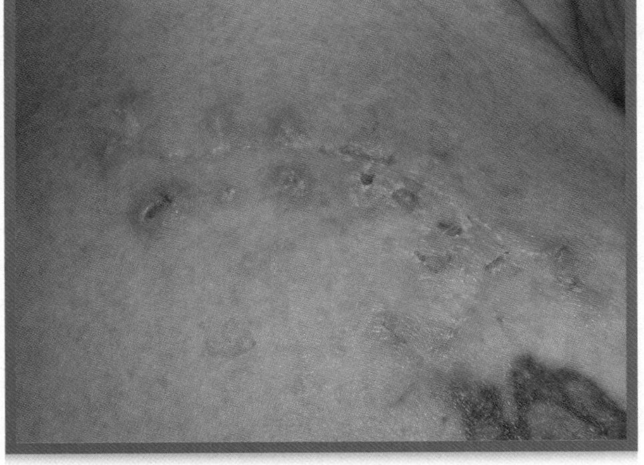

Rotation flaps provide the ability to recruit large areas of tissue with a wide vascular base for defect closure. This flap can be thought of as the closure of a triangular defect by rotating adjacent skin around a rotation point into the defect. The biggest advantage of these flaps over other flaps is that they have a particularly wide base and resulting excellent blood supply. Their primary disadvantage is that they require extensive cutting beyond the primary defect to develop the flap, increasing the length of the scar and the risk of nerve damage or bleeding.

Rotation flaps are well suited to closing defects on the nose, glabella, upper nasal dorsum, or nasolabial sulci. Small to midsize cheek defects can also easily be repaired using simple rotation flaps. Two simultaneous rotation flaps can be created when extra tissue is required. The bilateral rotation flap can be made with two mirror image rotation flaps that meet at the defect. This flap is similar to the A-to-T-plasty and the O-to-Z-plasty.

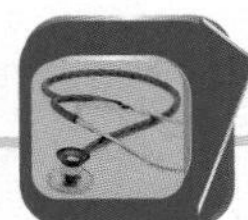

Equipment

- Surgical tray instruments are listed in Appendix G. Consider adding skin hooks to gently handle the skin flaps. Have at least three fine (mosquito) hemostats to assist with hemostasis while developing large skin flaps.
- Suggested suture removal times are listed in Appendix J, and a suggested anesthesia tray that can be used for this procedure is listed in Appendix F. All instruments can be ordered through local surgical supply houses.

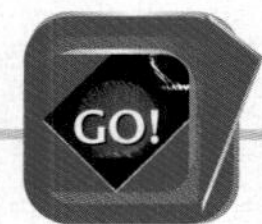

Indications

- Closure of skin defects that require minimum skin removal, or where skin may be under tension from a variety of directions.
- This flap work best for partial-thickness defects of the face, neck, and back.

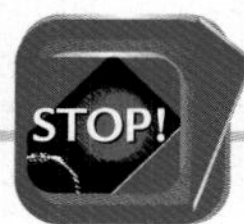

Contraindications (Relative)

- Areas with poor blood flow.
- Uncooperative patient.
- Wounds best closed by other methods.
- Presence of cellulitis, bacteremia, or active infection.
- Heavy smokers and insulin-dependent diabetics present an increased risk of complications.

The Procedure

Step 1. The rotation flap can be visualized as starting with an isosceles triangular defect to remove a lesion. The two sides of the triangle, which are equal in length, are longer than the third side, or defect base. This creates a narrow triangle with an acute angle opposite the defect's base. The long side of the triangle opposite the rotation flap will become one of the borders of the flap after defect closure.

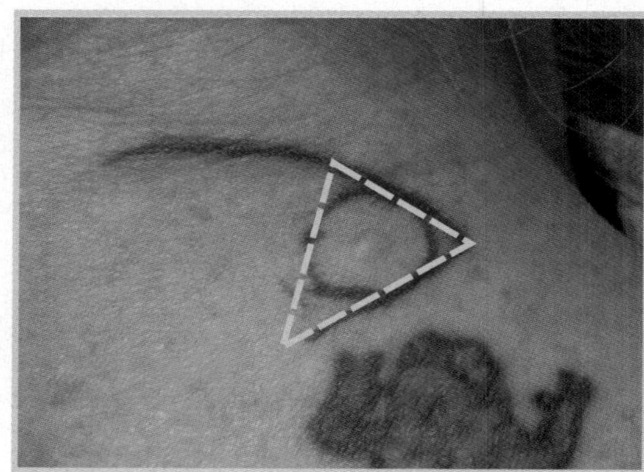

Step 1

Step 2. The base of the triangle is incorporated into a semicircular arc, which will be rotated to close the defect. Larger defects require more rotation from adjacent tissue. Generally, the length of the flap's border should be three to four times the length of the base of the triangle defect. Make the incision for the arc so that the final closure line is as parallel as possible to the lines of least skin tension and/or on an anatomic border.

- **PEARL:** The flap can always be enlarged if sufficient motion is not possible.

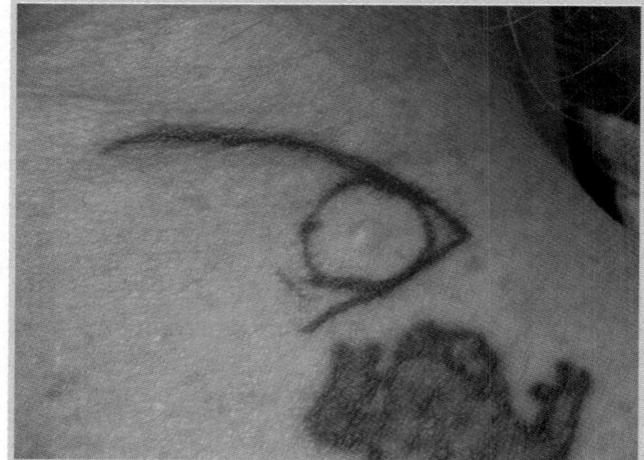

Step 2

Step 3. Perform a field block that extends well past the edges of the incisions and the entire flap. Prep the skin with povidone-iodine or chlorhexidine solution, and allow it to dry (see Appendix E: Skin Preparation Recommendations).

- **PEARL:** Prep a wide area so that an undraped area is not inadvertently exposed if the drape slides a little.

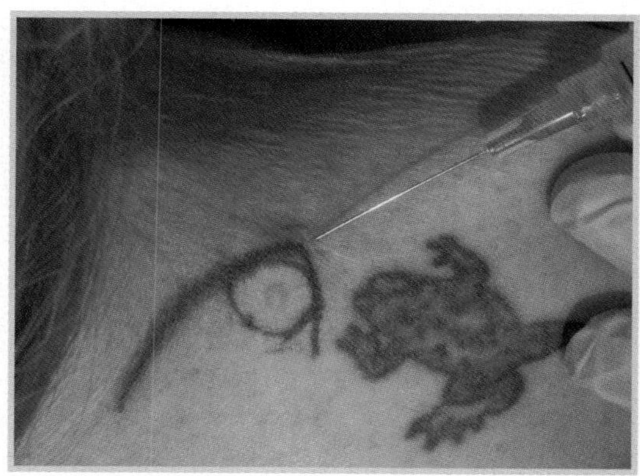

Step 3

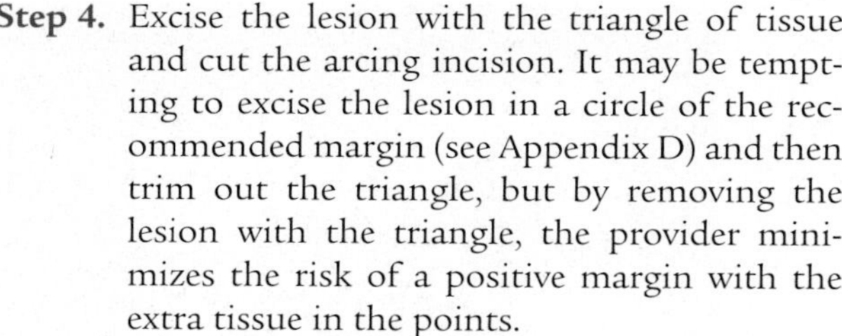

Step 4. Excise the lesion with the triangle of tissue and cut the arcing incision. It may be tempting to excise the lesion in a circle of the recommended margin (see Appendix D) and then trim out the triangle, but by removing the lesion with the triangle, the provider minimizes the risk of a positive margin with the extra tissue in the points.

- **PEARL:** Surgical defects are typically round. A larger round defect may be closed without the creation of a triangle defect by undermining the flap and cutting the point of the flap off in a curve to match the edge of the defect.

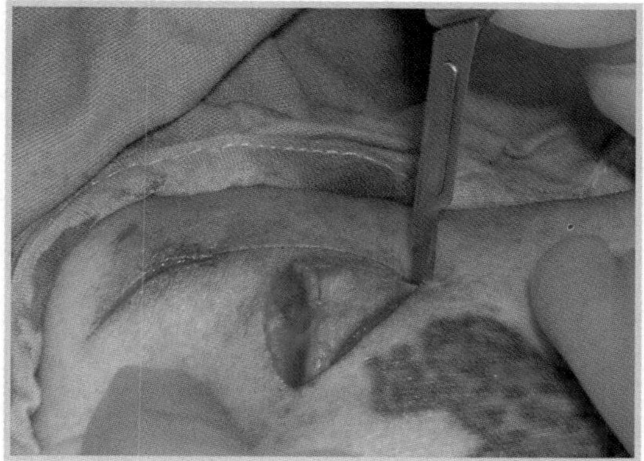

Step 4

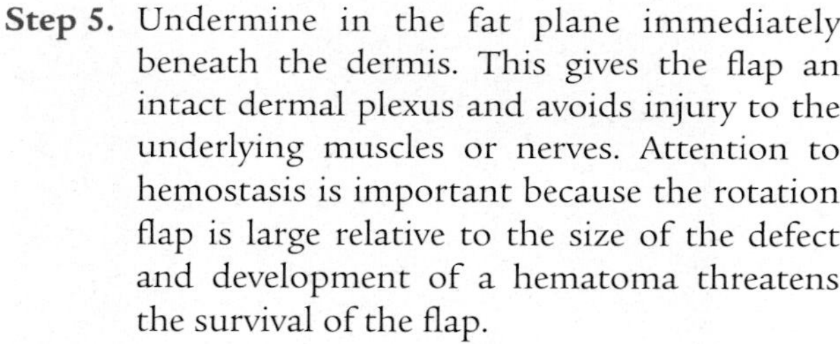

Step 5. Undermine in the fat plane immediately beneath the dermis. This gives the flap an intact dermal plexus and avoids injury to the underlying muscles or nerves. Attention to hemostasis is important because the rotation flap is large relative to the size of the defect and development of a hematoma threatens the survival of the flap.

- **PEARL:** The flap pedicle should be placed inferiorly so that gravity aids in lymphatic and venous drainage.

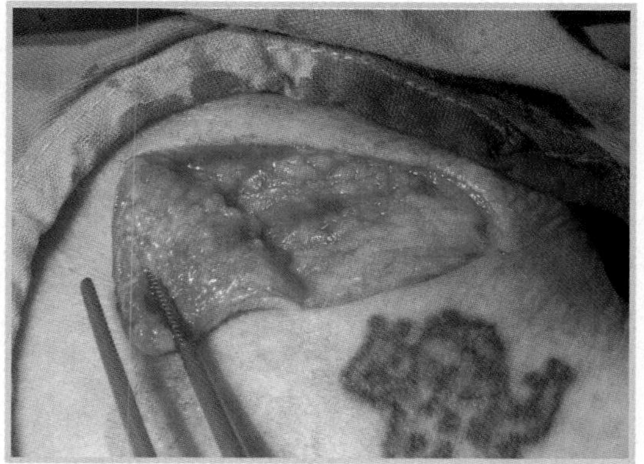

Step 5

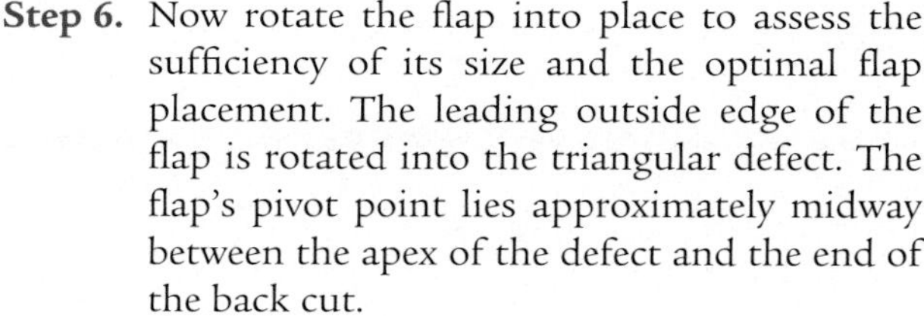

Step 6. Now rotate the flap into place to assess the sufficiency of its size and the optimal flap placement. The leading outside edge of the flap is rotated into the triangular defect. The flap's pivot point lies approximately midway between the apex of the defect and the end of the back cut.

- **PEARL:** A tacking suture (to be removed later) can be placed to assess flap motion and placement.

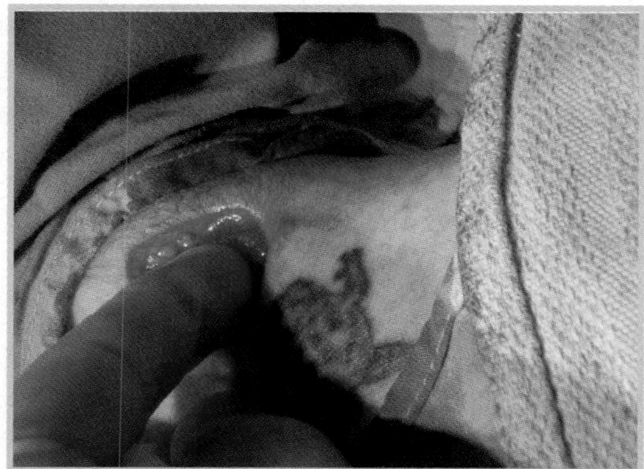

Step 6

Step 7. Place a corner suture to attach the tip of the flap to the corner of the defect. See Chapter 39.

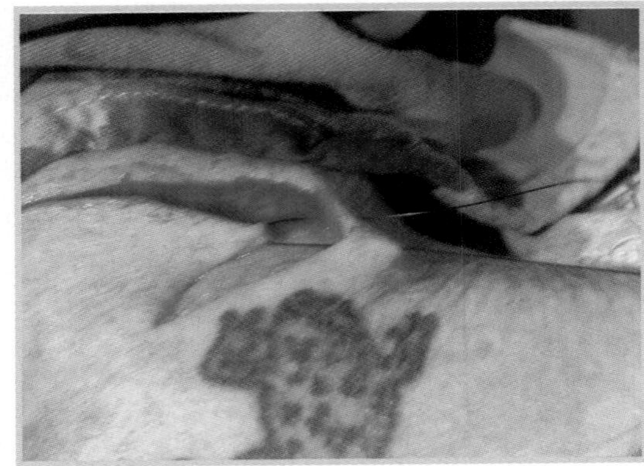

Step 7

Step 8. Use simple interrupted sutures to approximate the rest of the closure. See Chapter 38.

- **PEARL:** If tension is present in the flap, consider placing buried sutures to reduce the tension.

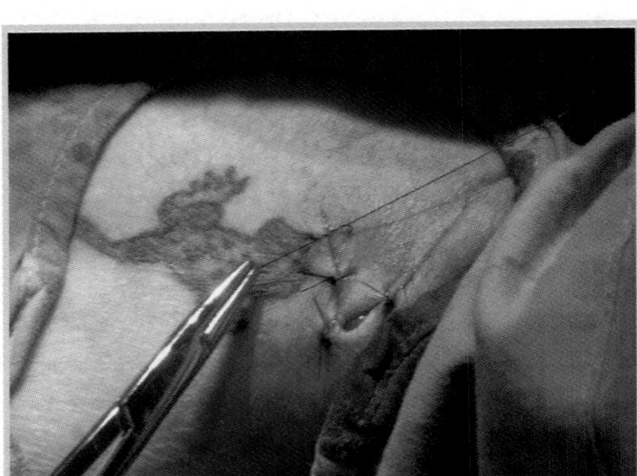

Step 8

Step 9. After rotation and suturing of tissue into the defect, a standing cone is often created at the distal end of the rotation flap. This deformity can often be managed with a Burow triangle repair (see Chapter 46). Apply antibacterial ointment and a pressure bandage.

- **PEARL:** Little mechanical benefit is gained in increasing flap length beyond a 90-degree arc. Increased undermining and increased arc radius gives small benefits on closing tension.
- **PITFALL:** The Burow triangle should not be taken into the pedicle of the flap itself because this diminishes the blood supply; rather, it should be moved away from the flap.

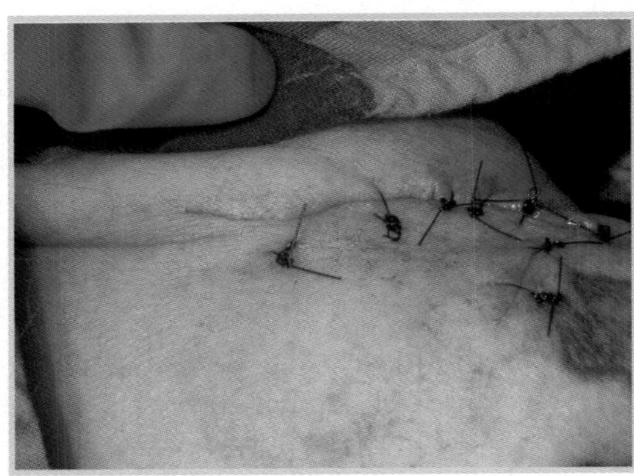

Step 9

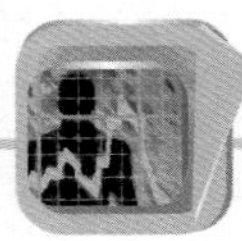

Complications

- Pain, infection, and bleeding
- Nonunion of skin edges
- Scar formation

- Tissue sloughing (usually due to excess tension or the blood supply being disrupted by undermining)
- Sensory changes (often subside with time)
- Flap necrosis and sloughing
- Distortion of neighboring landmarks

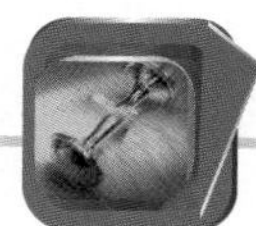

Pediatric Considerations

Generally, pediatric skin has excellent blood flow and heals very well. However, pediatric patients often find it difficult to sit or lie still during lengthy procedures. The patient's maturity and ability to cooperate should be considered before deciding to attempt any outpatient procedure.

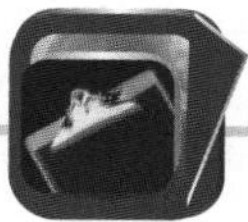

Postprocedure Instructions

Have the patient keep the bandage on and the wound dry for the first 24 hours. After that, it can be cleaned with hydrogen peroxide or gently washed with soap and water as needed. An antibiotic ointment and bandage should be reapplied until the patient returns or for 2 weeks. Have the patient report signs of infection. Schedule a return appointment for suture removal (see Appendix J).

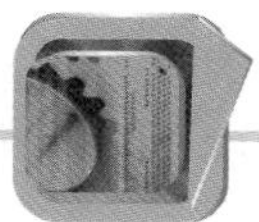

Coding Information

These codes encompass excision or repair, or both, by adjacent transfer or rearrangement, including Z-plasty, W-plasty, V-Y-plasty, rotation flaps, advancement flaps, and double-pedicle flaps. When applied to traumatic wounds, the defect must be developed by the surgeon because the closure requires it, and these codes should not be used for direct closure of a defect that incidentally results in the configuration of one of the flaps or plasties. If the configurations result incidentally from the laceration shape, closure should be reported using simple repair codes. All of the following codes are for adjacent tissue transfer or rearrangement, and they refer to defects in the trunk or the following sites: scalp, arms, or legs (SAL); forehead, cheeks, chin, mouth, neck, axillae, genitalia, hands, or feet (FCCMNAGHF); and eyelids, nose, ears, or lips (ENEL).

CPT Code	Description	2008 Average 50th Percentile Fee	Global Period
14000	Trunk ≤10 cm^2	$1,062.00	90
14001	Trunk 10.1–30.0 cm^2	$1,400.00	90
14020	SAL ≤10 cm^2	$1,222.00	90
14021	SAL 10.1–30.0^2	$1,684.00	90
14040	FCCMNAGHF ≤10 cm^2	$1,551.00	90
14041	FCCMNAGHF 10.1–30.0 cm^2	$1,757.00	90
14060	ENEL ≤10 cm^2	$1,841.00	90
14061	ENEL 10.1–30.0 cm^2	$2,254.00	90
14300	Any unusual or complicated area >30 cm^2	$2,749.00	90

CPT is a registered trademark of the American Medical Association.
2008 average 50th Percentile Fees are provided courtesy of 2008 MMH-SI's copyrighted Physicians' Fees and Coding Guide.
SAL, scalp, arms, or legs; FCCMNAGHF, forehead, cheeks, chin, mouth, neck, axillae, genitalia, hands, or feet; ENEL, eyelids, nose, ears, or lips.

Bibliography

Calhoun KH, Seikaly H, Quinn FB. Teaching paradigm for decision making in facial skin defect reconstructions. *Arch Otolaryngol Head Neck Surg.* 1998;124(1):60–66.

Cook TA, Israel JM, Wang TD, et al. Cervical rotation flaps for midface resurfacing. *Arch Otolaryngol Head Neck Surg.* 1991;117(1):77–82.

Green RK, Angelats J. A full nasal skin rotation flap for closure of soft-tissue defects in the lower one-third of the nose. *Plast Reconstr Surg.* 1996;98(1):163–166.

Jackson IT. Local flap reconstruction of defects after excision of nonmelanoma skin cancer. *Clin Plast Surg.* 1997;24(4):747–767.

Larrabee WF Jr, Sutton D. The biomechanics of advancement and rotation flaps. *Laryngoscope.* 1981;91(5):726–734.

Millman B, Klingensmith M. The island rotation flap: a better alternative for nasal tip repair. *Plast Reconstr Surg.* 1996;98(7):1293–1297.

Murtagh J. The rotation flap. *Aust Fam Physician.* 2001;30(10):973.

Myers B, Donovan W. The location of the blood supply in random flaps. *Plast Reconstr Surg.* 1976;58(3):314–316.

Patterson HC, Anonsen C, Weymuller EA, et al. The cheek-neck rotation flap for closure of temporozygomatic-cheek wounds. *Arch Otolaryngol.* 1984;110(6):388–393.

Schrudde J, Beinhoff U. Reconstruction of the face by means of the angle-rotation flap. *Aesthetic Plast Surg.* 1987;11(1):15–22.

Spector JG. Surgical management of cutaneous carcinomas at the inner canthus. *Laryngoscope.* 1985;95(5):601–607.

Whitaker DC. Random-pattern flaps. In: Wheeland RG, ed. *Cutaneous Surgery*. Philadelphia: WB Saunders; 1994.

2008 MAG Mutual Healthcare Solutions, Inc.'s Physicians' Fee and Coding Guide. Duluth, Georgia. MAG Mutual Healthcare Solutions, Inc. 2007.

CHAPTER 55

Scalp Repair Techniques

Robert W. Smith, MD, MBA, FAAFP
Vice Chair for Education, Department of Family Medicine
University of Pittsburgh School of Medicine, Pittsburgh, PA

E. J. Mayeaux, Jr., MD, DABFP, FAAFP
Professor of Family Medicine, Professor of Obstetrics and Gynecology
Louisiana State University Health Sciences Center, Shreveport, LA

Because the scalp contains one of the richest vascular supplies in the body, traumatic or surgical wounds there present special challenges for bleeding control. When scalp bleeding cannot be controlled with pressure, other emergent interventions must be applied often without sophisticated equipment. Scalp bleeding in the elderly can be especially brisk and life threatening. Two emergent field methods to control scalp bleeding and to approximate tissues are presented in this chapter: the hair-tying technique and the fishing line technique. A rapid hemostatic suture technique is described for management in controlled settings. These techniques are suitable for situations when hemostasis is immediately required.

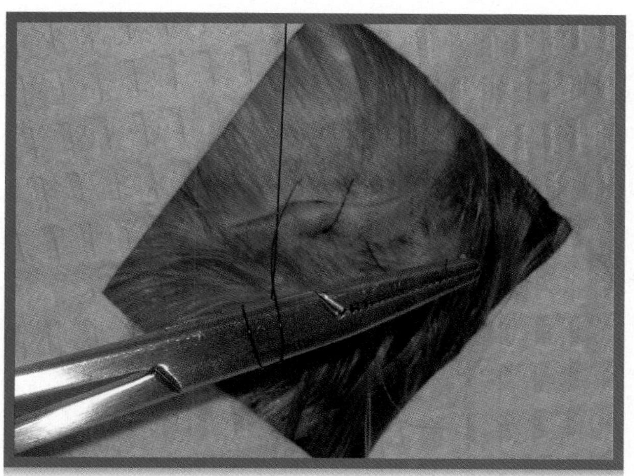

There are five layers to the scalp: the skin, subcutaneous tissue, musculoaponeurotic layer (i.e., galea), loose aponeurotic tissue, and periosteum. Hair roots are easily identified and must not be damaged when moving scalp wound edges. If undermining is required to close a wound, it should be performed close to the fat-galea junction, not near the lower dermis. Fibrous bands called *retinacula* in the subcutaneous layer provide support for blood vessels keeping them open when they are cut. This adds to the bleeding from scalp wounds.

A single layer closure can usually be performed in the office or emergency room setting as the deep scalp tissues often are adherent to the skin. Large needles and large-diameter suture materials (e.g., 3-0 Prolene with FS-1 cutting needle) are selected for use on the scalp as they grasp a greater amount of tissue and, when tied, firmly to assist in hemostasis. Excessive trimming of a macerated wound can create wider wounds and excessive tension.

Although many physicians have been instructed not to place crossing or “locking” stitches in skin, the scalp suturing technique demonstrated in this chapter involves placement of a skin suture that crosses. Although crossing sutures are appropriately avoided in many body locations to prevent avascular necrosis, the highly vascular scalp rarely experiences blood flow problems and necessitates a reliable hemostatic suture.

The musculoaponeurotic layer contains muscle between two facial layers in the forehead and occipital regions. The muscle is absent on the top of the head, and the two fascial layers fuse into the fibrous sheet known as the galea. The space beneath the galea is known as the danger space as hematomas or infections can accumulate beneath the galea. Anesthesia is always administered above the galea because the nerves are superficial to it, hematomas (and abscess) can be avoided and the fluid will not dissect to other areas such as the periorbital tissues as it would if it were injected more deeply.

If defects are found in the galea, they should be closed with interrupted absorbable sutures to prevent wounds with retracted skin edges and larger, thicker final scars. Tissue loss in the galea may require special intervention, because closure is difficult without scoring the surrounding galea. This will provide some stretch to help cover the defect. Pressure bandages or drains can be used to minimize subgaleal fluid accumulation.

It is not recommended to remove hair when performing scalp repair. Shaving the scalp is associated with higher skin infection rates, and patients often are unhappy with the short term cosmesis. Hair can be taped away from a wound or tincture of benzoin can be used to chemically hold hair away from a surgical site.

Although tissue glues are valuable on many areas of the body, they are more difficult to utilize and may not often provide adequate hemostasis on the scalp for larger wounds. Smaller wounds, however, can be managed by the hair apposition technique (HAT). One study demonstrated good cosmetic and functional outcomes with scalp closure using tissue glue in association with this technique. The sides of the wound are brought together using a single twist of hair and the hair was secured with the glue. The study demonstrated superior patient acceptance and less scarring with this closure technique.

When performing elective procedures on the scalp (e.g., biopsy), 2% Lidocaine with epinephrine should be utilized for anesthesia. This will control bleeding and providing adequate anesthesia for the entire procedure.

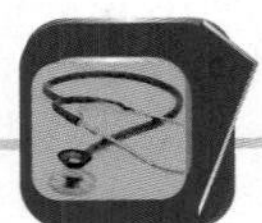

Equipment

- The standard instruments used for office surgery are also used for scalp repair techniques (see Appendix G).
- Suggested suture removal times are listed in Appendix J.
- A suggested anesthesia tray that can be used for this procedure is listed in Appendix F.
- Skin preparation recommendations appear in Appendix E: Skin Preparation Recommendations.
- Large sutures with large needles should be available
- For field use, a large bore needle, fishing line, hairspray and epoxy can be utilized.

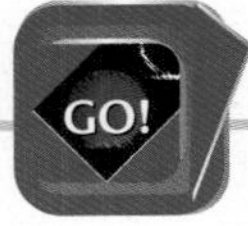

Indications

- Scalp lacerations
- Surgical wounds of the scalp

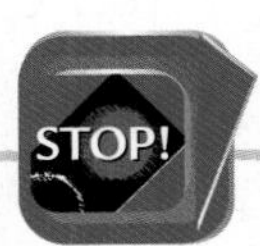

Contraindications

- Patient with other conditions of greater life threat that require stabilization
- Suspicion of underlying skull fracture
- Evidence of foreign body in the wound which cannot be removed

The Procedure

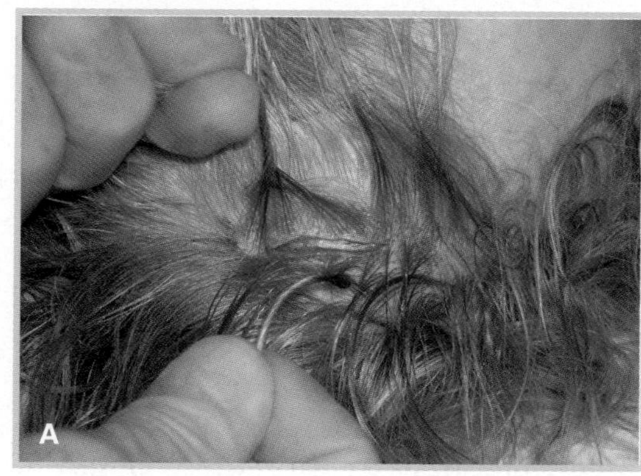

Step 1. On-field First Aid can be performed for bleeding scalp wounds by twisting nearby hair and then tying the hair over the top of the wound. If a spectator or observer has hair spray, vigorously spray the tied hair to maintain the knot until arrival at a medical facility.

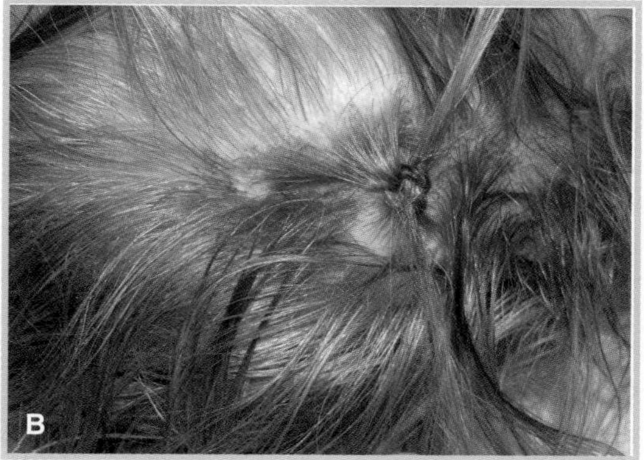

Step 1

Step 2. Keep a large hypodermic needle in the tackle box. If a laceration occurs in the field, the needle can be threaded through both wound edges.

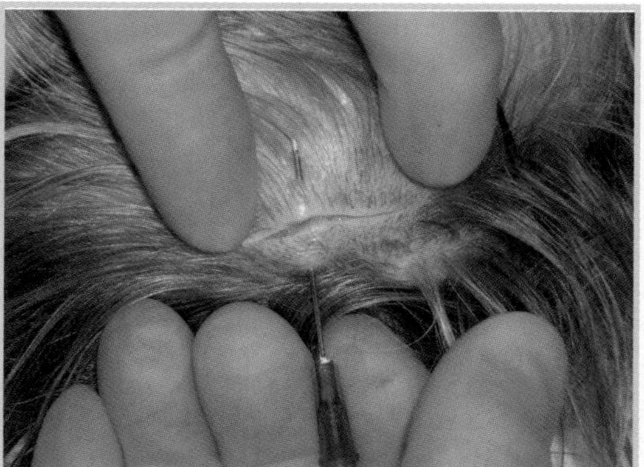

Step 2

Step 3. Fishing line can then be threaded through the needle.

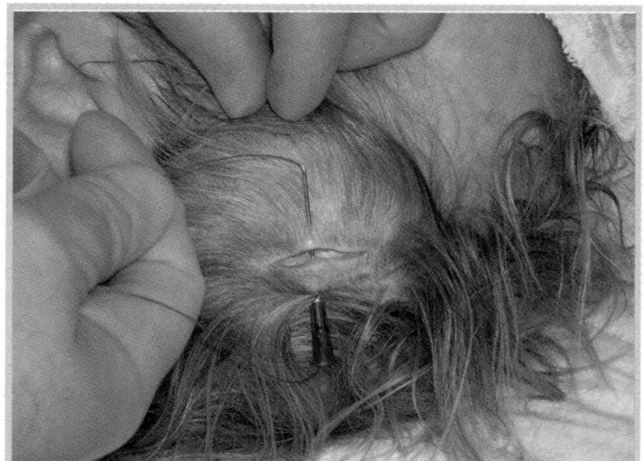

Step 3

Step 4. The needle is withdrawn with the line remaining within both wound edges.

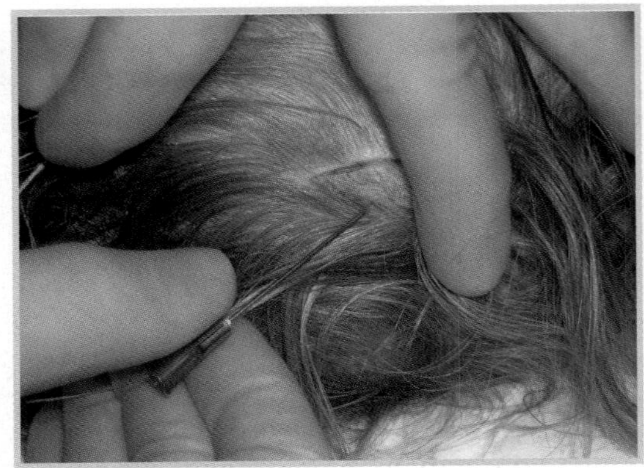

Step 4

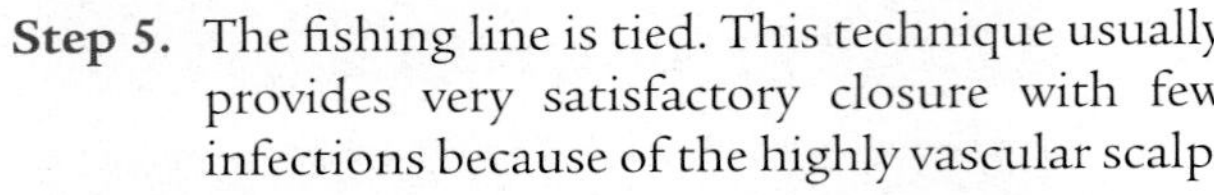

Step 5. The fishing line is tied. This technique usually provides very satisfactory closure with few infections because of the highly vascular scalp.

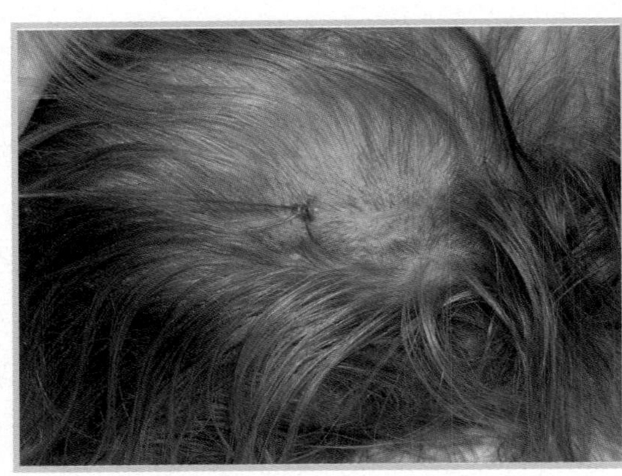

Step 5

Step 6. When giving anesthesia before repair of a scalp laceration, it is often less painful to inject through the laceration than doing a field block through uninjured skin.

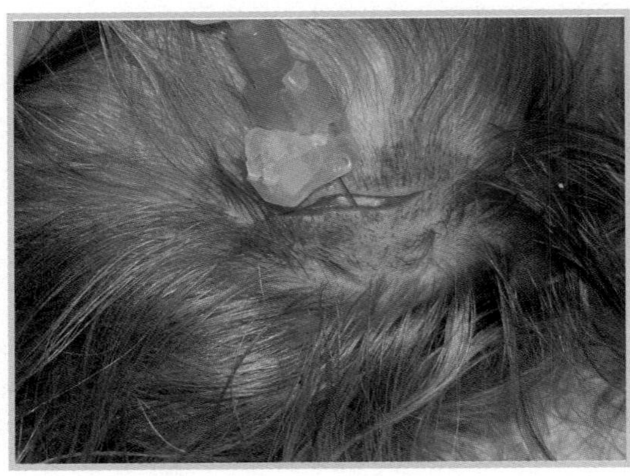

Step 6

Step 7. Closure of a galeal defect in the base of a scalp wound is achieved with a figure-of-eight pattern using absorbable suture (see next steps). If there is tissue loss of the galea, consider scoring the galea to provide relaxation.

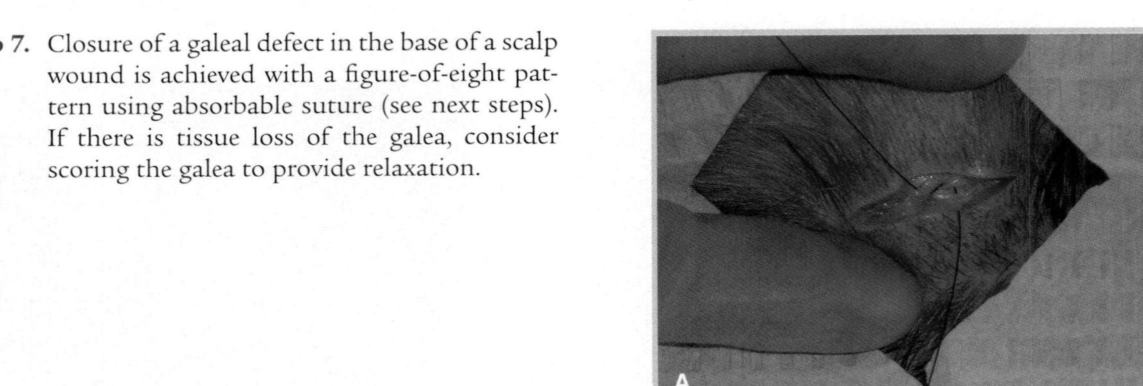

- **PITFALL:** When scoring the galea is required, the work is often done under sterile conditions.

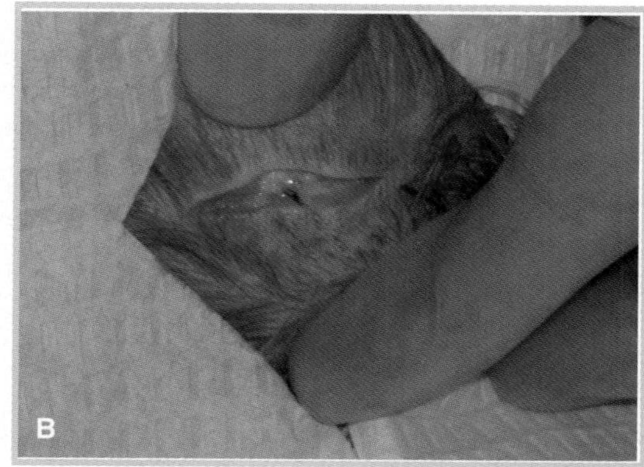

Step 7

Step 8. The hemostatic scalp suture is a simple, figure-of-eight closure. The suture is passed from the right side of the wound to the left side but not tied.

- **PEARL:** A smaller 4-0 nylon suture may be more appropriate in children.
- **PEARL:** Ensuring that the wound is clear of all debris will reduce complications in the post procedure period.

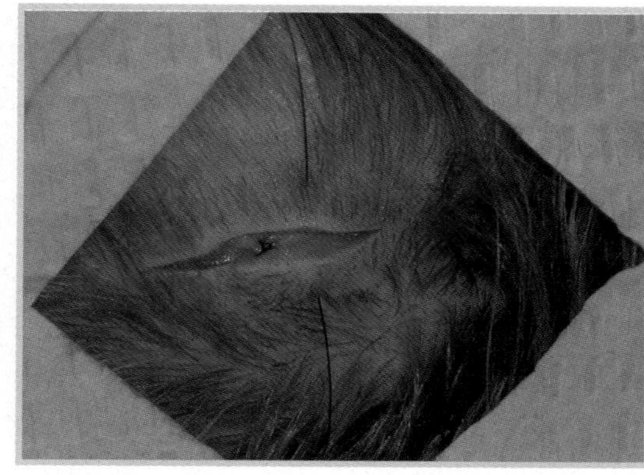

Step 8

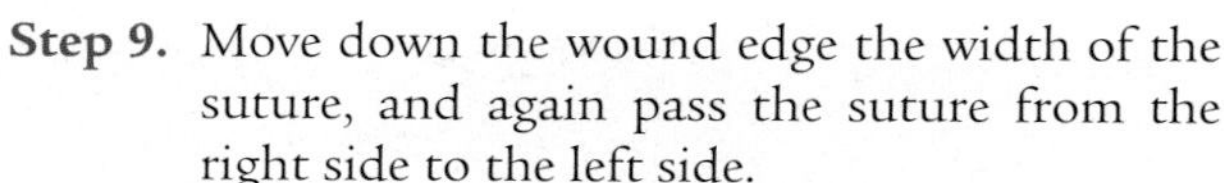

Step 9. Move down the wound edge the width of the suture, and again pass the suture from the right side to the left side.

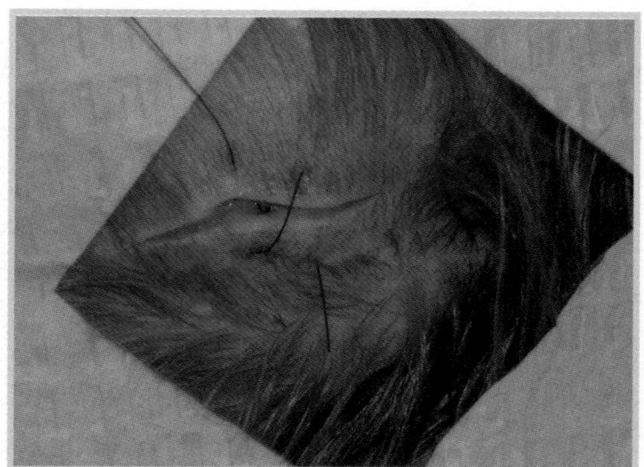

Step 9

Step 10. Tie the suture, with the suture strings crossing over the top of the wound in an X-shape configuration.

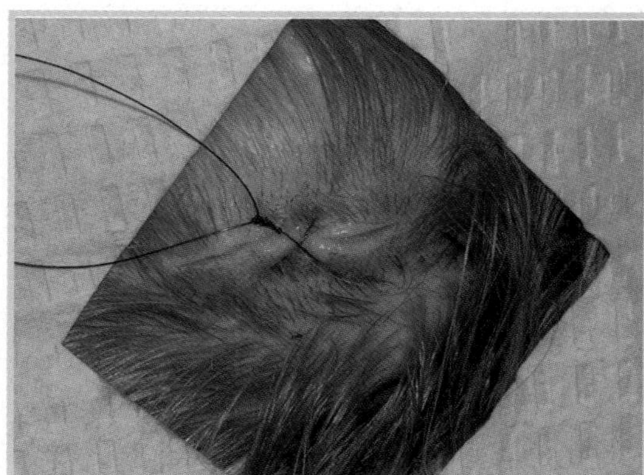

Step 10

Step 11. If the clinician does not like the suture crossing over the top of the wound, the suture can be made to cross beneath the surface. Pass from the right side of the wound to far down the left side of the wound. Do not tie the suture ends.

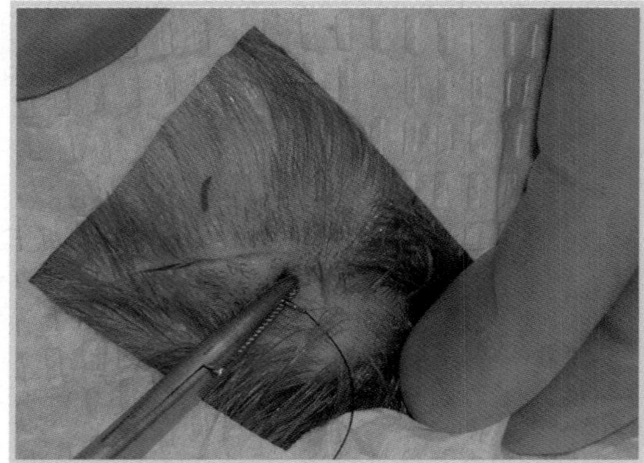

Step 11

Step 12. Then pass from far down the right side of the wound to the near point on the left side.

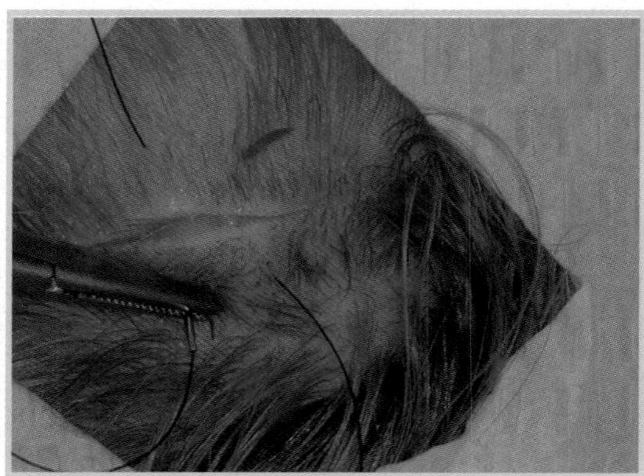

Step 12

Step 13. The suture should exit the skin on the left side across from where it first entered on the right side. Tie the suture, with the crossing of the suture threads beneath the wound.

- **PEARL:** A pressure bandage can be placed to reduce the likelihood of hematoma.
- **PEARL:** Cleansing blood and debris from the surrounding hair at the time of the procedure will make the patient less likely to want to wash his or her hair immediately upon going home.

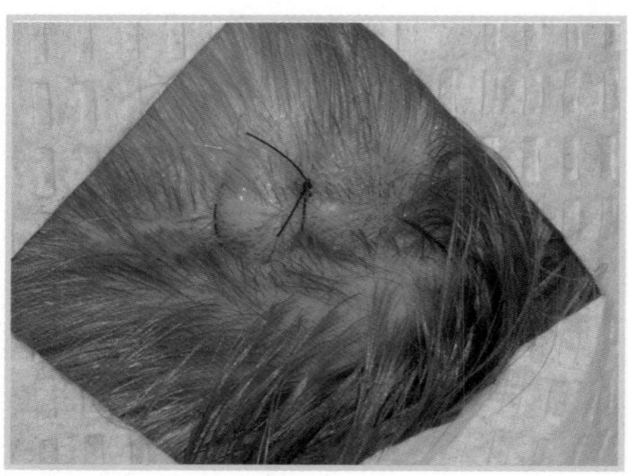

Step 13

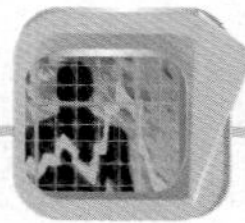

Complications

- Excessive bleeding
- Infection
- Abscess (rare)
- Scarring
- Permanent hair loss

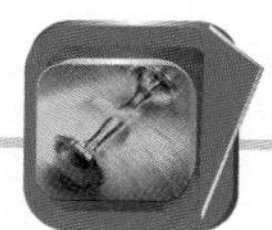

Pediatric Considerations

Assure the parent or guardian that there are appropriate numbers of personnel available to safely hold the child while the intervention is taking place. Do not attempt to suture the scalp while dealing with a "moving target" or close approximation will not take place and a more significant scar will occur. Proper approximation at the right level requires direct visualization of layers. A smaller 4-0 nylon suture may be more appropriate in children.

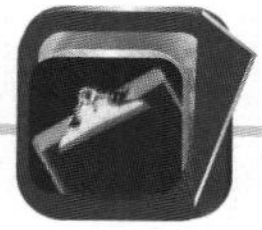

Postprocedure instructions

Routine instructions on follow-up for signs of significant head injury should be given to the patient and/or parent. The patient should not get the wound wet for at least 48 hours, as this will increase the likelihood of macerated wound edges and infection. Beyond that, every effort must be made to keep the wound dry.

Suture removal should be scheduled in 7 days for most scalp repairs.

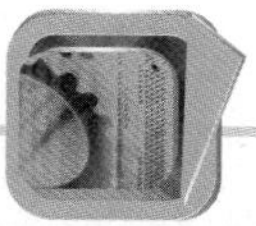

Coding Information and Supply Sources

CPT Code	Description	2008 Average 50th Percentile Fee	Global Period
12001	Simple repair SNAGTEHF ≤2.5 cm	$220.00	10
12002	Simple repair SNAGTEHF 2.6–7.5 cm	$235.00	10
12004	Simple repair SNAGTEHF 7.6–12.5 cm	$285.00	10
12005	Simple repair SNAGTEHF 12.6–20.0 cm	$408.00	10
12006	Simple repair SNAGTEHF 20.1–30.0 cm	$506.00	10
12007	Simple repair SNAGTEHF >30.0 cm		10
12011	Simple repair FEENLMM ≤2.5 cm	$240.00	10
12013	Simple repair FEENLMM 2.6–5.0 cm	$288.00	10
12014	Simple repair FEENLMM 5.1–7.5 cm	$351.00	10
12015	Simple repair FEENLMM 7.6–12.5 cm	$449.00	10
12016	Simple repair FEENLMM 12.6–20.0 cm	$585.00	10
12017	Simple repair FEENLMM 20.1–30.0 cm	$743.00	10
12018	Simple repair FEENLMM >30.0 cm		10
12020	Tmt. of superficial wound dehiscence, simple closure	$397.00	10

Patient Education Handout

A patient education handout, "Scalp Laceration Repair," can be found on the book's Web site.

Bibliography

Alexander JW, Fischer JE, Boyajian M, et al. The influence of hair-removal methods on wound infections. *Arch Surg.* 1983;118:347–352.

Bennett RG. *Fundamentals of Cutaneous Surgery*. St. Louis: CV Mosby; 1988:113–115.
Bernstein G. The far-near/near-far suture. *J Dermatol Surg Oncol.* 1985;11:470.
Brown JS. *Minor Surgery: A Text and Atlas*, 3rd ed. London: Chapman & Hall; 1997:76–77.
Davies MJ. Scalp wounds. An alternative to suture. *Injury.* 1988;19:375–376.
Frechet P. Minimal scars for scalp surgery. *Dermatol Surg.* 2007;33(1):45–55.
Howell JM, Morgan JA. Scalp laceration repair without prior hair removal. *Am J Emerg Med.* 1988;6:7–10.
Hock MO, Ooi SB, Saw SM, et al. A randomized controlled trial comparing the hair apposition technique with tissue glue to standard suturing in scalp lacerations (HAT study). *Ann Emerg Med.* 2002;40:19–26.
Stegman SJ, Tromovitch TA, Glogau RG. *Basics of Dermatologic Surgery*. Chicago: Year Book Medical Publishing; 1982:62.
Wardrope J, Smith JAR. *The Management of Wounds and Burns*. Oxford: Oxford University Press, 1992:162–163.
Zuber TJ. *The Illustrated Manuals and Videotapes of Soft-tissue Surgery Techniques*. Kansas City: American Academy of Family Physicians; 1998.
Zukin DD, Simon RR. *Emergency Wound Care: Principles and Practice*. Rockville, MD: Aspen Publishers; 1987:77–79.
2008 MAG Mutual Healthcare Solutions, Inc.'s Physicians' Fee and Coding Guide. Duluth, Georgia. MAG Mutual Healthcare Solutions, Inc. 2007.

CHAPTER 56

Skin Tag Removal

E. J. Mayeaux, Jr., MD, DABFP, FAAFP

Professor of Family Medicine, Professor of Obstetrics and Gynecology
Louisiana State University Health Sciences Center, Shreveport, LA

Skin tags, or acrochordons, are 1- to 2-mm skin growths commonly encountered on the neck, axilla, groin, or inframammary areas. The lesions develop on skin surfaces that rub together or that chronically rub against clothing. Skin tags are histologically classified as fibromas, with hyperplastic epidermis connected to the skin on a connective tissue stalk. At least one fourth of all adults exhibit skin tags, with one half of these occurring in the axilla. The lesions usually begin as tiny, flesh-colored or light brown excrescences. As the lesions enlarge, they can rub on clothing and commonly develop added pigmentation. Not all polypoid lesions are skin tags; nevi, angiomas, and even melanomas can appear polypoid.

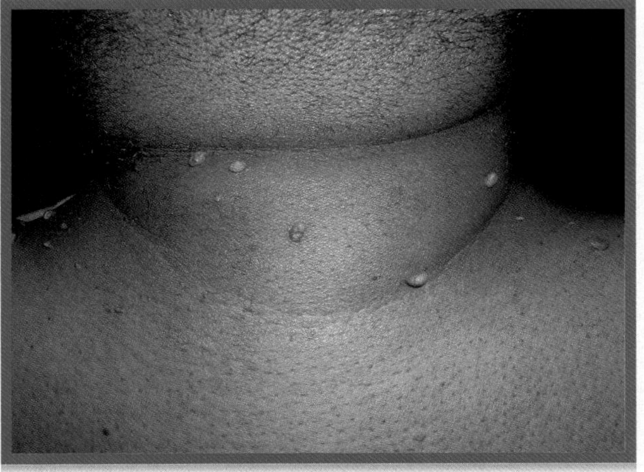

Skin tags increase in frequency from the second to fifth decade but generally do not increase significantly in number until after 50 years of age. There is a familial tendency for development of skin tags. Perianal skin tags may be associated with Crohn disease. Skin tags also may increase during the second trimester of pregnancy and may regress during the postpartum period. An association with type 2 diabetes mellitus also has been observed. Skin tags in adults historically have been associated with the presence of adenomatous colonic polyps, but studies in the primary care setting have failed to confirm such an association.

Fibroepitheliomatous polyps are larger, similar lesions commonly found on the trunk, eyelids, neck, and perineum. Fibroepitheliomatous polyps often have a baglike end on a narrow stalk and can grow quite large. Both acrochordons and fibroepitheliomatous polyps can be easily removed with the office techniques described here. Commonly used options for removal of skin tags include scissoring, sharp excision, ligature strangulation, electrosurgical destruction, or a combination of treatment modalities, including chemical or electrocauterization of the wound. These methods may employ local anesthesia, especially if the lesion is broad-based.

Electrosurgical excision is commonly employed for skin tags. The technique is hemostatic and is beneficial for removal of lesions, especially in noncosmetic areas (e.g., groin, axilla) or on the eyelids, where chemical hemostatic agents usually are avoided. The downside of electrosurgery for skin tags is the time required for equipment setup, the odor created during the procedure, and the need for anesthesia when using this technique. Cryosurgery avoids the need for anesthesia. However, the time required to perform cryosurgical destruction is greater than with other methods, and this method may be more painful.

Scissor excision is considered by many authorities to be the optimal removal technique for skin tags. Most small tags can be removed without the need for anesthesia, and scissor removal permits rapid removal of numerous lesions. It is not uncommon to remove 100 or more lesions at a single session, although some insurance companies cap payment at 45 to 65 tags per session. Because residual scarring depends on the depth of dermal injury, scarring can be minimized with scissor removal. Histologic assessment is offered to patients but may not be necessary if the experienced clinician removes small, characteristic tags. Application of antibiotic ointment usually promotes rapid (moist) healing of the site.

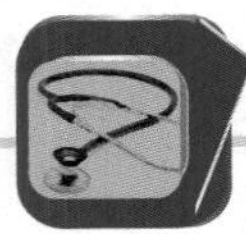

Equipment

- Required instruments depend on method selected for removal. If scissors removal is chosen, a pair of new, sharp, curved iris scissors should be available. If cryosurgery or electrosurgical excision is performed, see Chapters 24 and 34 for descriptions of the needed equipment. Skin preparation recommendations appear in Appendix E.

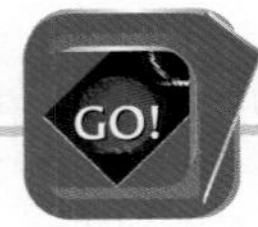

Indications

- Removal of superficial, polypoid growths on characteristic surfaces of the neck, groin, and eyelids

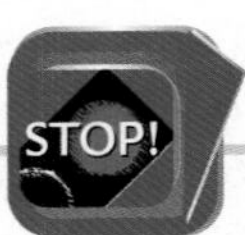

Contraindications

- Pigmented skin lesions (especially flat lesions) generally should not be destroyed because of the possibility of the lesion being a melanoma. If there is any concern about an unusual appearance of a lesion or confusion about whether a lesion is a skin tag, the lesion should have a full-thickness biopsy and histologic assessment.
- Fibroepitheliomas (often called large skin tags) often have a larger arterial supply that will require bleeding control and possibly suture closure.

The Procedure

Scissors Removal

Step 1. Most lesions can be rapidly removed without anesthetic. A simple anesthesia is chilling the skin with an ice cube before excising the lesion. The ice cube can be advanced to the next lesion while cutting the current lesion for efficient removal of multiple lesions.

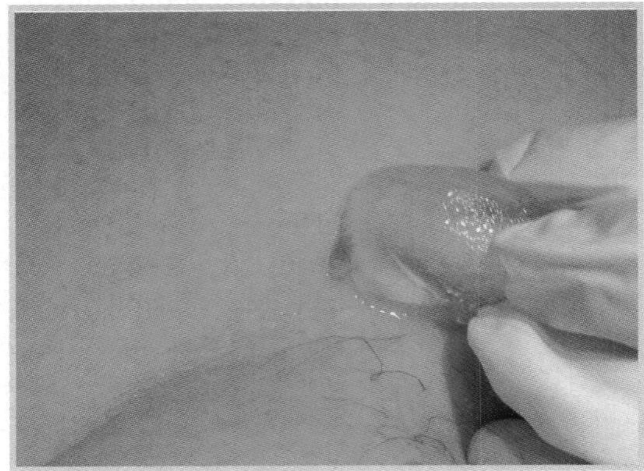

Step 1

Alternatively, when lesions are large or have a wide base (>2 mm), consider administering lidocaine cream or a small bleb of 1% lidocaine with epinephrine beneath the lesion.

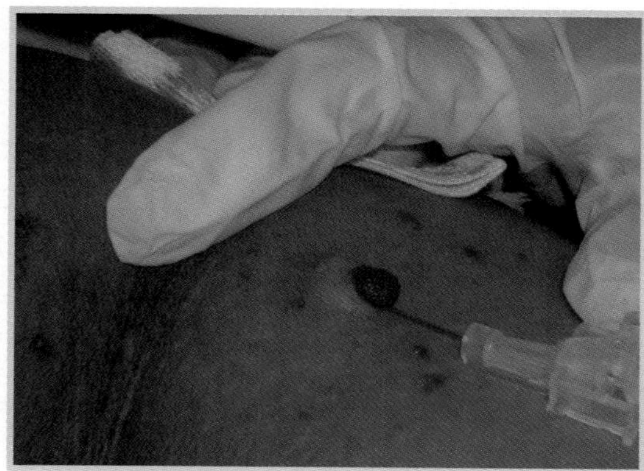

Picture courtesy of Dr. Jeff German.

Figure 1

Step 2. Use the nondominant hand to stretch skin to allow quicker removal with less pain. The nondominant thumb and index finger should forcefully stretch the skin surface to provide countertraction and to stretch pain fibers.

- PITFALL: It is easier to remove tags that are elevated with forceps. However, forceps pull up normal tissue beneath the tag, producing more scarring because of the deeper dermal injury. Dark-skinned individuals develop much more hypopigmentation and even keloid formation at skin tag removal sites when forceps are used. Avoid the use of forceps and learn to elevate the lesions in the blades of the scissors.

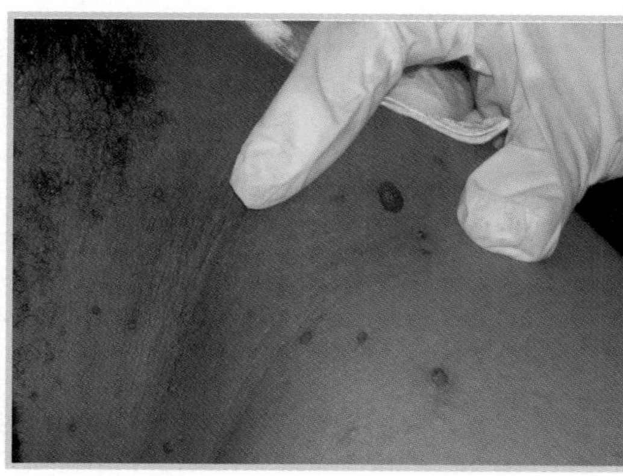

Step 2

Step 3. Use sharp, new, iris scissors. The tips of iris scissors are not best for cutting. Place the lesion into the blades of the scissors, at least one fourth of the way back from the tips. Wedge the closing blades of the scissors beneath the lesion, making sure no surrounding skin is caught between the blades.

- PITFALL: Straight iris scissors are often preferred by experienced clinicians, but may inadvertently pull surrounding tissue into the blades of the scissors. Curved iris scissors are easier to use for novice practitioners and may minimize the risk of removing excessive tissue.

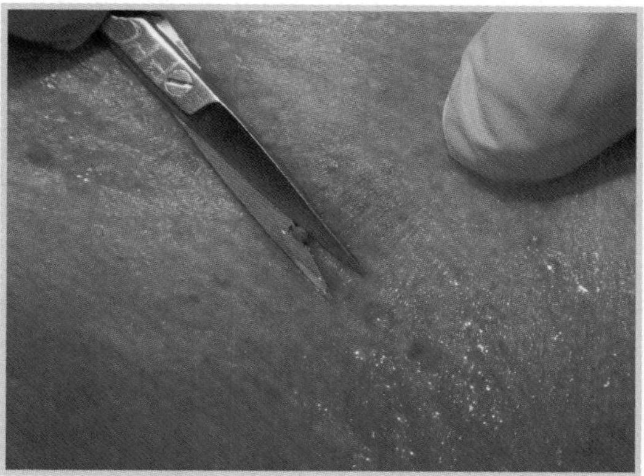

Step 3

Step 4. Rapidly cut the skin tag free. Apply Monsel solution (i.e., ferric subsulfate) or aluminum chloride solution to the wound base for hemostasis.

- PEARL: Talk to the patient during the procedure because "verbal anesthesia" usually helps. For instance, tell the patient to take a deep breath as the skin tag is cut.
- PEARL: Silver nitrate provides good hemostasis in this setting but runs the risk of depositing black silver salts under the skin (tattooing), which may later be confused as a developing melanoma.

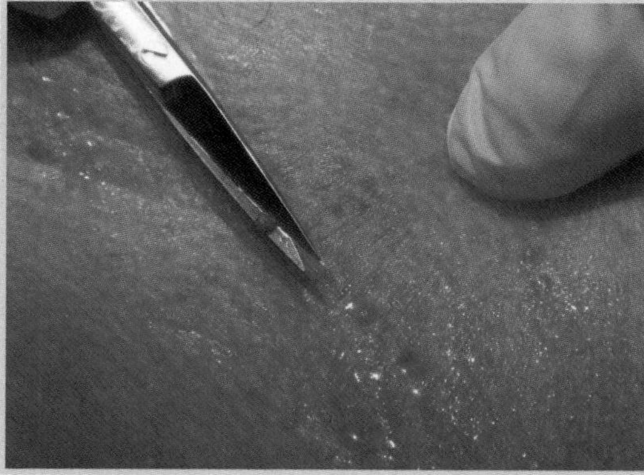

Step 4

Electrosurgical Removal

Step 1. Alternatively, the base of the lesion can be anesthetized, and an electrosurgical loop is placed over the lesion. Grasp the lesion with forceps, apply current to the loop, and pass the loop through the base of the lesion. Feather the base if any of the lesion remains. See Chapter 34.

- **PITFALL:** Avoid full-thickness or deep cuts or burns, because greater scarring is produced.

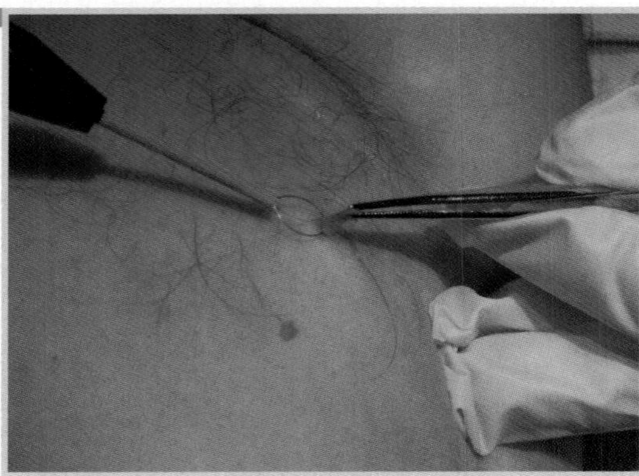

Step 1

Cryosurgical Removal

Step 1. Alternatively, the skin tag may be frozen. Pour liquid nitrogen into a disposable polystyrene cup. Cover the handle of the forceps with a folded 4×4-inch gauze to protect the fingers. Then dip the forceps into the liquid nitrogen until it becomes frosted. Pinch the lesion between the tips of the cold forceps until it turns frosty white. Keep the forceps on for an additional 15 seconds and repeat the process.

- **PEARL:** Benign lesions will fall off within 1 week and usually heal without problems.
- **PITFALL:** This method is slow and primarily used when only a few lesions are present.

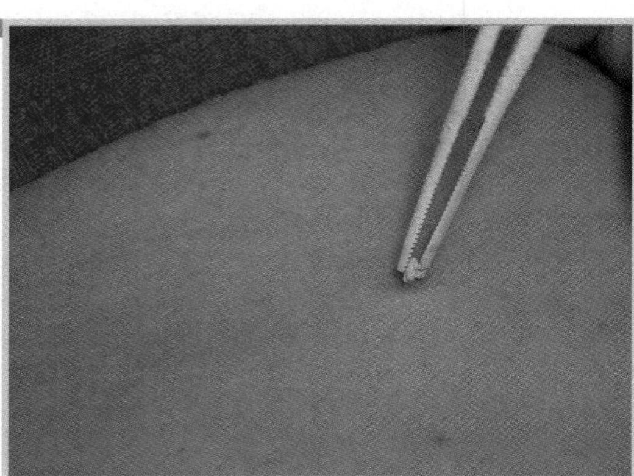

Picture courtesy of Dr. Russell Roberts.

Step 1

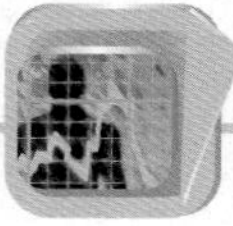

Complications

- Bleeding
- Infection
- Scarring

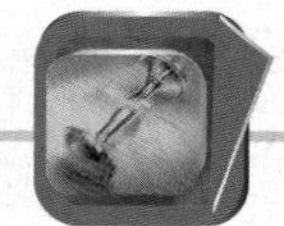

Pediatric Considerations

Skin tags are rare in childhood and, when found, may indicate the presence of other disorders such as nevoid basal cell carcinoma syndrome. Generally, pediatric skin has excellent blood flow and heals very well. However, pediatric patients often find it difficult to sit or lie still during even mildly painful procedures. The patient's maturity and ability to cooperate should be considered before deciding to attempt any outpatient procedure.

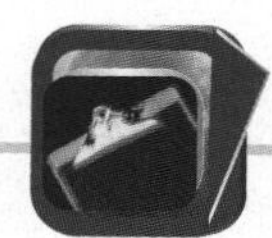

Postprocedure Instructions

Instruct the patient to gently wash the area the next day. Have the patient clean and dry the area well after washing, and use a small amount of antibiotic ointment to promote moist healing.

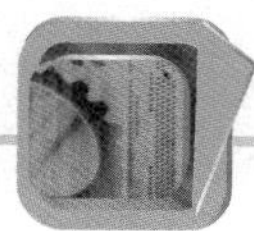

Coding Information and Supply Sources

CPT Code	Description	2008 Average 50th Percentile Fee	Global Period
11200	Removal (any method) of up to 15 multiple tags, any area	$126.00	10
11201	Removal of each additional 10 lesions (list separately)	$61.00	10

2008 average 50th Percentile Fees are provided courtesy of 2008 MMH-SI's copyrighted Physicians' Fees and Coding Guide.

Patient Education Handout

A patient education handout, "Skin Tags," can be found on the book's companion Web site,

Bibliography

Bennett RG. *Fundamentals of Cutaneous Surgery.* St. Louis: Mosby; 1988:692.

Chiritescu E, Maloney ME. Acrochordons as a presenting sign of nevoid basal cell carcinoma syndrome. *J Am Acad Dermatol.* 2001;44:789–794.

Coleman WP, Hanke CW, Alt TH, et al. *Cosmetic Surgery of the Skin: Principles and Techniques.* St. Louis: Mosby; 1997.

Habif TP. *Clinical Dermatology: A Color Guide to Diagnosis and Therapy.* 3rd ed. St. Louis: Mosby; 1996.

Kuwahara RT, Huber JD, Ray SH. Surgical pearl: forceps method for freezing benign lesions. *J Am Acad Dermatol.* 2000;43:306–307.

Kwan TH, Mihm MC. The skin. In: Robbins SL, Cotran RS, eds. *Pathologic Basis of Disease.* 2nd ed. Philadelphia: WB Saunders; 1979:1417–1461.

Parry EL. Management of epidermal tumors. In: Wheeland RG, ed. *Cutaneous Surgery.* Philadelphia: WB Saunders; 1994:683–687.

Usatine RP, Moy RL, Tobnick EL, et al. *Skin Surgery: A Practical Guide.* St. Louis: Mosby; 1998.

Zuber TJ. The illustrated manuals and videotapes of soft-tissue surgery techniques. Kansas City: American Academy of Family Physicians; 1998.

2008 MAG Mutual Healthcare Solutions, Inc.'s Physicians' Fee and Coding Guide. Duluth, Georgia. MAG Mutual Healthcare Solutions, Inc. 2007.

CHAPTER 57

Shave Biopsy

E. J. Mayeaux, Jr., MD, DABFP, FAAFP

Professor of Family Medicine, Professor of Obstetrics and Gynecology
Louisiana State University Health Sciences Center, Shreveport, LA

Shave biopsy is one of the most widely used procedures performed in primary care practice. The technique is used to obtain tissue for histologic examination and is useful for removing superficial lesions in their entirety. Pedunculated lesions above the skin surface are particularly well suited for this removal technique, but flat lesions that are high in the dermis and do not extend beneath the dermis also can be removed by shave technique. Horizontal slicing is performed at the level of the dermis, avoiding injury to the subcutaneous tissues. Cosmetic results generally are good, with the least noticeable scars occurring when lesions are removed from concave surfaces such as the nasolabial fold.

Four techniques are commonly employed for shave biopsy. A no. 15 scalpel blade held horizontally in the hand can provide good control of depth. The ease of the scalpel technique makes it a frequent choice of inexperienced physicians. Horizontal slicing with a flexed razor blade is a time-honored method for shave biopsy. This technique is used less frequently because of the potential for injury from the large, exposed cutting surface. Scissors (e.g., iris scissors) can be effectively used to remove elevated lesions. Scissors removal of flat lesions can be more difficult. Radiosurgical loop removal is effective, although novice practitioners tend to create deeper, "scoop" defects in the dermis beneath the lesion being removed.

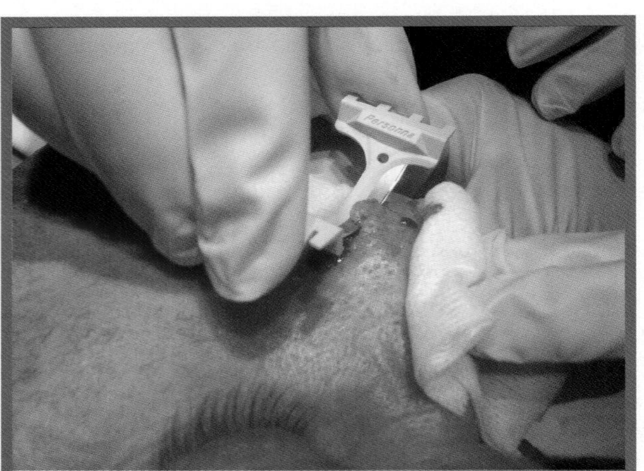

Shave biopsy is performed deep enough to remove the lesion but shallow enough to prevent significant damage to the deep dermis. The deeper the damage in the skin, the more likely scar formation will leave a noticeable, hypopigmented scar. If a scoop defect is created, the edges can be feathered (i.e., smoothed) to blend the color change into the surrounding skin (see Chapter 20). Depressed scars can result after this technique, especially from areas where there is extensive muscle tension on the skin, such as the chin or perioral areas.

Many physicians recommend not performing shave biopsy on pigmented lesions. If a lesion should turn out to be a melanoma on biopsy, using a technique that cuts through the middle of the lesion can create major problems for determining depth, prognosis, and therapy for the lesion. Some clinicians argue that the shave technique can be performed on melanomas and that the old adage of not shaving a pigmented lesion can be dropped. Most still recommend caution, and it is our recommendation that excisional biopsy (see Chapters 27 and 49) should be used for any pigmented lesion that is suspected to be a melanoma.

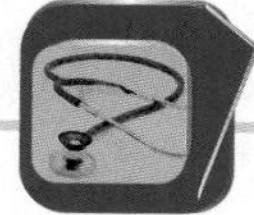

Equipment

- Instruments for simple biopsies are found in Appendix G and can be ordered through local surgical supply houses.
- A suggested anesthesia tray that can be used for this procedure is listed in Appendix F.
- Skin preparation recommendations are shown in Appendix E.

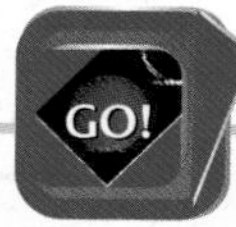

Indications

- Lesions amenable to shave excisional technique include acrochordons (i.e., skin tags), angiomas, fibromas, basal cell carcinomas (i.e., well-defined, small, primary and not recurrent, and in low-risk sites), dermatofibromas, keratoacanthomas, cutaneous horns, molluscum contagiosum, nonpigmented nevi (e.g., intradermal nevi), papillomas, warts, syringomas, venous lakes, cherry angiomas, stucco keratoses, seborrheic keratoses, actinic keratoses, rhinophymas, sebaceous hyperplasia, porokeratosis, neurofibromas, and dermatosis papulosa nigra.

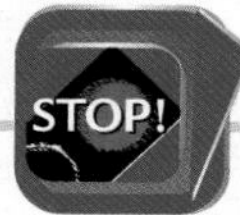

Relative Contraindications

- Pigmented nevi
- Skin appendage lesions (e.g., cylindromas, epidermoid cysts—should be full thickness)
- Subcutaneous lesions (pathology often missed by shave technique)
- Epidermal nevi (removal requires full-thickness excision)
- Infection at the site (relative)
- Severe bleeding disorders (relative)
- Patients on warfarin or clopidogrel (relative)

The Procedure

Step 1. Prepare the site with isopropyl alcohol, povidone-iodine, or chlorhexidine gluconate. For removal of a flat (sessile) lesion, local anesthetic is placed beneath the lesion in an intradermal location (see Chapter 1). The fluid raises the lesion upward, allowing easier removal. Administration of local anesthetic thickens the skin, making it less likely that the shave will penetrate the dermis into the subcutaneous fat.

- **PEARL:** Mask, gown, and sterile gloves are generally not necessary.

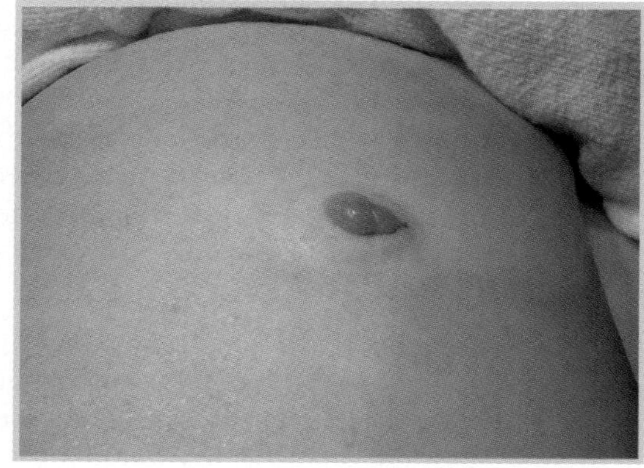

Step 1

- **PITFALL:** Unintentional penetration into the fat (i.e., yellow fat in the base of the wound) should prompt transforming the biopsy site into a sterile surgical wound. The wound should have the edges incised vertically, and the wound should be closed with sutures.

Step 2. A no. 15 blade is held horizontal in the dominant hand while the nondominant hand stabilizes surrounding skin or the lesion. The blade is brought across the base of the lesion with a back-and-forth movement until the lesion is removed, leaving a shallow crater in the dermis.

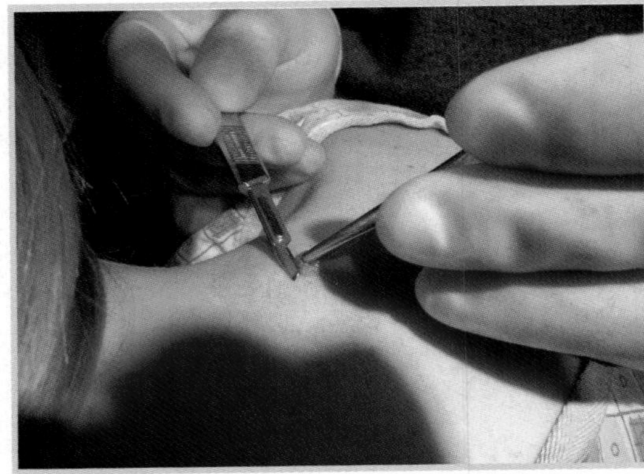

Step 2

Step 3. Biopsy can be performed with a razor blade (Dermablade) held in the hand, with tension applied to the two sides to create some curvature. The sharp surface is brought beneath the lesion for removal within the dermis.

- **PEARL:** Lesion removal can sometimes be facilitated by elevating and squeezing the surrounding skin.
- **PITFALL:** The large, exposed, cutting surface of the razor blade and the hand tension required to maintain curvature of the blade provide great potential for injury. Some surgeons no longer advocate use of razor blades for shave biopsy because of this potential for injury.

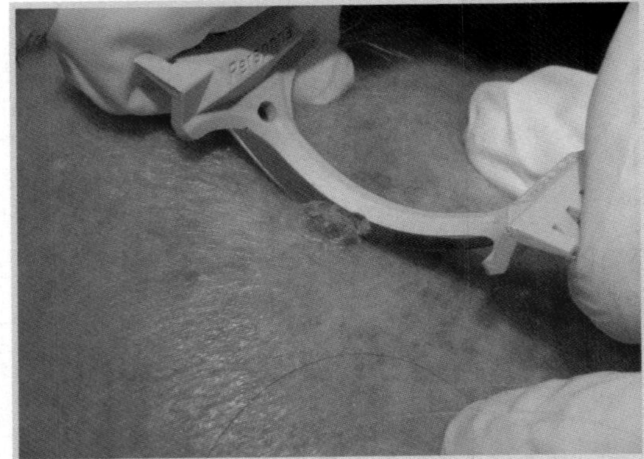

Step 3

Step 4. Small, pedunculated lesions can be removed easily with the scissors technique. The skin is stretched with the nondominant hand, and the lesion is removed with sharp iris scissors. Small lesions can be removed without local anesthesia or with 30 second application of ice if the pain receptors within the skin are stretched.

- **PITFALL:** The scissors must be flush with the skin surface to prevent leaving a residual stump, but no extra skin should be included within the scissor blades to prevent unintentional cutting of surrounding skin.

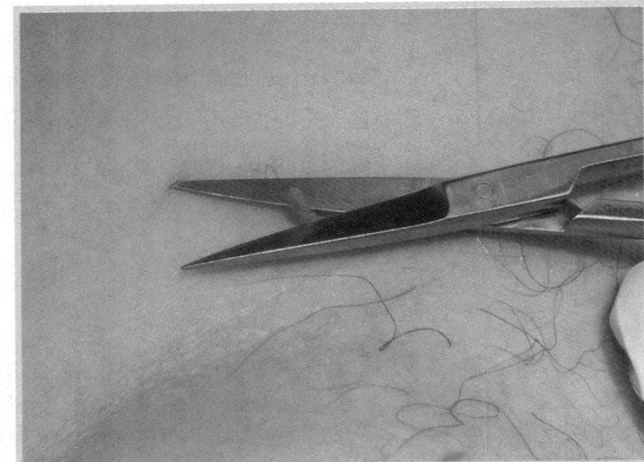

Step 4

Step 5. Radiosurgical loop excision can be used to perform a shave biopsy (see Chapter 34). After anesthesia is placed, the loop or bent wire is activated and moved back and forth across the lesion until it is excised. The radiosurgical current can be set to provide hemostasis to the wound base if needed.

- **PITFALL:** Novice physicians tend to scoop with the loop. The loop must be brought under the lesion horizontally, and the lesion must not be excessively elevated to prevent large scoop defects from this technique.

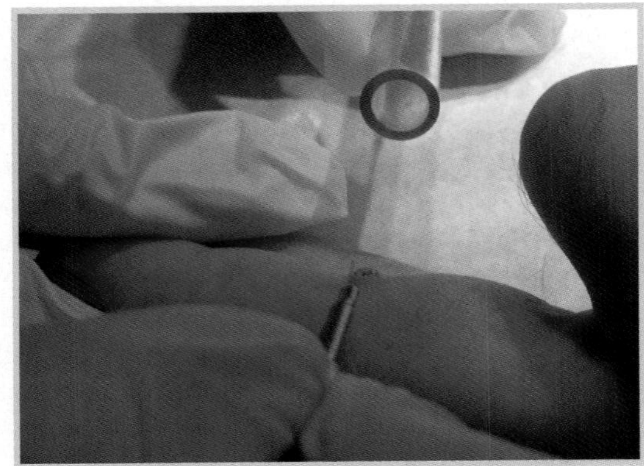

Step 5

Step 6. The wound base can be treated with pressure, coagulation, fulguration, 10% to 20% percent aluminum chloride, or ferric subsulfate (i.e., Monsel's solution) for hemostasis. All of these methods should be applied to a dry wound bed, so the blood must be wiped away and the treatment applied immediately thereafter. Antibiotic ointment and a bandage are then applied.

- PITFALL: Ferric subsulfate can rarely produce permanent discoloration or "tattooing" of the skin. Consider using a 35% to 85% aluminum chloride solution on the faces of fair-skinned (light-complected) individuals to avoid this complication.

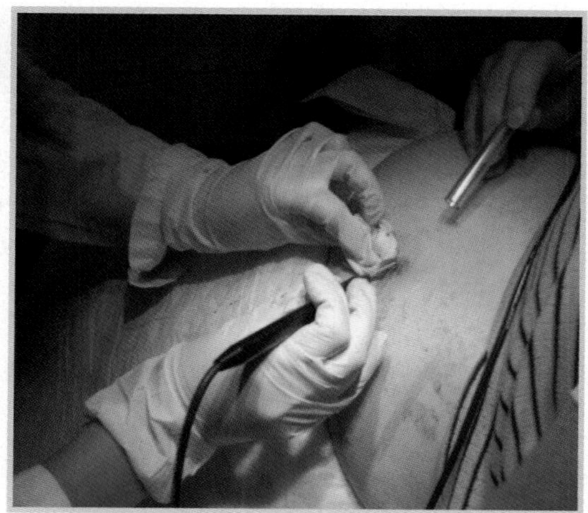

Step 6

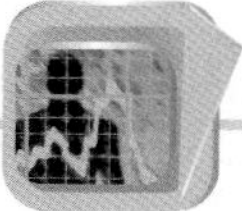

Complications

- Bleeding
- Infection
- Scar formation

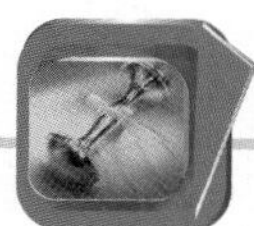

Pediatric Considerations

Generally, pediatric skin has excellent blood flow and heals very well. However, pediatric patients often find it difficult to sit or lie still during lengthy procedures. The patient's maturity and ability to cooperate should be considered before deciding to attempt any out-patient procedure. Sometimes it is necessary to sedate the patient to repair the laceration (see Chapter 122). The maximum recommended dose of lidocaine in children is 3 to 5 mg/kg, or 7 mg/kg when combined with epinephrine. Neonates have an increased volume of distribution, decreased hepatic clearance, and doubled terminal elimination half-life (3.2 hours).

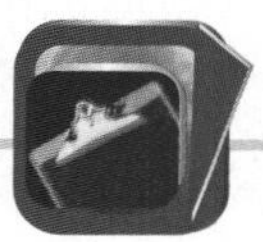

Postprocedure Instructions

Have the patient use a small amount of antibiotic ointment and cover the wound with a small bandage. Instruct the patient to gently wash the area after 1 day. Have the patient dry the area well after washing and use a small amount of antibiotic ointment to promote moist healing. Instruct the patient not to pick at or scratch the wound.

Histologic evaluation of the shave specimen should be reported to the patient. If the evaluation of a benign growth reveals that the specimen margin was positive, the lesion can probably be closely followed or re-excised. Specimens that reveal positive margins for malignancy should prompt re-excision. If a shave specimen is reported to contain melanoma, consider referral to a subspecialist in skin cancer.

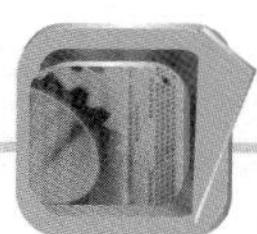

Coding Information and Supply Sources

The following coding information is for shaving of epidermal or dermal lesions, including lesions on mucous membranes (MM). The codes are for single lesion removal.

CPT Code	Description	2008 Average 50th Percentile Fee	Global Period
11300	Trunk, arm, or leg lesion <0.6 cm	$112.00	0
11301	Trunk, arm, or leg lesion 0.6–1.0 cm	$149.00	0
11302	Trunk, arm, or leg lesion 1.1–2.0 cm	$185.00	0
11303	Trunk, arm, or leg lesion >2.0 cm	$224.00	0
11305	Scalp, neck, hands, feet, or genitalia lesion <0.6 cm	$114.00	0
11306	Scalp, neck, hands, feet, or genitalia lesion 0.6–1.0 cm	$161.00	0
11307	Scalp, neck, hands, feet, or genitalia lesion 1.1–2.0 cm	$198.00	0
11308	Scalp, neck, hands, feet, or genitalia lesion >2.0 cm	$228.00	0
11310	Face, ears, eyelids, nose, lips, or MM lesion <0.6 cm	$145.00	0
11311	Face, ears, eyelids, nose, lips, or MM lesion 0.6–1.0 cm	$190.00	0
11312	Face, ears, eyelids, nose, lips, or MM lesion 1.1–2.0 cm	$223.00	0
11313	Face, ears, eyelids, nose, lips, or MM lesion >2.0 cm	$281.00	0

CPT is a registered trademark of the American Medical Association.
2008 average 50th Percentile Fees are provided courtesy of 2008 MMH-SI's copyrighted Physicians' Fees and Coding Guide.

- Hemostatic agents such as ferric subsulfate are available from surgical supply houses or the resources listed in Appendix G.
- For practitioners wishing to perform shave biopsy with a razor blade, the disposable DermaBlade (Personna Medical, American Razor Company, Stauton, VA) enhances safety by allowing the operator to grasp the sure-grip teeth to the sides instead of directly handling the blade.
- Radiosurgical generators; electrodes for dermatologic, gynecologic, plastic surgery, or ear, nose, and throat uses; smoke evacuators; and other accessories are available from
  - Ellman International, 1135 Railroad Avenue, Hewlett, NY 11557-2316 (phone: 800-835-2316; www.ellman.com)
  - Wallach Surgical Devices, 235 Edison Road, Orange, CT 06477 (phone: 203-799-2002; www.wallachsd.com).

Bibliography

Fewkes JL, Sober AJ. Skin biopsy: the four types and how best to do them. *Prim Care Cancer.* 1993;13:36–39.

Habif TP. *Clinical Dermatology: A Color Guide to Diagnosis and Therapy*, 3rd ed. St. Louis: Mosby, 1996:815.

Huerter CJ. Simple biopsy techniques. In: Wheeland RG, ed. *Cutaneous Surgery* Philadelphia: WB Saunders, 1994:159–170.

Pariser RJ. Skin biopsy: lesion selection and optimal technique. *Mod Med.* 1989;57:82–90.

Phillips PK, Pariser DM, Pariser RJ. Cosmetic procedures we all perform. *Cutis.* 1994;53:187–191.

Russell EB, Carrington PR, Smoller BR. Basal cell carcinoma: a comparison of shave biopsy versus punch biopsy techniques in subtype diagnosis. *J Am Acad Dermatol.* 1999;41:69–71.

Skin biopsy. Accessed: September 9, 2007. Available at: www.melanomacenter.org/diagnosing/typesskinbiopsies.html.

Stegman SJ, Tromovitch TA, Glogau RG. *Basics of Dermatologic Surgery*. Chicago: Year Book Medical; 1982.

Swanson NA. *Atlas of Ccutaneous Surgery*. Boston: Little, Brown; 1987:14–15.

Usatine RP, Moy RL, Tobinick EL, et al. *Skin Surgery: A Practical Guide*. St. Louis: Mosby; 1998; 55–76.

Zalla MJ. Basic cutaneous surgery. *Cutis.* 1994;53:172–186.

Zitelli JA. Wound healing by secondary intention: a cosmetic appraisal. *J Am Acad Dermatol.* 1983;9:407–415.

Zuber TJ. Dermal electrosurgical shave excision. *Am Fam Physician.* 2002;65:1883–1886, 1889–1890, 1895, 1899–1900.

Zuber TJ. Skin biopsy techniques: when and how to perform shave and excisional biopsy. *Consultant.* 1994;34:1515–1521.

2008 MAG Mutual Healthcare Solutions, Inc.'s Physicians' Fee and Coding Guide. Duluth, Georgia. MAG Mutual Healthcare Solutions, Inc. 2007.

CHAPTER 58

Tangential Laceration Repair

E. J. Mayeaux, Jr., MD, DABFP, FAAFP

Professor of Family Medicine, Professor of Obstetrics and Gynecology
Louisiana State University Health Sciences Center, Shreveport, LA

Some soft tissue injuries are caused by tangential forces that produce oblique, nonvertical, or beveled wound edges. If these beveled edges are sutured in standard fashion, an unsightly ledge of tissue often results. Uneven edges cast a shadow on vertical surfaces, and the shadow magnifies the appearance of the scar. Proper management of tangential lacerations, especially on cosmetically important areas such as the face, is essential for optimal results.

Angled or beveled wounds have a broad edge (base side) and a shallow edge. The shallow edge may heal with minimal tissue loss if the wound angle is near vertical. The distal portion (i.e., nearest the center of the wound) of the shallow edge often necroses with more pronounced wound edge angulation because of inadequate blood supply to the epidermis and upper dermis. If the shallow edge is so thin as to appear transparent at the time of injury, subsequent necrosis is almost guaranteed. A markedly shallow edge contracts and rolls inward if taped or sutured without modification.

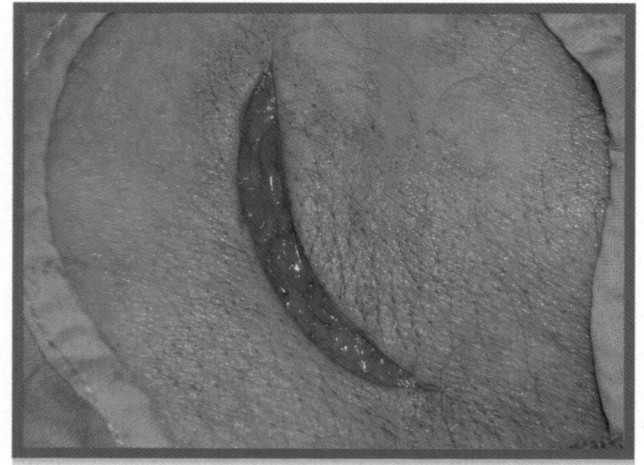

Tangential lacerations on the hand are commonly produced by glass fragments resulting from a glass breaking while being washed in the sink. Tangential lacerations on the head and face frequently result from glancing blows. Elderly individuals often experience tangential skin wounds (i.e., skin tears) on the extremities from even minimal contact. Skin tears in the elderly represent a special management situation. Because suturing skin tears on the extremities does not appear to improve outcomes, taping is recommended in the elderly and in persons with very poor blood flow.

A simple repair technique for tangential wounds involves taking a large, deep bite from the broad edge and a small bite from the shallow edge. Historically, tangential lacerations have been treated by transforming the beveled edges to vertical edges. Debridement of the wound edges is tedious and time consuming, and extensive removal of tissue on the face should be approached with caution. Despite these negative factors, the effort to transform wound edges can provide gratifying cosmetic and functional results.

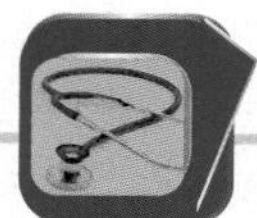

Equipment

- Instruments for simple, interrupted, skin suture placement are found in Appendix G and can be ordered through local surgical supply houses.
- Suture materials can be ordered from Ethicon, Somerville, NJ (http://ecatalog.ethi con.com/EC_ECATALOG/ethicon/default.asp).
- A suggested anesthesia tray that can be used for this procedure is listed in Appendix F.

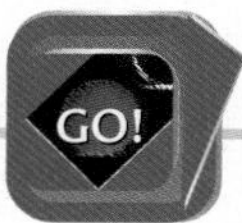

Indications

- Wounds with beveled (nonvertical) edges

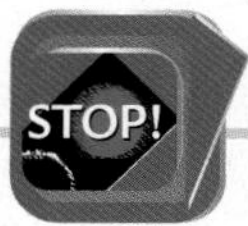

Contraindications (Relative)

- Skin tears in elderly individuals
- Severe bleeding disorders
- Extreme illness that would make wound healing difficult
- Cellulitis in the tissues to be incised
- Conditions that may interfere with wound healing (collagen vascular diseases, smoking, renal insufficiency, diabetes mellitus, nutritional status, obesity, chemotherapeutic agents, and corticosteroids)
- Disorders of collagen synthesis such as Ehlers-Danlos syndrome and Marfan syndrome that affect wound healing
- Concurrent medications that may increase the likelihood of intraoperative bleeding (aspirin, other nonsteroidal anti-inflammatory drugs, warfarin)
- Uncooperative patient

The Procedure

Step 1. An angulated skin wound will have reduced blood supply to the distal portion of the shallow wound edge, often resulting in necrosis of the shallow edge.

- PITFALL: If a tangential wound is approximated with a simple suture (i.e., equal bites through each wound edge), an inverted or depressed scar often results.

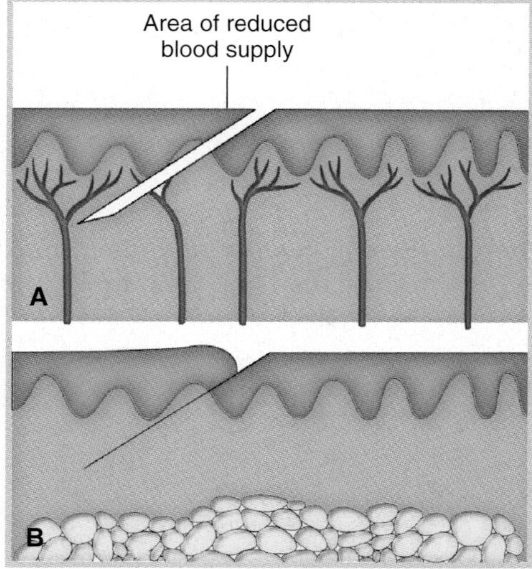

Step 1

Step 2. When repairing a tangential skin wound, take a large, deep bite with the suture needle through the broad edge and a small (2-mm) bite through the shallow edge. This path of the suture thread promotes eversion of the shallow edge and helps with the final appearance of the wound.

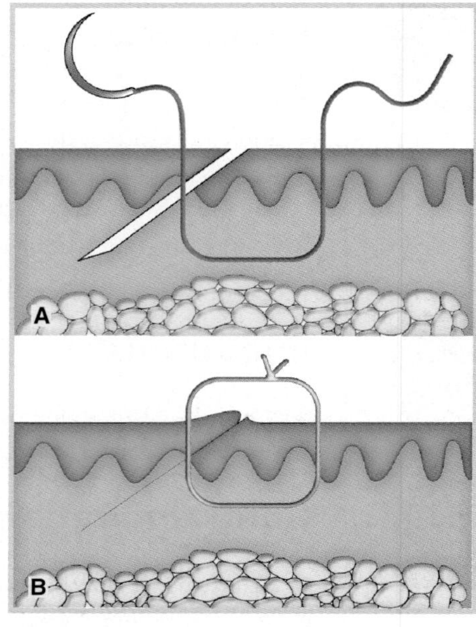

Step 2

Step 3. A C-shaped wound with beveled edges is often produced by a tangential injury. Use a scalpel to create vertical wound edges and undermine the edges to produce low-tension approximation.

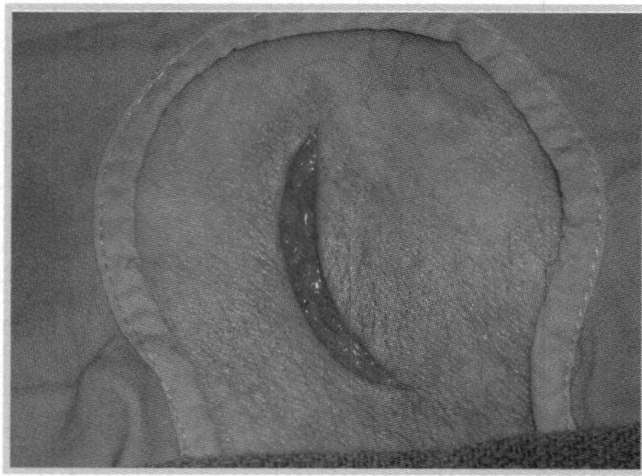

Step 3

Step 4. Place the first suture in the middle of the wound.

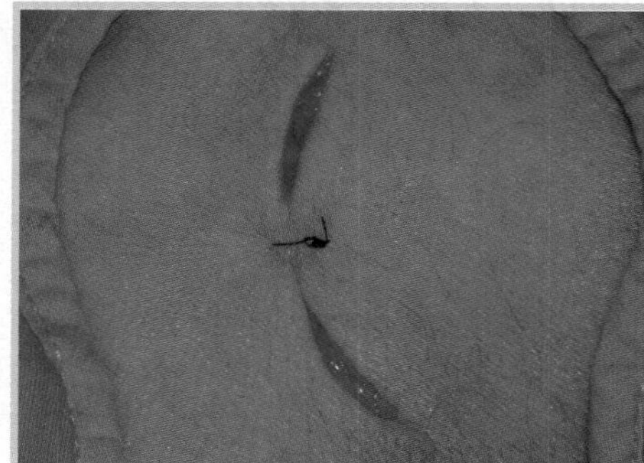

Step 4

Step 5. Place another simple interrupted suture at half of the remaining distance of the unapproximated defect.

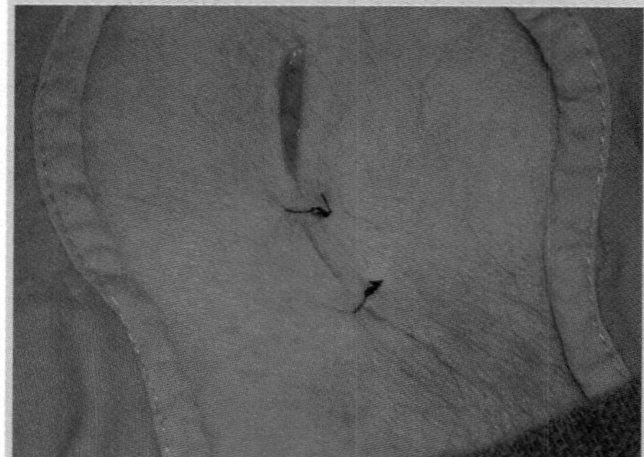

Step 5

Step 6. Continue placing simple interrupted sutures at half of the remaining distance of the unapproximated defect until the suture line is closed.

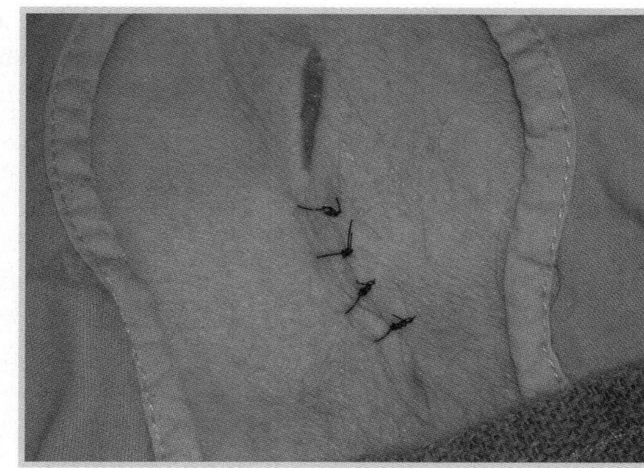

Step 6

Step 7. Alternatively, if a section requiring closure is better approximated with two additional sutures instead of three, place two additional sutures, each at one-third the total distance to finish the suture line.

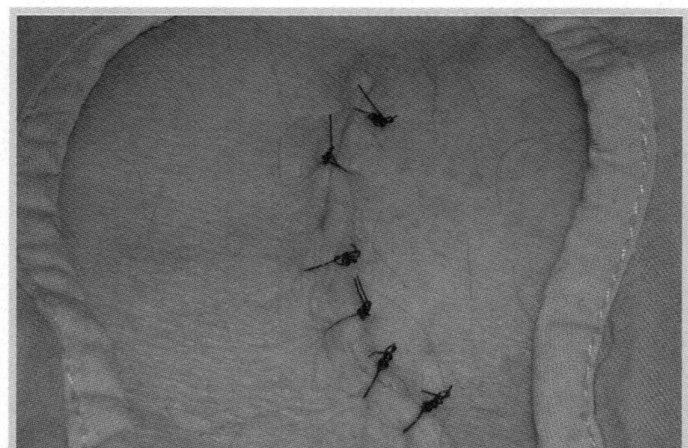

Step 7

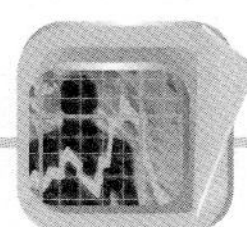

Complications

- Pain, infection, and bleeding
- Nonunion of skin edges
- Scar formation
- Incomplete excision of lesion

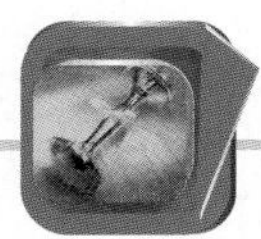

Pediatric Considerations

Generally, pediatric skin has excellent blood flow and heals very well. However, pediatric patients often find it difficult to sit or lie still during lengthy procedures. The patient's maturity and ability to cooperate should be considered before deciding to attempt any outpatient procedure. Sometimes it is necessary to sedate the patient to repair the laceration (see Chapter 122). The maximum recommended dose of lidocaine in children is 3 to 5 mg/kg, and 7 mg/kg when combined with epinephrine. Neonates have an increased volume of distribution, decreased hepatic clearance, and doubled terminal elimination half-life (3.2 hours).

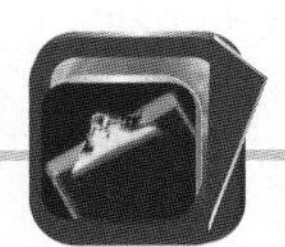

Postprocedure Instructions

Instruct the patient to gently wash an area that has been stitched after 1 day, but not to put the wound into standing water for two to three days. Have the patient dry the area well after washing and use a small amount of antibiotic ointment to promote moist healing. Recommend wound elevation to help lessen swelling, reduce pain, and speed healing. Instruct the patient not to pick at, break, or cut the stitches. Have them cover the wound with a nonocclusive dressing for two to three days. A simple Band-Aid will suffice for many small lacerations. The dressing should be left in place for at least 48 hours, after which time most wounds can be opened to air. Scalp wounds can be left open if small, but large head wounds can be wrapped circumferentially with rolled gauze.

Most uncontaminated wounds do not need to be seen by a provider until suture removal, unless signs of infection develop. Highly contaminated wounds should be seen for follow-up in 2 to 3 days. Give discharge instructions to the patient regarding signs of wound infection.

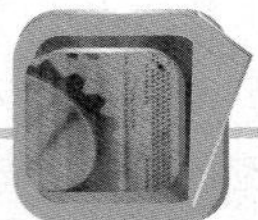

Coding Information and Supply Sources

All codes listed are for superficial wound closure using sutures, staples, or tissue adhesives with or without adhesive strips on the skin surface. If a layered closure is required, use intermediate closure codes 12031 to 12057 or complex repair codes 13100 to 13160.

Add together the lengths of wounds in the same classification and anatomic sites. Use separate codes for repairs from different anatomic sites. Debridement is considered a separate procedure only when gross contamination requires prolonged cleansing or when appreciable amounts of devitalized or contaminated tissue are removed.

Simple repair is included in the codes reported for benign and malignant lesion excision (see Chapter 49). The billing chart cites the following wound locations: scalp, neck, axillae, external genitalia, trunk, extremities, hands, and feet (SNAGTEHF) and face, ears, eyelids, nose, lips, and mucous membranes (FEENLMM).

CPT Code	Description	2008 Average 50th Percentile Fee	Global Period
12001	Simple repair SNAGTEHF ≤2.5 cm	$220.00	10
12002	Simple repair SNAGTEHF 2.6–7.5 cm	$235.00	10
12004	Simple repair SNAGTEHF 7.6–12.5 cm	$285.00	10
12005	Simple repair SNAGTEHF 12.6–20.0 cm	$408.00	10
12006	Simple repair SNAGTEHF 20.1–30.0 cm	$506.00	10
12007	Simple repair SNAGTEHF >30.0 cm		10
12011	Simple repair FEENLMM ≤2.5 cm	$240.00	10
12013	Simple repair FEENLMM 2.6–5.0 cm	$288.00	10
12014	Simple repair FEENLMM 5.1–7.5 cm	$351.00	10
12015	Simple repair FEENLMM 7.6–12.5 cm	$449.00	10
12016	Simple repair FEENLMM 12.6–20.0 cm	$585.00	10
12017	Simple repair FEENLMM 20.1–30.0 cm	$743.00	10
12018	Simple repair FEENLMM >30.0 cm		10
12020	Treatment of superficial wound dehiscence, simple closure	$397.00	10

CPT is a registered trademark of the American Medical Association.
2008 average 50th Percentile Fees are provided courtesy of 2008 MMH-SI's copyrighted Physicians' Fees and Coding Guide.
SNAGTEHF, scalp, neck, axillae, external genitalia, trunk, extremities, hands and feet;
FEENLMM, face, ears, eyelids, nose, lips, and mucous membranes.

Bibliography

Bennett RG. *Fundamentals of Cutaneous Surgery*. St. Louis: CV Mosby; 1988:355–444.

Dushoff IM. A stitch in time. *Emerg Med*. 1973;5:21–43.

Lammers RL, Trott AL. Methods of wound closure. In: Roberts JR, Hedges JR, eds. *Clinical Procedures in Emergency Medicine*, 3rd ed. Philadelphia: WB Saunders; 1998:560–598.

Perry AW, McShane RH. Fine tuning of the skin edges in the closure of surgical wounds: controlling inversion and eversion with the path of the needle—the right stitch at the right time. *J Dermatol Surg Oncol*. 1981;7:471–476.

Stein A, Williamson PS. Repair of simple lacerations. In: Driscoll CE, Rakel RE, eds. *Patient Care Procedures for Your Practice*. Los Angeles: Practice Management Information Corporation; 1991:299–306.

Williamson P. Office Procedures. Philadelphia: WB Saunders; 1955:215–223.

Wilson JL, Kocurek K, Doty BJ. A systemic approach to laceration repair. *Postgrad Med*. 2000;107: 77–88.

Zuber TJ. Wound management. In: Rakel RE, ed. *Saunders Manual of Medical Practice*. Philadelphia: WB Saunders; 1996:1007–1008.

Zukin DD, Simon RR. *Emergency Wound Care: Principles and Practice*. Rockville, MD: Aspen Publishers; 1987:63–76.

2008 MAG Mutual Healthcare Solutions, Inc.'s Physicians' Fee and Coding Guide. Duluth, Georgia. MAG Mutual Healthcare Solutions, Inc. 2007.

CHAPTER 59

T-plasty

E. J. Mayeaux, Jr., MD, DABFP, FAAFP

Professor of Family Medicine, Professor of Obstetrics and Gynecology
Louisiana State University Health Sciences Center, Shreveport, LA

The T-plasty (A-T-plasty, O-T flap) can be thought of as half of a double advancement flap. The basic technique involves creating a triangular-shaped defect superimposed over the primary circular excision to be closed. The flap is constructed by making an incision along the base of the imagined triangular defect and then joining the two basal tips of the triangle with the midpoint of the base. Two large pedicles are created to allow good blood flow to the distal portions of the flap. The pedicles slide along the incision line to close the triangular defect. This results in an inverted T-shaped closure. The lines of tension are created by the rotation of the skin recruited. The tension created is mostly in a 15-degree arc along the lines that bisect the angles formed by the horizontal and vertical incisions.

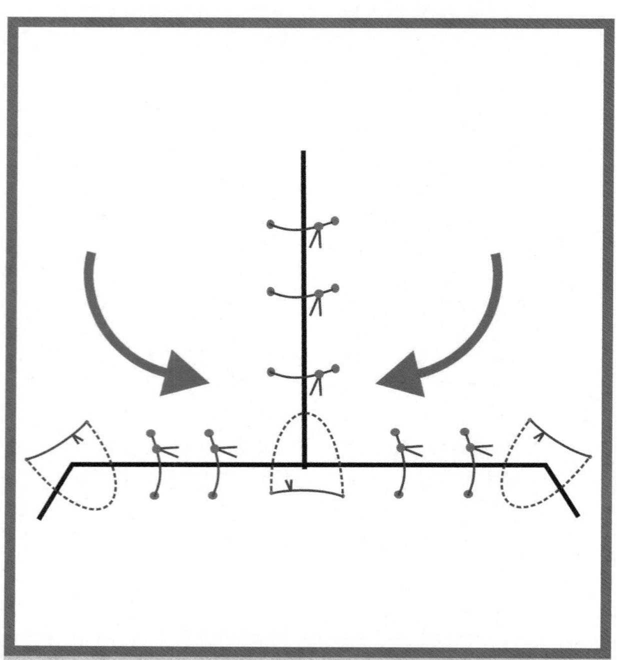

Dog ears are frequently encountered at the ends of the flaps after closure of the triangular defect. Burow triangle repair (see Chapter 46) is sometimes needed on each end of the incision line opposite the original triangular defect. The Burow wedge triangles allow the pedicles to move easier. To avoid unnecessary or excessive tissue removal, Burow wedge triangles should not be excised until after the pedicles have been sutured. If a dog ear appears at the apex of the triangle where the two pedicles meet, it can be corrected by removing the extraneous tissue.

The dimensions of the imaginary triangle that guides the formation of this flap will obviously vary depending on the size of the defect, the size of the standing cone that is formed, and the proximity of adjacent structures. The optimal design (to minimize closure tension) for a T-plasty includes a triangle height that is twice the excision defect diameter, base extensions of one defect diameter on each side, and three defect diameters (measured from the center of the defect) of undermining.

The T-plasty is valuable when distortion of a structure adjacent to one edge of a defect is undesirable, or the defect is at or near long anatomic boundaries. When this is the case, the base of the flap is placed along the border of the edge to be preserved. This method prevents the violation of important structures and allows scars to be relatively well hidden. This flap is particularly useful on the forehead, where the base incision can be concealed along the eyebrow or hairline; on the chin, where the base incision can be concealed along the mental crease; and on the lip, where the base incision can be concealed along the vermilion border. However, when using this flap on the lip, the surgeon must take care to avoid secondary movement, which may distort the free margin of the vermilion border.

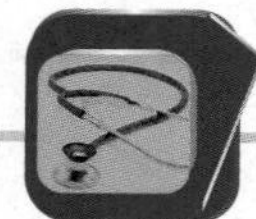

Equipment

- Surgery tray instruments are listed in Appendix G. Consider adding skin hooks to gently handle the skin flaps. Have at least three fine (mosquito) hemostats to assist with hemostasis while developing large skin flaps.
- Suggested suture removal times are listed in Appendix J, and a suggested anesthesia tray that can be used for this procedure is listed in Appendix F. All instruments can be ordered through local surgical supply houses.

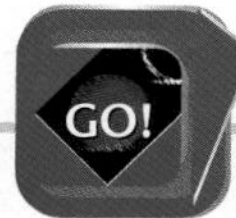

Indications

- Closure of lower eyelid defects: The T-plasty will reduce the risk of depression of the lower eyelid, compared to a fusiform excision.
- Closure of preauricular defects: A long incision line is created parallel to the ear, and the two pedicles are created on the cheek.
- Closure of upper lip defects: Red-colored tissue located inside the vermilion border is not used for repair of lip defects outside of the vermilion border. The A-to-T flap can be used effectively to close a defect at this site.
- Closure of lateral nasal ala defects: If an incision cannot be extended into the nasal ala, a T-closure may be performed by lining up the long incision line with the nasolabial fold.
- Closure of upper eyebrow defects: Fusiform excision of lesions just above the eyebrow can result in cosmetically unacceptable elevation of the eyebrow.

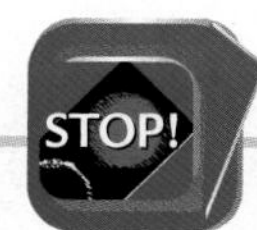

Contraindications

- Poor skin vascular supply
- Diseases causing poor vascular supply to the skin (e.g., atherosclerotic heart disease, diabetes, smoking, collagen vascular disease, prior irradiation, severe anemia, anticoagulation)
- History of poor wound healing, hypertrophic scarring, or keloid formation
- Uncooperative patient
- Presence of cellulitis, bacteremia, or active infection

The Procedure

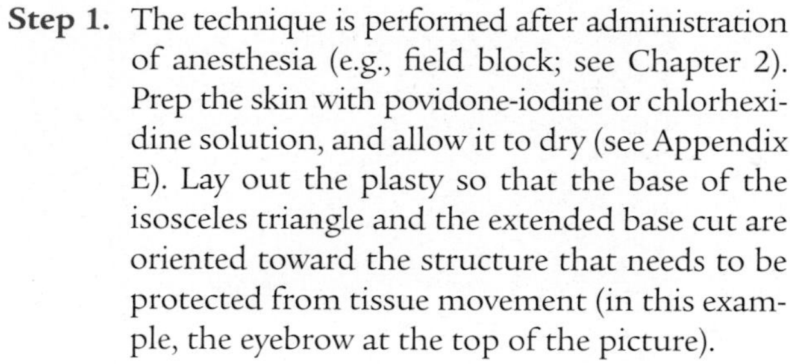

Step 1. The technique is performed after administration of anesthesia (e.g., field block; see Chapter 2). Prep the skin with povidone-iodine or chlorhexidine solution, and allow it to dry (see Appendix E). Lay out the plasty so that the base of the isosceles triangle and the extended base cut are oriented toward the structure that needs to be protected from tissue movement (in this example, the eyebrow at the top of the picture).

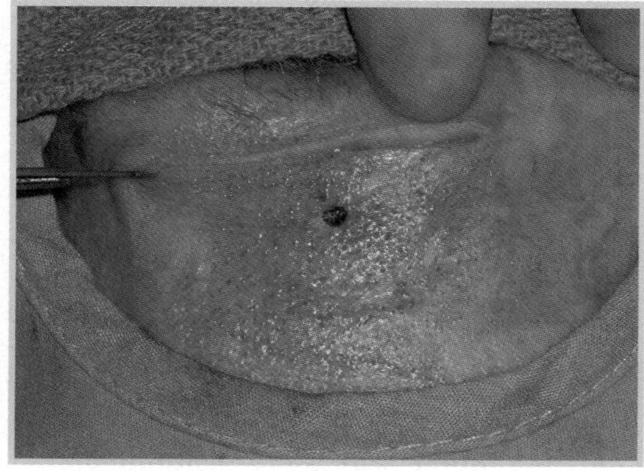

Step 1

- **PEARL:** Prep a wide area so that an undraped area is not inadvertently exposed if the drape slides a little.

Step 2. The original circular defect is planned based on the size of the lesion plus an appropriate margin (see Appendix D). The planned circular defect is then converted into a triangular defect.

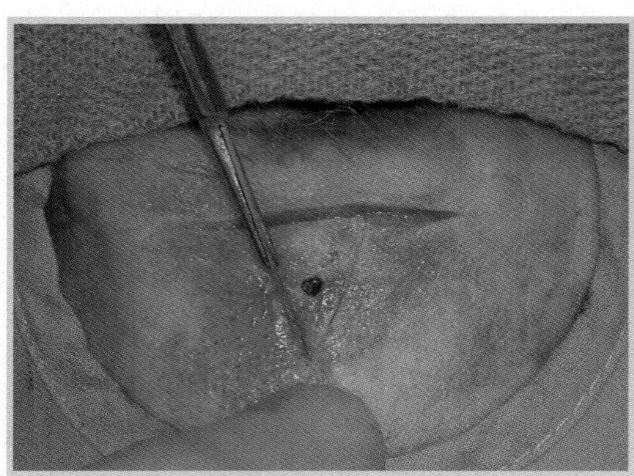

Step 2

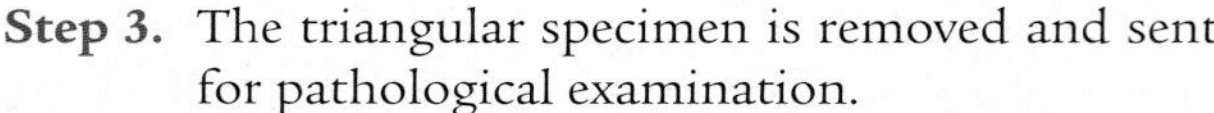

Step 3. The triangular specimen is removed and sent for pathological examination.

- **PITFALL:** Some providers excise the circular defect first, then cut out the triangle. However, when the lesion is excised with the entire triangle, the extra tissue on the excision margin minimizes the risk of a margin that is positive for disease.

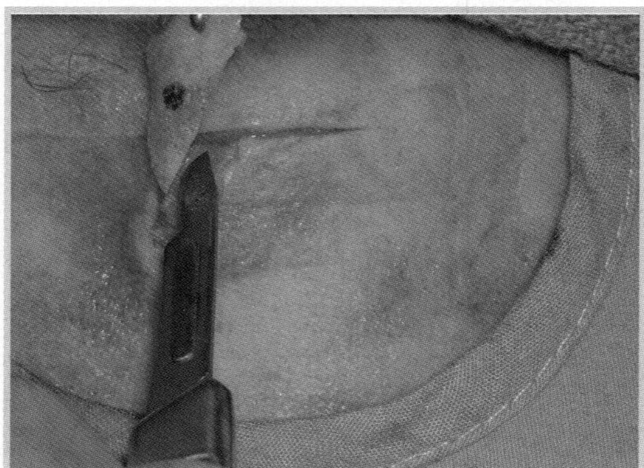

Step 3

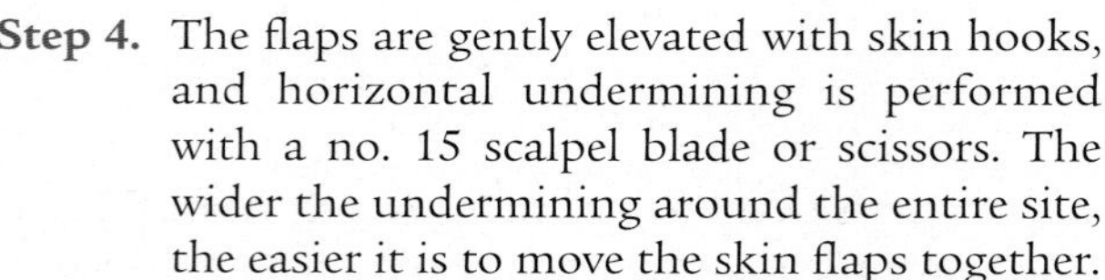

Step 4. The flaps are gently elevated with skin hooks, and horizontal undermining is performed with a no. 15 scalpel blade or scissors. The wider the undermining around the entire site, the easier it is to move the skin flaps together.

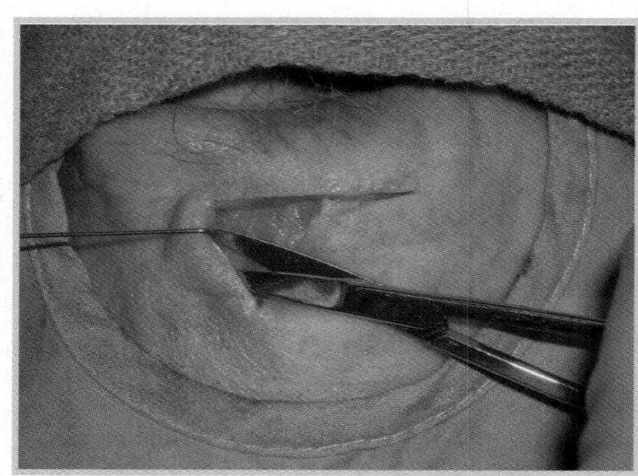

Step 4

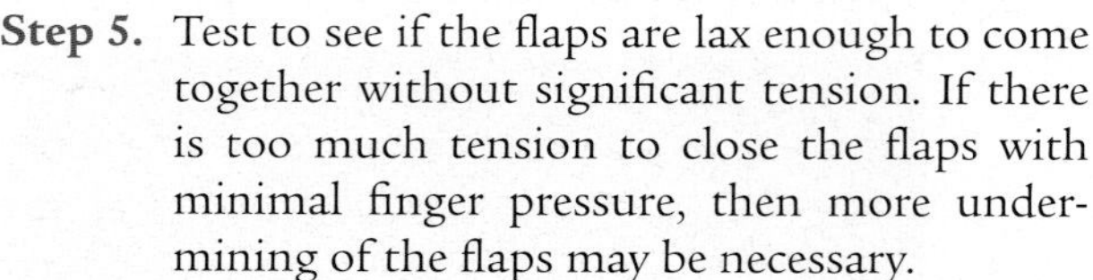

Step 5. Test to see if the flaps are lax enough to come together without significant tension. If there is too much tension to close the flaps with minimal finger pressure, then more undermining of the flaps may be necessary.

- **PITFALL:** If the flaps are well undermined and still do not close with minimal pressure, check the overall length of the flaps. In the optimally designed T-plasty, the base extensions should equal one defect diameter on each side, and there should be three defect diameters (measured from the center of the defect) of undermining.

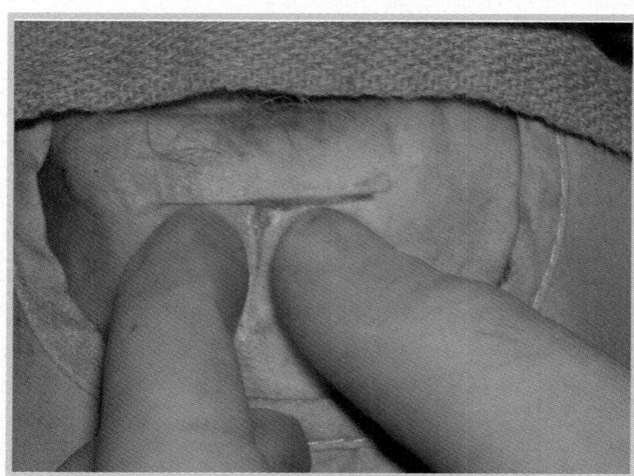

Step 5

Step 6. Slide the two pedicles to the center, and anchor the pedicles to the long incision line and to each other. Place a corner stitch.

- **PEARL:** Make sure the corner stitch is placed in the middle of the base cut. If the center stitch is displaced to either side, the skin tones may not match as well and the dog ear will be more pronounced on one side.

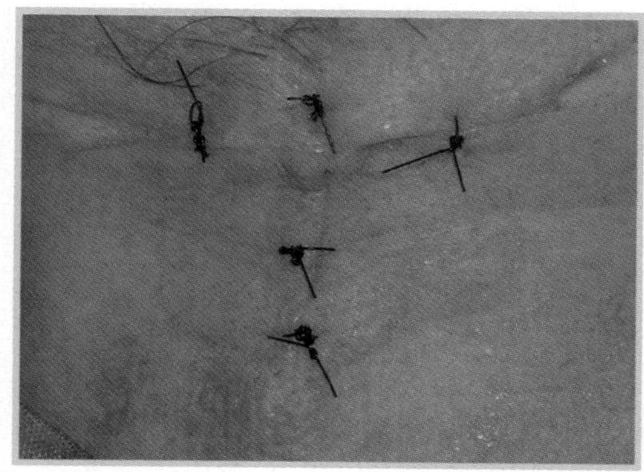

Step 6

Step 7. If tissue has bunched at the end of the incision lines, Burow wedge triangle excisions are performed to correct the dog ears (see Chapter 46).

- **PITFALL:** Sometimes a corner stitch cannot be used to close the flap tips. A corner stitch is typically employed to close the two flap tips. However, an anatomic obstruction may limit the amount of space available to perform a corner stitch. Occasionally, it may be necessary to tape the corner down, rather than place a corner stitch.

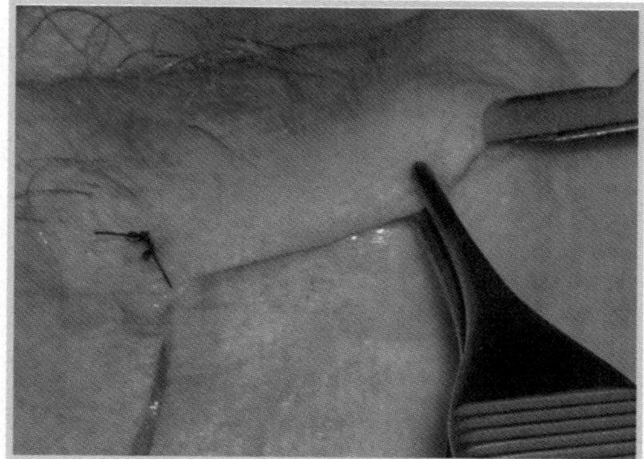

Step 7

Step 8. Finish the closure with simple interrupted sutures.

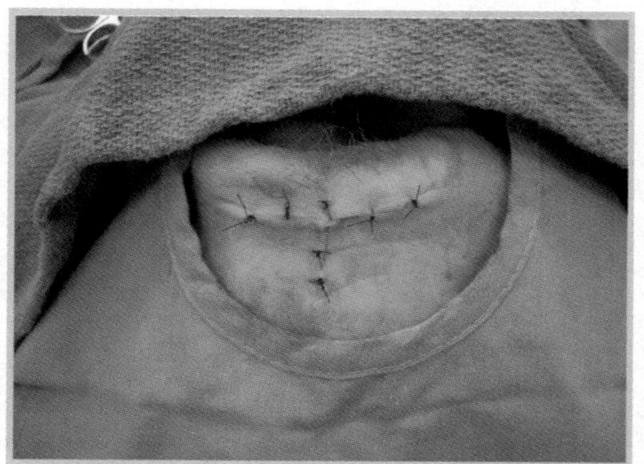

Step 8

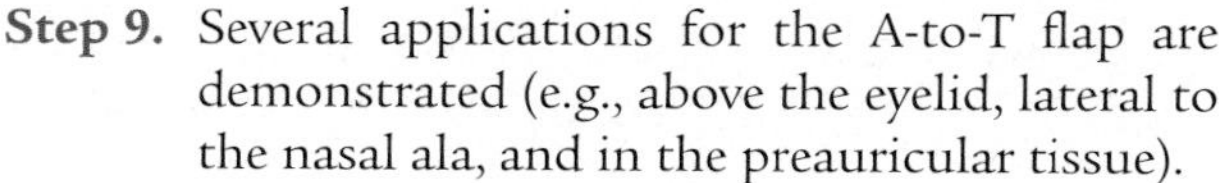

Step 9. Several applications for the A-to-T flap are demonstrated (e.g., above the eyelid, lateral to the nasal ala, and in the preauricular tissue).

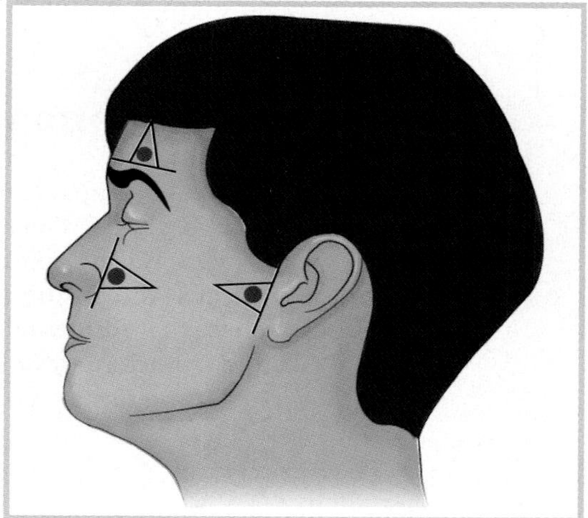

Step 9

Step 10. A triangular defect on the lower eyelid has an extended incision line. The pedicles are undermined, and the flaps are centered. There may not be enough room to place a corner suture outside the edge of the eyelid.

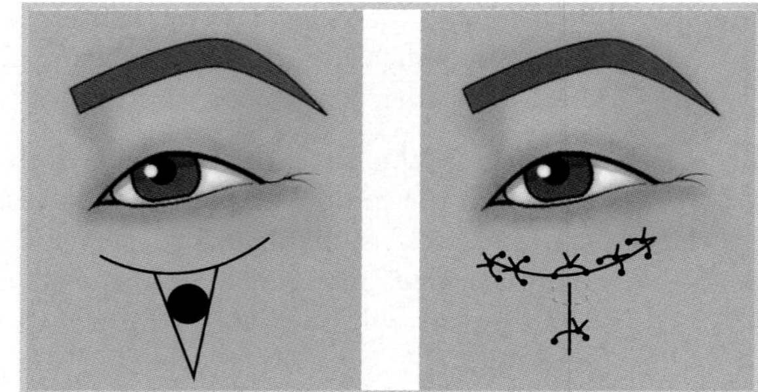

Step 10

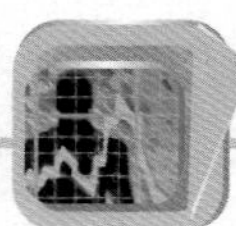

Complications

- Pain, infection, and bleeding
- Nonunion of skin edges
- Scar formation
- Sensory changes (often subside with time)
- Flap necrosis
- Hematoma formation

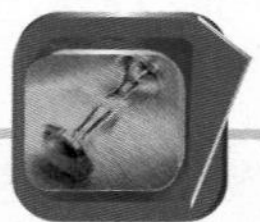

Pediatric Considerations

Generally, pediatric skin has excellent blood flow and heals very well. However, pediatric patients often find it difficult to sit or lie still during lengthy procedures. The patient's maturity and ability to cooperate should be considered before deciding to attempt any outpatient procedure.

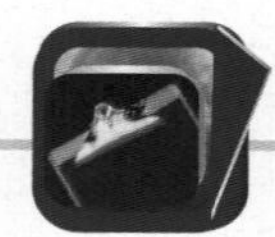

Postprocedure Instructions

Apply topical antibiotics and a pressure dressing after the procedure. Have the patient keep the bandage on and the wound dry for the first 24 hours. After that, it can be cleaned with hydrogen peroxide or gently washed with soap and water as needed. An antibiotic ointment and bandage should be reapplied until the patient returns or for 2 weeks. Have the patient report signs of infection. Schedule a return appointment for suture removal (see Appendix J).

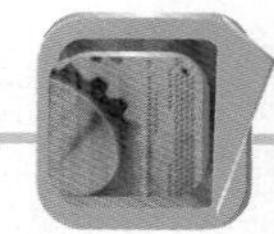

Coding Information

These codes encompass excision or repair, or both, by adjacent transfer or rearrangement, including Z-plasty, W-plasty, V-Y-plasty, rotation flaps, advancement flaps, and double-pedicle flaps. When applied to traumatic wounds, the defect must be developed by the surgeon because the closure requires it, and these codes should not be used for direct closure of a defect that incidentally results in the configuration of one of the flaps or plasties. If the configurations result incidentally from the laceration shape, closure should be reported using simple repair codes.

CPT Code	Description	2008 Average 50th Percentile Fee	Global Period
14000	Trunk $\leq$10 cm^2	$1,062.00	90
14001	Trunk 10.1–30.0 cm^2	$1,400.00	90
14020	SAL $\leq$10 cm^2	$1,222.00	90
14021	SAL 10.1–30.0^2	$1,684.00	90
14040	FCCMNAGHF $\leq$10 cm^2	$1,551.00	90
14041	FCCMNAGHF 10.1–30.0 cm^2	$1,757.00	90
14060	ENEL $\leq$10 cm^2	$1,841.00	90
14061	ENEL 10.1–30.0 cm^2	$2,254.00	90
14300	Any unusual or complicated area >30 cm^2	$2,749.00	90

CPT is a registered trademark of the American Medical Association.
2008 average 50th Percentile Fees are provided courtesy of 2008 MMH-SI's copyrighted Physicians' Fees and Coding Guide.
SAL, scalp, arms, or legs; FCCMNAGHF, forehead, cheeks, chin, mouth, neck, axillae, genitalia, hands, or feet; ENEL, eyelids, nose, ears, or lips.

Bibliography

Chernosky ME. Scalpel and scissors surgery as seen by the dermatologist. In: Epstein E, Epstein E Jr., eds. *Skin Surgery*. 6th ed. Philadelphia: Saunders; 1987:88–127.

Krishnan R, Garman M, Nunez-Gussman J, et al. Advancement flaps: A basic theme with many variations. *Dermatol Surg*. 2005;31(8):987–994.

Larrabee WF, Sutton D. The biomechanics of advancement and rotation flaps. *Laryngoscope*. 1981;91:726–734.

Stegman SJ, Tromovitch TA, Glogau RG. *Basics of Dermatologic Surgery*. Chicago: Year Book Medical; 1982:87.

Stevens C, Tan L, Kassir R, et al. Biomechanics of A-to-T flap design. *Laryngoscope*. 1999;109:113–117.

Swanson NA. *Atlas of Cutaneous Surgery*. Boston: Little Brown; 1987:96–97.

Wheeland RG. Reconstruction of the lower lip and chin using local and random-pattern flaps. *J Dermatol Surg Oncol*. 1991;17:605–615.

2008 MAG Mutual Healthcare Solutions, Inc.'s Physicians' Fee and Coding Guide. Duluth, Georgia. MAG Mutual Healthcare Solutions, Inc. 2007.

CHAPTER 60

V-to-Y-plasty

E. J. Mayeaux, Jr., MD, DABFP, FAAFP

Professor of Family Medicine, Professor of Obstetrics and Gynecology
Louisiana State University Health Sciences Center, Shreveport, LA

The V-to-Y-plasty is an easy-to-learn technique commonly used in plastic surgical practice. In this technique, an incision is made in a triangular pattern, and the triangular-shaped flap is advanced to cover the defect in the Y shape. The double V-to-Y-plasty involves a fusiform-shaped incision with two triangular-shaped pedicles that are advanced to the center of the defect and closed in the shape of two Ys, with the upper arms connected. The V-to-Y-plasty is an island pedicle flap. Although most local flaps rotate into a wound from nearby tissues, bringing the blood supply with the intact portion of the flap, island pedicle flaps receive the blood supply from below, in the capillaries immediately beneath the dermis. This capillary supply must not be disrupted by undermining the tissue when creating an island pedicle flap.

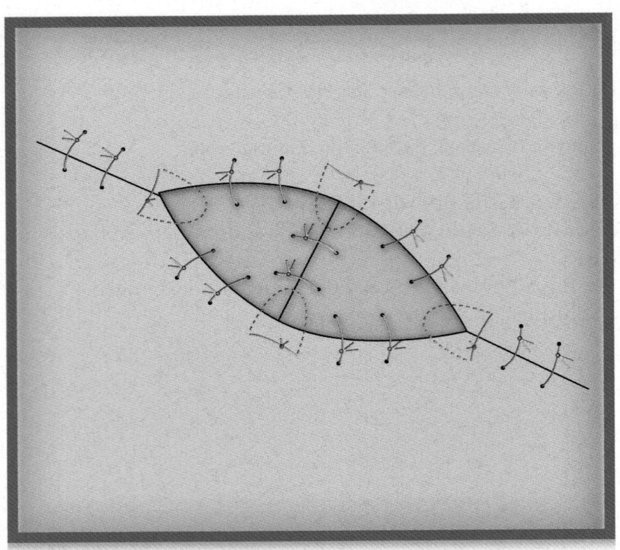

Although the V-to-Y-plasty is a common procedure in covering skin defects, it has limited use in areas of poorer subcutaneous blood flow, such as the lower extremities. It works very well on the face, neck, and back. The V-to-Y-plasty may also be used to repair fingertip amputation, in which case the V-to-Y-plasty flap technique works best when the injury leaves more pulp than nail bed. The V-to-Y-plasty technique preserves the normal contours of the dorsal finger, helps pad the fingertip, and preserves normal sensation. It allows most patients to regain sensation and two-point discrimination in the fingertip. The cosmetic results are usually excellent, with good contour and fingertip padding preserved.

The V-to-Y-plasty may also be used to alleviate the tension caused by a contracted scar in the skin or on a skin structure. In this scenario, the arms of the Y are cut around the contracted scar and away from the skin area or structure being distorted. The V flap is not undermined or moved, but natural tissue recoils will pull the lesion so as to relieve tension in the skin. Then the Y-shaped suture line is created.

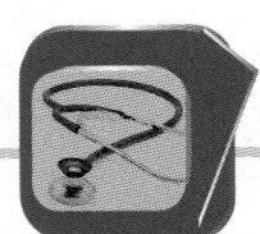

Equipment

- Surgery tray instruments are listed in Appendix G. Consider adding skin hooks to gently handle the skin flaps. Have at least three fine (mosquito) hemostats to assist with hemostasis while developing large skin flaps.

- Suggested suture removal times are listed in Appendix J, and a suggested anesthesia tray that can be used for this procedure is listed in Appendix F. All instruments can be ordered through local surgical supply houses.

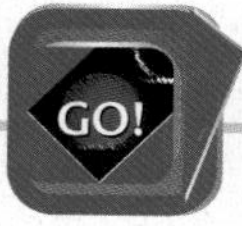

Indications

- Closure of skin defects that require minimal skin removal, or where skin may be under tension from a variety of directions.

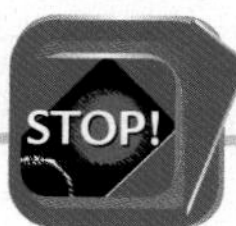

Contraindications (Relative)

- Poor blood flow areas
- Uncooperative patient
- Wounds best closed by other methods
- Presence of cellulitis, bacteremia, or active infection

The Procedure

Step 1. The layout of the double V-to-Y-plasty is based on the fusiform excision. Measure and mark the extent of the excision, including appropriate surgical margins (see Appendix D). Lay out the fusiform shape with the usual 3:1 length-to-width ratio, with the long axis parallel with the lines of least skin tension (see Appendix B: Lines of Lesser Skin Tension (Langer)). Square the ends of the planned triangular flaps.

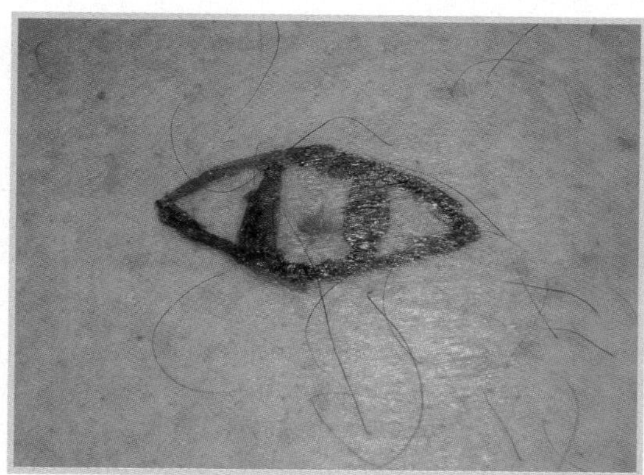

Step 1

Step 2. Prep the skin with povidone-iodine or chlorhexidine solution, and allow it to dry (see Appendix E). Incise the outline of the fusiform incision. Skin incisions are made through the full thickness of the skin. Do not undermine the flap itself, because the blood supply for this island pedicle flap comes from the pedicle beneath. The flap based on the fusiform shape usually has enough mobility to allow for closure of the defect.

- **PEARL:** Prep a wide area so that an undraped area is not inadvertently exposed if the drape slides a little.

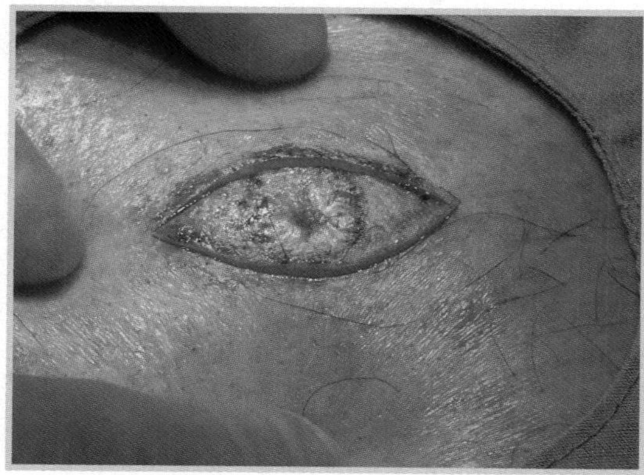

Step 2

Step 3. Finish excising the lesion (with its surgical margins) by making two straight incisions perpendicular to the long axis of the fusiform.

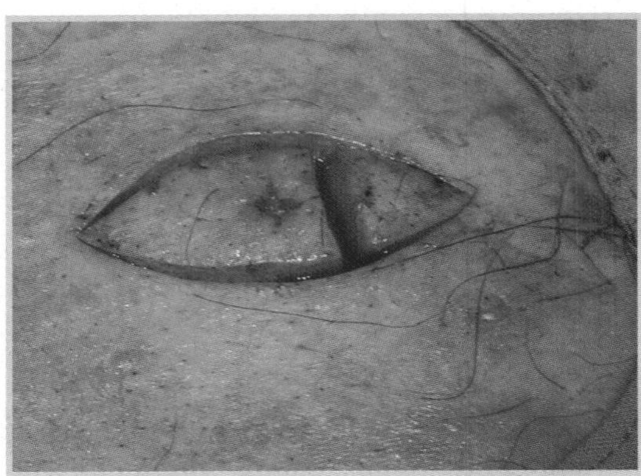

Step 3

Step 4. Remove the specimen and place in a specimen container to send it for pathologic examination. Clamp or tie off any bleeding at the base of the excision.

- PITFALL: Bleeding from the flap base will impede healing and promote flap necrosis.

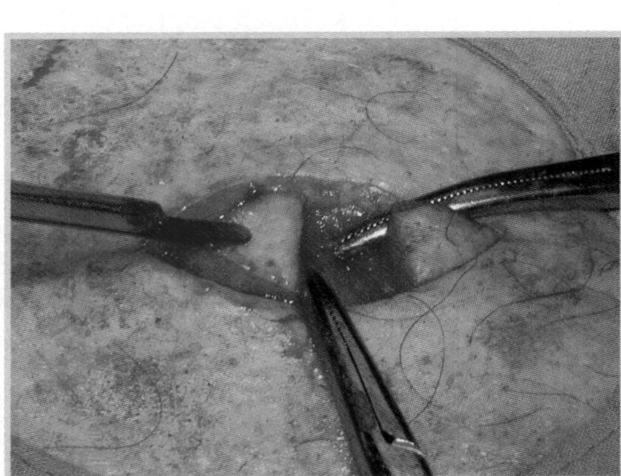

Step 4

Step 5. Make sure the dermis around the pedicles is completely bisected.

- PITFALL: Do not undermine the flap itself, because the blood supply for this flap comes from the pedicle beneath. If the pedicle is undermined for any reason, convert the procedure to a fusiform excision.

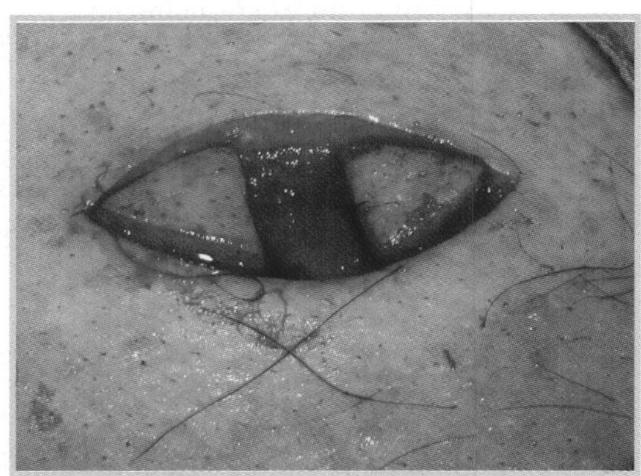

Step 5

Step 6. Start the closure by suturing the two straight margins together in the center of the defect using a simple interrupted suture or vertical mattress suture. See Chapters 38 and 43.

- **PEARL:** The use of loupe magnification may assist the performance of this technique; a 4-0 to 5-0 suture will produce fewer suture marks.

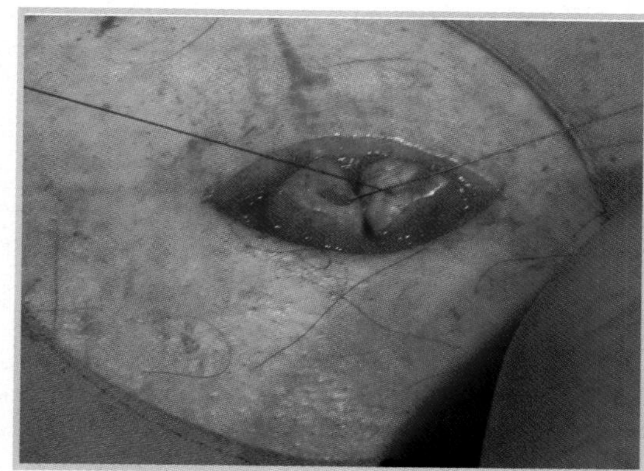

Step 6

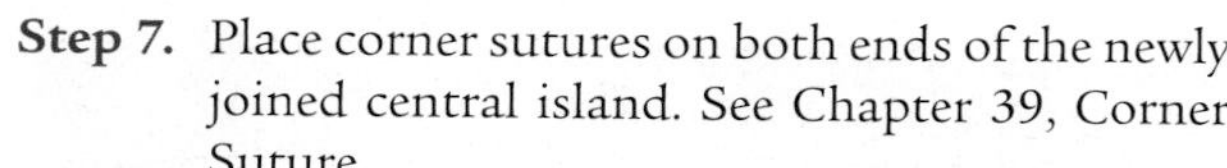

Step 7. Place corner sutures on both ends of the newly joined central island. See Chapter 39, Corner Suture.

- **PITFALL:** Make sure to maintain the same depth in the dermis throughout each corner suture.

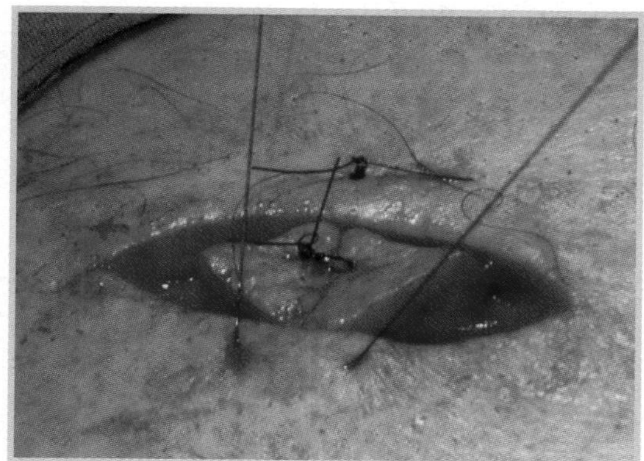

Step 7

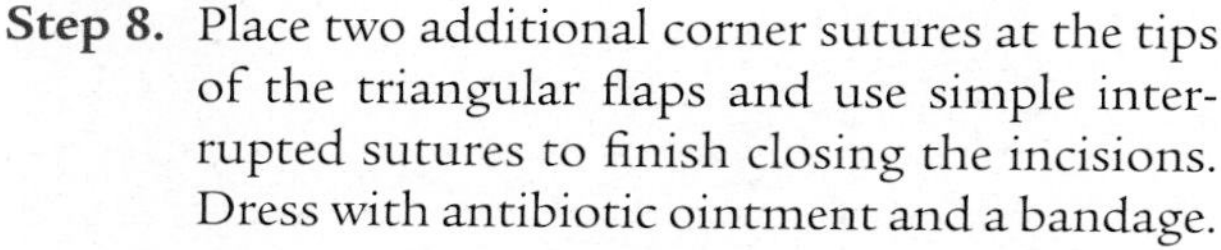

Step 8. Place two additional corner sutures at the tips of the triangular flaps and use simple interrupted sutures to finish closing the incisions. Dress with antibiotic ointment and a bandage.

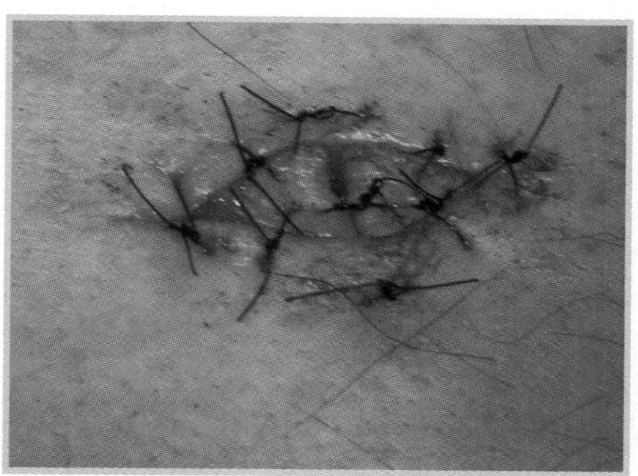

Step 8

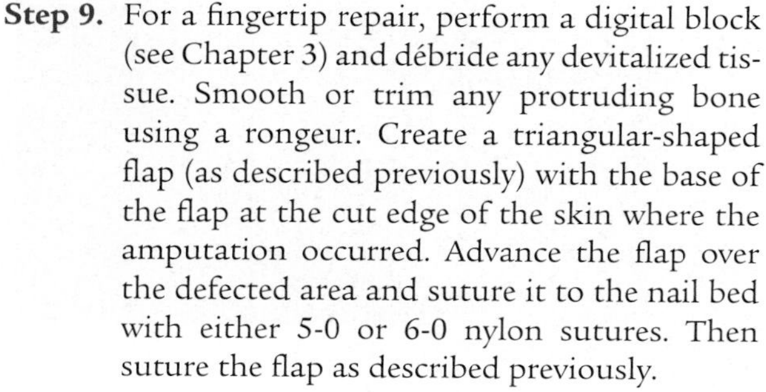

Step 9. For a fingertip repair, perform a digital block (see Chapter 3) and débride any devitalized tissue. Smooth or trim any protruding bone using a rongeur. Create a triangular-shaped flap (as described previously) with the base of the flap at the cut edge of the skin where the amputation occurred. Advance the flap over the defected area and suture it to the nail bed with either 5-0 or 6-0 nylon sutures. Then suture the flap as described previously.

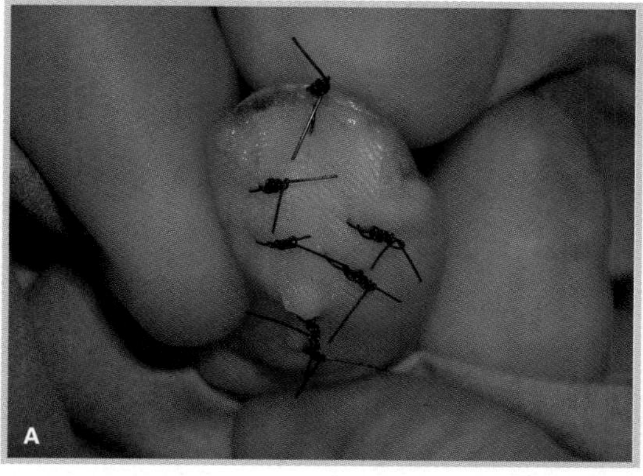

A

- **PEARL:** The flap should be as wide as the greatest width of the amputation.

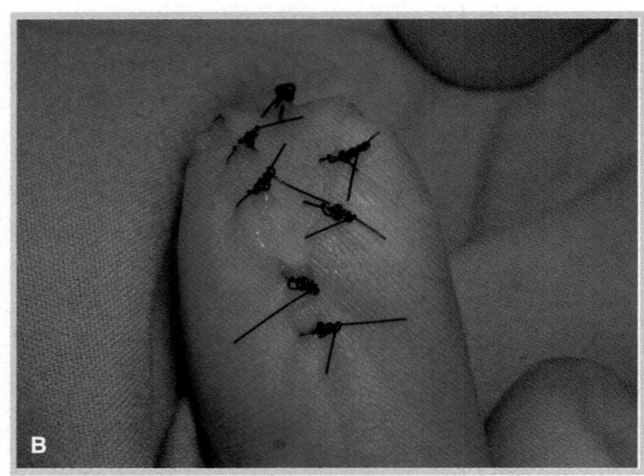

Step 9

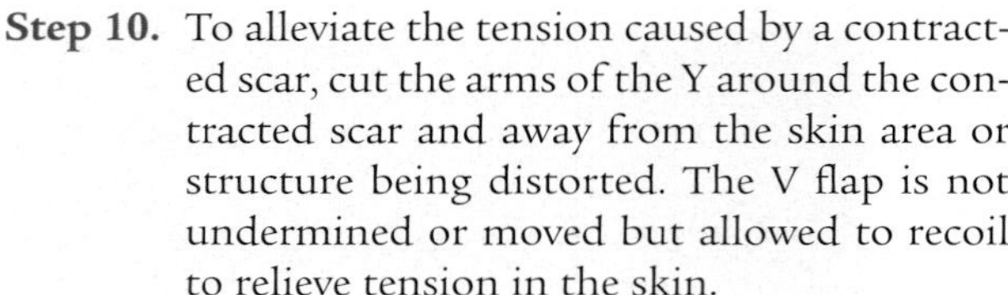

Step 10. To alleviate the tension caused by a contracted scar, cut the arms of the Y around the contracted scar and away from the skin area or structure being distorted. The V flap is not undermined or moved but allowed to recoil to relieve tension in the skin.

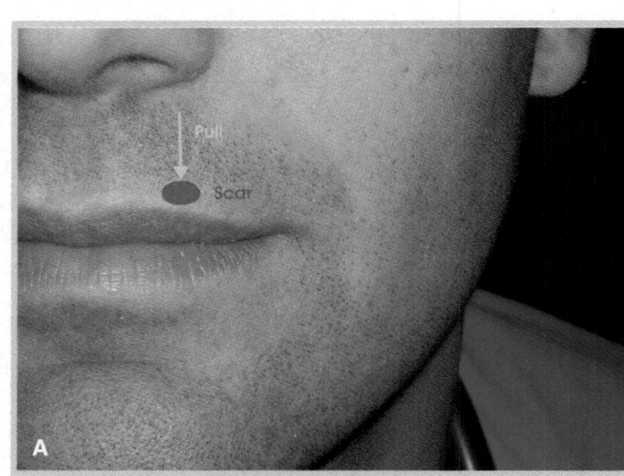

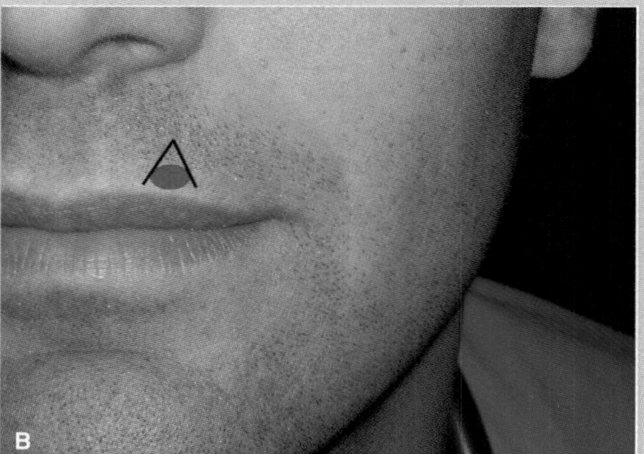

Then the Y-shaped suture line is created as described before.

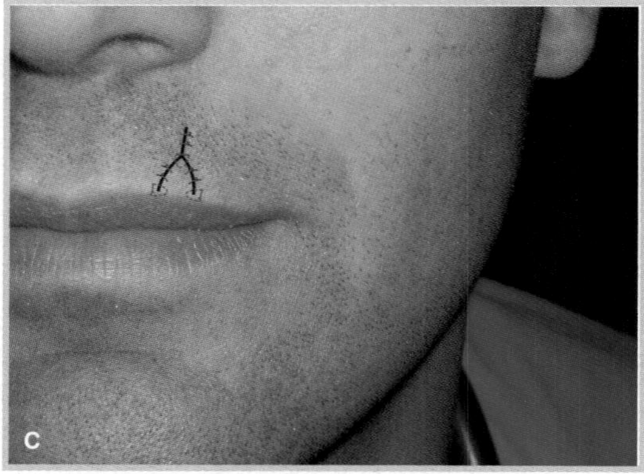

Step 10

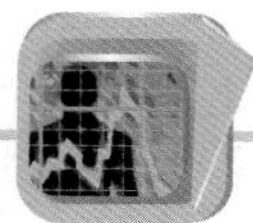

Complications

- Pain, infection, and bleeding
- Nonunion of skin edges
- Scar formation
- Tissue sloughing, usually due to excess tension or the blood supply being disrupted by undermining
- Sensory changes, which often subside with time

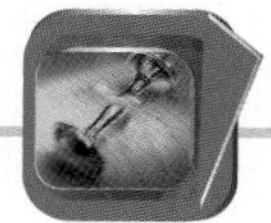

Pediatric Considerations

Generally, pediatric skin has excellent blood flow and heals very well. However, pediatric patients often find it difficult to sit or lie still during lengthy procedures. The patient's maturity and ability to cooperate should be considered before deciding to attempt any outpatient procedure.

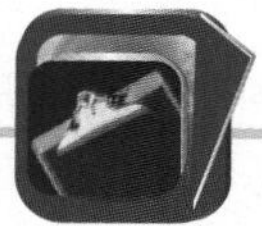

Postprocedure Instructions

Have the patient keep the bandage on and the wound dry for the first 24 hours. After that, it can be cleaned with hydrogen peroxide or gently washed with soap and water as needed. An antibiotic ointment and bandage should be reapplied until the patient returns or for 2 weeks. Have the patient report signs of infection. Schedule a return appointment for suture removal (see Appendix J).

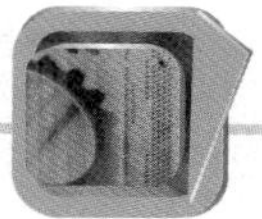

Coding Information

These codes encompass excision or repair, or both, by adjacent transfer or rearrangement, including Z-plasty, W-plasty, V-to-Y-plasty, rotation flaps, advancement flaps, and double-pedicle flaps. When applied to traumatic wounds, the defect must be developed by the surgeon because the closure requires it, and these codes should not be used for direct closure of a defect that incidentally results in the configuration of one of the flaps or plasties. If the configurations result incidentally from the laceration shape, closure should be

CPT Code	Description	2008 Average 50th Percentile Fee	Global Period
14000	Trunk $\leq$10 cm^2	$1,062.00	90
14001	Trunk 10.1–30.0 cm^2	$1,400.00	90
14020	SAL $\leq$10 cm^2	$1,222.00	90
14021	SAL 10.1–30.0^2	$1,684.00	90
14040	FCCMNAGHF $\leq$10 cm^2	$1,551.00	90
14041	FCCMNAGHF 10.1–30.0 cm^2	$1,757.00	90
14060	ENEL $\leq$10 cm^2	$1,841.00	90
14061	ENEL 10.1–30.0 cm^2	$2,254.00	90
14300	Any unusual or complicated area >30 cm^2	$2,749.00	90

CPT is a registered trademark of the American Medical Association.
2008 average 50th Percentile Fees are provided courtesy of 2008 MMH-SI's copyrighted Physicians' Fees and Coding Guide.
SAL, scalp, arms, or legs; FCCMNAGHF, forehead, cheeks, chin, mouth, neck, axillae, genitalia, hands, or feet; and ENEL, eyelids, nose, ears, or lips.

reported using simple repair codes. All of the following codes are for adjacent tissue transfer or rearrangement, and they refer to defects in the trunk or the following sites: scalp, arms, or legs (SAL); forehead, cheeks, chin, mouth, neck, axillae, genitalia, hands, or feet (FCCMNAGHF); and eyelids, nose, ears, or lips (ENEL).

Bibliography

Baker SR. Reconstructive surgery for skin cancer. In Rigel DS, Friedman RJ, Dzubow LM, et al., eds. *Cancer of the Skin*. New York: Elsevier; 2005:573–592.

Dautel G, Corcella D, Merle M. Reconstruction of fingertip amputations by partial composite toe transfer with short vascular pedicle. *J Hand Surg [Br]*. 1998;23:457–464.

Dilek ON, Bekerecioglu M. Role of simple V-Y advancement flap in the treatment of complicated pilonidal sinus. *Eur J Surg*. 1998;164:961–964.

Jackson EA. The V-Y plasty in the treatment of fingertip amputations. *Am Fam Physician*. 2001;64:455–458.

Kapetansky KI. Double pendulum flaps for whistling deformities in bilateral cleft lips. *Plast Reconstr Surg*. 1971;47:321–324.

Kutler W. Clinical notes, suggestions and new instruments: A new method for finger tip amputations. *JAMA*. 1947;133:29–30.

Lee HB, Kim SW, Lew DH, et al. Unilateral multilayered musculocutaneous V-Y advancement flap for the treatment of pressure sore. *Plast Reconstr Surg*. 1997;100:340–345.

Maruyama Y, Iwahira Y, Ebihara H. V-Y advancement flaps in the reconstruction of skin defects of the posterior heel and ankle. *Plast Reconstr Surg*. 1990;85:759–761.

Nilson RZ, Dockery GL. V-Y plasty and its variants. *J Am Podiatr Med Assoc*. 1995;85:22–27.

Parry S, Park R, Park C. Fasciocutaneous V-Y advancement flap for repair of sacral defects. *Ann Plast Surg*. 1989;22:543–546.

Rosenthal EA. Treatment of fingertip and nail bed injuries. *Orthop Clin North Am*. 1983;14:675–697.

Zook EG, Van Beak AL, Russel RC, et al. V-Y advancement flap for facial defects. *Plast Reconstr Surg*. 1980;65:786–789.

Zuber TJ. *Advanced Soft Tissue Surgery*. Kansas City: American Academy of Family Physicians; 1999:80–85.

2008 MAG Mutual Healthcare Solutions, Inc.'s Physicians' Fee and Coding Guide. Duluth, Georgia. MAG Mutual Healthcare Solutions, Inc. 2007.

CHAPTER 61

Z-plasty

E. J. Mayeaux, Jr., MD, DABFP, FAAFP
Professor of Family Medicine, Professor of Obstetrics and Gynecology
Louisiana State University Health Sciences Center, Shreveport, LA

Historically, Z-plasty has been a commonly taught and used technique in plastic surgery. It is a type of transposition flap that incorporates principles of both advancement and rotation flaps in its design and execution. Many variations of Z-plasty have been developed, but this chapter focuses on the more common, basic 60-degree Z-plasty technique. The procedure uses the transposition of two triangular flaps to produce a Z-shaped wound. The main indication for performing Z-plasty is to change the direction of a wound so that it aligns more closely with the resting skin tension lines, or so that a scar runs through (instead of across) a joint line. Because the technique increases the length of skin available in a desired direction, Z-plasty also is used to correct contracted scars across flexor creases. The 60-degree Z-plasty lengthens the total scar by 75%.

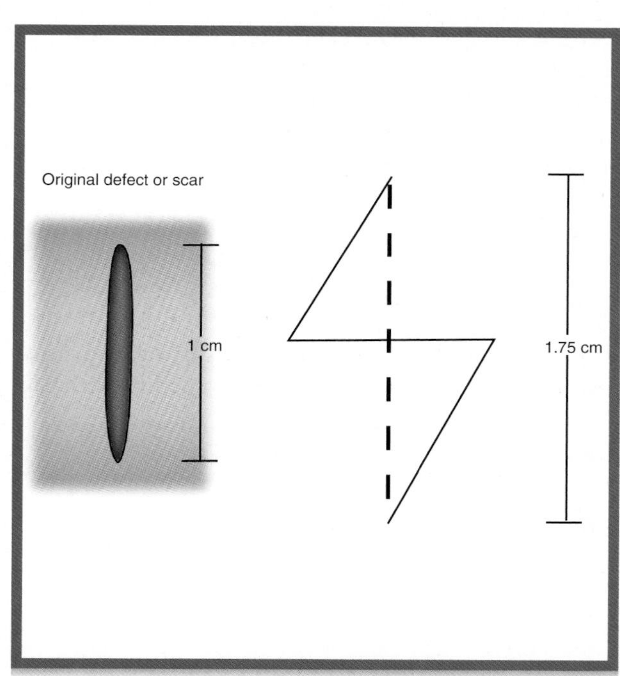

The key to a well-designed Z-plasty is symmetry. The length of each lateral limb and the central limb must all be equal. Also the two lateral limb–central limb angles must always be mirror images. This allows the subsequently developed flaps to be easily interchanged. A 60-degree angle between the central limb and the lateral limbs produces the best outcome. This creates two 30–60–90-degree right triangles, which rotates the central line 90 degrees when the flaps are transposed. The two-dimensional geometry dictates that the point-to-point length of the final scar is equal to the square root of three times the length of the original scar or incision.

When considering the use of a Z-plasty, some physicians theoretically object to the creation of a wound that is three times as long as the original wound in the final maximal length (i.e., the two diagonal arms are as long as the central wound). Although the creation of long wounds is generally discouraged, a well-designed Z-plasty can significantly improve the cosmetic and functional outcome. Z-plasty can be performed on a fresh wound that is counter to the resting skin tension lines, although some experts recommend simple closure of the wound and then Z-plasty at a later date to revise scars that are problematic. Physicians with the opportunity to frequently perform Z-plasty observe generally favorable functional and cosmetic outcomes.

When performing a Z-plasty, the skin surgeon must practice meticulous attention to technique. When possible, advise the patient to stop taking anticoagulants or aspirin before the surgery. Prophylactic antibiotics may be considered for use in patients with diabetes and in other immunocompromised patients, but data supporting the efficacy of this approach are lacking. The "trapdoor effect," elevation of central tissue resulting from a downward contraction of a surrounding scar, may be avoided by employing sufficient undermining of tissues surrounding the flap site. Multiple contiguous Z-plasties may be used to break up a long scar line.

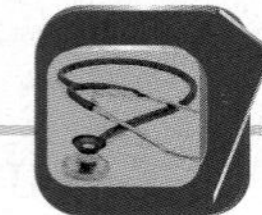

Equipment

- Surgery tray instruments are listed in Appendix G. Consider adding skin hooks to gently handle the skin flaps. Have at least three fine (mosquito) hemostats to assist with hemostasis while developing large skin flaps.
- Suggested suture removal times are listed in Appendix J, and a suggested anesthesia tray that can be used for this procedure is listed in Appendix F. All instruments can be ordered through local surgical supply houses.

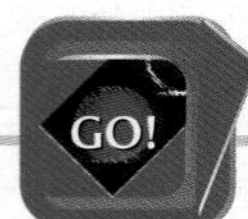

Indications

- Revision of contractures or scars that cross flexor creases and result in bowstring-type scars (e.g., vertical scars over the flexor creases of the proximal interphalangeal joints of the hands)
- Revision of scars that traverse concavities (e.g., across a deep nasolabial fold, a vertical scar that traverses between the lower lip and the chin)
- Redirection of wounds that are perpendicular to joint lines or the lines of least skin tension (i.e., reorient to a direction that will produce a cosmetically superior result)
- Creation of wound irregularity (i.e., improved cosmetic results with a line that is broken up or zigzag versus a long, straight line that is less appealing)
- Repositioning of poorly positioned tissues that produce a trapdoor effect (i.e., rearranging a circular scar that is causing the central tissue to raise upward)

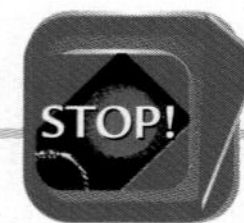

Contraindications

- Poor skin vascular supply
- Diseases causing poor vascular supply to the skin (e.g., atherosclerotic heart disease, diabetes, smoking, collagen vascular disease, prior irradiation, severe anemia, anticoagulation)
- History of poor wound healing, hypertrophic scarring, or keloid formation
- Uncooperative patient
- Presence of cellulitis, bacteremia, or active infection

The Procedure

Step 1. The original wound or scar is perpendicular to the line of the nasolabial fold. Contraction of the scar will produce an obvious scar. Prep and drape the area (see Appendix E, Skin Preparation Recommendations). Administer a field block (see Chapter 2, Field Block Anesthesia).

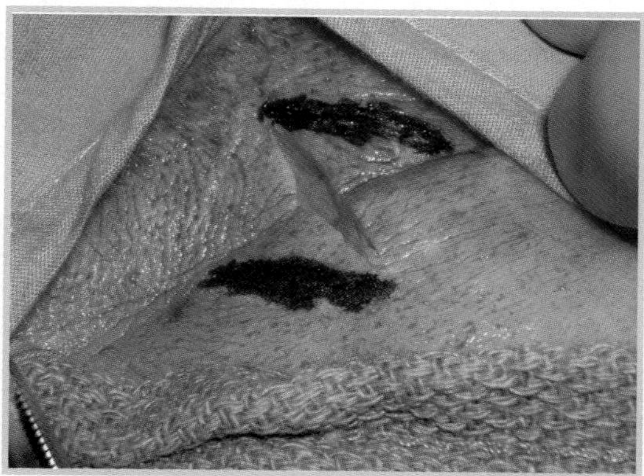

Step 1

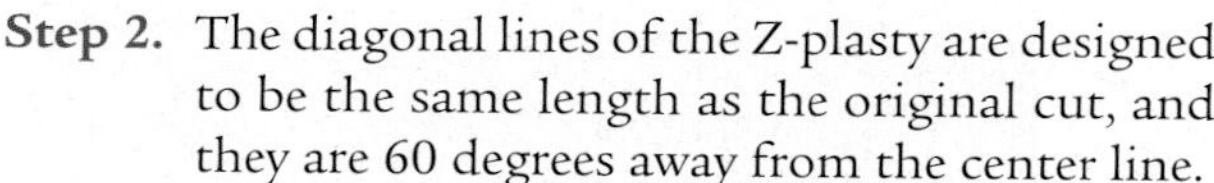

Step 2. The diagonal lines of the Z-plasty are designed to be the same length as the original cut, and they are 60 degrees away from the center line.

- PITFALL: Novice providers occasionally make the error of performing their first Z-plasty with the arms on the same side of the central wound. Drawing the proposed Z-plasty helps prevent this problem.
- PITFALL: Many providers unintentionally incise the diagonal lines at 45-degree angles, rather than 60-degree angles. Flaps in a 45-degree Z-plasty are easier to transpose but only rotate the direction of the original defect by 60 to 70 degrees (rather than 90 degrees with a 60-degree Z-plasty).

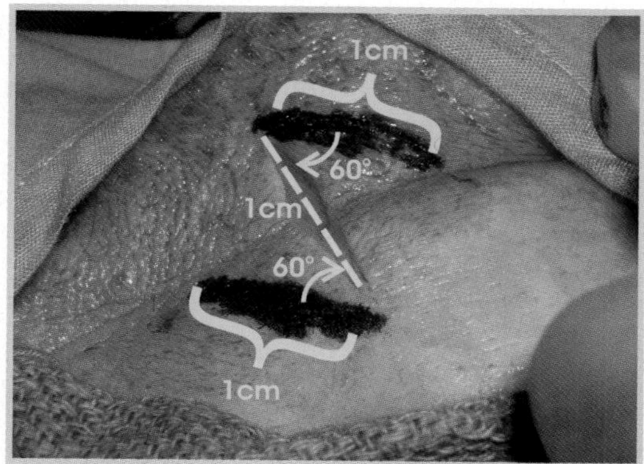

Step 2

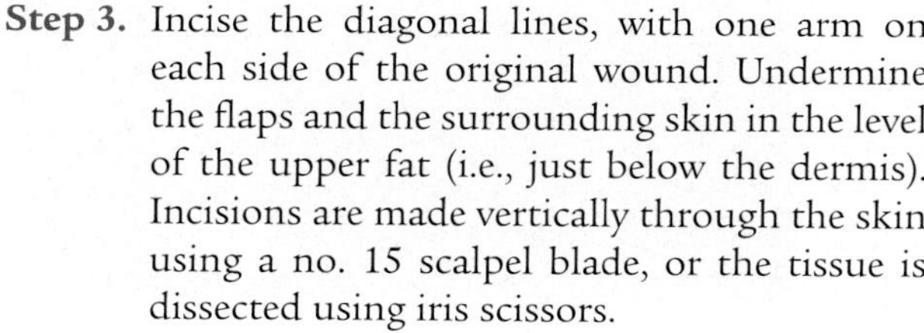

Step 3. Incise the diagonal lines, with one arm on each side of the original wound. Undermine the flaps and the surrounding skin in the level of the upper fat (i.e., just below the dermis). Incisions are made vertically through the skin using a no. 15 scalpel blade, or the tissue is dissected using iris scissors.

- PITFALL: Failure to undermine extensively makes the transposition very difficult. Liberal undermining is beneficial.
- PITFALL: Undermine the flaps just below the dermal-fat junction. If too much subcutaneous tissue is attached to the flap, a poorer cosmetic result may result.

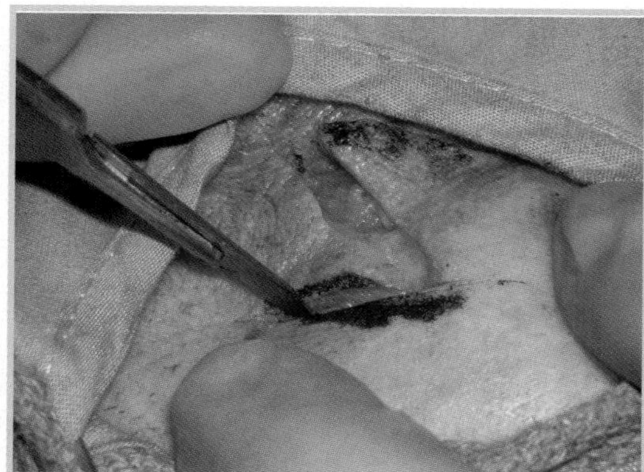

Step 3

Step 4. Transpose the flaps. The upper right flap from above is pulled down and rotated 90-degrees to become the bottom (left-pointing) flap, and the lower left flap from above is pulled up and rotated ninety-degrees to become the upper (right-pointing flap. Note that the ventral line is now in line with the nasolabial fold.

- **PITFALL:** Handle the flaps gently, grasping the skin with skin hooks or Adson forceps without teeth. Many physicians transpose the flaps with toothed forceps, causing tears or damage to the flaps and adding unnecessary scarring.

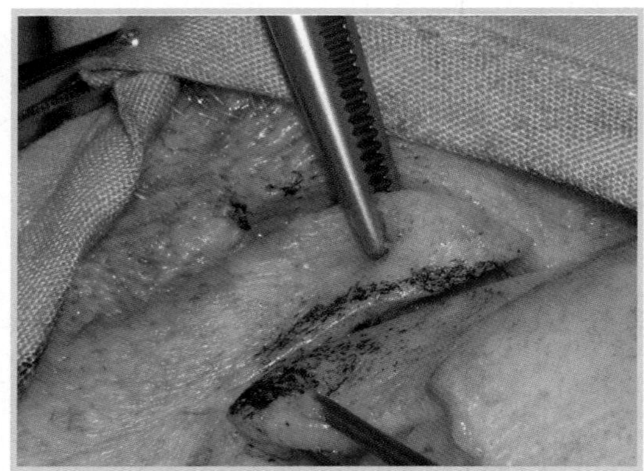

Step 4

Step 5. Place corner stitches in the corners of each flap.

- **PEARL:** Consider half-buried, horizontal mattress sutures in place of the simple interrupted sutures (see Chapter 39).
- **PITFALL:** Almost all 60-degree Z-plasties performed on human skin result in some pouching upward, or dog-ear formation, at the base of the flap after transposition. They will usually flatten with time, resulting in a good cosmetic outcome.

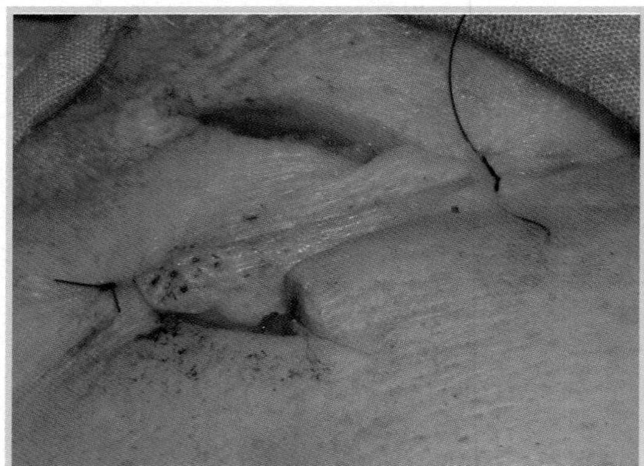

Step 5

Step 6. Place simple interrupted sutures to finish closing the suture lines. Keep the stitches on the diagonals to a minimum, and do not place the diagonal stitches near the corners.

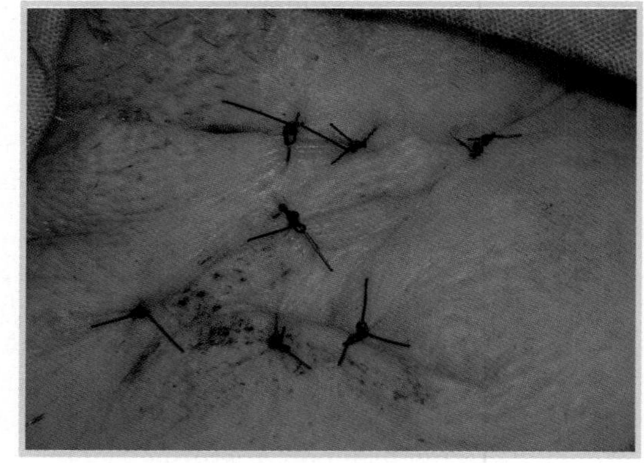

Step 6

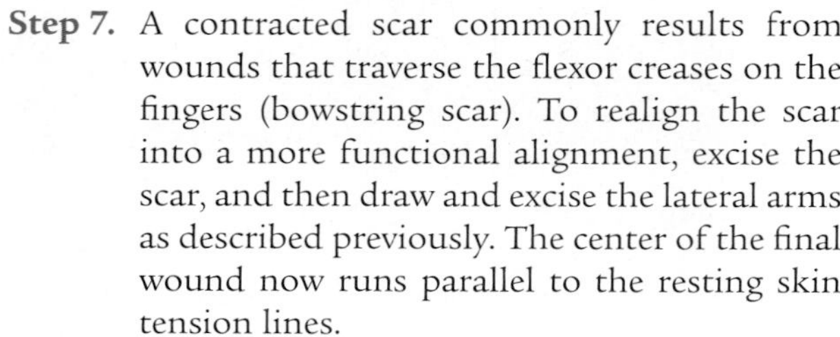

Step 7. A contracted scar commonly results from wounds that traverse the flexor creases on the fingers (bowstring scar). To realign the scar into a more functional alignment, excise the scar, and then draw and excise the lateral arms as described previously. The center of the final wound now runs parallel to the resting skin tension lines.

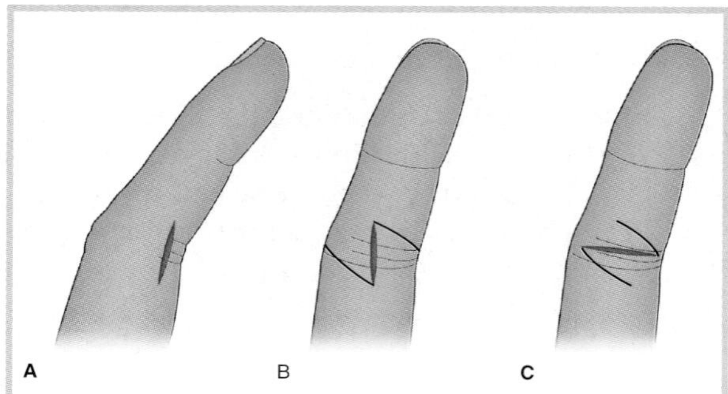

Step 7

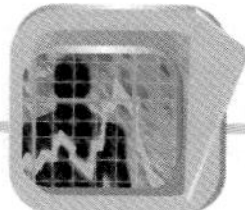

Complications

- Pain, infection, and bleeding
- Nonunion of skin edges
- Scar formation
- Sensory changes, which often subside with time
- Flap necrosis
- Hematoma formation
- Sloughing of the flap caused by high wound tension
- Trapdoor effect
- Increased scar length and two additional required incisions

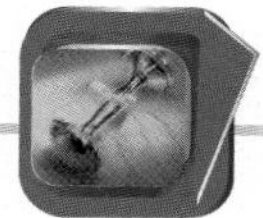

Pediatric Considerations

Generally, pediatric skin has excellent blood flow and heals very well. However, pediatric patients often find it difficult to sit or lie still during lengthy procedures. The patient's maturity and ability to cooperate should be considered before deciding to attempt any outpatient procedure.

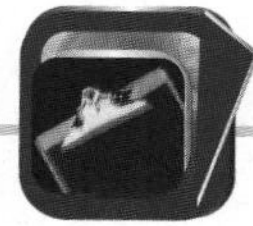

Postprocedure Instructions

Apply topical antibiotics and a pressure dressing after the procedure. Have the patient keep the bandage on and the wound dry for the first 24 hours. After that, it can be cleaned with hydrogen peroxide or gently washed with soap and water as needed. An antibiotic ointment and bandage should be reapplied until the patient returns or for 2 weeks. Have the patient report signs of infection. Schedule a return appointment for suture removal (see Appendix J, Recommended Suture Removal Times).

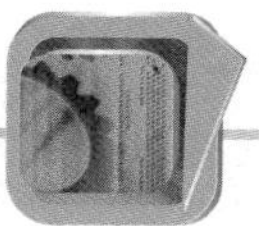

Coding Information

These codes encompass excision or repair, or both, by adjacent transfer or rearrangement, including Z-plasty, W-plasty, V-to-Y-plasty, rotation flaps, advancement flaps, and double-

CPT Code	Description	2008 Average 50th Percentile Fee	Global Period
14000	Trunk ≤10 cm^2	$1,062.00	90
14001	Trunk 10.1–30.0 cm^2	$1,400.00	90
14020	SAL ≤10 cm^2	$1,222.00	90
14021	SAL 10.1–30.0^2	$1,684.00	90
14040	FCCMNAGHF ≤10 cm^2	$1,551.00	90
14041	FCCMNAGHF 10.1–30.0 cm^2	$1,757.00	90
14060	ENEL ≤10 cm^2	$1,841.00	90
14061	ENEL 10.1–30.0 cm^2	$2,254.00	90
14300	Any unusual or complicated area >30 cm^2	$2,749.00	90

CPT is a registered trademark of the American Medical Association.
2008 average 50th Percentile Fees are provided courtesy of 2008 MMH-SI's copyrighted Physicians' Fees and Coding Guide.
SAL, scalp, arms, or legs; FCCMNAGHF, forehead, cheeks, chin, mouth, neck, axillae, genitalia, hands, or feet; and ENEL, eyelids, nose, ears, or lips.

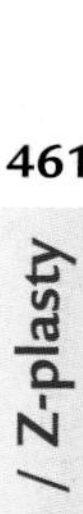

pedicle flaps. When applied to traumatic wounds, the defect must be developed by the surgeon because the closure requires it, and these codes should not be used for direct closure of a defect that incidentally results in the configuration of one of the flaps or plasties. If the configurations result incidentally from the laceration shape, closure should be reported using simple repair codes.

Patient Education Handout

A patient education handout, "Scar Repair using a Z-plasty," can be found on the book's companion Web site, .

Bibliography

Borges AF, Alexander JE. Relaxed skin tension lines, Z-plasties on scars, and fusiform excision of lesions. *Br J Plast Surg.* 1962;15:242–254.

Dingman, R. O. Some application of the Z-plastic procedure. *Plast Reconstr Surg.* 1955;16:246.

Dzubow LM. Z-plasty mechanics. *J Dermatol Surg Oncol.* 1994;20:108.

Furnas DW, Fischer GW. The Z-plasty: biomechanics and mathematics. *Br J Plast Surg.* 1971;24:144.

Gahankari D. Z-plasty template: an innovation in Z-plasty fashioning. *Plast Reconstr Surg.* 1996;97:1196–1199.

Hudson DA. Some thoughts on choosing a Z-plasty: the Z made simple. *Plast Reconstr Surg.* 2000;106:665–671.

Johnson SC, Bennett RG. Double Z-plasty to enhance rhombic flap mobility. *J Dermatol Surg Oncol.* 1994;20:128–132.

Lesavoy MA, Weatherley-White RCA. The integument. In: Hill GJ, ed. *Outpatient Surgery.* 3rd ed. Philadelphia: WB Saunders; 1988:123–148.

McCarthy JG. Introduction to plastic surgery. In: McCarthy JG, ed. *Plastic Surgery*. Philadelphia: WB Saunders; 1990:1–68.

McGregor A. The Z-plasty. *Br J Plast Surg.* 1966;19:82.

Micali G, Reali UM. Scars: traumatic and factitial. In: Parish LC, Lask GP, eds. *Aesthetic Dermatology*. New York: McGraw-Hill; 1991:84–95.

Robson MC, Zachary LS. Repair of traumatic cutaneous injuries involving the skin and soft tissue. In: Georgiade GS, Georgiade NS, Riefkohl R, et al., eds. *Textbook of Plastic, Maxillofacial, and Reconstructive Surgery*. 2nd ed. Baltimore: Williams & Wilkins; 1987:129–140.

Rohrich RJ, Zbar RI. A simplified algorithm for the use of Z-plasty. *Plast Reconstr Surg.* 1999;103:1513–1517.

Salam GA, Amin JP. The basic Z-Plasty. *Am Fam Physician*. 2003;67:2329–32.

Sclafini AP, Parker AJ. Z-plasty. E-medicine. Available at http://www.emedicine.com/ENT/topic652.htm

Stegman SJ, Tromovitch TA, Glogau RG. *Basics of Dermatologic Surgery*. Chicago: Year Book Medical Publishing; 1982.

Stegman SJ. Fifteen ways to close surgical wounds. *J Dermatol Surg.* 1975;1:25–31.

Zuber TJ. *Skin Biopsy, Excision, and Repair Techniques*. Kansas City, MO: American Academy of Family Physicians; 1998:52–61.

2008 MAG Mutual Healthcare Solutions, Inc.'s Physicians' Fee and Coding Guide. Duluth, Georgia. MAG Mutual Healthcare Solutions, Inc. 2007.

SECTION SIX

Nail Procedures

CHAPTER 62

Digital Mucous Cyst Removal

E. J. Mayeaux, Jr., MD, DABFP, FAAFP
Professor of Family Medicine, Professor of Obstetrics and Gynecology
Louisiana State University Health Sciences Center, Shreveport, LA

Digital mucous (myxoid) cysts are flesh-colored nodules that appear on fingers between the distal interphalangeal (DIP) joint and the proximal nail fold. Also known as digital myxoid cysts, the lesions are usually 3 to 12 mm in diameter, solitary, and more common on the dominant hand. The cysts typically appear just lateral to the midline. The lesions are more common in middle-aged to older adults and rarely are encountered on the toes. Women are affected twice as often as men. The lesions would be better described as pseudocysts because they lack a true epithelial lining.

Two different types of cysts have been identified. One type is associated with degenerative arthritis of the DIP joint and can appear similar to ganglions or synovial cysts. These lesions often have an identifiable stalk that can be traced back to the joint. The second type is independent of the joint and arises from metabolic derangement of the soft tissue fibroblasts. These lesions are associated with the localized production of hyaluronic acid.

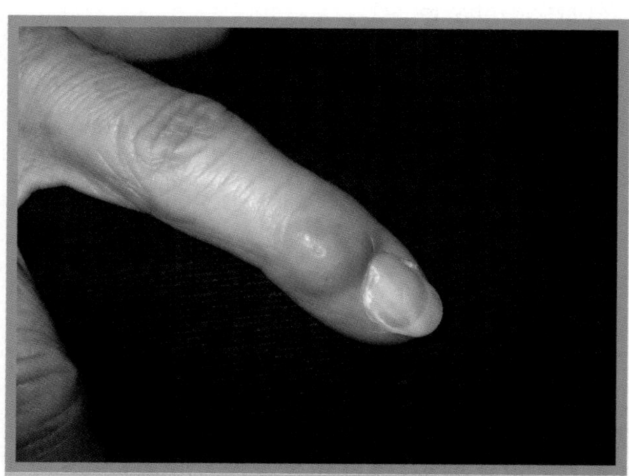

Patients may be asymptomatic or report pain, tenderness, or nail deformity associated with the lesion. Nail ridging is observed in up to one third of patients; a prior history of trauma may be reported by those younger than 40 years of age. One longitudinal study found that the cysts occasionally regress spontaneously.

Asymptomatic lesions may remain stable for years and can be observed without treatment. Many different treatment regimens have been suggested for symptomatic digital mucous cysts. Aggressive surgery with removal of the cyst and underlying osteophytes may produce the fewest recurrences. Osteophyte removal alone (without cyst removal) also appears effective. Osteophyte removal has been associated with higher cost and complications of joint stiffness, loss of motion, and nail deformity.

Simpler treatment interventions also have been advocated. Repeated needling of the cyst can provide cure rates in up to 70% of cases. At least two to five punctures appear to be necessary for cyst resolution, and patients can be provided with sterile needles for home treatment. Aspiration and injection of an equal mixture of 0.2 mL of 1% lidocaine

(Xylocaine) and 0.2 mL of triamcinolone acetonide (Kenalog, 10 mg/mL) has been advocated historically, but the high rate of recurrence limits this technique.

Cryosurgical, chemical, or electrosurgical ablation of the cyst base is effective in eradicating the cyst. If freezing is employed, repeated freeze–thaw–freeze technique appears superior to a single freeze. Even with proper cryosurgical technique, there is a 10% to 15% recurrence rate. Carbon dioxide lasers also are being used to ablate the cyst base. A simple office excision technique is described in this chapter. Because infection is a common complication of mucous cyst treatments, some providers recommend prophylactic antibiotics for 3 days postoperatively.

Historically, sclerotherapy was considered an appropriate method of treatment. However, sclerotherapy is now considered a dangerous approach because of the potential for extravasation of the chemical into the joint or tendon sheath with resultant scarring.

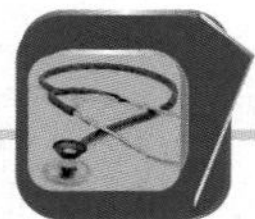

Equipment

- A standard office surgery tray, as described in Appendix G, should be available for the excision procedure.
- A suggested anesthesia tray that can be used for this procedure is listed in Appendix F.

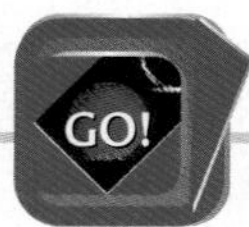

Indications

- Symptomatic nodules on the dorsum of the finger between the DIP joint and proximal nail fold

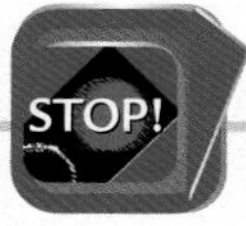

Contraindications (Relative)

- Uncooperative patient
- Presence of cellulitis, bacteremia, or active infection
- Heavy smokers and insulin-dependent diabetics (increased risk of complications)

The Procedure

Needling

Step 1. Clean the skin surface with an alcohol wipe, and enter the cyst with a 25-gauge needle. Pass the needle through the wall of the cyst 5 to 10 times. Multiple needle sticks separated by days may be superior to multiple sticks during one session. The patient may be trained to repeat the procedure at home.

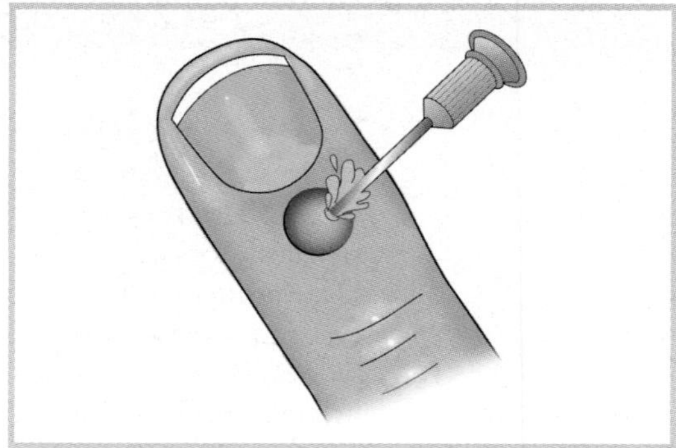

Step 1

Step 2. Clear, jelly-like contents will protrude and can be squeezed from the cyst.

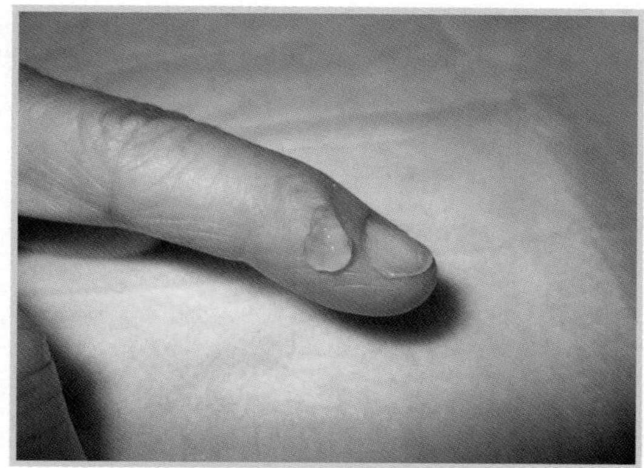

Courtesy of Dr. Scott Bergeaux.

Step 2

Ablation of the Cyst Base

Step 1. After the application of local or digital block anesthesia (see Chapters 1 and 3), shave off the skin and cyst roof using a horizontally held no. 15 scalpel blade. Apply the cryosurgery probe to the cyst base, and create an ice ball that extends outward onto 2 to 3 mm of the normal-appearing surrounding skin. Alternatively, spray the base with a liquid nitrogen sprayer to the same diameter. Use the freeze–thaw–freeze technique.

- PITFALL: Avoid prolonged freezing of the tissues, because notching of the proximal nail fold may develop. The length of the freeze is based on the observed size of the ice ball.

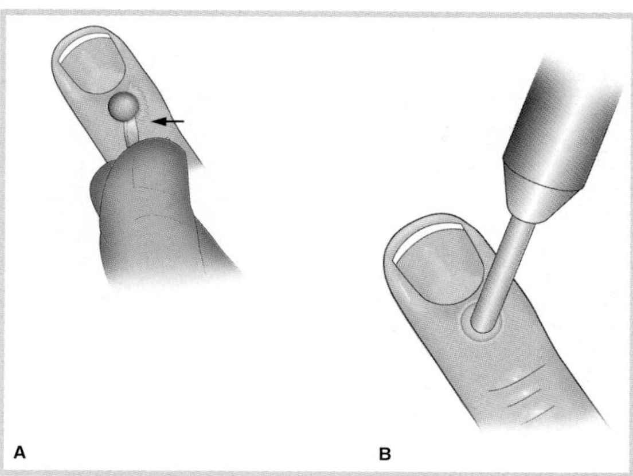

Step 1

Excision

Step 2. After digital anesthesia, the skin over the cyst is excised, and the cyst is dissected and excised from the surrounding tissues.

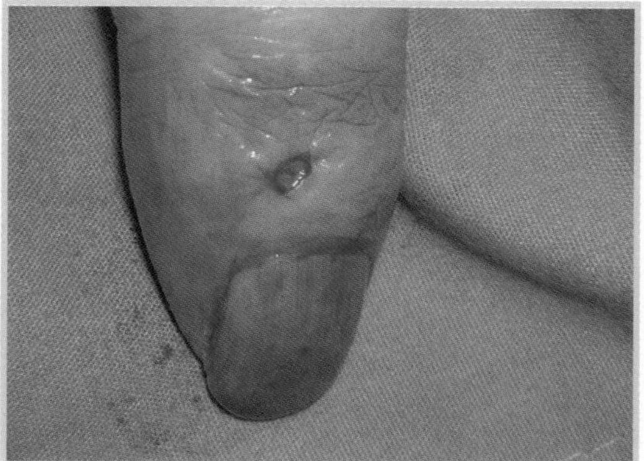

Step 2

Step 3. Incise a V-shaped base to this circular defect, creating a defect shaped like an ice cream cone.

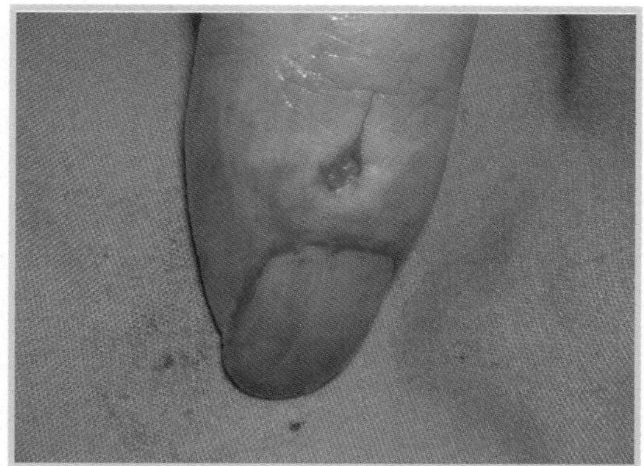

Step 3

Step 4. A small, inverted U-shaped rotation flap is incised and undermined from nearby skin on the dorsum of the finger.

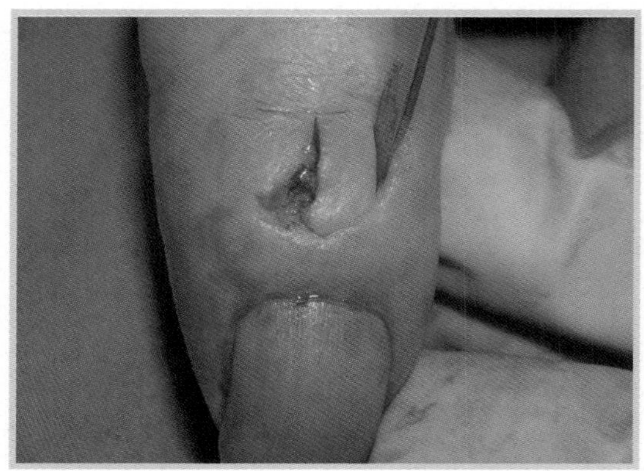

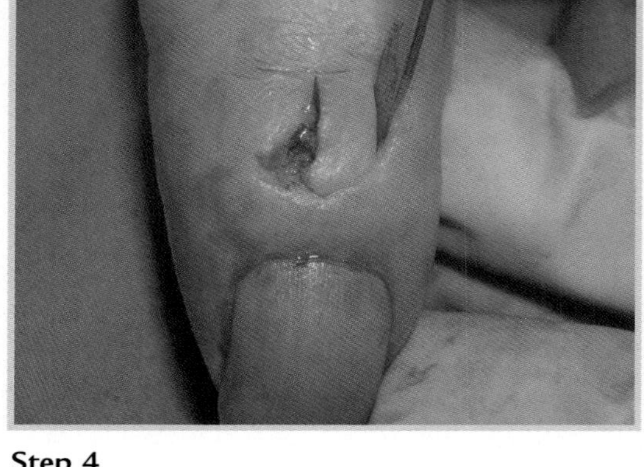

Step 4

Step 5. The flap may be moved over the defect and preferably left to heal to the wound bed. Note that suturing the flap may be preferable, because the larger wound produces scarring that may help to reduce cyst recurrence.

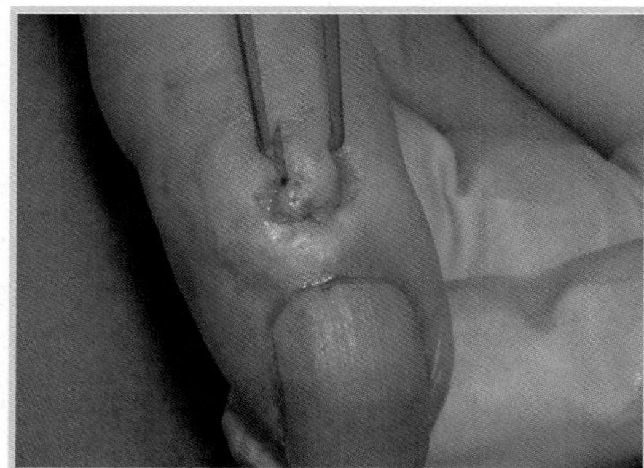

Step 5

Step 6. Often, the flap does not center over the wound, or excessive bleeding may occur. A single stitch on one or both sides of the flap can help alleviate these problems. Antibiotic ointment and splinting are provided after the procedure.

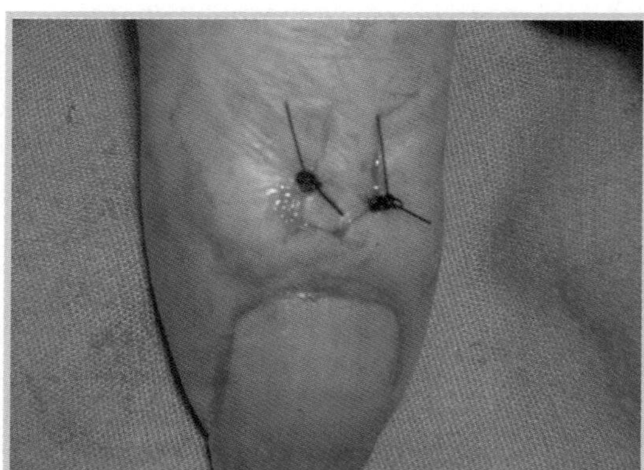

Step 6

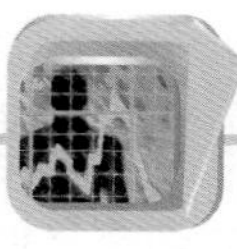

Complications

- Notching of the proximal nail fold
- Cyst recurrence
- Scarring of the nail matrix with nail dystrophy
- Local depigmentation after steroid injection
- Radial or ulnar deviation of the DIP joint
- Tendon injury
- DIP septic arthritis
- Persistent swelling
- Pain or numbness

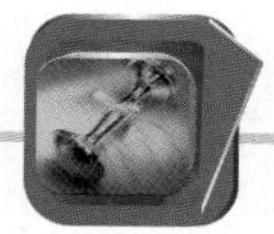

Pediatric Considerations

Digital mucous cysts are rare in childhood.

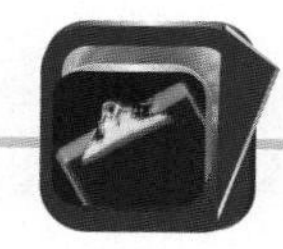

Postprocedure Instructions

Antibiotic ointment and a light gauze dressing are placed after cyst treatments. Gentle active range of motion is allowed, and sutures usually are removed after 2 weeks.

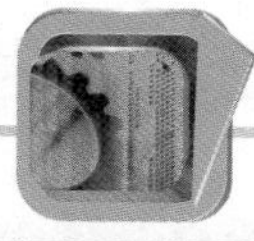

Coding Information and Supply Sources

CPT Code	Description	2008 Average 50th Percentile Fee	Global Period
20612	Aspiration or injection of ganglion cyst, any site	$135.00	0
26160	Excision of lesion of tendon sheath or joint capsule (mucous cyst)	$1,050.00	90

CPT is a registered trademark of the American Medical Association.
2008 average 50th Percentile Fees are provided courtesy of 2008 MMH-SI's copyrighted Physicians' Fees and Coding Guide.

Instrument and Materials Ordering

- A standard office surgery tray, as described in Appendix G, should be available for the excision procedure.
- A suggested anesthesia tray that can be used for this procedure is listed in Appendix F.
- Skin preparation recommendations appear in Appendix E.

Bibliography

Bennett RG. *Fundamentals of Cutaneous Surgery*. St. Louis: CV Mosby; 1988:754–756.

Dodge LD, Brown RL, Niebauer JJ, et al. The treatment of mucous cysts: long-term follow-up in sixty-two cases. *J Hand Surg Am.* 1984;9:901–904.

Epstein E. A simple technique for managing digital mucous cysts. *Arch Dermatol.* 1979;115:1315–1316.

Fritz GR, Stern PJ, Dickey M. Complications following mucous cyst excision. *J Hand Surg Br.* 1997;22:225–225.

Haneke E, Baran R. Nails: surgical aspects. In: Parish LC, Lask GP, eds. *Aesthetic Dermatology*. New York: McGraw-Hill; 1991:236–241.

Hernandez-Lugo AM, Dominguez-Cherit J, Vega-Memije AE. Digital mucoid cyst: the ganglion type. *Intl Dermatol.* 1999;38:531–538.

Salasche SJ. Myxoid cysts of the proximal nail fold: a surgical approach. *J Dermatol Surg Oncol.* 1984;1035–1039.

Singh D, Osterman AL. Mucous cyst. E-medicine. Available at http://www.emedicine.com/orthoped/topic520.htm. Accessed February 21, 2002.

Sonnex TS. Digital myxoid cysts: a review. *Cutis.* 1986;37:89–94.

Zuber TJ. Office management of digital mucous cysts. *Am Fam Physician.* 2001;64:1987–1990.

2008 MAG Mutual Healthcare Solutions, Inc.'s Physicians' Fee and Coding Guide. Duluth, Georgia. MAG Mutual Healthcare Solutions, Inc. 2007.

CHAPTER 63

Nail Avulsion and Matrixectomy

E. J. Mayeaux, Jr., MD, DABFP, FAAFP

Professor of Family Medicine, Professor of Obstetrics and Gynecology
Louisiana State University Health Sciences Center, Shreveport, LA

Nail avulsion is a commonly performed procedure in which all or a portion of the nail plate is removed from the nail bed. Avulsions may be done for both diagnostic and therapeutic indications. Avulsing the nail plate allows examination and visualization of lesions in the underlying nail bed and matrix. Nail avulsions are sometimes performed when treating onychomycosis to relieve pain from collection of subungual debris. Avulsions are most frequently done for ingrown and incurved nails.

Ingrown nails (onychocryptosis) is a common problem encountered in primary care practice. Individuals with ingrown nails often present in the second or third decades of life with pain, drainage, and difficulty walking. Ingrown nails are due to abnormal fit of the nail plate in the lateral groove, resulting in a foreign body reaction that produces edema, infection, and granulation tissue. This propensity may be exacerbated by the factors shown in Table 63-1. Some ingrown nails exhibit a laterally pointing spicule of nail that digs into the lateral tissue.

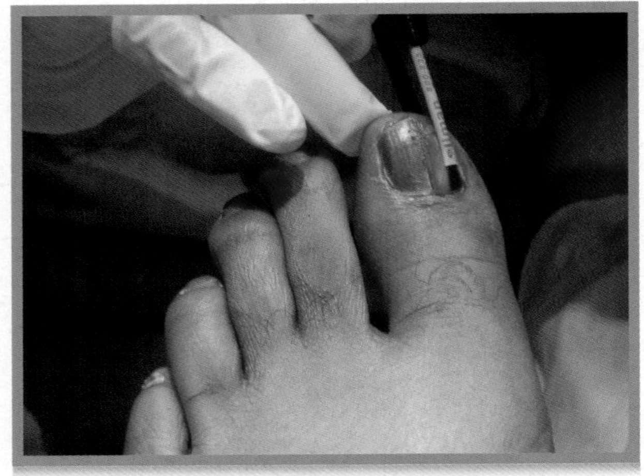

Three stages have been described for the progression of ingrown nails. In stage I, the lateral nail fold exhibits erythema, mild edema, and pain when pressure is applied. In stage II, individuals experience increased symptoms, drainage, and infection. Stage III is characterized by magnified symptoms, the presence of granulation tissue in the lateral nail fold, and lateral wall hypertrophy.

Many management options have been proposed for ingrown nails. Soaks, topical or systemic antibiotics, and insertion of a cotton wick into the lateral nail groove have all been used for stage I disease (Table 63-2). Surgical intervention is advocated for stage II and more often for stage III disease. Historically, simple nail avulsion or wedge resection of the distal corner of the nail has been performed. Because ingrown nails represent an abnormal lateral nail groove fit, removal of more than the lateral one fourth of the nail is unnecessary. High recurrence rates are associated with these simple nail excision procedures.

Matrixectomy of the lateral nail matrix is required to permanently ablate lateral nail-forming tissue and to narrow the width of the nail plate to better fit the lateral nail fold.

TABLE 63-1. Factors Associated with Ingrown Nails

Improperly trimmed nails or torn distal nails
Hyperhidrosis
Excessive external pressure from improperly fitting footwear or poor stance and gait
Trauma to the nail unit
Subungual neoplasms or skeletal abnormalities
Diabetes mellitus
Obesity
Nail changes of the elderly, including onychogryphosis and onychomycosis

Many physicians prefer to perform chemical matrixectomy with sodium hydroxide or more commonly with phenol. Phenol produces adequate nail bed ablation, but it is associated with a pungent odor, lateral nail fold damage, excessive wound discharge, and infection. Electrosurgical ablation of the nail bed is a highly successful alternative that produces less discharge. Special high-frequency-unit matrixectomy electrodes with one coated side can be used to avoid injury to the overlying normal tissue of the proximal nail fold (i.e., cuticle) while ablating the nail bed. Laser matrixectomy is another option, but it is less attractive (to most primary care practices) because of the high capital and upkeep costs.

The granulation tissue produced by the foreign body reaction can produce lateral wall hypertrophy. Because this tissue is abnormal, some physicians advocate removal at the time of nail surgery. Removal of lateral wall hypertrophy can be accomplished with scalpel excision or with electrosurgical excision or ablation. Tissue removal can produce a scooped-out defect in the lateral tissue at the time of surgery. This defect fills in over several weeks as the remaining normal lateral tissue grows to the newly formed lateral nail edge.

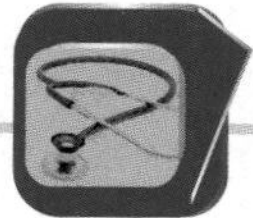

Equipment

- Syringe (3 mL or 5 mL) with long (1- or 1.5-inch) 25- or 27-gauge needle
- Local anesthetic without epinephrine
- Narrow periosteal elevator (nail elevator)
- Sterile scissors with straight blades (or nail splitter)

TABLE 63-2. Management Options for Ingrown Toenails

Warm water soaks
Cotton-wick insertion in the lateral groove corner
Debridement (debulking) of the lateral nail groove
Silver nitrate cauterization of the hypertrophied lateral nail tissue
Complete nail avulsion
Partial nail avulsion
Wedge resection of the distal nail edge
Partial nail avulsion with phenol matricectomy, sodium hydroxide matricectomy, laser matricectomy, or electrosurgical matricectomy
Surgical excision of nail plate, nail bed, and matrix

- Two straight hemostats
- Alcohol swabs
- Sterile gauze and tubular gauze dressing
- Topical antibiotic ointment
- Phenol solution (88%) and a radiofrequency electrosurgical unit with a Teflon-insulated matrix tip or a low-frequency unit with a needle tip (if performing a matrixectomy)

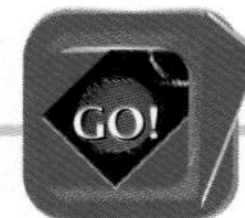

Indications

- Onychocryptosis (ingrown nail), especially stage II or stage III
- Onychomycosis (fungal infection of the nail) when pressure on the nail causes pain)
- Onychogryposis (deformed, curved nail)
- Pincer nails

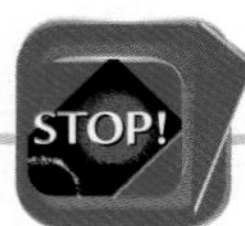

Contraindications (Relative)

- Diabetes mellitus.
- Peripheral vascular disease, especially if digital ischemia exists.
- Coagulopathy or bleeding diathesis.
- Uncooperative patient.
- Overt bacterial infection of the operative site is a relative contraindication to matrixectomy. However, most "infected" ingrown nails do not contain bacteria; they have a sterile inflammatory reaction to the trauma.

The Procedure

Step 1. Position the patient in the supine position, with the knees flexed and the foot flat on the table or the leg extended and the foot hanging off the end of the table. The physician wears nonsterile gloves. Perform a digital block as described in Chapter 3. After adequate time has elapsed (5 to 10 minutes), test the patient's ability to sense pain in the digit.

- **PEARL:** Some physicians prefer to place a tourniquet (a rubber band or Penrose drain placed around the digit and held with a hemostat) in an attempt to limit bleeding during the procedure. There is no evidence this actually works, and many providers perform the procedure without this step with identical outcomes.

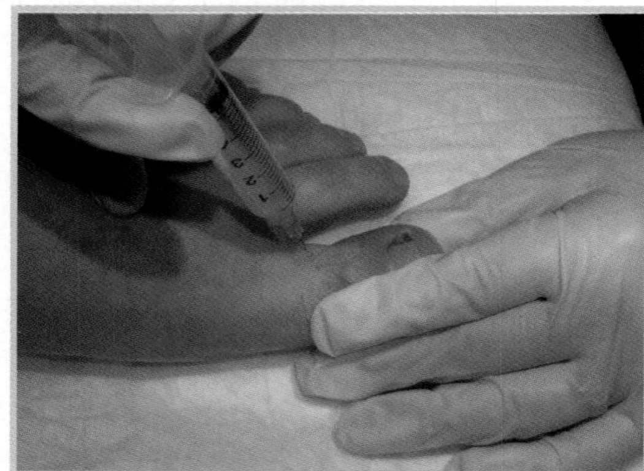

Step 1

- **PEARL:** When checking the patient's ability to sense pain in the digit, ask them if they "feel pain," not if they "feel anything." Remember, local anesthetics do not block touch receptors.
- **PITFALL:** If using a tourniquet, avoid pulling the rubber band too tightly and damaging the tissues. Limit the amount of time that the tourniquet is placed. It is advisable to withdraw the tourniquet after 10 minutes of application to limit vascular injury from interrupted blood flow to the digit.

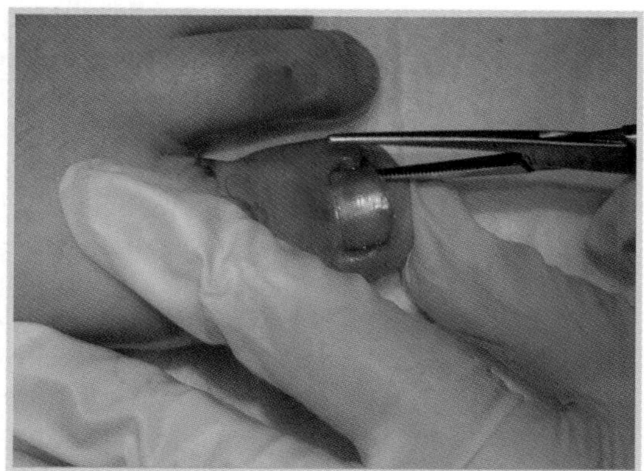

Step 2

Step 2. Prep the toe (see Appendix E). Free the lateral nail plate from the overlying proximal nail fold (i.e., cuticle). A Freer septum elevator or hemostat can be used to lift the cuticle off the nail plate. Create a tunnel between the nail plate and bed with the elevator or one jaw of a hemostat to allow passage of a nail splitter and removal of the lateral one fifth to one third of the nail.

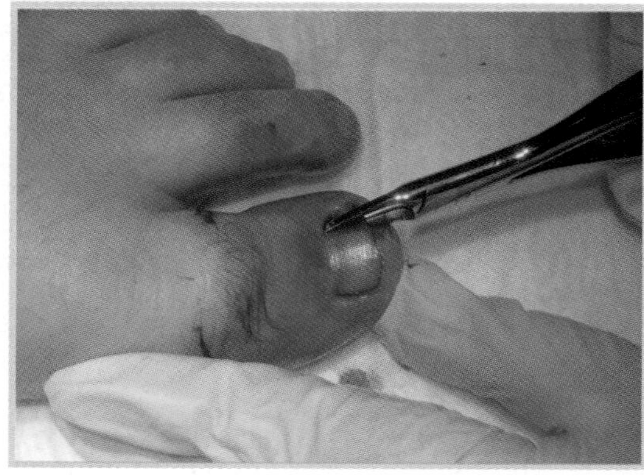

Step 3

Step 3. If performing a partial nail avulsion, cut the nail with nail splitters or bandage scissors, placing the thin blade beneath the distal (free) edge of the nail. Cut the nail straight back beneath the proximal nail fold. As the proximal edge of nail is cut, a "give" is often felt by the operator.

- **PITFALL:** Avoid damaging the nail bed when cutting the nail plate. If the scissors are used, the blade placed beneath the nail plate can traumatize the nail bed. Advance the scissors by cutting just with the tips of the scissors, and angle the tips of the scissors upward away from the nail bed.
- **PITFALL:** Do *not* cut the ventral fold, because this area may be slow to heal.

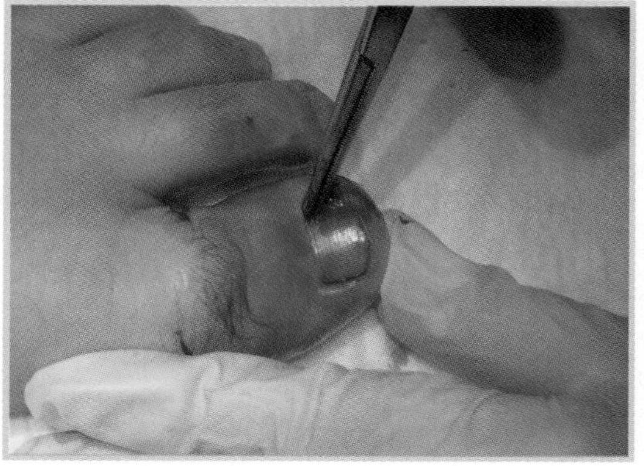

Step 4

Step 4. Grasp the lateral nail with straight hemostats and lift the nail out using a side-to-side rocking combined with a twisting motion that pulls outward and laterally. Part or all of the nail plate may be removed in this manner.

- **PITFALL:** Grasp as much of the lateral nail in the hemostats before attempting withdrawal. If just the end of the nail plate is grasped, the nail frequently breaks on removal.

Step 5. After the nail has been removed, examine the lateral sulcus beneath the proximal nail fold to ensure no pieces of nail remain within the corner. Also examine the part of the nail removed. If part of the nail plate is missing, it must be found and removed or it will slow healing and cause pain.

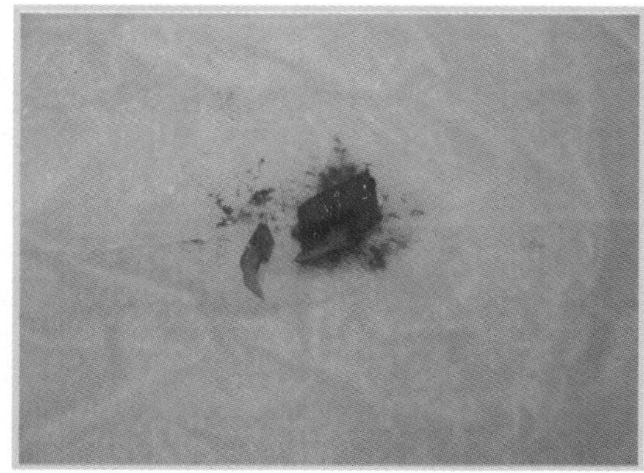

Step 5

Step 6. Matrixectomy can be performed chemically or electrosurgically, as demonstrated here. Place the electrode over the lateral nail bed with the Teflon-coated portion upward. Lift the electrode about 1 mm, creating a small gap. Make sure the lateral horn of the matrix is ablated by moving the electrode laterally beneath the proximal nail fold. Activate the electrode for 3 to 10 seconds, gently bouncing the electrode against the nail bed to produce ablation of the tissue. A short sizzling sound and a small puff of smoke may be seen. A properly treated nail bed appears white after thermal ablation.

- **PITFALL:** Avoid prolonged activation of the electrode against the nail bed. Prolonged burning can damage the deep tissues (i.e., extensor tendon insertion beneath the nail bed) and cause excessive time (months) for healing.
- **PITFALL:** If the lateral horn of the matrix is not destroyed, a new spicule of nail will grow into the new lateral nail fold, with recurrence of symptoms in the months after the procedure.

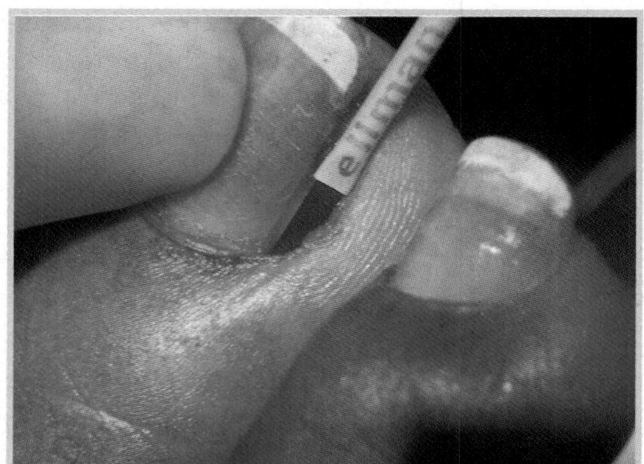

Step 6

Step 7. If needed, the hypertrophied lateral tissue can be cut away or ablated with an electrode or scalpel. Place a thin film of antimicrobial ointment on the exposed nail bed and cover it with a nonadherent dressing. Wrap the digit with 1- or 2-inch rolled gauze. Disposable surgical slippers or open toe shoes can be worn by the patient on leaving the office.

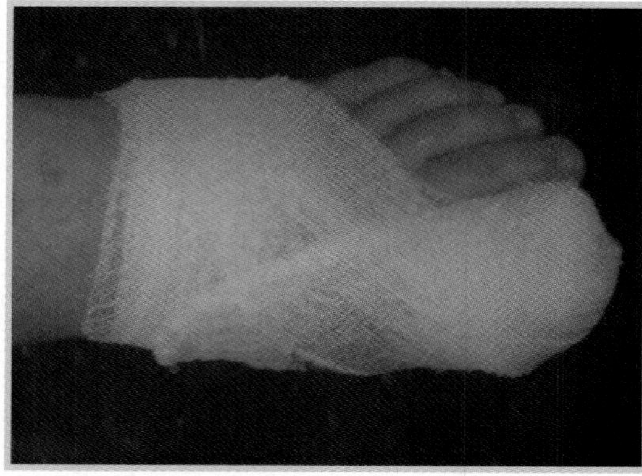

Step 7

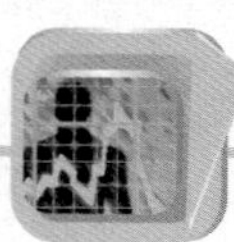

Complications

- Infections (treat with soaks and appropriate antibiotics).
- Regrowth of nail and return of symptoms. (The regrowth rate following phenol cauterization is 4% to 25%; for radiofrequency, <5%.)
- Permanent loss of nail plate (mainly with bilateral matrixectomy).
- Damage to underlying structures due to excessive application of electrosurgical matrixectomy.

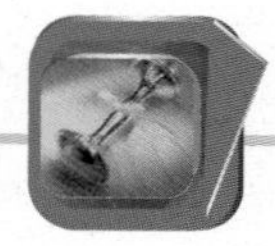

Pediatric Considerations

The conditions that lead to this procedure are rare in the preadolescent population. Adolescent patients are treated in the same manner as adults.

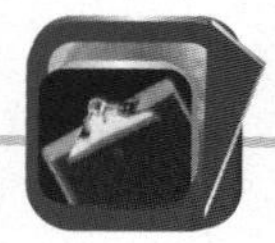

Postprocedure Instructions

The foot should be rested and preferably elevated during the first 12 to 24 hours. Because matrixectomy ablates the nerve endings of the nail bed, pain should be minimal when it is used. Nonsteroidal anti-inflammatory drugs (NSAIDs) may be used for discomfort.

The dressing should be changed in 24 hours, at which point normal ambulation may fully resume. The toe should be soaked and cleaned in warm water to help remove the bandage, and topical antibiotics may be recommended until healing is complete. The dressing change should be repeated daily. Tell the patient to expect a sterile exudate from the nail bed for several weeks. Emphasize proper nail hygiene to the patient.

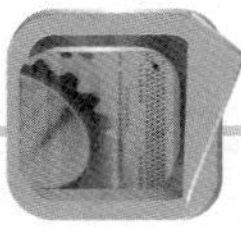

Coding Information and Supply Sources

Code 11750 is most commonly reported when partial avulsion and matrixectomy are performed for permanent nail removal. Simple avulsion without matrixectomy is reported with 11730 or 11730 and 11732.

CPT Code	Description	2008 Average 50th Percentile Fee	Global Period
11730	Avulsion of a single nail plate, partial or complete, simple	$121.00	0
11732	Avulsion of each additional nail plate	$85.00	0
11750	Excision of nail and nail matrix, partial or complete	$375.00	10
11765	Wedge excision of skin of nail fold	$169.00	10

CPT is a registered trademark of the American Medical Association.
2008 average 50th Percentile Fees are provided courtesy of 2008 MMH-SI's copyrighted Physicians' Fees and Coding Guide.

The Freer septum elevator, bandage scissors or nail splitters, and hemostats are available from surgical supply stores or instrument dealers. Disposable surgical slippers are available from surgical supply houses. Matrixectomy electrodes and electrosurgical equipment are available from Ellman International, Hewlett, NY (phone: 1-800-835-5355; Web site: http://www.ellman.com). A suggested anesthesia tray that can be used for this procedure is listed in Appendix G.

Patient Education Handout

A patient education handout, "Ingrown Toenail," can be found on the book's companion Web site.

Bibliography

Appenheimer AT. Treatment of ingrown toenail. *Patient Care.* 1987;21:119–125.

Brown JS. *Minor Surgery: A Text and Atlas.* London: Chapman & Hall; 1997:224–235.

Ceilley RI, Collison DW. Matrixectomy. *J Dermatol Surg Oncol.* 1992;18:728–734.

Clark RE, Madani S, Bettencourt MS. Nail surgery. *Dermatol Clin.* 1998;16:145–164.

Clark RE, Tope WD. Nail surgery. In: Wheeland RG, ed. *Cutaneous Surgery.* Philadelphia: WB Saunders; 1994:375–402.

Daniel CR III. Basic nail plate avulsion. *J Dermatol Surg Oncol.* 1992;18:685–688.

Fishman HC. Practical therapy for ingrown toenails. *Cutis.* 1983;32:159–160.

Gillette RD. Practical management of ingrown toenails. *Postgrad Med.* 1988;84:145–158.

Hettinger DP, Valinsky MS, Nuccio G, et al. Nail matrixectomies using radio wave technique. *J Am Podiatr Med Assoc.* 1991;81:317–321.

Leahy AL, Timon CI, Craig A, et al. Ingrowing toenails: improving treatment. *Surgery* 1990;107:566–567.

Onumah N, Scher RK. Nail surgery. Emedicine Web site. Available at http://www.emedicine.com/derm/topic818.htm. Accessed September 18, 2002.

Quill G, Myerson M. A guide to office treatment of ingrown toenails. *Hosp Med.* 1994;30:51–54.

Zuber TJ. Ingrown toenail removal. *Am Fam Physician.* 2002;65:2547–2550, 2551–2552, 2554, 2557–2558.

Zuber TJ. *Office Procedures.* Kansas City: American Academy of Family Physicians; 1998:123–130.

2008 MAG Mutual Healthcare Solutions, Inc.'s Physicians' Fee and Coding Guide. Duluth, Georgia. MAG Mutual Healthcare Solutions, Inc. 2007.

CHAPTER 64

Nail Plate and Nail Bed Biopsy

E. J. Mayeaux, Jr., MD, DABFP, FAAFP

Professor of Family Medicine, Professor of Obstetrics and Gynecology
Louisiana State University Health Sciences Center, Shreveport, LA

A nail plate or nail bed biopsy is a direct means of diagnosis when routine clinical and laboratory methods fail to distinguish nail conditions. Nail bed biopsy can prevent misdiagnosis or delay in the diagnosis of potentially serious or disfiguring conditions such as subungual tumors. Occasionally, a biopsy can be therapeutic. Nail biopsy can provide rapid information that can guide therapy for inflammatory and infectious nail disorders, and it may prevent the unnecessary use of potentially hazardous, empirically applied medications.

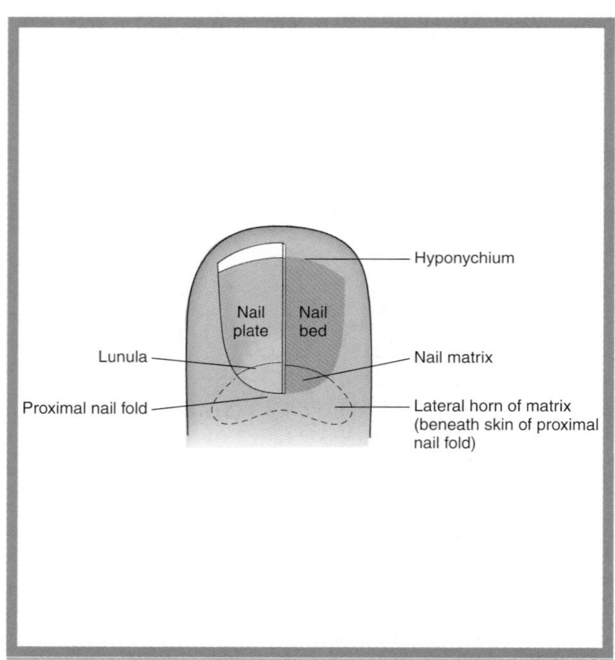

Nail bed biopsy is easily performed in an office setting. The technique uses skills similar to those incorporated in skin biopsy of other sites. Despite the safety of the procedure, the potential for patient discomfort and permanent nail dystrophy discourages many providers from performing the technique. Proper patient selection and education is important to a successful outcome. Patients should be informed about the slow healing after a nail bed biopsy. Mean fingernail growth is 3 mm per month, and mean toenail growth is 1 mm per month.

A correct understanding of nail anatomy and physiology is important to a successful outcome. Some guiding principles for the performance of nail bed biopsy are listed in Table 64-1. The nail bed adheres the nail plate, and biopsies of the nail bed usually heal without significant scarring. A 2- or 3-mm punch biopsy through the nail plate can provide accurate information about the nail bed. The nail matrix is the nail-forming tissue, and biopsies of the nail matrix can produce permanent dystrophy. Certain conditions are best diagnosed from a nail matrix biopsy, including unexplained longitudinal melanonychia, nail dystrophy involving the entire nail plate, and tumors of the nail matrix.

To prevent formation of a split nail deformity after biopsying the nail matrix, avoid transecting the matrix. The curvature of the lunula should be maintained, because this curvature is important to the proper contour of the nail. The superior surface of the nail plate is formed in the proximal matrix, and the underside of the nail is formed in the distal matrix. Biopsy should be performed in the distal matrix whenever possible. The

TABLE 64-1. Principles Guiding Nail Bed Biopsy

When the information can be obtained from another site, avoid biopsy of the nail matrix.
Avoid transecting the nail matrix, to prevent a split nail deformity.
Suture defects in the matrix when possible.
When possible, perform a distal rather than proximal matrix biopsy.
Retain the distal curvature of the nail matrix.

Adapted from Rich P. *J Dermatol Surg Oncol.* 1992;18:673–682.

thickness of the nail is determined by the length of the matrix. Tissue loss in the matrix can produce permanent, focal thinning of the nail plate.

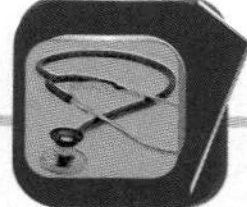

Equipment

- The punch biopsy instrument (trephine) has a plastic, pencil-like handle and a circular scalpel blade. The blade attaches to the handle at the hub of the instrument.
- Basic setup for this procedure includes local anesthesia (1 to 3 mL of anesthetic), the punch biopsy instrument, and sharp iris scissors to cut the specimen free. If the specimen cannot be lifted using the anesthesia needle, Adson pickups without teeth may be used to lift the specimen.
- Suggested suture removal times are listed in Appendix J. A suggested anesthesia tray that can be used for this procedure is listed in Appendix F. Skin preparation recommendations appear in Appendix E.

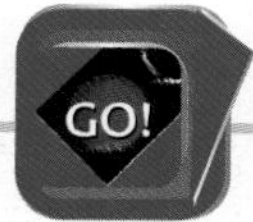

Indications

- Diagnosis and removal of subungual tumors: warts, glomus tumors, enchondromas, fibromas, and squamous cell carcinomas. (Consider a radiograph to assess bony involvement by the mass.)
- Diagnosis or exclusion of acral lentiginous melanoma in a patient with longitudinal melanonychia.
- Identification of an inflammatory nail condition (e.g., lichen planus, psoriasis).
- Alleviation of a painful nail condition (e.g., glomus tumor pain).
- Histologic identification of an undiagnosed nail condition.

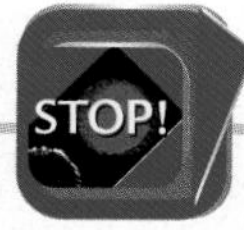

Contraindications

- Uncooperative patient
- Coagulopathy or bleeding diathesis
- Presence of diabetes, peripheral vascular disease, or active connective tissue disease

The Procedure

Anatomy of the nail is depicted.

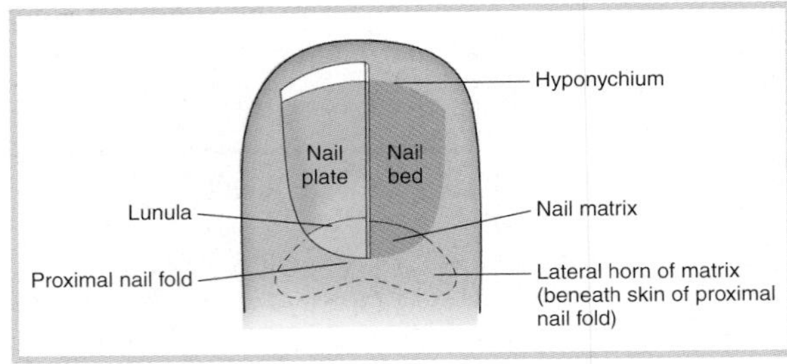

Figure 1

Step 1. Perform a digital block to provide anesthesia (see Chapter 3). Prep the skin with povidone-iodine or chlorhexidine solution, and allow it to dry (see Appendix E).

- **PEARL:** Prep a wide area so that an undraped area is not inadvertently exposed if the drape slides a little.

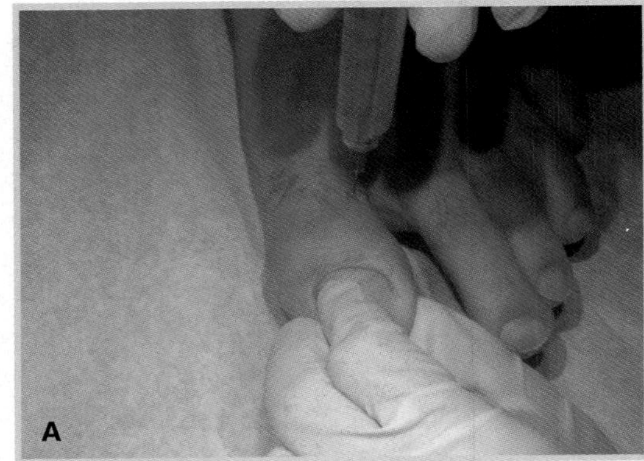

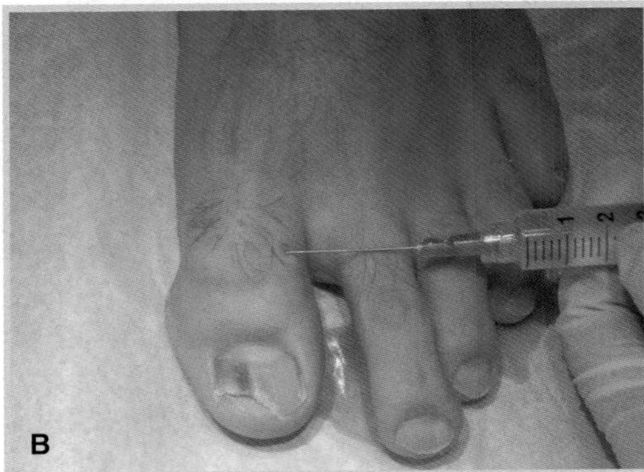

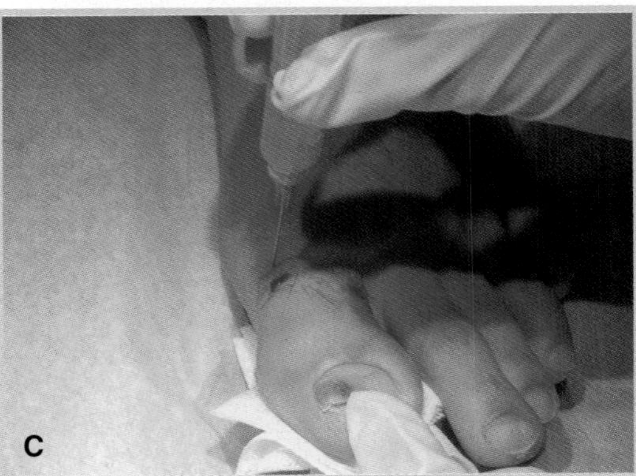

Step 1

Step 2. For a nail plate biopsy, place a 3- to 6-mm punch trephine flat against the nail plate, and rotate with downward pressure until the blade cuts through the nail. The provider should feel a sudden pressure drop-off or "give."

Step 2

Step 3. The nail plate often is removed with the punch.

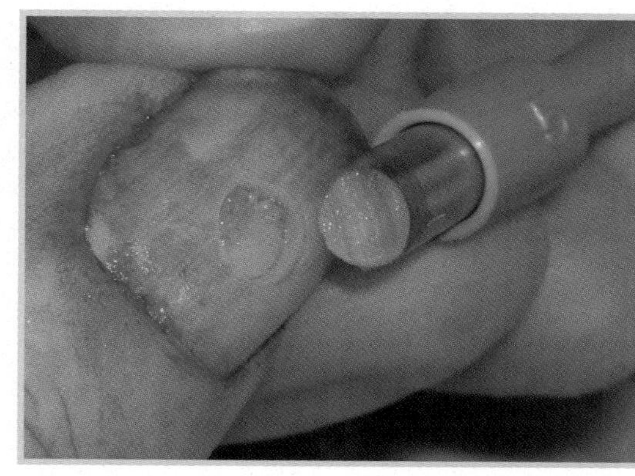

Step 3

Step 4. If the nail plate remains in the cut made by the punch, use a needle to lift it out.

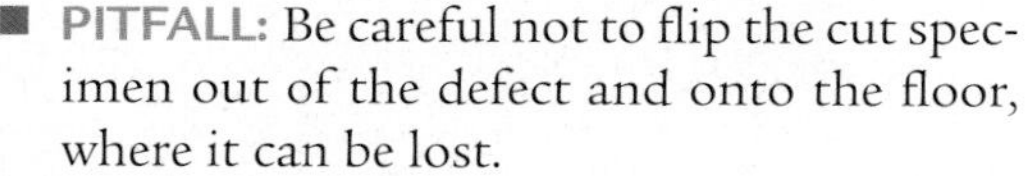

- **PITFALL:** Be careful not to flip the cut specimen out of the defect and onto the floor, where it can be lost.

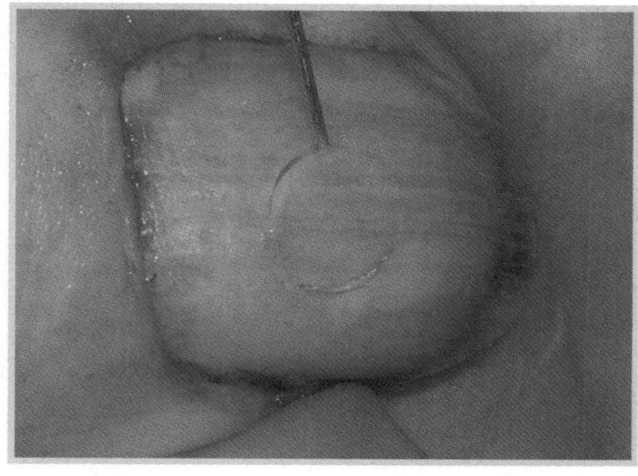

Step 4

Step 5. The technique of nail bed biopsy can be performed with or without nail plate avulsion. With the double-punch technique for nail bed biopsy, a 5- or 6-mm punch is used to first remove a section of the nail plate as described previously. After the nail bed is exposed with the large punch or by nail plate avulsion, a 3-mm punch is then used in the center of the previously created window in the nail plate to obtain a specimen of the nail bed.

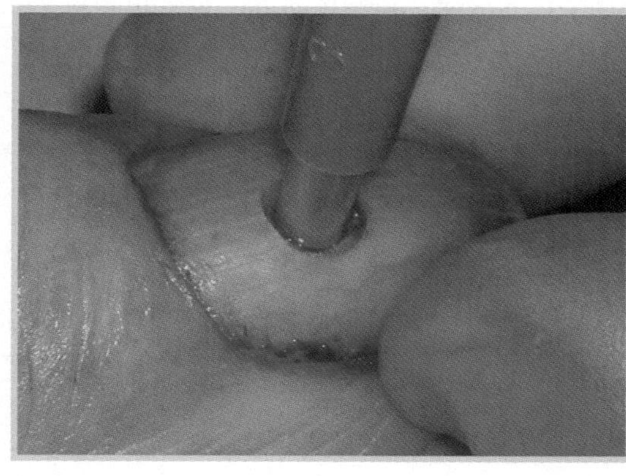

Step 5

Step 6. The specimen may then be removed with a needle or with pickups. Monsel solution can be used for hemostasis, and the site heals by secondary intention.

- **PITFALL:** Do not damage the nail bed when using the larger punch to remove the nail plate. Proceed slowly and carefully until the instrument just passes through the nail plate.

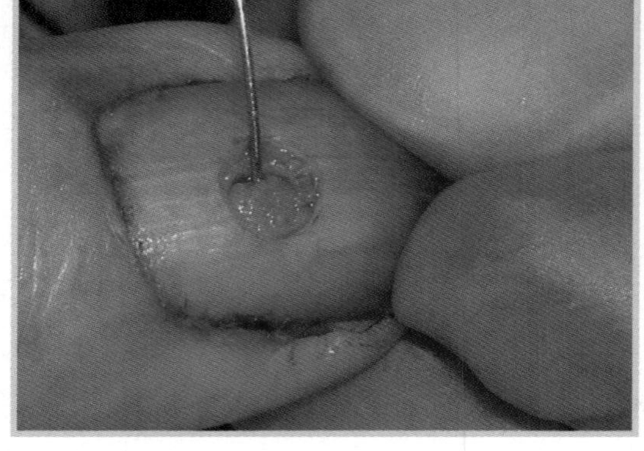

Step 6

Nail Matrix Biopsy

Step 7. After a digital block and prep, the proximal nail fold is separated from the nail plate using a Freer septum elevator, a blunt probe, or hemostats.

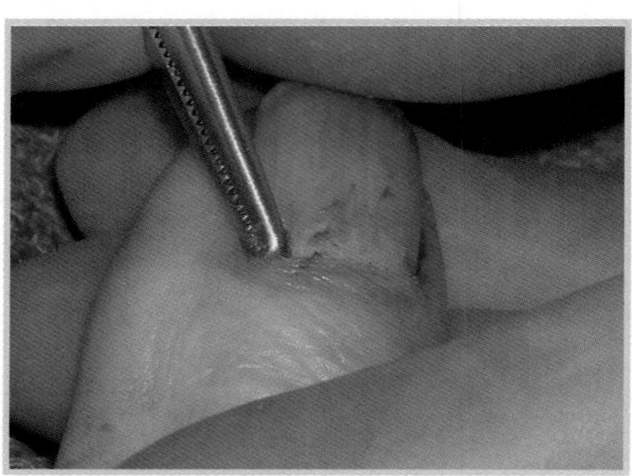

Step 7

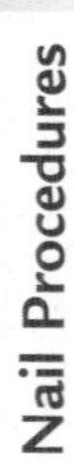

Step 8. Make lateral incisions in the proximal nail fold (5 mm toward the distal interphalangeal joint).

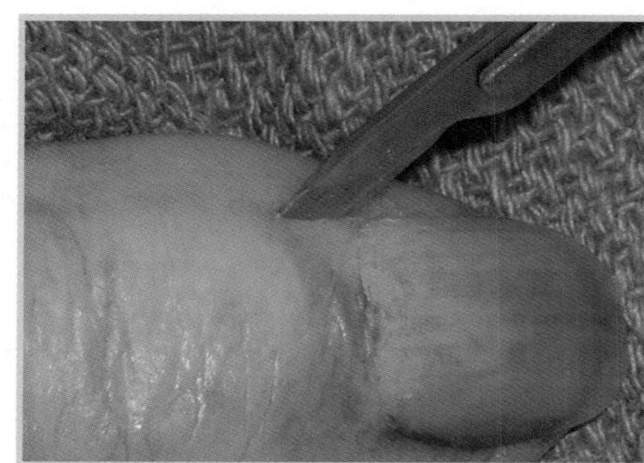

Step 8

Step 9. Now the proximal nail fold may be reflected.

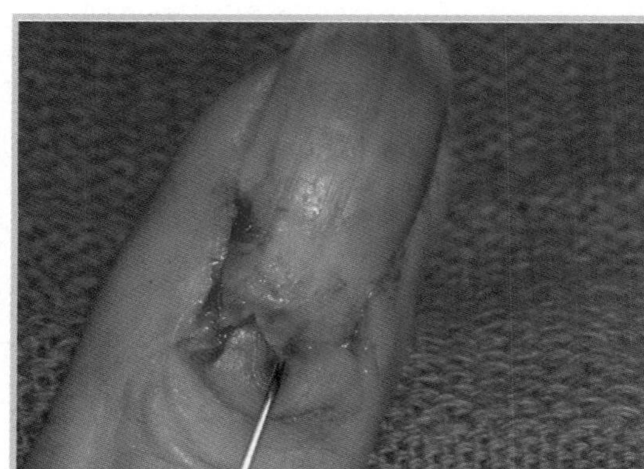

Step 9

Step 10. The nail plate is gently separated from underlying tissues, and the plate is placed on the surgery tray.

- **PEARL:** Incising the ventral fold before removing the nail plate allows the nail plate to protect the underlying nail matrix during incision.

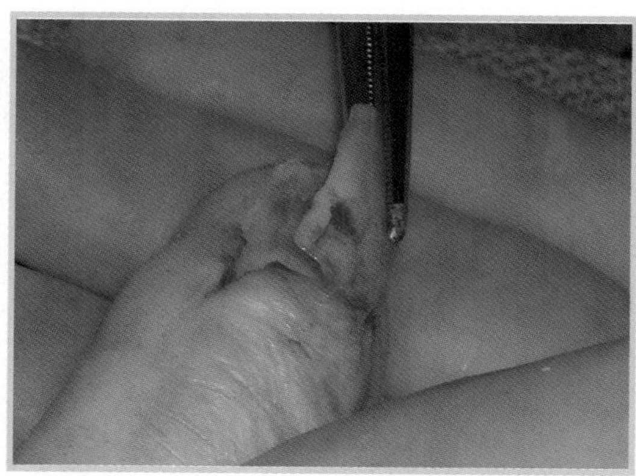

Step 10

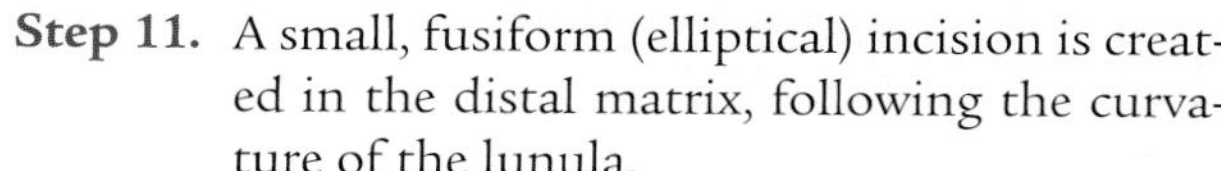

Step 11. A small, fusiform (elliptical) incision is created in the distal matrix, following the curvature of the lunula.

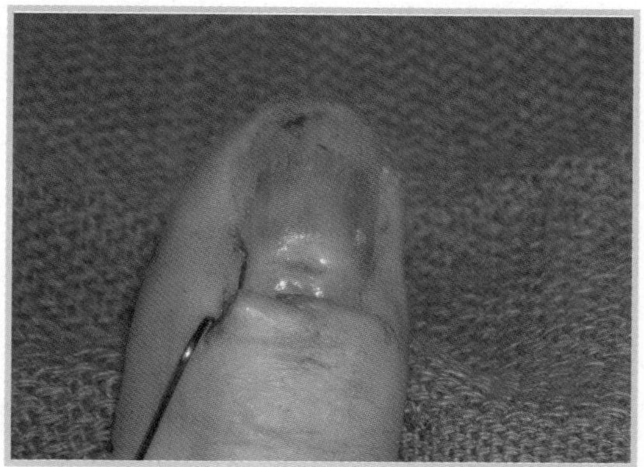

Step 11

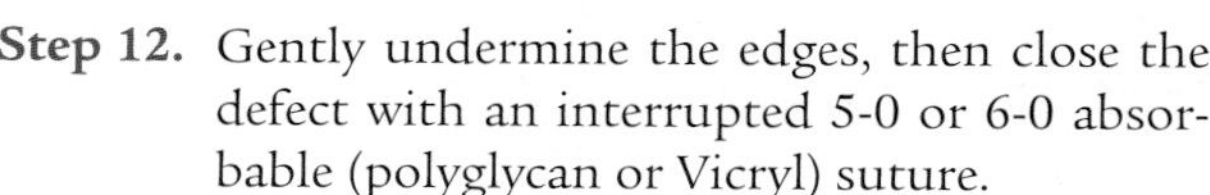

Step 12. Gently undermine the edges, then close the defect with an interrupted 5-0 or 6-0 absorbable (polyglycan or Vicryl) suture.

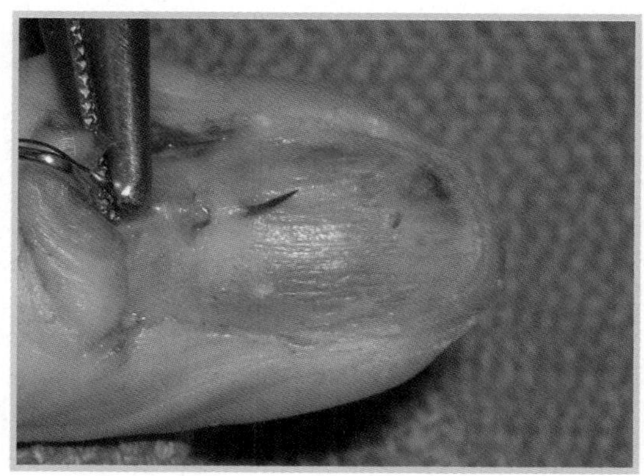

Step 12

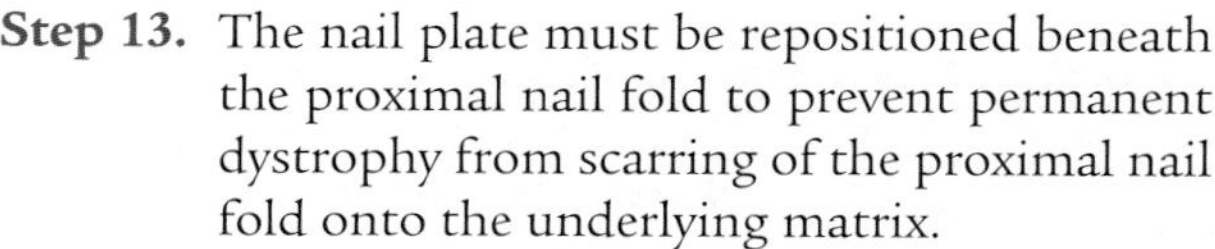

Step 13. The nail plate must be repositioned beneath the proximal nail fold to prevent permanent dystrophy from scarring of the proximal nail fold onto the underlying matrix.

- **PITFALL:** The nail plate may be unintentionally discarded during the procedure. Other materials, such as petroleum-impregnated gauze, plastic nails, or nonadherent or plastic dressings, can be used to separate the proximal nail fold from the nail matrix for 1 to 2 weeks after the procedure.

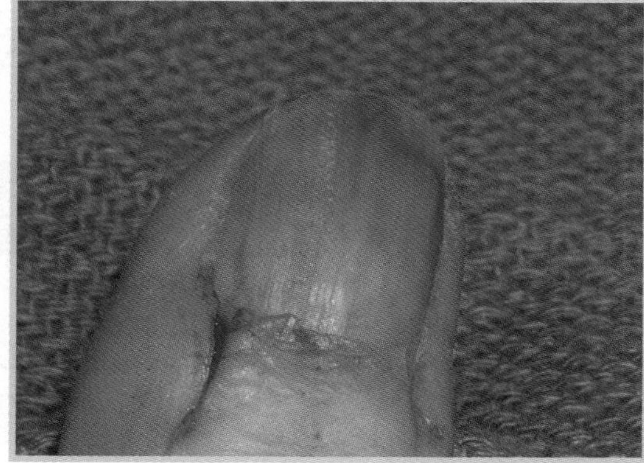

Step 13

Step 14. A 5-0 nylon suture can be used to close the incisions in the proximal nail fold. Some practitioners prefer to anchor the nail plate by suturing it to lateral tissues.

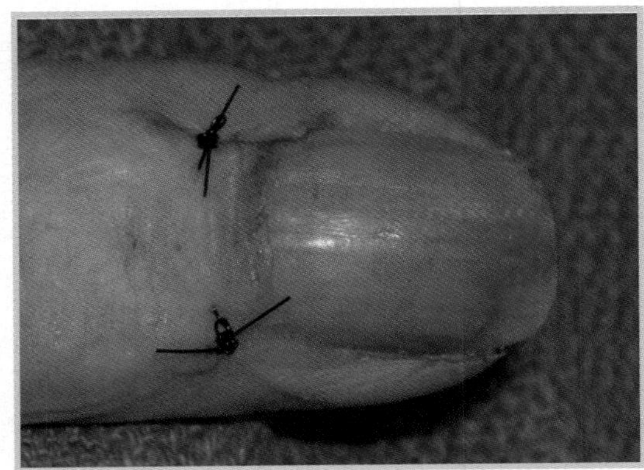

Step 14

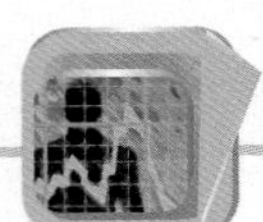

Complications

- Onycholysis
- Nail deformity (often nail splitting)
- Infection

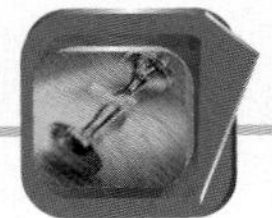

Pediatric Considerations

The procedure in children is essentially the same. Younger children may not be able to hold still, so restraining them may be necessary. Consider procedural sedation for nail bed exploration or repair (see Chapter 122).

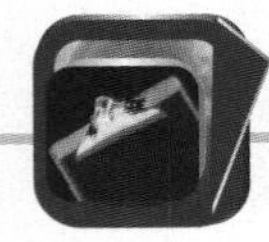

Postprocedure Instructions

The site should be kept covered with a sterile gauze dressing while the wound continues to drain (1 to 2 days for trephination). The dressing should be changed daily. If the nail matrix was repaired, the removed nail should be dressed and repositioned beneath the proximal nail fold to prevent permanent dystrophy from scarring of the proximal nail fold onto the underlying matrix. Some practitioners prefer to anchor the nail plate by suturing it to lateral tissues. Other materials, such as petroleum-impregnated gauze, plastic nails, or nonadherent or plastic dressings, can be used to separate the proximal nail fold from the nail matrix for 1 to 2 weeks after the procedure.

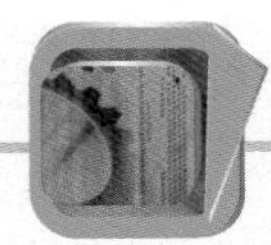

Coding Information and Supply Sources

CPT Code	Description	2008 Average 50th Percentile Fee	Global Period
11755	Biopsy of nail unit (nail plate, bed, or folds)	$188.00	0

Disposable punch biopsy instruments and suture material can be obtained from surgical supply houses or from dermatology suppliers such as Delasco (Web site: http://www.delasco.com). The Freer septum elevator is available from sellers of surgical instruments.

Bibliography

Baran R, Haneke E. Surgery of the nail. In: Epstein E, Epstein E Jr, eds. *Skin Surgery*. 6th ed. Philadelphia: WB Saunders; 1987:534–547.

Clark RE, Madani S, Bettencourt MS. Nail surgery. *Dermatol Clin.* 1998;16:145–164.

Clark RE, Tope WE. Nail surgery. In: Wheeland RG, ed. *Cutaneous Surgery*. Philadelphia: WB Saunders; 1994:375–402.

De Berker DA, Dahl MG, Comaish JS, et al. Nail surgery: an assessment of indications and outcome. *Acta Verereol (Stockh).* 1996;76:484–487.

Grammer-West NY, Corvette DM, Giandoni MB. Clinical pearl: nail plate biopsy for the diagnosis of psoriatic nails. *J Am Acad Dermatol.* 1998;38:260–262.

Haneke E, Baran R. Nails: surgical aspects. In: Parish LC, Lask GP, eds. *Aesthetic Dermatology*. New York: McGraw-Hill; 1991:236–247.

Rich P. Nail biopsy indications and methods. *J Dermatol Surg Oncol.* 1992;18(8):673–682.

Rich P. Nail biopsy: indications and methods. *Dermatol Surg.* 2001;27:229–234.

Siegle RJ, Swanson NA. Nail surgery: a review. *J Dermatol Surg Oncol.* 1982;8:659–666.

Tosti A, Piraccini BM. Treatment of common nail disorders. *Dermatol Clin.* 2000;18:339–348.

Van Laborde S, Scher RK. Developments in the treatment of nail psoriasis, melanonychia striata, and onychomycosis. *Dermatol Clin.* 2000;18:37–46.

Zuber TJ. *Skin Biopsy, Excision, and Repair Techniques.* Kansas City: American Academy of Family Physicians; 1998:70–75.

2008 MAG Mutual Healthcare Solutions, Inc.'s Physicians' Fee and Coding Guide. Duluth, Georgia. MAG Mutual Healthcare Solutions, Inc. 2007.

CHAPTER 65

Subungual Hematoma Drainage

E. J. Mayeaux, Jr., MD, DABFP, FAAFP

Professor of Family Medicine, Professor of Obstetrics and Gynecology
Louisiana State University Health Sciences Center, Shreveport, LA

Subungual hematoma is a common injury, usually caused by a blow to a distal phalanx, such as crushing a finger in a doorjamb or stubbing a toe. The blow causes bleeding of the nail matrix or nail bed, with subsequent subungual hematoma formation. The traumatic accumulation of blood beneath the nail plate can create an excruciatingly painful injury. The often pulsatile pain is caused by increased pressure of the blood within a closed space adjacent to the sensitive nail bed and matrix. Subungual hematomas frequently manifest with a blue-black discoloration that can extend beneath part or all of the nail surface. The pain of a subungual hematoma can be dramatically and instantaneously relieved by drainage.

Trephination provides a simple technique to evacuate hematomas. Various techniques have been advocated, including the use of heated paper clips, scalpel blades, dental burrs, and cautery units. Because the nail plate has no sensation, anesthesia generally is not required. Care should be exerted with any trephination instrument, because downward pressure increases pain. The use of a hot-tipped cautery unit is advocated because it burns a hole through nail plate without the need for much downward pressure or mining. The examiner must be prepared to lift up immediately on passage through the nail plate to avoid injury to the sensitive nail bed.

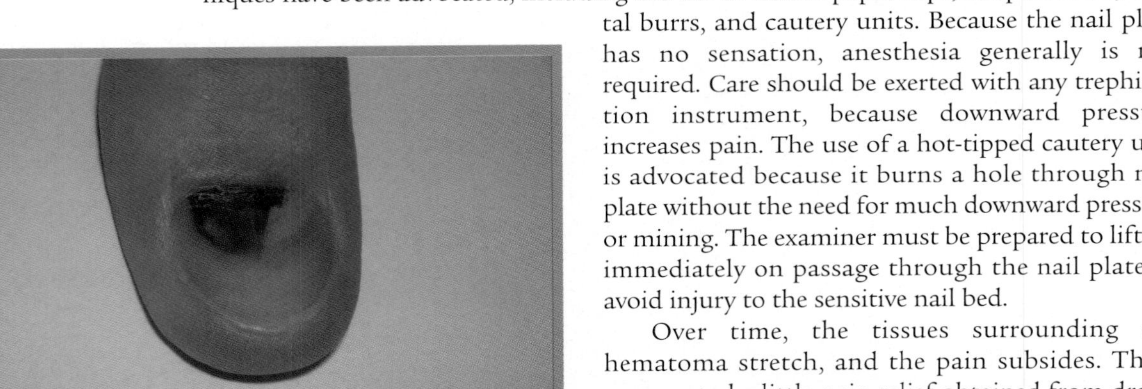

Over time, the tissues surrounding the hematoma stretch, and the pain subsides. There appears to be little pain relief obtained from draining a hematoma after about 48 to 72 hours following the initial injury. The discoloration of a subungual hematoma will grow out with the nail and be replaced with normal-appearing tissues.

Up to 25% of all subungual hematomas are associated with a fracture of the distal phalanx. Fractures are more likely to be present in patients with hematomas involving at least 50% of the nail bed, and some providers advocate routine x-ray examination, especially in children. If fracture is identified, 60% of those nails will have a laceration large enough to warrant closure with a small, absorbable suture. The major incentive to nail bed exploration and laceration repair is to prevent permanent nail dystrophy or deformity from a step-off or separated laceration.

Appropriate management of a subungual hematoma seeks to provide pain relief, recognizes associated injuries, and promotes regrowth of a functionally normal and cosmetically acceptable nail. Historically, it was recommended that hematomas involving more than 25% to 50% of the nail surface be explored. Nail plate removal and nail bed exploration was advocated to optimize the cosmetic outcome. The routine practice of nail bed exploration has been questioned by several studies; it appears that the practice is justified only when a laceration is through the nail plate or through either of the lateral nail folds. If no laceration is detected, it is probably safe to evacuate the hematoma, although 1 in 12 patients still may experience residual nail change.

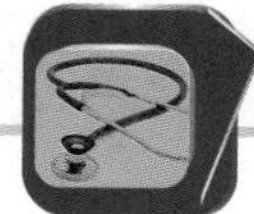

Equipment

- Fine-tipped battery cautery units
- Needle, 19 gauge
- A suggested surgical tray that can be used for laceration repair is listed in Appendix G
- A suggested anesthesia tray that can be used for this procedure is listed in Appendix F

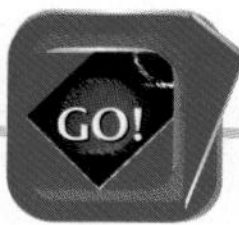

Indications

- Severe pain with a subungual hematoma after acute traumatic injury

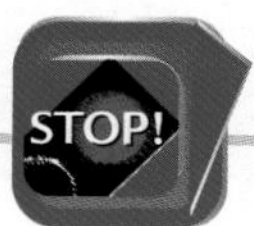

Contraindications

- Patient is no longer experiencing pain at rest (after 48 to 72 hours)
- Subungual ecchymosis (pain resolves after 30 minutes; only mild bleeding occurs)
- Blood collection without trauma (tumors such as glomus tumors, keratoacanthomas, and Kaposi sarcoma may manifest initially as a subungual hematoma)
- Subungual band of pigmentation (most likely represents nontraumatic benign or malignant pigmentation)

The Procedure

Step 1. Restrain the digit (and the child if he or she is uncooperative). Clean the nail with a prep solution (see Appendix E). Hold the fine-tipped cautery vertically over the center of the hematoma. Activate the cautery, and burn through the nail plate.

- **PITFALL:** As the nail plate is traversed, blood may spurt upward as the pressure is released. The provider should wear personal protective gear and make sure he or she is not directly over the device, where the risk of contamination is greatest.

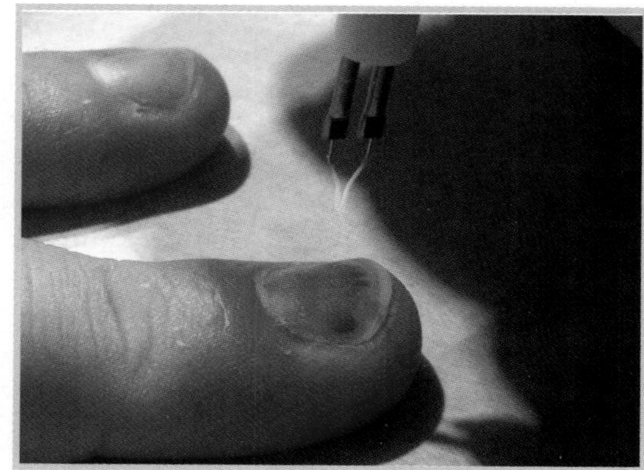

Step 1

Step 2. As soon as the subungual space is entered, the operator must be prepared to pull up and not allow the hot tip to touch down on the highly sensitive nail bed.

- **PEARL:** Create a hole large enough for continued drainage, which can occur for 1 to 2 days after the injury.

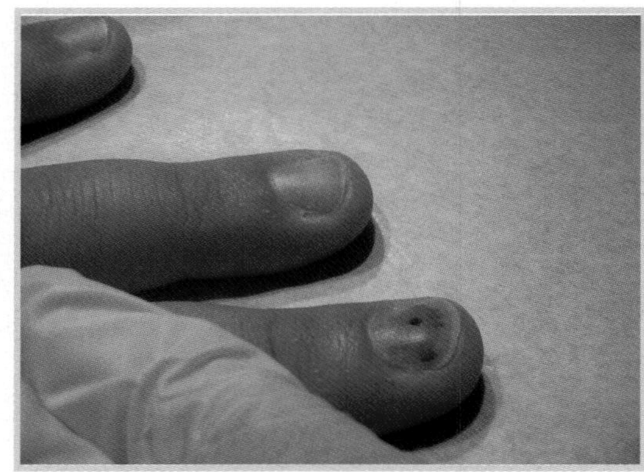

Step 2

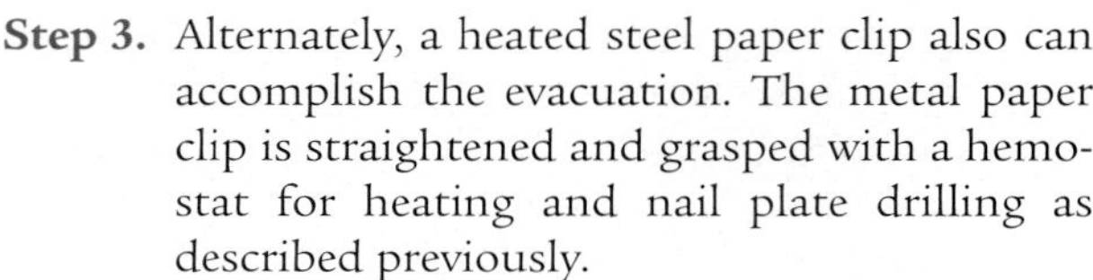

Step 3. Alternately, a heated steel paper clip also can accomplish the evacuation. The metal paper clip is straightened and grasped with a hemostat for heating and nail plate drilling as described previously.

- **PITFALL:** Avoid heating coated paper clips, which can produce a malodorous plume and burns from the molten coating. Avoid copper paper clips, which can melt.

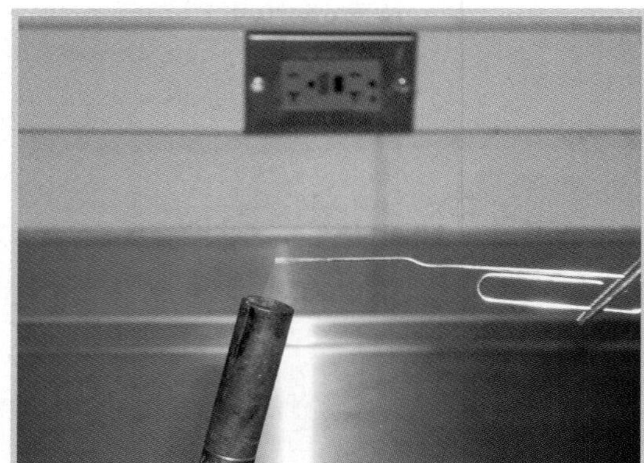

Step 3

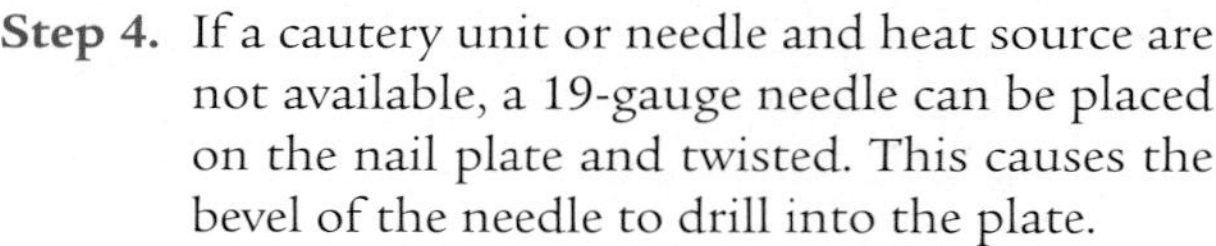

Step 4. If a cautery unit or needle and heat source are not available, a 19-gauge needle can be placed on the nail plate and twisted. This causes the bevel of the needle to drill into the plate.

- **PITFALL:** Be careful to stop drilling as soon as blood starts draining to prevent the needle from contacting the nail bed.

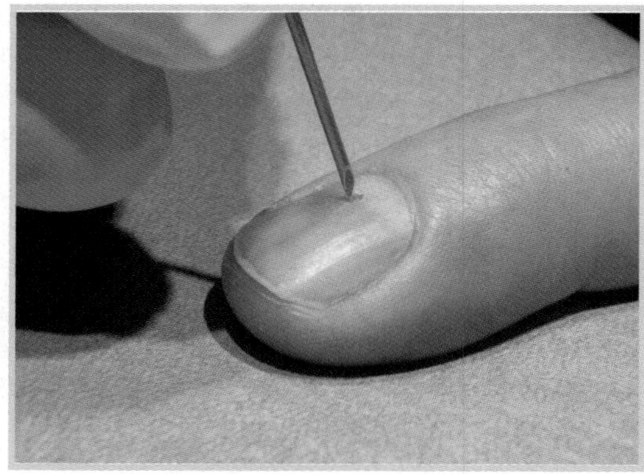

Step 4

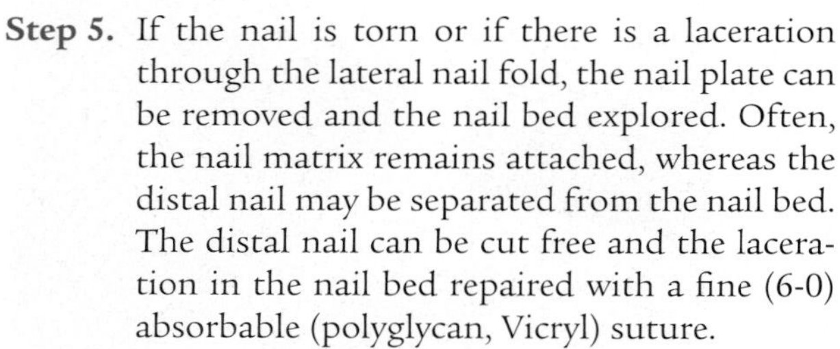

Step 5. If the nail is torn or if there is a laceration through the lateral nail fold, the nail plate can be removed and the nail bed explored. Often, the nail matrix remains attached, whereas the distal nail may be separated from the nail bed. The distal nail can be cut free and the laceration in the nail bed repaired with a fine (6-0) absorbable (polyglycan, Vicryl) suture.

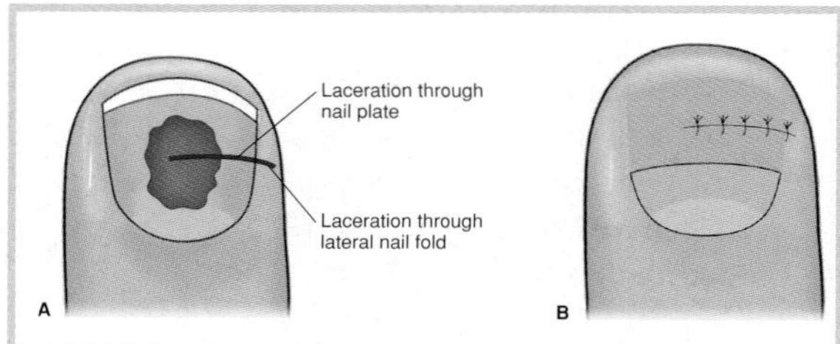

Step 5

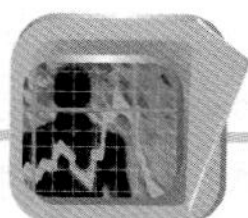

Complications

- Onycholysis
- Nail deformity (often nail splitting)
- Infection
- Inadvertent burns

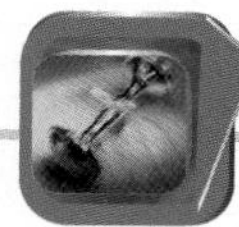

Pediatric Considerations

The procedure in children is essentially the same. Younger children may not be able to hold still, so restraining them may be necessary. Consider procedural sedation for nail bed exploration or repair (see Chapter 122).

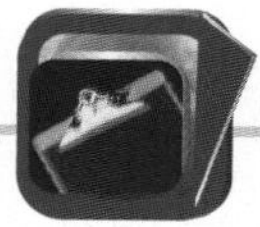

Postprocedure Instructions

The site should be kept covered with a sterile gauze dressing while the wound continues to drain (1 to 2 days for trephination). The dressing should be changed daily.

If the nail plate was removed, instruct the patient to soak the digit in clean water twice daily. After the soaks, apply a topical antibiotic ointment and a dry sterile bandage or adhesive bandage.

If the nail matrix was repaired, the removed nail should be dressed and repositioned beneath the proximal nail fold to prevent permanent dystrophy from scarring of the proximal nail fold onto the underlying matrix. Some practitioners prefer to anchor the nail plate by suturing it to lateral tissues. Other materials, such as petroleum-impregnated gauze, plastic nails, or nonadherent or plastic dressings, can be used to separate the proximal nail fold from the nail matrix for 1 to 2 weeks after the procedure.

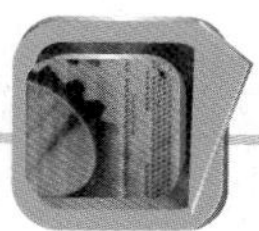

Coding Information and Supply Sources

When evacuation of a hematoma is performed, usually only code 11740 is reported.

CPT Code	Description	2008 Average 50th Percentile Fee	Global Period
11740	Evacuation of subungual hematoma	$80.00	0
11730	Avulsion of a single nail plate, partial or complete, simple	$121.00	0
11732	Avulsion of each additional nail plate	$85.00	0
11760	Repair of nail bed	$408.00	10

CPT is a registered trademark of the American Medical Association.
2008 average 50th Percentile Fees are provided courtesy of 2008 MMH-SI's copyrighted Physicians' Fees and Coding Guide.

Supply Sources

- Fine-tipped battery cautery units are available from Aaron Medical (high-temperature cautery AA01, http://www.hospitalnetwork.com) or from Advanced Meditech International (thermal cautery CH-HI, about $35 each; phone: 1-800-635-2452; http://www.ameditech.com).

Patient Education Handout

A patient education handout, "Subungual Hematoma (Bleeding under nail)," can be found on the book's companion Web site.

Bibliography

Aronson S. Evacuation of a subungual hematoma. *Hosp Med.* 1995;31:47–48.

Baran R, Haneke E. Surgery of the nail. In: Epstein E, Epstein E Jr, eds. *Skin Surgery*. 6th ed. Philadelphia: WB Saunders; 1987:534–547.

Brown JS. *Minor Surgery: A Text and Atlas*. 3rd ed. London: Chapman & Hall, 1997:327–328.

Buttaravoli P, Stair T. *Minor Emergencies: Splinters to Fractures*. St. Louis: Mosby; 2000:413–415.

Clark RE, Madani S, Bettencourt MS. Nail surgery. *Dermatol Clin*. 1998;16:145–164.

Clark RE, Tope WD. Nail surgery. In: Wheeland RG, ed. *Cutaneous Surgery*. Philadelphia: WB Saunders; 1994:375–402.

Driscoll CE. Drainage of a subungual hematoma. *Patient Care.* 1991;25:113–114.

Fieg EL. Management of nail bed lacerations [Letter]. *Am Fam Physician*. 2002;65:1997B–1998.

Helms A, Brodell RT. Surgical pearls: prompt treatment of subungual hematoma by decompression. *J Am Acad Dermatol.* 2000;42:508–509.

Roser SE, Gellman H. Comparison of nail bed repair versus nail trephination for subungual hematomas in children. *J Hand Surg Am.* 1999;24:1166–1170.

Zuber TJ. *Skin Biopsy, Excision, and Repair Techniques*. Kansas City: American Academy of Family Physicians; 1998:76–81.

2008 MAG Mutual Healthcare Solutions, Inc.'s Physicians' Fee and Coding Guide. Duluth, Georgia. MAG Mutual Healthcare Solutions, Inc. 2007.

CHAPTER 66

Paronychia Surgery

E. J. Mayeaux, Jr., MD, DABFP, FAAFP
Professor of Family Medicine, Professor of Obstetrics and Gynecology
Louisiana State University Health Sciences Center, Shreveport, LA

Paronychia is a superficial infection or abscess of the tissues bordering the nails (i.e., nail folds). It is one of the most common infections of the hand. The infections develop when a disruption occurs between the seal of the proximal nail fold and the nail plate. Excessive contact with moisture or chronic irritants may predispose an individual to the development of a paronychia. Trauma such as nail biting, manicure, a splinter or thorn in the distal edge of the nail, or a hangnail removal may also predispose a patient to a paronychia.

Acute paronychia manifests with rapid development of erythema and swelling in the proximal or lateral nail fold. Infection with *Staphylococcus aureus*, *Streptococci*, or *Pseudomonas* species is most common. Acute paronychia may follow a manicure or placement of sculptured nails, and it often produces tenderness and throbbing pain.

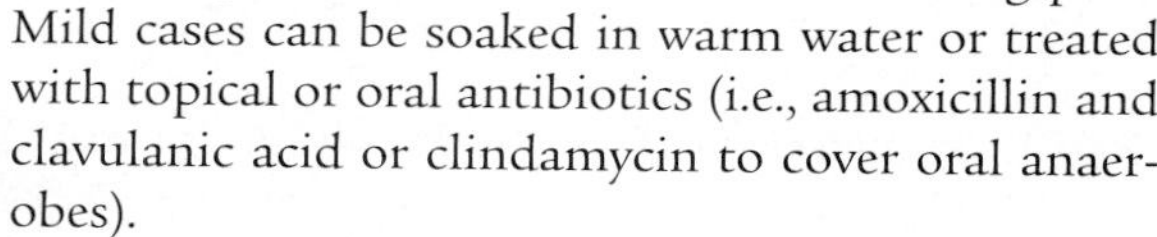

Mild cases can be soaked in warm water or treated with topical or oral antibiotics (i.e., amoxicillin and clavulanic acid or clindamycin to cover oral anaerobes).

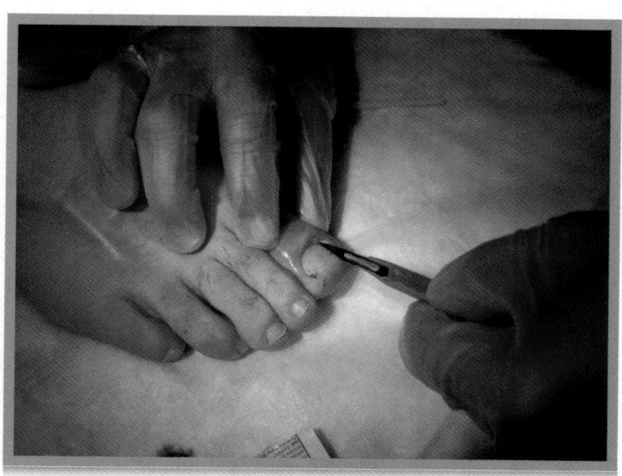

Chronic paronychia by definition must have been present for at least 6 weeks. These lesions often develop insidiously, and they may be associated with low-grade infections with *Candida albicans*. Chronic paronychia is common in bakers, bartenders, dishwashers, or thumb suckers who expose their hands to repeated or prolonged moisture and irritation. Women in the middle reproductive years are most commonly affected, with some series reporting female-to-male ratios of 10:1. Secondary nail plate changes may be found, including onycholysis (i.e., separation), lateral greenish brown discoloration, and transverse ridging.

Elimination of the offending activities or agents and treatment with antifungal agents (such as miconazole or ketoconazole) and topical or oral corticosteroids are advocated for chronic paronychia. Although medical therapy is the mainstay of treatment for chronic paronychia, surgical therapy may provide benefit for nonresponders. The most common surgical technique used to treat chronic paronychia is called eponychial marsupialization. Advanced cases of acute paronychia should be incised and drained. Advanced cases of paronychia result in disappearance of the cuticle with retraction of the proximal nail fold from the underlying nail plate.

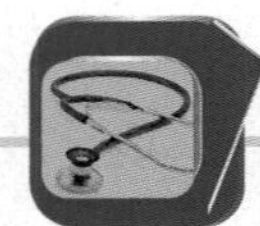

Equipment

- A recommended anesthesia tray is shown in Appendix F.
- A typical surgical tray is shown in Appendix G.

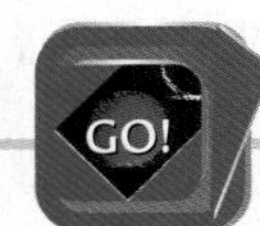

Indications

- Abscess formation or severe pain in acute paronychia
- Lack of response to medical therapy and avoidance of moisture and irritation
- Deformity (i.e., loss of the proximal nail fold) in chronic paronychia

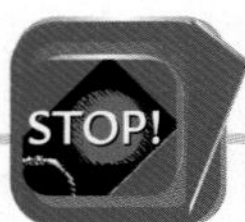

Contraindications

- Unfamiliarity of the practitioner with the techniques
- Bleeding diathesis or coagulopathy
- Chronic paronychia surgery in an unreliable patient or person unable to provide wound care

The Procedure

Step 1. A digital block is commonly performed (see Chapter 3) before surgery, although some practitioners prefer no anesthesia or a paronychia block when treating acute paronychia. The paronychia block uses a small (27- to 30-gauge) needle inserted from the lateral side near the distal interphalangeal joint, proximal to the paronychia. Administer between 1 and 3 mL of 1% lidocaine at this site.

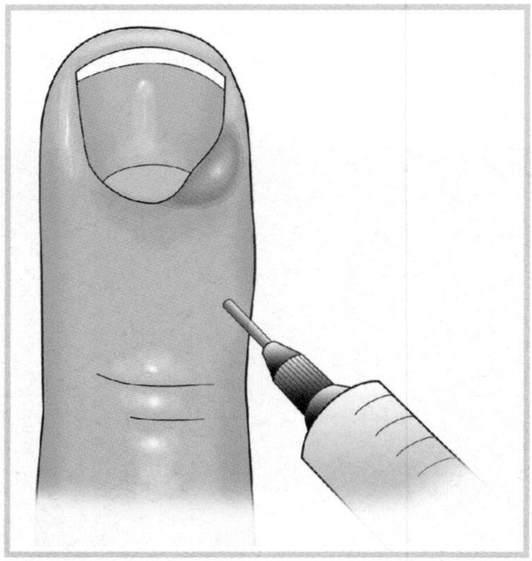

Step 1

Step 2. Swelling of the proximal and lateral nail fold is associated with this abscess of an acute paronychia. A no. 11 scalpel blade is laid flat on top of the nail plate, with the tip of the blade directed to the center of the abscess or fluctuance. The blade is guided quickly but gently into the nail surface under the nail fold, and then the tip is elevated, pulling the nail fold upward.

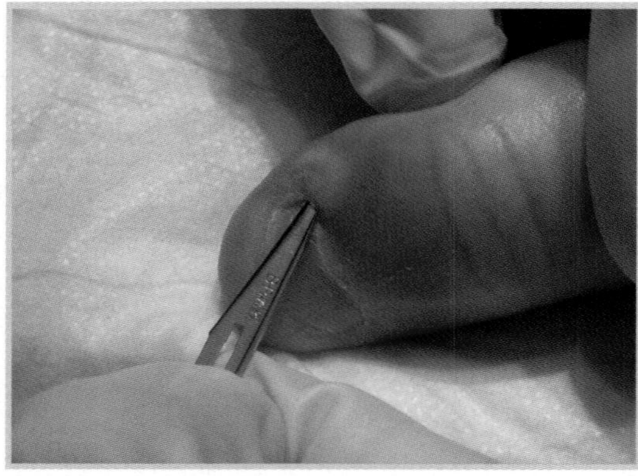

Step 2

Step 3. The nail plate acts as a fulcrum; pushing down on the back of the blade (or blade handle) causes the tip to elevate. A large amount of pus may drain on top of the nail plate. Pus can be squeezed from beneath the nail and through the small opening. This technique has the advantage of the absence of a skin incision.

- PITFALL: Failure to elevate the tissue sufficiently may permit pus to remain in the site. Because the opening over the nail plate is small and does not involve an incision, the site can reseal, and the abscess can redevelop. Several sites along the nail fold may require elevation to ensure adequate drainage, and the patient should be reexamined in 2 days to check for reformation of the paronychia.

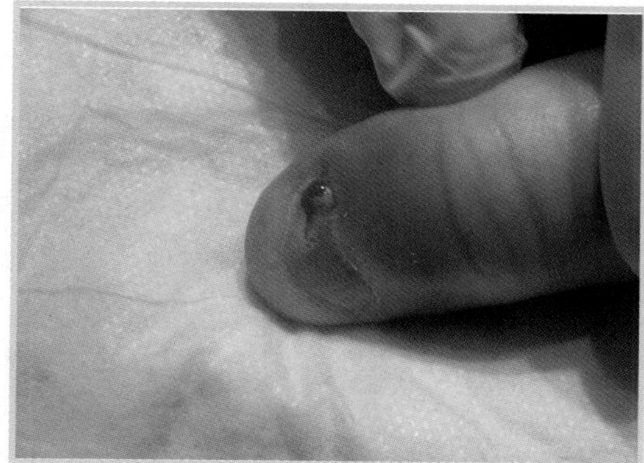

Step 3

Step 4. Recalcitrant chronical paronychia can be treated with excision of the proximal nail fold. After a digital block, a Freer septum elevator or the jaw of a hemostat is used to separate the proximal nail fold from the nail plate.

- PEARL: The flat elevator may then position beneath the proximal nail fold to protect underlying tissues during the excision.

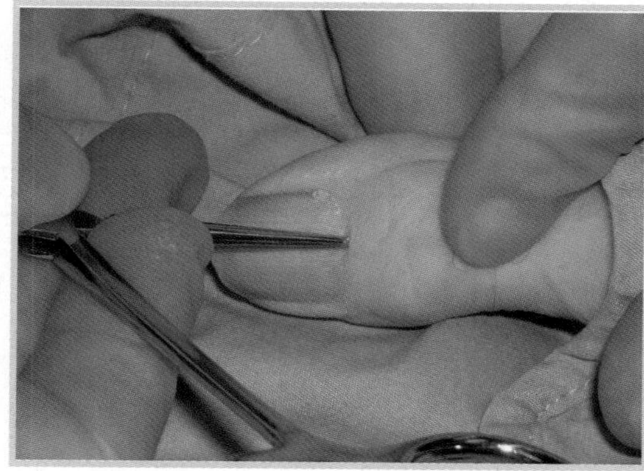

Step 4

Step 5. A crescent-shaped, full-thickness incision is made in the proximal nail fold. The incision extends from one lateral nail fold to the other.

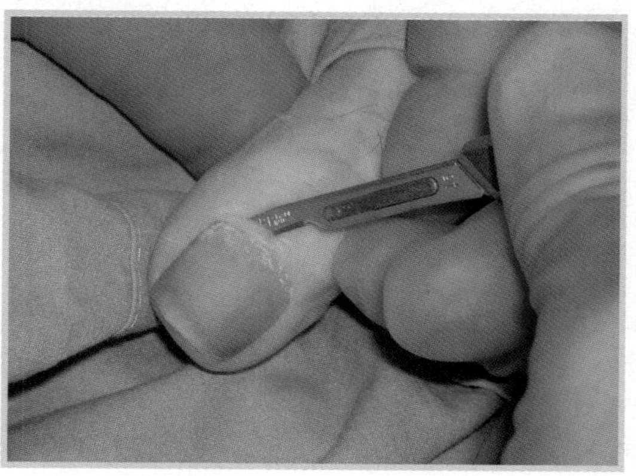

Step 5

Step 6. The island of skin to be removed is 3–5 mm wide, incorporates the entire swollen portion of the proximal nail fold, and extends to just proximal to the proximal nail plate. The side heals by secondary intention after about 2 months, with the resulting nail revealing a more visible lunula.

- PITFALL: Meticulous wound care is required after this procedure, and the surgery is appropriate only for patients who are able and willing to provide this care. Some physicians apply a combination antifungal and steroid ointment at night and antibiotic ointment during the day until the wound heals.

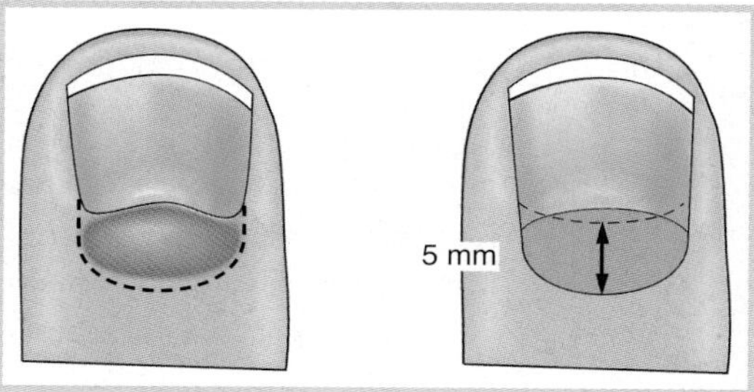

Step 6

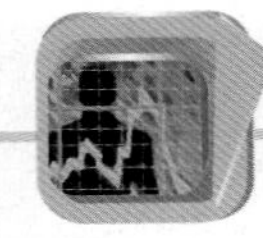

Complications

- Paronychial infections may spread
- Felon
- Secondary ridging, thickening, and discoloration of the nail
- Nail loss (rare)

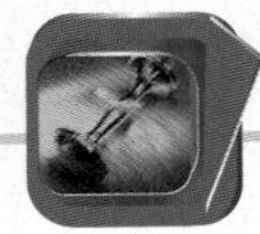

Pediatric Considerations

Children who bite their nails are more prone to paronychia. Behavioral modification may be necessary to prevent recurrences.

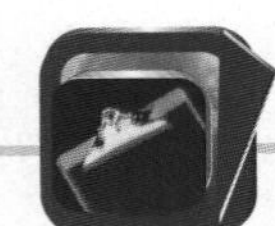

Postprocedure Instructions

The dressing should be removed in 48 hours. Then start warm water soaks four times a day for 15 minutes with gentle massage to express any collected pus. Between soakings, an adhesive bandage should be placed over the nail area. Antibiotic therapy is usually not necessary.

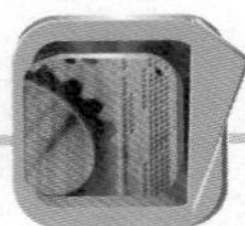

Coding Information and Supply Sources

CPT Code	Description	2008 Average 50th Percentile Fee	Global Period
10060	I&D of single or simple abscess	$167.00	10
10061	I&D of multiple or complex abscesses	$293.00	10

CPT is a registered trademark of the American Medical Association.
2008 average 50th Percentile Fees are provided courtesy of 2008 MMH-SI's copyrighted Physicians' Fees and Coding Guide.
I&D, incision and drainage.

Common ICD-9 Codes

Paronychia finger	681.02
Paronychia toe	681.11
Paronychia chronic	681.9

Instrument and Materials Ordering

- Instruments used for paronychia surgery, such as no. 11 scalpel blades, can be obtained from local surgical supply houses.
- Freer septum elevators can be purchased from surgical instrument dealers or through surgical supply houses.
- A suggested anesthesia tray that can be used for this procedure is listed in Appendix F.

Patient Education Handout

A patient education handout, "Paronychia," can be found on the book's Web site.

Bibliography

Clark RE, Madani S, Bettencourt MS. Nail surgery. *Dermatol Gin.* 1998;16:145–164.

Clark RE, Tope WD. Nail surgery. In: Wheeland RG, ed. *Cutaneous Surgery*. Philadelphia: WB Saunders; 1994:375–402.

Dahdah MJ, Scher RK. Nail diseases related to nail cosmetics. *Dermatol Clin.* 2006 Apr;24(2):233–239.

Goodheart HP. Infections: paronychia and onychomycosis. *Womens Health Prim Care.* 1998;1:232–237.

Haneke E, Baran R. Nails: surgical aspects. In: Parish LC, Lask GP, eds. *Aesthetic Dermatology*. New York: McGraw-Hill; 1991:236–247.

Lee S, Hendrickson ME. Paronychia. E-medicine. Available at http://www.emedicine.com/derm/topic798.htm. Accessed June 20, 2002.

Mayeaux EJ. Nail disorders. *Prim Care.* 2000;27:333–351.

Parungao AJ. A swollen, draining thumb. *Am Fam Physician*. 2002;65:105–106.

Rich P. Nail disorders: diagnosis and treatment of infectious, inflammatory, and neoplastic nail conditions. *Med Clin North Am.* 1998;82:1171–1183.

Roberge RJ, Weinstein D, Thimons MM. Perionychial infections associated with sculptured nails. *Am J Emerg Med.* 1999;17:581–582.

Rockwell PG. Acute and chronic paronychia. *Am Fam Physician*. 2001;63:1113–1116.

Shaw J, Body R. Incision and drainage preferable to oral antibiotics in acute paronychial nail infection? *Emerg Med J*. 2005;22;813–814.

Tosti A, Piraccini BM. Treatment of common nail disorders. *Dermatol Clin.* 2000;18:339–348.

2008 MAG Mutual Healthcare Solutions, Inc.'s Physicians' Fee and Coding Guide. Duluth, Georgia. MAG Mutual Healthcare Solutions, Inc. 2007.

SECTION SEVEN

Gynecology and Urology

CHAPTER 67

Bartholin Gland Cyst and Abscess Treatment

E. J. Mayeaux, Jr., MD, DABFP, FAAFP

Professor of Family Medicine, Professor of Obstetrics and Gynecology
Louisiana State University Health Sciences Center, Shreveport, LA

Bartholin gland cysts or abscesses develop in approximately 2% of all women. These lesions can cause extreme pain and limitation of activity because of expansion or infection. The glands' secretions provide some moisture for the vulva but are not needed for sexual lubrication. Removal of a Bartholin gland does not compromise the vestibular epithelium or sexual functioning.

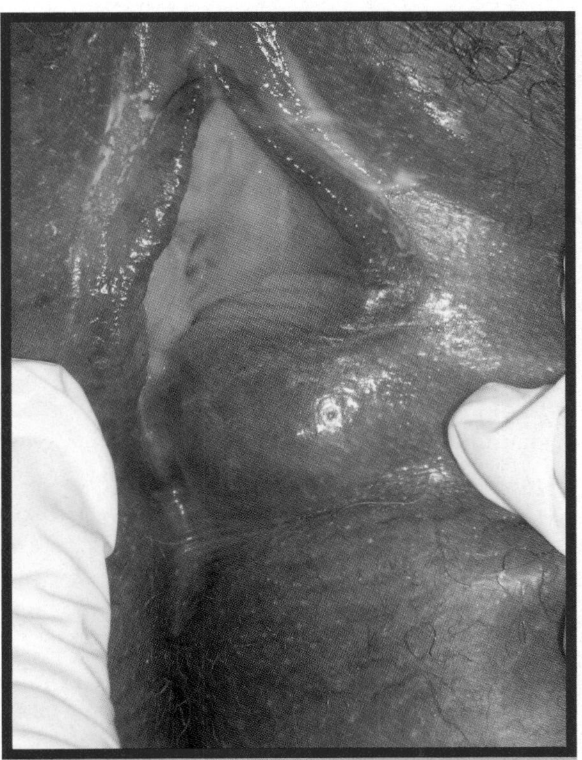

The Bartholin glands are located at 5 o'clock and 7 o'clock at the vaginal introitus and normally cannot be palpated. Bartholin gland cysts develop from dilation of the duct after blockage of the duct orifice. These lesions usually are 1 to 3 cm in diameter and asymptomatic. When symptoms occur, the patient may report vulvar pain, dyspareunia, inability to engage in sports, and pain during walking or sitting.

When the Bartholin cyst become an abscess, patients may experience severe dyspareunia, difficulty in walking or sitting, and vulvar pain. Patients can develop a large, tender mass in the vestibular area with associated vulvar erythema and edema. The abscess usually develops over 2 to 4 days and can become larger than 8 cm in diameter. The condition can be so painful that the patient is incapacitated. The abscess tends to rupture and drain after 4 to 5 days.

The best method for treating a cyst or abscess is one that preserves physiologic function with a minimum of scarring. Simple incision and drainage has a recurrence rate of 70% to 80%. When treating an abscess, obtain cultures for chlamydia and gonorrhea, and prescribe oral broad-spectrum antibiotics. Diabetic patients are more susceptible to necrotizing infections and need careful observation. Consider inpatient management of women with severe infections.

Simple incision and drainage provides prompt symptomatic relief, but recurrence is common. Treatment is not contraindicated in pregnant women, although the increase in blood flow to the pelvic area during pregnancy may lead to excessive bleeding from the procedure. If treatment is necessary because of an abscess, local anesthesia and most broad-spectrum antibiotics are safe.

In 1964, Dr. B. A. Word introduced a simple fistulization technique using a small, inflatable, self-sealing, bulb-tipped catheter. Early abscesses can be treated with sitz baths until the abscess points, making incision and definitive treatment easier. Instruct the patient to return in 4 weeks for a follow-up examination or sooner if she experiences discomfort, swelling, or other symptoms of infection. Patients may use ibuprofen (400 to 800 mg taken every 6 hours) for discomfort in the immediate postoperative period, and they should refrain from intercourse during the healing time to prevent displacement of the catheter. The catheter is removed by deflating the balloon, and over time, the resulting orifice will decrease in size and become unnoticeable.

Other options for treatment of a Bartholin gland abscess include the marsupialization or "window" procedure, carbon dioxide laser excision, and surgical excision. The marsupialization procedure is a relatively straightforward procedure that can be performed in the office, emergency department, or outpatient surgical suite in about 15 minutes using local anesthesia. It can be used as primary treatment or can be used if a cyst or abscess recurs after treatment with a Word catheter. The recurrence rate after marsupialization is 10% to 15%.

A cyst that has recurred several times despite office-based treatment may require excision. Excision of a Bartholin gland cyst is an outpatient surgical procedure that probably should be performed in an operating suite by an experienced physician because of the possibility of copious bleeding from the underlying venous plexus. Excision is usually performed under general anesthesia or with a pudendal block. It can result in intraoperative hemorrhage, hematoma formation, secondary infection, and dyspareunia as a result of scar tissue formation.

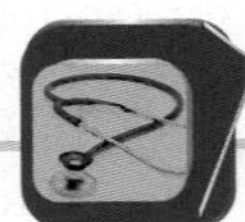

Equipment

- Prep solution (see Appendix E)
- Anesthetic solution

Word Catheter Technique

- Word catheter
- 18- or 20-gauge needle and 5-mL syringe plus water or gel for inflation of catheter tip
- No. 11 scalpel
- Hemostat (for breaking up loculations)
- Culture media for gonorrhea, chlamydia, and routine cultures
- Silver nitrate sticks
- Gauze pads

Marsupialization

- No. 11 scalpel
- Delayed-absorbable suture (3-0 or 4-0) on small cutting needle
- Small needle driver
- Scissors
- Hemostats
- Forceps
- Culture media
- Silver nitrate sticks
- Gauze pads

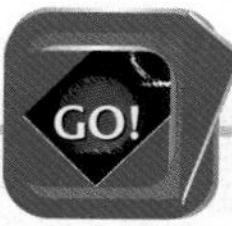

Indications

- Enlarged or painful Bartholin cyst or abscess

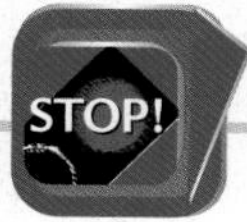

Contraindications

- Surgery on an acutely, severely inflamed abscess (relative contraindication)
- Asymptomatic cysts (relative contraindication)
- Latex allergy (e.g., to Word catheter)

The Procedure

Word Catheter

Step 1. Explain the procedure of fistulization with a Word catheter and obtain informed consent. Test the device by inserting the needle into the center of the base of the Word catheter and inflate the bulb.

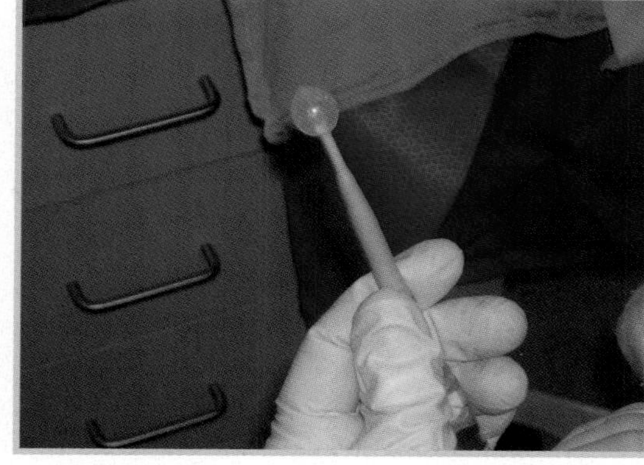

Step 1

Step 2. Apply field block anesthesia (see Chapter 2) and prep the area (see Appendix E).

- **PITFALL:** Inject under and around the abscess, not into it. Lidocaine injected into the cavity is trapped and cannot provide anesthesia. Injection into the abscess can cause increased internal pressure and outward rupture of the abscess.
- **PEARL:** It may cause less pain to simply incise without anesthesia an abscess that has very attenuated overlying skin.

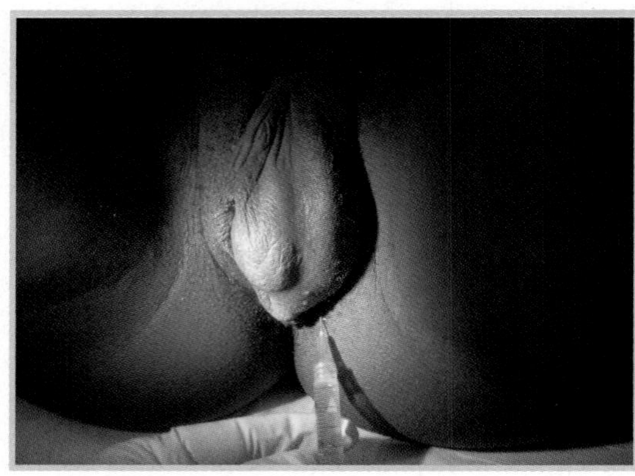

Step 2

Step 3. Use a stab incision with a no. 11 scalpel blade to make a 1.0- to 1.5-cm-deep opening into the cyst, preferably just inside or, if necessary, just outside the hymenal ring. Consider testing abscess contents for chlamydia and gonorrhea.

- **PITFALL:** Do not make the incision on the outer labium minus or labium majus. The resulting scar may cause pain, a poor cosmetic result, or a permanent fistula.
- **PITFALL:** Do not extend the incision beyond the width of the blade, or the catheter will require a retention stitch.

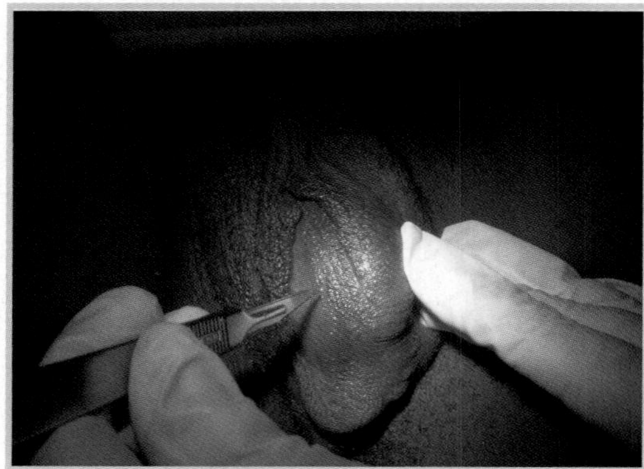

Step 3

Step 4. Break up loculations with a hemostat or similar instrument.

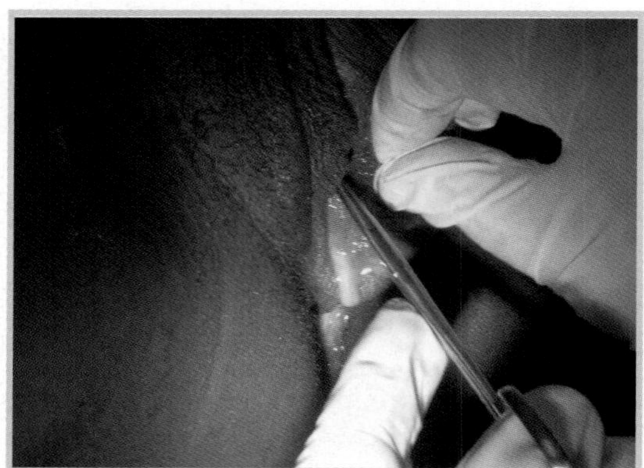

Step 4

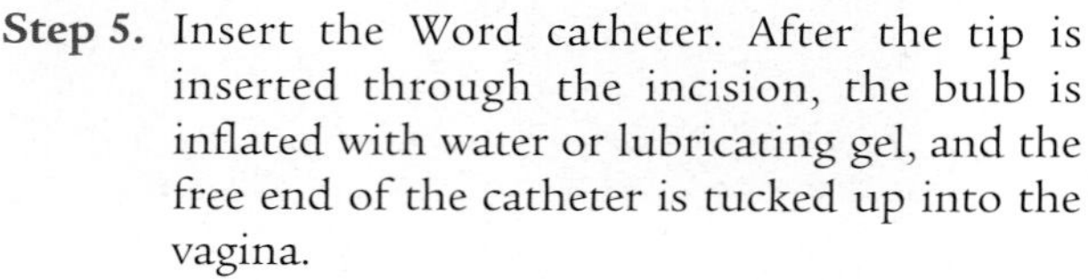

Step 5. Insert the Word catheter. After the tip is inserted through the incision, the bulb is inflated with water or lubricating gel, and the free end of the catheter is tucked up into the vagina.

- **PITFALL:** Use water or gel rather than air to prevent premature deflation of the balloon.

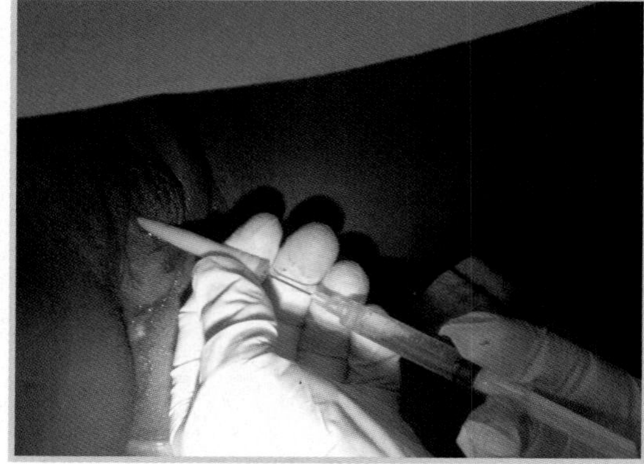

Step 5

Step 6. Leave the catheter in place for up to 4 weeks to permit complete epithelialization of the new tract. The patient may take daily baths or showers and gently cleanse the area with soap and water. Contact the patient if tests for sexually transmitted diseases are positive.

- **PITFALL:** The catheter frequently falls out. Placement of a vaginal suture into vulvar skin and tied to the catheter can help hold those that recurrently fall out.

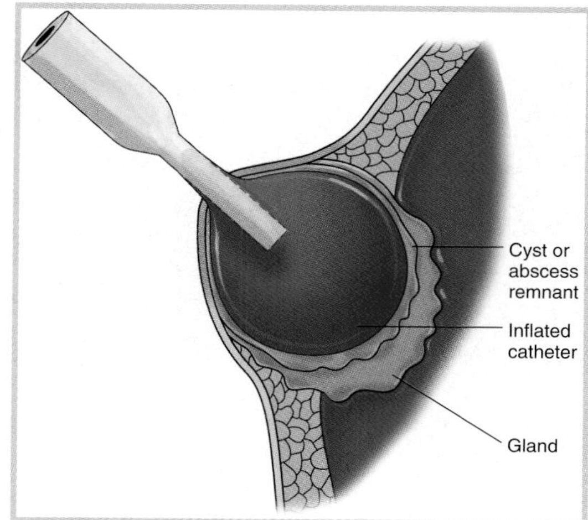

Step 6

Marsupialization

Step 1. For marsupialization, wash the area with povidone-iodine solution, and make a fusiform incision adjacent to the hymenal ring.

- **PITFALL:** Do not make the incision on the outer labium minus or labium majus. The resulting scar may cause pain, a poor cosmetic result, or a permanent fistula.

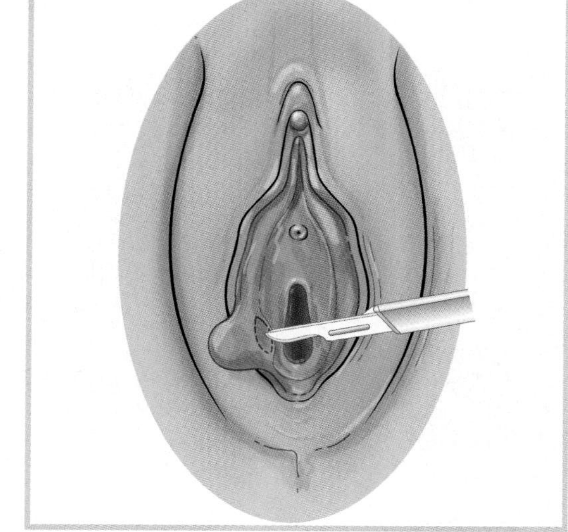

Step 1

Step 2. The incision should measure about 2 cm long and should be deep enough to enter the cyst. Remove an oval wedge of vulvar skin and the underlying cyst wall. The cyst or abscess will drain once it has been unroofed. Break up loculations inside the cyst, if present.

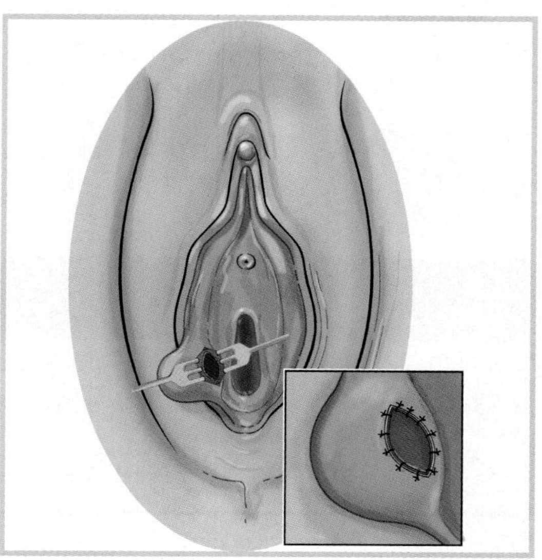

Step 2

Step 3. Suture the cyst wall to the adjacent vestibular skin using interrupted 3-0 or 4-0 absorbable (Vicryl) sutures. The new tract will slowly shrink over time and epithelialize, forming a new, larger duct orifice.

- **PITFALL:** If bleeding occurs, use suture placement or direct pressure for hemostasis of the skin edge.

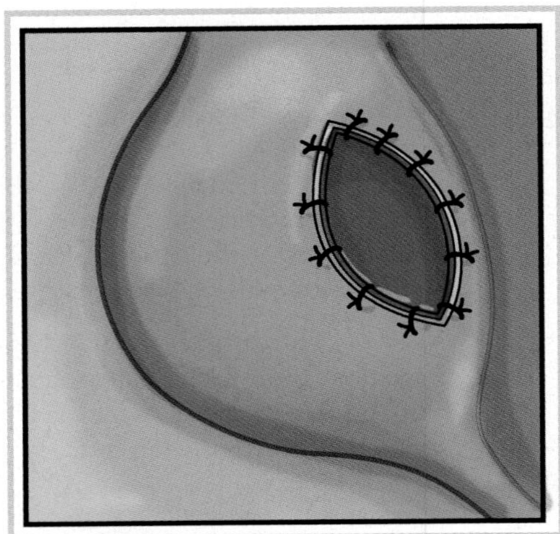

Step 3

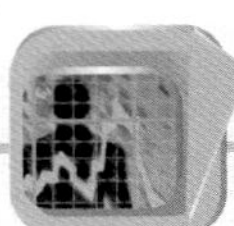

Complications

- Nonhealing
- Recurrent abscess
- Scarring
- Septic shock (with incision of abscess)

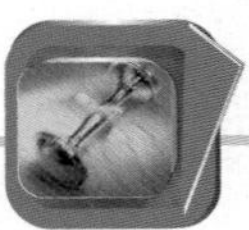

Pediatric Considerations

This problem is rarely encountered in the pediatric population.

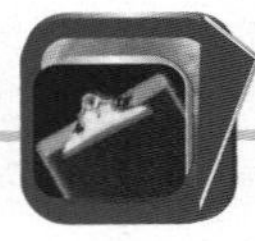

Postprocedure Instructions

The patient should avoid tub baths and intercourse until the tissues heal. The patient can resume other usually activities.

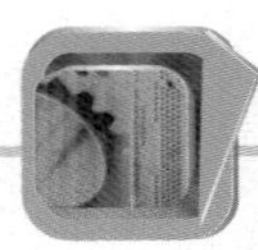

Coding Information and Supply Sources

CPT Code	Description	2008 Average 50th Percentile Fee	Global Period
56420	I&D of abscess of Bartholin gland	$340.00	10
56440	Marsupialization of Bartholin gland cyst	$872.00	10
56740	Excision of Bartholin's gland or cyst	$992.00	10

CPT is a registered trademark of the American Medical Association.
2008 average 50th Percentile Fees are provided courtesy of 2008 MMH-SI's copyrighted Physicians' Fees and Coding Guide.
I&D, incision and drainage.

Supply Sources

- A standard office surgical tray used for simple surgical procedures is described in Appendix G.
- A suggested anesthesia tray that can be used for this procedure is listed in Appendix F.
- Word catheters may be ordered from Milex Products, Inc., Chicago, 11 (phone: 1-800-621-1278; http://www.milexproducts.com) or from your local Milex dealer.

Patient Education Handout

A patient education handout, "Bartholin Gland Cysts and Abscesses," can be found on the book's Web site.

Bibliography

Andersen PG, Christensen S, Detlefsen GU, et al. Treatment of Bartholin's abscess: marsupialization versus incision, curettage and suture under antibiotic cover: a randomized study with 6 months' follow-up. *Acta Obstet Gynecol Scand.* 1992;71:59–62.

Bleker OP, Smalbraak DJ, Schutte ME. Bartholin's abscess: the role of *Chlamydia trachomatis. Genitourin Med.* 1990;66:24–25.

Brook I. Aerobic and anaerobic microbiology of Bartholin's abscess. *Surg Gynecol Obstet.* 1989;169:32–34.

Curtis JM. Marsupialisation technique for Bartholin's cyst. *Aust Farre Physician.* 1993;22:369.

Davies JA, Rees E, Hobson D, et al. Isolation of *Chlamydia trachomatis* from Bartholin's ducts. *Br J Vener Dis.* 1978;54:409–413.

Downs MC, Randall HW. The ambulatory surgical management of Bartholin duct cysts. *J Emerg Med.* 1989;7:623–626.

Hill DA, Lense JJ. Office management of Bartholin gland cysts and abscesses. *Am Earn Physician.* 1998;57:1611–1616.

Lee YH, Rankin JS, Alpert S, et al. Microbiological investigation of Bartholin's gland abscesses and cysts. *Am J Obstet Gynecol.* 1977;129:150–153.

Monaghan JC. Fistulization for Bartholin's gland cysts. *Patient Care.* 1991;5:119–122.

Omole F, Simmons BJ, Hacker Y. Management of Bartholin's duct cyst and gland abscess. *Am Fam Physician.* 2003;68:135–140.

Wren MW. Bacteriological findings in cultures of clinical material from Bartholin's abscess. *J Clin Pathol.* 1977;30:1025–1027.

Yavetz H, Lessing JB, Jaffa AJ, et al. Fistulization: an effective treatment for Bartholin's abscesses and cysts. *Acta Obstet Gynecol Scand.* 1987;66:63–64.

2008 MAG Mutual Healthcare Solutions, Inc.'s Physicians' Fee and Coding Guide. Duluth, Georgia. MAG Mutual Healthcare Solutions, Inc. 2007.

CHAPTER 68

Cold Knife Conization of the Uterine Cervix

Racheal Whitaker, MD
Assistant Professor of Obstetrics and Gynecology
Louisiana State University Health Sciences Center, Shreveport, LA

Cervical conization refers to the surgical excision of a cone-shaped portion of the uterine cervix surrounding the endocervical canal and including the entire transformation zone and all or most of the cervical canal. It has been used for years for both diagnosis and treatment of cervical intraepithelial neoplasia. Screening for cervical dysplasia using cytology has resulted in a significant decrease in the incidence and mortality of cervical cancer. Once a patient has had an abnormal Papanicolaou (Pap) smear, the clinician should move forward to colposcopy with directed biopsies in an attempt to establish a histologic diagnosis. Conization of the cervix is indicated for the following: an unsatisfactory colposcopy (i.e., the entire squamocolumnar junction or the full extent of lesions cannot be visualized); colposcopic biopsy shows a lesion that is CIN (cervical intraepithelial neoplasia) II or CIN III and is not amenable to less invasive measures; cytologic and/or histologic findings are suggestive of possible invasive disease; recurrent disease after more conservative therapy; and discrepancy between the Pap results and colposcopic findings.

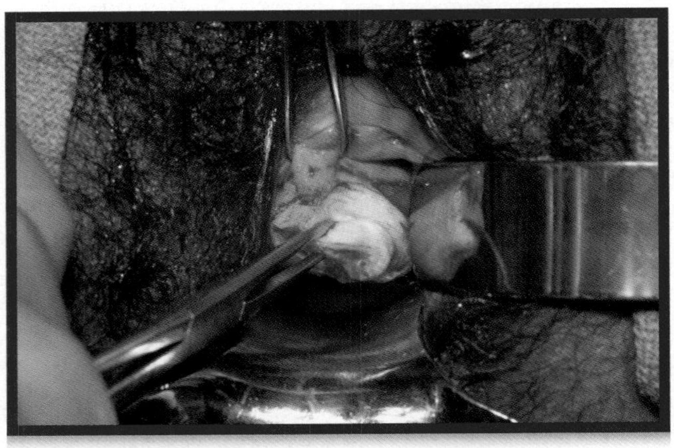

Anesthesia for the procedure may be regional or general. There are a number of ways to perform cervical conization, including laser, LEEP (loop electrosurgical excision procedure), and cold knife cone (CKC). This chapter focuses on cold knife conization.

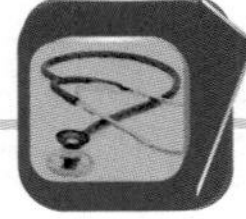

Equipment

- Urinary catheter
- Weighted speculum
- Right-angle retractor

- Single-tooth tenaculum
- Long-handled scalpel
- No. 11 blade
- Allis clamps
- Electrocautery unit
- Mayo scissors
- Kevorkian endocervical curette
- Delayed absorbable sutures (optional)
- Absorbable gelatin sponge (Gelfoam) (optional)

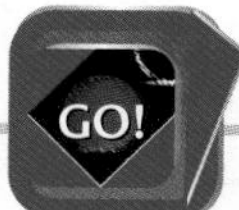

Indications

- Colposcopy is unsatisfactory:
  - Entire TMZ (transformation zone) cannot be visualized
  - Entire lesion cannot be visualized and/or extends into the cervical canal beyond the ability to visualize
- Cytologic and/or histologic findings show possible invasive disease.
- Two-grade difference is found between the Pap results and the colposcopic findings (e.g., the Pap shows high-grade squamous intraepithelial lesion [HSIL], but the colposcopy is normal).
- Biopsy shows microinvasion.
- Positive endocervical curettage (ECC) has been performed.
- Adenocarcinoma in situ is present.

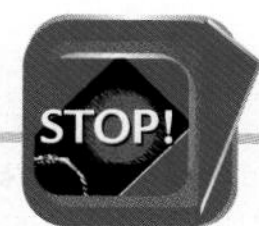

Contraindications

- Pregnancy (relative): conization should be done only in the case of cervical cancer and should be performed by a gynecological oncologist.
- Cervical cancer is beyond stage IA1.

The Procedure

Step 1. Place the patient in the dorsal lithotomy position in candy cane stirrups.

- **PITFALL:** Do not do a digital vaginal exam at this time because it may cause bleeding and obscure the field.

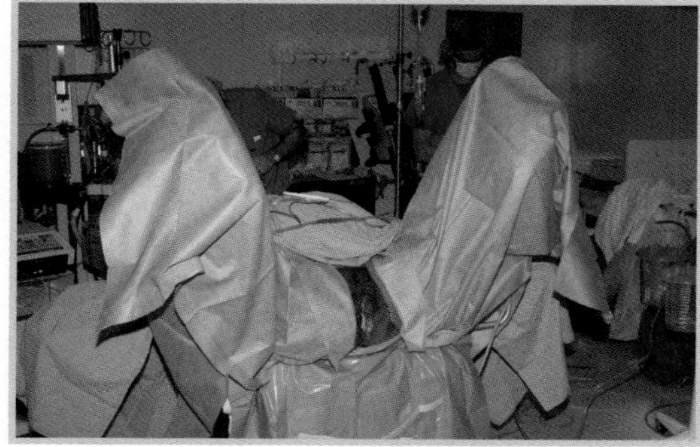

Step 1

Step 2. Perform a colposcopy with 3% to 5% acetic acid or Lugol's solution and examine the cervix. Some clinicians choose not to do this when there is a colposcopic diagram available that shows the areas of dysplasia. See Chapter 71, Colposcopy and Directed Cervical Biopsy.

- **PEARL:** Be gentle when preparing the cervix and vagina to prevent trauma to the cervix that may lead to difficulty in histologic interpretation of the cervix.

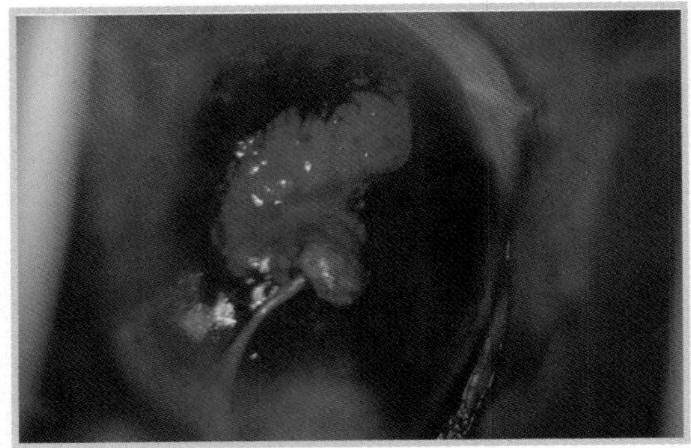

Step 2

Step 3. Grasp the anterior lip of the cervix, and inject diluted vasopressin or epinephrine into the cervical stroma just lateral to the area that is to be coned.

- **PITFALL:** Always let the anesthesiologist know when you inject a vasoconstrictor.
- **PEARL:** Some clinicians place absorbable sutures at 3 o'clock and 9 o'clock positions in the cervix at the cervicovaginal junction to impede flow to the cervical branches of the uterine arteries. One must take care not to place the sutures too deep so that they will not be inadvertently cut during excision.

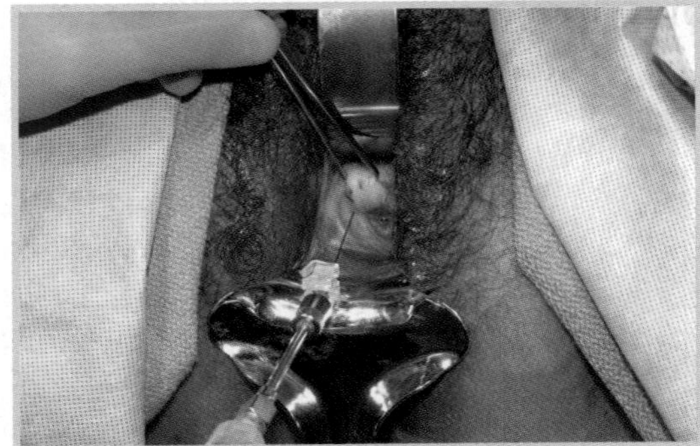

Step 3

Step 4. Use a long-handled scalpel with a no. 11 blade to make a circumferential incision just lateral to the TMZ. Start posteriorly, and insert the scalpel blade at the desired depth, angling toward the endocervical canal. It is also reasonable to make a superficial circumferential incision initially and then go deep.

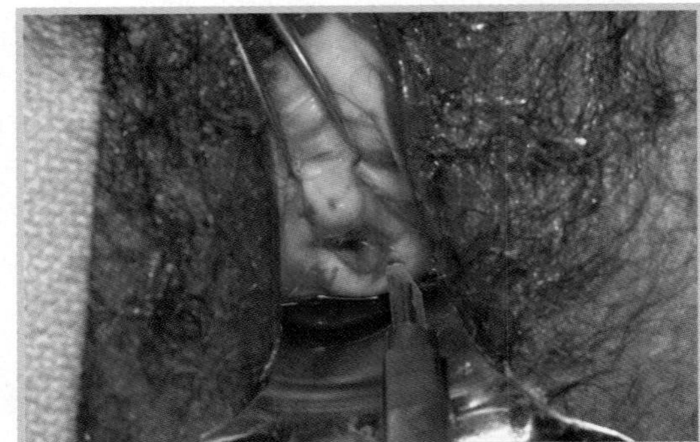

Step 4

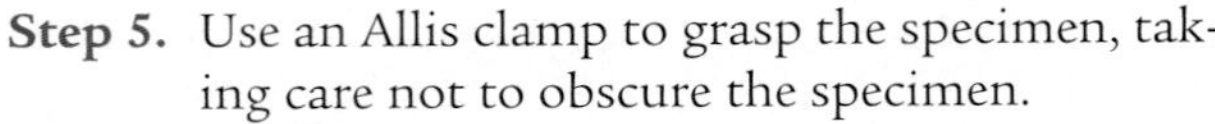

Step 5. Use an Allis clamp to grasp the specimen, taking care not to obscure the specimen.

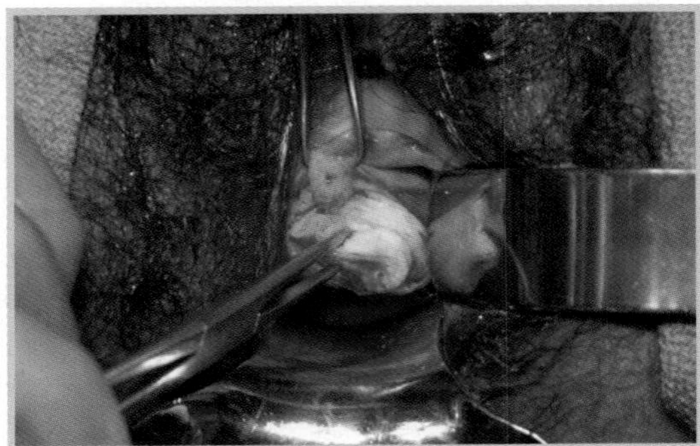

Step 5

Step 6. With either Mayo scissors or a scalpel, completely excise the specimen. Label the specimen with a stitch so that the pathologist will be properly oriented (e.g., place a stitch at 12 o'clock).

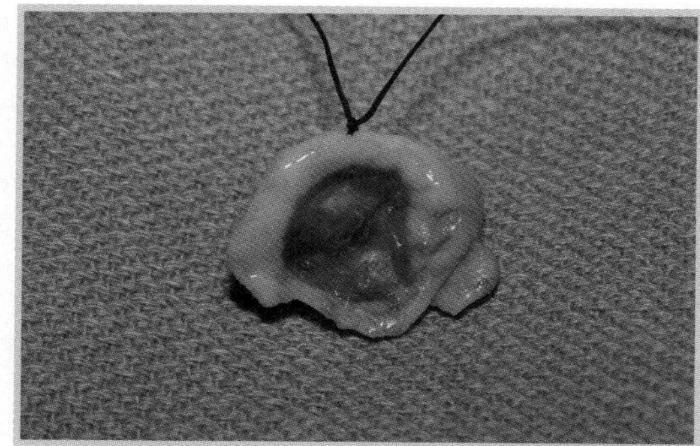

Step 6

Step 7. Perform a curettage of the endocervix to exclude residual disease. The cone bed can be made hemostatic with electrocautery. Some clinicians place Gelfoam in the cone bed when sutures are used. The ends of the suture are then tied over the Gelfoam.

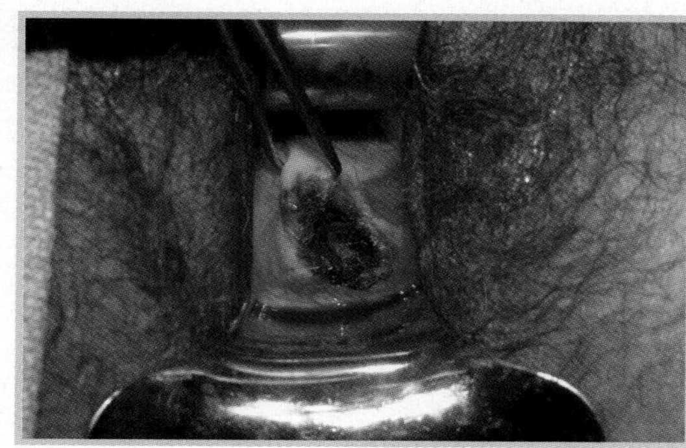

Step 7

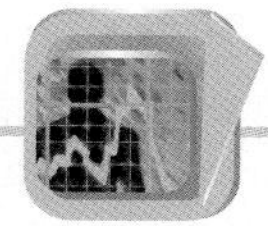

Complications

Immediate

- Bleeding (intraoperative or postoperative)
- Infection
- Uterine perforation

Long Term

- Cervical stenosis
- Cervical incompetence

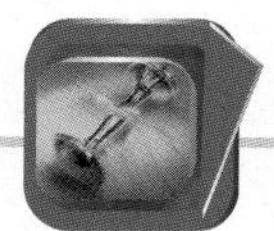

Pediatric Considerations

Advanced cervical dysplasia and especially cancer are very rare in the pediatric population. However, the indications and procedure are similar, except CIN2 and diagnostic mismatches may be followed with colposcopy in the adolescent population.

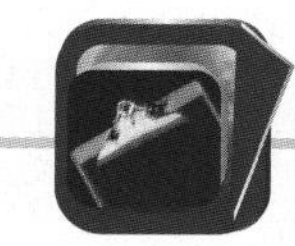

Postprocedure Instructions

The patient is instructed to place nothing into her vagina (tampons, douching, intercourse) for 4 weeks. She should also avoid immersing herself in water (e.g., by taking a bath or swimming) for 4 weeks.

Pain from the procedure is minimal and very seldom requires narcotics. A discharge is normal and may last for up to 4 weeks. Patients with no surgical complications may return to work within a day of surgery.

Assessment of cervical cytology and colposcopy are performed 4 to 6 months postoperatively. Specimens should not be obtained before 3 months because the inflammation makes pathology difficult to interpret.

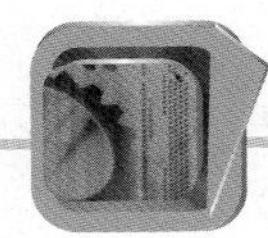

Coding Information and Supply Sources

CPT Code	Description	2008 Average 50th Percentile Fee	Global Period
57520	Conization of the cervix, w/wo fulguration, w/wo D&C, w/wo repair, cold knife or laser	$1,230.00	90

Typical gynecological instruments may be obtained from surgical supply houses and hospital supply sources, and many are listed in Appendix H.

Patient Education Handout

A patient education handout, "Conization of the Cervix," can be found on the book's companion Web site.

Bibliography

Berek SJ, Hacker NF. *Practical Gynecologic Oncology.* Philadelphia: Lippincott Williams & Wilkins, 2004.

Clinical Management Guidelines for Obstetrician-Gynecologist. Washington, DC: American College of Obstetricians and Gynecologists; 2005. ACOG Practice Bulletin 66.

Hoffman M, Mann W. Procedures for cervical conization: technique and outcome. http://www.utdol.com/. Accessed December 6, 2007.

Reich O, Pickel H, Lahousen M, et al. Cervical intraepithelial neoplasia III: long-term outcome after cold-knife conization with clear margins. *Obstet Gynecol.* 2001;97(3):428–430.

Webb M. Mayo Clinic Manual of Pelvic Surgery. Webb M (ed.). Philadelphia: Lippincott Williams & Wilkins, 2000.

Wright TC Jr, Cox JT, Massad LS, et al. Consensus guidelines for the management of women with cervical cytological abnormalities and cervical cancer precursors, part I: cytological abnormalities. *JAMA.* 2002;287(18):2120–2129.

Wright TC, Cox JT, Massad LS, et al. Consensus guidelines for the management of women with cervical intraepithelial neoplasia. *Amer J Obstet Gynecol.* 2003;189:295–304.

2008 MAG Mutual Healthcare Solutions, Inc.'s Physicians' Fee and Coding Guide. Duluth, Georgia. MAG Mutual Healthcare Solutions, Inc. 2007.

CHAPTER 69

Cervical Polyp Removal

E.J. Mayeaux, Jr., MD, DABFP, FAAFP

Professor of Family Medicine, Professor of Obstetrics and Gynecology
Louisiana State University Health Sciences Center, Shreveport, LA

Cervical polyps are pedunculated tumors that commonly arise from the mucosa of the endocervical canal. They are usually red and have a soft, spongy structure. Cervical polyps are common and are most often seen in perimenopausal and multigravid women in the third through fifth decades of life. The cause of most polyps is unknown, but they are associated with increasing age, inflammation, trauma, and pregnancy.

The histology of cervical polyps is similar to that of the endocervical canal, with a single tall columnar cell layer and occasional cervical glands. Vascular congestion, edema, and inflammation are frequently present. Many endocervical polyps demonstrate squamous metaplasia, which may cytologically and colposcopically mimic dysplasia. Squamous dysplasia and cancer may originate on cervical polyps, but malignant degeneration is rare. However, if a polyp is discovered after an atypical Papanicolaou (Pap) smear, the polyp should be sent for pathologic study, especially if it contains any acetowhite epithelium.

TABLE 69-1. Differential Diagnosis

Endometrial polyp
Prolapsed myoma
Incomplete spontaneous abortion
Leiomyosarcoma
Squamous papilloma
Sarcoma
Cervical malignancy

Polyps are often asymptomatic and are typically found at the time of the routine gynecologic examination. They may be single or multiple and may vary in size from a few millimeters to several centimeters. Rarely, the pedicle can become so elongated that the polyp protrudes from the vaginal introitus. There may be vaginal discharge associated with cervical polyps, especially if the polyp becomes infected. Ulceration of the tip and vascular congestion often result in postcoital or dysfunctional uterine bleeding. Larger polyps may bleed periodically, producing intermenstrual spotting and postcoital bleeding. Valsalva straining also may stimulate bleeding. Symptoms may be exactly the same as in the early stages of cervical cancer.

An association exists between cervical and endometrial polyps. Postmenopausal women with cervical polyps have a higher incidence of coexisting endometrial polyps that is unrelated to hormone replacement therapy. Patients on tamoxifen therapy have a very high association of cervical polyps with endometrial polyps and probably should be evaluated with dilatation and curettage. However, most physicians perform simple polypectomy in the office if the patient is otherwise asymptomatic. The differential diagnosis for cervical polyps is shown in Table 69-1.

Because most polyps are benign, they may be removed or observed on routine examinations. They are often twisted off during routine examinations to reduce the incidence of inflammation and incidental bleeding. Polyps may also be removed during dilatation and curettage, by hysteroscopic wire or snare, by electrocautery, during a loop electrosurgical excisional procedure, or by surgical excision.

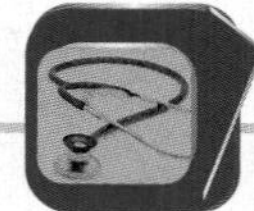

Potential Equipment

- Ring forceps
- Cervical curette
- Kogan's endocervical speculum
- Cervical biopsy forceps
- Monsel's solution

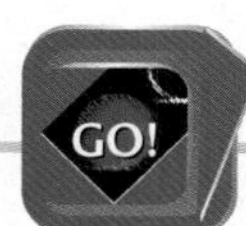

Indications

- Removal of polyps is usually indicated to prevent irritation, vaginal discharge, and bleeding.

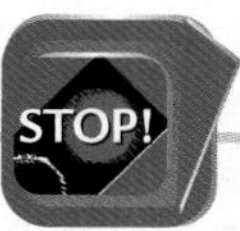

Contraindications

- During pregnancy, the cervix is highly vascularized, and polyps should be observed if they are stable and appear benign. They should be removed only if they are causing bleeding.
- Severe bleeding disorders
- Local infection

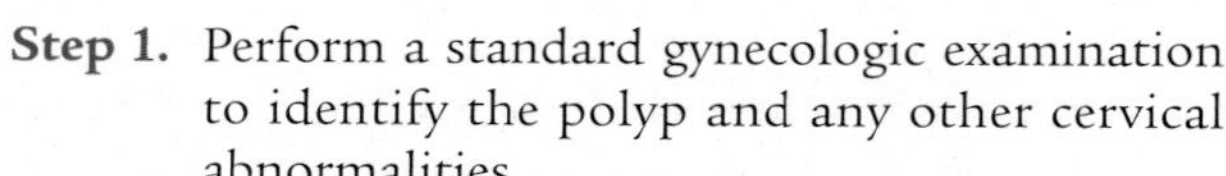

The Procedure

Step 1. Perform a standard gynecologic examination to identify the polyp and any other cervical abnormalities.

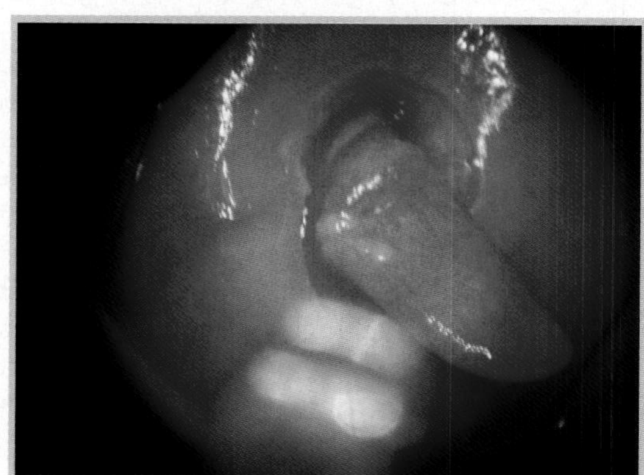

Step 1

Step 2. Attempt to identify the base of the polyp and ensure it originates from the cervical canal.

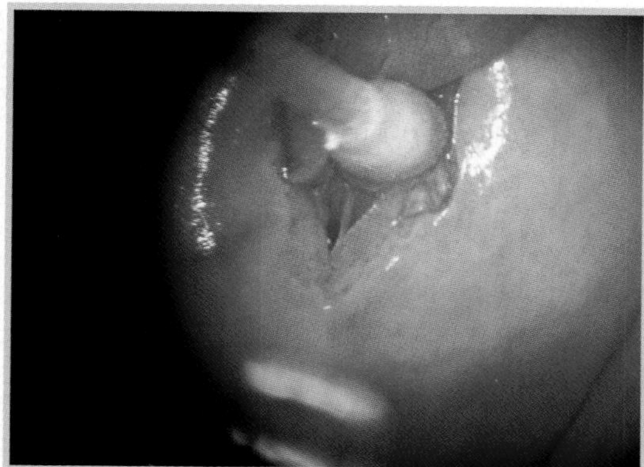
Step 2

Step 3. If the base of the polyp can not be readily identified, consider using Kogan's endocervical speculum to move the polyp and identify the base.

- **PEARL:** When the base is identified, the endocervical speculum may be closed on the polyp and used to remove it.

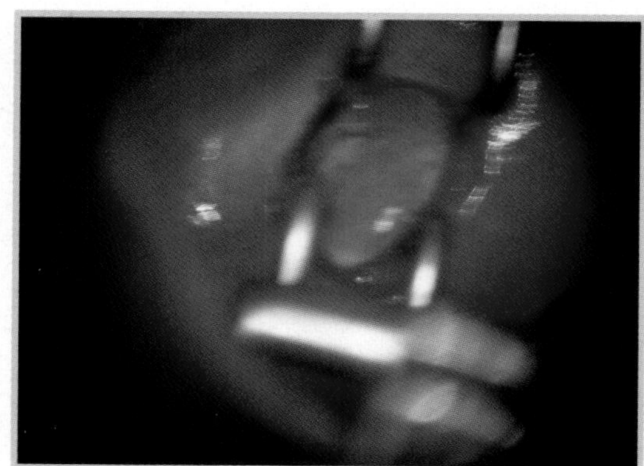
Step 3

Step 4. Gently grasp the polyp with ring forceps or the endocervical speculum, apply slight traction, and twist repeatedly until it falls off.

- **PITFALL:** Be sure to identify the location of the base of the polyp to exclude the possibility of an endometrial polyp, which may produce extensive bleeding. If the pedicle extends too deeply to be easily visualized, a Kogan endocervical speculum and colposcopic magnification are often helpful.

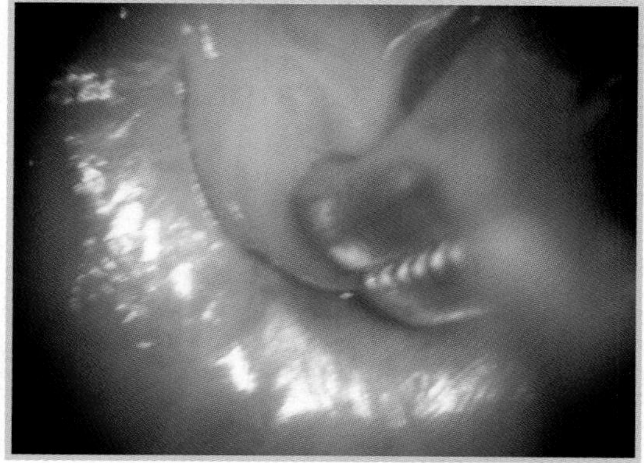
Step 4

Step 5. Alternatively, a small polyp may be scraped off in its entirety with a sharp curette or biopsied off with a Tischler biopsy forceps. Bleeding is usually self-limited but can be controlled with pressure, Monsel's solution, or cautery.

- **PITFALL:** If multiple polyps, irregular bleeding, or ongoing tamoxifen therapy is noted, it may be prudent to remove the polyps while performing dilatation and curettage.

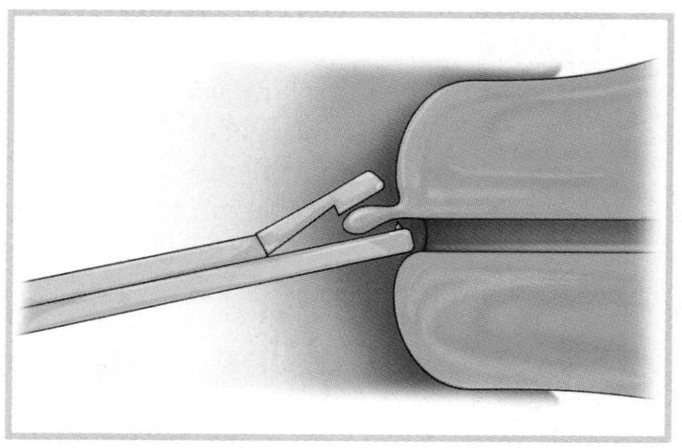
Step 5

Step 6. Inspect the cervical os to make sure the entire polyp was removed. If a significant amount of the base of the polyp remains, it may be scraped off with a curette.

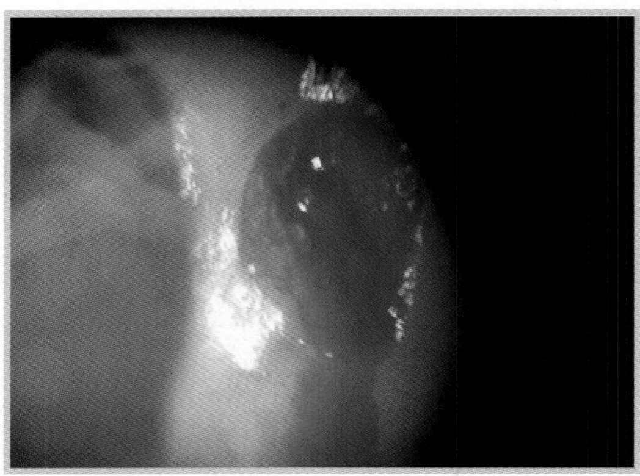

Step 6

Step 7. If a significant amount of bleeding is present, Monsel's paste may be applied for hemostasis.

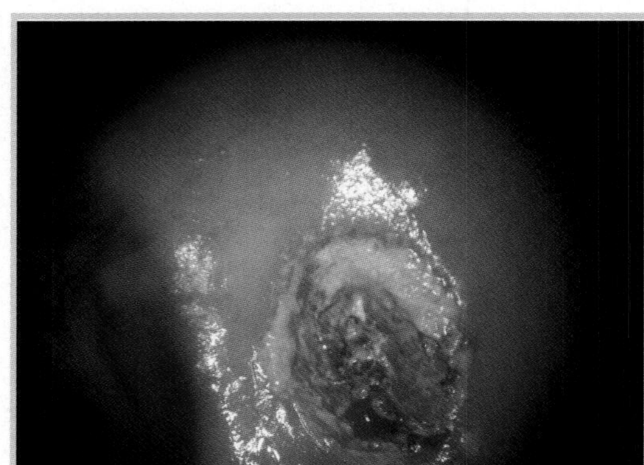

Step 7

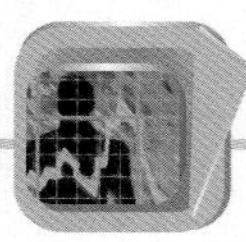

Complications

- Typically none
- Bleeding
- Regrowth

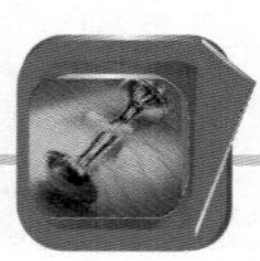

Pediatric Considerations

This procedure is almost never necessary or performed in the pediatric population.

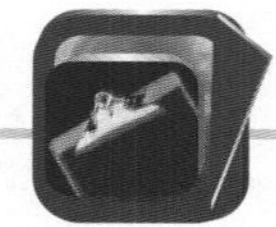

Postprocedure Instructions

After removal of a polyp, the patient should avoid sexual intercourse, douching, and tampon usage for several days. A follow-up examination may be done in 1 to 2 weeks to check for problems, if desired. If active bleeding occurs, the patient should be seen immediately. Examination to check for regrowth should be performed at routine gynecologic visits. Unfortunately, recurrence is common.

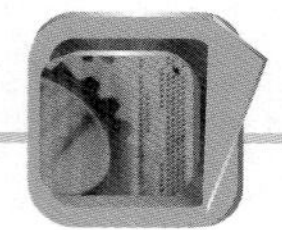

Coding Information and Supply Sources

There is no separate CPT code for cervical polyp removal. Some practitioners report polypectomy with 57500 (cervix uteri biopsy) or 57505 (endocervical curettage). If the colposcope is used to identify the polyp base, 57452 can be used to report services.

The medical equipment such as Ring forceps, curettes, Kogan's endocervical speculums, and cervical biopsy forceps may be ordered from:

- Cooper Surgical, Shelton, CT (phone: 800-645-3760 or 203-929-6321; www.coopersurgical.com)
- Olympus America, Inc., Melville, NY (phone: 800-548-555 or 631-844-5000; www.olympusamerica.com)
- Utah Medical Products, Inc., Mid-vale, UT (phone: 800-533-4984 or 801-566-1200; www.utahmed.com)
- Wallach Surgical Devices, Inc., Orange, CT (phone: 203-799-2000 or 800-243-2463; www.wallachsurgical.com)

Patient Education Handout

A patient education handout, "Cervical Polyp" can be found on the book's Web site.

Bibliography

Abramovici H, Bornstein J, Pascal B. Ambulatory removal of cervical polyps under colposcopy. *Int J Gynaecol Obstet.* 1984;22:47–50.

Coeman D, Van Belle Y, Vanderick G, et al. Hysteroscopic findings in patients with a cervical polyp. *Am J Obstet Gynecol.* 1993;169:1563–1565.

David A, Mettler L, Semm K. The cervical polyp: a new diagnostic and therapeutic approach with CO2 hysteroscopy. *Am J Obstet Gynecol.* 1978;130:662–664.

Di Naro E, Bratta FG, Romano F, et al. The diagnosis of benign uterine pathology using transvaginal endohysterosonography. *Clin Exp Obstet Gynecol.* 1996;23:103–107.

Golan A, Ber A, Wolman I, et al. Cervical polyp: evaluation of current treatment. *Gynecol Obstet Invest.* 1994;37:56–58.

Goudas VT, Session DR. Hysteroscopic cervical polypectomy with a polyp snare. *J Am Assoc Gynecol Laparoscopists.* 1999;6:195–197.

Hillard GD. Case for diagnosis: cervical polyp. *Mil Med.* 1978;143:618, 631.

Khalil AM, Azar GB, Kaspar HG, et al. Giant cervical polyp: a case report. *J Reprod Med.* 1996;41:619–621.

Lee WH, Tan KH, Lee YW. The aetiology of postmenopausal bleeding—a study of 163 consecutive cases in Singapore. *Singapore Med J.* 1995;36:164–168.

Neri A, Kaplan B, Rabinerson D, et al. Cervical polyp in the menopause and the need for fractional dilatation and curettage. *Eur J Obstet Gynecol Reprod Biol.* 1995;62:53–55.

Vilodre LC, Bertat R, Petters R, et al. Cervical polyp as risk factor for hysteroscopically diagnosed endometrial polyps. *Gynecol Obstet Invest.* 1997;44:191–195.

2008 MAG Mutual Healthcare Solutions, Inc.'s Physicians' Fee and Coding Guide. Duluth, Georgia. MAG Mutual Healthcare Solutions, Inc. 2007.

CHAPTER 70

Endometrial Biopsy

E.J. Mayeaux, Jr., MD, DABFP, FAAFP
Professor of Family Medicine, Professor of Obstetrics and Gynecology
Louisiana State University Health Sciences Center, Shreveport, LA

Endometrial biopsy (EMB) is a safe and effective method for diagnosing various endometrial abnormalities. It provides a minimally invasive assessment of the endometrium that may be used as an alternative to dilatation and curettage or hysteroscopy. Modern suction catheters have made this outpatient technique easy to learn and perform. It provides part of a cost-effective diagnostic workup for abnormal uterine bleeding, and may be considered part of an evaluation that could include hysteroscopy, dilatation and curettage, or transvaginal ultrasonography. Although a negative study is reassuring, further evaluation is warranted if a patient demonstrates continued abnormal bleeding.

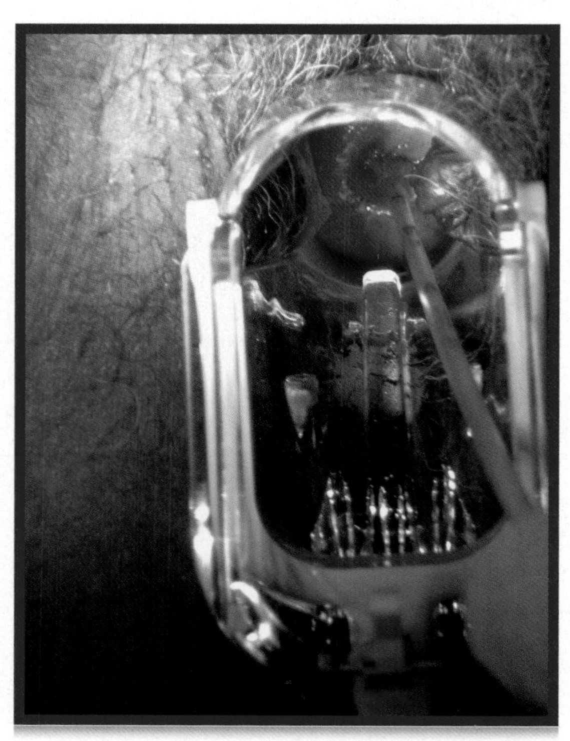

Catheter-type EMBs are safe. Uterine perforations are rare unless the device is forced. Postoperative infection is rare but may be prevented with the use of prophylactic antibiotic therapy such as doxycycline (100 mg) administered twice daily for 4 days after the procedure. The patient may also be premedicated with a nonsteroidal anti-inflammatory drug (NSAID) such as ibuprofen (600 to 800 mg) the night before and morning after or at least 1 hour before the procedure to decrease the cramping associated with the sampling. Bacterial endocarditis prophylaxis is no longer recommended (see Appendix C). Intraoperative and postoperative cramping is a frequent side effect of the procedure.

Some physicians prefer to apply a tenaculum and give slight countertraction toward the operator. Although a tenaculum helps stabilize the cervix, it also causes additional pain and bleeding. It may also be used to straighten a markedly anteverted or retroverted uterus and may make the procedure safer in this setting. If used, it should be applied to the anterior lip of the cervix (not in the os), with the teeth in a horizontal plane.

Because of the stenosis of the cervical os that develops in low-estrogen states, it can be difficult to perform an EMB in postmenopausal women. Elderly women can have a laminaria (i.e., thin piece of dried, sterile seaweed) placed in the cervix in the morning and then return in the afternoon to have the swollen (now moistened) laminaria removed immediately before the procedure. A cervical dilator may also be used when the EMB catheter cannot be passed through the internal os in postmenopausal women.

Topical benzocaine solution (i.e., Hurricaine solution) may be applied to the cervix to decrease the pain from entry of the curette into the uterus. A cervical or paracervical block also may be used. For a cervical block, inject 1% to 2% lidocaine with epinephrine submucosally in the center of each cervical quadrant. Anesthesia may be applied at any time during the procedure. Some data suggest that instilling 5 mL of 2% lidocaine into the uterine cavity before endometrial biopsies significantly decreases the pain of the EMB.

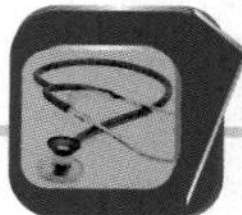

Equipment

- Catheter-type devices
  - Unimar PIPELLE (Pipelle de Cornier), which can be ordered from CooperSurgical, Inc., Shelton, CT. Phone: 1-800-243-2974. Web site: http://www.coopersurgical.com/.
  - Wallach Endocell Endometrial Cell Sampler (20-piece box), which can be ordered from Wallach Surgical Devices, Inc., 235 Edison Road, Orange, CT 06477. Phone: 203-799-2000; fax: 203-799-2002. E-mail: wallach@wallachsurgical.com. http://wallach@wallachsurgical.com/.

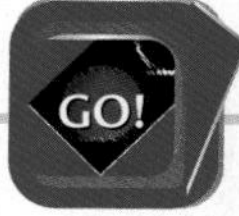

Indications

- Examination for abnormal uterine bleeding (to rule out endometrial hyperplasia or cancer)
- Workup for atypical glandular endometrial cells seen on the Papanicolaou (Pap) smear
- Monitor unopposed estrogen therapy for the development of hyperplasia
- Endometrial dating
- Infertility evaluation
- Postmenopausal bleeding

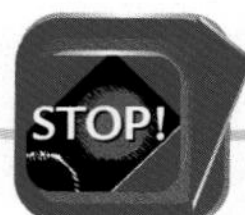

Contraindications

- Pregnancy or suspected pregnancy
- Acute pelvic inflammatory disease
- Acute cervical or vaginal infections
- Uncooperative patient (relative contraindication)
- Pregnancy
- Clotting disorders (coagulopathy)
- Cervical cancer
- Morbid obesity (relative)
- Severe pelvic relaxation with uterine descensus (relative)
- Severe cervical stenosis (relative)

The Procedure

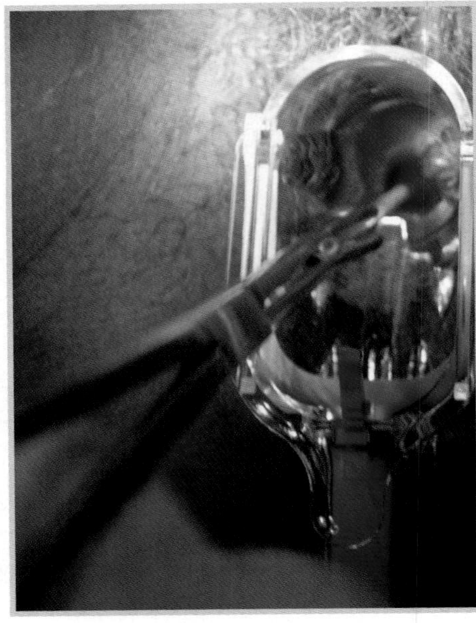

Step 1

Step 1. Explain the procedure, and obtain informed consent. Perform a pelvic examination. Determine the size and position of the uterus. Apply povidone-iodine to the ectocervix (if not allergic) and external os with a swab or cotton ball.

- PITFALL: Check for masses or structural abnormalities, cervical stenosis, or signs of infection that may make the procedure more difficult or impossible.

Step 2. Sound the uterus (normal depth is 6 to 9 cm) if desired. Some devices are graduated and may be used in place of a sound.

- PITFALL: When inserting a sound, apply firm, steady forward pressure to pass through the tightly closed internal os of the upper cervix. Be prepared to immediately pull back after the internal os is penetrated, or the tip of the sound can be thrust forward against the upper uterus and perforate the opposing wall. Perforations also can occur through the thin lower uterine segment. Placement of a tenaculum in difficult cases and straightening of the uterocervical angle can help reduce perforation after the sound passes through the internal os.

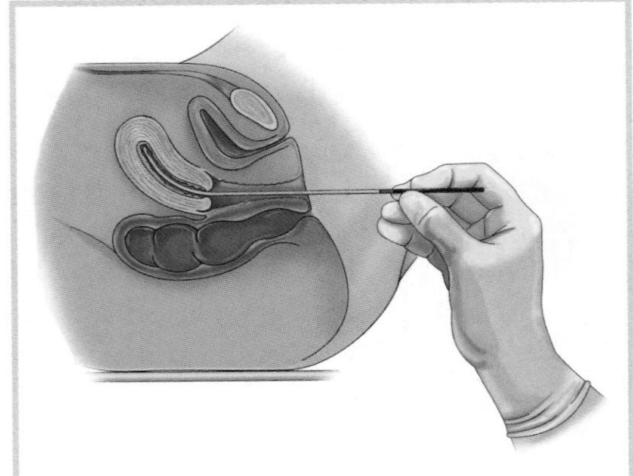

Step 2

Step 3. With the central piston fully inserted into the sheath (do not pull out), the endometrial sampler is inserted into the os until it reaches the fundus. Note the depth of insertion. Do not touch the end of the device that is to be inserted or allow it to touch the patient except at the os.

- PITFALL: If strong resistance is encountered, consider repeat sounding the uterus. If still unable to enter the endometrial cavity with the EMB catheter, abort the procedure. Forcing the catheter may result in uterine perforation.
- PITFALL: If the catheter bends excessively, apply a small amount of torque to the catheter. This causes it to flex less.

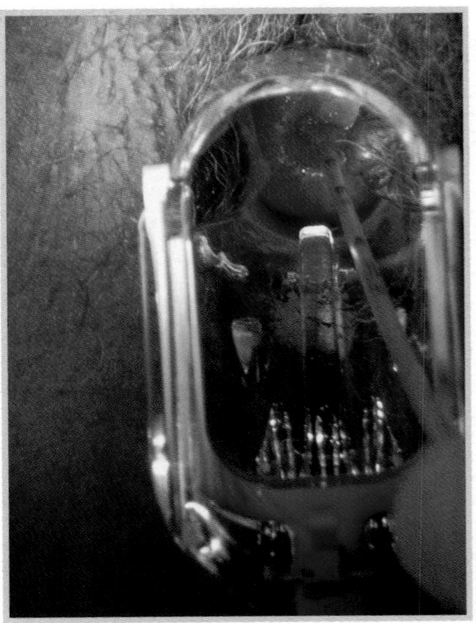

Step 3

Step 4. Holding the sheath steady, pull back on the piston until it stops. This creates negative pressure inside the curette. Leave the piston fully retracted.

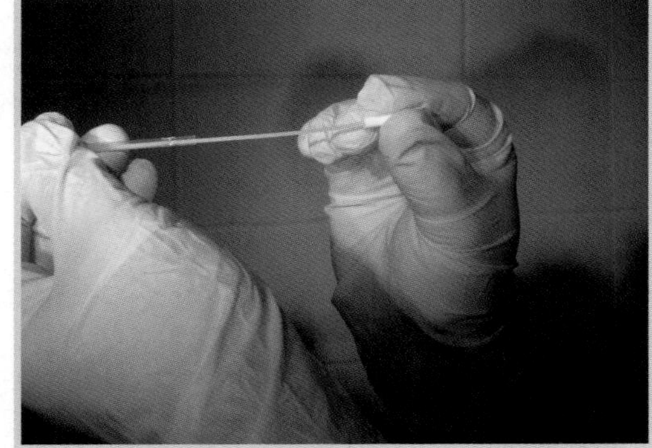

Step 4

Step 5. Roll or twirl the sheath laterally between the thumb and fingers while simultaneously moving the sheath tip back and forth between the fundus and internal os. Tissue should move into the sheath as the operation progresses. Complete the maneuver three or four times to obtain the sample.

- PITFALL: Do not allow the hole in the tip to emerge from the cervix, or all of the suction will be lost.

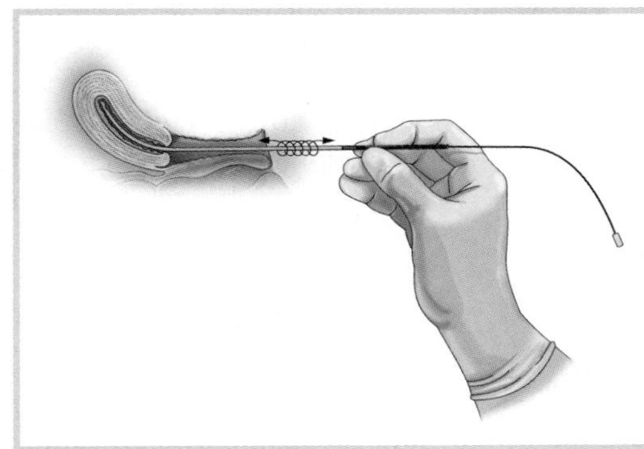

Step 5

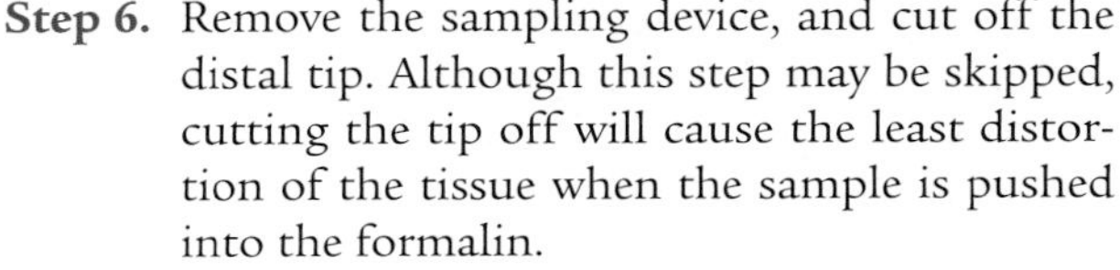

Step 6. Remove the sampling device, and cut off the distal tip. Although this step may be skipped, cutting the tip off will cause the least distortion of the tissue when the sample is pushed into the formalin.

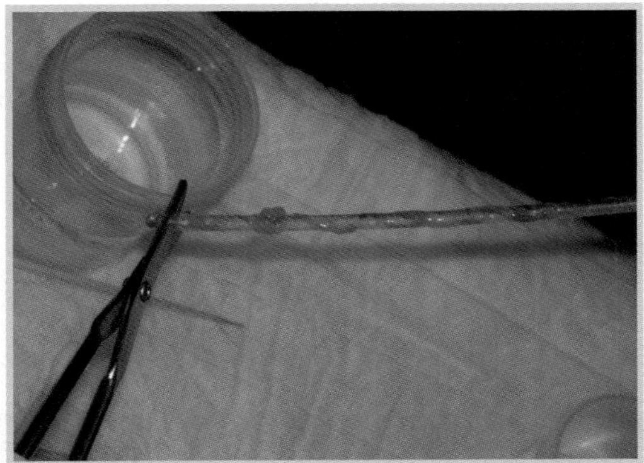

Step 6

Step 7. Slowly push the piston completely into the sheath to expel the sample into the fixative. Remove the speculum, and allow the patient to sit up and rest before dressing.

- PITFALL: Do not force the tissue out of the sampling hole without cutting the tip off because this may distort the histologic sample.

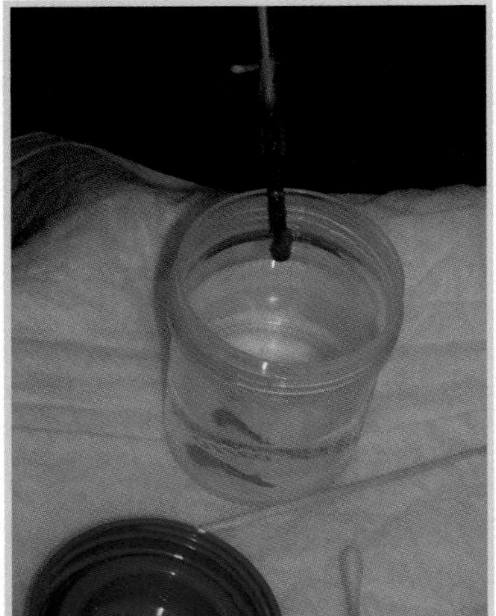

Step 7

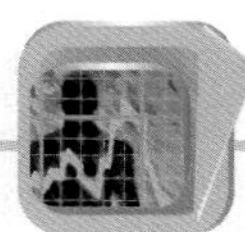

Complications

- Pain (especially cramping)
- Spotting
- Infection

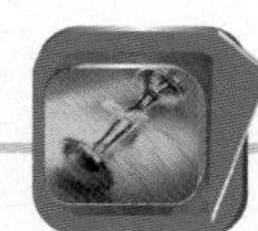

Pediatric Considerations

This procedure is rarely performed in the pediatric population.

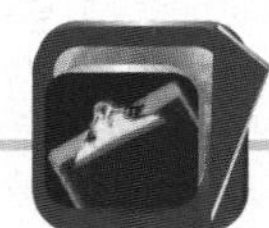

Postprocedure Instructions

Instruct the patient to take a NSAID or acetaminophen if they have any discomfort after the procedure. Explain that some vaginal bleeding or spotting is common following the procedure. Have the patient call if she experiences heavy bleeding, pain in the lower abdomen or vagina, or a foul-smelling vaginal discharge. Finally, tell the patient not to place anything in her vagina and to avoid intercourse for 1 week following the procedure.

Follow-up is often dictated by the test results.

- Atrophic endometrium: Hormonal therapy may be considered for patients with atrophic endometrium. Persistent vaginal bleeding should warrant further diagnostic workup.
- Cystic or simple hyperplasia: Progresses to cancer in fewer than 5% of patients. Most individuals with simple hyperplasia *without atypia* can be managed with medroxyprogesterone (Provera), 10 mg daily for 5 days to 3 months, or with close followup.
- Atypical hyperplasia: Considered a premalignant lesion that can progress to cancer in 30% to 45% of women. A dilation and curettage (D&C) procedure to exclude the presence of endometrial carcinoma is recommended.
- Endometrial carcinoma: Consider referral to a gynecologic oncologist for definitive surgical therapy.

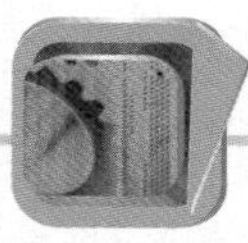

Coding Information and Supply Sources

CPT Code	Description	2008 Average 50th Percentile Fee	Global Period
58100	Endometrial sampling (biopsy), with or without endocervical sampling, without cervical dilatation, any method	$287.00	0
58110	Endometrial sampling (biopsy) in conjunction with a colposcopy	$163.00	ZZZ
57800	Dilation of cervical canal, instrumental	$185.00	0
59200	Insertion of cervical dilator, laminaria	$292.00	0

ZZZ, code related to another service and is always included in the global period of the other service.
CPT is a registered trademark of the American Medical Association.
2008 average 50th Percentile Fees are provided courtesy of 2008 MMH-SI's copyrighted Physicians' Fees and Coding Guide.

Patient Education Handout

A patient education handout, "Endometrial Biopsy," can be found on the book's companion Web site.

Bibliography

Archer DF, Lobo RA, Land HF, et al. A comparative study of transvaginal uterine ultrasound and endometrial biopsy for evaluating the endometrium of postmenopausal women taking hormone replacement therapy. *Menopause*. 1999;6:201–208.

Bakour SH, Khan KS, Gupta JK. Controlled analysis of factors associated with insufficient sample on outpatient endometrial biopsy. *Br J Obstet Gynecol*. 2000;107:1312–1314.

Bayer SR, DeCherney AH. Clinical manifestations and treatment of dysfunctional uterine bleeding. *JAMA*. 1993;269:1823–1828.

Cicinelli E, Didonna T, Schonauer LM, et al. Paracervical anesthesia for hysteroscopy and endometrial biopsy in postmenopausal women: a randomized, double-blind, placebo-controlled study. *J Reprod Med*. 1998;43:1014–1018.

Dijkhuizen FP, Mol BW, Brolmann HA, et al. The accuracy of endometrial sampling in the diagnosis of patients with endometrial carcinoma and hyperplasia: a meta-analysis. *Cancer*. 2000;89:1765–1772.

Mishell DR Jr, Kaunitz AM. Devices for endometrial sampling: a comparison. *J Reprod Med*. 1998;43:180–184.

Oriel KA, Schranger S. Abnormal uterine bleeding. *Am Fam Physician*. 1999;60:1371–1380.

Tahir MM, Bigrigg MA, Browning JJ, et al. A randomized controlled trial comparing transvaginal ultrasound, outpatient hysteroscopy and endometrial biopsy with inpatient hysteroscopy and curettage. *Br J Obstet Gynaecol*. 1999;106:1259–1264.

Trolice ME, Fishburne C Jr, McGrady S. Anesthetic efficacy of intrauterine lidocaine for endometrial biopsy: a randomized double-masked trial. *Obstet Gynecol*. 2000;95:345–347.

Zuber TJ. Endometrial biopsy. *Am Fam Physician*. 2001;63:1131–1135, 1137–1141.

2008 MAG Mutual Healthcare Solutions, Inc.'s Physicians' Fee and Coding Guide. Duluth, Georgia. MAG Mutual Healthcare Solutions, Inc. 2007.

CHAPTER 71

Colposcopy and Directed Cervical Biopsy

E. J. Mayeaux Jr., MD, DABFP, FAAFP

Professor of Family Medicine, Professor of Obstetrics and Gynecology
Louisiana State University Health Sciences Center, Shreveport, LA

The Papanicolaou (Pap) smear is a commonly employed screening test for dysplasia and cancer of the uterine cervix. Colposcopy is the diagnostic test to evaluate patients with an abnormal cervical cytologic smear or an abnormal-appearing cervix. The main goal of colposcopy is to highlight the areas of greatest abnormality in cervical intraepithelial neoplasia (CIN) or vaginal intraepithelial neoplasia (VAIN) for directed biopsy. It entails the use of a field microscope to examine the cervix after application of acetic acid (and possibly Lugol iodine) to temporarily stain the cervix and vagina. The cervix and vagina are examined under magnification, and all abnormal areas are identified. The transformation zone (TZ) is the area of the cervix extending from the original (prepubertal) squamocolumnar junction (SCJ) to the current SCJ. This and other benign colposcopic findings are listed in Table 71-1. An atypical TZ is defined as one with findings suggesting cervical dysplasia or neoplasia.

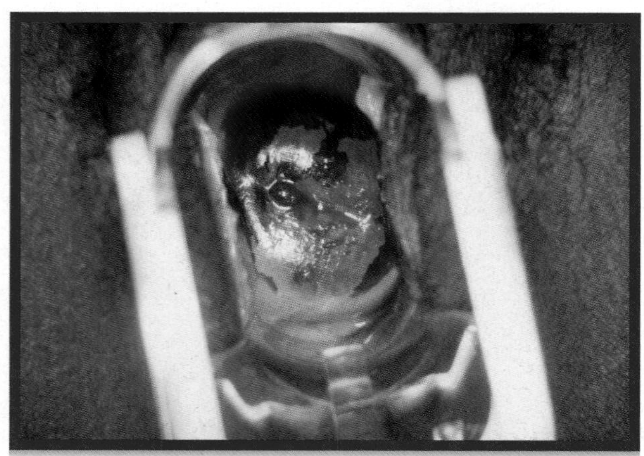

When performing a colposcopic exam, assure your patient that you will attempt to minimize pain, because this is often a consuming worry for patients. Although studies show that the sharpness of the instruments is the most important factor in the pain of a biopsy, many physicians apply topical 20% benzocaine (i.e., Hurricane solution) to decrease pain . This topical anesthetic is effective in 30 to 45 seconds. Know the pregnancy status of your patient. A nonsteroidal anti-inflammatory drug (NSAID) such as ibuprofen (800 mg) may be administered the night before and morning of the procedure unless contraindications to the drug exist.

The goal of colposcopy is to identify and biopsy the most abnormal-appearing areas in abnormal lesions. This requires that the borders of all lesions be seen in their entirety. Colposcopy is considered satisfactory if the entire TZ (including the entire SCJ) is examined and the extent of all lesions is seen. Directed biopsies of the most severe

TABLE 71-1. Benign Colposcopic Findings

Site or Condition	Findings
Original squamous epithelium	The original squamous epithelium is a featureless, smooth, pink epithelium that has no features suggesting columnar epithelium, such as gland openings or Nabothian cysts. This epithelium is considered always squamous and was not transformed from columnar to squamous.
Columnar epithelium	The columnar epithelium is a single-cell layer and mucus-producing tissue that extends between the endometrium and the squamous epithelium. Columnar epithelium appears red and irregular with stromal papillae and clefts. With acetic acid application and magnification, columnar epithelium has a grapelike or sea anemone appearance. It is mostly found in the endocervix.
Squamocolumnar junction (SCJ)	Generally, a clinically visible line is seenon the ectocervix or within the distal endocervical canal that demarcates endocervical tissue from squamous or squamous metaplastic tissue.
Squamous metaplasia	It is the normal physiologic process whereby columnar epithelium matures into squamous epithelium. At the squamocolumnar junction, it appears as a "ghost white" or white-blue film with application of acetic acid. It is usually sharply demarcated toward the cervical os and has very diffuse borders peripherally.
Transformation zone (TZ)	The geographic area between the original squamous epithelium (before puberty) and the current squamocolumnar junction may contain gland openings, Nabothian cysts, and islands of columnar epithelium surrounded by metaplastic squamous epithelium.
Vaginocervicitis	Cervicitis may cause abnormal Papanicolaou (Pap) smear results and make colposcopic assessment more difficult. Many authorities recommend treatment before biopsy when a sexually transmitted disease is strongly suspected.
Traumatic erosion	Traumatic erosions are most commonly caused by speculum insertion and too vigorous Pap smears, but they can also result from irritants such as tampons, diaphragms, and intercourse.
Atrophic epithelium	Atrophic vaginal or cervical epithelium may cause abnormal Pap smears. Colposcopists often prescribe estrogen for 2 to 4 weeks before a colposcopy to "normalize" the epithelium before the examination. This is thought to be safe even if dysplasia or cancer is present because the duration of therapy is short and these lesions do not express any more estrogen receptors than a normal cervix.
Nabothian cysts	Nabothian cysts are areas of mucus-producing epithelium that are "roofed over" with squamous epithelium. They do not require any treatment. They provide markers for the transformation zone because they are in squamous areas but are remnants of columnar epithelium.

lesions are performed, leading to a tissue diagnosis of the disease present. If the entire SCJ or the limits of all lesions cannot be completely visualized (unsatisfactory examination), a diagnostic conization with a cold knife cone, laser cone, or loop electrosurgical excisional procedure (LEEP) cone is necessary in nonadolescent patients. The uncooperative patient and the patient with a severely flexed uterus with inadequate visualization are common potential causes of unsatisfactory colposcopy. Lesions that are more likely to be missed or underread by colposcopic examination include endocervical lesions, extensive lesions that are difficult to sample, and necrotic lesions.

TABLE 71-2. Parameters Used to Grade Severity of Cervical Dysplasia

Less Severe (more normal)	More Severe (more dysplastic)
Mild acetowhite epithelium	Intensely acetowhite
No blood vessel pattern	Punctation
No blood vessel pattern or punctation	Mosaic
Diffuse vague borders	Sharply demarcated borders
Normal surface contour of the cervix	Abnormal contour or "humped up"
Normal iodine reaction (dark)	Iodine-negative epithelium (yellow)

Abnormal Findings

Leukoplakia is typically an elevated, white plaque on the cervical or vaginal mucosa, seen before the application of acetic acid. It results from a thick keratin layer that obscures the underlying epithelium. It may also represent exophytic human papilloma virus (HPV) disease or may signal severe dysplasia or cancer. Although it may be associated with benign findings, it generally warrants a biopsy.

Acetowhite lesions are transient, white-appearing areas of epithelium after the application of acetic acid (Table 71-2). Acetowhite changes correlate with areas of higher nuclear density in the tissue. Because both benign and dysplastic lesions may turn acetowhite, several features must be examined to estimate the severity. Assess the lesion's margins, including the sharpness of the margin and the angularity of the contour of the margin. The margins of high-grade CIN are straighter and sharper compared with the vague, feathery, geographic borders of CIN 1 or HPV disease. Higher-grade lesions also turn white more slowly, are a dull or thick-appearing white, and may never turn yellow or totally lose their acetowhite effect. When high-grade CIN coexists in the same lesion with a lower-grade lesion, the higher-grade lesion often manifests with a sharply defined internal margin or border (i.e., border-within-a-border pattern).

With increasing levels of CIN, desmosomes (i.e., intracellular bridges) that attach the epithelium to the basement membrane are often lost, producing an edge that easily peels. This loss of tissue integrity should raise the suspicion of high-grade dysplasia. The extreme expression of this effect is the ulceration that sometimes forms with invasive disease. High-grade CIN lesions are usually adjacent to the SCJ. Higher-grade lesions often appear dull and less white than most low-grade lesions, which are usually snowy white with a shiny surface. Invasive lesions may lose the acetowhite effect altogether. Nodular elevations and ulceration may indicate high-grade disease or invasive cancer.

Increases in local factors, such as tumor angiogenesis factor or vascular endothelial growth factor, cause growth of abnormal surface vasculature, producing punctation, mosaic, and frankly abnormal (atypical) vessels. However, most high-grade lesions do not develop any abnormal vessels. ***Punctation*** is a stippled appearance of small capillaries seen end-on, often found within the acetowhite area, appearing as fine to coarse, red dots. Coarse punctation represents increased caliber vessels that are spaced at irregular intervals and is more highly associated with increasing levels of dysplasia.

The ***mosaic pattern*** is an abnormal pattern of small blood vessels suggesting a confluence of "tiles" or a "chicken-wire pattern" with reddish borders. It represents capillaries that grow on or near the surface of the lesion that form partitions between blocks of proliferating epithelium. It develops in a manner very similar to punctation and is often found in the same lesions. A coarse mosaic pattern is more highly associated with increasing levels of dysplasia.

Atypical vessels are atypical, irregular surface vessels that have lost their normal arborization or branching pattern. They represent an exaggeration of the abnormalities of punctation and mosaic, and increasing severity of the lesion. They are indicative of CIN3 or invasive cancer. These vessels are usually nonbranching, appear with abrupt courses and patterns, and often appear as commas, corkscrews, coarse parallel vessels, or spaghetti.

Lugol iodine staining (i.e., Schiller test) may be used when further clarification of potential biopsy sites is necessary. It need not be used in all cases, but the sharp outlining afforded by Lugol iodine can be dramatic and very helpful. It darkly stains epithelium containing glycogen, such as normal mature squamous epithelium. Lugol solution is often very helpful on the vagina and proximal vulva (i.e., nonkeratinized skin). It can be used to examine the entire vagina and cervix for glycogen-deficient areas, which correlate with HPV or dysplasia in nonglandular mucosa. High-grade lesions uniformly reject iodine because of the absence of glycogen and produce a beige to mustard-yellow effect.

Grading Lesions

Carefully note the shape, position, and characteristics of all lesions to draw a picture of the lesions and biopsy sites after the procedure is completed. Do not let the finding of vessels divert you from carefully observing acetowhite and border changes, because the areas with vessel abnormalities may not be the most abnormal areas on the cervix. Classically, the parameters in Table 71-2 are used to grade severity, and the more advanced findings indicate more severe dysplasia.

Leukoplakia is usually a very good sign (i.e., condylomata) or a very bad sign (i.e., high-grade CIN or squamous cell carcinoma). Abnormal vessels are always suspicious because they may indicate cancer. When multiple areas of dysplasia are present, the areas of highest-grade dysplasia are usually most proximal to the SCJ. With all other things being equal, the presence of vessel atypia in any lesion implies more severe dysplasia.

Large, high-grade lesions that cover three or four quadrants of the cervix should be carefully evaluated for the possibility of unsuspected invasive cancer. Although many lesions have vascular abnormalities, some invasive lesions are densely acetowhite and avascular. They may also manifest as ulcerative lesions. Lesions that extend >5 mm into the cervical os have an increased risk of higher-grade disease beyond the limits of the examination. Studies have shown that the more biopsies taken, the more likely significant disease will be discovered.

It is debatable whether endocervical curettage (ECC) or brushing (ECB) adds any useful information to a clearly satisfactory colposcopy, because of the high false-positive and false-negative rates. Patients in whom there is not a clear view of the cervical canal, who have had previous treatment, who gave evidence of glandular dysplasia, or who have no ectocervical lesions that explain their abnormal Pap smears should have an ECC or ECB. An ECC or ECB can be performed before or after taking biopsies, with the decision based on whether bleeding will obscure subsequent biopsy sites. Following curettage, the ECC sample appears as a coagulum of mucus, blood, and small tissue fragments. Use ring forceps or a cytobrush to gently retrieve the sample. In addition to retrieving the ECC, a cytobrush can be used to evaluate the endocervical canal. A short drinking straw placed over a cytobrush can act as a sheath to protect the brush from contamination from ectocervical disease.

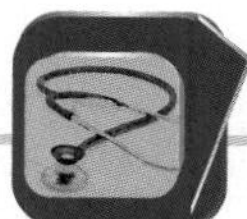

Equipment

- A colposcope is typically defined as a stereoscopic binocular field microscope with a long focal length and powerful light source. Modern colposcopes permit magnification between 2× and 40×, although most routine colposcopic work can be done at 10× to 15× magnification. Some scopes have a single fixed magnification level. Others have a series of par-focal lenses or a smooth zoom capability that allows for easy adjustment of the magnification via knob or rotor.
- Interchangeable eyepieces with various levels of magnification are available. Some eyepieces can be individually adjusted to compensate for variance in an individual user's vision. A diopter scale on the side can identify these. Eyepieces can be adjusted in a manner similar to microscopes to adjust to each colposcopist's interpupillary distance.
- The usual working distance (focal length) of a colposcope is 30 cm. Most scopes also have a fine focus handle that is attached to a machine screw under the mounting

bracket for the colposcope head. Applying pressure to this handle to subtly control the alignment of the scope and twisting it produces very gradual forward or backward movements of the head for exquisite fine focus control.

- A flexible articulating arm or overhead boom colposcope can be mounted on a stable base (with or without wheels), the wall, or an examination table. A column- or stick-mounted scope can easily be moved.
- A colposcope usually has a powerful light source, with a rheostat to adjust the level of illumination. The colposcope should be equipped with a green or blue filter (red-free filter). These filters remove red light, thereby enhancing vascular detail by making the blood vessels appear dark.

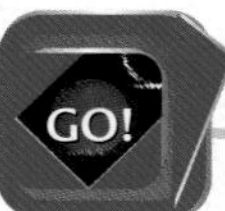

Indications

- Atypical squamous cells cannot rule out high grade disease (ASC-H), low-grade squamous epithelial lesion (LSIL), high-grade squamous epithelial lesion (HSIL), or atypical glandular cells (AGUS)
- Repeated Pap smears with atypical squamous cells
- Repeated Pap smears consistent with LSIL in a patient younger than 21 years of age
- Pap smear with repeated unexplained inflammation
- Abnormal-appearing cervix or abnormal-feeling cervix (by palpation)
- Patients with a history of intrauterine diethylstilbestrol (DES) exposure

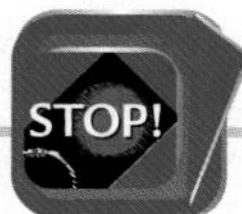

Contraindications (Relative)

- Active cervical or vaginal infection, because it can lower test sensitivity and increase bleeding (relative contraindication)
- Severe bleeding disorders
- Late pregnancy or active labor

The Procedure

Step 1. Prepare your patient, obtain informed consent (see Appendix A), and answer her questions. If a bimanual examination was not done with the Pap smear, perform it now. Examine the vulva for obvious condylomata or other lesions. Warm the speculum with water, and gently insert it. Consider using a vaginal sidewall retractor, a Penrose drain, or latex glove thumb in obese, pregnant, or multiparous women with vaginal redundancy.

- PITFALL: Repeating the Pap smear is often unnecessary, and even a correctly performed Pap smear may irritate the cervix and cause bleeding.

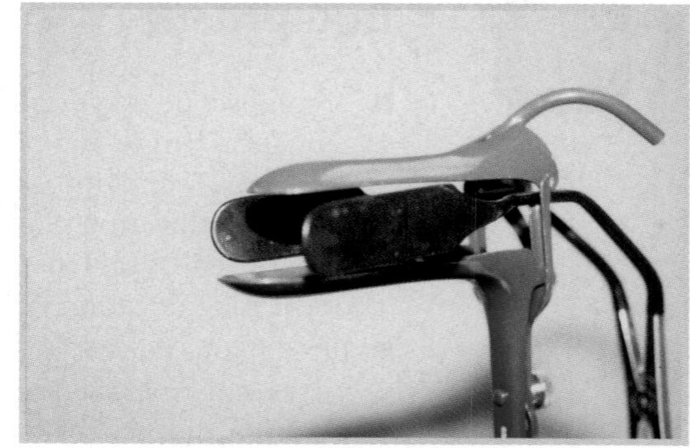

Step 1

Step 2. Place the patient in the dorsal lithotomy position. Insert a speculum and position the colposcope to observe the cervix. Gross focus is achieved by moving the scope toward or away from the cervix.

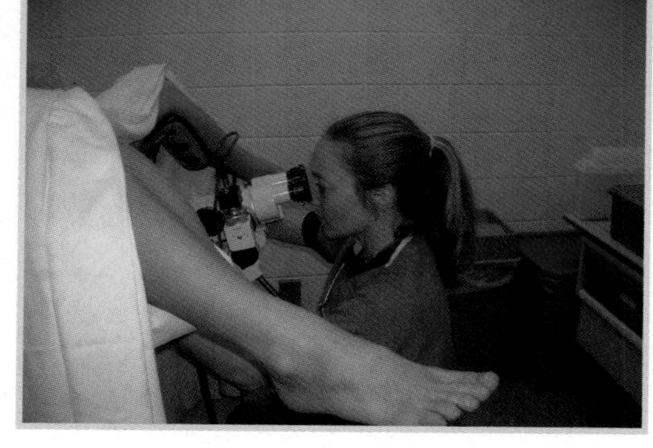

Step 2

Step 3. Fine focus is achieved by knobs, handles, or motorized foot pedals that incrementally move the head of the scope forward or backward. In this illustration, the fine focus knob is controlled by the left hand.

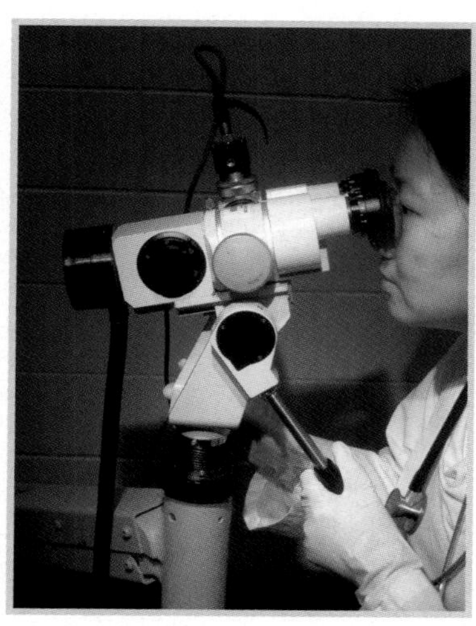

Step 3

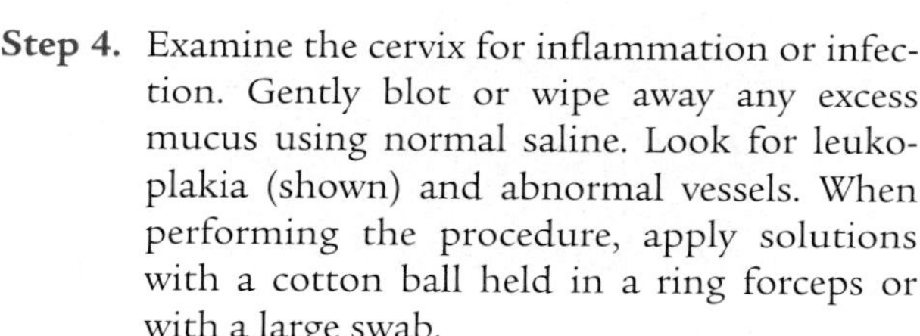

Step 4. Examine the cervix for inflammation or infection. Gently blot or wipe away any excess mucus using normal saline. Look for leukoplakia (shown) and abnormal vessels. When performing the procedure, apply solutions with a cotton ball held in a ring forceps or with a large swab.

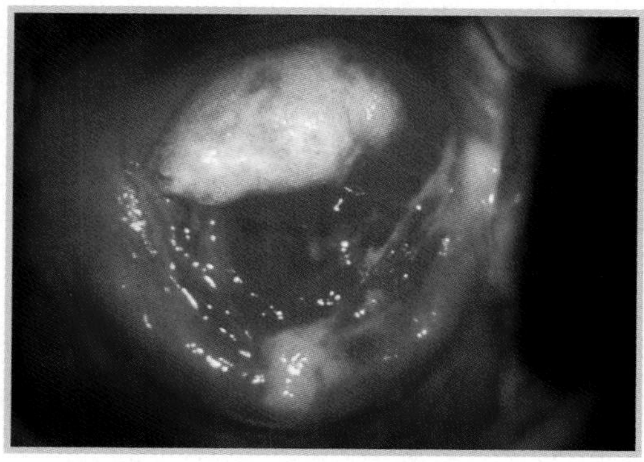

Step 4

Step 5. Apply 5% acetic acid. Repeat the application every 2 to 5 minutes, as necessary. Examine the cervix, starting with low power and using white light. Determine if the colposcopy is satisfactory by identifying the squamocolumnar junction (SCJ, shown) and the extent of any lesions identified.

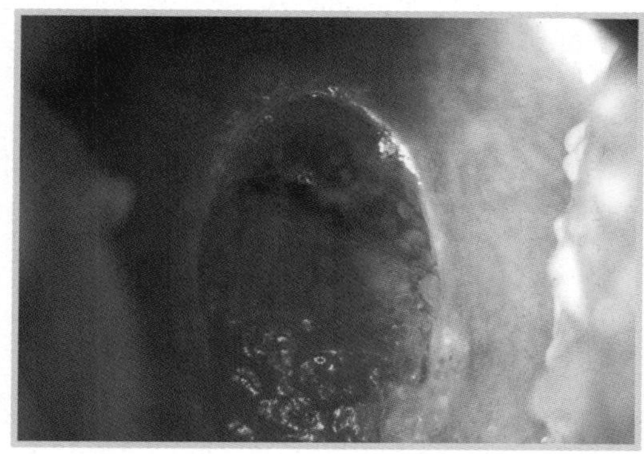

Step 5

Step 6. A cotton-tipped applicator soaked in vinegar may be used to move the SCJ or evert the os to examine the SCJ.

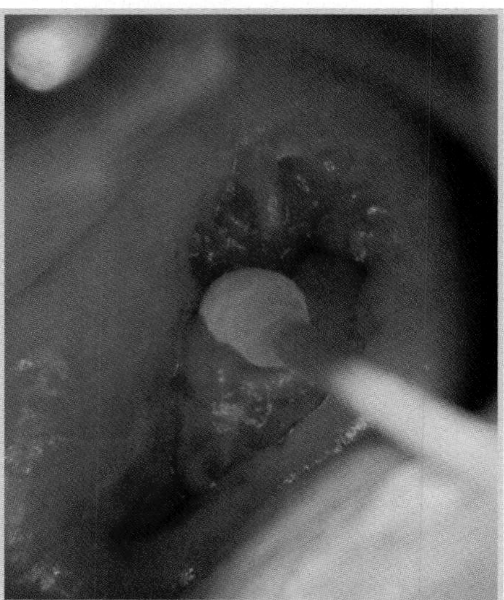
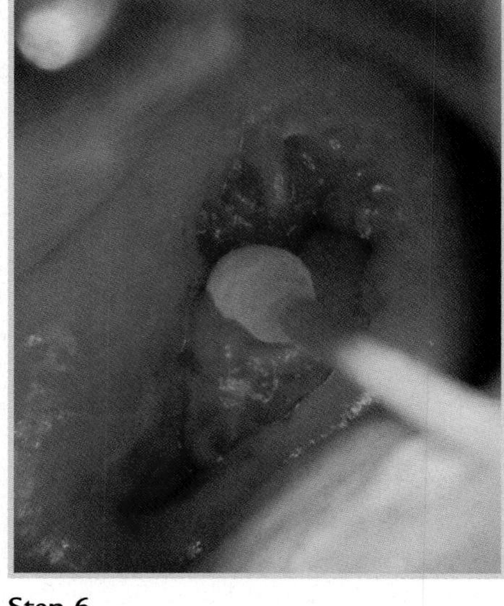

Step 6

Step 7. A Kogan endocervical speculum can greatly aid the examination of the distal endocervical canal. Use a vinegar-soaked Q-tip to help manipulate the cervix and SCJ into view, as necessary.

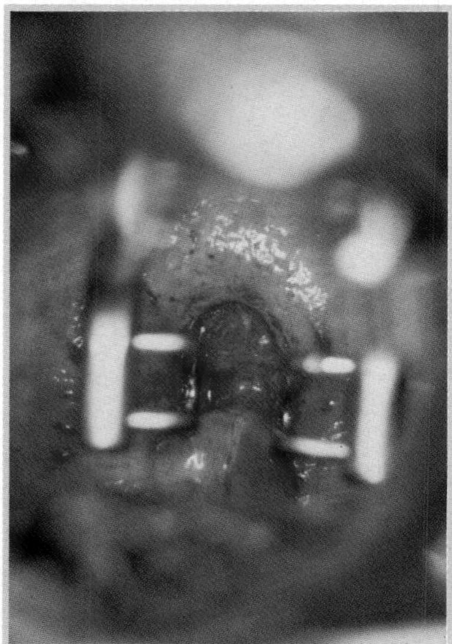

Step 7

Step 8. Use higher magnification and the red-free (green) filter to carefully document any abnormal vascular patterns, such as this acetowhite lesion with course punctation.

- PITFALL: Calling the solution *acetic acid* may increase the patient's perception of burning; describing the solution as *vinegar* is preferable.
- PITFALL: A tenaculum is almost never necessary to move the cervix and may cause cervix-obscuring bleeding.

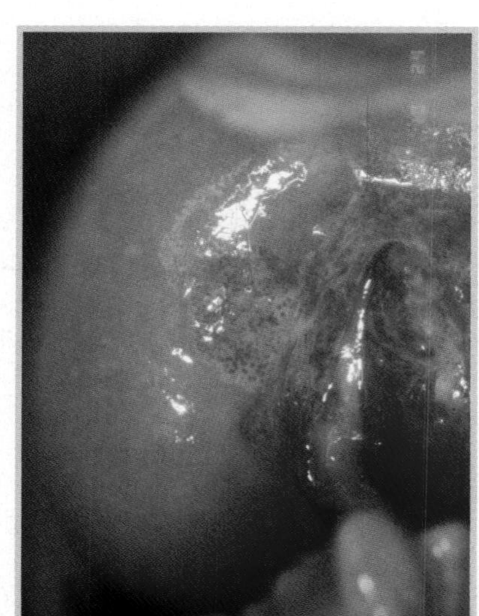

Step 8

Step 9. Also note if the cervix exhibits any mosaic pattern.

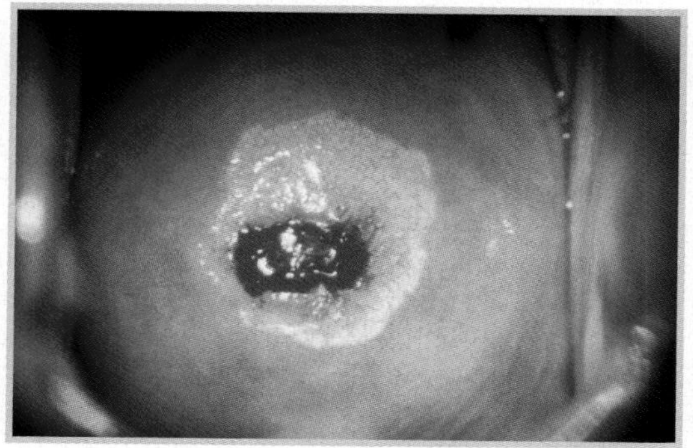

Step 9

Step 10. Be sure to identify any areas with frankly abnormal blood vessels, which raises the suspicion of cancer. These vessels may take the form of nonbranching vessels, commas, corkscrews, or coarse punctation.

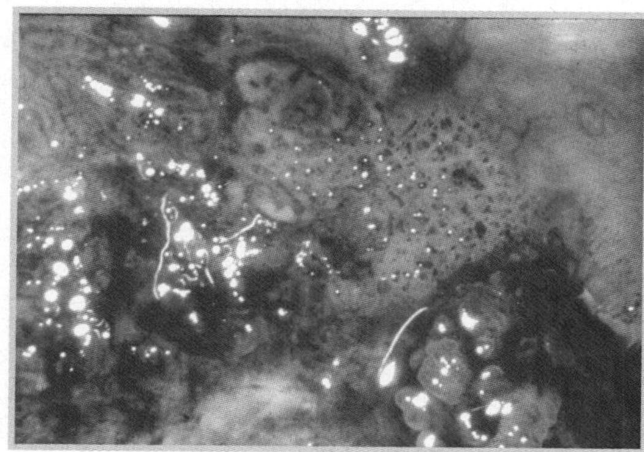

Step 10

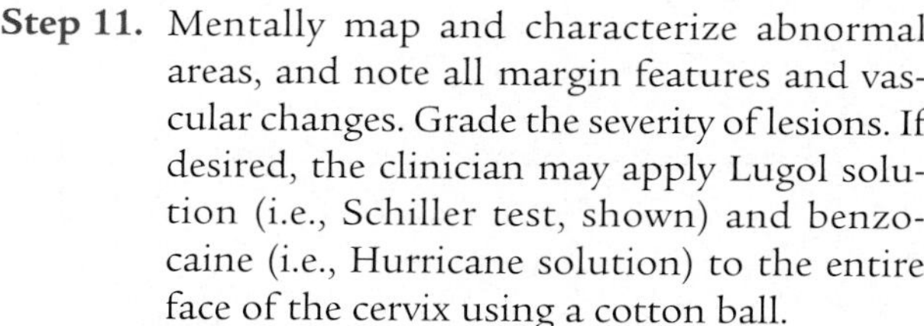

Step 11. Mentally map and characterize abnormal areas, and note all margin features and vascular changes. Grade the severity of lesions. If desired, the clinician may apply Lugol solution (i.e., Schiller test, shown) and benzocaine (i.e., Hurricane solution) to the entire face of the cervix using a cotton ball.

- **PITFALL:** Unsatisfactory colposcopy with cytologic evidence of dysplasia usually requires cervical cone biopsy for further evaluation.
- **PITFALL:** Make sure the patient is not allergic to iodine (shellfish) or benzocaine before using these solutions.

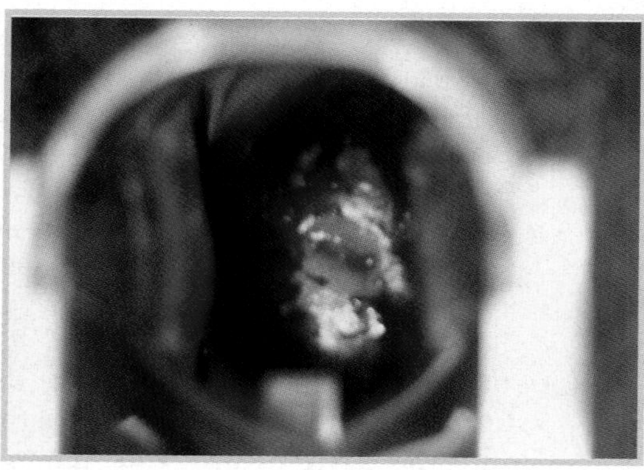

Step 11

Step 12. Perform an endocervical curettage if indicated. Use a Kevorkian curette (preferably without a basket), and scrape all walls of the canal, rotating the curette twice through 360 degrees of rotation. Place the curette into the canal until resistance is felt (Figure A), push it against the canal while pulling it out (stop short of the external os) (Figure B), and then push it back in with a slight (approximately 10-degree) twist to sample the next strip of canal with the next outward stroke (Figure C). After removing the curette, use ring forceps or a cytobrush to gently retrieve the sample.

- **PITFALL:** Do not do an ECC on pregnant patients.

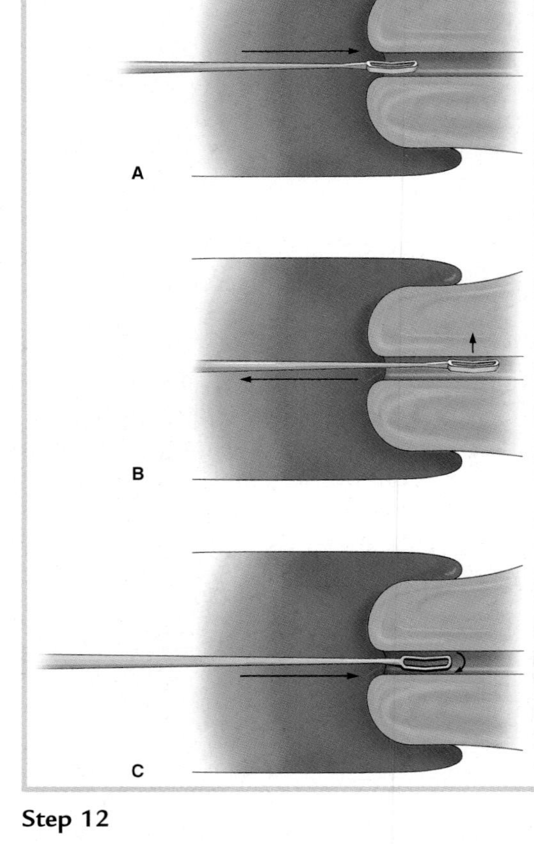

Step 12

Step 13. Alternatively, a cytobrush can be used to retrieve an ECB sample of the endocervical canal. A sheath or short drinking straw may be placed over a cervical Pap smear brush (i.e., pipe-cleaner-type brush) to act as a sheath to protect the brush from contamination by the ectocervix while the device is being introduced or withdrawn. Place the brush inside the straw, and place the straw against the os (Figure A). Advance the brush into the cervical canal, and spin it around five times (Figure B).

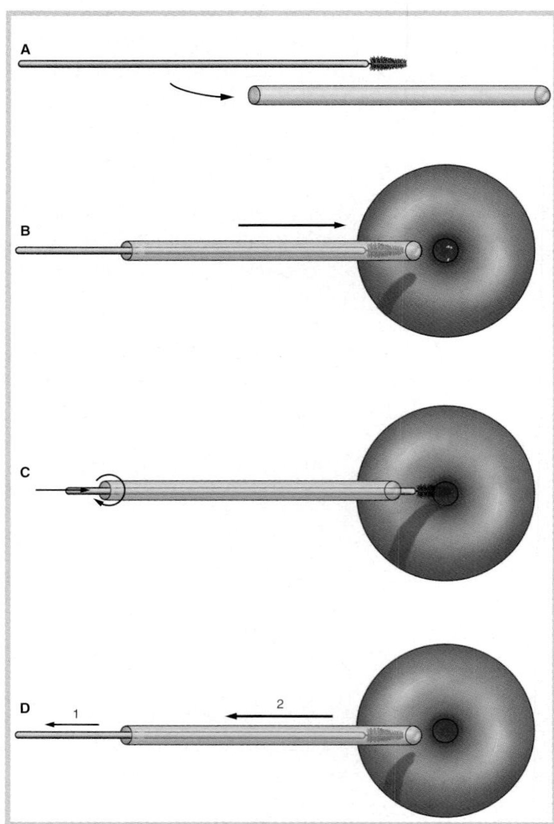

Step 13

Step 14. Withdraw the brush back into the straw, and remove the straw and brush from the vagina.

- **PEARL:** The bush should appear bloody when the procedure is done correctly. If only mucus is present on the brush, an inadequate sample was used.

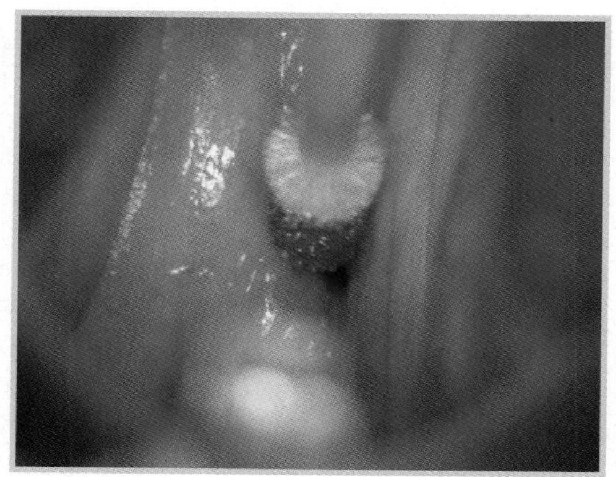

Step 14

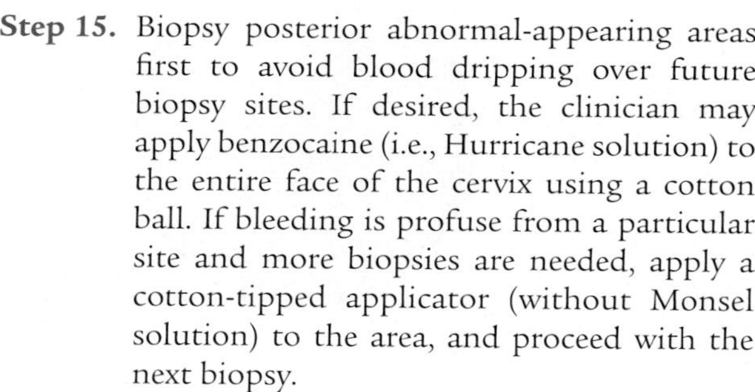

Step 15. Biopsy posterior abnormal-appearing areas first to avoid blood dripping over future biopsy sites. If desired, the clinician may apply benzocaine (i.e., Hurricane solution) to the entire face of the cervix using a cotton ball. If bleeding is profuse from a particular site and more biopsies are needed, apply a cotton-tipped applicator (without Monsel solution) to the area, and proceed with the next biopsy.

- **PEARL:** The cervix can be manipulated with a cotton-tipped applicator or hook if necessary to provide an adequate angle for biopsy.
- **PEARL:** It is not necessary to include normal margins with biopsy samples.
- **PITFALL:** Beginning colposcopists often place samples from different biopsy sites in different bottles, subsequently correlating them with colposcopic impressions. Separate specimens can increase costs and generally are not necessary, because the entire TZ is treated based on the worst biopsy result found.

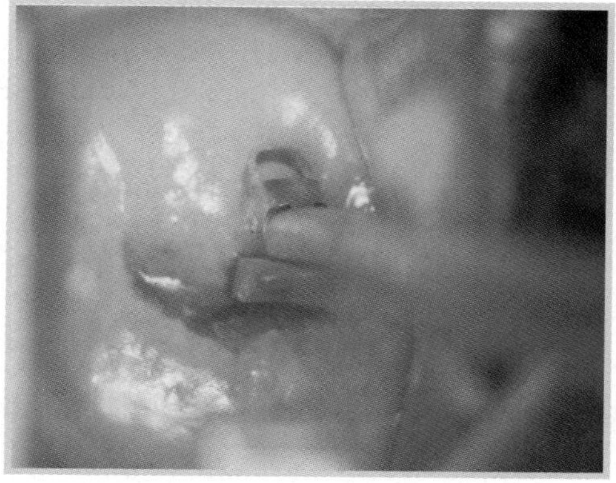

Step 15

Step 16. Align the forceps radially from the os, so that the fixed jaw of the forceps is placed on the most posterior part of the site (Figure A). Note that the fixed position is away from the os for a lesion on the outside edge (above) and within the os when the lesion is on the inside curve (below). The jaws should be centered over the area to be biopsied (Figure B). Biopsies should be approximately 3 mm deep and should include all areas with vessel atypism.

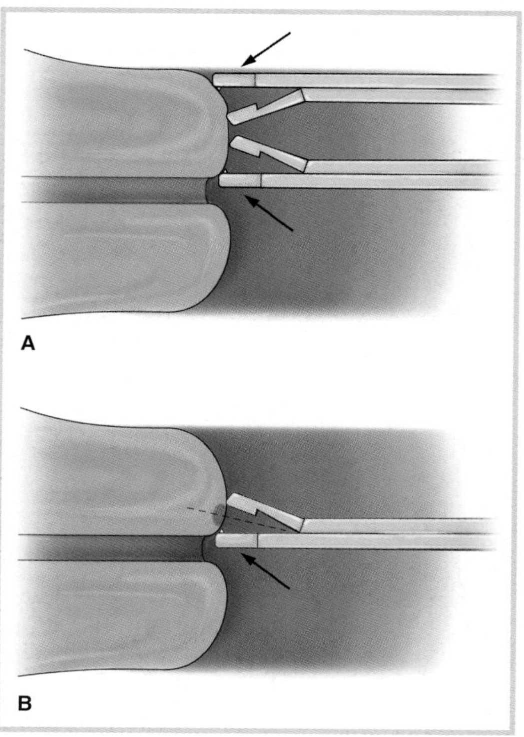

Step 16

Step 17. Apply pressure and Monsel solution if needed (after all biopsies are completed) to bleeding sites.

- **PITFALL:** Do not apply Monsel solution until all biopsies are completed.
- **PITFALL:** Swab out the excess Monsel solution and blood debris, which appears as a coffee-ground-like black substance that eventually will pass and may cause alarm (and late-night phone calls).

Step 18. Gently remove the speculum, and view the vaginal wall collapse around the receding blades of the speculum. Inspect for any abnormal areas on the vagina or vulva. Carefully draw and label a picture of lesions and biopsy sites. Correlate the pictures with the submitted samples, if placed in different containers. Note whether the colposcopy was satisfactory.

- **PITFALL:** Post-procedure fainting and light-headedness are not uncommon. Have the patient rest supine for at least several minutes and then sit up slowly.

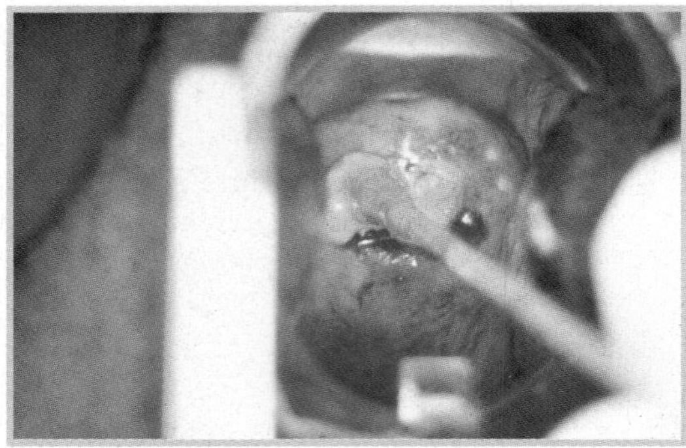

Step 17

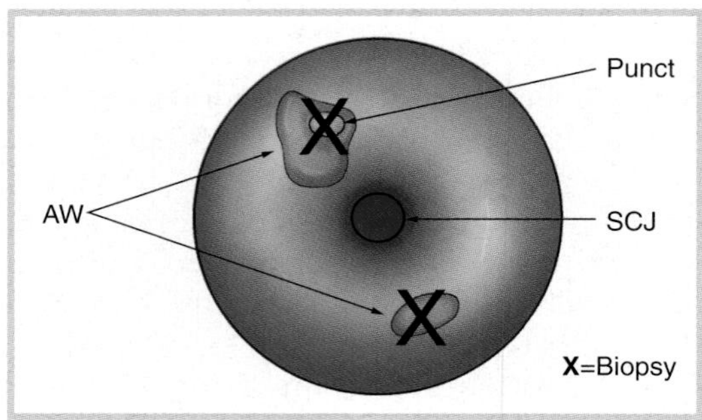

Step 18

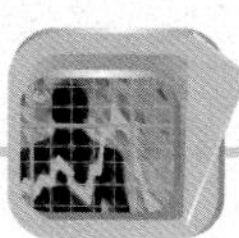

Complications

- Vasovagal responses postprocedure
- Bleeding or spotting
- Infection (very rare)
- Uterine cramping

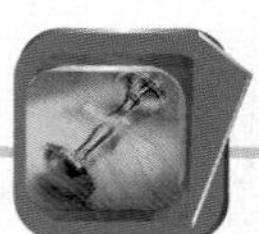

Pediatric Considerations

Colposcopy is rarely indicated in children. Most professional societies recommend starting cervical cytologic screening 3 years after initiation of sexual intercourse or age 21 years, whichever comes first. Because of the lower risk of cancer in adolescents, the indications for colposcopy and treatment of cervical dysplasia are more conservative. Check the American Society for Colposcopy and Cervical Pathology Web site at http://ASCCP.org for the latest evidence-based recommendations.

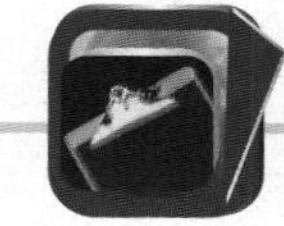

Postprocedure Instructions

After a colposcopy, advise patients to avoid douching, intercourse, or tampons for 1 to 2 weeks (or until the return visit). Instruct patients to return if they experience a foul vaginal odor or discharge, pelvic pain, or fever. Tylenol, ibuprofen, or naproxen sodium may be used for cramps. The follow-up visit is usually in 1 to 3 weeks to discuss pathology results and plan treatment, if necessary. With the high regression rate of CIN 1, patients should be followed with serial Pap smears or colposcopy if adequate follow-up can be ensured. CIN 2 and 3 lesions are usually treated with cervical cryotherapy, LEEP, or laser vaporization, although CIN 2 lesions may be followed with serial Pap smears and colposcopy in adolescents. Be concerned if a significant discrepancy is found between the colposcopic impression, Pap smear cytology, and biopsy histology, especially if the biopsy reports are significantly less severe than the Pap cytology. A discrepancy of two grades should be considered significant and a contraindication to ablative therapy. If the discrepancy cannot be explained or corrected on a repeat colposcopy, conization is usually indicated.

Cervical conization (i.e., cold cone, laser, or LEEP cone) is indicated in adult patients if the ECC or ECB sample reveals dysplasia, dysplasia visually extends into the cervical canal more than 3 or 4 mm, or the colposcopic results are unsatisfactory. There is a higher risk of poor outcomes if ablative therapies are used when disease is present in the endocervical canal. Positive ECC or ECB findings are sometimes a result of contamination with dysplastic lesions at the verge of the os, but this should not be assumed.

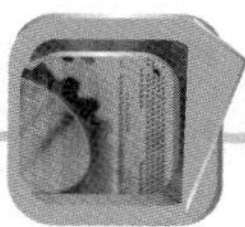

Coding Information and Supply Sources

CPT Code	Description	2008 Average 50th Percentile Fee	Global Period
56820	Colposcopy of vulva	$347.00	0
56821	Colposcopy of vulva with biopsy	$473.00	0
57420	Colposcopy of entire vagina, including cervix	$371.00	0
57421	Colposcopy of entire vagina with biopsy	$503.00	0
57452	Colposcopy of cervix or upper vagina	$327.00	0
57454	Colposcopy of cervix with biopsy, ECC	$437.00	0
57455	Colposcopy of cervix with biopsy	$376.00	0
57456	Colposcopy of cervix with ECC	$358.00	0
57460	Colposcopy of cervix with LEEP biopsy	$1,012.00	0
57461	Colposcopy of cervix with LEEP cone	$1,098.00	0
57500	Cervical biopsy alone, single/multiple, or excision	$307.00	0
57505	ECC alone (not part of dilatation and curettage)	$270.00	10

Common ICD-9 Codes

078.11	Condyloma acuminatum
233.3	Carcinoma in situ of other and unspecified female genital organs
622.0	Erosion and ectropion of cervix
622.2	Leukoplakia of cervix (uteri)
622.7	Mucous polyp of cervix
623.1	Leukoplakia of vagina (abnormal-appearing cervix)
795.00	AGUS (all types) Papanicolaou smear
795.01	ASCUS unspecified (favor benign) Papanicolaou smear
795.02	ASC-H (favor high-grade disease or dysplasia) Papanicolaou smear
795.03	LSIL Papanicolaou smear
795.04	HSIL Papanicolaou smear
795.05	Positive high-risk HPV—also use HPV code (079.4)
V10.41	Personal history of malignant neoplasm of cervix uteri
V15.89	High risk for cervical dysplasia: early onset of sexual activity (age <16 years), multiple sexual partners (>4/lifetime), history of STDs (inc. HIV), <3 negative or no Pap smear within previous 7 years, DES or daughters of women who took DES during pregnancy.

SUPPLIERS

- A 20% solution of benzocaine (i.e., Hurricane solution) can be obtained at Beutlich Pharmaceuticals LP, 1541 Shields Drive, Waukegan IL, 60085. Phone: 847-473-1100 or 1-800-238-8542. Web site: http://www.beutlich.com/products.htm.

Colposcopes and Instruments

- Cooper Surgical, Shelton, CT. Phone: 1-800-645-3760 or 203-929-6321. Web site: http://www.coopersurgical.com.
- Olympus America, Inc., Melville, NY. Phone: 1-800-548-555 or 631-844-5000. Web site: http://www.olympusamerica.com.
- Utah Medical Products, Inc., Mid-vale, UT. Phone: 1-800-533-4984 or 801-566-1200. Web site: http://www.utahmed.com.
- Wallach Surgical Devices, Inc., Orange, CT. Phone: 203-799-2000 or 1-800-243-2463. Web site: http://www.wallachsurgical.com.
- Acetic acid (3% to 5%) and normal saline can be obtained from a supermarket (i.e., white vinegar) or from a medical supply source.

Monsel solution (i.e., ferric subsulfate) performs best when it has a thick, toothpaste-like consistency. It can be bought this way or produced by allowing the stock solution to sit exposed to the air in a small open container. This allows evaporation and thickening of the agent, a process that can be enhanced by placing the open container in a warm place, such as on top of a refrigerator. The resulting paste texture can be maintained by keeping the paste in a closed container and by adding small amounts of Monsel solution whenever the paste becomes excessively thick.

Patient Education Handout

Patient education handouts, "Colposcopy" and "Postcolposcopy Instructions," can be found on the book's companion Web site.

Bibliography

Brotzman GL, Apgar BS. Cervical intraepithelial neoplasia: current management options. *J Fam Pract.* 1994;39:271–278.

Ferris DG, Harper DM, Callahan B, et al. The efficacy of topical benzocaine gel in providing anesthesia before cervical biopsy and endocervical curettage. *J Low Genital Tract Disease.* 1997;1:221–227.

Ferris DG, Willner WA, Ho JJ. Colposcopes: a critical review. *J Fam Pract.* 1991;33:506–515.

Greimel ER, Gappmayer-Locker E, Girardi FL, et al. Increasing women's knowledge and satisfaction with cervical cancer screening. *J Psychosom Obstet Gynecol.* 1997;18:273–279.

Hoffman MS, Sterghos S Jr, Gordy LW, et al. Evaluation of the cervical canal with the endocervical brush. *Obstet Gynecol.* 1993;82:573–577.

McCord ML, Stovall TG, Summitt RL, et al. Discrepancy of cervical cytology and colposcopic biopsy: is cervical conization necessary? *Obstet Gynecol.* 1991;77:715–719.

Newkirk GR, Granath BD. Teaching colposcopy and androscopy in family practice residencies. *J Fam Pract.* 1990;31:171–178.

Reid R, Campion MJ. HPV-associated lesions of the cervix: biology and colposcopic features. *Clin Obstet Gynecol.* 1989;32:157–179.

Reid R, Scalzi P. Genital warts and cervical cancer, VII: an improved colposcopic index for differentiating benign papillomaviral infections from high-grade cervical intraepithelial neoplasia. *Am J Obstet Gynecol.* 1985;153:611–618.

Sadan O, Frohlich RP, Driscoll JA, et al. Is it safe to prescribe hormonal contraception and replacement therapy to patients with premalignant and malignant uterine cervices? *Gynecol Oncol.* 1986;34:159–163.

Schiffman MH, Bauer HM, Hoover RN, et al. Epidemiological evidence showing that human papillomavirus infection causes most cervical intraepithelial neoplasia. *J Natl Cancer Inst.* 1994;85:958–964.

Stafl A, Wilbanks GD. An international terminology of colposcopy: report of the nomenclature committee of the International Federation of Cervical Pathology and Colposcopy. *Obstet Gynecol.* 1991;77:313–334.

Wright TC, Massad LS, Dunton CJ, et al. 2006 consensus guidelines for the management of women with abnormal cervical cancer screening tests. *Am J Obstet Gynecol.* 2007;197(4):346–355.

Wright TC Jr, Massad LS, Dunton CJ, et al., for the 2006 American Society for Colposcopy and Cervical Pathology-sponsored Consensus Conference. 2006 consensus guidelines for the management of women with cervical intraepithelial neoplasia or adenocarcinoma in situ. *Am J Obstet Gynecol.* 2007;197:340–345.

2008 MAG Mutual Healthcare Solutions, Inc.'s Physicians' Fee and Coding Guide. Duluth, Georgia. MAG Mutual Healthcare Solutions, Inc. 2007.

CHAPTER 72

Fitting Contraceptive Diaphragms

Sandra M. Sulik, MD, MS, FAAFP

Associate Professor Family Medicine

SUNY Upstate and St. Joseph's Family Medicine Residency, Fayetteville, NY

Contraceptive diaphragms provide effective, reversible, episodic contraception without hormonal influence. The device consists of a shallow, cup-shaped, latex or silicone sheet anchored to a circular outer spring that is contained in the rim. A diaphragm acts as a physical barrier that prevents sperm from entering the cervix and holds spermicide in place as an additional barrier. Diaphragms are always used in combination with spermicides, which usually contain nonoxynol-9 as their active ingredient, but preparations with octoxynol-9 also are available.

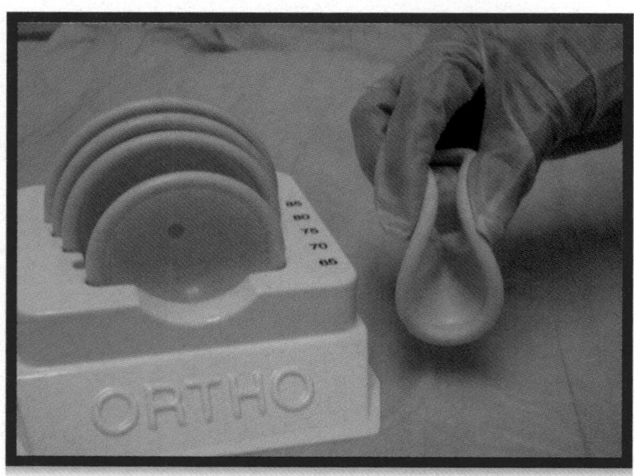

Latex diaphragms are available by prescription from most pharmacies. Silicone diaphragms must be ordered from the manufacturer. They range in size from 50 to 105 mm in diameter; the 65- to 80-mm sizes are the most commonly prescribed. The diaphragm must be fitted by the practitioner in the office. Sizing must be rechecked 6 weeks after the birth of a child, after a 20-lb weight gain or loss, and annually. Avoid devices that are too large (i.e., uncomfortable or press excessively on the urethra) or too small (i.e., easily displaced or expelled). When the diaphragm is pinched, the device folds into an arc. This allows the posterior edge to easily slip behind the cervix and facilitates insertion. Diaphragms require a high level of patient motivation and compliance to be effective, and they may be used in combination with condoms to help prevent transmission of human immunodeficiency virus (HIV). They remain popular because they do not use hormones, and most patients and their partners cannot feel them when they are properly fitted.

Diaphragms can be ordered in silicone (Milex) or latex (Ortho). The latex-allergic patient should use the silicone diaphragm only. Patients should be educated that oil-based lubricants may dissolve the latex and cause contraceptive failure. The diaphragm should be cleaned after every use with mild soap and water, gently dried, and stored in a protective container. The user should never apply powders on the device and should always inspect for holes or damage before use. Urinary tract infections may be more common in diaphragm users, but voiding after intercourse may help avoid this complication.

The contraceptive diaphragm has a failure rate between 13% and 23%. Younger users (<25 years) and patients who have intercourse more than four times each week may have a higher failure rate. Diaphragms may be inserted up to 6 hours before intercourse, and they must be removed 6 to 24 hours after intercourse. Use of a spermicide with the diaphragm is recommended, although studies have failed to prove that spermicide enhances the effectiveness of the diaphragm. Additional spermicide must be applied intravaginally with an applicator before any additional episodes of intercourse. When using these contraceptive methods, the possibility of system failure or patient noncompliance must be anticipated. Many patients can benefit from discussion about emergency contraception when a barrier method is decided on and periodically thereafter.

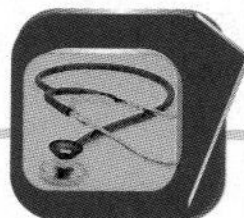

Equipment

- Items for a gynecologic examination (Appendix H: Instruments and Materials in a Standard Gynecological Tray)
- Diaphragm fitting rings or diaphragms for fitting

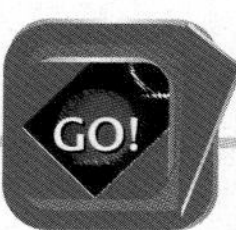

Indications

- Nonhormonal, reversible contraception
- Intolerance to hormonal contraception
- Desire for sexually transmitted disease (STD) protection

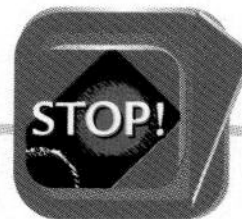

Contraindications

- Vaginal stenosis
- Uterine prolapse
- History of toxic shock syndrome
- Congenital vaginal abnormalities (septum)
- Patient <6 weeks postpartum
- Vaginal cysts
- Use of petroleum-based products that may damage latex diaphragms
- Drug allergies to the spermicides

The Procedure

Step 1. Explain the diaphragm-fitting procedure, and obtain informed consent. With the patient in the dorsal lithotomy position, perform a pelvic examination to rule out disease and identify atypical anatomy. During the bimanual examination, place the middle finger into the posterior cul-de-sac. Use the thumb to mark the point where the symphysis pubis abuts the index finger.

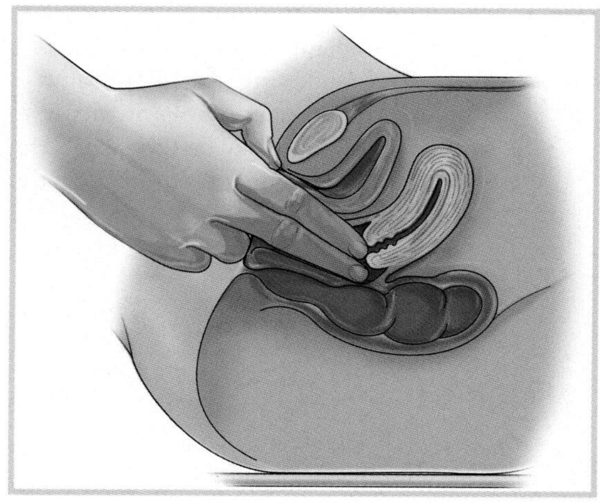

Step 1

Step 2. The distance from the tip of the middle finger to the point marked on the index finger is the approximate diameter of the diaphragm. The fitting ring or diaphragm is selected by measuring the marked length or by placing the ring against the measurement fingers.

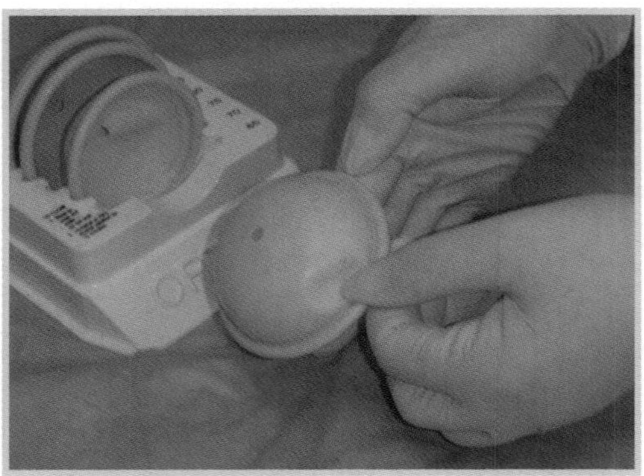
Step 2

Step 3. Insert the diaphragm after using a water-soluble lubricant on the rim of the device. Fold the device in half, spread the labia open, and the insert the device in a downward fashion toward the posterior fornix. The diaphragm will spring open. Check placement by sweeping the finger around the rim of the diaphragm to ensure it completely covers the cervix and reaches the posterior fornix. The anterior rim should be one finger's breadth from the symphysis pubis.

- **PEARL:** Check size by trying a larger or smaller diaphragm and compare the fit.
- **PITFALL:** Discomfort or excessive pressure on the urethra indicates the device is too large, and a device that is easily displaced or expelled is probably too small.
- **PITFALL:** Have the patient perform a Valsalva maneuver (i.e., cough). If the diaphragm is displaced or comes out, select the next larger size, and try again.

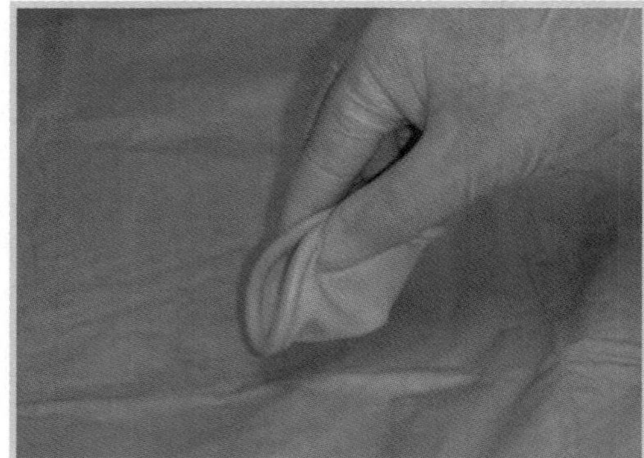
Step 3

Step 4. The diaphragm is removed by hooking the index finger under the ring behind the symphysis and pulling.

- **PEARL:** When properly fitted, the patient should not feel any discomfort and should be comfortable during intercourse.
- **PITFALL:** Caution the patient not to puncture the diaphragm with a long or ragged fingernail.

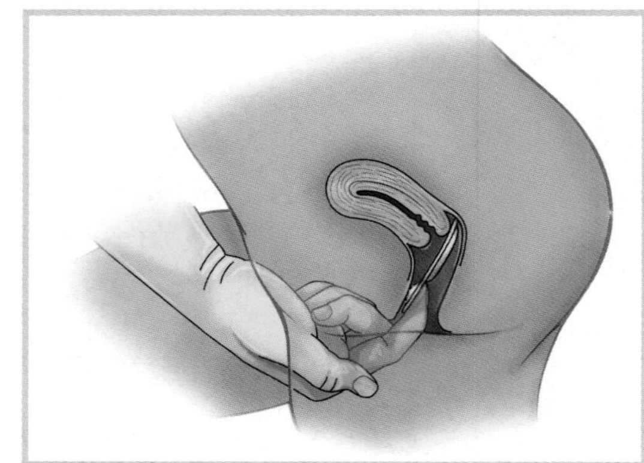
Step 4

Step 5. The woman should practice inserting (with water-soluble lubricant), checking for placement, and removing the diaphragm in the office. A diaphragm that is difficult for the woman to remove may be too small. Have her walk around and make sure the diaphragm stays in place.

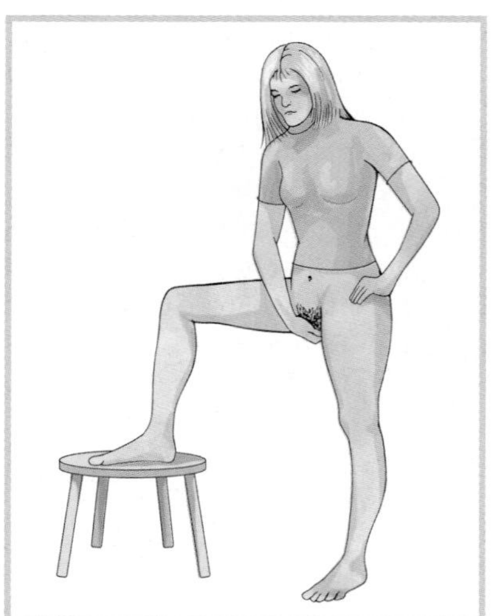
Step 5

Step 6. Teach the patient to hold the diaphragm up to the light to look for holes, so she can do it every time she plans to insert the diaphragm.

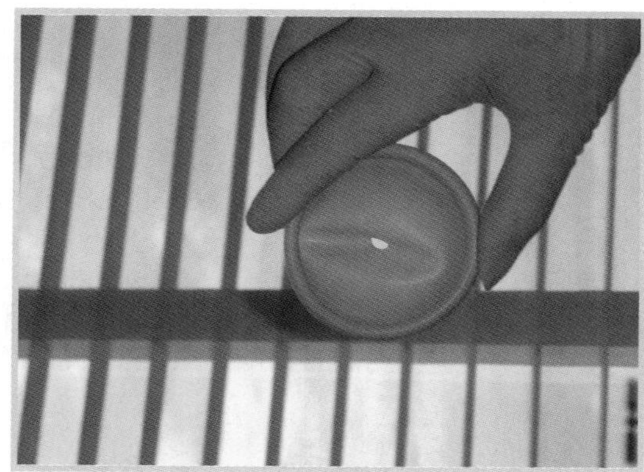

Step 6

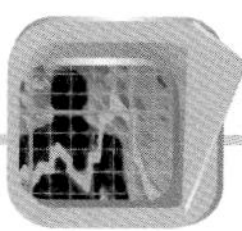

Complications

- Increased risk of urinary tract infection
- Toxic shock syndrome: 2.4 cases per 100,000 women (occurs almost exclusively when the diaphragm has been left in place >24 hours)

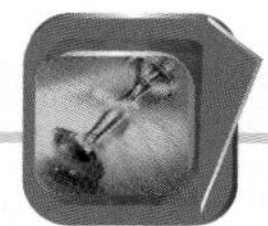

Pediatric Considerations

This procedure is not used in children. Although not commonly used in adolescents, the procedure is the same.

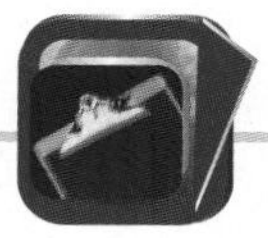

Postprocedure Instructions

The patient should be comfortable inserting and removing her diaphragm before she leaves the office. She should also be instructed to place approximately 1 teaspoon of spermicidal jelly in the dome of the diaphragm before insertion and that she can use a small amount of spermicidal jelly on the rim as a lubricant. She should be reminded that the diaphragm can be inserted any time before intercourse but it must stay in place for a minimum of 6 hours and up to 24 hours after intercourse. If repeated acts of intercourse occur, additional spermicide should be placed in the vagina but the diaphragm should not be taken out before the 6 hours. The patient should also be comfortable checking the diaphragm to make sure it is inserted properly and that her cervix can be felt through the dome of the cervix. Once the diaphragm is removed, it should be washed with soap and water and stored in the plastic case.

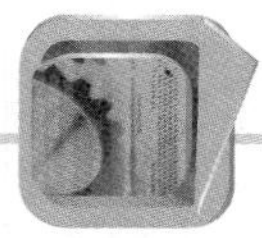

Coding Information and Supply Sources

CPT Code	Description	2008 Average 50th Percentile Fee	Global Period
57170	Diaphragm or cervical cap fitting with instructions	$169.00	0

CPT is a registered trademark of the American Medical Association.

2008 average 50th Percentile Fees are provided courtesy of 2008 MMH-SI's copyrighted Physicians' Fees and Coding Guide.

Suppliers

Diaphragms (e.g., Ortho-flex) are dispensed by prescription from pharmacies.

Fitting rings or diaphragm-fitting kits may be obtained from Ortho-McNeil Pharmaceuticals:

- Ortho-McNeil Pharmaceutical Company, 1000 Route 202 South, Raritan, NJ 08869-0602. Phone: 1-800-682-6532. Web site: http://www.ortho-mcneil.com.

Silicone diaphragms:

- Milex Products, Inc., 4311 N. Normandy, Chicago, IL 60634. Phone: 1-800-621-1278; fax: 1-800-972-0696. Web site: http://www.milexproducts.com.

Patient Education Handout

A patient education handout, "The Contraceptive Diaphragm," can be found on the book's companion Web site.

Bibliography

Allen RE. Diaphragm fitting. *Amer Fam Physician*. 2004;69(1):97–100.

Bulut A, Ortayli N, Ringheim K, et al. Assessing the acceptability, service delivery requirements, and use-effectiveness of the diaphragm in Colombia, Philippines, and Turkey. *Contraception*. 2001;63:267–275.

Cook L, Nanda K, Grimes D, et al. Diaphragm versus diaphragm with spermicides for contraception. Cochrane Database of Systematic Reviews 2003, Issue 1. Art. No.: CD002031. DOI: 10. 1002/14651858. CD002031.

DelConte, A. Contraception. In: Curtis MG, Hopkins MP, Overholt S, eds. *Glass's Office Gynecology*. 6th ed. Philadelphia: Lippincott Williams & Wilkins; 2006:347–383.

Fihn SD, Latham RH, Roberts P, et al. Association between diaphragm use and urinary tract infections. *JAMA*. 1986;25:240–245.

Grady MR, Haywood MD, Yagi J. Contraceptive failure in the United States: estimates from the 1982 National Survey of Family Growth. *Fam Plan Perspect*. 1986;18:200.

Hatcher RA, Stewart F, Trussel J, et al. *Contraceptive Technology*. 15th ed. New York: Iverting; 1992.

Hooton TM, Hillier S, Johnson C, et al. *Escherichia coli* bacteriuria and contraceptive method. *JAMA*. 1991;265:64–69.

Hooton TM, Scholes D, Stapleton AE, et al. A prospective study of asymptomatic bacteriuria in sexually active young women. *N Engl J Med*. 2000;343:992–997.

Mauck C, Callahan M, Weiner DH, et al. A comparative study of the safety and efficacy of FemCap, a new vaginal barrier contraceptive, and the Ortho All-Flex diaphragm. *Contraception*. 1999;60:71–80.

Speroff L, Darney P. *A Clinical Guide for Contraception*. 2nd ed. Baltimore: Williams & Wilkins; 1996.

2008 MAG Mutual Healthcare Solutions, Inc.'s Physicians' Fee and Coding Guide. Duluth, Georgia. MAG Mutual Healthcare Solutions, Inc. 2007.

CHAPTER 73

Cervical Cryotherapy

E. J. Mayeaux, Jr., MD, DABFP, FAAFP

Professor of Family Medicine, Professor of Obstetrics and Gynecology
Louisiana State University Health Sciences Center, Shreveport, LA

Cryotherapy is a time-proven, ablative method of treating lower grades of cervical dysplasia. The procedure is easy to learn, perform, and apply in outpatient settings. It works by freezing and killing abnormal tissue, which then sloughs off, and new tissue grows in its place. The tip of the cryoprobe is cooled by a refrigerant gas that is fed into the hollow cryoprobe under pressure. The gas then rapidly expands, absorbing heat in the process. The temperature of a nitrous oxide probe tip falls to −65°C to −85°C. A water-soluble lubricant is applied to the probe to act as a thermocouple with the irregular surface of the cervix. This produces a more uniform freeze. A rapid freeze followed by a slow thaw maximizes cryonecrosis, and a freeze–thaw–refreeze cycle is more effective than a single freeze.

After the cryoprobe is placed in contact with the cervix and activated, a ring of frozen tissue, or ice ball, extends outward. The depth of freeze approximates the lateral spread of the freeze. Cell death occurs when the temperature falls to <−10°F. However, there is a ring of tissue (i.e., thermal injury or recovery zone) that freezes but does not reach the −10°F necessary for cell death. This is why it is necessary to freeze well beyond the margins of any lesions. Studies have demonstrated that endocervical crypt (gland) involvement of cervical intraepithelial neoplasia (CIN) may penetrate up to 3.8 mm into the cervix. A freeze that causes cell death to 4 mm should effectively eradicate 99.7% of lesions with gland involvement. Current recommendations are to produce an ice ball with a 5-mm lateral spread to accomplish this goal.

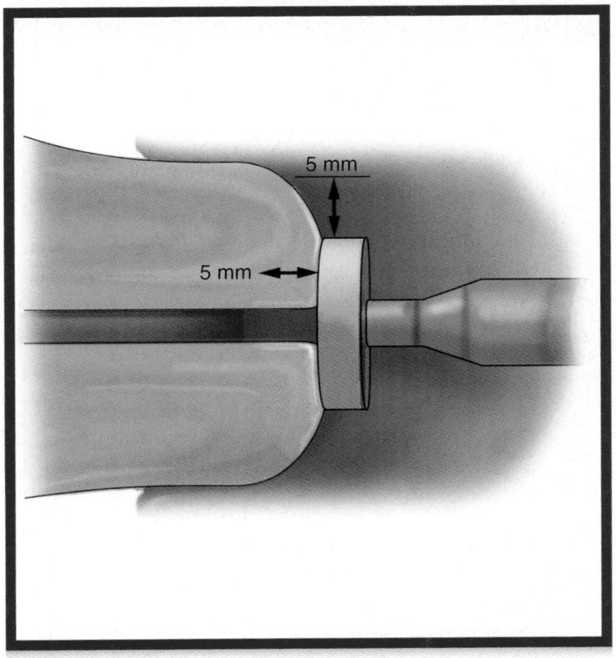

The cryotherapy appointment should be scheduled when the patient is not experiencing heavy menstrual flow. Select the largest speculum that the patient can comfortably tolerate, and open the blades and the front end of the speculum as widely as possible without discomfort. If collapsing side walls are a problem, place a condom with the tip cut off, the thumb from a very large rubber glove with the tip cut off, or one half of a Penrose drain over the speculum. Alternatively, tongue blades or sidewall retractors may be placed to improve exposure.

The choice of treatment modality for cervical dysplasia is at the discretion of the health-care provider. It is well established that cold knife conization increases a woman's risk of future preterm labor, low-birth-weight infant, and cesarean section. Several large retrospective series have now reported that women who have undergone a loop excision procedure (LEEP) or laser conization are also at increased risk for future preterm delivery, low-birth-weight infant, and premature rupture of membranes. The recent American Society for Colposcopy and Cervical Pathology (NCI/ASCCP) consensus guidelines note that, although cryotherapy studies have not shown these adverse effects on pregnancy outcome, it is difficult to measure small effects on pregnancy outcome. Therefore, some experts recommend cervical cryotherapy over LEEP for treatment of appropriately selected reproductive-age women. Advantages and disadvantages of cryotherapy appear in Table 73-1.

No anesthetic is required before cryotherapy because the procedure is relatively painless, although some cramping may occur. Some physicians recommend the use of nonsteroidal anti-inflammatory drugs to decrease cramping. Submucosal injection of 1% lidocaine with epinephrine (1:100,000) can be administered to decrease local pain.

The most common minor complication occurs if the probe touches the vaginal side wall and adheres to it. This causes pain, and bleeding may occur from the injured vaginal mucosa. Occasionally, a patient may experience an undue amount of pain and cramping, which is usually associated with a high level of anxiety. If this can be anticipated, a paracervical block before cryotherapy, oral or intramuscular administration of benzodiazepines

TABLE 73-1. Advantages and Disadvantages of Cervical Cryotherapy

Advantages	Disadvantages
Easily performed in the outpatient setting with relatively simple and inexpensive equipment	Women experience a heavy discharge for several weeks following cryotherapy.
Quick and easy to learn and to perform	Uterine cramping often occurs during therapy but rapidly subsides.
Serious injuries and complications are rare	Bleeding and infection are rare problems during the reparative period.
Minimal chance of heavy bleeding during or after the procedure	Cervical stenosis may occur.
Can be performed in a short time and does not interfere with other activities such as work or school later in the day	Unlike excisional therapies, there can be no histologic examination of the entire lesion. However, the cost of histologic examination is avoided.
No anesthetic is required. The procedure is relatively painless, although cramping may occur.	Future Pap smears and colposcopy may be more difficult. The squamocolumnar junction has a tendency to migrate deeper into the cervical os, making it difficult to sample the endocervix.
Least expensive and most widely available form of treatment for CIN	Possible higher failure rates than other cervical procedures for high-grade disease.

(e.g., 1 mg of lorazepam [Ativan] given intramuscularly), or intravenous sedation may be chosen for relief. These measures are seldom required.

Rarely, a patient may experience a vasovagal reaction. Allowing the patient to rest on the examination table after the procedure and to get up slowly is usually sufficient to overcome this problem. There has been a reported case of anaphylaxis due to cold urticaria. Some concern has been raised about occupational exposure to vented NO_2 gas following cryotherapy, but the scientific evidence for harm is very weak.

The patient should refrain from sexual intercourse and tampon use for 3 weeks after cryotherapy to allow the cervix to re-epithelialize. Excessive exercise also should be discouraged to lessen the chance of bleeding after treatment.

Most patients experience a heavy and often odorous discharge for the first month after cryotherapy. About one half of women rate the postprocedure discharge and its odor worse than a normal period. This discharge results from the sloughing of dead tissue and exudate from the treatment site. Routine cervical eschar debridement does not shorten the duration or amount of discharge and offers no significant advantage. Amino acids/sodium propionate/urea cervical cream (Amino-Cerv) cream may be prescribed if a heavy discharge is present after the procedure, although there is no scientific evidence of efficacy. Approximately one third of patients restrict their activities because of side effects of the procedure.

The first follow-up Papanicolaou (Pap) smear should not be performed for 6 months. Cytology can be very confusing if sampled during the sloughing or regenerative phases, which take at least 3 months to complete. If the first two follow-up smears are normal, Pap smears can be repeated every 6 months until two normal tests are obtained. Most recurrences take place within 2 years of treatment. Annual smears may be recommended after 2 years. An alternative follow-up schedule involves replacing the initial and each annual Pap smear with a colposcopic examination. Unfortunately, patient compliance with serial cytology follow-up is suboptimal.

If any of the follow-up tests are positive, restart the workup as if there was a newly diagnosed, first-time dysplasia. Colposcopy with directed biopsy is usually indicated. Unfortunately, colposcopy after cryotherapy may be more difficult because of migration of the squamocolumnar junction deeper into the cervical os. Other treatment methods (usually LEEP) are preferred if persistent disease is discovered.

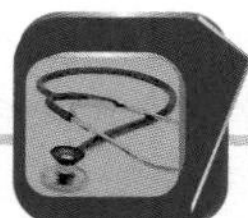

Equipment

- The device consists of a gas tank containing nonexplosive, nontoxic gases (usually nitrous oxide but sometimes carbon dioxide).
- A 20-lb gas cylinder is preferable to the 6-lb E-type tank, because the former has a more efficient pressure release curve.
- Liquid nitrogen has been used in the past, but it is difficult to control and is not recommended.
- Tanks are usually obtained from local suppliers.
- Appropriately sized vaginal specula.
- Adequate light source.
- Cervical probes in a variety of sizes.
- Water-soluble lubricant.

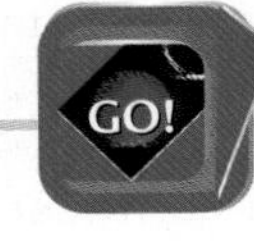

Indications

- Treatment of biopsy-proven cervical intraepithelial neoplasia 2 and 3 lesions
- Cervical intraepithelial neoplasia (CIN) 1 lesions persistent for 2 or more years, especially in women who do not wish to have children

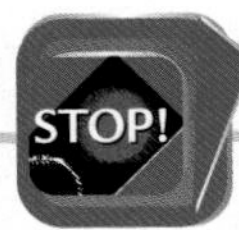

Contraindications

- An unsatisfactory colposcopic examination.
- A lesion that extends more than 3 or 4 mm into the cervical os because the area of destruction may not reliably penetrate beyond this level.
- A positive endocervical curettage.
- A lesion that covers more than two quadrants of the cervix.
- A lesion that cannot be completely covered by the cryoprobe.
- CIN 3 lesions (relative contraindication). There may be a higher recurrence rate compared with LEEP for CIN 3 level lesions, possibly because of the greater depth of glandular involvement with CIN 3.
- A mismatch of cytologic, histologic, and colposcopic findings greater than two histologic grades.
- Pregnancy.
- Active cervicitis.
- Some physicians recommend using an excisional therapy (e.g., LEEP) for recurrent dysplasia after ablative therapy.
- Adenocarcinoma in situ (should have cold knife conization).
- Unsatisfactory colposcopy.
- Lesion not fully visible or extending beyond the range of the cryotherapy probe.
- Biopsy consistent with or suspicious for invasive carcinoma.

The Procedure

Step 1. Informed consent is obtained. Perform a pregnancy test if there is any doubt about the patient's pregnancy status. Make sure that there is adequate pressure in the tank; usually, the needle is in the "green zone" on the pressure gauge.

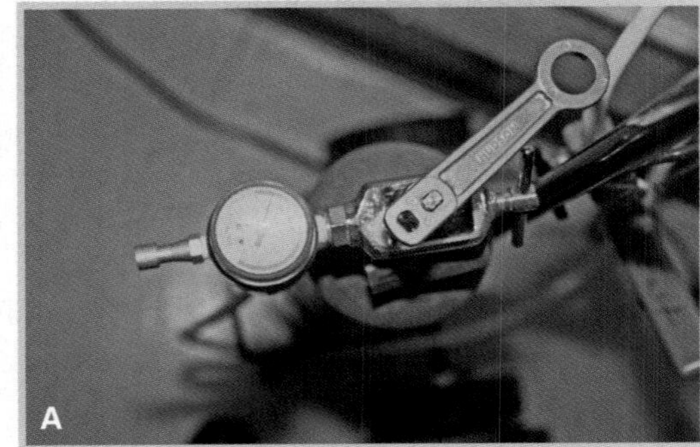

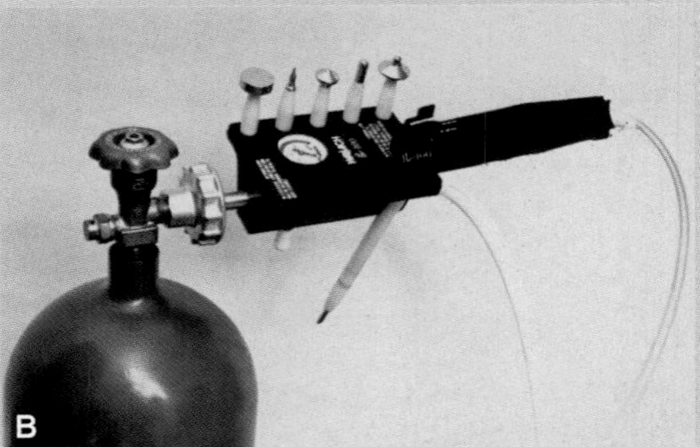

Step 1

Step 2. Place the patient in the dorsal lithotomy position, and place a vaginal speculum. If collapsing side walls are a problem, use a condom with the tip cut off, the thumb from a very large rubber glove with the tip cut off, or one half of a Penrose drain over the speculum, or use tongue blades or sidewall retractors to improve exposure.

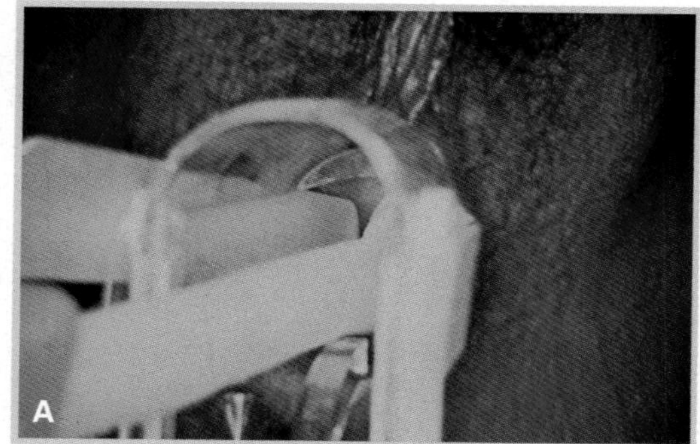

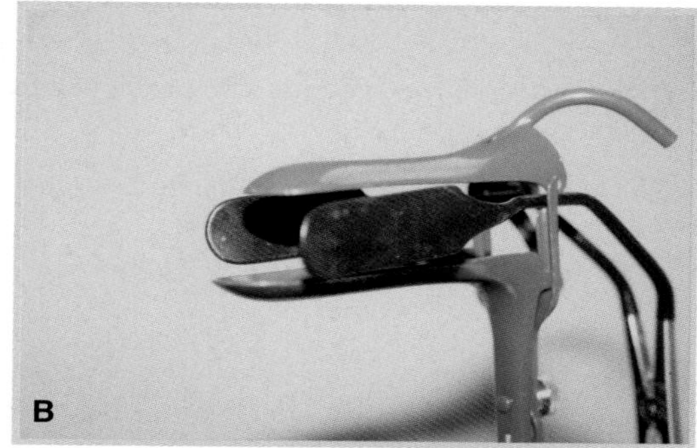

Step 2

Step 3. Select a probe that adequately covers the entire lesion and the entire transformation zone. Use only flat-ended or short nipple-tipped probes, not probes with long endocervical extensions, because they cause more cervical stenosis.

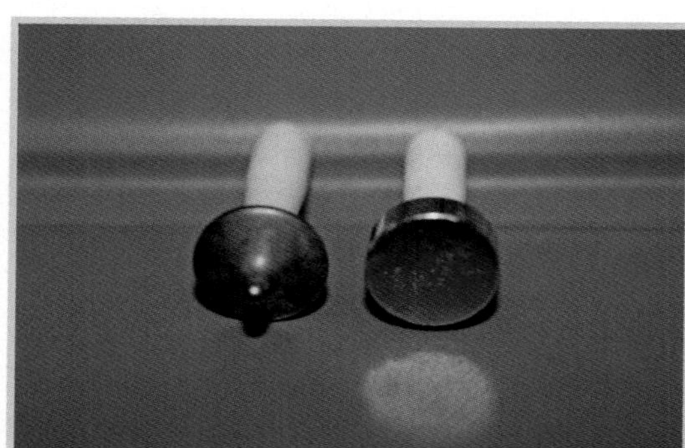

Step 3

Step 4. Apply a water-soluble lubricant to the probe to act as a thermocouple with the irregular surface of the cervix.

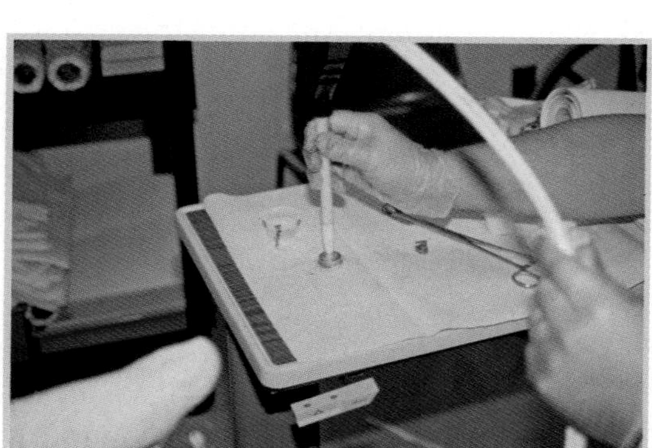

Step 4

Step 5. Apply the probe firmly to the cervix, and make sure that it is not touching the side walls of the vagina. Start the freeze by pulling the cryogun trigger on the single-trigger device or pressing the freeze button on the two-button device.

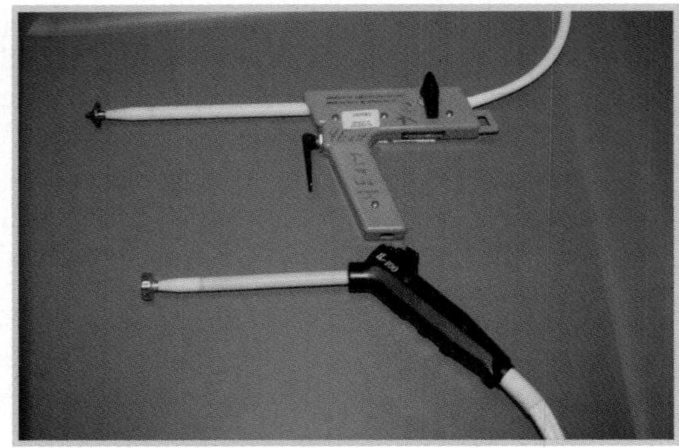

Step 5

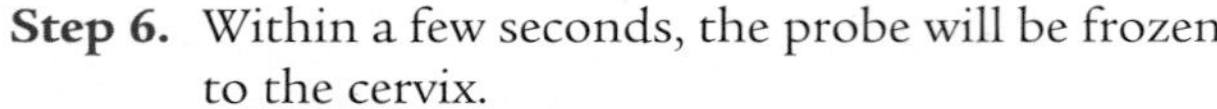

Step 6. Within a few seconds, the probe will be frozen to the cervix.

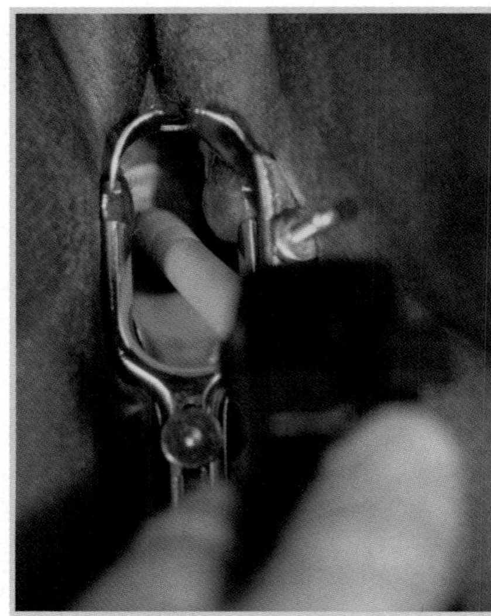

Step 6

Step 7. Using very light backward pressure on the cryogun, gently draw the cervix forward a few millimeters into the vagina, where probe contact with the side walls is less likely.

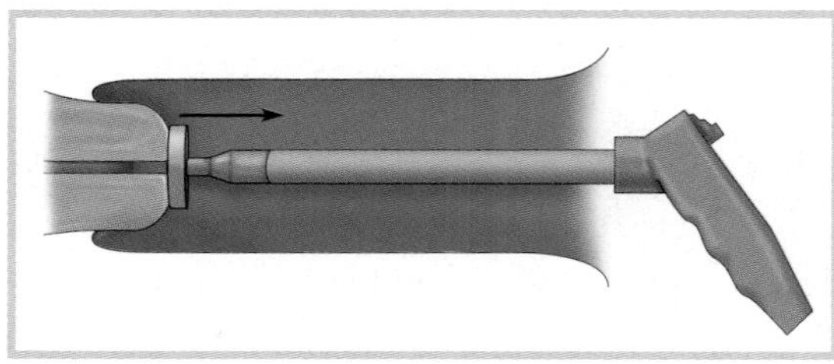

Step 7

Step 8. A rim of ice should form and grow to a width of at least 5 mm in all quadrants.

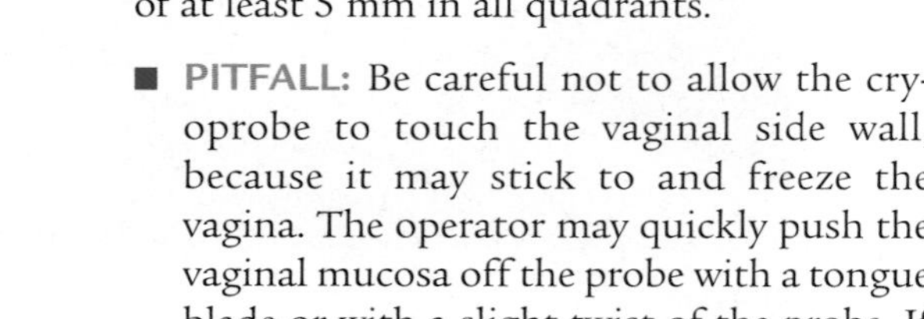

- **PITFALL:** Be careful not to allow the cryoprobe to touch the vaginal side wall, because it may stick to and freeze the vagina. The operator may quickly push the vaginal mucosa off the probe with a tongue blade or with a slight twist of the probe. If this is not done quickly, it will become more difficult as the freeze deepens, and

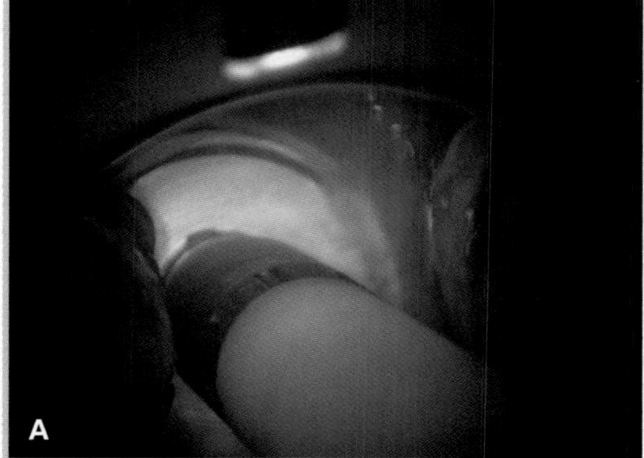

A

more vaginal mucosa will be destroyed. The operator should defrost the probe just enough to release the sidewall and then continue the freeze.

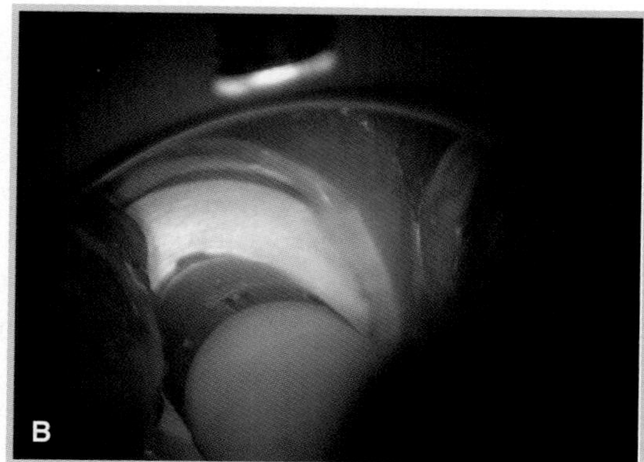

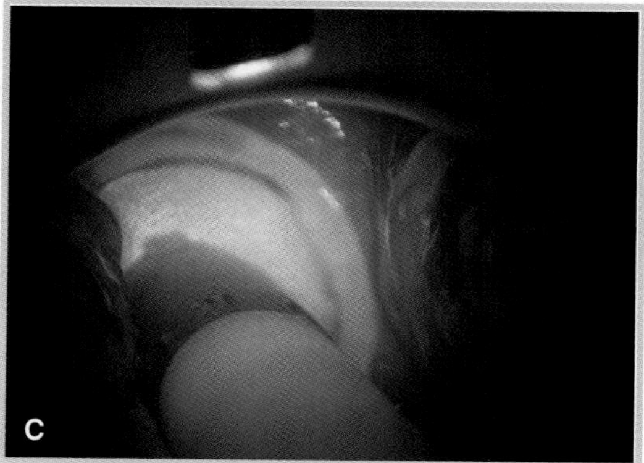

Step 8

Step 9. Discontinue the freeze. Release the Cryogun trigger or press the defrost button. Wait until the probe visibly defrosts before attempting to disengage it from the cervix. The end of the cervix should appear frozen and white. The cervix should be allowed to regain its pink color (usually in about 5 minutes).

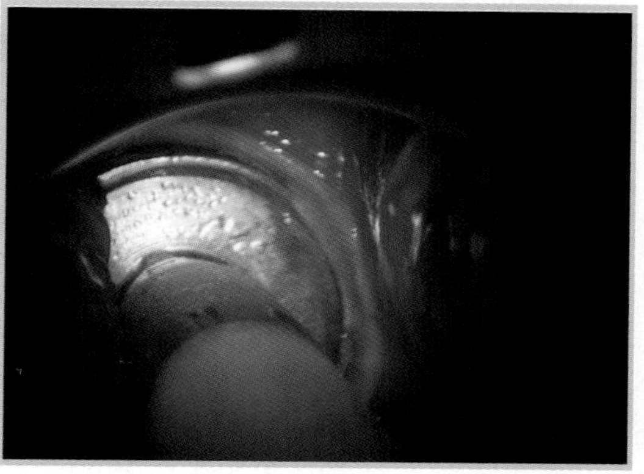

Step 9

Step 10. Repeat the freeze sequence as described. The second freeze is usually faster. After the freeze is completed, disengage the probe and remove the speculum. The patient may get up, get dressed, and leave as soon as she is ready.

- PITFALL: Fainting and light-headedness are not uncommon. Have the patient rest supine for at least several minutes and then sit up slowly.

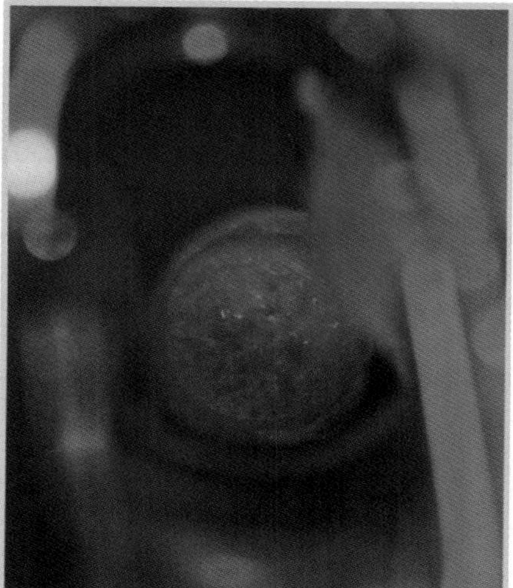

Step 10

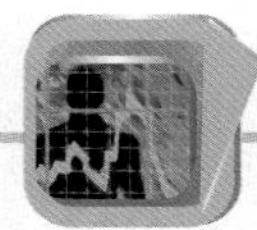

Complications

- Women will experience a heavy discharge for several weeks after cryotherapy. Amino-Cerv cream (one applicator high in the vagina Qhs for 10 days) may be used after therapy in an attempt to decrease the discharge, although this use is not well studied. Cervical eschar debridement does *not* shorten the length or amount of discharge.
- Bleeding and infection (rare).
- Undergoing cryotherapy of the uterine cervix increases the risk that a follow-up colposcopic examination will be inadequate. The squamocolumnar junction has a tendency to migrate deeper into the cervical os, making it difficult to sample the endocervix. This is especially true of older nipple-tipped probes, which are not currently recommended.
- Development of carcinoma after cryotherapy (failure of therapy).
- Anaphylactoid reaction to the cold exposure.
- Theoretical concerns about reduced fertility include the induction of cervical stenosis, a detrimental effect on cervical mucus, cervical incompetence, and tubal dysfunction secondary to ascending infection. No strong clinical evidence supports any of these concerns.

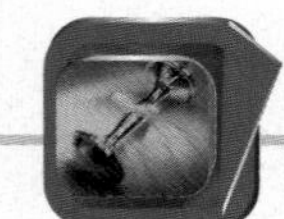

Pediatric Considerations

Because Pap smear screening is not recommended until a patient has been sexually active for 3 years or is 21 years of age, this procedure is not commonly performed in the pediatric population. Also, treatment recommendations are much more conservative in this population.

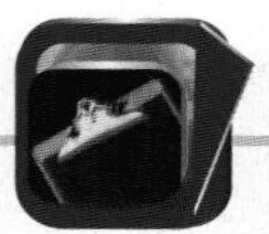

Postprocedure Instructions

Instruct the patient to refrain from sexual intercourse, douching, and tampon use for 2 to 4 weeks. A discharge is expected for 3 to 6 weeks, but it may last up to 2 months. The patient should report any significant bleeding or malodorous vaginal discharge. A follow-up Pap smear with or without colposcopy should be scheduled for 6 months later.

Patients may be followed with Pap smears or colposcopy, or both, every 6 months until two negative exams are obtained. Routine yearly screening may then be resumed, although the patient is at high risk for developing lower genital tract dysplasia for at least 20 years. Any sign of recurrence requires repeat colposcopic examination.

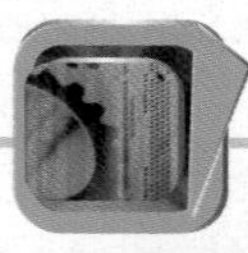

Coding Information and Supply Sources

CPT Code	Description	2008 Average 50th Percentile Fee	Global Period
57511	Cryotherapy of uterine cervix	$377.00	10

ICD-9 Codes

622.10	Dysplasia of cervix (uteri) unspecified
622.11	CIN 1: mild dysplasia of cervix (uteri)
622.12	CIN 2: moderate dysplasia of cervix (uteri)
233.1	CIN 3: severe dysplasia of cervix (uteri) (CIS)

SUPPLIES

Appendix H lists standard gynecologic instruments. Cryotherapy units may be obtained from these suppliers:

- Cooper Surgical, Shelton, CT. Phone: 1-800-645-3760 or 203-929-6321. Web site: http://www.coopersurgical.com.
- Ellman International, Inc., Hewlett, NY. Phone: 1-800-835 5355 or 516-569-1482. Web site: http://www.ellman.com.
- Olympus America, Inc., Melville, NY. Phone: 1-800-548-555 or 631-844-5000. Web site: http://www.olympusamerica.com.
- Utah Medical Products, Inc., Mid-vale, UT. Phone: 1-800-533-4984 or 801-566-1200. Web site: http://www.utahmed.com.
- Wallach Surgical Devices, Inc., Orange, CT. Phone: 1-800-243-2463 or 203-799-2000. Web site: http://www.wallachsurgical.com.
- Welch Allen, Skaneateles Falls, NY. Phone: 1-800-535-6663 or 315-685-4100. Web site: http://www.welchallyn.com.

Patient Education Handout

A patient education handout, "Cervical Cryotherapy," can be found on the book's companion Web site.

Bibliography

ACOG.: ACOG practice bulletin number 66: Management of abnormal cervical cytology and histology. *Obstet Gynecol.* 2005;106(3):645–664.

Anderson ES, Husth M. Cryosurgery for cervical intraepithelial neoplasia: 10-year follow-up. *Gynecol Oncol.* 1992;45:240–242.

Benedet JL, Miller DM, Nickerson KG, et al. The results of cryosurgical treatment of cervical intraepithelial neoplasia at one, five, and ten years. *Am J Obstet Gynecol.* 1987;157:268–273.

Charles EH, Savage EW. Cryosurgical treatment of cervical intraepithelial neoplasia: analysis of failures. *Gynecol Oncol.* 1980;9:361–369.

Dunton CJ. Cryotherapy: evidence-based interventions and informed consent. *J Fam Pract.* 2000;49(8):707–708.

Ferris DG, Ho JJ. Cryosurgical equipment: a critical review. *J Fam Pract.* 1992;35:185–193.

Harper DM, Mayeaux EJ Jr, Daaleman TP, et al. Healing experiences after cervical cryosurgery. *J Fam Pract.* 2000;49:701–706.

Harper DM, Mayeaux EJ Jr, Daaleman TP, et al. The natural history of cervical cryosurgical healing. *J Fam Pract.* 2000;49:694–699.

Hemmingsson E, Stendahl U, Stenson S. Cryosurgical treatment of cervical intraepithelial neoplasia with follow-up of five to eight years. *Am J Obstet Gynecol.* 1981;139:144–147.

Hemmingsson E. Outcome of third trimester pregnancies after cryotherapy of the uterine cervix. *Br J Obstet Gynecol.* 1982;89:275–277.

Kleinberg MJ, Straughn JM, Stringer JS, et al. A cost-effectiveness analysis of management strategies for cervical intraepithelial neoplasia grades 2 and 3. *Am J Obstet Gynecol.* 2003;188(5):1186–1188.

Mitchel MF, Tortolero-Luna G, Cook E, et al. A randomized clinical trial of cryotherapy, laser vaporization, loop electrosurgical excision for treatment of squamous intraepithelial lesions of the cervix. *Obstet Gynecol.* 1998;92:737–744.

Montz FJ. Management of high-grade cervical intraepithelial neoplasia and low-grade squamous intraepithelial lesion and potential complications. *Clin Obstet Gynecol.* 2000;43(2):394–409.

Richart M, Townsend DE, Crisp W, et al. An analysis of "long-term" follow-up results in patients with cervical intraepithelial neoplasia treated by cryosurgery. *Am J Obstet Gynecol.* 1980;137:823–826.

Sammarco MJ, Hartenbach EM, Hunter VJ. Local anesthesia for cryosurgery of the cervix. *J Reprod Med.* 1993;38:170–172.

Schantz A, Thormann L. Cryosurgery for dysplasia of the uterine ectocervix: a randomized study of the efficacy of the single- and double-freeze techniques. *Acta Obstet Gynecol Scand.* 1984;63:417–420.

Spitzer M. Fertility and pregnancy outcome after treatment for cervical intraepithelial neoplasia. *J Low Genital Tract Dis.* 1998;2:225–230.

Stienstra KA, Brewer BE, Franklin LA. A comparison of flat and conical tips for cervical cryotherapy. *J Am Board Fam Bract.* 1999;12:360–366.

Weed JC, Curry SL, Duncan ID, et al. Fertility after cryosurgery of the cervix. *Obstet Gynecol.* 1978;52:245–246.

Wright TC, Massad LS, Dunton CJ, et al. 2006 consensus guidelines for the management of women with abnormal cervical cancer screening tests. *Am J Obstet Gynecol.* 2007;197(4):346–355.

Wright TC Jr, Massad LS, Dunton CJ, et al.2006 consensus guidelines for the management of women with cervical intraepithelial neoplasia or adenocarcinoma in situ. *Am J Obstet Gynecol.* 2007;197:340–345.

2008 MAG Mutual Healthcare Solutions, Inc.'s Physicians' Fee and Coding Guide. Duluth, Georgia. MAG Mutual Healthcare Solutions, Inc. 2007.

CHAPTER 74

Dilation and Curettage (D&C)

Ya'aqov M. Abrams, MD

Assistant Professor, Department of Family Medicine, University of Pittsburgh, Chief of Staff, Department of Family Medicine, Magee Womens Hospital, Pittsburgh, PA

Dilation and curettage (D&C) can be used as a therapeutic or diagnostic procedure. Although D&C has in some cases been replaced by hysteroscopy, in carefully selected patients D&C is useful in treating persistent vaginal bleeding that is unresponsive to hormonal manipulation and can be used in the diagnostic approach to vaginal bleeding.

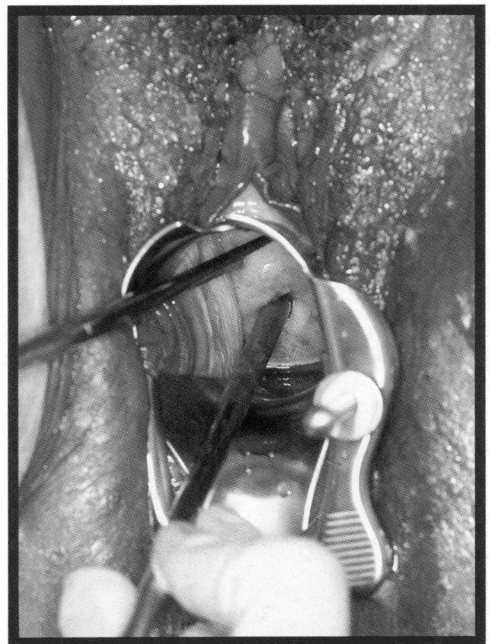

D&C should be used to treat heavy and life-threatening bleeding from missed or incomplete abortion. However, before 8 weeks gestation and if bleeding from a spontaneous abortion is light or not prolonged, observation of the patient for several weeks to see if the patient spontaneously completes the abortion is acceptable. If a gravid uterus is more than 10 to 12 weeks in size, D&C should be done because it is unlikely that the patient will complete expulsion of the products of conception (POC), and retained POC may result in infection or prolonged bleeding. Between 8 and 12 weeks, the choice between expectant and surgical management is based on weighing the severity of bleeding and the patient's preference.

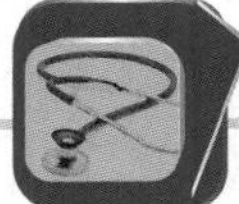

Equipment

- Consent for procedure (see Appendix A)
- Method of sedation
  - If done in the office or outpatient surgery, pretreat with oral benzodiazepine such as diazepam 10 mg 1 hour before the procedure.
  - If done in an operating room, the patient will receive intravenous (IV) sedation and oxygen.
- Sterile bivalve or weighted speculum
- Topical antiseptic (see Appendix E)

- Syringe, 10 mL
- Lidocaine (1%) without epinephrine
- Spinal needle, 22 g
- Cervical curette
- Single-toothed tenaculum
- Malleable uterine sound
- Hegar cervical dilators
- Teflon-treated gauze for collection of endocervical curettage specimens
- Suction with trap for uterine contents
- Stone forceps for removal of polyps
- Sharp uterine curette
- Suction curettes

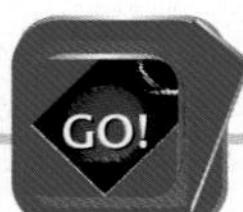

Indications

- Treatment of missed or incomplete abortion
- Treatment of dysfunctional uterine bleeding not responsive to hormonal manipulation
- Diagnosis of dysfunctional uterine bleeding (DUB) after failed endometrial biopsy
- Diagnosis and treatment of postmenopausal bleeding

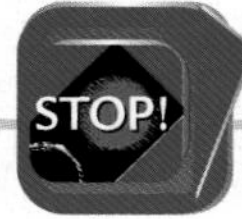

Contraindications

- Perimenarchal DUB because of the high risk of Asherman syndrome, which is due to the denuded basal endometrium
- Active uterine infection or pelvic inflammatory disease
- Coagulopathy

The Procedure

Step 1. Check the patient's hemoglobin before starting the procedure. If the hemoglobin is <8 g, order a type and screen, and perform the procedure in the operating room. Check the blood type and Rh in pregnant patients, and treat Rh negative patients with RhoGAM 300 mcg intramuscularly once. Examine the patient under anesthesia to determine uterine position and size. Record the uterine size in terms of weeks of gestation. Insert the speculum. The speculum should be large enough to prevent the vaginal walls from bowing into the operative field.

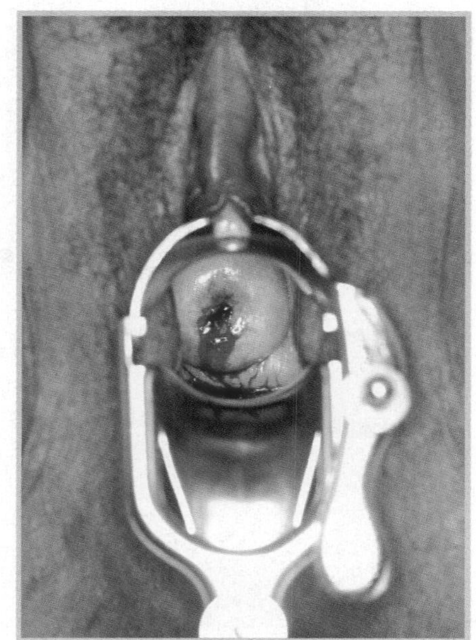

Step 1

Step 2. Grasp the cervix at 12 o'clock with the tenaculum.

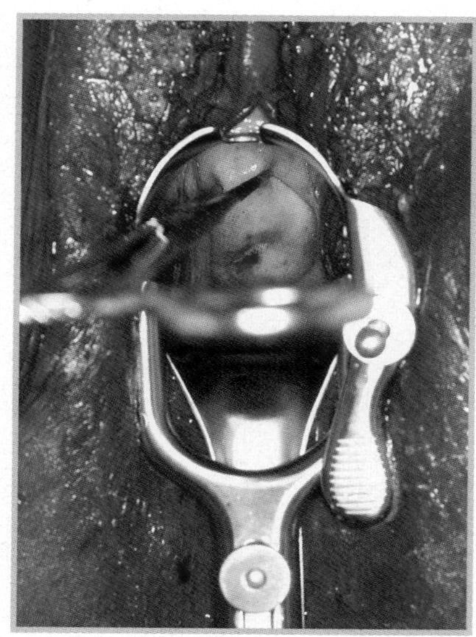

Step 2

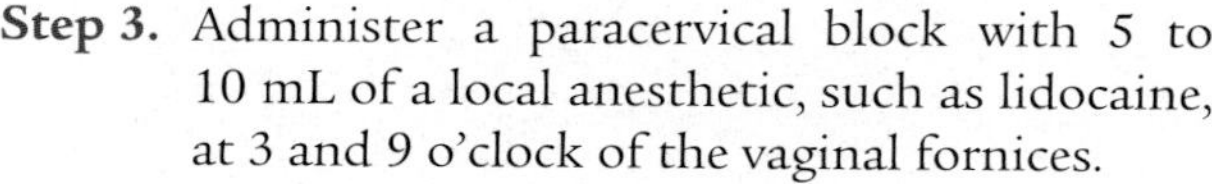

Step 3. Administer a paracervical block with 5 to 10 mL of a local anesthetic, such as lidocaine, at 3 and 9 o'clock of the vaginal fornices.

- **PITFALL:** As with all injections, aspirate before injecting in order to avoid intravascular injection of local anesthetic.

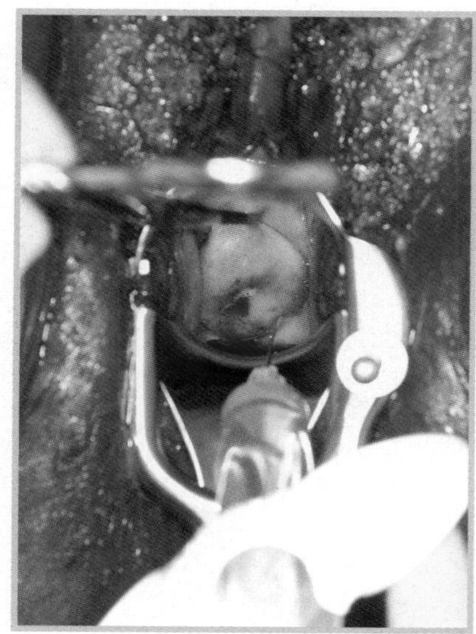

Step 3

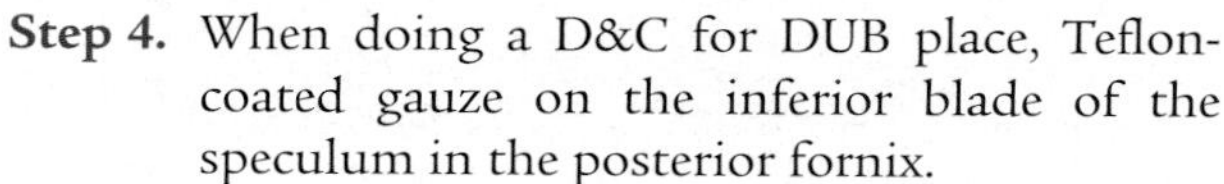

Step 4. When doing a D&C for DUB place, Teflon-coated gauze on the inferior blade of the speculum in the posterior fornix.

- **PEARL:** The gauze will absorb blood and prevent the loss of sometimes scant endometrial curettings.

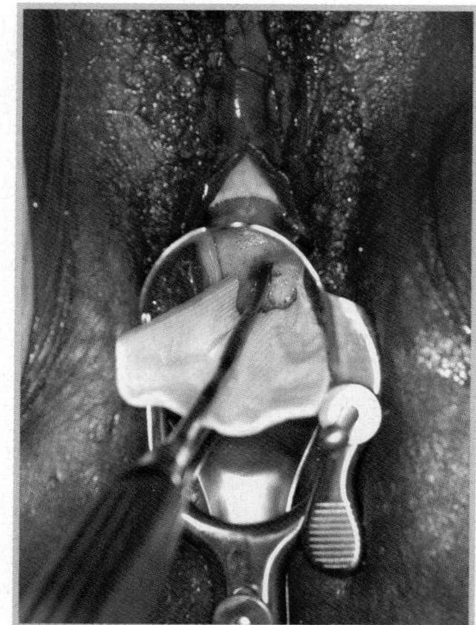

Step 4

Step 5. Perform an endocervical curettage (ECC). Curettings should be placed onto the gauze and transferred to a fixative solution.

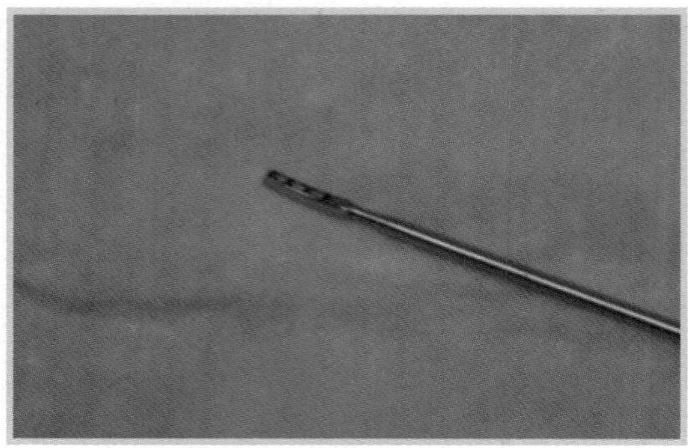

Step 5

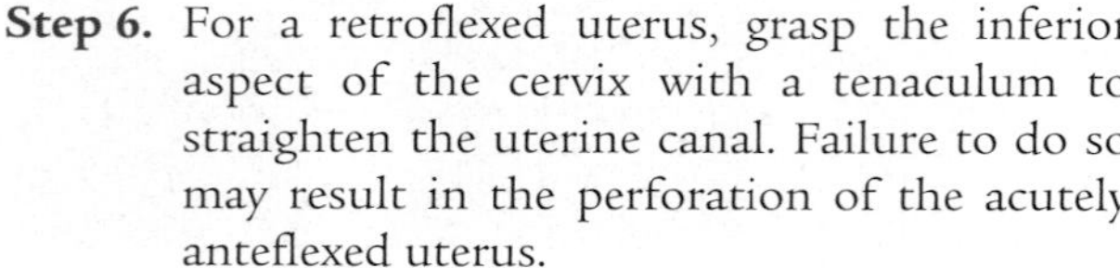

Step 6. For a retroflexed uterus, grasp the inferior aspect of the cervix with a tenaculum to straighten the uterine canal. Failure to do so may result in the perforation of the acutely anteflexed uterus.

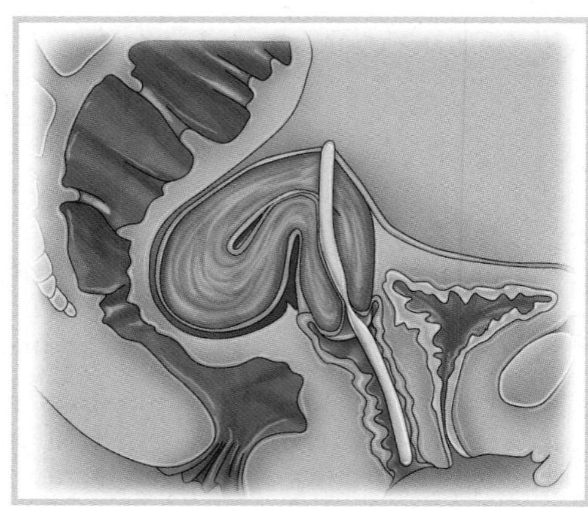

Step 6

Step 7. For an anteverted uterus, grasp the superior aspect of the cervix to straighten out the canal. Do not place the tenaculum through the cervical os. Failure to do so may result in the perforation of the retroflexed uterus.

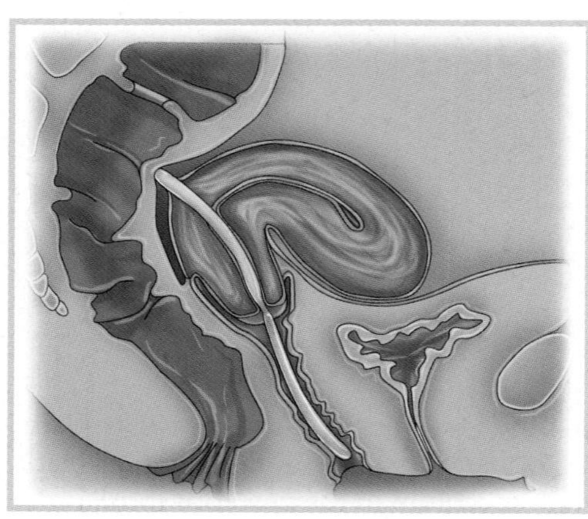

Step 7

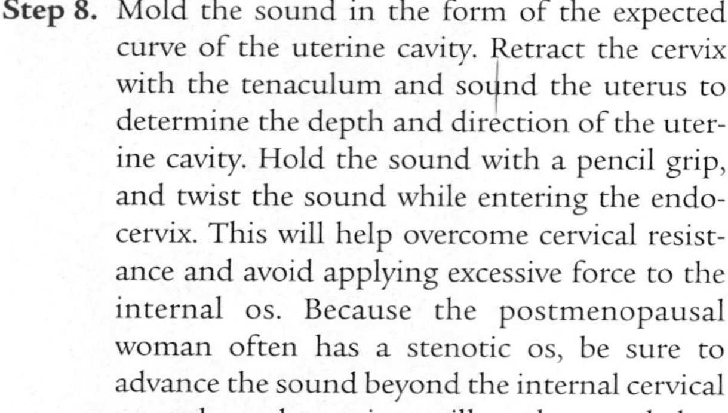

Step 8. Mold the sound in the form of the expected curve of the uterine cavity. Retract the cervix with the tenaculum and sound the uterus to determine the depth and direction of the uterine cavity. Hold the sound with a pencil grip, and twist the sound while entering the endocervix. This will help overcome cervical resistance and avoid applying excessive force to the internal os. Because the postmenopausal woman often has a stenotic os, be sure to advance the sound beyond the internal cervical os or the endometrium will not be sampled.

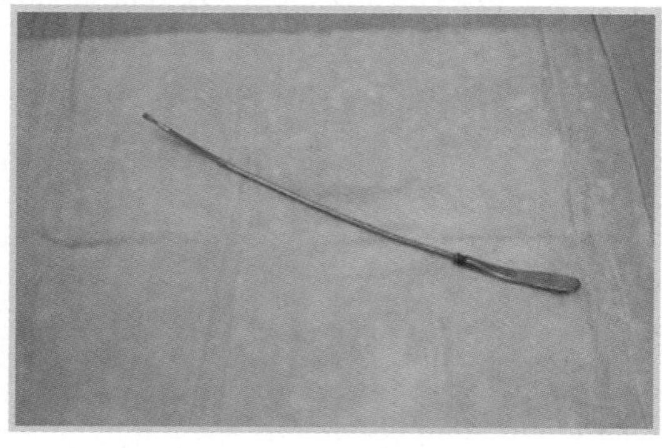

Step 8

Step 9. While retracting the cervix with the tenaculum, dilate the cervix with Hegar dilators, and start with the smallest dilator. Hold the dilator with a pencil grip. In the setting of DUB, dilation to 8 to 9 mm is usually sufficient. In the treatment of missed or incomplete abortion, the amount of dilation in millimeters should equal the uterine size in weeks. One should use the largest curette that can be easily advanced through the dilated cervix.

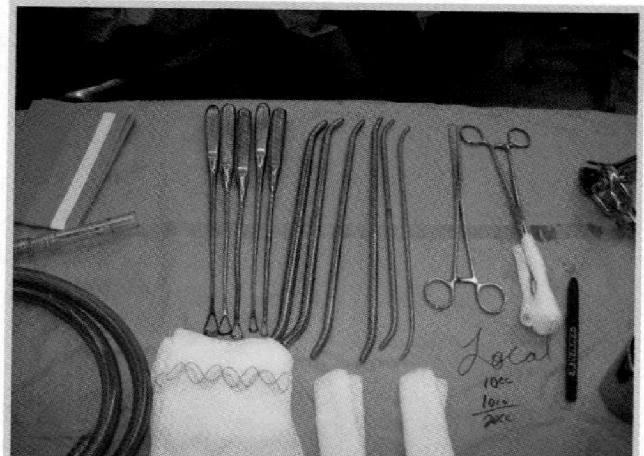

Step 9

D&C for DUB

Step 10. Explore the uterine cavity with stone forceps to search for uterine polyps. Explore the dome, lateral, anterior, and posterior walls of the uterus.

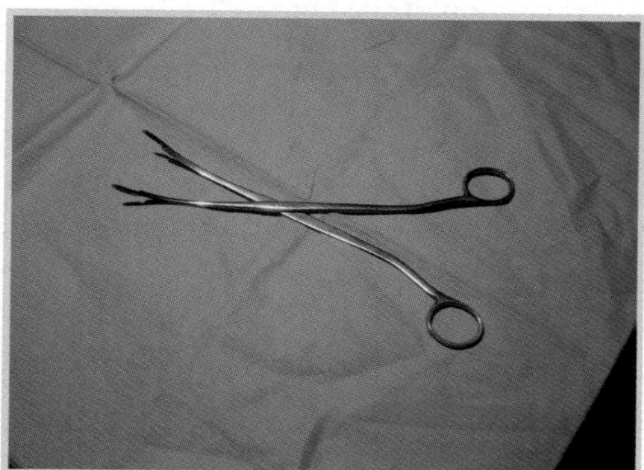

Step 10

Step 11. Choose a medium-sized sharp curette.

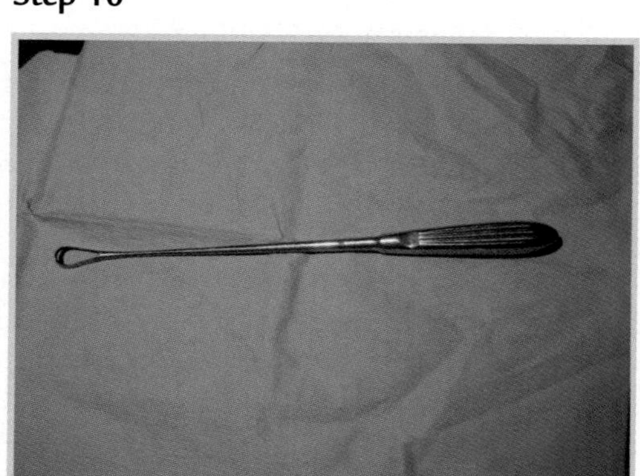

Step 11

Step 12. Insert into the uterus while holding the curette in a pencil grip. Curette the anterior, posterior, lateral walls, and dome of uterus. When a rough sandpaper sensation is palpable through the curette, the endometrium has been sufficiently curetted. Place the curettings onto the gauze pad, and transfer the sample to a fixative solution.

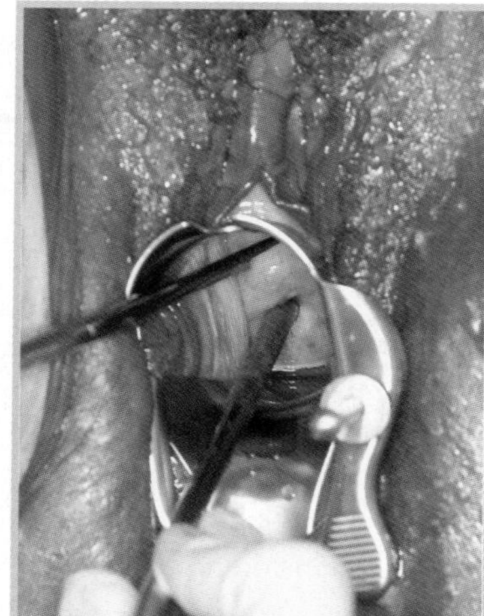

Step 12

D&C for Missed or Incomplete Abortion

Step 13. Attach a suction curette to suction tubing while keeping the O-ring away from the hole in the curette to prevent suction from forming. The size of the suction curette in millimeters should approximately equal the size of the uterus in weeks of gestation.

- **PEARL:** When doing a D&C for a uterus >13 weeks size, ultrasound guidance should be used to verify complete evacuation of the uterus.

Step 14. Gently advance curette through the cervix to the depth of the uterus estimated by uterine sound. Have an assistant activate the suction. Then close the hole with the O-ring on the curette and curette the uterus as with a sharp curette.

- **PITFALL:** Do not remove the curette from the cervix while the suction is active.
- **PEARL:** Always check the curettings to assure that there is no fat, which would suggest the possibility of uterine perforation and visceral injury.

Step 15. When the suction curettage is complete, raise the O-ring to allow the POC to be suctioned into the suction trap. If all POC are not removed with the suction curettage, perform sharp curettage as described previously and repeat suction curettage of the uterus. Observe the patient for uterine bleeding after completion of the procedure. Clean the vaginal vault of all blood because patients can be very concerned if they discharge a large amount of blood after standing. Check the tenaculum site for bleeding, and apply silver nitrate or a suture if the ectocervix is bleeding actively. Remove the speculum.

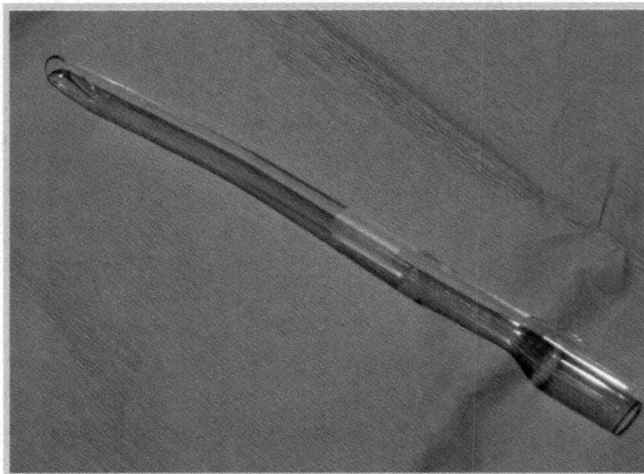

Step 13

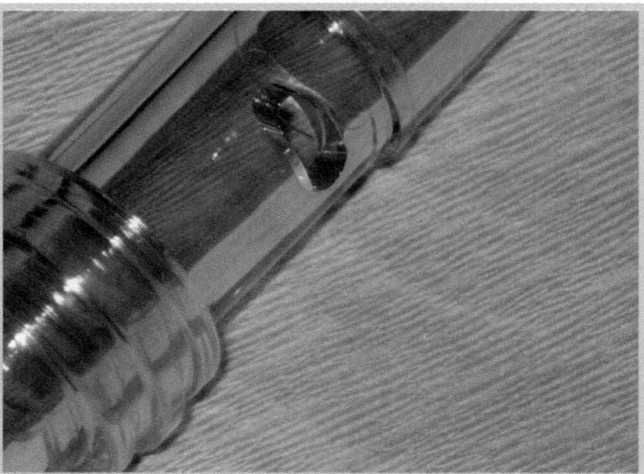

Step 14

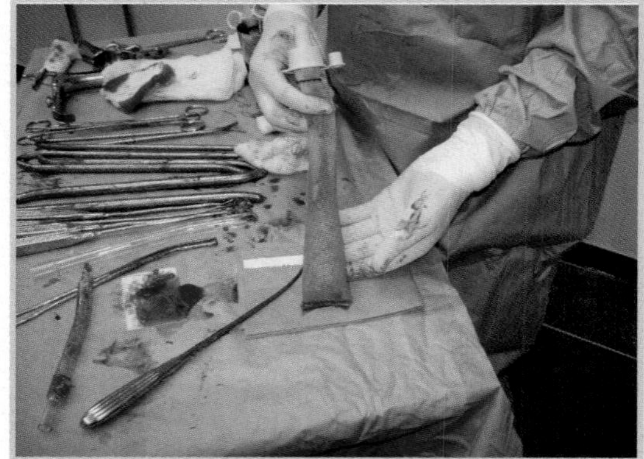

Step 15

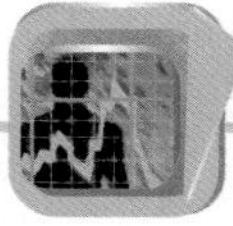

Complications

- Uterine perforation: lateral perforation can lead to intraperitoneal hemorrhage and broad ligament hematoma.
- Bleeding.
- Infection, including peritonitis, abscess, and endometritis. There is controversy over whether or not to prophylactically treat with antibiotics after a D&C, but most physicians do not.

- Trauma to abdominal viscera, including the bowel, omentum, mesentery, ureter, or fallopian tube.
- Asherman syndrome.

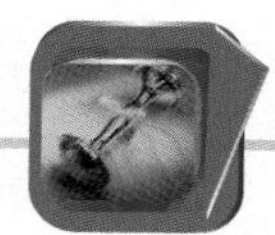

Pediatric Considerations

Although it may be tempting to use D&C in a menarchal patient who is having heavy anovulatory bleeding, the endometrium in young girls is often denuded by bleeding. A D&C is more likely to cause scaring (Asherman syndrome) that may result in permanent infertility.

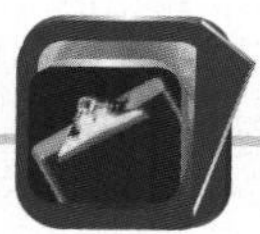

Postprocedure Instructions

Properly complete a pathology request form. For DUB patients, the ECC and endometrial portions should be labeled separately. In the case of missed and incomplete abortion, submit specimens for routine pathology and genetic analysis. Genetic abnormalities are common in spontaneous abortion, and it is important not to miss a molar pregnancy.

Observe the patient in the office or recovery room for at least 1 hour after the procedure. Monitor her vital signs and development of pain or vaginal bleeding.

Pain management is often accomplished using nonsteroidal anti-inflammatory drugs (NSAIDs). Be aware, however, that uterine cramping after D&C for pregnancy-related problems can be intense.

Inform the patient that postprocedure bleeding should be lighter than the patient's usual menses. Set a follow-up appointment for 1 week after the procedure to check bleeding and the patient's status.

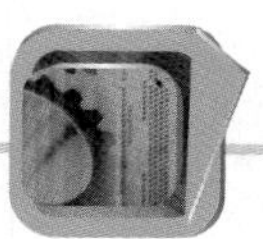

Coding Information and Supply Sources

CPT Code	Description	2008 Average 50th Percentile Fee	Global Period
58120	Endometrial tissue retrieval	$977.00	10

CPT is a registered trademark of the American Medical Association.
2008 average 50th Percentile Fees are provided courtesy of 2008 MMH-SI's copyrighted Physicians' Fees and Coding Guide.

ICD-9 Codes

626	Disorders of menstruation and other abnormal bleeding from genital tract
627	Menopausal and premenopausal bleeding
627.1	Postmenopausal bleeding
632	Missed abortion
634	Spontaneous abortion

Suppliers

- McKesson Medical-Surgical, One Post Street, San Francisco, CA 94104. Phone: 1-800-283-1558. Web site: http://www.mckesson.com/en_us/McKesson.com/.
- PSS World Medical, Inc., 4345 Southpoint Boulevard, Jacksonville, FL 32216. Phone: 904-332-3000. Web site: http://www.pssd.com/pss/index.htm

Patient Education Handout

Patient education handouts, "Dysfunctional Uterine Bleeding," "Spontaneous Abortion or Miscarriage," and "Postprocedure Dilation and Curettage," can be found on the book's companion Web site.

Bibliography

Chen BA, Creinin A, Mitchell D. Contemporary management of early pregnancy failure. *Clin Obstet Gynecol.* 2007;50(1):67–88.

Harris LH, Dalton VK, Johnson TR. Surgical management of early pregnancy failure: history, politics, and safe, cost-effective care. *Am J Obstet Gynecol.* 2007;196(5):445.e1–5.

Nanda K, Peloggia A, Grimes D, et al. Expectant care versus surgical treatment for miscarriage. Cochrane Database of Systematic Reviews (2):CD003518; 2006.

Rock JA, Jones III HW. *TeLinde's Operative Gynecology*. 9th ed. Philadelphia: Lippincott Williams & Wilkins. 461–478.

Ramphal SR, Moodley J. Best practice and research in clinical obstetrics and gynaecology. *Emerg Gynaecol.* 2006;20(5):729–750.

2008 MAG Mutual Healthcare Solutions, Inc.'s Physicians' Fee and Coding Guide. Duluth, Georgia. MAG Mutual Healthcare Solutions, Inc. 2007.

CHAPTER 75

Hysteroscopic Female Sterilization with Microinsert (Essure)

Jay M. Berman, MD, FACOG
Assistant Professor, Wayne State University School of Medicine
Department of OB/GYN
Hutzel Women's Hospital, Detroit, MI

Female sterilization is one of the most common methods of birth control used in the United States, accounting for approximately 22% of users. Until recently, female sterilization was a hospital or surgery center procedure, either performed postpartum at the time of delivery or shortly after or as an interval procedure performed more than 6 weeks after a delivery.

In November 2002, the U.S. Food and Drug Administration approved the sale of the first hysteroscopic sterilization method available in the United States. This device is called the Essure microinsert. The device is constructed from Nitinol (nickel titanium), stainless steel, platinum, and PET (polyethylene terephthalate) fibers. The wound-down insert is 4 cm long and 0.8 mm in diameter. When released from the delivery system, the outer coil expands to 1.5 to 2.0 mm in diameter to anchor the microinsert in the fallopian tube.

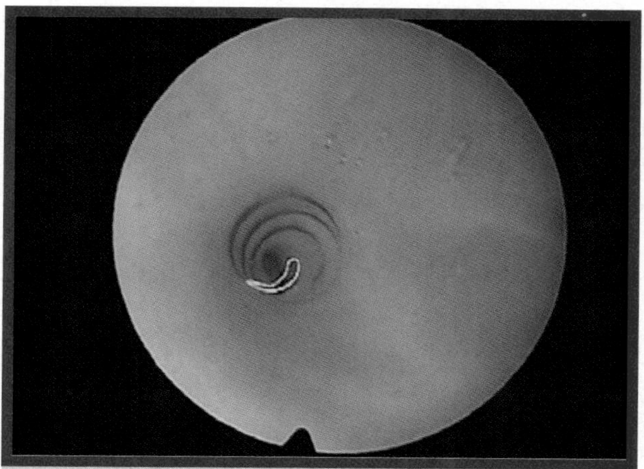

The approval of this device has been heralded as the start of a new age in female sterilization. The Essure procedure is safe, simple, and effective and can be performed in the hospital, ambulatory surgery center, or office setting. Patients can frequently choose their location and type of anesthetic. Local, local and sedation, and general anesthesia are all options for anesthesia during Essure microinsert placement. The vast majority of patients will return to normal activities in 0 to 2 days.

Recently, the manufacturer of the Essure microinsert released a third-generation device with a simplified delivery and deployment system. The new device is identified by its purple handle and has an even faster time of insertion. Average operating time for an experienced user is about 4 minutes. Several other devices are undergoing trials, but as of this writing, none have been approved for use in the United States.

The majority of patients who desire permanent sterilization are between 30 and 45 years. This age group also has a large group of women with menorrhagia. It is tempting to offer simultaneous endometrial ablation for these women. However, the package labeling is clear that simultaneous endometrial ablation with the balloon device is not indicated. Anecdotally, this author has collected more than 70 cases of simultaneous hysteroscopic sterilization and endometrial ablation with freely circulating hot water (HTA, Boston Scientific) with no significant complications. The key issue for the package labeling is the ability to obtain a satisfactory hysterosalpingogram (HSG) at 3 months. In addition, payment from insurance carriers for procedures done on the same day is usually less than satisfactory.

Prior to scheduling a hysteroscopic sterilization procedure with Essure microinserts, all patients need contraceptive counseling, especially because 49% of pregnancies in the United States are unintended (U.S. Centers for Disease Control data). Visualization of the endometrial cavity is facilitated by timing procedures in the early luteal phase. Treatment with oral contraceptives or medroxyprogesterone (Depo-Provera) also improves visualization. This has the added benefit of providing the needed contraception until the HSG is completed at 3 months.

One of the most significant benefits of this technique is its high efficacy of 99.74% at 5 years. It provides this high efficacy with no incision and without general anesthesia in an outpatient setting. It is safe for patients who are poor candidates for laparoscopic surgery or hormonal contraceptives. It also requires less time lost from work and family.

Prior to the date of the procedure, informed consent should be obtained from the patient. Also in some states, a separate state-mandated form must be signed >30 and <180 days before the procedure. The need for contraception until the confirmatory HSG at 3 months should be reviewed and emphasized.

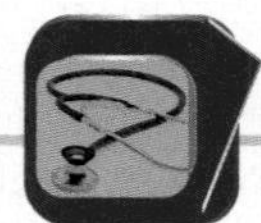

Equipment

- Urine pregnancy test.
- Premedication with a nonsteroidal anti-inflammatory drug (NSAID) of the provider's choice (suppositories, oral medicine, or intramuscular injection).
- Atropine (0.5 to 1.0 mg) can be given intravenously, subcutaneously, or intramuscularly. Initial single doses in adults vary from around 0.5 to 1 mg for bradycardia associated with vagal reaction.
- Standard gynecological equipment tray including tenaculum and dilators.
- Stirrups.
- Weighted speculum, Graves speculum, or Graves speculum with open side.
- Single-tooth tenaculum (two).
- Gimpelson tenaculum for patulous cervix or endoloop for patulous cervix.
- Sterile gauze, 2 × 2 inches or 4 × 4 inches.
- Betadine.
- Operating hysteroscope sheath with 5-French or larger channel.
- 30-degree hysteroscope lens (12-degree or 0-degree will not work with lateral tubes).
- Tubing and drapes for hysteroscope system being used.
- Normal saline, 1- or 3-L bags warmed to reduce tubal spasm.
- Sterile gloves.
- Local anesthetic for paracervical block (bupivacaine or lidocaine).
- Control-top syringe and 22-g spinal needle.
- Essure systems, two minimum. Additional units should be available in case of malfunction or inadvertent contamination.
- Patient ID card supplied with Essure package.

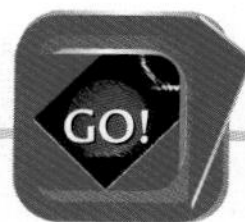

Indications

- Patient who desires to end fertility permanently (must be older than 21 in most states)
- Younger than 45 years of age, although this is a personal choice of patient and physician
- Inability to tolerate general anesthesia
- Medical conditions that make pregnancy and/or general anesthetics dangerous
- Previous abdominal surgeries that increase the risk of complications
- Willing to use another form of birth control for 3 months and undergo an HSG to confirm placement and tubal occlusion

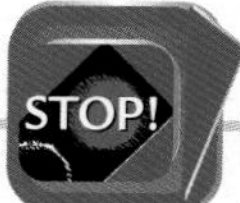

Contraindications

- Unsure about desire to end fertility
- Patients in whom only one microinsert can be placed
- Patients with previous tubal ligation
- Patients with unicornuate uterus
- Known or suspected pregnancy
- Pregnancy less than 6 weeks prior to placement
- Active or recent pelvic infection
- Known allergy to contrast media
- Known allergy to nickel confirmed by skin test
- Inability to follow-up or refusal to have confirmatory HSG
- Immunosuppressive therapy with systemic corticosteroids, chemotherapy, or other agents such as tumor necrosis factor (TNF) blockers (relative contraindication, as the therapy is expected to negatively affect tissue response)

The Procedure

Step 1. On the day of the procedure, patients are instructed to refrain from food and drink from midnight until the time of surgery. If taking any other medications, they should take them as usual with a sip of water, except for anticoagulants. Depending on the venue and anesthetic, patients should be given an oral NSAID or a parenteral NSAID 30 to 45 minutes prior to the procedure. Patients are placed in the dorsal lithotomy position or stirrups, and the vagina is prepped with povidone-iodine solution (if not allergic). An electric examination table is helpful but not required in the office setting.

- **PEARL:** Anticoagulated patients should be managed with the patient's primary provider, depending on the anticoagulant and the underlying medical disorder.
- **PEARL:** Routine catheterization of the bladder is not required but may be necessary if there has been a long wait or the patient has received excessive intravenous fluids.

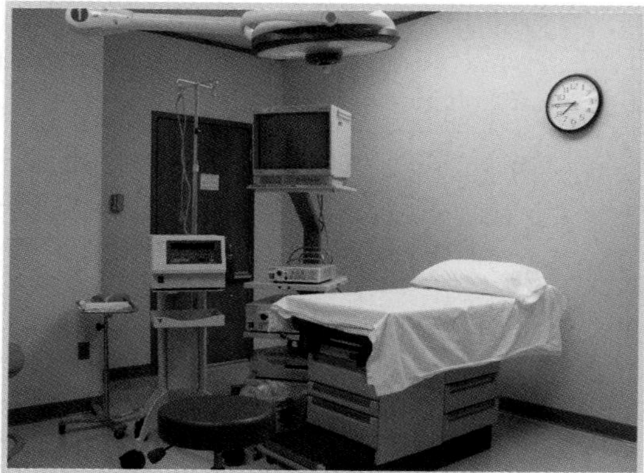

Step 1

Step 2. A weighted or bivalve speculum is inserted, and the cervix is visualized. The anterior lip of the cervix is grasped with a single-tooth tenaculum, and the paracervical block is placed (see Chapter 82). If no resistance to injection is met, the needle may be intraperitoneal, and the block will not be effective. If very strong resistance is felt, the needle is too deep in the cervix, again resulting in decreased effectiveness.

- PITFALL: The key to successful local anesthetic is placing it properly and waiting for it to work prior to stimulating the surgical site. Begin assembling the other equipment only after placing the anesthetic. It takes about 3 minutes to assemble the hysteroscope and prepare for the next portion of the procedure, just about the time needed for local anesthetic to be effective.

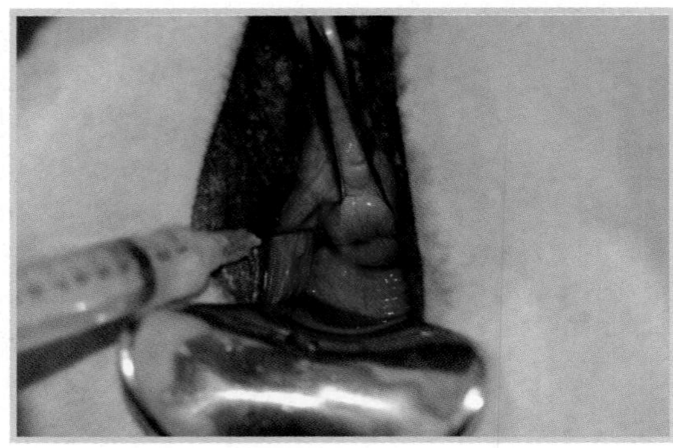

Step 2

Step 3. The hysteroscope used for this procedure should have 30-degree lenses and a 5-French operating channel. The 30-degree lenses facilitate placement of microinserts in laterally located tubes. The outside diameter of the sheath is approximately 5.5 mm (16.5 French). Normal saline solution is the distending medium of choice because of its safety and low cost. A 1-L bag should be adequate in most circumstances. Three-liter bags are just as cost-effective, and if the cervix is patulous, more fluid may be needed. Once the anesthetic has taken effect, the hysteroscope is inserted into the cervical os, and the fluid is started. Most of the women undergoing this procedure do not require dilatation. It is important to visualize the endocervical canal and endometrial cavity while advancing the hysteroscope to decrease the chance of perforation.

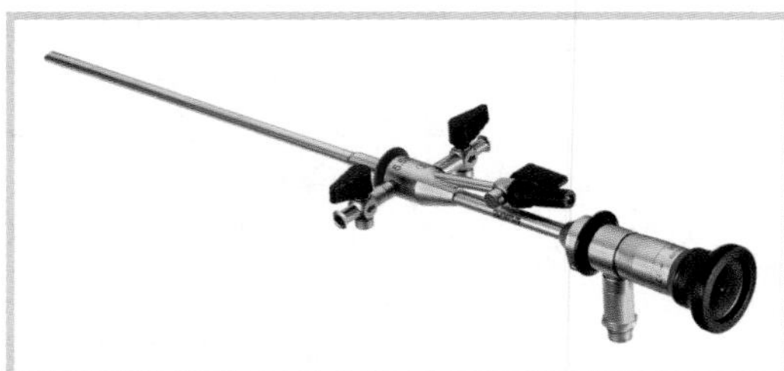

Step 3

- PITFALL: Cold solution increases pain and tubal spasm. This can be greatly reduced by heating the solution to body temperature. Care must be taken not to make the solution hot enough to cause a burn.
- PITFALL: The uterine sound is not necessary and indeed increases the risk of perforation. It is not possible to continue this procedure if perforation is diagnosed.

Step 4. As the hysteroscope is advanced, the endocervical canal and endometrial cavity should be thoroughly examined. Both tubal ostia should be identified and note taken of any abnormalities, including polyps, fibroids, and the thickness of the endometrium, because these abnormalities can interfere with proper placement of the microinserts. It may be possible to remove polyps and then complete the procedure. Fibroids will not generally be amenable to treatment on the spot but may require separate procedures. Any areas where hyperplasia or cancer is suspected should be biopsied, and the Essure should be delayed until a diagnosis is made. After the endometrial cavity is visualized and both tubal ostia seen, the micro-insert package can be opened. Insert the DryFlow introducer into the 5-French working channel.

- **PITFALL:** It is important not to open the Essure microinsert package until the endometrial cavity is visualized and both tubal ostia confirmed. If both tubal ostia cannot be seen or the endometrium is too thick, then the procedure should be cancelled and possibly rescheduled.
- **PITFALL:** Note which device is being used. The following steps are for the new ESS305 system with the purple handle, not for the previous version with the white handle.
- **PEARL:** The valve in the introducer prevents fluid from splashing back. The fluid no longer needs to be turned off during catheter insertion.

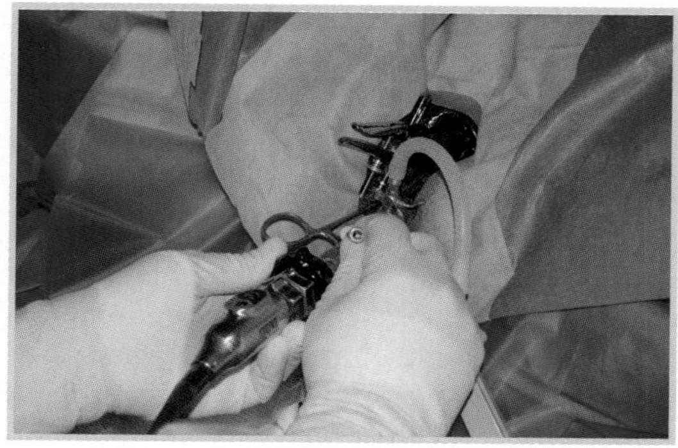

Step 4

Step 5. Insert the Essure catheter carefully into the introducer.

- **PITFALL:** Note that the tip of the Essure is curved. Do not attempt to straighten the tip, because the curve is important for guiding it into the tubal ostia. The dominant hand should manipulate the catheter and the nondominant hand should hold the hysteroscope.

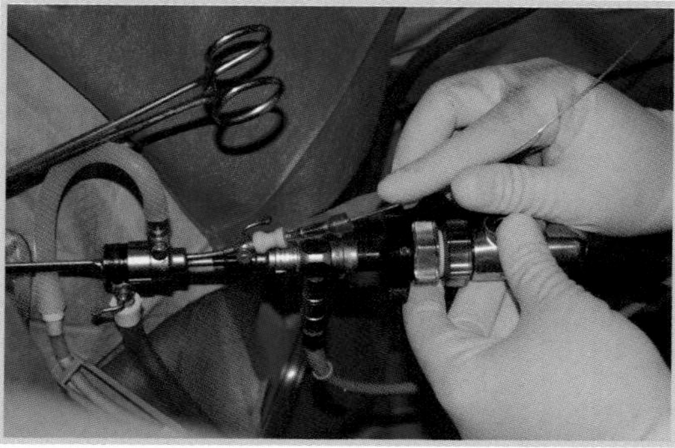

Step 5

Step 6. Move the hysteroscope close to the tubal ostia. Advance the delivery catheter into the tube until the black positioning marker is at the ostium. Catheter guidance may require rotating the hysteroscope for a better view of the ostium. The catheter should be manipulated close to the introducer to avoid bending it. It is helpful to have an assistant hold the handle while the operator advances the catheter.

- **PEARL:** Consider starting with the right tubal ostia. This makes it easier to keep track of which side was done first and to find the opposite side.
- **PITFALL:** If the catheter flexes while advancing, moving the hysteroscope closer to the ostium will make the catheter act stiffer.
- **PEARL:** To place the catheter in lateral tubes, it is necessary to turn 30 degrees

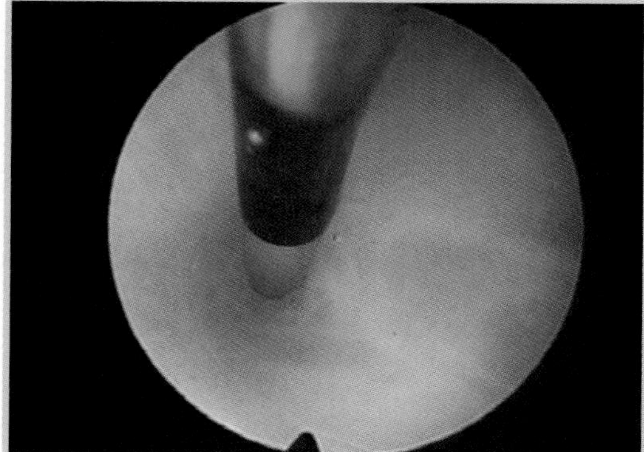

Step 6

away from the ostium; that is, turn the lightpost toward the ostium, not away from it. This is counterintuitive to most hysteroscopists, but it is necessary for successful placement.

Step 7. At this point, it is extremely important that the operator hold the hysteroscope and handle in the same (usually nondominant) hand. The dominant hand should then carry out the maneuvers to deploy the microinsert. Most of the difficulties seen in teaching this procedure come from not adhering to this rule.

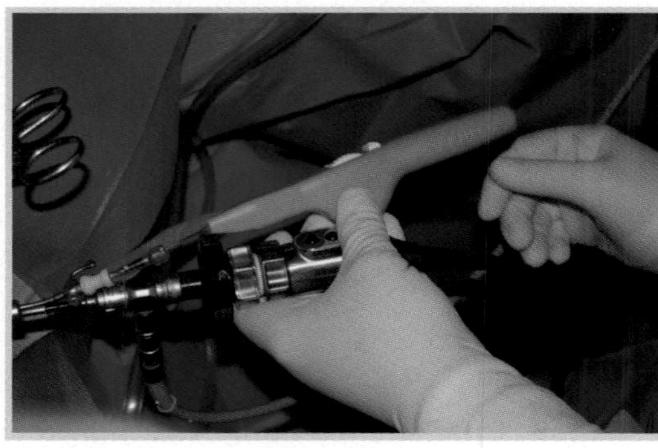

Step 7

Step 8. Once the operator is happy with the position, the thumb wheel is rolled back. The black positioning marker moves toward the operator until the thumb wheel reaches a hard stop.

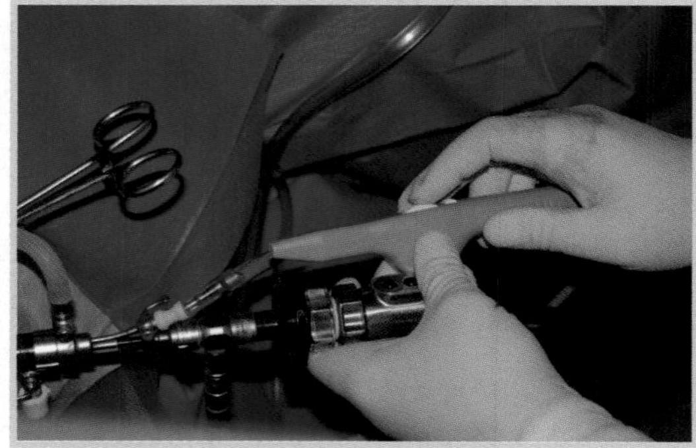

Step 8

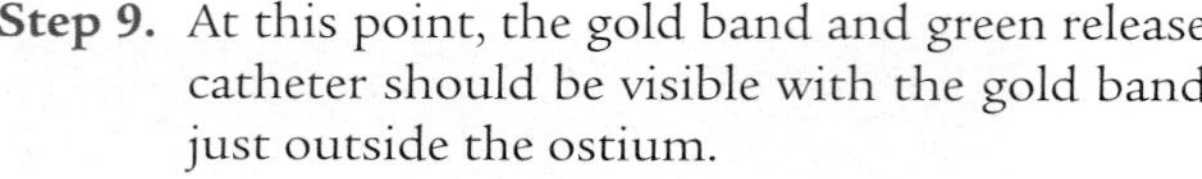

Step 9. At this point, the gold band and green release catheter should be visible with the gold band just outside the ostium.

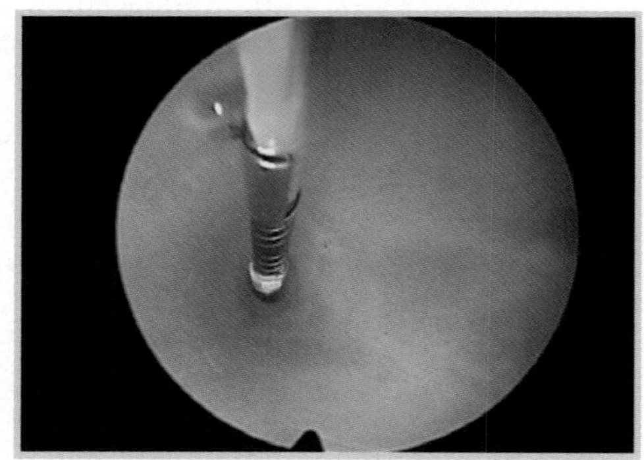

Step 9

Step 10. Depress the button on the purple handle to initiate deployment. The microinsert will not yet deploy, allowing final positioning.

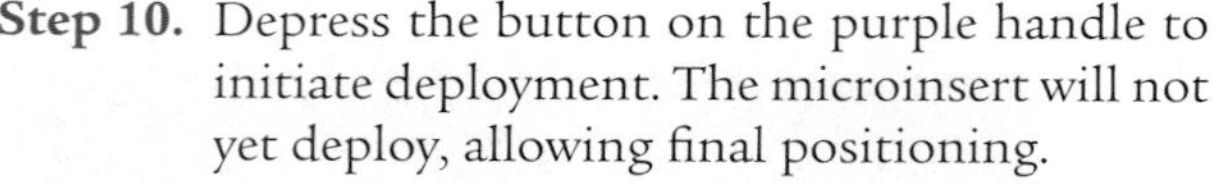

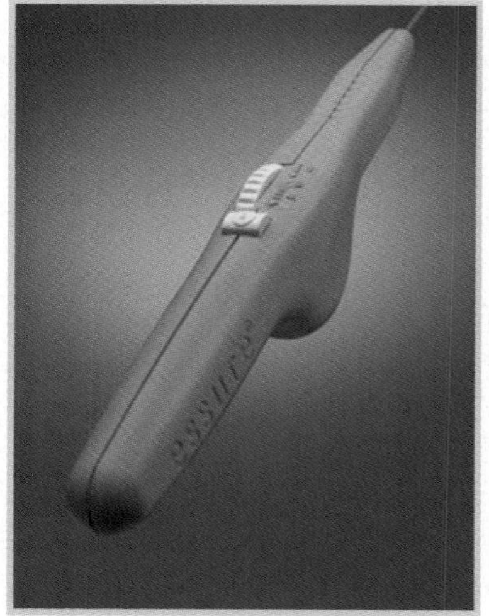

Step 10

Step 11. Roll the thumb wheel back again to a hard stop; this expands and detaches the microinsert. The thumb wheel should be rolled backward at about one click per second; this allows full control of the procedure. This detaches the release catheter from the insert. This procedure for the ESS305 is greatly simplified from the previous version.

Step 12. There should be two to four coils visible at the ostium marking optimal placement. Up to 15 coils can be visible for acceptable placement. If more than 15 coils are visible, the microinsert should be removed with a hysteroscopic grasper and another one inserted. Document the placement and the number of proximal coils in the cavity. Withdraw the catheter, and repeat with second catheter for contralateral ostium. When completed, remove all of the instruments, note condition of tenaculum site, and perform a sponge count. Office patients can lie down or sit in a lounge chair for approximately 20 minutes until ready for discharge. Surgery center or hospital patients should be discharged as per their normal protocols.

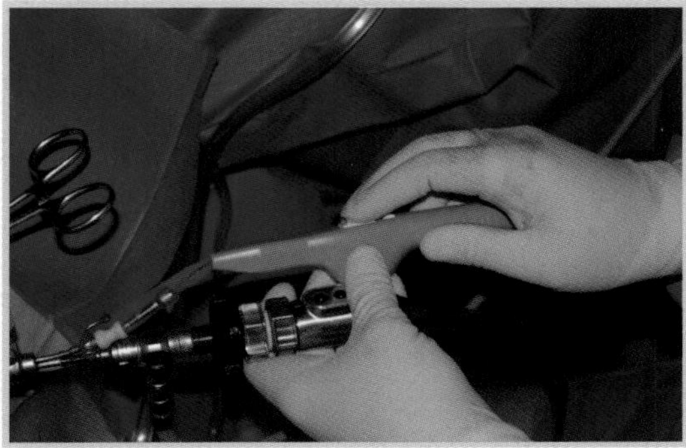

Step 11

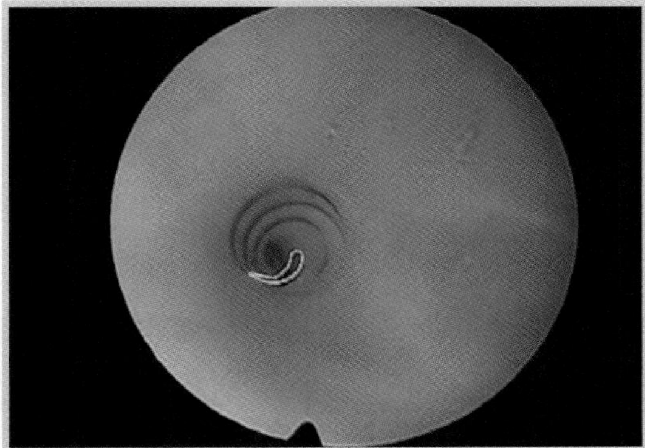

Step 12

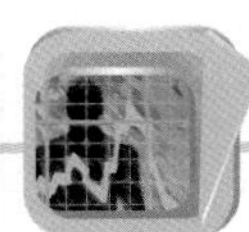

Complications

- Transient cramping
- Pain
- Nausea and vomiting
- Bleeding or spotting
- Tubal perforation
- Expulsion or migration of microinsert
- Uterine perforation

A perforation is diagnosed in several ways. Most commonly, there is loss of visualization, and increasing flow or pressure does not improve the situation. Rarely, the peritoneal cavity or ovaries are visualized. If either of these is noted, the procedure should be terminated immediately and the patient observed closely. It would be rare to require surgery for these situations because no energy source has been applied to the peritoneal cavity. A repeat procedure can be scheduled in month.

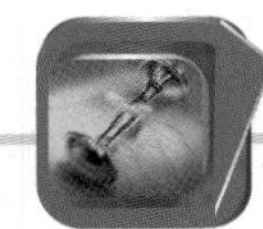

Pediatric Considerations

In general, the Essure microinsert is not applicable to the pediatric population. There are a small number of individuals who might benefit from this procedure because of developmental abnormalities that carry a risk of pregnancy. The need for sterilization in this group should only be after careful consultation with parents and pediatric specialists.

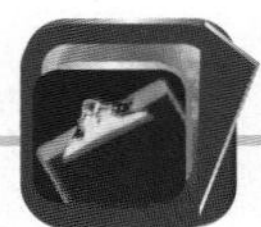

Postprocedure Instructions

Prior to discharge, review with the patient the need for additional contraception until the HSG is performed and confirms bilateral placement and occlusion. After the procedure, patients can resume normal activities as soon as they wish, and intercourse can resume as soon as the spotting stops, usually 7 to 10 days. Patients should be seen for a postoperative visit in 1 to 2 weeks. At that time, a referral slip or appointment should be made for the HSG, and the instructions should be repeated. Because most primary providers do not perform HSG, the provider should make arrangements with a radiology group to provide this service. The HSG for Essure confirmation has different requirements than those done for infertility. A complete description is available at http://www.essuremd.com. It is in the best interests of the provider to make this document available to the radiologist who will be providing this service.

Inform the patient that the Essure microinserts have been tested and found to be safe to use in magnetic resonance imaging/magnetic resonance angiography (MRI/MRA) units.

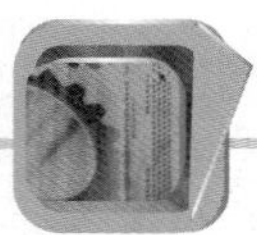

Coding Information and Supply Sources

CPT Code	Description	2008 Average 50th Percentile Fee	Global Period
58565	Hysteroscopy, surgical; with bilateral fallopian tube cannulation to induce occlusion by placement of permanent implants	$2,319.00	90
58340	Catheterization and introduction of saline or contrast material for saline infusion sonohysterography (SIS) or hysterosalpingography	$657.50	0
74740	Hysterosalpingography, radiologic supervision and interpretation	$219.00	XXX
74740-26	Hysterosalpingography, radiologic supervision and interpretation	$98.00	XXX

CPT is a registered trademark of the American Medical Association.
2008 average 50th Percentile Fees are provided courtesy of 2008 MMH-SI's copyrighted Physicians' Fees and Coding Guide.

ICD-9 Codes

V25.2 Admission for sterilization

Hysterosalpingogram Testing (Use Both in This Order)

V67.09 Follow-up examination following other surgery
V26.51 Tubal ligation status

Suppliers

The procedure kit, consisting of two introducers and two devices, is available only from Conceptus, Mountain View, CA. Web site: http://www.conceptus.com.

Office hysteroscopy equipment is available from Olympus, Karl Storz, Richard Wolf, ACMI, or any number of small manufacturers.

Patient Education Handout

A patient education handout, "Essure Hysteroscopic Sterilization," can be found on the book's companion Web site.

Bibliography

Chandra A. Surgical sterilization in the United States: prevalence and characteristics, 1965–95. *Vital Health Stat.* 1998;23(20).

Chern B, Siow A. Initial Asian experience in hysteroscopic sterilization using the Essure permanent birth control device. *BJOG.* 2005;112:1322–1327.

Connor V. Contrast infusion sonography to assess microinsert placement and tubal occlusion after Essure. *Fert Steril.* 2006;85:1791–1793.

Cooper J, Carignan C, Cher D, et al. Microinsert nonincisional hysteroscopic sterilization. *Obstet Gynecol.* 2003;102:59–67.

Essure. Prescribing and procedural information. http:// www.Essuremd.com. Accessed October 2007.

Kerin J, Carignan C, Cher D. The safety and effectiveness of a new hysteroscopic method for permanent birth control: results of the first Essure PBC clinical study. *Aust NZ J Obstet Gynaecol.* 2001;41:364–370.

Kerin J, Cooper J, Price T, et al. Hysteroscopic sterilization using a micro-insert device: results of a multicenter phase II study. *Hum Reprod.* 2003;18:1223–1230.

Kerin J, Munday D, Ritossa M, et al. Essure hysteroscopic sterilization: results based on utilizing a new coil catheter delivery system. *J Am Assoc Gynecol Laparosc.* 2004;11:388–1193.

Thiel J, Suchet I, Lortie K. Confirmation of Essure micro-insert tubal coil placement with conventional and volume-contrast imaging three-dimensional ultrasound. *Fertil Steril.* 2005;84:504–508.

Valle R, Carignan C, Wright T, et al. Tissue response to the STOP microcoil transcervical permanent contraceptive device: results from a prehysterectomy study. *Fertil Steril.* 2001;76:974–980.

2008 MAG Mutual Healthcare Solutions, Inc.'s Physicians' Fee and Coding Guide. Duluth, Georgia. MAG Mutual Healthcare Solutions, Inc. 2007.

CHAPTER 76

Treatment of Noncervical Human Papillomavirus Genital Infections

Nancy R. Berman MSN, APRN, BC
Nurse Practitioner, Northwest Internal Medicine Associates
Division of the Millennium Medical Group, PC, Southfield, Michigan

Human papillomavirus (HPV) is the most common sexually transmitted infection in the United States. There are approximately 30 anogential types of HPV, and they are grouped into low and high risk according to their association with cervical cancer. Though most people who are sexually active will be infected with HPV at some point, the virus will usually be cleared by an immune response and will never be detected by the individual or in screening. Cervical cancer is caused by persistence of high-risk types of HPV, and this is preventable through the use of HPV vaccines, cervical screening, and treatment.

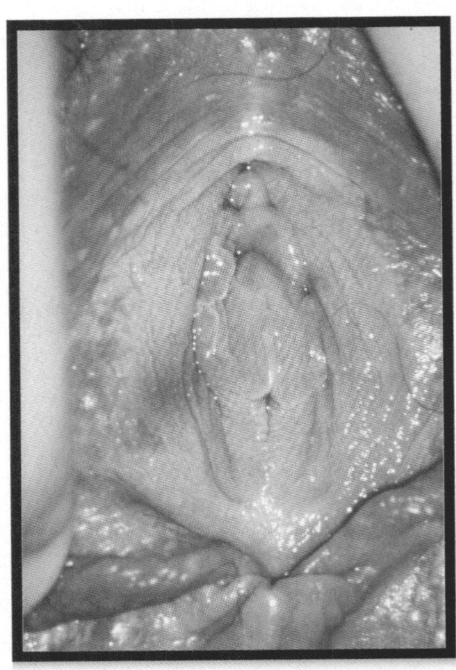

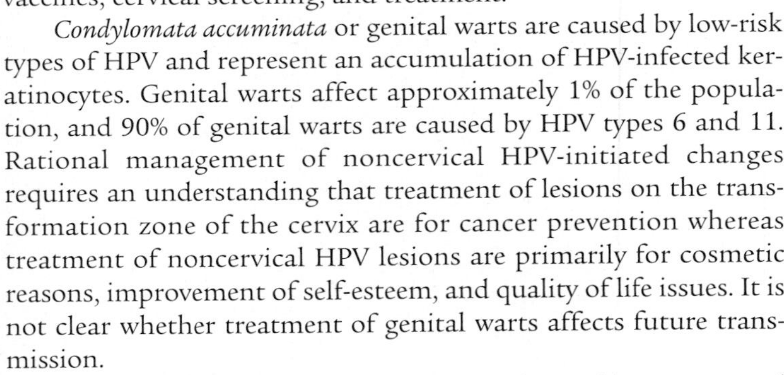

Condylomata accuminata or genital warts are caused by low-risk types of HPV and represent an accumulation of HPV-infected keratinocytes. Genital warts affect approximately 1% of the population, and 90% of genital warts are caused by HPV types 6 and 11. Rational management of noncervical HPV-initiated changes requires an understanding that treatment of lesions on the transformation zone of the cervix are for cancer prevention whereas treatment of noncervical HPV lesions are primarily for cosmetic reasons, improvement of self-esteem, and quality of life issues. It is not clear whether treatment of genital warts affects future transmission.

The quadravalent HPV vaccine (Gardasil, Merck) was approved by the U.S. Food and Drug Administration (FDA) in June 2006 for young girls and women from 9 to 26 and is recommended by numerous organizations including the American College of Ob/Gyn, the American Academy of Pediatrics, and the American

Academy of Family Physicians. The vaccine creates immunogenicity for HPV types 6, 11, 16, and 18 with noninfectious viruslike particles and an aluminum adjuvant. The vaccine will not treat existing HPV infection, but it will not make pre-existing disease worse. Prevaccine HPV testing is not required, and at this time there are not any FDA-approved type-specific HPV tests in clinical practice.

External genital warts can usually be diagnosed by their gross clinical appearance as they are visible to the naked eye. After the application of 5% acetic acid, genital warts may be easier to identify because of acetowhitening. The only indication for applying acetic acid to the genital skin is to aid in the differential diagnosis of obvious lesions. After the application of acetic acid, the skin may turn diffusely white. This may represent subclinical HPV infection or could be due to microtrauma or inflammation, it and does not require treatment (see Figure 1). There is not an indication to look for subclinical HPV infection in the absence of visible clinical disease.

External genital warts may first appear or worsen in pregnancy. They should be treated around the 32nd week of pregnancy as recurrence in pregnancy is common. Cesarean section is indicated only if the warts physically obstruct the pelvic outlet. Though neonatal exposure to maternal HPV may cause the rare condition of recurrent laryngeal papillomatosis, there are not any published prospective studies that support the use of cesarean section for the prevention of this problem, and the Centers for Disease Control and Prevention clearly recommends against it.

TABLE 76-1. Factors Influencing Modality of Treatment of Condylomata Acuminata

- Patient preference
- Cost
- Patient resources including the ability for the patient to return for office visits
- Location of warts
  - Internal on mucous membrane
    - Proximal to the Hart line
    - Soft, fleshy
    - Responds well to destructive therapy
  - External
    - Distal to the Hart line
    - Fleshy
    - Keratotic (thickened)
    - May be more difficult to clear with destructive therapy
    - May require repeated visits
  - How extensive the warts are
  - Whether the patient is pregnant

The treatment plan for genital warts requires communication between the practitioner and the patient. It is important to stress that there is not always one treatment that will successfully clear warts, and for some people, recurrence will continue to be a problem. The treatment choices include both practitioner-applied (Table 76-2) and patient-applied (Table 76-3)

TABLE 76-2. Treatment Options That are Patient Applied

Imiquimod (Aldara, Graceway Pharmaceuticals Bristol, TN)

- Immune modulator
- Pregnancy class B
- Only treatment that may both clear and prevent the recurrence of disease
- Induces multiple subtypes of interferon: alfa, several cytokines, tumor necrosis factor, and interleukins
- Activates natural killer cells, T-cells, polymorphonuclear neutrophils, and macrophages
- For external use
- May clear keratotic or fleshy condylomata
- May be used as a debulking therapy for large disease volume
- Approved for 16 weeks of application
- Apply at bedtime three times a week
- Open sachet
  - Apply by fingertip
  - May require application by "feel" and not visualization by patient
- Mild to moderate skin irritation may occur and "drug holiday" may be taken if necessary until patient is comfortable to resume application
- Clearance rates of 72% for women and 33% for men
- Wart reduction rates of more than 50% for women and 70% for men

Podophyllotoxin (Condylox, Watson Pharmaceuticals Corona, CA)

- 0.5% gels, solutions, or cream
- Purified resin of active component of podophyllin
- Better standardized and safer than podophyllin
- Works by inhibition of nuclear division at metaphase
- Success rates vary from 44% to 88%
- Apply twice/day for 3 successive days and then a rest period for 4 days
- Repeat on a weekly basis for as long as 4 weeks or until resolution of warts

Sinecatechins 15% Ointment (Veregen, C.P.M. Contract Pharma GmbH & Co. KG Gedlkirchen-Westerham, Germany)

- FDA approved for 18 and older men and women for treatment of external genital and perianal warts.
- Mixture of eight catechins derived from the water extract of green tea (*Camellia sinensis*).
- Applied topically TID.
- May reduce the expression of HPV gene products E6 and E7, which lead to the induction of HPV-induced cell growth and neoplasia.
- May also inhibit proinflammatory enzymes and proteases such as COX-2.
- In studies, a wart clearance of 50% was observed for 77.6% (15% ointment) of all patients in the studies.
- Local skin reactions included erythema, edema, and erosion peaking at 2–4 weeks with a gradual decrease by the end of treatment.

TABLE 76-3. Treatment Options That are Provider Applied

Loop Electrosurgical Excisional Procedure (LEEP)

- Can be used to treat perineal condylomata in male and female patients.
- Excisional procedure that produces a specimen for histologic evaluation.
- Loops used for the removal of external lesions are typically smaller and shorter than standard cervical loops and are selected to allow easy removal of the lesion.
- The power setting must be high enough to allow easy passage with low tissue drag through the lesion and epidermis.
- The smoke evacuator should be activated before performing LEEP.
- Anesthesia can be obtained with 1% to 2% lidocaine with epinephrine (except on the penis, where epinephrine generally is avoided).
- Follow-up protocols vary.
  - Typically, patients return in 2 weeks to 1 month for follow-up unless there is unexpected pain or infection.
  - Late bleeding has been reported in 4% of patients treated for vaginal lesions and can usually be controlled with Monsel solution or fulguration.
- Infections is an uncommon complication that is usually controlled with topical (and rarely, systemic) antibiotics.
- Hypopigmentation and hypertrophic scars are rarely reported.
- Success rates for treating noncervical lesions with LEEP are in the range of 90% to 96%.

Cryotherapy

- Works by freezing and killing abnormal tissue, which then sloughs off and new tissue grows in its place.
- Local injection or topical anesthetic cream may be used but generally is unnecessary.
- Recalcitrant lesions can be rated with a freeze–thaw–refreeze technique to increase efficacy.
- Follow-up for retreatment is usually every 2 weeks until the lesion is resolved.
- The procedure does involve some pain during freezing and healing.
- Local infection and ulceration has been anecdotally reported.
- The success rate for cryotherapy is 71% to 79%.

Trichloroacetic Acid and Bichloracetic Acid

- Works by physically destroying tissue.
- Quickly inactivated after contact with tissue, therefore toxicity is not a problem.
- May be used on internal and external disease including on the vagina, vulva, and perianal skin.
- Apply every 1 to 3 weeks until the lesions resolve.
- Success rates are highest on warts that arise from mucous membrane and are soft and fleshy and are on internal skin (proximal to the Hart line).
- Lower rate of clearance and greater number of treatments required for warts that are keratotic (thickened) and arise from external skin (distal to the Hart line).
- Depth of treatment is difficult to control.
- Avoid overapplication, which can lead to penetration through the dermis and result in slow-healing ulcerations and scar formation.
- Pain can result from extensive or deep level of penetration of therapy.
- Pain medication may be offered for very extensive treatment.
- The response rate is between 50% and 81% and a higher rate of success is seen with the treatment of disease that is soft, fleshy, and internal.

Podophyllin

- Podophyllin resin is derived from the root of the "may apple plant."
- Commonly formulated as a 25% concentration in tincture of benzoin though concentrations may vary greatly.
- Arrests cellular replication of warts by inhibiting mitosis especially in rapidly growing tissue.

(*continued*)

TABLE 76-3. Treatment Options That are Patient Applied (*Continued*)

- No longer used commonly in clinical practice because newer options are available.
- Absorption through the mucosa occurs quite readily and is therefore contraindicated in pregnant women because it is considered teratogenic.
- Apply directly to the skin using a cotton tip applicator and primarily to small amounts of disease.
- Reapply weekly for 4 to 6 weeks or until wart resolution.
  - Pitfall: The drug can cause hepatotoxicity, neurotoxicity, or even death so the amount used should be limited, and it should primarily be used on keratotic skin.
  - Podophyllin may produce histopathologic changes that mimic epithelial atypia. If warts are biopsied after the recent application of podophyllin, it is important to advise the pathologist that podophyllin has recently been used.

therapies. If warts are left untreated, they may regress spontaneously, persist, or increase in size or number. The majority of individuals will remain free of warts after 9 months from initial onset, but those who continue to develop new warts have refractory disease. The choice of therapy does not generally affect whether new disease develops other than with imiquimod cream, which clears warts by immune modulation and creates immune memory that may prevent recurrence for that individual.

There are many options available for the treatment of genital warts, and the decision should be guided by patient preference. Practitioners should be familiar with at least one patient- applied therapy and one provider-applied therapy. There may be a need to utilize more than one therapy for the same individual but generally not at the same time. There is not necessarily a best treatment for any individual, but it should be based on the assessment of the patient's individual preference and capabilities (Table 76-4), disease distribution, and resources.

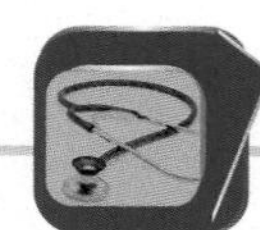

Equipment

Selection of equipment is individualized according to the practitioner's training and practice site. Additionally, treatment plans are determined by disease distribution and extent and patient preference and resources.

- Large cotton swabs.
- Small cotton swabs.
- Large mirror.
- High-frequency electrosurgical (LEEP) generator.
- Small, short loops for LEEP.
- Local anesthesia.
- Lidocaine (1% to 2%) with and without epinephrine.

TABLE 76-4. Teaching Patients Self-Application of Medication

- Patient will need to verbalize comfort with self-application.
- Use a mirror to allow patient to visualize the location of warts.
- Determine whether patient is able to reach areas for treatment.
- Recommend that patients use medication sparingly on first applications and observe for tolerance.
- Recommend that the patient soaks in water before application and then rubs area of disease with a towel before applying medication.
- Area should be washed with soap and water in the morning after application.

- Monsel solution.
- Smoke evacuator.
- Virus filtering mask.
- Syringes, 3 cc.
- Small-gauge needles, preferably dental needles.
- Povidone-iodine prep.
- Formalin containers.
- Cryotherapy cylinders.
- Portable cryosurgical units.
- Trichloroacetic acid (TCA).
- Bichloracetic acid (BCA).
- Podophyllin.
- Scissors.
- Pickup.
- Scalpel.
- Gauze pads.
- Cryotherapy equipment: a variety is available to meet the needs of practitioners. Equipment choice is based on such factors as cost, number of cases performed, and ease of use. Small thermos containers are an efficient way to store the liquid nitrogen.
- Self-contained portable cryosurgical units using liquid nitrogen may also be used. The device is designed to deliver constant operating pressure to ensure consistent and accurate freezing. Units range in price from $600 to $800.

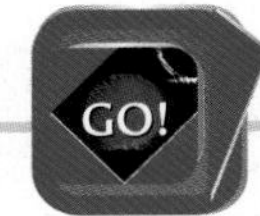

Indications

- Elimination of obvious, symptomatic, or troublesome external genital warts and vaginal warts
- Careful observation to determine the clinical diagnosis of genital warts and biopsy when indicated for presentations that are unclear
- Debulking HPV lesions before vaginal delivery to prevent bleeding and tearing of vaginal or perineal tissues

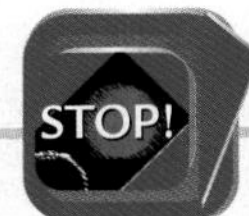

Contraindications

- Clinician experience and equipment determines the treatment choice.
- Imiquimod is not indicated for use on occluded mucous membranes, the uterine cervix, or in children.
- Imiquimod is not recommended for use in pregnancy.
- Imiquimod may damage condoms or diaphragms.
- Podofilox is not recommended for use in the vagina, urethra, perianal area, or cervix. It has not been studied for pregnancy, but its parent compound is contraindicated in pregnancy.
- LEEP is not recommended for penile, vaginal, and the anal verge.
- TCA and BCA are not recommended for use on the cervix or in the urinary meatus. Care must be taken when using around the clitoral hood. Use in the vagina is possible with significant care to avoid deep penetration of the mucous membrane.

The Procedure

Step 1. Assess the genital skin on the male or female for the presence of grossly visible lesions. Determine whether there are any lesions that require biopsy for definitive diagnosis or whether there are clinically apparent benign lesions. See Table 76-5.

TABLE 76-5. Differential Diagnosis for Condylomata Acuminata

CONDITION	DIAGNOSTIC CHARACTERISTICS
Condyloma latum (syphilis)	Broad-based smooth papules; test with rapid plasma reagin (RPR), Venereal Disease Research Laboratory (VDRL), micro hemagglutination-Treponema pallidum (MHA-TP), or fluorescent treponemal antibody absorbed (FTA–ABS) test
Common skin lesions	Seborrheic keratoses, nevi, angiomas, skin tags, and pearly penile papules
Neoplasms	Vulvar or vaginal intraepithelial neoplasia, bowenoid papulosis, and malignant melanoma
Buschke–Lowenstein tumor (i.e., giant condyloma)	A low-grade, locally invasive malignancy; appears as a fungating condyloma
Molluscum contagiosum	Waxy, umbilicated papules

Step 2. Any lesion that appears atypical, is pigmented red or white before acetic acid, or is resistant to previous therapy should be biopsied to rule out cancer or precancer. There is no widely accepted screening test for the diagnosis of external HPV lesions except physical examination.

- **PITFALL:** Failure to identify precancerous lesions can delay definitive treatment.

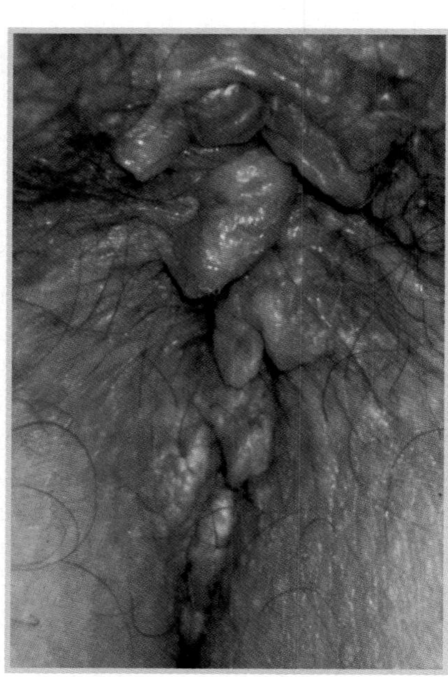

Courtesy of Richard Reid.

Step 2

Step 3. It is important to avoid overdiagnosis of normal variants including pearly papules on the male penis and papillomatosis on the female vulva. This normal variant of papillomatosis is distinguished from condyloma lesions in that the papillary projections of condyloma arise from a common base and each papular projection in papillomatosis arises directly from the epithelium.

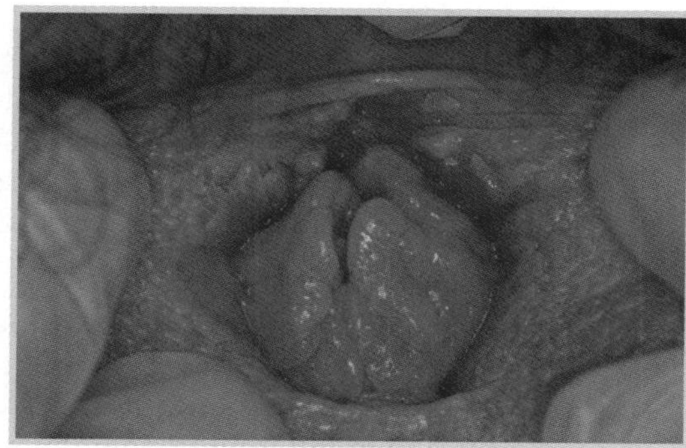

Courtesy of Richard Reid.

Step 3

Step 4. If genital warts are diagnosed, begin to determine a plan of treatment based on their location anatomically, their characteristics, and whether provider- or patient-applied therapy will be used. Soft, fleshy warts and in particular those that are internal arising from mucous membrane may respond well to provider-applied destructive therapies such as acid treatments. Those warts that arise from squamous epithelium distal to the Hart line may be thicker because they arise from more keratotic epithelium. Those warts may require many office visits for destructive therapy, which leads to more patient cost and inconvenience. Patients may want to reconsider self-applied therapy in that case or if after repeated office visits the warts are not clearing.

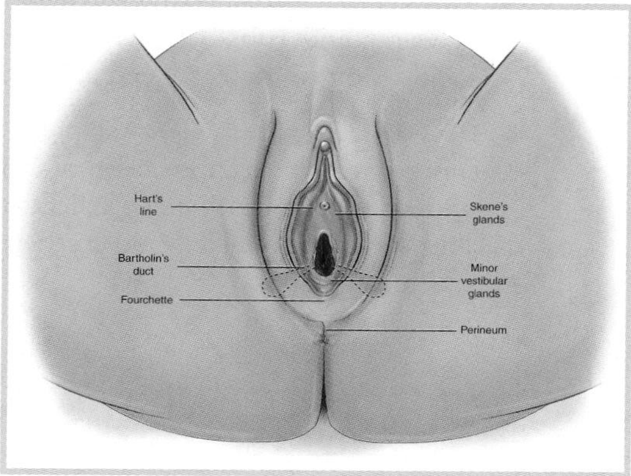

Step 4

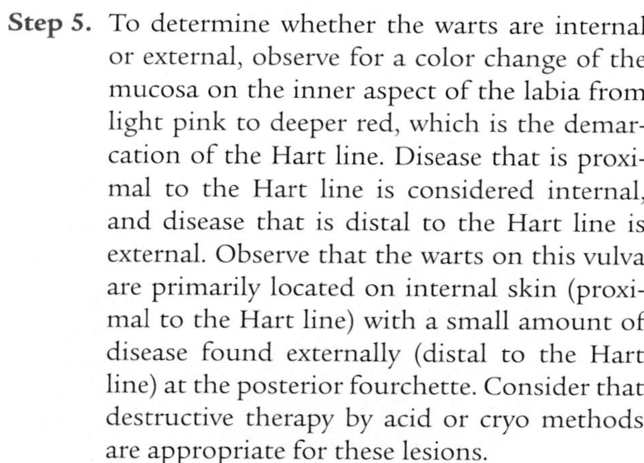

Step 5. To determine whether the warts are internal or external, observe for a color change of the mucosa on the inner aspect of the labia from light pink to deeper red, which is the demarcation of the Hart line. Disease that is proximal to the Hart line is considered internal, and disease that is distal to the Hart line is external. Observe that the warts on this vulva are primarily located on internal skin (proximal to the Hart line) with a small amount of disease found externally (distal to the Hart line) at the posterior fourchette. Consider that destructive therapy by acid or cryo methods are appropriate for these lesions.

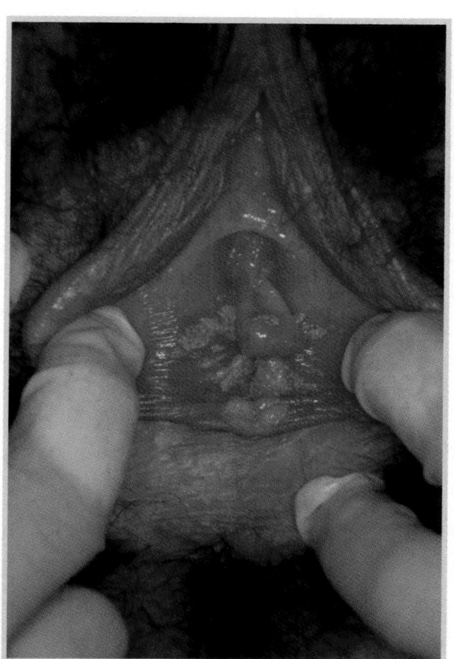

Courtesy of Richard Reid.

Step 5

Step 6. Observe whether warts are located distal to the Hart line and are external in origin and whether they are fleshy or keratotic because the choice of therapy will be different. Choosing destructive therapy for these warts would likely be appropriate because they are fleshy.

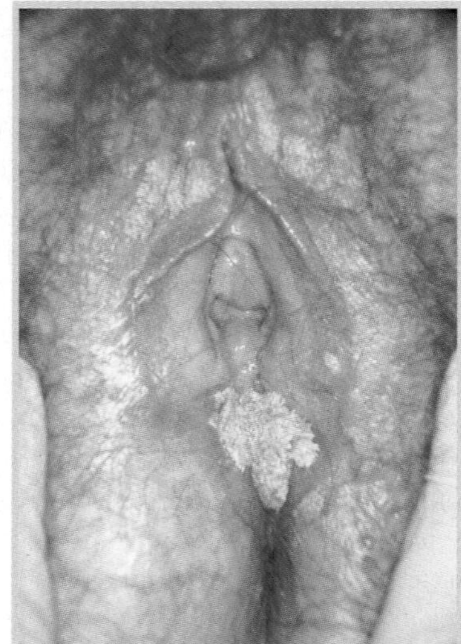

Courtesy of Richard Reid.

Step 6

Step 7. Note whether the external warts are more keratotic (thickened) and might be more resistant to destructive therapy. Consider debulking by a patient-applied therapy such as imiquimod and that excisional methods may become necessary.

- **PEARL:** Recommend that the patient soaks in water and rubs area with towel before application to increase mediation efficacy.
- **PITFALL:** Recommend that patient takes care to avoid overapplication of cream. If a patient applies too much medication to the skin, he or she may develop erythema, pain, and ulceration.

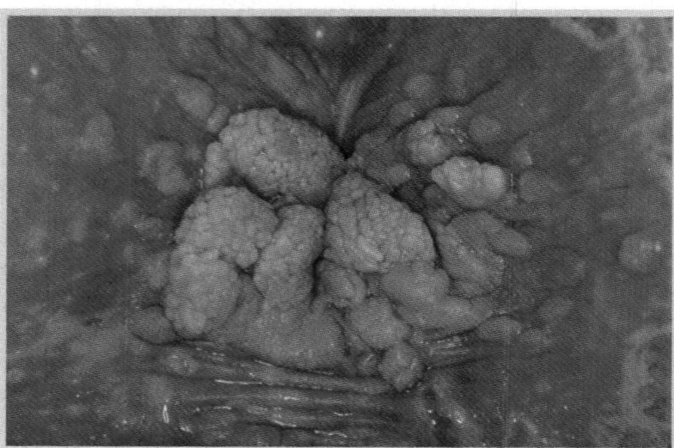

Courtesy of Richard Reid.

Step 7

LEEP Therapy

Step 8. Determine whether your practice setting will allow for the use of more expensive methods for excision of warts such as LEEP.

- **PEARL:** If your practice is using radiofrequency (RF) generators for other purposes, it is often cost-effective to use them for dermatologic applications with proper training.

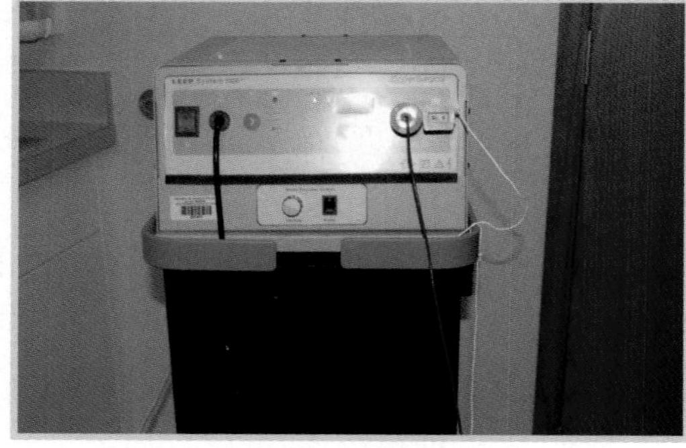

Step 8

Step 9. If LEEP equipment is available, use the medium-sized flat loop or small dermatologic loop or wire. It is important to pull the loop just above the base of the lesion and to avoid overpenetration of the dermis, which would lead to scarring. A gradual back and forth motion

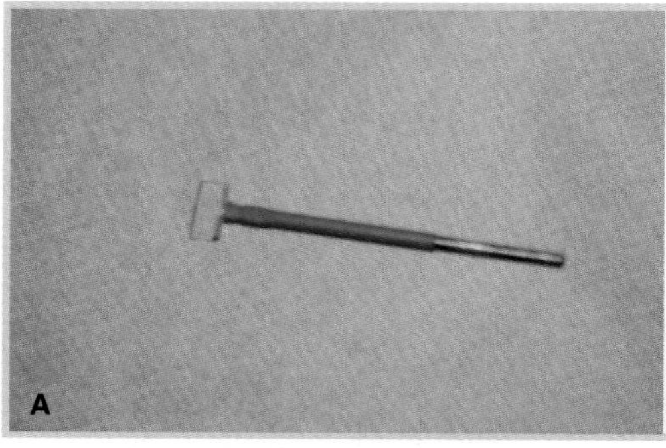

A

can produces a gently sloping excision with good cosmesis. A ball electrode may be used to stop minor bleeding.

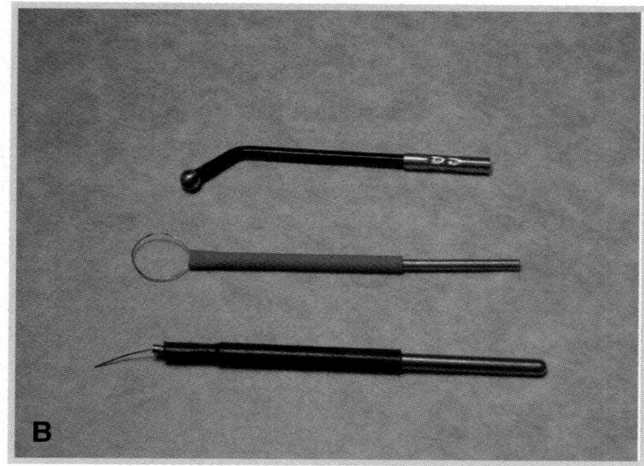

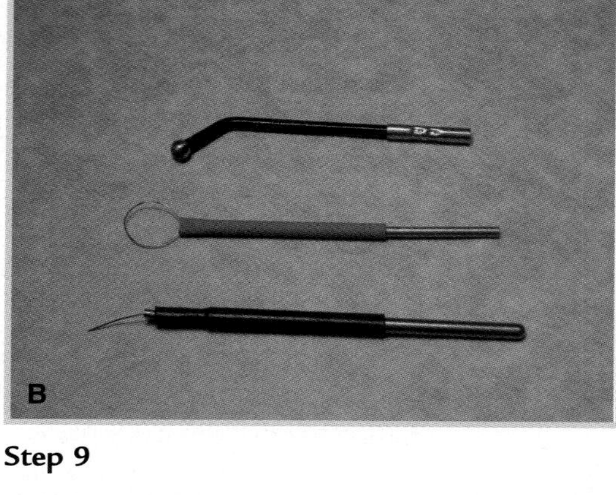

Step 9

Step 10. To remove a lesion with LEEP, first inject anesthetic under the site.

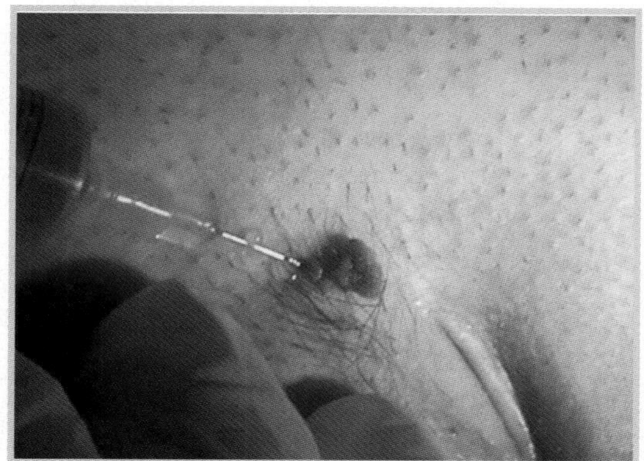

Step 10

Step 11. With the operator's hand resting against the patient for stability, the loop or "square" loop is introduced just *above* the base of the lesion and pulled completely through to debulk it.

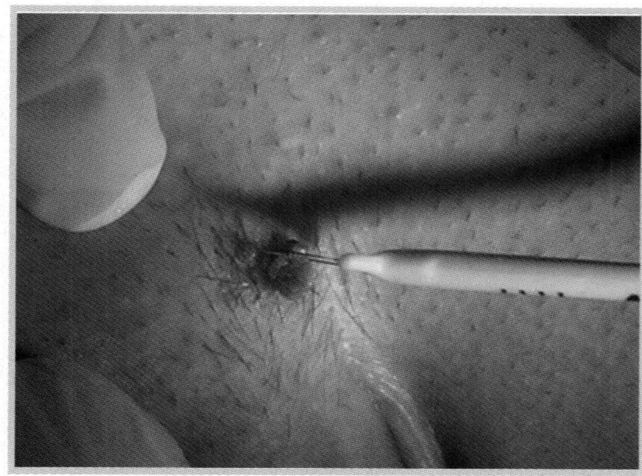

Step 11

Step 12. After debulking the lesion, the remaining lesion should be carefully shaved down to the dermis.

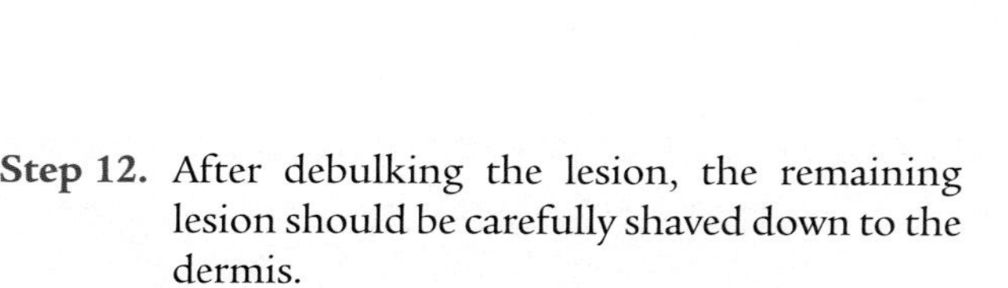

- PITFALL: Care should be taken to not penetrate the dermis during the shave excision. A proper shave site has gently sloping sides, dermis at the base, and no subcutaneous fat showing through.

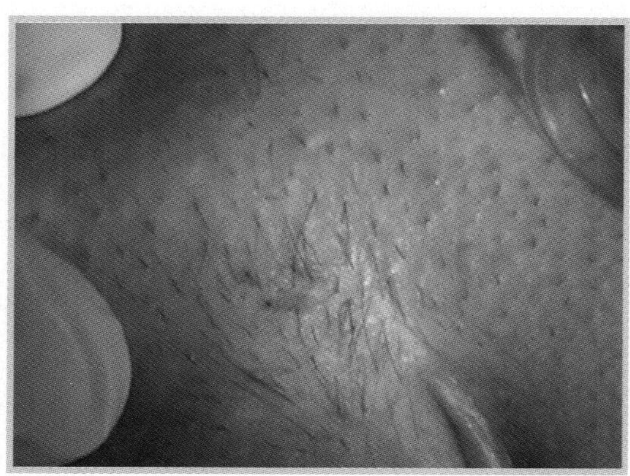

Step 12

Cryotherapy

Step 13. Alternatively, cryotherapy may be used. A variety of cryotherapy equipment is available to meet the needs of practitioners. Liquid nitrogen can be purchased and stored in large Dewer drums with small supplies brought into individual examination rooms in foam cups.

- **PITFALL:** Small vacuum-flask containers are an efficient way to store the liquid nitrogen, but applicators should not be dipped back into the flask after touching the patient, because some viruses may survive in the liquid nitrogen.

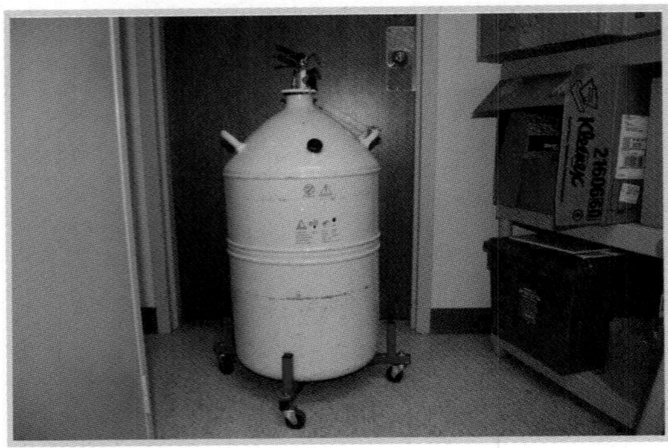

Step 13

Step 14. Large, cotton-tipped applicators for liquid nitrogen are easy to use and require little skill. If using a standard long-handled, cotton-tipped applicator, increase the size of the cotton head by pulling wisps of cotton off of a cotton ball and loosely rolling them onto the applicator. Dip the applicator into liquid nitrogen for 5 to 10 seconds, and then place it on the lesion until a 2-mm ice ball forms beyond the edges of the lesion. Repeat the application once the ice ball thaws. Therapy is repeated at 2-week intervals until the lesion resolves.

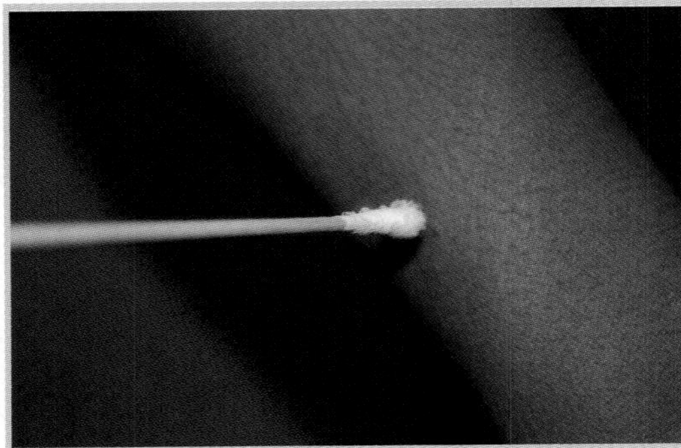

Step 14

Step 15. Alternatively, use a portable cryosurgical unit. An ice ball is created, and care is taken to avoid extending treatment beyond the area of the lesion. After the thaw, there may be a repeat of creating an ice ball.

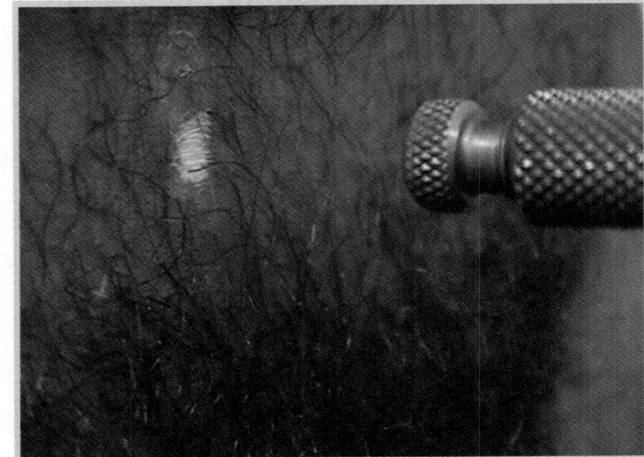

Courtesy of Ali Moiin.

Step 15

Topical Application

Step 16. TCA, BCA (DCA), or in limited cases podophyllin may be used for external lesions with care to avoid dripping excessive solution on the skin. TCA or BCA may be used on internal lesions, except on the cervix. The cotton swab should be pulled over the bottle neck to reduce the amount of solution that is brought over to the patient. Advise the

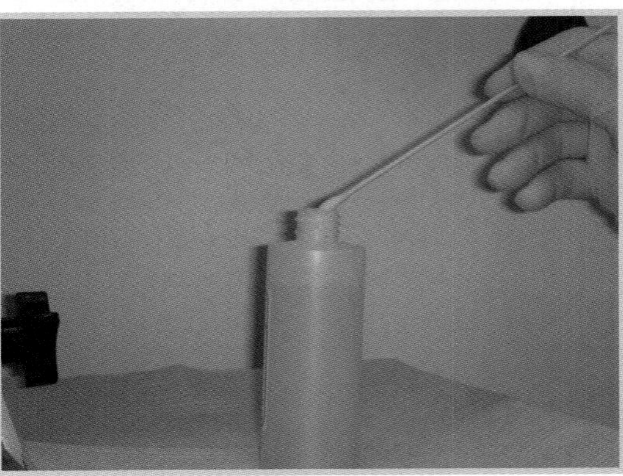

Step 16

patient that when acid is used, a burning sensation may occur, but this will usually go away in a few minutes. Treating internal skin will usually create greater pain than treating keratotic warts on external skin.

- **PITFALL:** If the swab is dripping with TCA or BCA, there will be risk of excessive treatment and potential for deep burns.

Step 17. The swab is used to paint the acid to the areas of disease. There is no need to use protective substances on the surrounding skin. The same swab may be used to treat multiple areas as long as there is an obvious whitening effect from the treatment with acid.

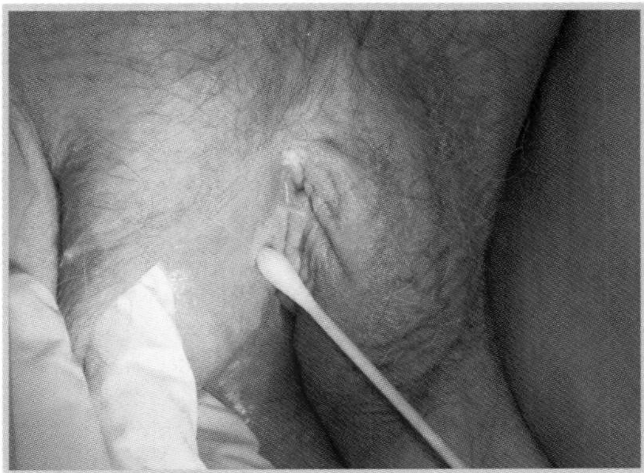

Step 17

Step 18. Large areas of extensive disease may be treated with acid. When treating an area this large, a dilute solution of half water and half acid may be used.

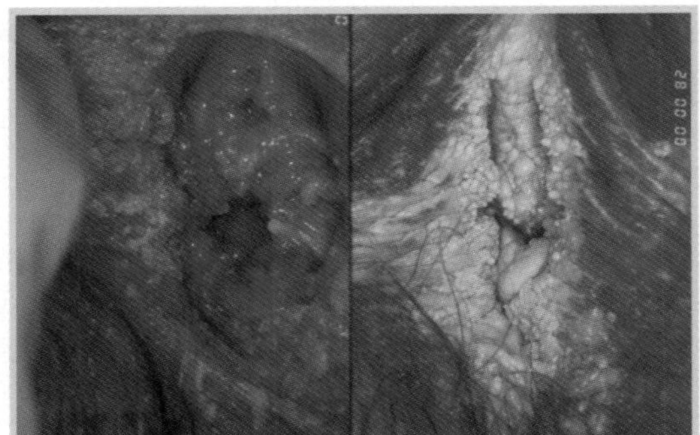

Courtesy of Richard Reid.

Step 18

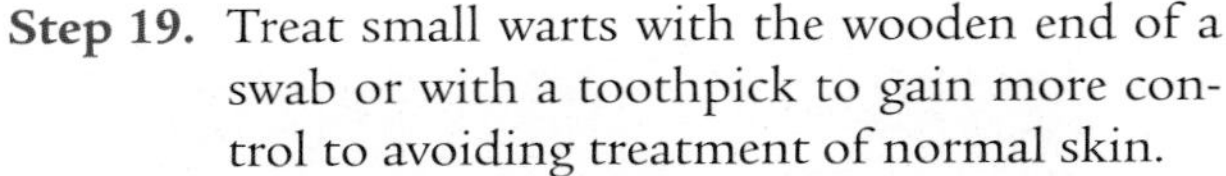

Step 19. Treat small warts with the wooden end of a swab or with a toothpick to gain more control to avoiding treatment of normal skin.

- **PITFALL:** Solution will be wicked up the applicator beyond the end. Be careful not to lay the length of the applicator against normal skin.

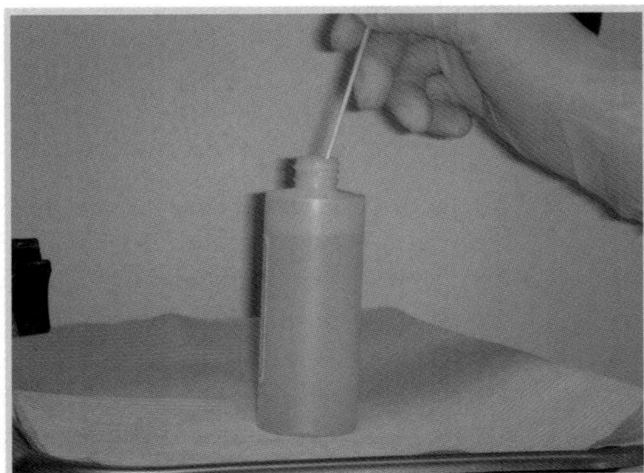

Step 19

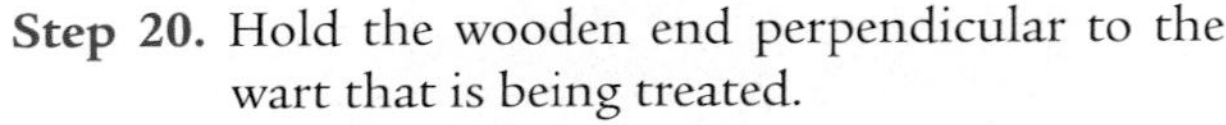

Step 20. Hold the wooden end perpendicular to the wart that is being treated.

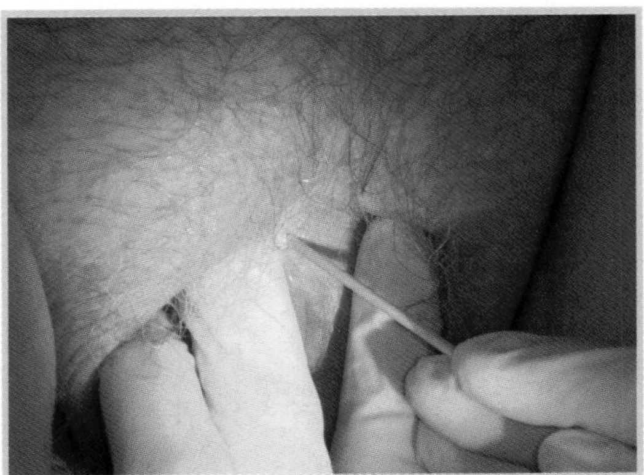

Step 20

Step 21. Watch for the whitening of the treated area to verify there has been sufficient treatment.

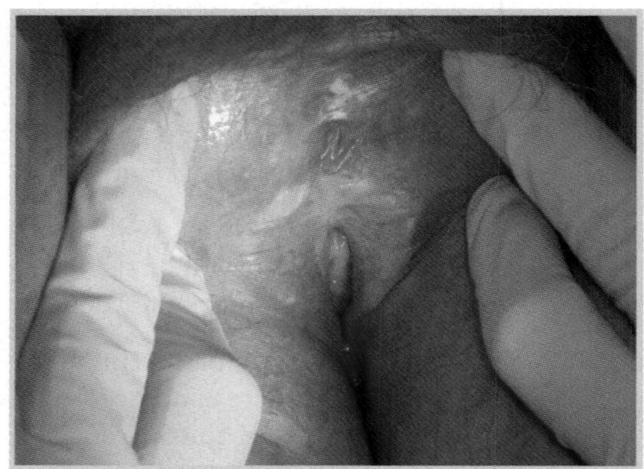

Step 21

Mechanical Excision

Step 22. Shave biopsy removal of external genital warts by scissors or scalpel excision can be a simple, effective treatment. It will also produce tissue for histologic evaluation if needed. The area must be anesthetized (see Chapter 1). Stabilize the area between the thumb and index finger. Using a no. 15 blade, shave the lesion flush with the level of the normal tissue. Apply Monsel solution (i.e., ferric subsulfate), pressure, or cautery to stop bleeding.

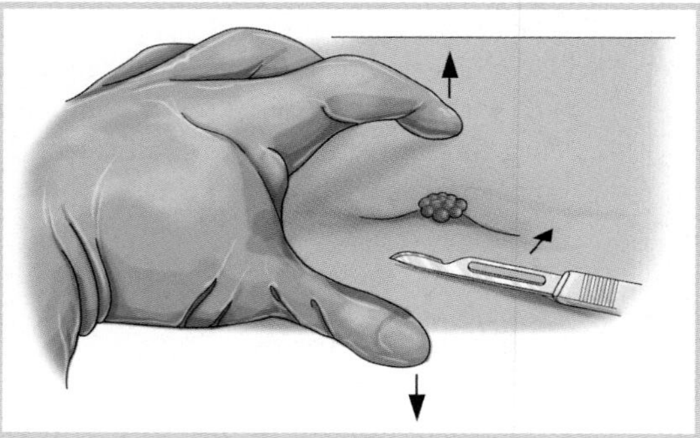

Step 22

- **PITFALL:** Care should be taken to not penetrate the dermis during the shave excision, because this can induce scarring.

Step 23. Alternatively, scissors are especially good for exophytic, pedunculated lesions. With the jaws of the scissors partially closed, bring the smallest point of the opening up against the base of the lesion. As soon as the scissors start cutting the skin, gently lift the lesion upward with the blades of the scissors as you are cutting. This keeps the cut in a shallow plane that prevents formation of a deep crater.

- **PITFALL:** Avoid deep penetration to reduce the risk of scarring.

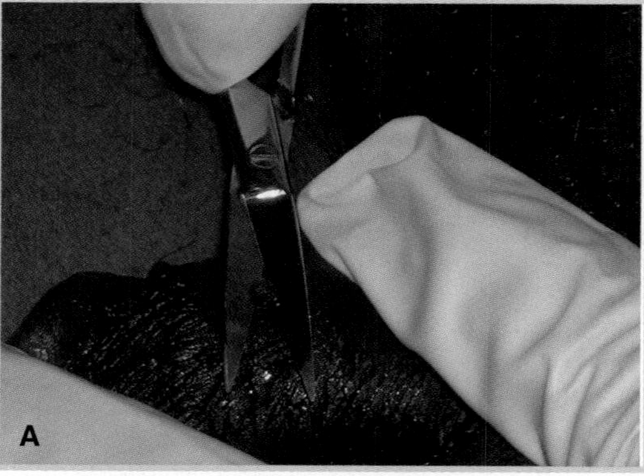

A

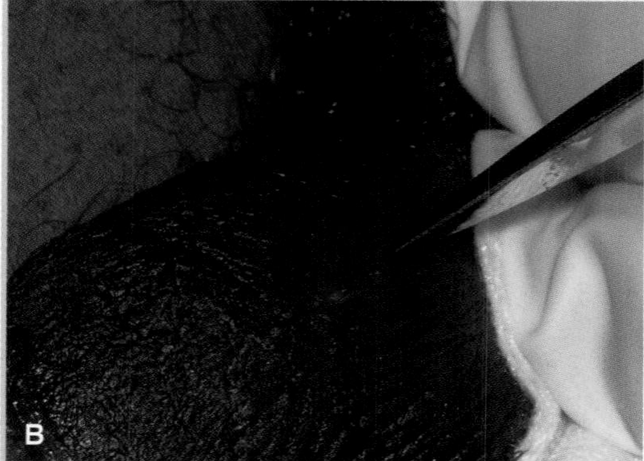

B

Step 23

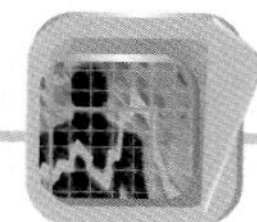

Complications

- Pain, infection, and bleeding
- Ulceration and depigmentation
- Scar formation
- Incomplete excision of lesion

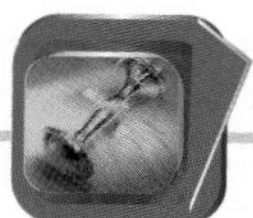

Pediatric Considerations

Genital warts may be seen in children and may be considered a sign of abuse, although this is not always the case. Clinicians may consider referral for treatment and reporting when appropriate. Imiquimod has not been studied in children.

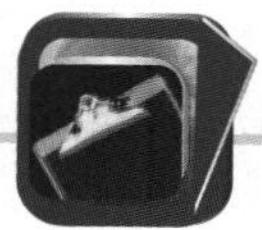

Postprocedure Instructions

After excision of warts, skin may be washed gently. No special care is needed, and the treatment sites should not be bandaged. The patient should be advised to report any increased pain, redness, bleeding, or drainage from the site.

After TCA or BCA, patients should be advised that it is unpredictable as to when or if warts will clear after treatment and return visits will likely be necessary. The patient will need to schedule follow-up appointments as indicated for surgically treated disease or for repeated treatments.

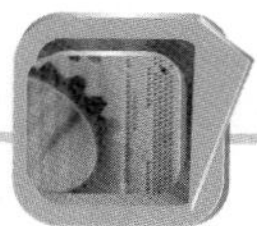

Coding Information and Supply Sources

In addition to the codes in the following chart, you may also consider using benign excision from the genitalia codes (11420 to 11426) or malignant excision from the genitalia codes (11620 to 11626), depending on the pathology findings.

CPT Code	Description	2008 50th Percentile Fee	Global Period
56501	Destruction of lesions of the vulva, simple	$300.00	10
56515	Destruction of lesions of the vulva, extensive	$839.00	10
56605	Biopsy of vulva or perineum, 1 lesion	$249.00	0
56606	Biopsy of vulva or perineum, each additional lesion	$174.00	ZZZ
57061	Destruction of lesions of the vagina, simple	$412.00	10
57065	Destruction of lesions of the vagina, extensive	$1,127.00	10
57100	Biopsy of vaginal mucosa, simple	$268.00	0
57105	Biopsy of vagina, extensive and requiring suture closure	$533.00	10
57135	Excision of vaginal cyst or tumor	$792.00	10

ZZZ, code related to another service and is always included in the global period of the other service.
CPT is a registered trademark of the American Medical Association.
2008 average 50th Percentile Fees are provided courtesy of 2008 MMH-SI's copyrighted Physicians' Fees and Coding Guide.

Instrument and Materials Ordering

Imiquimod (Aldara) and podophyllotoxin (Condylox) are prescription medications that are available through pharmaceutical suppliers and by prescription.

Cryosurgical gun applicators, tank units, and handheld devices can be obtained from

- Wallach Surgical, 235 Edison Road, Orange, CT 06477. Phone: 203-799-2000. Web site: http://www.wallach.com/.
- Brymill Cryogenic Systems, 105 Windermere Avenue, Ellington, CT 06029-3858. Phone: 1-800-777-2796. Web site: http://www.brymill.com/.
- Delasco, 608 13th Ave., Council Bluffs, IA USA 51501-6401. Phone: 1-800-831-6273; fax: 1-800-320-9612. E-mail: questions@delasco.com. Web site: http://www.delasco.com/pcat/1/Cryosurgery/.
- Liquid nitrogen cryoguns can be obtained from national medical supply houses such as the Henry Schein medical catalog. Liquid nitrogen can usually be obtained from local suppliers.

Suppliers for LEEP include

- Cooper Surgical, Shelton, CT. Phone: 1-800-645-3760 or 203-929-6321. Web site: http://www.coopersurgical.com.
- Ellman International, Inc., Hewlett, NY. Phone: 1-800-835 5355 or 516-569-1482. Web site: http://www.ellman.com.
- Olympus America, Inc., Melville, NY. Phone: 1-800-548-555 or 631-844-5000. Web site: http://www.olympusamerica.com.
- Utah Medical Products, Inc., Mid-vale, UT. Phone: 1-800-533-4984 or 801-566-1200. Web site: http://www.utahmed.com.
- Wallach Surgical Devices, Inc., Orange, CT. Phone: 203-799-2000 or 1-800-243-2463. Web site: http://www.wallachsurgical.com.

Patient Education Handout

A patient education handout, "Treatment of Condylomata Accuminata (Genital Warts)," can be found on the book's companion Web site.

Bibliography

Bergman A, Bhatia NN, Broen E. Cryotherapy for the treatment of genital condylomata during pregnancy. *J Reprod Med.* 1984;29:432–435.

Center for Disease Control and Prevention (CDC). 2006. Sexually transmitted disease treatment guidelines. Morbidity and Mortality Weekly Report 2006: 55(RR-11). http://www.cdc.gov/std/treatment/.

Centers for Disease Control and Prevention. Human papillomavirus: HPV information for clinicians. November 2006.

Ferris DG, Cox JT, O'Connor DM, et al. Management of lower genital tract neoplasia: treatment of external genital warts. In *Modern Colposcopy, Textbook and Atlas*. 2nd ed. Dubuque, IA: Kendal/Hunt; 2004:613–621.

Ferris DG, Cox JT, O'Connor DM, et al. The biology and significance of human papillomavirus infection. In *Modern Colposcopy, Textbook and Atlas*. 2nd ed. Dubuque, IA: Kendal/Hunt; 2004:89–123.

The FUTURE II Study Group, Quadrivalent vaccine against HPV to prevent high-grade-cervical lesions. *N Engl J Med.* 2007;356:1915–1927.

Gartland SM, Hernandex-Avila M, Wheeler CM, et al. Quadrivalent vaccine against human papillomavirus to prevent anogenital diseases. *NEJM*. 2007;3546:19.

Manhart LE, Koutsky LA. Do condoms prevent genital HPV infection, external genital HPV infection, external genital warts, or cervical neoplasia? A meta-analysis. *Sex Trans Dis.* 2002;29:725–735.

Stockfleth E, Beutner K, Thielert C, et al. Polyphenon E ointment in the treatment of external genital warts. *J European Acad Dermatol Vener.* 2005;p19(Suppl 2):FC06.8, 116.

2008 MAG Mutual Healthcare Solutions, Inc.'s Physicians' Fee and Coding Guide. Duluth, Georgia. MAG Mutual Healthcare Solutions, Inc. 2007.

CHAPTER 77

Fine-Needle Aspiration of the Breast

E. J. Mayeaux Jr., MD, DABFP, FAAFP

Professor of Family Medicine, Professor of Obstetrics and Gynecology
Louisiana State University Health Sciences Center, Shreveport, LA

Fine-needle aspiration (FNA) cytology is a rapid, safe, inexpensive, and relatively atraumatic method of sampling both cystic and solid breast masses. It is commonly performed in the office setting by a primary care clinician, surgeon, or cytopathologist. FNA can reliably diagnose benign and malignant conditions (Table 77-1) and has a false-negative rate for experienced practitioners of 3% to 5%. The accuracy of the procedure somewhat depends on the skill of the clinician in performing the biopsy and of the pathologist in reading the smear. FNA may also be used to assess recurrent masses after lumpectomy.

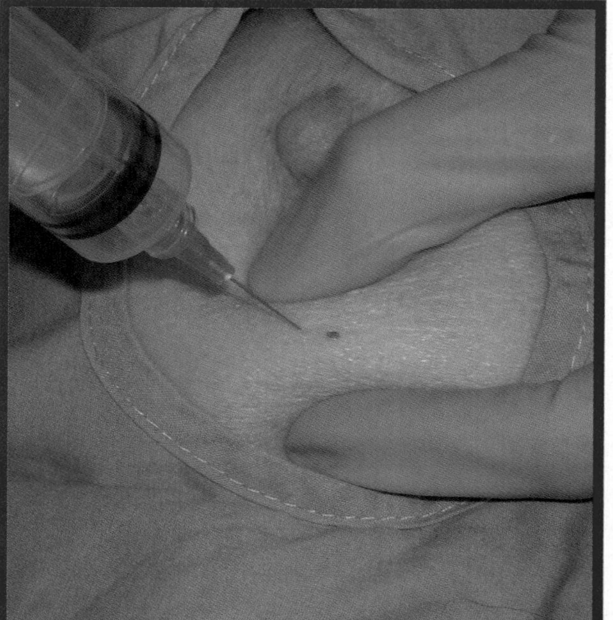

Compared with open surgical biopsy, needle biopsy causes less trauma and cosmetic disfigurement. It is performed as an outpatient procedure with local anesthetic. For benign lesions, establishing a definitive diagnosis obviates unnecessary surgical excision and the psychosocial and resource costs associated with protracted follow-up. A definitive diagnosis of cancer allows the patient to make an informed choice concerning follow-up and to obtain counseling prior to surgery. It also facilitates in the planning of multimodal treatment.

One of the major benefits of using FNA on a breast mass is the ability to determine whether a lesion is cystic or solid. Typically, mammography cannot distinguish between a cystic or solid lesion. However, when the needle is inserted into the lesion and negative pressure is applied, fluid is readily obtained from a cyst. After the cyst is drained, the site should be examined to exclude a persisting mass, which would require a biopsy to rule out the presence of cystic carcinoma. If the cyst completely disappears, the patient should be reexamined in 1 month. If the cyst recurs, it can be drained one additional time and re-examined in another month. If it recurs a second time, the patient should be referred for excision of the lesion to exclude cystic carcinoma.

TABLE 77-1. **Approximate Frequency of Common Findings in Women with Breast Lumps**

Finding	Frequency (%)
Fibrocystic changes	40
No disease	30
Miscellaneous benign changes	13
Cancer	10
Fibroadenoma	7

FNA, like all breast diagnostic techniques, is imperfect. However, the triple diagnostic technique of clinical breast examination, FNA, and mammography can provide very useful information for the woman, especially when all three techniques suggest the lesion is benign. This allows many clinicians to reassure the patient with simple outpatient testing. Lesions that appear suspicious on any of the triple diagnostic tests should be referred for biopsy (Table 77-2).

When a mass is discovered, the breast can be re-examined at the optimal time of the menstrual cycle (i.e., days 4 to 10 of the cycle immediately after the menstrual period). Mammography is usually performed before that office visit if the woman is of an appropriate age. If FNA is performed before mammography, allow at least 2 weeks to elapse before attempting mammography, so that any hematoma at the site is not erroneously described as a malignancy. Mammographically identified, nonpalpable lesions should not be approached with FNA in the office setting.

The basic principle of FNA involves moving a 22- to 25-gauge needle back and forth within a lesion, under suction from a 10- to 20-mL syringe, to shave and aspirate small cores of tissue samples from the lesion. Devices are available to make it easier for the clinician to maintain suction during the sampling process. A simple 20-mL syringe and needle also may be used, but this is considered inferior because effort and attention must be diverted from the movement of the needle to maintaining suction. Skin anesthesia often is unnecessary for FNA, but local 1% lidocaine or local cold therapy may be used if desired. Sterile drapes are usually unnecessary.

Recommended follow-up protocols for FNA results are shown in Table 77-3. When inadequate smears are obtained, the procedure can easily be repeated, often resulting in a satisfactory specimen. However, if an adequate sample cannot be obtained, the clinician should vigorously pursue other biopsy options because cancers may be missed, especially lobular cancer and ductal carcinoma in situ. Infection is rare, and prophylaxis for bacterial endocarditis is not required.

TABLE 77-2. **Common Morphologic Features of Invasive Cancer**

- Focal lesions extending progressively in all directions
- Lesions adherent (fixed) to the deep chest wall fascia
- Lesions extending to the skin and producing retraction and dimpling
- Lymphatic blockage producing skin thickening, lymphedema, and peau d'orange (orange peel) changes
- Main ductal involvement producing nipple retraction
- Widespread infiltration of the breast producing acute redness, swelling, and tenderness (i.e., inflammatory carcinoma)

Adapted from Cotran RS, Kumar V, Robbins SL, et al. *Robbins Pathologic Basis of Disease*. Philadelphia: WB Saunders, 1994:1089–1111.

TABLE 77-3. Breast Needle Aspiration Cytology of Solid Lesions and Recommended Follow-up

RESULT	SUGGESTED FOLLOW-UP
Scant or insufficient cells for diagnosis	Repeat needle aspiration or biopsy if clinical suspicion is high, or use guided biopsy
Benign—fibroadenoma	Reassurance or symptomatic treatment if cellular changes are not complex or associated with atypical hyperplasia
Benign—fibrocystic	Symptomatic treatment if not associated with atypical hyperplasia
Benign—other (includes fat necrosis, lipoma, inflammation,papilloma, and other benign ductal epithelium)	Reassurance and clinical follow-up
Atypical cells	Clinical follow-up can be considered reactive or degenerative atypia (seen in fibrocystic change); mammogram and biopsy for most atypia (especially if severe atypia)
Suspicious for malignancy	Surgical referral and biopsy
Malignant cells	Surgical referral and biopsy

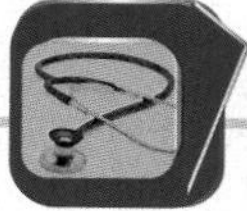

Equipment

Please see the follow appendixes for supply information:

- Appendix A: Informed Consent
- Appendix C: Bacterial Endocarditis Prevention Recommendations
- Appendix E: Skin Preparation Recommendations
- Appendix I: Suggested Tray for Soft Tissue Aspiration and Injection Procedures
  - Two sterile plain evacuated blood tubes
  - Needles, 21, 22, 23 gauge
  - Syringe of appropriate size
  - Pistol grip device if desired
  - Slides with frosted ends (three or four)
  - Glass cover slips or extra slides for smearing the specimens
  - Gauze pads, 4 × 4 inches
  - Sterile gloves
  - Alcohol, povidone-iodine, or chlorhexidine swabs
  - Syringe (1 mL) with 30-gauge needle and 1% lidocaine for anesthesia

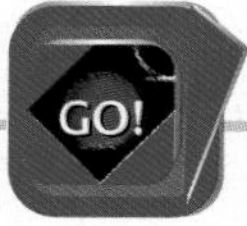

Indications

- Presence of a palpable mass in the breast

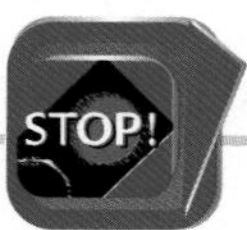

Contraindications

- Local infection
- Absence of a qualified cytopathologist capable of interpretation of the FNA slides
- Lack of clinician training with the procedure
- Severely immunocompromised patients (relative contraindication)

The Procedure

Step 1. Several devices may be used for the FNA procedure. A 21-gauge butterfly with extension tubing can be attached to any device or syringe and used with a nurse applying the back pressure and the clinician focusing full attention on the needle tip. The mechanical movement for the Cameco pistol syringe (shown) is produced by motion of the arm and elbow. This device allows for easy application of extensive suction and good control of the syringe and needle.

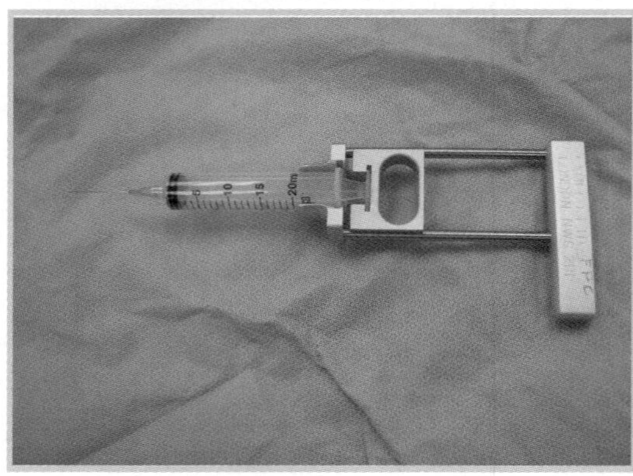

Step 1

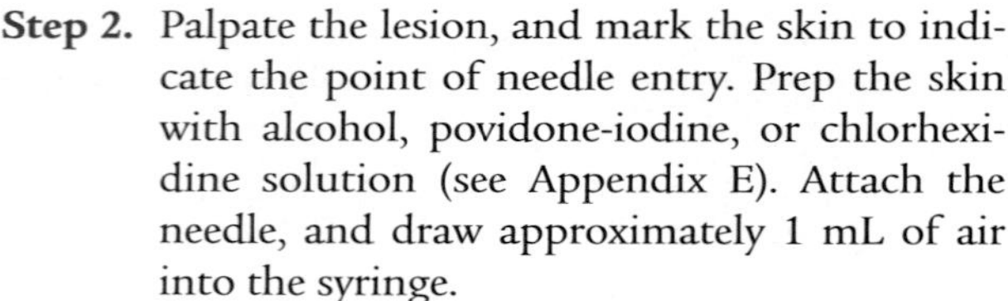

Step 2. Palpate the lesion, and mark the skin to indicate the point of needle entry. Prep the skin with alcohol, povidone-iodine, or chlorhexidine solution (see Appendix E). Attach the needle, and draw approximately 1 mL of air into the syringe.

- PITFALL: Avoid injecting air because this may cause a vascular air embolus.

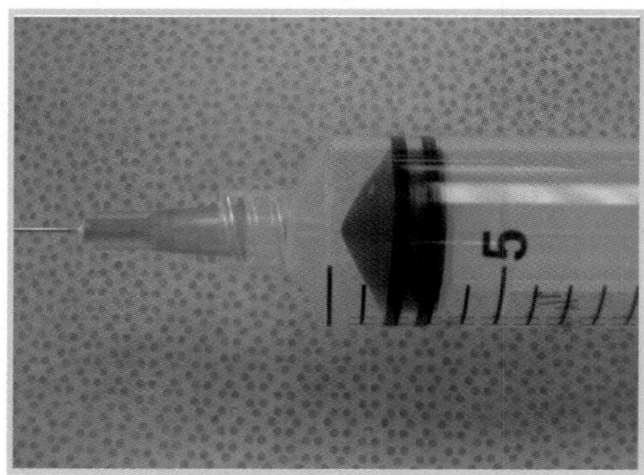

Step 2

Step 3. Use the nondominant hand to surround and stabilize the lesion. Surrounding the lesion allows the sensory portion of the fourth and fifth fingers to feel the needle tip enter the lesion as the lesion moves against these fingers. Rarely, the glove may need to be removed from the nondominant hand if it interferes with palpation of the lesion. Make sure the patient understands why the glove is being removed.

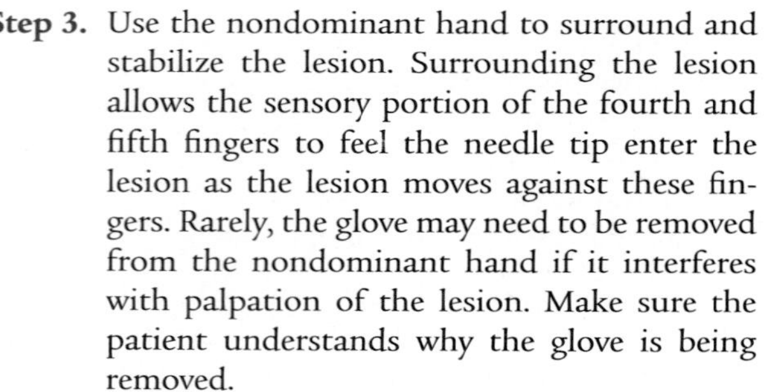

- PITFALL: Use care to avoid putting the needle tip through the breast and into the examiner's hand.
- PITFALL: Isolating the lesion by using the nondominant hand to press the lesion down against the chest wall increases the risk of a pneumothorax.

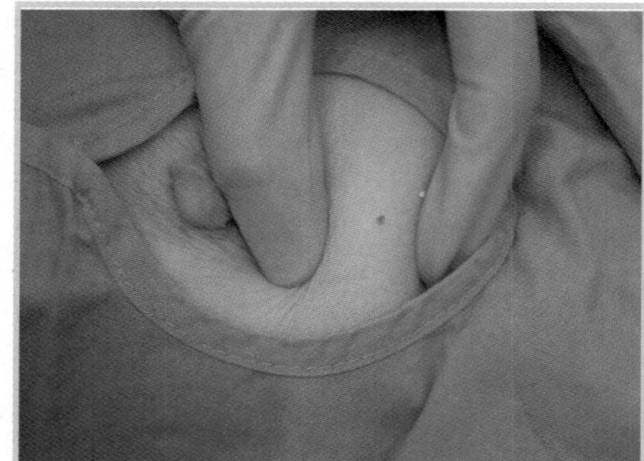

Step 3

Step 4. Insert the needle into the lesion, and withdraw the plunger to create a vacuum. If the lesion is a cyst, the fluid will usually flow easily into the syringe. Withdraw all of the fluid and palpate the area to be sure the lesion is completely gone. If residual lesion is present, consider an open biopsy. If the cyst completely disappears and the fluid is not bloody, the fluid does not have to be sent for analysis. Otherwise, submit the fluid on slides or in a sterile (without anticoagulant) blood collection tube.

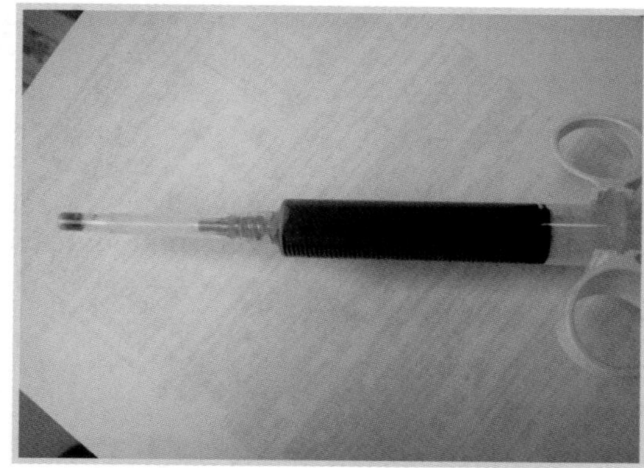

Step 4

Step 5. If the lesion is solid, make 10 to 20 up-and-down passes, keeping the needle in the lesion. The sample will fill the needle and possibly part of the hub. With the needle still in the lesion, return the plunger to the resting position to release the suction. Then withdraw the needle from the skin.

- PITFALL: Do not let the needle come out of the skin while a vacuum is present in the syringe. This causes the sample to be drawn up into the syringe, where it may be difficult to remove.
- PITFALL: It is not necessary to change the angle of the needle during the FNA, because it is the passage of the needle into the center of a lesion and the subsequent back-and-forth motion of the needle tip around the initial needle pass that allow shaved fragments of cells to enter the syringe. Moving the needle tip off this initial path in the center of the lesion often results in the needle moving out of the lesion and causes undue errors.

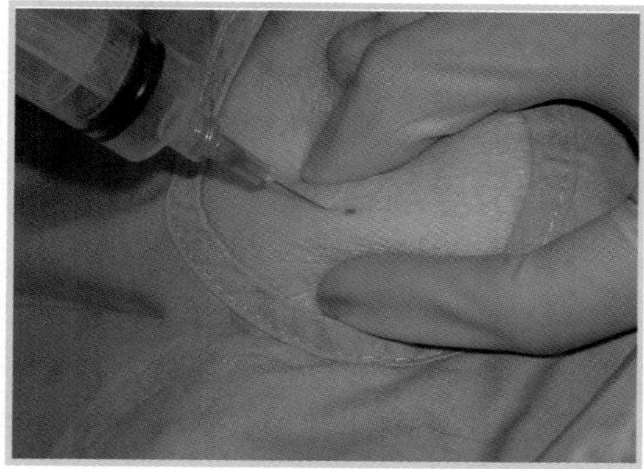

Step 5

Step 6. With the needle pointed downward, use the air in the syringe to deposit the sample into monolayer preservative or onto the slide.

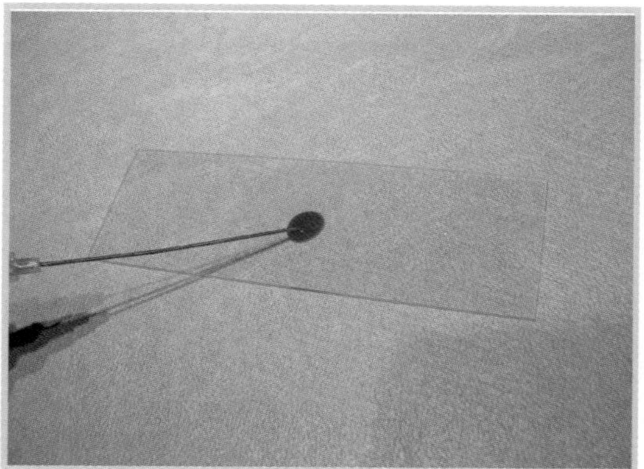

Step 6

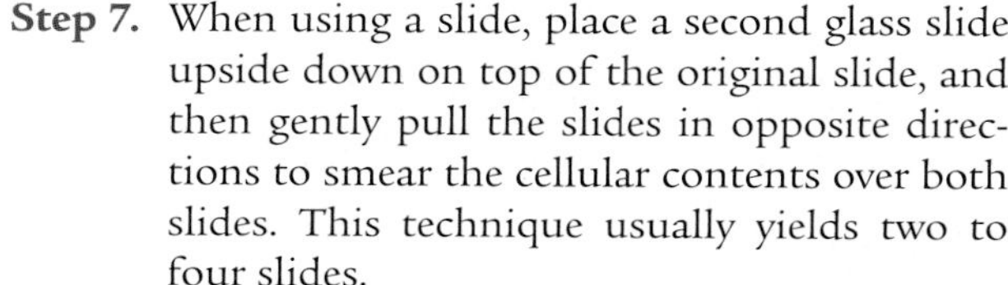

Step 7. When using a slide, place a second glass slide upside down on top of the original slide, and then gently pull the slides in opposite directions to smear the cellular contents over both slides. This technique usually yields two to four slides.

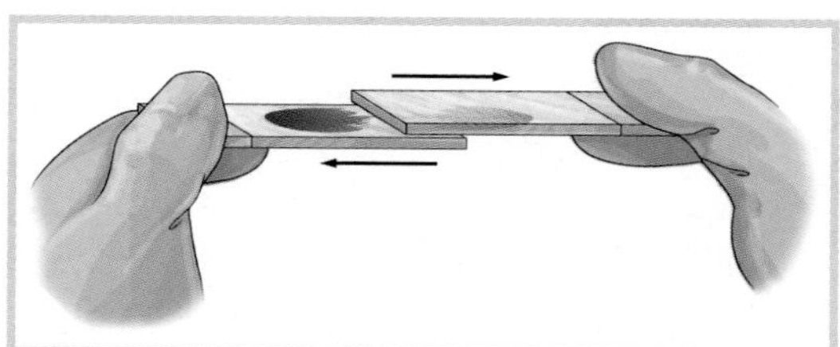

Step 7

Step 8. Apply spray fixative as when obtaining a Papanicolaou smear. If a solid-core specimen is expressed from the needle (rare), wash it from the slide into a vial of preservative, and submit it for histologic examination. Remove the syringe from the needle, replace it with a fresh one, and repeat the procedure if desired.

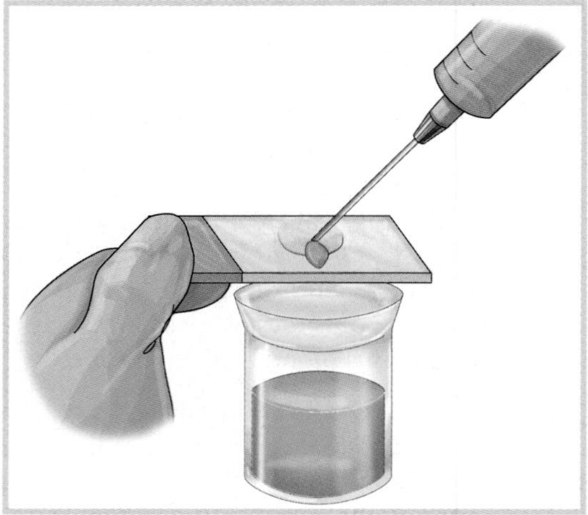

Step 8

Step 9. Apply compression to the aspiration site with a gauze pad for 5 to 10 minutes to help minimize bruising. Place several folded gauze pads under a snug brassiere to form a compression dressing.

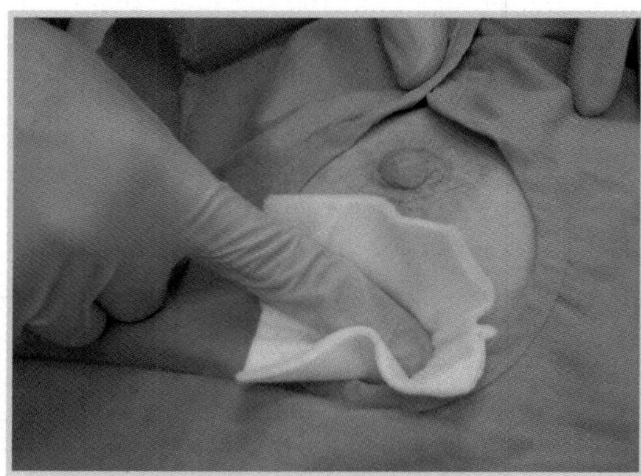

Step 9

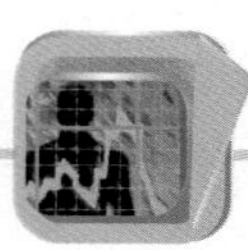

Complications

- The major risk of the FNA procedure is failure to place the needle tip into the lesion. Significant complications of FNA, such as pneumothorax, are rare. Some patients experience mild soreness, hematoma formation, and skin discoloration. The patient with controlled anticoagulation may safely undergo FNA if parameters are in the therapeutic range and adequate site compression is used after the procedure to avoid hematoma. All patients undergoing FNA of breast lesions should wear a supportive brassiere after the procedure.

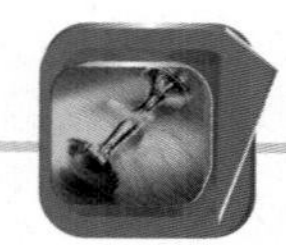

Pediatric Considerations

This procedure is usually not performed in the pediatric age groups.

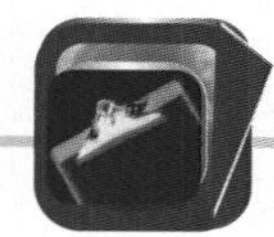

Postprocedure Instructions

Instruct the patient to leave the pressure dressing in place for at least several hours to prevent hematoma formation. A small ice pack can be applied to the FNA site for 15 to 60 minutes after the procedure if desired. The samples are sent for cytologic or histologic analysis using staining and simple microscopy or a monolayer system. Arrange for a follow-up visit to discuss results.

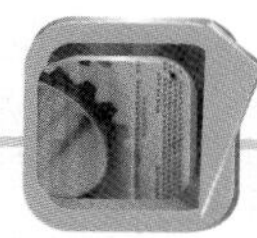

Coding Information and Supply Sources

CPT CODE	DESCRIPTION	2008 AVERAGE 50TH PERCENTILE FEE	GLOBAL PERIOD
19000	Aspiration drainage of a breast cyst; one cyst	$201.00	0
19001	Aspiration drainage of a breast cyst; each additional cyst	$111.00	0
10021	FNA without imaging guidance	$227.00	XXX

XXX, global concept does not apply.
CPT is a registered trademark of the American Medical Association.
2008 average 50th Percentile Fees are provided courtesy of 2008 MMH-SI's copyrighted Physicians' Fees and Coding Guide.

Common ICD9 Codes

174.0	Malignant neoplasm of female breast; nipple and areola
174.4	Malignant neoplasm of female breast; upper/outer quadrant
174.6	Malignant neoplasm of female breast; axillary tail
174.9	Malignant neoplasm of breast (female) unspecified
217	Benign neoplasm of breast: connective tissue, glandular tissue, soft parts. Excludes adenofibrosis, benign cyst of breast, fibrocystic disease, skin of breast
610.0	Solitary cyst of breast
610.1	Diffuse cystic mastopathy
610.2	Fibroadenosis of breast
611.0	Inflammatory disease of breast: abscess or mastitis (acute) (chronic) (non-puerperal) of areola, breast, mamillary fistula

Suppliers

- The Cameco syringe pistol ($286) is available from Precision Dynamics Corporation, 13880 Del Sur Street, San Fernando, CA 91340-3490. Phone: 1-800-772-1122. Web site: http://www.pdcorp.com, although this item is not on their Web site.
- Morton Medical Ltd., 262a Fulham Road, London SW10 9EL. Phone, UK only: 0207 352 1297; phone outside of the UK: +44 207 352 1297. Web site: http://www.morton-healthcare.co.uk/products_index.htm

Note that the FNA-21 fine-needle aspiration device from CooperSurgical has been discontinued.

Patient Education Handout

A patient education handout, "Fine-Needle Aspiration Biopsy of the Breast," can be found on the book's companion Web site.

Bibliography

Al-Kaisi N. The spectrum of the "gray zone" in breast cytology. *Acta Cytol.* 1994;38:898–908.

Conry C. Evaluation of a breast complaint: is it cancer? *Am Fam Physician.* 1994;49:445–450, 453–454.

Erickson R, Shank JC, Gratton C. Fine-needle breast aspiration biopsy. *J Fam Pract.* 1989;28:306–309.

Frable W. Thin-needle aspiration biopsy. *Am J Clin Pathol.* 1976;6:168–182.

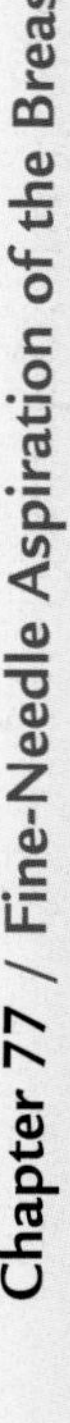

Hamburger JI. Needle aspiration for thyroid nodules: skip ultrasound—do initial assessment in the office. *Postgrad Med.* 1988;84:61–66.

Hammond S, Keyhani-Rofagha S, O'Toole RV. Statistical analysis of fine-needle aspiration cytology of the breast: a review of 678 cases plus 4,265 cases from the literature. *Acta Cytol.* 1987;3:276–280.

Ku NNK, Mela NJ, Fiorica JV, et al. Role of fine needle aspiration cytology after lumpectomy. *Acta Cytol.* 1994;38:927–932.

Layfield LJ, Chrischilles EA, Cohen MB, et al. The palpable breast nodule. *Cancer.* 1993;72: 1642–1651.

Lee KR, Foster RS, Papillo JL. Fine-needle aspiration of the breast: importance of the aspirator. *Acta Cytol.* 1987;3:281–284.

Lever JV, Trott PA, Webb AJ. Fine-needle aspiration cytology. *J Clin Pathol.* 1985;3:1–11.

Stanley MW. Fine-needle aspiration biopsy: diagnosis of cancerous masses in the office. *Postgrad Med.* 1989;85:163–172.

Vural G, Hagmar B, Lilleng R. A one-year audit of fine needle aspiration cytology of breast lesions. *Acta Cytol.* 1995;39:1233–1236.

2008 MAG Mutual Healthcare Solutions, Inc.'s Physicians' Fee and Coding Guide. Duluth, Georgia. MAG Mutual Healthcare Solutions, Inc. 2007.

CHAPTER 78

Implanon (Etonogestrel Implant)

Sandra M. Sulik, MD, MS, FAAP
Associate Professor Family Medicine
SUNY Upstate and St. Joseph's Family Medicine Residency, Fayetteville, NY

Implanon is single-rod etonogestrel progestin implant approved for use in the United States in 2006. As of April 2007, Implanon is currently marketed in more than 30 countries with approximately 2.5 million implants inserted since its inception in 1998.

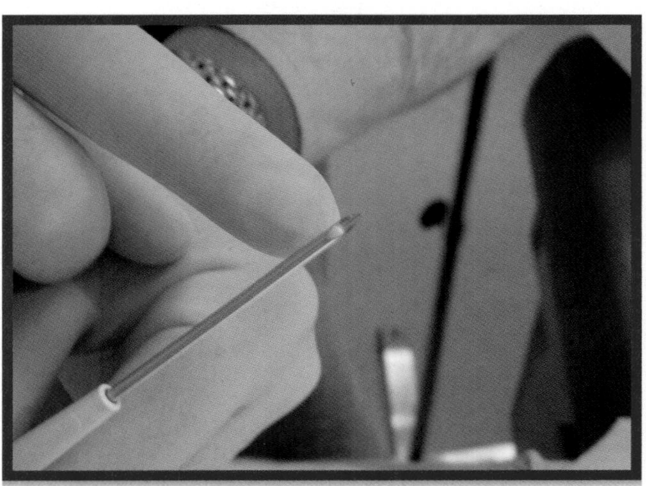

The rod is effective for up to 3 years. It is inserted using a preloaded, sterile, single-use applicator. The Implanon is inserted subdermally in the inner aspect of the nondominant upper arm. The rod is placed in the groove between the biceps and triceps in the sulcus bicipitalis medialis. It is easily accessible but not easily seen.

The Implanon rod is 4 cm in length and 2 mm in diameter. It is composed of a solid core of ethylene vinyl acetate (EVA) with crystals of etonogestrel (ENG) imbedded within the core. The rod contains 68 mg of etonogestrel releasing 60 to 70 μg/day initially, which decreases to 40 to 45 μg/day after a few weeks and then decreases to 25 to 30 μg/day by the end of the third year. Implanon is not radio-opaque and therefore cannot be seen on x-ray or computer tomography (CT) scans. It is easily detectable by ultrasound using a high-frequency linear-array transducer or by magnetic resonance imagery (MRI).

Six pregnancies have been reported in 20,648 cycles of Implanon use, with a cumulative Pearl Index of 0.38 pregnancies per 100 woman years of use. The effectiveness of Implanon in overweight women was not evaluated in the original studies, as women heavier than 130% of their ideal body weight were not included. Serum concentrations of etonogestrel (ENG) are inversely related to body weight and decrease with time after insertion; therefore it is possible that with time Implanon may be less effective in overweight women.

Implanon works by two main mechanisms: inhibition of ovulation and increased viscosity of cervical mucus. It is quickly reversible, with undetectable serum concentrations of etonogestrel noted within the first week of removal. Return to ovulation within 3 months of removal occurs in more than 90% of women.

The most common side effect seen in women with Implanon is bleeding. It is crucial that women be counseled prior to insertion that spotting and bleeding will occur. The total number of bleeding and spotting days is similar to or better than what most women have with normal menstrual cycles; however, it is more irregular and less predictable. Dysmenorrhea improves significantly with Implanon. Other side effects include weight gain (2.3%), emotional lability (2.3%), headache (1.6%), acne (1.3%), and depression (1.0%). Most discontinuations occur within the first year as a result of bleeding or spotting. No significant effects have been noted in breastfeeding women with either production of breast milk or growth and development of infants.

Timing of insertion is crucial.

- If no preceding hormonal contraceptive use in the past month, insert during days 1 to 5 of the menstrual cycle.
- If switching from combination methods, insert anytime during the 7 days of the last active combined dose.
- Any day when switching from a progestin-only pill (do not skip any dose).
- Same day as implant or intrauterine system is removed.
- On the day when the next contraceptive injection would be due.
- Within 5 days following a first trimester abortion.
- Between 3 to 4 weeks following childbirth or second trimester abortion.
- After the fourth postpartum week if exclusively breastfeeding.

A back-up method of contraception is not needed if insertion occurs as described. If deviating from the recommended timing of insertion, rule out pregnancy and use a back-up method of contraception for 7 days after Implanon is inserted.

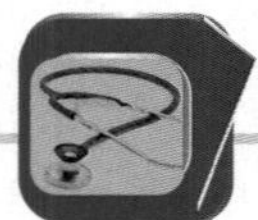

Equipment

- Sterile drapes
- Antiseptic swabs
- Gauzes, 2 × 2 inches
- Alcohol pad
- Syringe (3 cc) with 1% lidocaine
- No. 11 scalpel
- Pressure dressing
- Adhesive bandage
- Surgical pen
- Tape measure
- Implanon device

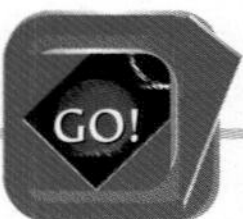

Indications

- Any woman desiring long-acting, reversible contraception
- Smoking women older than age 35 who desire contraception
- Women who desire contraception but have a contraindication to use of estrogen

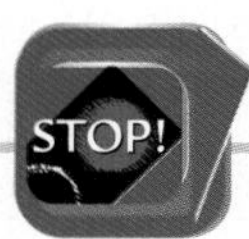

Contraindications

- Known or suspected pregnancy
- Current or past history of thrombotic disease

- Hepatic tumors or active liver disease
- Undiagnosed abnormal genital bleeding
- Known, suspected, or history of breast cancer
- Hypersensitivity to any of the components of Implanon

It is not recommended for women who require chronic use of drugs that are potent inducers of hepatic enzymes.

Contraceptive effectiveness may be reduced when co-administered with antibiotics, antifungals, anticonvulsants, and any drugs that increase the metabolism of contraceptive steroids

It is unknown whether anti-HIV protease inhibitors affect Implanon.

Herbal products containing St. John's wort may reduce effectiveness.

The Procedure

Implanon Insertion

Step 1. The patient should be properly counseled and provided with the appropriate patient education materials. The patient package insert with consent form should be reviewed. Check the expiration date on the Implanon package. Place the patient in a supine position with her nondominant arm flexed at the elbow and externally rotated.

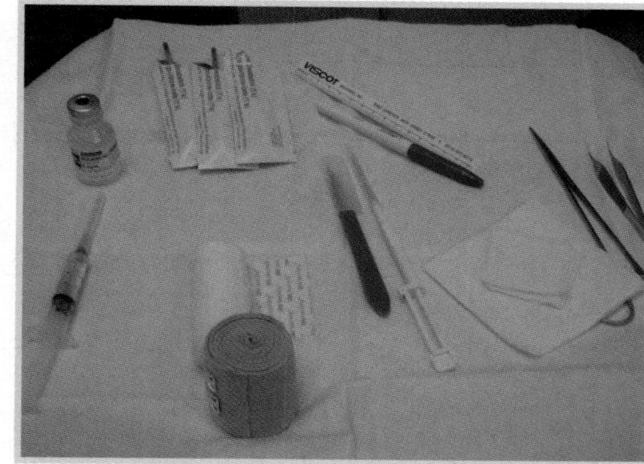

Step 1

Step 2. Identify the insertion site, which is 6 to 8 cm above the elbow crease at the inner side of the arm overlying the groove between the biceps and triceps. Mark the insertion site and make a second mark 6 to 8 cm above the first.

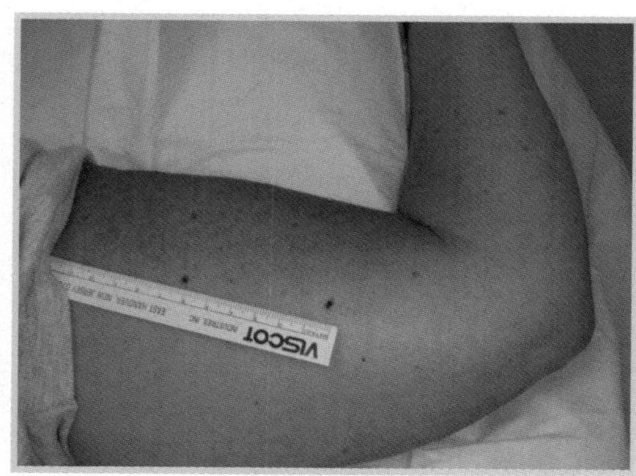

Step 2

Step 3. Clean the insertion site with povidone-iodine or chlorhexidine solution, and then inject a small amount of anesthetic just under the skin along the planned insertion canal. Raise a small weal, then inject the full distance where the rod will be inserted.

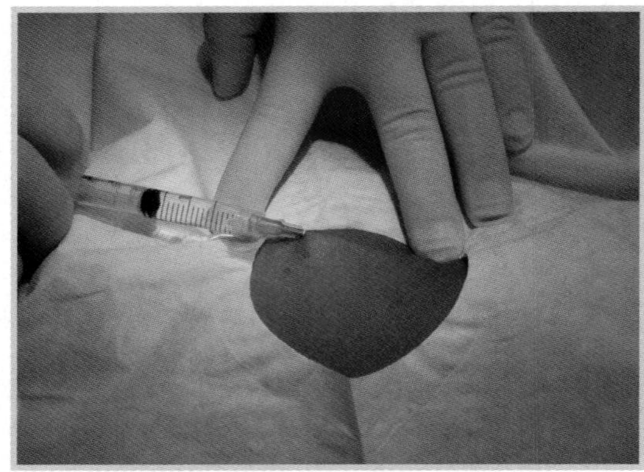
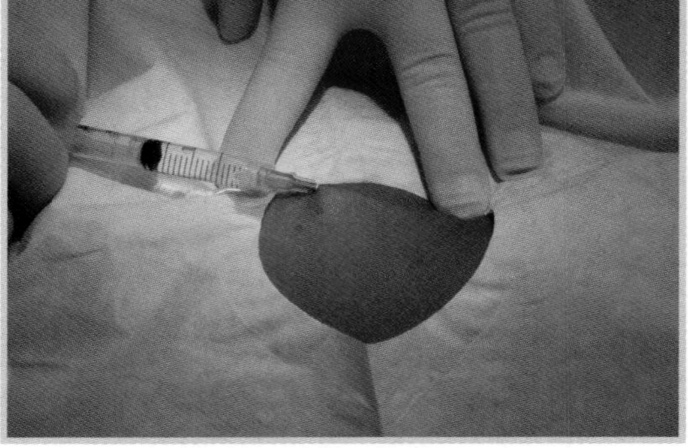

Step 3

Step 4. Carefully remove the Implanon sterile applicator from its blister pack. Keep the tip of the applicator up in order to keep the Implanon rod within the applicator. Identify the tip of the rod.

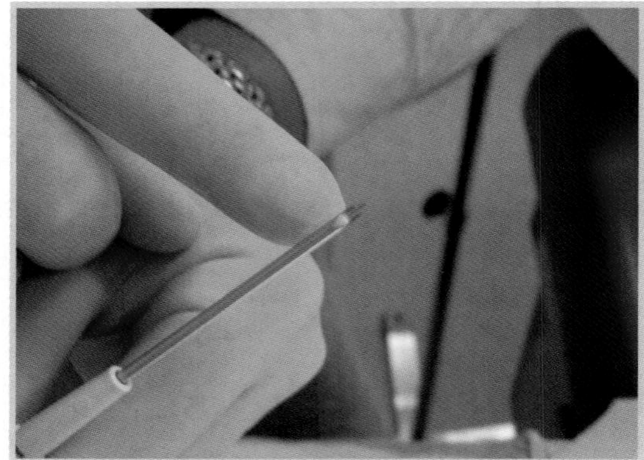

Step 4

Step 5. Gently tap the reverse end of the applicator to ensure that the entire rod is back within the applicator.

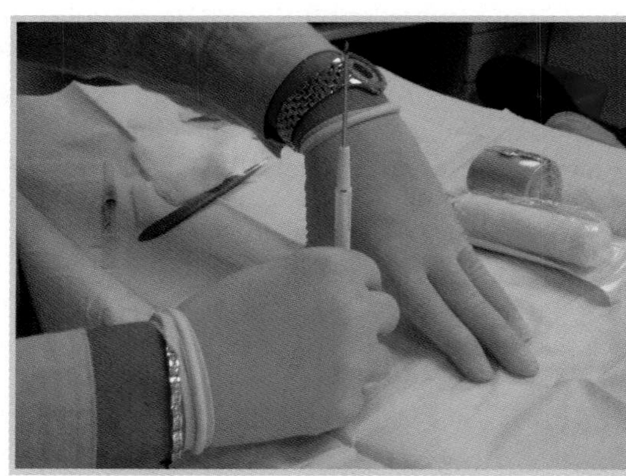

Step 5

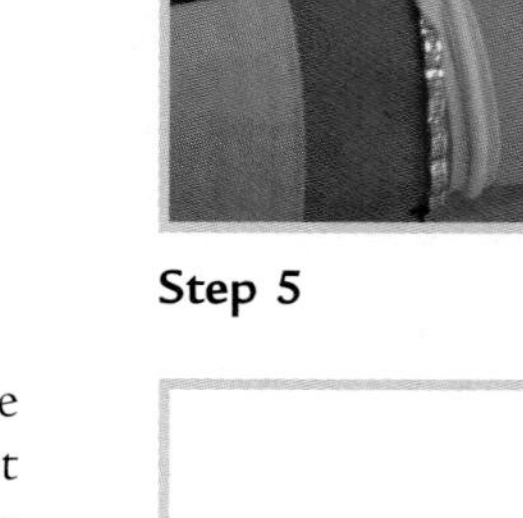

Step 6. Stretch the skin at the insertion site with the thumb and index finger of your nondominant hand. Insert the needle tip, beveled side up, no greater than a 20-degree angle just until the skin has been penetrated.

- **PEARL:** It is helpful to puncture the skin with the tip of a no. 11 scalpel blade before inserting the applicator tip.

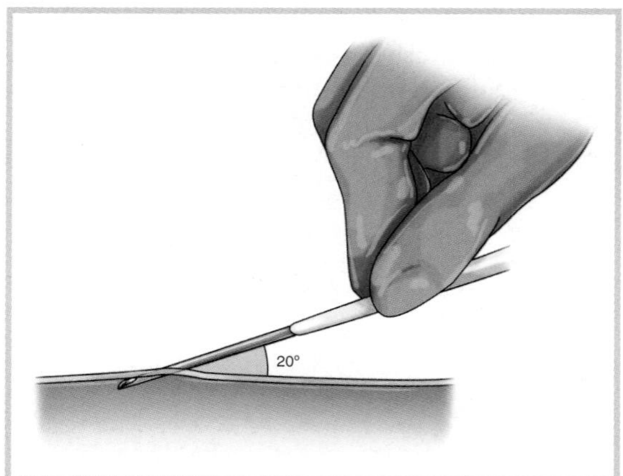

Step 6

Step 7. Once the tip is inserted, the applicator should be lowered to the horizontal plane. Lift or tent the skin with the tip of the needle while gently inserting the needle to its full length.

- **PEARL:** If the needle is angled too deeply or too superficially, simply pull the needle back a bit and redirect to the subdermal plane.

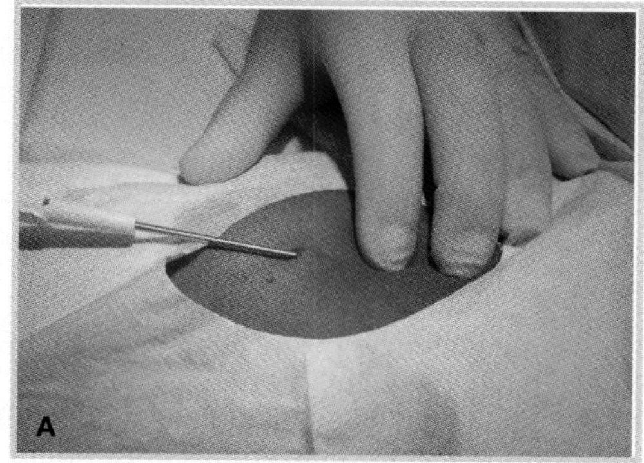

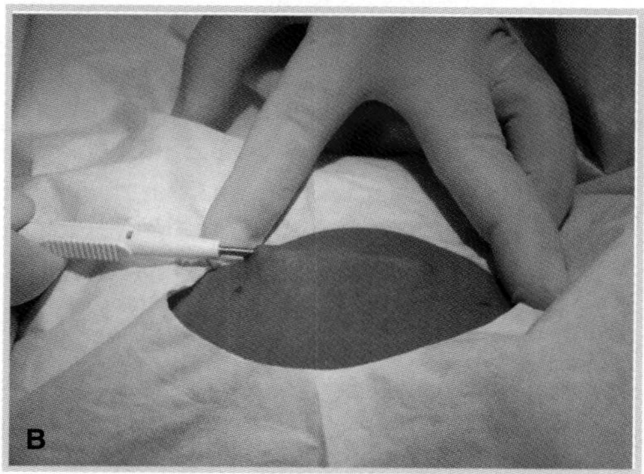

Step 7

Step 8. Break the seal of the applicator by pressing the obturator support and turn the obturator 90 degrees in either direction with respect to the cannula. Fix or hold the obturator in place on the patient's arm with your nondominant hand. Using your other hand, slowly retract the needle (cannula) back along the full length of the obturator.

- **PEARL:** You may need to push firmly on the obturator to break the seal. You will hear a "click" as the seal is broken. Once the seal is broken, the obturator should rotate freely.
- **PITFALL:** The procedure is similar to inserting a copper intrauterine device (IUD), where the obturator is fixed and cannula is withdrawn. *Do not push the obturator*—this will force the implant further up the arm in the incorrect place.

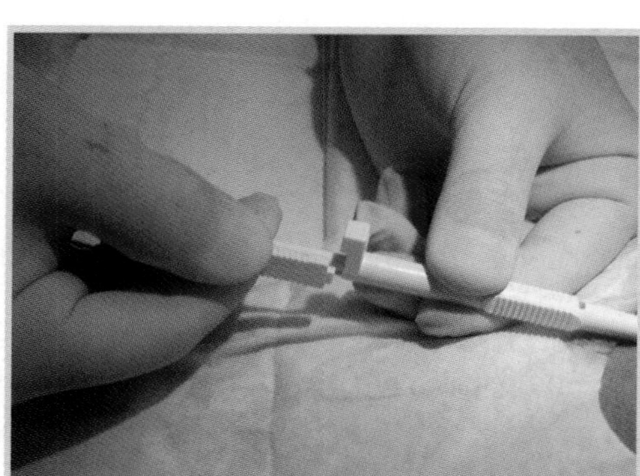

Step 8

Step 9. Check the obturator and look for the grooved tip visible inside the needle opening.

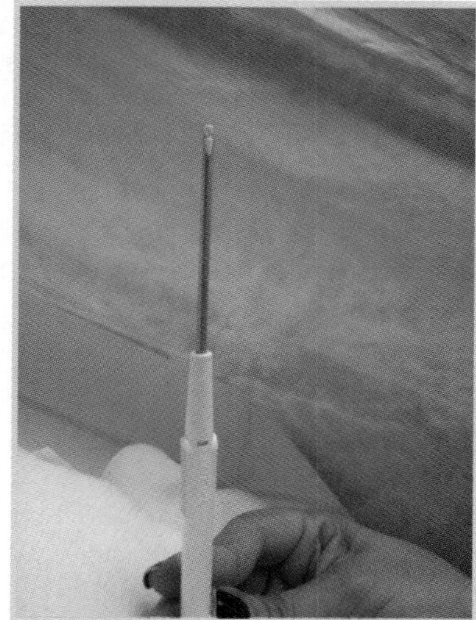

Step 9

Step 10. Palpate the implant to verify it is in the correct position. Have patient palpate the implant as well to confirm its position.

- **PEARL:** If the implant is not palpable, confirm its presence in the arm with high-frequency linear array transducer (>10 MHz) ultrasound or if necessary with MRI.
- **PEARL:** If the implant is not palpable, instruct the patient to use a back-up method until the presence of the Implanon has been confirmed.

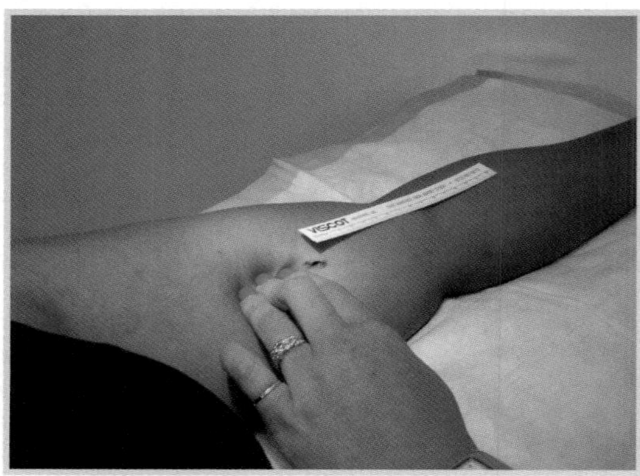

Step 10

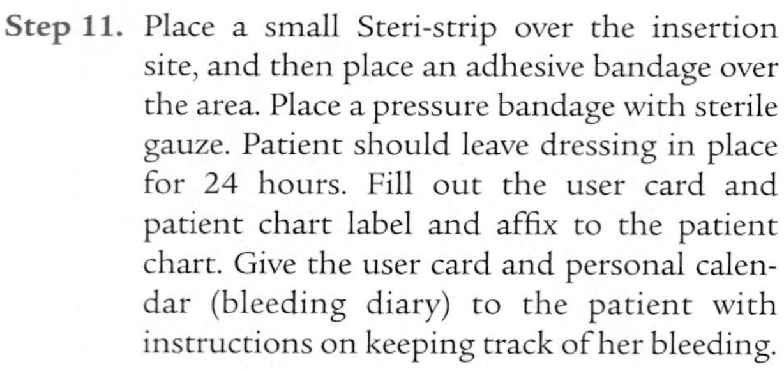

Step 11. Place a small Steri-strip over the insertion site, and then place an adhesive bandage over the area. Place a pressure bandage with sterile gauze. Patient should leave dressing in place for 24 hours. Fill out the user card and patient chart label and affix to the patient chart. Give the user card and personal calendar (bleeding diary) to the patient with instructions on keeping track of her bleeding.

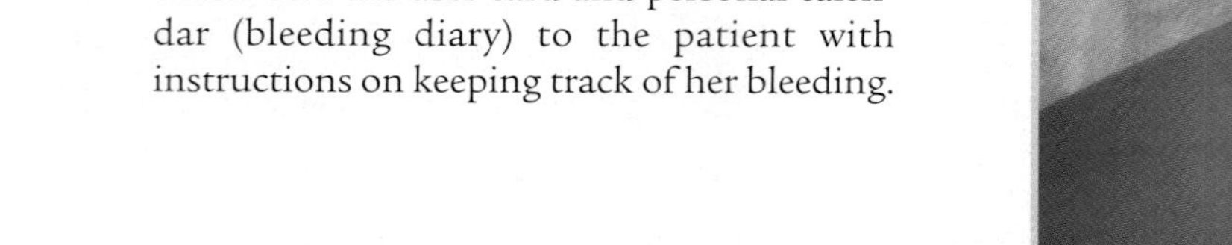

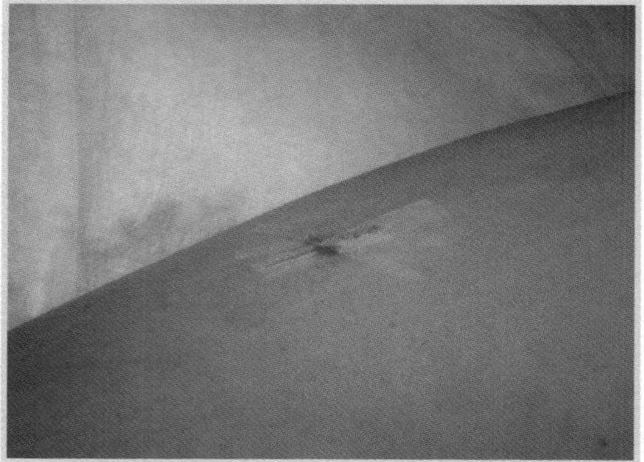

Step 11

Implanon Removal

Step 1. Locate the implant by palpating the arm and mark the end closest to the elbow. Clean the area with antiseptic solution. Inject a small but sufficient amount of 1% lidocaine just underneath the base of the implant (usually 0.5 cc is enough).

- **PITFALL:** If unable to palpate the implant, localize the implant using ultrasound or MRI. Ultrasound should be performed with a linear array transducer with at least 10 MHz or higher frequency. Remove as soon as possible after localization has been determined.
- **PITFALL:** It is important to inject just under the implant to prevent obscuring the implant and making it more difficult to remove.

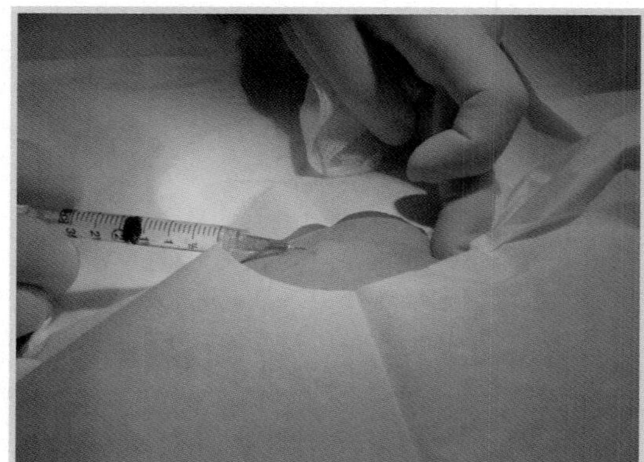

Step 1

Step 2. Press down on the end of the implant closet to the axilla. Make a 2 to 3 mm incision in the arm (in a longitudinal direction) at the tip of the implant near the elbow. (The incision should be made at the tip of the implant and extend just below it.)

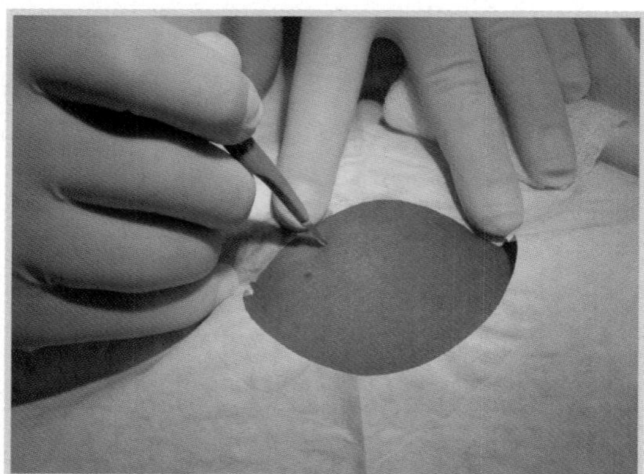

Step 2

Step 3. Gently push the implant toward the incision until the tip is visible. Grasp the implant with a mosquito forceps and gently pull out.

- PITFALL: If the implant is encapsulated, gently dissect to remove the capsule then grasp the implant and remove.

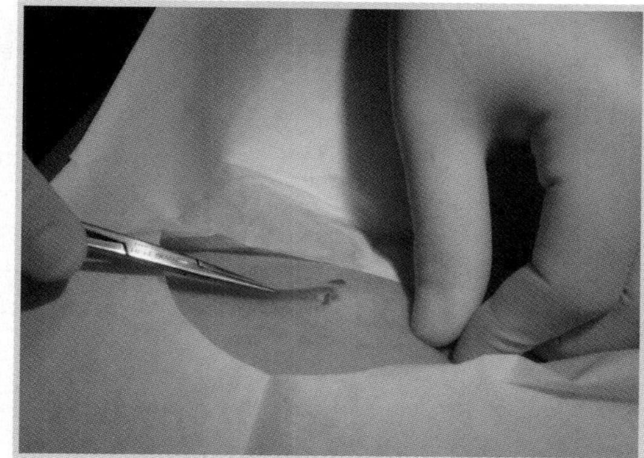

Step 3

Step 4. If the tip is not visible after gently pushing it toward the incision, insert a curved forceps into the incision and grasp the implant.

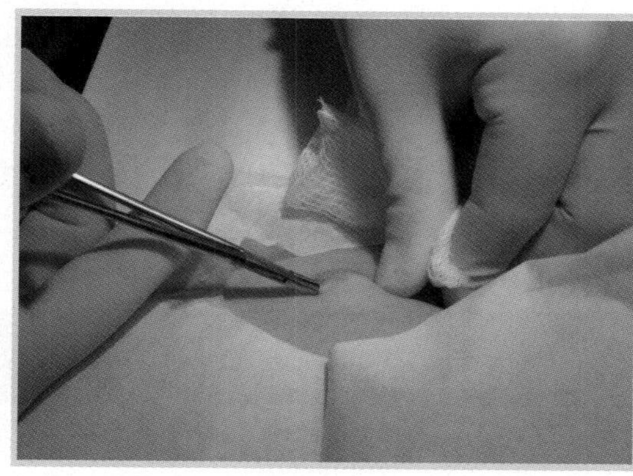

Step 4

Step 5. Flip the forceps and use a second pair of forceps to localize the implant and dissect the capsule off the implant, then gently remove. If another Implanon is desired, a new implant can be placed in the same arm through the same incision. Close the incision with a Steri-strip and apply an adhesive bandage. Place gauze with a pressure dressing over the incision.

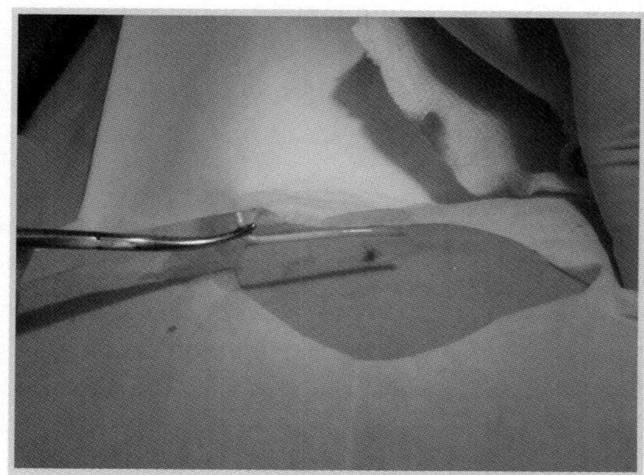

Step 5

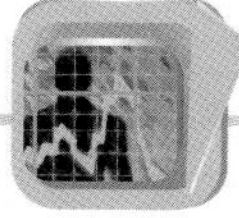

Complications

- Deep insertion: difficult localization and removal
- Mistimed insertion: pregnancy
- Broken/bent implant: difficult removal
- Multiple insertions: increased risk of side effects
- Noninsertion: pregnancy
- Bleeding/spotting
- Infection
- Bruising

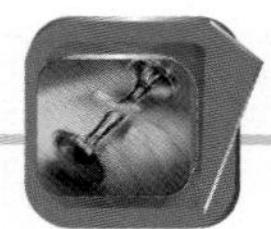

Pediatric Considerations

Progestin-only contraceptive methods are preferred methods for breastfeeding women. The effect of Implanon with breastfeeding has been studied in a nonrandomized group comparative study with copper IUD and Implanon. Approximately 0.2% of the maternal dose of etonogestrel is excreted in the breast milk. There was no change in the length of time breastfeeding or the quantity of breast milk in either group. There is no data on bone mass in adolescents to date.

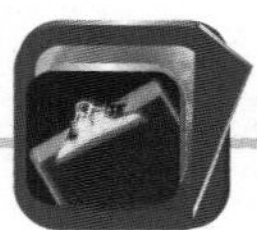

Postprocedure Instructions

The provider should instruct the patient to leave the pressure dressing in place for 24 hours. Minimal pain is usually associated with insertion, but the patient can be instructed to use acetaminophen or ibuprofen if needed. No back-up method is necessary if inserted at the appropriate time of the cycle.

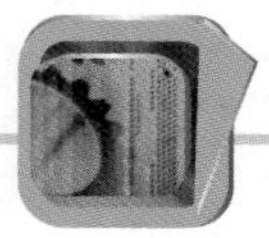

Coding Information and Supply Sources

CPT Code	Description	2008 Average 50th Percentile Fee	Global Period
11981	Insertion, nonbiodegradable drug delivery implant	$335.00	XXX
11982	Removal, nonbiodegradable drug delivery implant	$364.00	XXX
11983	Removal, with reinsertion, nonbiodegradable drug delivery implant	$520.00	XXX
11975	Insertion, implantable contraceptive capsules	$333.00	
11976	Removal, implantable contraceptive capsules	$366.00	0
11977	Removal, with reinsertion, implantable contraceptive capsules	$546.00	XXX

XXX, global concept does not apply.
CPT is a registered trademark of the American Medical Association.
2008 average 50th Percentile Fees are provided courtesy of 2008 MMH-SI's copyrighted Physicians' Fees and Coding Guide.

S-Code

Etonogestrel implant, 68 mg $653.75

Some offices use the 11981–83 codes, whereas others use 11975–77 depending on the type of office setting.

The kit cost $523.00 direct to the provider and $675.00 for patient acquisition via a prescription at a pharmacy.

Diagnosis Codes

V25.5 Encounter for contraceptive management, insertion of implantable subdermal contraceptive

V25.43	Encounter for contraceptive management, surveillance of previously prescribed contraceptive method (checking, reinsertion, or removal of contraceptive device), implantable subdermal contraceptive
V48.52	Other postprocedural states, presence of contraceptive device subdermal contraceptive implant

Patient Education Handout

A patient education handout, "Implanon," can be found on the book's companion Web site.

Bibliography

Affandi B. An integrated analysis of vaginal bleeding patterns in clinical trials of Implanon™. *Contraception*. 1998;58:99S–107S.

A new progestin implant (Implanon) for long-term contraception. *Med Lett Drugs Ther*. 2006; 48(1245):83–84.

Croxatto HB, Mäkäräinen L. Pharmacodynamics and efficacy of Implanon. *Contraception*. 1998; 58:91S–97S.

Edwards JE, Moore A. Implanon™: a review of clinical Studies. *Br J Fam Plann*. 1991;24(Suppl 4): 3–16.

Fraser IS. The challenges of location and removal of Implanon™ contraceptive implants. *J. Fam Plann Reprod Health Care*. 2006;32(3):151–152.

Implanon package insert. Roseland, NJ: Organon USA Inc.; 2006.

Kennedy H, Mumagahn M. Implanon: when is the ideal time to insert? *J Fam Plann Reprod Health Care*. 2001;27(3):158.

Mascarenhas L. Insertion and removal of Implanon: practical considerations. *Eur J Contracept Reprod Health Care*. 2000;5 (Suppl 2):29–34.

Reinprayoon D, Taneepanichskul S, Bunyavejchevin S, et al. Effects of the etonogestrel-releasing contraceptive implant (Implanon on parameters of breastfeeding compared to those of an intrauterine device. *Contraception*. 2000:62:239–246.

Thuriarajah K. Implanon insertion. *J Fam Plann Reprod Health Care*. 2006;32(4):268.

Walling M. How to remove impalpable Implanon implants. *J Fam Plann Reprod Health Care*. 2005;31(4):320–321.

2008 MAG Mutual Healthcare Solutions, Inc.'s Physicians' Fee and Coding Guide. Duluth, Georgia. MAG Mutual Healthcare Solutions, Inc. 2007.

CHAPTER 79

Intrauterine Device Insertion and Removal

Sandra M. Sulik, MD, MS, FAAFP

Associate Professor Family Medicine

SUNY Upstate and St. Joseph's Family Medicine Residency, Fayetteville, NY

The intrauterine device (IUD) is the most commonly used method of reversible contraception worldwide. However, it is used by only 1% of women in the United States who desire reversible contraception. The infrequent use in this country results from public fear of health risks, complicated and promoted by medicolegal factors.

The IUD was developed in the United States and was popular in this country until the mid-1970s, when the Dalkon Shield came into use and was associated with ascending uterine infections. This complication was not intrinsic to all IUDs, but was caused by use of a braided IUD string, that provided a path for bacteria to enter the uterus. This resulted in ascending infections, pelvic inflammatory disease, and infertility. The device was removed from the market in 1975. Although other IUDs, especially those containing copper, were safe and effective, litigation and other economic factors led to most of them being removed from the market in the early 1980s.

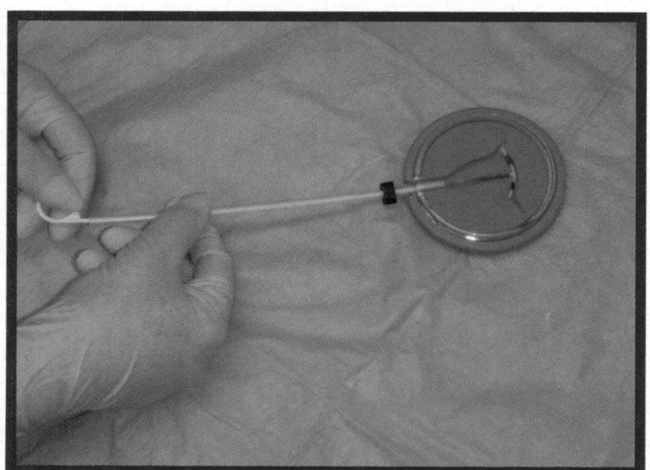

Currently there are two types of IUD's available in the United States. The ParaGard copper IUD (copper IUD) and the Mirena Intrauterine System (LNG IUS). The Copper T380A (ParaGard, Ortho-McNeil, Raritan, NJ), introduced in 1988, is now commonly used by primary care practitioners. It contains copper on a polyethylene T-shaped frame that is 32 mm wide and 36 mm long. It may be used for 10 years before replacement and has a failure rate of <1%. The Copper T380A is one of the most thoroughly studied IUDs. Careful patient selection, good patient education, and thorough informed consent have greatly reduced the medicolegal risk with this IUD. The Mirena IUS, a 5-year IUD containing levonorgestrel (Mirena, Berlex Laboratories, Montville, NJ) emerged on the U.S. market in the 1990s. The major advantage of this device is the reduction of bleeding after 6 months of use. Approximately 20% of women experience amenorrhea after 1 year of use.

The primary mechanism of action of the Copper T380A IUD is probably through the spermicidal effects of the copper. Sperm are damaged in transit, and few reach the ovum. Those that do ascend are generally in poor shape. There also may be alterations in cervical mucus produced by the IUD. IUDs also cause a foreign body inflammatory reaction. The levonorgestrel-releasing system provides pregnancy prevention by thinning the lining of the uterus, inhibition of sperm movement, and thickening of cervical mucus. There is minimal scientific evidence (despite more than 30 years of study) that the IUD is an abortifacient. However, if a patient is not able to accept this as a possible minimal mechanism of action, she may wish to consider an alternative form of birth control. IUDs have a lower actual failure rate in clinical use than oral contraceptives and most other reversible contraceptive methods (0.1% to 0.8% vs 5% for the combined oral contraceptive). Fertility usually returns promptly after removal of an IUD.

IUDs may be inserted any time after delivery, after abortion, or during the menstrual cycle. The advantages of insertion during a menstrual period include a possibly more open cervical canal, the masking of insertion-related bleeding, and the knowledge that the patient is not pregnant. Insertions can be more difficult when the cervix is closed between periods.

Insertion can be performed between 4 and 8 weeks postpartum without an increase in pregnancy rates, expulsion, uterine perforation, or removal for bleeding or pain. Insertion can even occur immediately after a vaginal delivery without an increased risk of infection, uterine perforation, postpartum bleeding, or uterine subinvolution if no infection is present. Expect a slightly higher expulsion rate compared with insertion 4 to 8 weeks postpartum. The IUD also can be inserted at the time of cesarean section, with the expulsion rate slightly lower than immediately after vaginal delivery. Insertion of an IUD in breast-feeding women is associated with a lower removal rate for bleeding or pain. An IUD can be inserted immediately after a first-trimester abortion, but the patient should wait after a second-trimester abortion until uterine involution occurs.

Patient satisfaction studies have revealed higher ratings for IUDs than for most other contraceptive methods. Increased menstrual bleeding and cramping is a typical side effect of IUD use. Bleeding causes removal of the T380A during the first year in 5% to 15% of patients. Nonsteroidal anti-inflammatory drugs often help reduce these problems.

Infections caused by IUDs usually occur within the first 20 days after insertion. The overall rate of infection is only 0.3%. Routine antibiotic prophylaxis is not needed for the insertion of an IUD. Cases of tuboovarian actinomycosis associated with IUD use have been reported. If this organism is reported on a Papanicolaou (Pap) smear in an asymptomatic patient, the IUD should be removed and may be replaced when a repeat Pap smear is negative.

The ectopic pregnancy rate with use of the IUD is lower than with no contraception (90% reduction in risk). However, if a patient becomes pregnant with an IUD in place, it is more likely that the pregnancy is ectopic. There is no increase in ectopic pregnancy with a history of prior IUD use. Intrauterine pregnancy with an IUD in place causes a 20-fold increased risk of developing life-threatening, second-trimester septic abortion. The IUD, therefore, should be removed as early as possible if intrauterine pregnancy occurs.

Spontaneous expulsion occurs in 5% of women during the first year, most often during the first menses after insertion. Partial expulsion or displacement is marked by lengthening of the IUD string. The IUD may be immediately reinserted if no infection is present (prophylactic antibiotics are recommended).

Displacement of the IUD may occur, and absence of the string on the patient's self examination is cause for further evaluation. Plain films of the abdomen can determine the presence of the IUD, and ultrasonography or hysteroscopy can be used to determine its location or to extract the device. If the device is in the abdominal cavity, laparoscopy is usually successful at removal. Uterine perforation may occur during insertion but is uncommon.

Patients with newly inserted IUDs should attempt to feel the strings before they leave the examining room. Give the patient the cut ends of the strings as a sample of what to feel. The patient should make a follow-up visit in 1 month to confirm presence of the IUD and to trim the string if it is too long. Palpation of the strings should be performed monthly by the patient to verify continuing presence of the IUD after each menstrual flow.

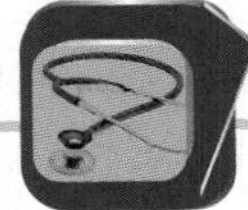

Equipment

- Speculum
- Exam gloves
- IUD or IUS
- Light source
- Iodine/Povidine solution in a small basin with cotton balls
- Ring forceps or long Kelly
- Cervical tenaculum
- Uterine sound
- Large absorbant swabs (Scopettes)
- Long-handled scissors
- Nonsterile gloves for bimanual exam and sterile for IUD insertion

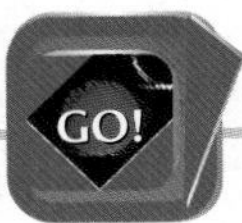

Indications

- Reversible contraception for patients in a monogamous relationship at low risk for STDs
- Consider for women with the following medical conditions:
  - Diabetes
  - Thromboembolism
  - Menorrhagia/dysmenorrhea (LNG IUS—off-label use)
  - Breast-feeding
  - Breast cancer (Copper IUD only)
  - Liver disease (Copper IUD only)
  - Severe dysmenorrhea/menorrhagia (LNG IUS)

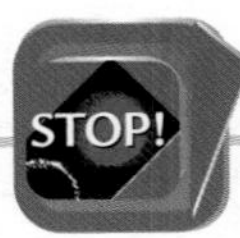

Contraindications

- Pregnancy
- Undiagnosed genital bleeding
- Wilson's disease and allergy to copper (copper IUD)
- Known or suspected cervical or uterine neoplasia
- Pelvic inflammatory disease/septic abortion present or within 3 months of insertion
- Severe dysmenorrhea or menorrhagia (copper IUD)
- An abnormally shaped uterus, or fibroids that distort the uterine cavity (the uterine cavity should sound to 6 to 10 cm)
- Sign of cervicitis or vaginitis on the day of insertion
- Patients at high risk for endocarditis (e.g., prosthetic valves, major valve abnormalities, shunt lesions)
- Use with great caution with anticoagulation (copper IUD)

The Procedure

Insertion of ParaGard Copper IUD

Step 1. Explain the IUD insertion procedure, and obtain informed consent. Review current Pap smear and culture results. American College of Obstetrics and Gynecology guidelines do not recommend checking cultures in low-risk women. If Pap is not current, repeat just prior to insertion of the IUD. Check urine pregnancy test prior to insertion of device. With the patient in the lithotomy position, perform a bimanual examination to determine the uterine size and position and to rule out structural abnormalities. Place a sterile speculum in the vagina, and swab the cervix with an antiseptic solution such as an iodine or benzalkonium preparation. Make sure the IUD package is intact and that all of the parts are present.

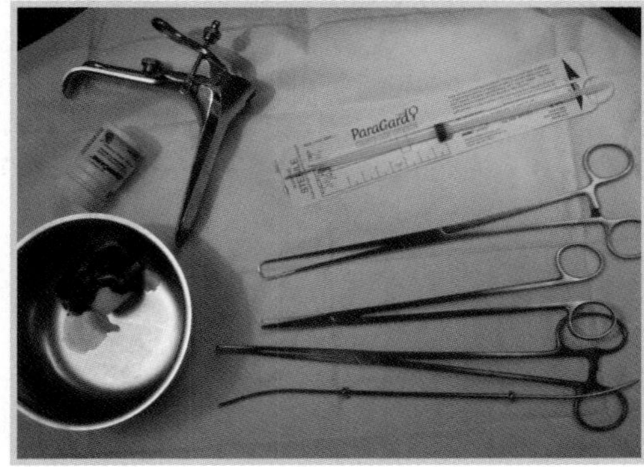

Step 1

Step 2. Using sterile technique, grasp the anterior lip of the cervix with a tenaculum and sound the uterus (should be between 6 and 10 cm). A paracervical block can be used to decrease the pain of the procedure. Inject 2% lidocaine just off the cervix at the 3- and 9-o'clock positions (or 4- and 10-o'clock positions if preferred).

- **PITFALL:** A paracervical block takes a few minutes for full effect. Wait 2 to 3 minutes following the injections before initiating the procedure.

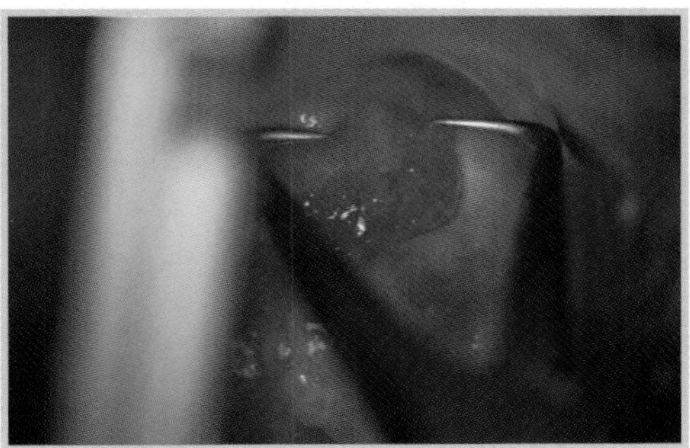

Step 2

Step 3. With sterile gloves or through the sterile wrapper, fold down the arms of the IUD into the insertion tube just enough to hold them in place during insertion. The phalange on the insertion tube is set to the distance of the sounding. This permits visual confirmation of when the top of the IUD reaches the fundus.

- **PITFALL:** Fold the arms right before or during the procedure. Prolonged bending of the arms causes them to release slowly and increases the likelihood of device expulsion.

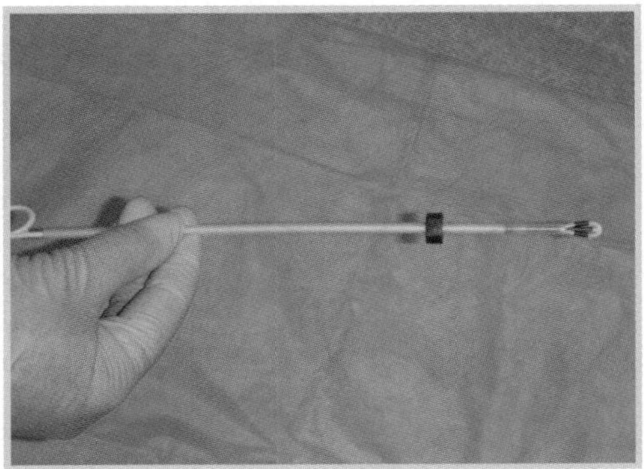

Step 3

Step 4. Insert the device into the uterine cavity until it meets resistance at the fundus, and then slightly withdraw (i.e., a few millimeters).

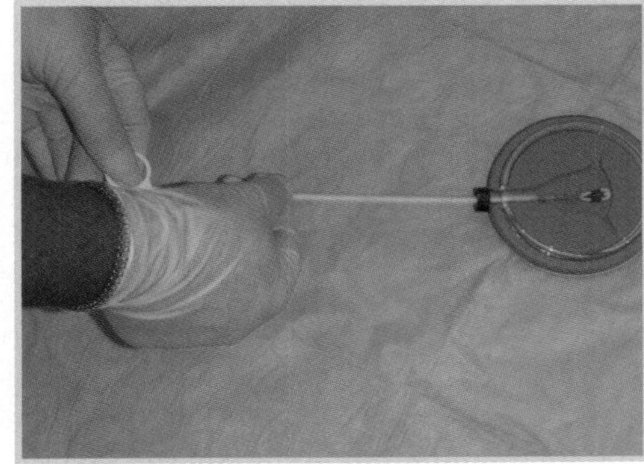

Step 4

Step 5. While holding the insertion rod in place, withdraw the insertion tube 1 to 2 cm to release the arms of the IUD in the horizontal plane of the uterus.

- **PITFALL:** Do not push the insertion rod upward to elevate the IUD. This practice is painful for the patient and increases the risk of perforation.

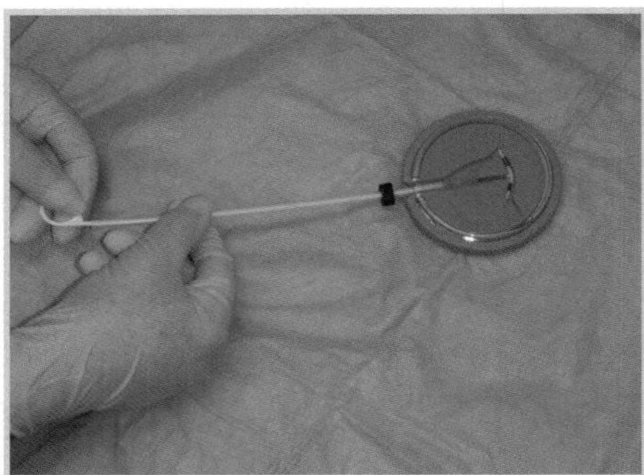

Step 5

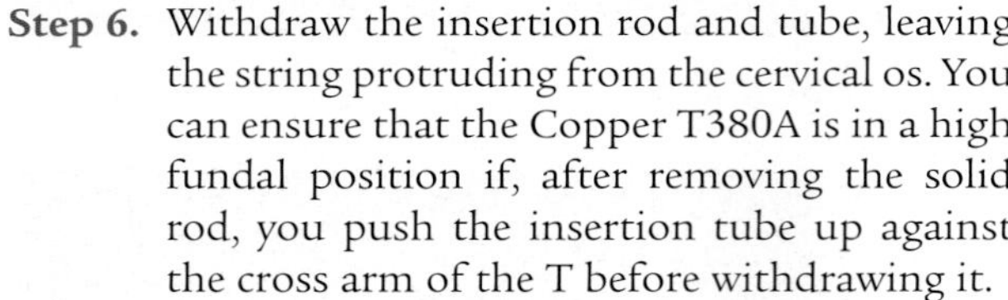

Step 6. Withdraw the insertion rod and tube, leaving the string protruding from the cervical os. You can ensure that the Copper T380A is in a high fundal position if, after removing the solid rod, you push the insertion tube up against the cross arm of the T before withdrawing it.

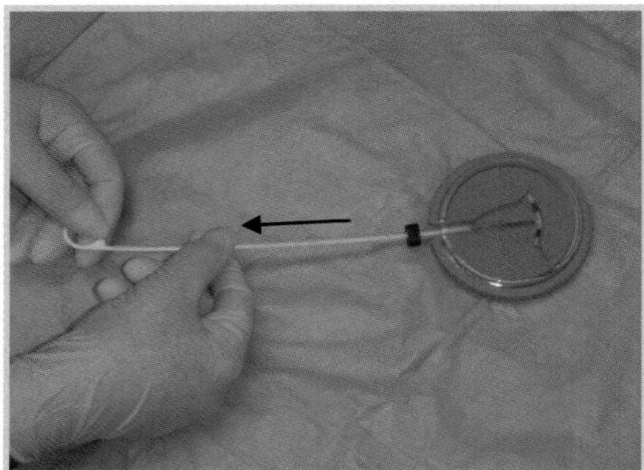

Step 6

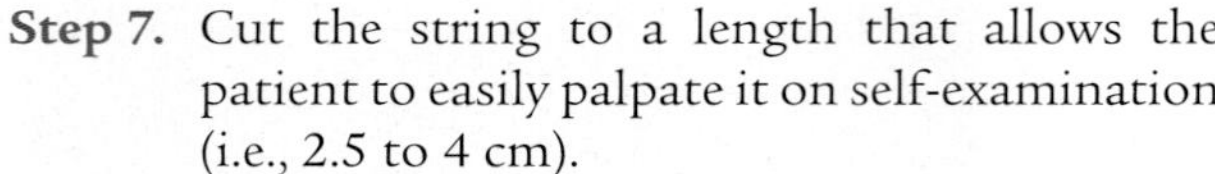

Step 7. Cut the string to a length that allows the patient to easily palpate it on self-examination (i.e., 2.5 to 4 cm).

- **PITFALL:** Do not cut the strings too short; err on the side of too long because the strings can always be cut again. If the strings are cut too short, they tend to impale the end of the glans penis and cause pain during intercourse.
- **PITFALL:** Despite proper placement, early expulsion is possible. Inform the patient of this possibility, and instruct her to return the IUD to your office. The manufacturer will provide a sterile replacement for reinsertion at no cost.

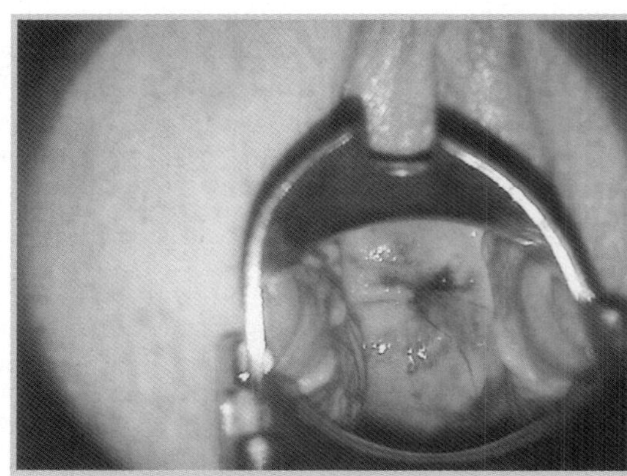

Step 7

Insertion of Mirena Intrauterine System

Step 8. Follow first two steps above. Mark the depth of the uterus with the green phalange on the intrauterine system (IUS). Free the strings from the IUS and pull down on the strings as you push the green slider towards the IUS.

- **PITFALL:** Make sure that the arms of the IUS are horizontal to the insertion device in order to assure proper loading. The entire tips of the IUS should be loaded into the device prior to insertion.

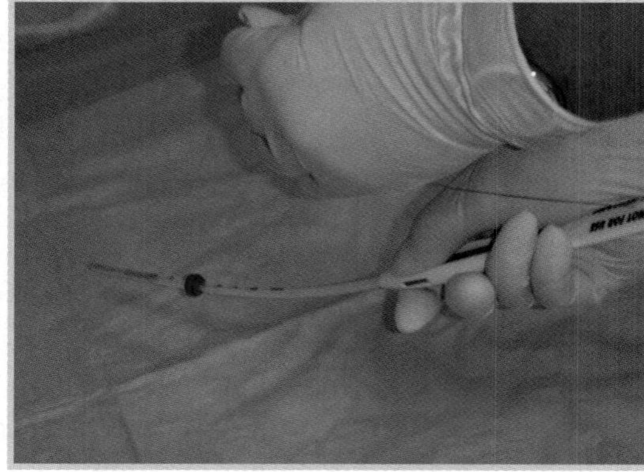

Step 8

Step 9. Using traction from the tenaculum, insert the IUS through the cervical os and to the depth marked on the IUS. Gently pull the entire system back 1 cm away from the cervix.

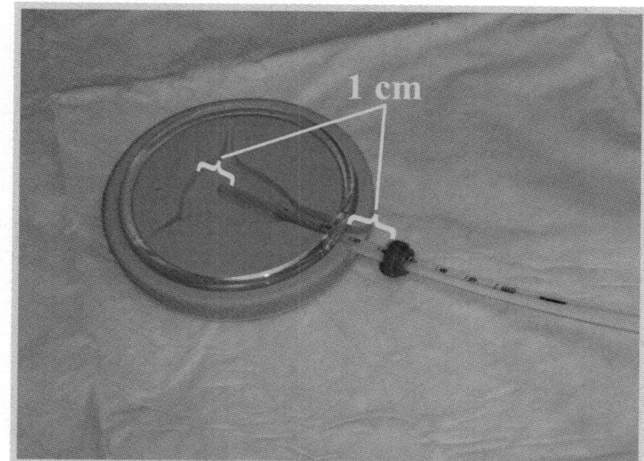

Step 9

Step 10. Release the slider (green phalange) to the marked position (only!) on the side of the device. (This releases the arms of the IUS.)

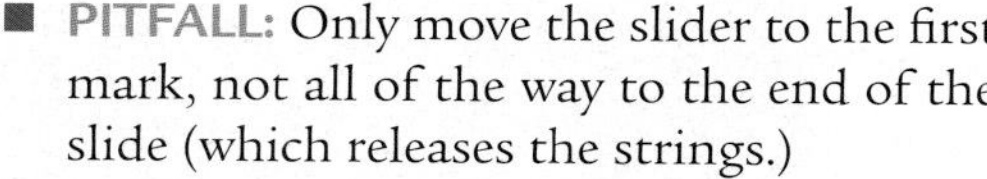

- PITFALL: Only move the slider to the first mark, not all of the way to the end of the slide (which releases the strings.)

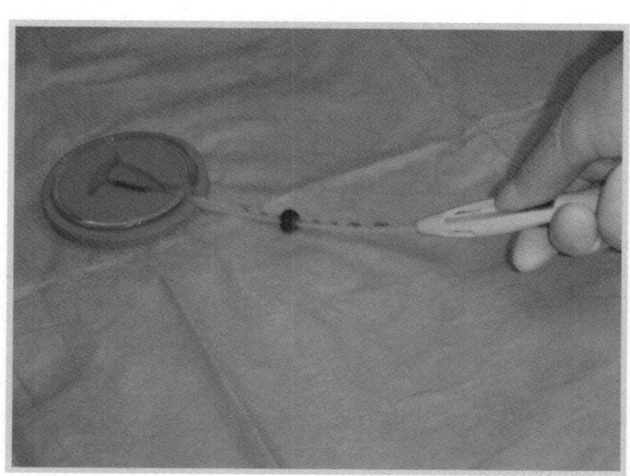

Step 10

Step 11. Then, advance the entire device back to the uterine depth marker on the IUS. This will place the IUS at the fundus of the uterus.

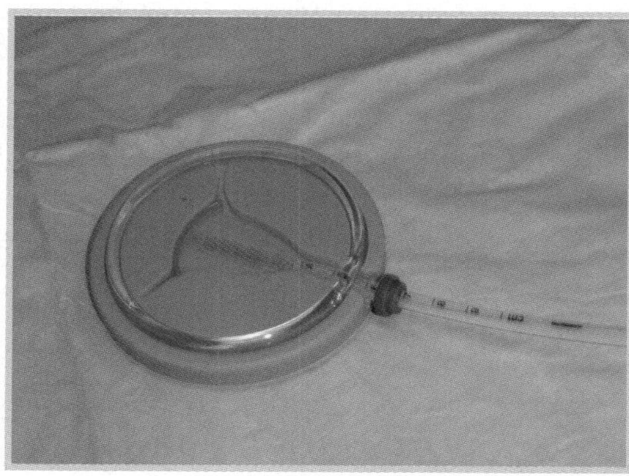

Step 11

Step 12. Pull the slider (green phalange) all the way back to release the string. Remove the inserter from the uterus. Cut the strings at a depth of 2.5 to 4 cm. Remove the tenaculum and speculum and instruct the patient in how to find the strings to check for placement.

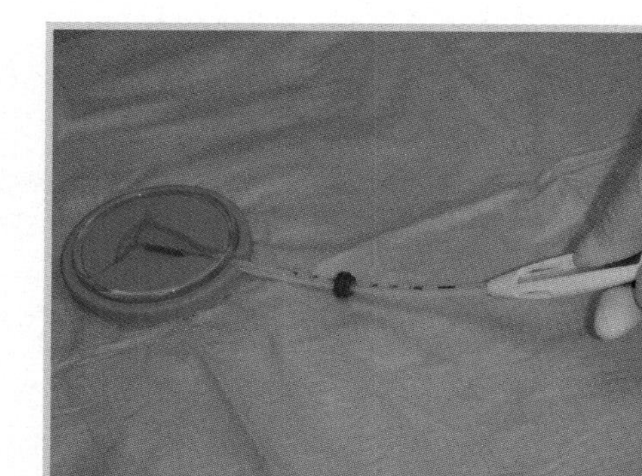

Step 12

IUD Removal

Step 13. Place a cervical speculum and find the IUD strings. Removal of an IUD usually can be accomplished by grasping the string with a ring forceps and exerting firm, steady traction (usually during the menstrual period).

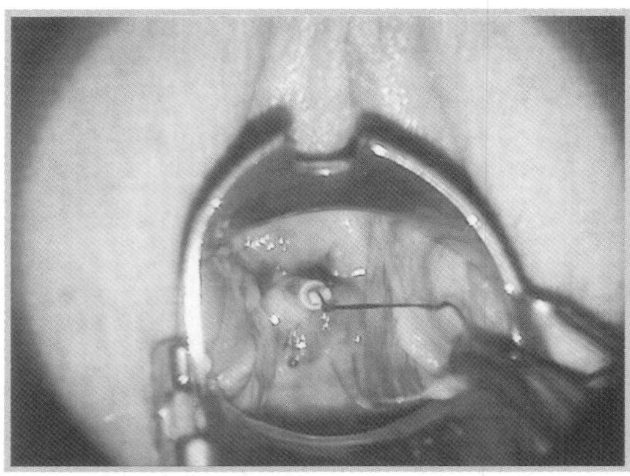

Step 13

Step 14. If strings cannot be seen, they can often be extracted from the cervical canal by rotating two cotton-tipped applicators or a Pap smear cytobrush in the endocervical canal.

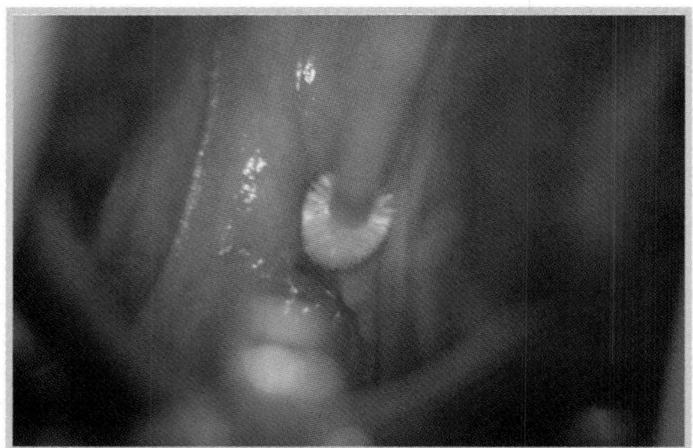

Step 14

Step 15. If IUD strings cannot be identified or extracted from the endocervical canal, a light plastic uterine sound should be passed into the endometrial cavity after administration of a paracervical block. The IUD can frequently be felt with the sound and localized against the anterior or posterior wall of the uterus. The device can then be removed using polyp- or alligator-type forceps directed to where the device was felt.

- **PITFALL:** Because there is a risk of perforation with this procedure, patients are often referred for hysteroscopic removal at this stage.

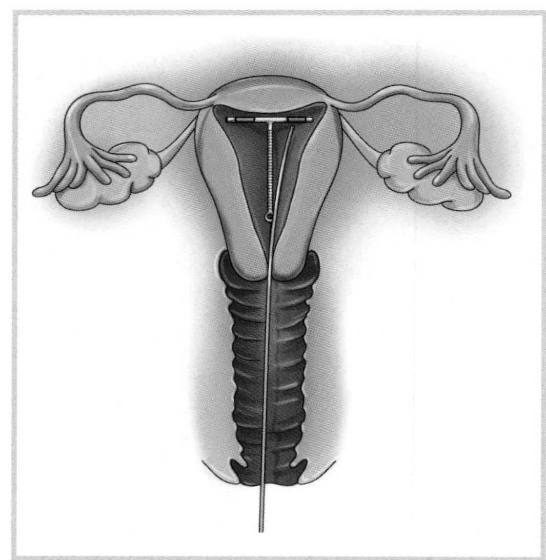

Step 15

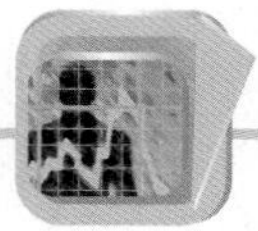

Complications

- Pregnancy (rare <1%)
- PID (only in the first 20 days after insertion)
- Perforation (extremely rare)
- Spontaneous expulsion (most occur within first 6 months)

- Lost IUD string (rule out pregnancy, look in endocervical canal)
- Actinomyces (usually asymptomatic, pull IUD and treat, replace IUD when actinomyces is no longer present on Pap)
- Uterine bleeding and cramping (usually within the first 3 months of insertion)

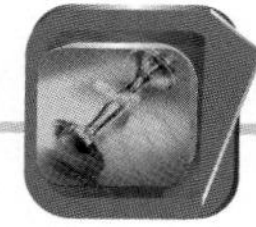

Pediatric Considerations

This procedure is not used in children. Although not commonly used in adolescents, the procedure is the same.

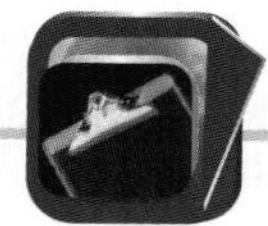

Postprocedure Instructions

Once the IUD insertion is complete, wipe off the strings and hand them to the patient to feel. Have the patient feel for the strings before she leaves the office. Explain that some spotting initially is normal. Give the patient the IUD handout that comes with each IUD package insert.

Remind the patient that routine Pap smears are still necessary and that the IUD will not protect from STDs; therefore, condoms should also be used. Review the signs of expulsions with the patient—severe cramping being the most important. Tell the patient to call if she cannot find the strings and to use a backup method until the presence of the IUD can be confirmed. Counsel the patient to report any excessive bleeding, malodorous discharge, unexplained fever, pain with intercourse, prolonged bleeding, amenorrhea, or prolonged pelvic pain.

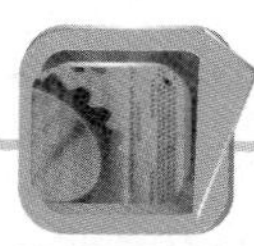

Coding Information and Supply Sources

CPT Code	Description	2008 Average 50th Percentile Fee	Global Period
58300	Insertion of IUD	$274.00	XXX
58301	Removal of IUD	$272.00	0
J7300	Charge for Copper IUD	XXX	XXX
J3490	Unclassified drug (Mirena)	XXX	XXX

CPT is a registered trademark of the American Medical Association.
2008 average 50th Percentile Fees are provided courtesy of 2008 MMH-SI's copyrighted Physicians' Fees and Coding Guide.
XXX global does not apply.

ICD-9-CM Diagnostic Codes

V 25-1 Encounter of contraceptive management, insertion of IUD
V2542 Intrauterine conceptive device, checking, reinsertion or removal of IUD

Instrument and Materials Ordering

ParaGard IUDs can be obtained from Ortho-McNeil Pharmaceuticals (phone: 1-800-322-4966). A physician can establish an account free of charge and place orders for the product. They may be ordered singly or in a box of five at a lower cost per unit.

Mirena may be ordered from Berlex Laboratories, Inc. (phone: 1-866-647-3646). Before any insertion, it is important to obtain training on the proper technique specific to Mirena. Training can be found at http://www.mirena-us.com or by writing Berlex Laboratories, Inc., 6 West Belt Road, Wayne, NJ 07470-6806.

Instruments and materials in a standard gynecological tray are listed in Appendix H: Instruments and Materials in a Standard Gynecological Tray.

Patient Education Handout

A patient education handout, **"Intrauterine Devices"** can be found on the book's Web site.

Bibliography

Croxatto HB, Ortiz ME, Valdez E. IUD mechanisms of action. In: Bardin CW, Mishell DR Jr, eds. *Proceedings of the Fourth International Conference on IUDs*. Boston: Butterworth-Heinemann; 1994.

Delbanco SF, Mauldon J, Smith MD. Little knowledge and limited practice: emergency contraceptive pills, the public, and the obstetrician-gynecologist. *Obstet Gynecol.* 1997;89:1006–1011.

Grimes DA, Schulz KF. Antibiotic prophylaxis for intrauterine contraceptive device insertion. *Cochrane Database Syst Rev* 2001;(2):CD001327.

Hill DA, Weiss NS, Voigt LF, et al. Endometrial cancer in relation to intra-uterine device use. *Int Cancer.* 1997;70:278–281.

Intrauterine Device. *ACOG Pract Bull.* 2005;59:1–10.

Mendelson MA. Contraception in women with congenital heart disease. *Heart Dis Stroke.* 1994;3:266–269.

Mishell DR Jr. Intrauterine devices: mechanisms of action, safety, and efficacy. *Contraception.* 1998;58(Suppl):45S–53S.

Nelson AL. The intrauterine contraceptive device. *Obstet Gynecol Clin North Am.* 2000;27:723–740.

Ramirez Hidalgo A, Pujol Ribera E. Use of the intrauterine device: efficacy and safety. *Eur J Contracept Rep Rod Health Care.* 2000;5:198–207.

Shelton JD. Risk of clinical pelvic inflammatory disease attributable to an intrauterine device. *Lancet.* 2001;357:443.

Speroff L, Darney P. *A Clinical Guide for Contraception*, (2nd ed.) Baltimore: Williams & Wilkins; 1996.

Thonneau P, Goulard H, Goyaux N. Risk factors for intrauterine device failure: a review. *Contraception.* 2001;64:33–37.

Trussell J, Koenig J, Ellertson C, et al. Preventing unintended pregnancy: the cost-effectiveness of three methods of emergency contraception. *Am J Public Health.* 1997;87:932–937.

Zimmer DE. Avoiding litigation in a new age of IUDs. *Obstet Gynecol Surv.* 1996;51:S56–S60.

2008 MAG Mutual Healthcare Solutions, Inc.'s Physicians' Fee and Coding Guide. Duluth, Georgia. MAG Mutual Healthcare Solutions, Inc. 2007.

CHAPTER 80

Loop Electrosurgical Excisional Procedure

E. J. Mayeaux, Jr., MD, DABFP, FAAFP
Professor of Family Medicine, Professor of Obstetrics and Gynecology
Louisiana State University Health Sciences Center, Shreveport, LA

Premalignant cervical lesions usually occur in women of or past child-bearing years. Until recently, the historical choices for treatment of these included cryosurgery, electrocoagulation, laser vaporization or conization, knife conization, and hysterectomy. The first three options are outpatient procedures and allow for the possibility of future pregnancies. However, because they are ablative therapies, no tissue is sent for pathologic inspection, raising the possibility of missing microinvasive or invasive cancer. Conization and hysterectomy produce tissue specimens with wide margins but usually require outpatient surgery or hospitalization with general anesthesia, and hysterectomy precludes future pregnancies. The loop electrosurgical excisional procedure (LEEP or LLETZ) allows outpatient treatment of cervical lesions, produces good pathology specimens, and has a low risk of interfering with child-bearing.

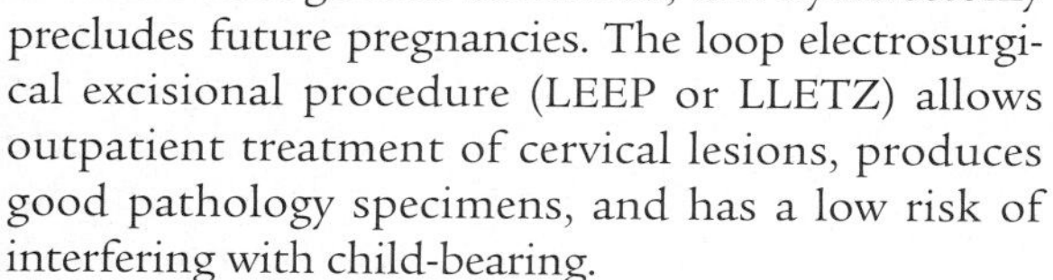

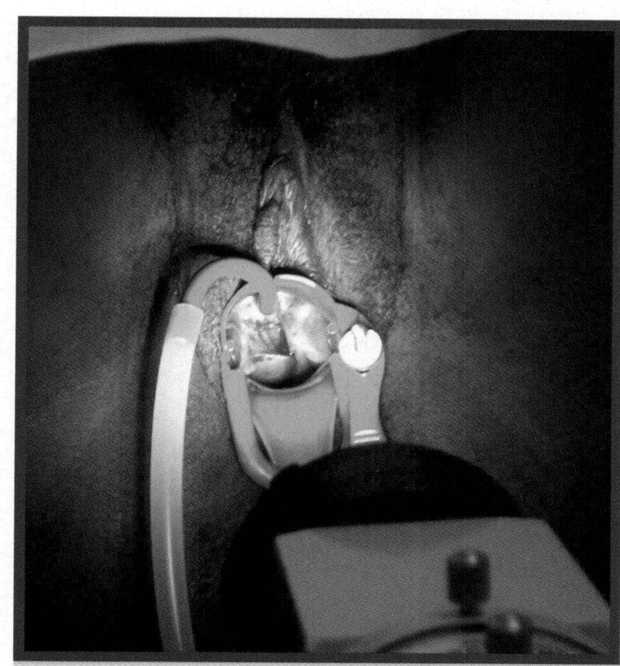

LEEP makes use of low-voltage and relatively high-frequency electric current. In pure cutting mode, high-frequency current is produced in a smooth, uninterrupted sine wave. The cutting effect is not produced by heating the wire. As the loop is introduced to the tissue, an arc occurs near the point of contact, causing the cells to be rapidly heated and exploded into steam. The steam envelope allows continued arcing, extending the cut. This produces a clean cut with little coagulation artifact. The transformation zone can be removed, with a good-quality specimen sent to the pathology department for examination.

In the coagulation mode, fulguration of tissue is produced with short bursts of high-peak-voltage current. This mode is often used with a ball electrode to achieve hemostasis. Most modern units can combine the amount of cutting and coagulation currents in blend modes. With all three operational modes, the current is quickly dispersed to the grounding electrode. The large surface area of the return electrode prevents high-charge density and prevents burns. An improperly applied return electrode can result in burns.

Efficacy and patient acceptance of LEEP compare favorably with other treatment methods for cervical intraepithelial neoplasia (CIN). Few studies directly compare treatment modalities with sufficient statistical power to draw conclusions. A prospective, randomized study by Mitchel et al. did not find any significant differences among cryotherapy, laser ablation, and LEEP. This study could only detect large differences, and it did show a trend toward better outcomes for CIN 3 with LEEP. General studies indicate LEEP is 91% to 98% effective in treating CIN. LEEP is also a well-tolerated procedure, with 85% of patients reporting no discomfort. Most patients who do report discomfort indicate that the degree of pain is mild.

LEEP is approximately 95% effective for treatment of immunocompetent women. Most recurrences happen within 1 year of treatment. The procedure provides an adequate specimen for pathologic study. Confirming complete removal of the lesion by observing specimen margins essentially eliminates the risk of missing microinvasive cancers. Despite removal of tissue, the transformation zone heals with a normal appearance in most patients, allowing for normal, long-term cytologic and colposcopic follow-up.

LEEP also offers the advantage of being a clinic procedure performed under local anesthesia. Treatment of even advanced lesions can be accomplished with the complete removal of the transformation zone or conization, with results comparable to knife conization. The cost of a LEEP unit is much less than laser equipment. In some cases, LEEP avoids the hospital and anesthesia costs of conization. By improving diagnostic accuracy, LEEP may prevent the human and financial cost of missing microinvasive cancer.

Patient Preparation

Patient preparation starts when the patient is informed she has dysplastic cervical cells on colposcopically directed biopsy. Basic education should be provided about cervical disease, treatment options, and the LEEP procedure. The patient may be given instructions to premedicate with a nonsteroidal anti-inflammatory drug the night before and the morning of the procedure if there are no contraindications. The optimal timing of the procedure is within 7 days of completion of the menstrual period to minimize the likelihood that the patient is pregnant. After cervical LEEP, there may be swelling sufficient to occlude the endocervical canal, which can lead to hematocolpos, with the need to drain the uterus.

Patient consent is mandatory, because every management strategy carries with it some element of risk. Among states and geographic regions, there is considerable variation on issues, such as who constitutes a minor and when parental consent must be received by the physician before treating a minor. Many states do not require parental informed consent before providing treatment to a minor with a sexually transmitted disease. Conditions related to human papillomavirus (HPV) infections, such as cervical dysplasia, fall within the latter guideline. The physician should record on the minor patient's chart any and all efforts to secure and receive informed consent.

Pregnancy Effects

Pregnancy rates after LEEP are comparable to those after laser therapy and better than rates after conization. It is well established that cold-knife conization increases a woman's risk of future preterm labor, low-birth-weight infant, and cesarean section. Several large retrospective series report that women who have undergone a loop excision procedure or a laser conization are also at increased risk for future preterm delivery, a low-birth-weight infant, and premature rupture of membranes. Although most studies of ablative methods have not shown these effects on pregnancy to be associated, it is difficult to measure small effects on pregnancy outcome. Therefore, some experts recommend cervical cryotherapy over LEEP for treatment of appropriately selected reproductive-age women (see Chapter 73).

See-and-Treat LEEP

See-and-treat LEEP refers to the practice of diagnosing and treating some patients in a single visit. This method is not widely performed in the United States and but is commonly used worldwide. It has been proposed for patients with evidence of high-grade dysplasia (not low-grade squamous intraepithelial lesions or HPV lesions) on Papanicolaou (Pap) smear cytology with visible lesions and an adequate colposcopic examination, or for highly unreliable patients not likely to follow up. It should not be used when colposcopic findings are equivocal or suggest invasive cancer. The major concern with this approach is that an excision procedure may be performed unnecessarily. Traditional colposcopy followed by treatment was been found to be more cost-effective than see-and-treat LEEP. The American Society for Colposcopy and Cervical Pathology 2006 evidence-based guidelines allow for an immediate loop electrosurgical excision or colposcopy with endocervical assessment managing nonpregnant, nonadolescent women with high-grade squamous intraepithelial lesions.

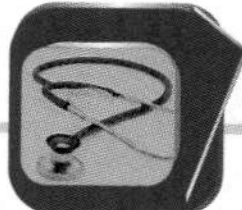

Equipment

- Electrosurgical generators used for LEEP are identical to ones used in dermatologic, laparoscopic, and urologic surgery. The alternating current output ranges between 100 and 5,000 kHz. At frequencies >100 kHz, cellular membrane depolarization does not occur, and there is no associated shock or muscular contraction.
- The amount of current used depends on the generator and the loop size. The relative cutting power needed is proportional to the amount of wire that comes into contact with the cervix. As the surface area of the cut increases, the amount of power needed to make the cut also increases. Larger or deeper cuts and larger loops require higher current settings. Drier or more keratinized skin also requires higher current settings. Setting the current too high results in increased thermal damage and increased risk of unintentional burns.
- Modern electrical generator features usually include isolated circuitry (i.e., unit automatically deactivates if any active electrode current is not returned through the patient electrode) and return electrode monitoring (i.e., warns if the return circuit is interrupted). Most generators allow switching between cutting and coagulation modes and can blend a cutting effect with a coagulation effect. These blend modes permit concomitant coagulation hemostasis and surgical excision of tissues. Blend modes represent a greater proportion of coagulation effect, which further minimizes bleeding but often increases thermal damage to the excised tissue. If a thermal artifact is present, evaluation of the specimen margin to exclude margin involvement by tumor becomes difficult.
- Most loops have an insulated shaft and crossbar to prevent accidental thermal injury. Common loop sizes range from 1 × 1 cm to 2.0 × 1.5 cm. The stainless steel or tungsten wire of the loop is approximately 0.2 mm thick. Ball electrodes ranging from 3 to 5 mm are used for fulguration. The probe is a monopolar output and requires the use of a grounding electrode. Return (patient) electrodes may be disposable adhesive gel pads or a reusable solid "antenna".
- A smoke evacuator to remove the plume produced during the procedure is essential. It filters airborne particles and coexisting microorganisms present in the plume. Several manufacturers have combined an electrosurgical unit with a smoke evacuator so that, when the generator is activated, the smoke evacuator also is automatically activated. Negative pressures from the smoke evacuator cause air to flow into the vagina, up the fixed tubing in the speculum, and through the evacuator tubing toward the equipment. This minimizes plume spillage into the treatment room. A series of microfilters help remove the carbon, odor, and viral particles generated. Because HPV has been isolated from similar laser plumes, clinicians usually wear micropore or submicron surgical masks.
- Most electrosurgical generator manufacturers recommend using insulated vaginal speculums to prevent secondary patient burns from conduction through the speculum to nonanesthetized vaginal and vulvar areas. Treat insulated speculums as if they were not insulated; do not touch them with an activated electrode! Nonconductive lateral wall retractors may assist with visualization to counteract lateral vaginal wall redundancy and protect the vaginal walls.

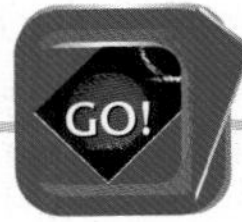

Indications

- Treatment of biopsy-proven CIN 2 and 3 lesion
- CIN 1 lesions persistent for 2 or more years, especially in women not desiring child-bearing
- Dysplasia deemed inappropriate for cryotherapy, such as large lesions not fitting beneath a cryotherapy probe
- Lesions extending >5 mm into the cervical canal, when the colposcopy is inadequate, or when the ECC is positive (LEEP conization)
- Cryotherapy failures, especially if the subsequent colposcopy is unsatisfactory
- An unresolvable biopsy–Pap smear or biopsy-impression mismatch (LEEP or LEEP conization)

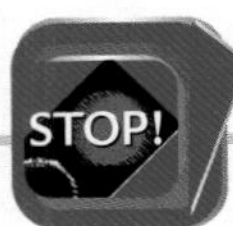

Contraindications

- HPV infection alone
- CIN 1 without evidence of high-grade dysplasia that is not persistent
- Vaginal lesions due to risk of perforation (relative contraindication)
- Clinically apparent invasive carcinoma
- Bleeding disorders
- Pregnancy
- Acute cervicitis (due to risk of spreading infection and increased bleeding)
- Uncooperative patient
- Being <3 months postpartum due to increased bleeding (relative contraindication)
- History of cervical conization with recurrence (relative contraindication)
- Markedly atrophic cervix (relative contraindication)
- Lesions that extend far laterally
- Suspected microinvasive or invasive cancer
- Adenocarcinoma in situ (often best treated with a cold-knife cone or hysterectomy)

The Procedure

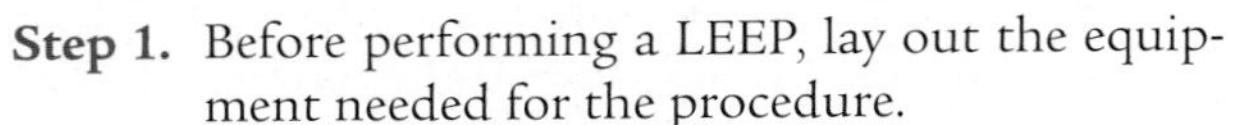

Step 1. Before performing a LEEP, lay out the equipment needed for the procedure.

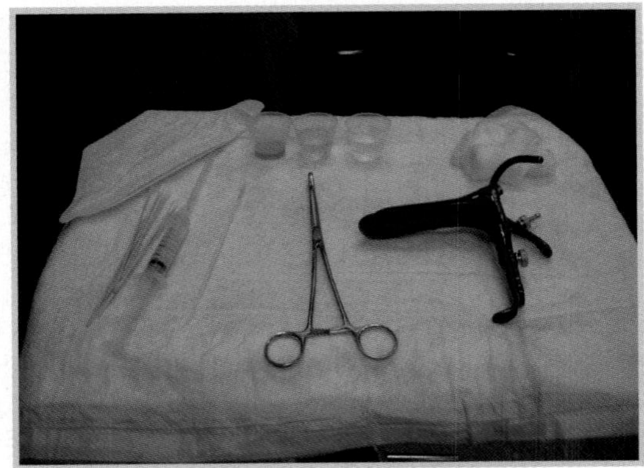

Step 1

Step 2. Inspect the components, including the speculum, LEEP unit, grounding system, and smoke evacuation system. Attach a return electrode is to the patient, usually on the upper leg or under the buttocks. Insert the speculum and smoke evacuation tubing.

- **PITFALL:** If using a side-wall retractor, avoid pinching the vagina between the retractor and the speculum. Slowly open the retractor, making sure the side wall does not become entrapped.

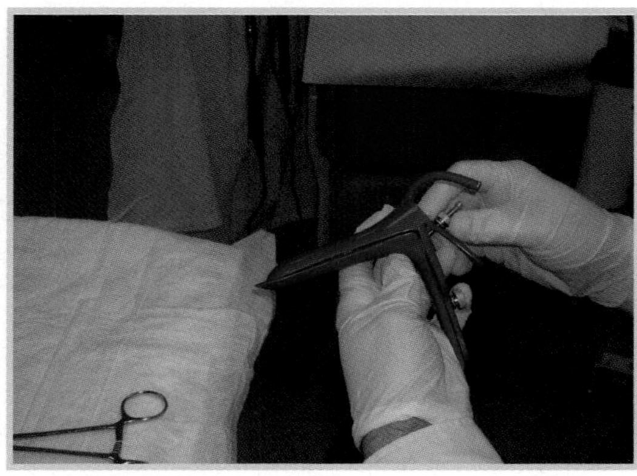

Step 2

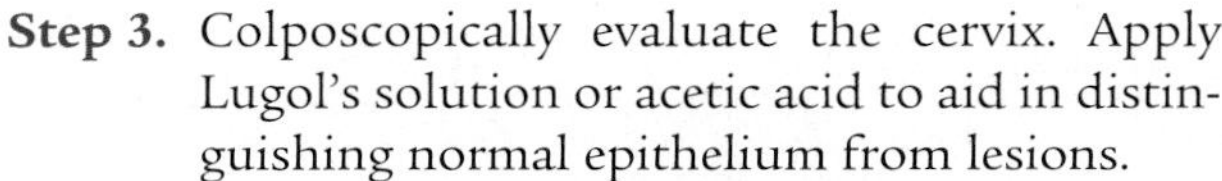

Step 3. Colposcopically evaluate the cervix. Apply Lugol's solution or acetic acid to aid in distinguishing normal epithelium from lesions.

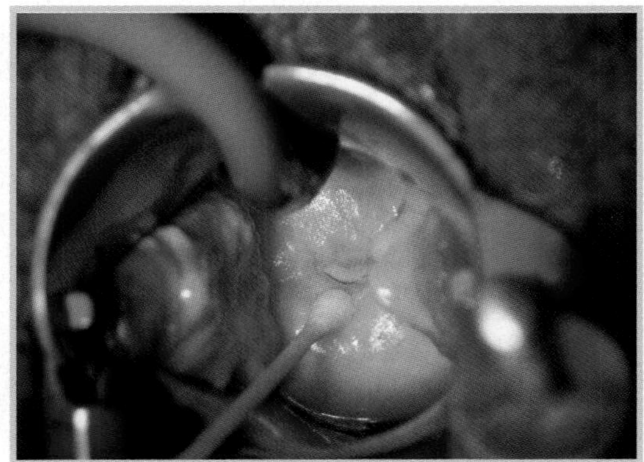

Step 3

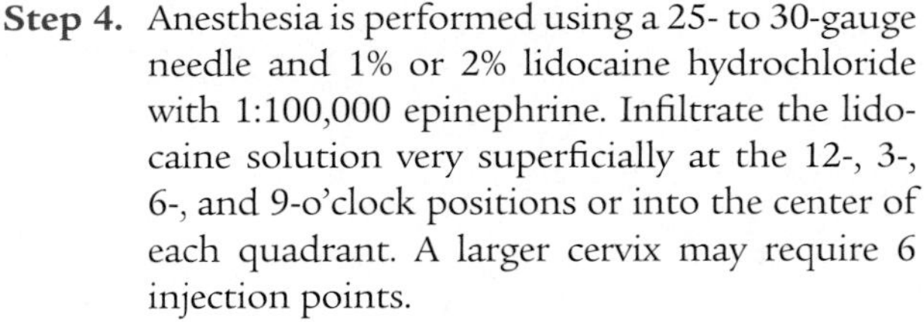

Step 4. Anesthesia is performed using a 25- to 30-gauge needle and 1% or 2% lidocaine hydrochloride with 1:100,000 epinephrine. Infiltrate the lidocaine solution very superficially at the 12-, 3-, 6-, and 9-o'clock positions or into the center of each quadrant. A larger cervix may require 6 injection points.

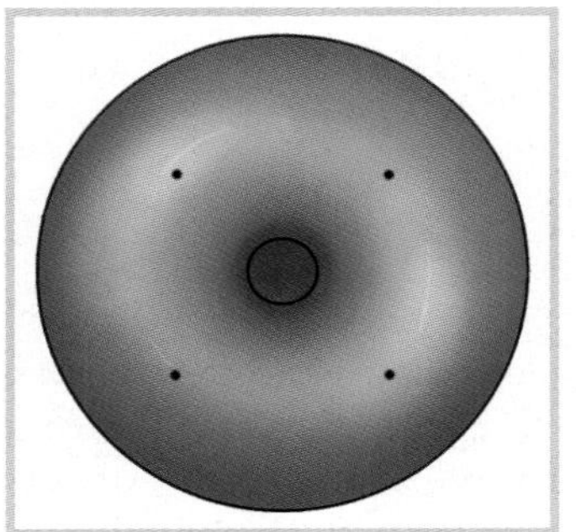

Step 4

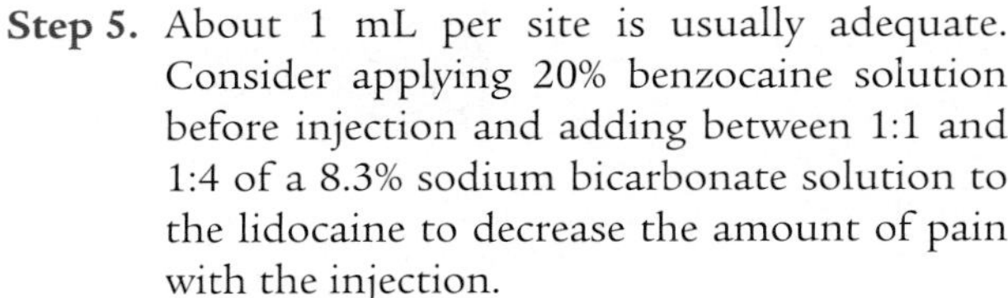

Step 5. About 1 mL per site is usually adequate. Consider applying 20% benzocaine solution before injection and adding between 1:1 and 1:4 of a 8.3% sodium bicarbonate solution to the lidocaine to decrease the amount of pain with the injection.

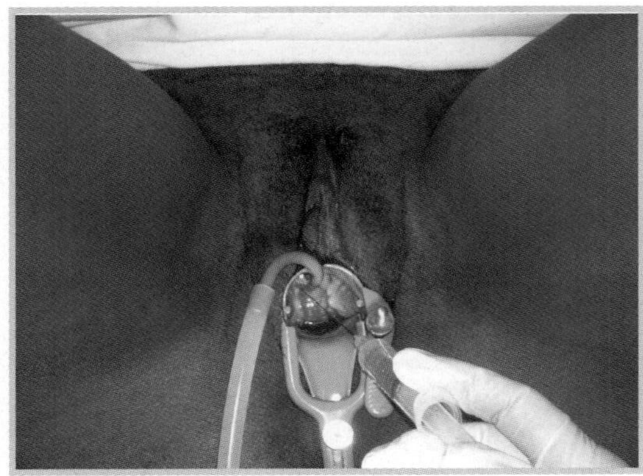

Step 5

Step 6. Choose a loop that allows excision of the entire transformation zone (usually 12 to 20 mm wide and 7 to 10 mm deep) in one or two passes without major risk of contact with the vaginal side wall. Ring forceps held against the cervix may be a useful size referent. Set the current (usually 40 to 60 watts or 4 to 6 on higher-frequency units), and set the unit to a blended or pure cutting mode. The loop is attached to a pencil-like base that is controlled with a finger or foot switch.

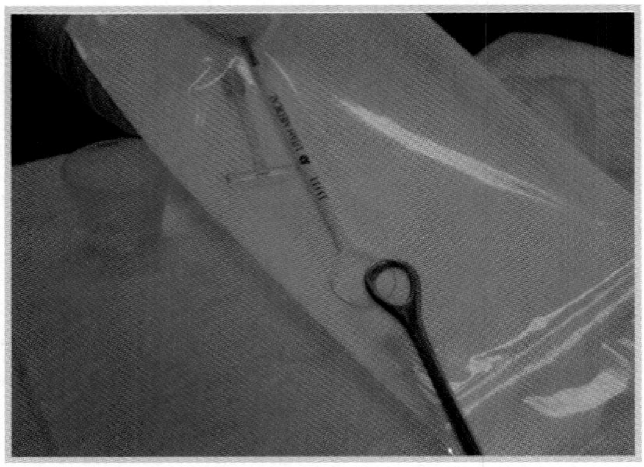

Step 6

Step 7. To excise tissue, the loop is held just above the surface of the cervix and 2 to 5 mm lateral to the lesion or edge of the transformation zone. Current is applied before the loop contacts the cervix. The loop is pushed into the tissue to a depth of about 7 to 8 mm, because maximal crypt involvement by CIN is approximately 4 mm, and you must account for the volume of injected anesthetic.

- PITFALL: If current is applied after contact is made, significant thermal injury will occur and the quality of the cut will be poor.
- PITFALL: Activate the loop only when looking at it. This avoids inadvertent alternate-site burns.

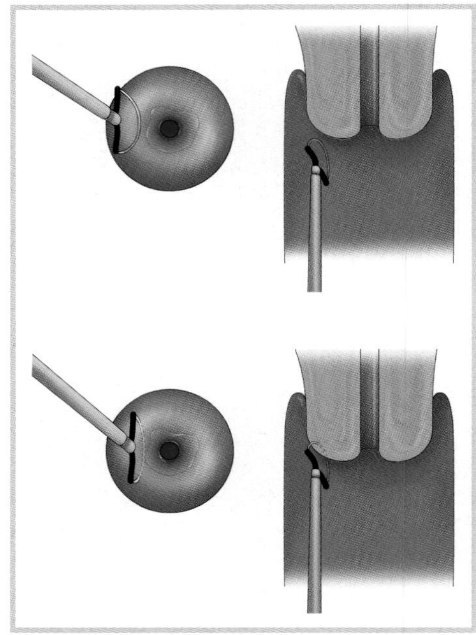

Step 7

Step 8. Draw the loop slowly through the tissue until the loop is 2 to 5 mm past the edge of the transformation zone on the opposite side. Remove the loop perpendicularly. The average cutting time is approximately 5 to 10 seconds.

- PITFALL: The excision should be done in a single, smooth motion with continuous current. Stopping the cutting current before the excision is completed causes extensive thermal injury and may damage the loop.

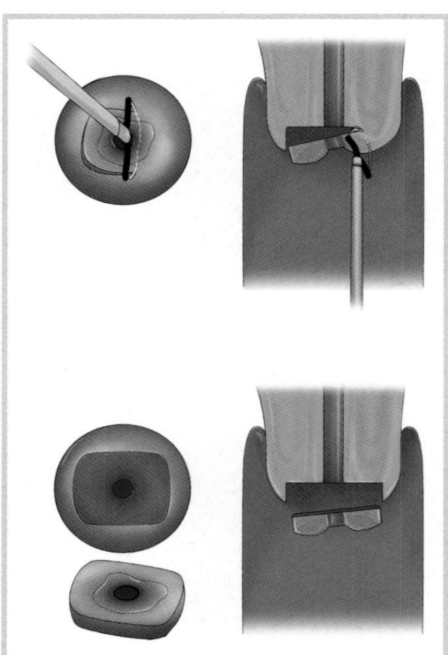

Step 8

Step 9. Remove the specimen with the loop or ring forceps and immediately place the specimen in formalin. Endocervical curettage (ECC) is recommended by many experts at this point, especially if one was not performed during the preceding colposcopy.

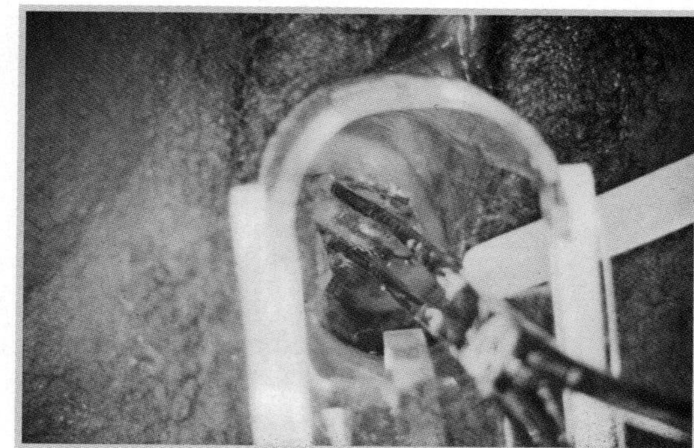

Step 9

Step 10. Superficial fulguration is usually applied to the entire crater (being careful to not fulgurate the cervical os) and to any spots of point hemorrhage. The normal edge of the defect (lateral margin) is always fulgurated.

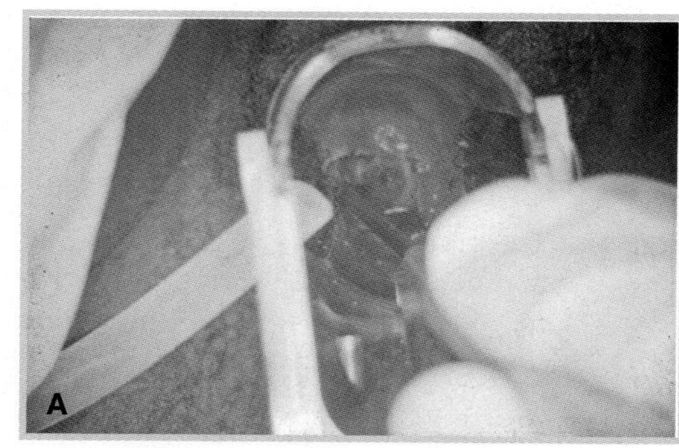

A

B

Step 10

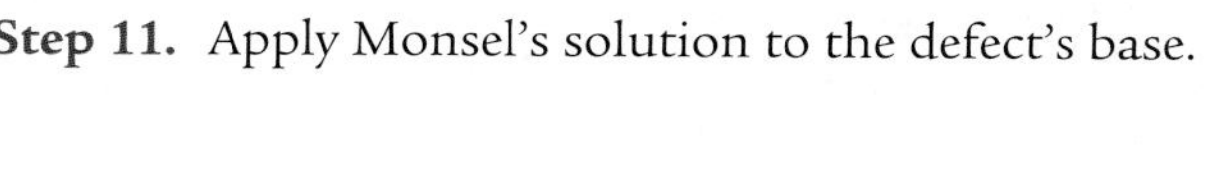

Step 11. Apply Monsel's solution to the defect's base.

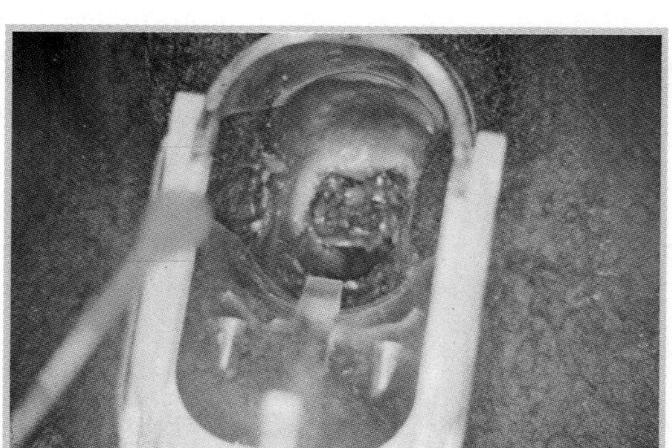

Step 11

Step 12. LEEP conization, also known as the "cowboy hat" procedure, can be performed when an excision into the canal is required. The technique is often used when a lesion extends into the endocervical canal. The cervix is anesthetized as described earlier, except that an additional 0.5 to 2 mL of lidocaine is infiltrated at the 6- and 12-o'clock positions around the os to a depth of approximately 1 cm.

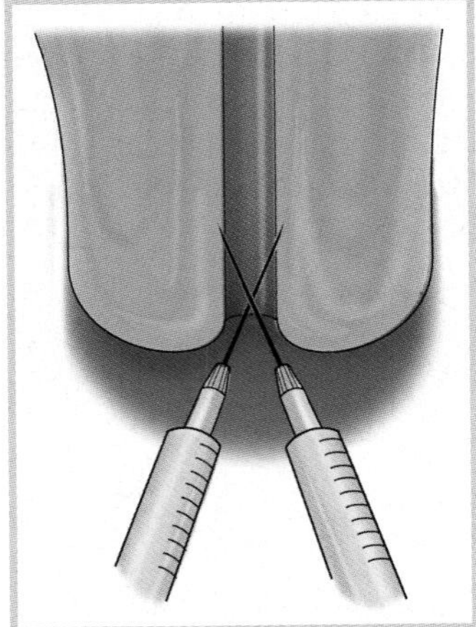

Step 12

Step 13. The transformation zone is excised in the manner described previously. Then, the distal endocervical canal can be excised an additional 9 to 10 mm, usually with a 10 × 10-mm loop or square electrode.

- **PITFALL:** Orientation of the specimen is necessary for the pathologist to be able to determine if the deep margin is involved with dysplasia.
- **PITFALL:** Avoid extending the excision into or past the internal cervical os. The depth of the remaining canal may be assessed after ectocervical excision by placing an instrument or sound into the canal.

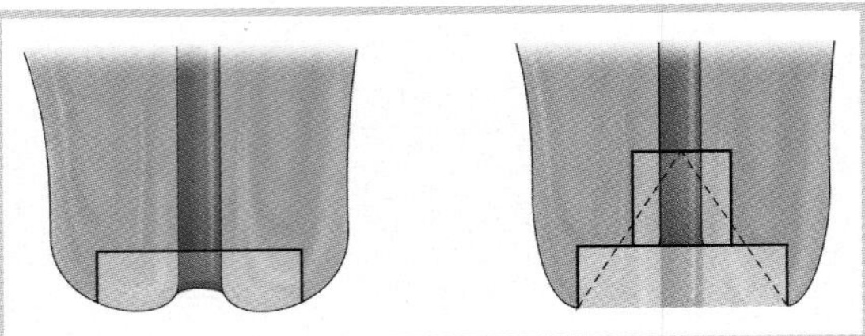

Step 13

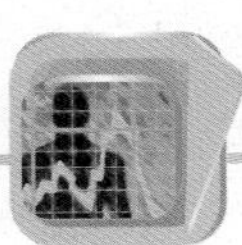

Complications

- Burns in the vaginal vault are usually caused by poor visualization or operator inexperience. There is also a risk of burns through alternate grounding sites or under the pad due to poor return electrode contact. Most of the latter two sources of burns have been eliminated with modern return electrode monitoring. When testing the loop before the procedure, avoid inadvertent contact with the patient.
- When excising the transformation zone with the LEEP procedure, perioperative bleeding is rare, especially with the use of fulguration and Monsel's solution.
- Significant late bleeding has been reported in 0% to 14% of patients who had LEEP therapy. Most did not require hospitalization and were treated with vaginal packing or suturing. This compares well with bleeding rates for laser therapy and for cryotherapy. Infection has been reported in 0% to 8% of patients.

- A less common complication found in larger studies was cervical stenosis (0.5% to 4% of cases). Rarely, cervical os obliteration was reported. These complications occurred mainly with multiple procedures and deep removal of extensive lesions. Two grams of intravaginal estrogen placed after LEEP conization in postmenopausal women protects against os stenosis and obliteration.
- The risk of incompetent cervix and sterility are included in informed consent by some practitioners for theoretical reasons, but there are no published clinical data to support this.
- LEEP conization has been found to have a higher complication rate than LEEP excision of the transformation zone.

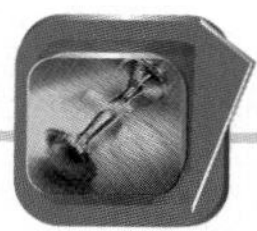

Pediatric Considerations

Because Pap smear screening is not recommended until a patient has been sexually active for 3 years or is 21 years of age, this procedure is not commonly performed in the pediatric population. Also, treatment recommendations are much more conservative in this population.

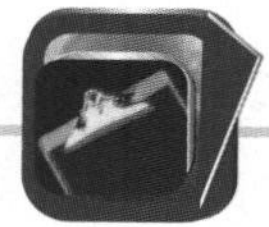

Postprocedure Instructions

Instruct the patient to refrain from sexual intercourse, douching, and tampon use for 2 to 4 weeks. A discharge is expected for 2 to 3 weeks, but it may last up to 6 weeks. The patient should report any significant bleeding or malodorous vaginal discharge. A follow-up Pap smear with or without colposcopy should be scheduled for 6 months later.

Patients are instructed to return for results of the pathologic examination. A report indicating no dysplasia should be interpreted as showing that the sample had a clear margin, not that no dysplasia was present. Small internal lesions may be missed by pathology. Patients with no dysplasia in the resection margins may be followed with Pap smears, colposcopy, or both every 6 months until two negative exams are obtained. Routine yearly screening may then be resumed, although the patient is at high risk for developing lower genital tract dysplasia for at least 20 years. Any sign of recurrence requires repeat colposcopic examination.

Because the recurrence rate with positive margins is about 25%, immediate retreatment is usually not necessary. A positive ECC result after a LEEP cone or LEEP procedure should have close follow-up, usually with colposcopy with directed biopsy and ECC, or referral for conization. It is important to check for recurrences deep in the os (i.e., skip lesions) and along the edge of the original LEEP cut. Patients with biopsy-proven recurrent lesions should be offered retreatment or hysterectomy. Women infected with human immunodeficiency virus (HIV) have high rates of recurrent and persistent CIN despite standard therapy, and low levels of CD4-positive T cells and margin involvement are risk factors for recurrence. The use of highly active antiretroviral therapy (HAART) is associated with a lower risk of recurrence, persistence, and progression of CIN.

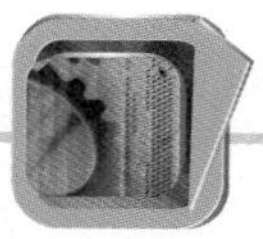

Coding Information and Supply Sources

CPT Code	Description	2008 Average 50th Percentile Fee	Global Period
57460	Colposcopy of cervix with LEEP biopsy	$1,012.00	0
57461	Colposcopy of cervix with LEEP conization	$1,098.00	0
57522	Conization of the cervix with LEEP	$1,178.00	90

2008 average 50th Percentile Fees are provided courtesy of 2008 MMH-SI's copyrighted Physicians' Fees and Coding Guide.

ICD-9 Codes

622.10	Dysplasia of cervix (uteri) unspecified
622.11	**CIN 1** – mild dysplasia of cervix (uteri)
622.12	**CIN 2** – moderate dysplasia of cervix (uteri)
233.1	**CIN 3** – severe dysplasia of cervix (uteri) (CIS)

Suppliers

LEEP units and associated materials may be obtained from:

- Cooper Surgical, Shelton, CT (phone: 800-645-3760 or 203-929-6321; www.coopersurgical.com)
- Ellman International, Inc., Hewlett, NY (phone: 1-800-835 5355 or 516-569-1482; www.ellman.com)
- Olympus America, Inc., Melville, NY (phone: 800-548-555 or 631-844-5000; www.olympusamerica.com)
- Utah Medical Products, Inc., Mid-vale, UT (phone: 800-533-4984 or 801-566-1200; www.utahmed.com)
- Wallach Surgical Devices, Inc., Orange, CT (phone: 203-799-2000 or 800-243-2463; www.wallachsurgical.com)

Patient Education Handout

Patient education handouts, **"The LEEP Procedure"** and **"LEEP Home Care Instructions"** can be found on the book's Web site.

Bibliography

Althuisius SM, Schornagel IJ, Dekker GA, et al. Loop electrosurgical excision procedure of the cervix and time of delivery in subsequent pregnancy. *Intl Gynaecol Obstet.* 2001;72:31–34.

Bigrigg A, Haffenden DK, Sheeham AL, et al. Efficacy and safety of large loop excision of the transformation zone. *Lancet.* 1994;343:32–34.

Buxton EJ, Luesley DM, Shafi MI, et al. Colposcopy directed punch biopsy: a potentially misleading investigation. *Br J Obstet Gynaecol.* 1991;98:1273–1276.

Duggan BD, Felix JC, Muderspach LI, et al. Cold-knife conization versus conization by the loop electrosurgical excision procedure: a randomized, prospective study. *Am J Obstet Gynecol.* 1999;180:276–282.

Felix JC, Muderspach LI, Duggan BD, et al. The significance of positive margins in loop electrosurgical cone biopsies. *Obstet Gynecol.* 1994;84:996–1000.

Ferris DG, Rainer BL, Pfenninger JL, et al. Electrosurgical loop excision of the cervical transformation zone: the experience of family physicians. *J Fam Pract.* 1995;41:337–344.

Gonzalez DI Jr, Zahn CM, Retzloff MG, et al. Recurrence of dysplasia after loop electrosurgical excision procedures with long-term follow-up. *Am J Obstet Gynecol.* 2001;184:315–321.

Holschneider CH, Ghosh K, Montz FJ. See-and-treat in the management of high-grade squamous intraepithelial lesions of the cervix: a resource utilization analysis. *Obstet Gynecol.* 1999;94:377–385.

Kyrgiou M, Koliopoulos G, Martin-Hirsch P, et al. Obstetric outcomes after conservative treatment for intraepithelial or early invasive cervical lesions: Systematic review and meta-analysis. *Lancet.* 2006;367:489–498.

Kyrgiou M, Tsoumpou I, Vrekoussis T, et al. The up-to-date evidence on colposcopy practice and treatment of cervical intraepithelial neoplasia: The Cochrane colposcopy and cervical cytopathology collaborative group (C5 group) approach. *Cancer Treat Rev.* 2006;32:516–523.

Kobak WH, Roman LD, Felix JC, et al. The role of endocervical curettage at cervical conization for high-grade dysplasia. *Obstet Gynecol.* 1995;85:197–201.

Mathevet P, Dargent D, Roy M, et al. A randomized prospective study comparing three techniques of conization: cold knife, LASER, and LEEP. *Gynecol Oncol.* 1994;54:175–179.

Mayeaux EJ Jr, Harper MB. Loop electrosurgical excisional procedure. *J Fam Pract.* 1993:36: 214–219.

Mitchel MF, Tortolero-Luna G, Cook E, et al. A randomized clinical trial of cryotherapy, laser vaporization, loop electrosurgical excision for treatment of squamous intraepithelial lesions of the cervix. *Obstet Gynecol.* 1998;92:737–744.

Murdoch JB, Morgan PR, Lopes A, et al. Histological incomplete excision of CIN after large loop excision of the transformation zone (LLETZ) merits careful follow up, not retreatment. *Br J Obstet Gynaecol.* 1992;99:990–993.

Naumann RW, Bell MC, Alvarez RD, et al. LLETZ is an acceptable alternative to diagnostic cold-knife conization. *Gynecol Oncol.* 1994;55:224–228.

Paraskevaidis E, Lolis ED, Koliopoulos G, et al. Cervical intraepithelial neoplasia outcomes after large loop excision with clear margins. *Obstet Gynecol.* 2000;95:828–831.

Prentice ME, Dinh TA, Smith ER, et al. The predictive value of endocervical curettage and loop conization margins for persistent cervical intraepithelial neoplasia. *J Low Genital Tract Dis.* 2000;4:155.

Sadler L, Saftlas A, Wang W, et al. Treatment for cervical intraepithelial neoplasia and risk of preterm delivery. *JAMA.* 2004;291:2100–2106.

Samson SL, Bentley JR, Fahey TJ, et al. The effect of loop electrosurgical excision procedure on future pregnancy outcome. *Obstet Gynecol.* 2005;105:325–332.

Sawchuck WS, Webber PJ, Lowy DR, et al. Infectious papillomavirus in the vapor of warts treated with carbon dioxide laser or electrocoagulation: detection and protection. *J Am Acad Dermatol.* 1989;21:41–49.

Spitzer M. Vaginal estrogen administration to prevent cervical os obliteration following cervical conization in women with amenorrhea. *J Low Genital Tract Dis* 1997;1:53–56.

Williams FS, Roure RM, Till M, et al. Treatment of cervical carcinoma in situ in HIV positive women. *Int J Gynaecol Obstet.* 2000;71:135–139.

Wright TC, Massad LS, Dunton CJ, et al. 2006 consensus guidelines for the management of women with abnormal cervical cancer screening tests. *Am J Obstet Gynecol.* 2007;197(4): 346–355.

Wright TC Jr, Massad LS, Dunton CJ, et al. 2006 consensus guidelines for the management of women with cervical intraepithelial neoplasia or adenocarcinoma in situ. *Am J Obstet Gynecol.* 2007;197:340–345.

2008 MAG Mutual Healthcare Solutions, Inc.'s Physicians' Fee and Coding Guide. Duluth, Georgia. MAG Mutual Healthcare Solutions, Inc. 2007.

CHAPTER 81

Office Hysteroscopy

Jay M. Berman, MD, FACOG

Assistant Professor, Wayne State University School of Medicine
Department of Obstetrics and Gynecology, Hutzel Women's Hospital, Detroit, MI

Valerie I. Shavell, MD

Resident, Department of Obstetrics and Gynecology
Wayne State University School of Medicine, Detroit, MI

The first hysteroscopic procedure was performed by Pantaleoni in 1869; however, the technique did not gain popularity until the 1970s. Outpatient hysteroscopy first became possible in the 1990s with the advent of newer hysteroscopes designed with a diameter of <5 mm. Office hysteroscopy is an invaluable procedure that enables direct visualization of the uterine cavity as well as localization of intrauterine pathology. The procedure may be performed for diagnostic or operative reasons. The primary purpose of office hysteroscopy is the evaluation of abnormal uterine bleeding.

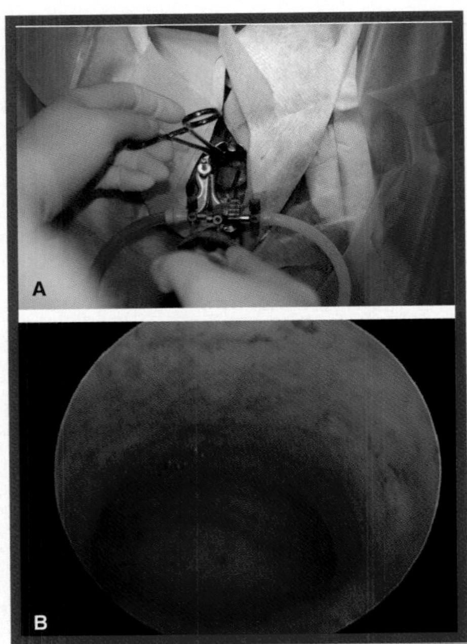

There are two varieties of office hysteroscopes. There are small, 4- to 5-mm rigid hysteroscopes and 3.1- to 3.5-mm flexible units. Both the rigid and the flexible hysteroscope may be utilized without difficulty in the office setting. The learning curve for the procedure is rather steep. Typically, only three to five procedures are needed for a provider to master the technique. The procedure is ordinarily completed within 15 to 30 minutes with very few complications. Valuable information can be gained from this safe and effective office procedure.

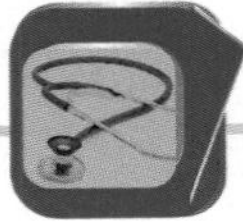

Equipment

- Hysteroscope (rigid or flexible), 30, 12, or 0 degree
- Hysteroscopic instruments (e.g., scissors, grasping forceps, biopsy forceps)
- Light source and light cord
- Camera (optional)
- Monitor (optional)
- Bags of normal saline (1 or 3 L), pressure cuff (80 to 150 mm Hg), and tubing
- Sterile gloves

- Cervical speculum (bivalve or weighted) in appropriate sizes
- Cervical tenaculum
- Small cervical dilators (only used if absolutely necessary)
- Sterile gauze, 2 × 2 or 4 × 4 inches
- Prep bowl and sterile povidone-iodine solution
- Local anesthetic for paracervical block (i.e., 1% lidocaine)
- Syringe and 22-gauge spinal needle
- Sterile drapes

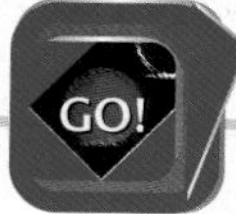

Indications

- Evaluation of abnormal uterine bleeding
- Diagnosis and treatment of intrauterine lesions (e.g., polyps, fibroids)
- Investigation of infertility or recurrent miscarriage
- Diagnosis and treatment of intrauterine adhesions or uterine septa
- Location and removal of intrauterine devices or foreign bodies
- Evaluation of endometrial hyperplasia
- Hysteroscopic sterilization (Essure)

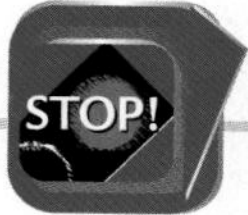

Contraindications

- Current pregnancy
- Heavy uterine bleeding
- Current pelvic inflammatory disease
- Cervical cancer

Procedure

Step 1. Assemble the required equipment in the examination or procedure room. The patient is placed in the dorsal lithotomy position on the procedure table, and the vagina is prepped with a sterile povidone-iodine solution using sterile gauze. Sterile drapes may be used but are not required. A pelvic examination is then performed.

- **PEARL:** Thirty minutes prior to the procedure, the patient may take ibuprofen (600 to 800 mg) or any other comparable nonsteroidal anti-inflammatory drug (NSAID) to decrease pain and cramping during the procedure.
- **PEARL:** Routine catheterization of the bladder is not required. Patients should be instructed to void just prior to starting the procedure.

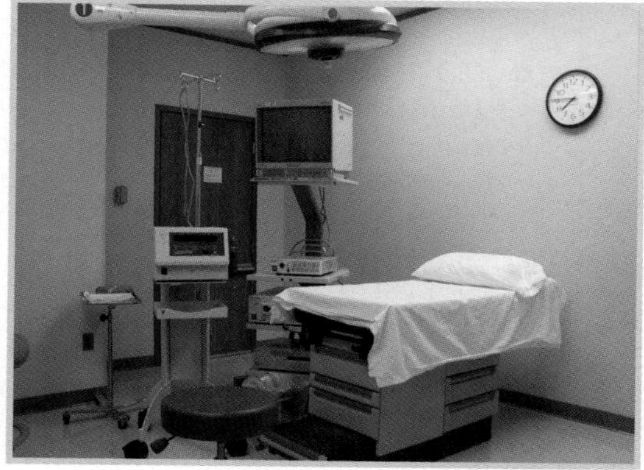

Step 1

Step 2. The cervix is visualized with the assistance of a bivalve or weighted speculum, and a tenaculum is used to grasp the anterior lip of the cervix. If desired, 1% lidocaine or other local anesthetic may be injected into the cervix to provide a paracervical block (refer to Chapter 82).

- **PEARL:** While you are waiting for the paracervical block to take effect, assemble the hysteroscope and begin the next step.
- **PEARL:** A 30-degree hysteroscope is necessary for the Essure procedure. Diagnostic procedures can be performed with 0-, 12-, or 30-degree hysteroscopes. The angle must be considered when inserting the scope and evaluating the cavity.

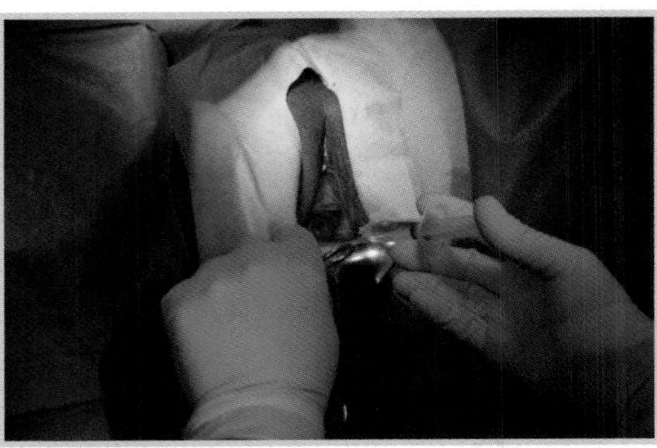

Step 2

Step 3. A 1- or 3-L bag of normal saline in an 80- to 150-mm Hg pressure cuff is attached to the hysteroscope. The saline is used to distend the uterine cavity, enabling visualization of the entire surface of the endometrium. A minimum of 30 mm Hg is needed to separate the uterine walls.

- **PEARL:** Other distending media may be used (e.g., Ringer's lactate, Hartmann's solution, Hyskon (32% dextran 70 in dextrose, CooperSurgical, Trumbull, CT), glycine, sorbitol, mannitol, or CO_2); however, normal saline is the distending media of choice because of its low cost and safety profile.
- **PITFALL:** CO_2 is convenient, cost-effective, and easy on instruments but cannot be used if there is any bleeding. It limits the provider to diagnostic procedures.
- **PEARL:** Most cavities can be assessed using gravity-fed saline on an intravenous (IV) pole. It is much easier to evaluate the endometrium with lower pressures. Flexible hysteroscopes can be used with saline solution in 50-cc syringes.
- **PITFALL:** Excessive pressure can result in significant absorption of fluid through the endometrium and out through the tubes. Use the least amount that will let you visualize the endometrium. Usually 50 to 80 mm Hg is adequate.

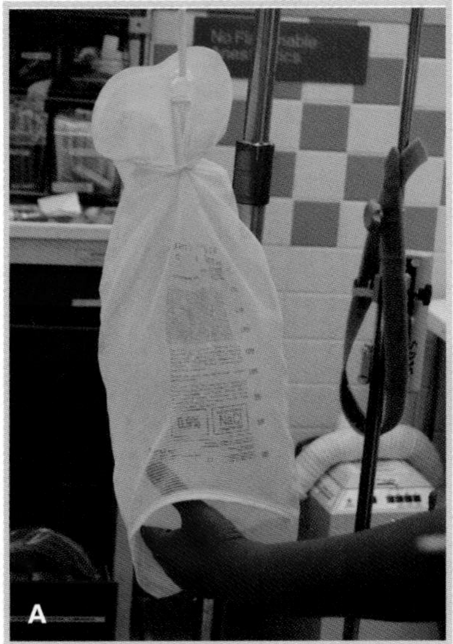

A

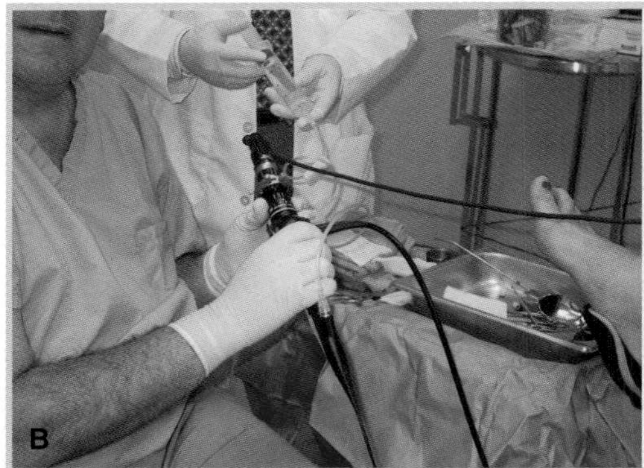

B

Step 3

Step 4. The hysteroscope is inserted into the endocervical canal. If necessary, a small cervical dilator is used to facilitate entry of the hysteroscope.

- **PITFALL:** Uterine sounds and dilators are usually not necessary for small 3- to 5.5-mm scopes. In fact, they lead to perforation and bleeding that make evaluation of the endometrium difficult to impossible. Do not use the sound.

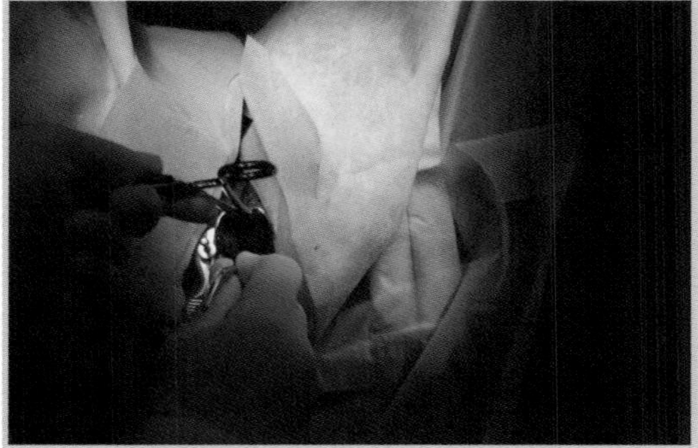

Step 4

- **PEARL:** Pratt dilators are marked in French (circumference). Hysteroscopes and sheaths are marked in millimeters (diameter). Working channels (operating channels) and instruments are marked in French. Only the smallest dilators are needed. A 5.5-mm sheath needs only a 15 Pratt (15-French) dilator. Flexible scopes (3.1 mm) rarely need a 9 Pratt (9-French) dilator.
- **PITFALL:** Failure to identify a retroverted uterus may result in inadvertent uterine perforation during cervical dilation or insertion of the hysteroscope. If perforation occurs, immediately terminate the procedure and observe the patient.

Step 5. The hysteroscope is introduced through the cervix into the uterine cavity with inflow turned on and a small amount of outflow if using a continuous flow hysteroscope. A panoramic view of the cavity is noted. Thoroughly inspect the endometrial cavity for abnormalities such as polyps, fibroids, septations, and adhesions. The endometrium should be thoroughly assessed for thickness and vascularity.

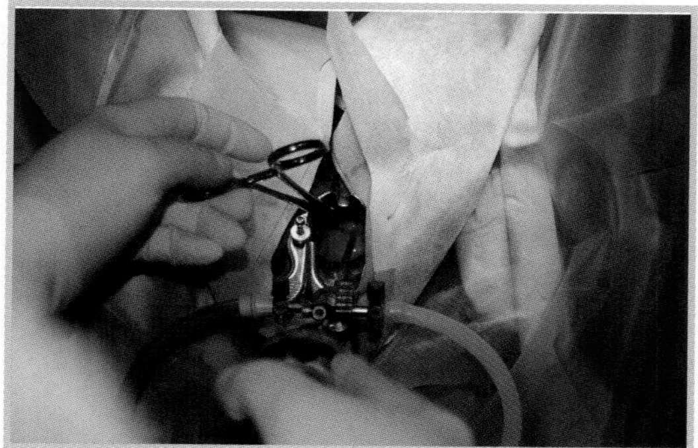

Step 5

- **PEARL:** Keep the camera in a vertical orientation as the scope is rotated. This is an absolute must to maintain visual orientation, especially if any operative procedures are contemplated.
- **PEARL:** Advancing the hysteroscope through the endocervical canal and into the endometrial cavity with visualization will decrease the chances of perforation.

Step 6. Advance the hysteroscope into the endometrial cavity and rotate the light cord to the right to view the right tubal ostium and corneal area.

- **PEARL:** Take advantage of the fore oblique angle of the hysteroscope and rotate the hysteroscope to view all areas. Do not angle the scope to view the entire endometrial cavity.
- **PITFALL:** It is easy to lose orientation in a large endometrial cavity, especially with large fibroids, polyps, or a thick endometrium. Return to the internal os and tubal ostia to regain orientation.
- **PEARL:** Use a standard protocol for evaluation. Start with the endocervical canal, internal os, panoramic uterine cavity, right cornu, anterior uterine wall, left cornu, posterior uterine wall. This necessitates turning a 12- or 30-degree scope to visualize each area. If using a pressure bag, repeat with decreased pressure to evaluate

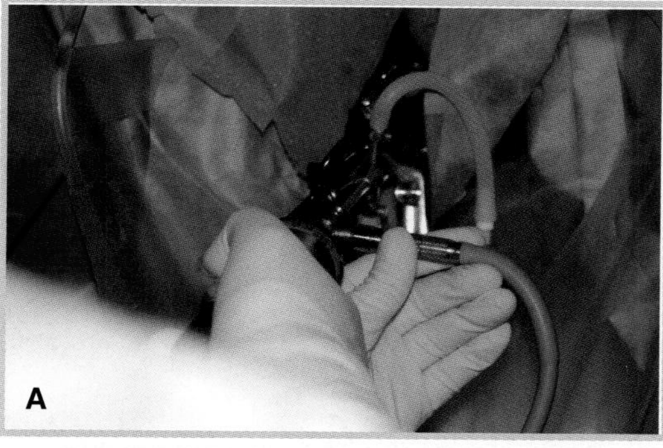

A

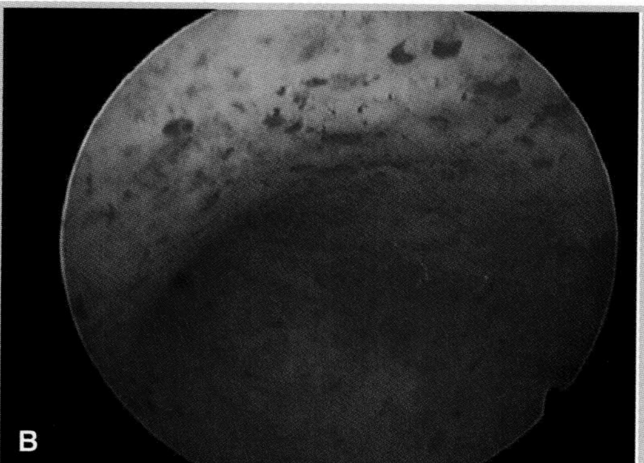

B

Step 6

endometrial thickness and contour. This may reveal hidden fibroids or polyps.

- **PITFALL:** Prolonged operative hysteroscopy may result in an excessive fluid deficit that can cause electrolyte abnormalities and pulmonary edema. Watch for nausea, confusion, seizures, and respiratory distress.

Step 7. Return to vertical and inspect the anterior endometrial cavity

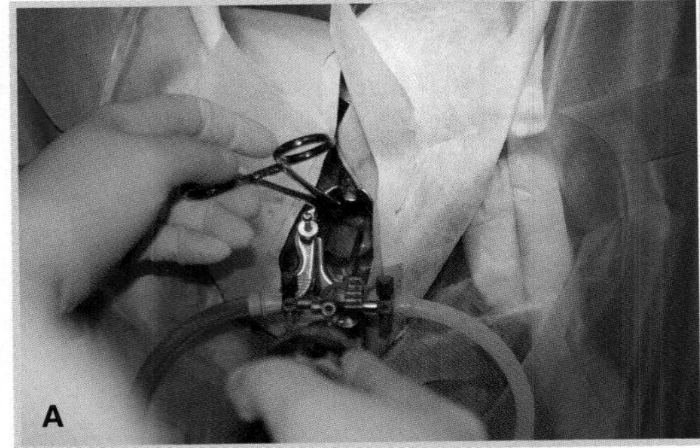

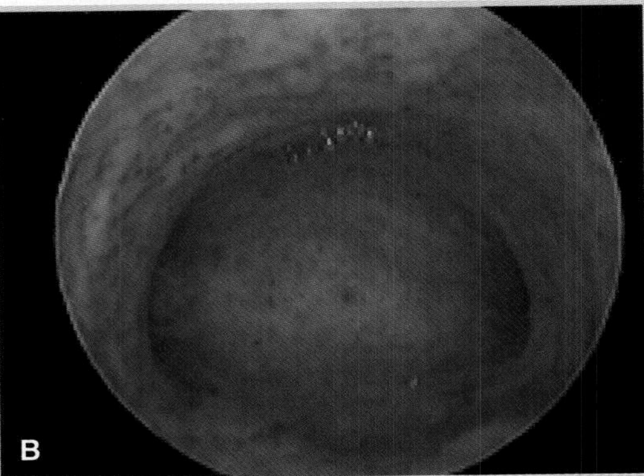

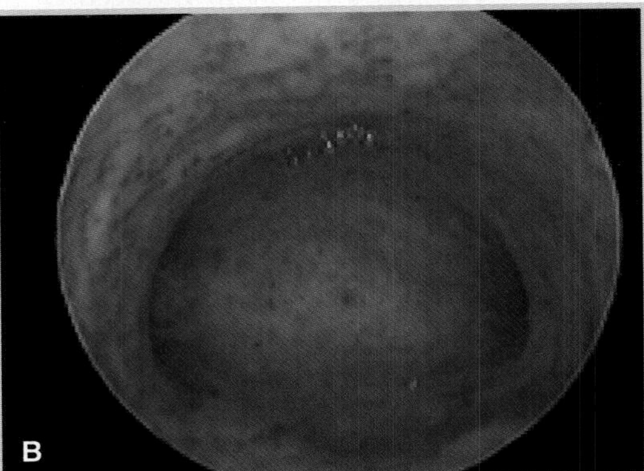

Step 7

Step 8. Rotate the hysteroscope to the left to view the left tubal ostium and corneal area.

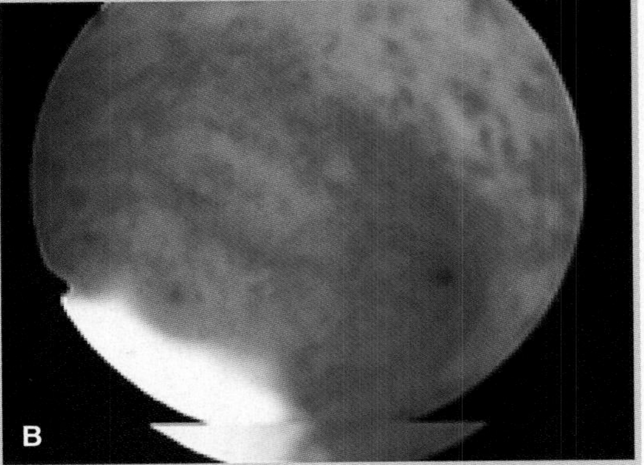

Step 8

Step 9. Rotate the hysteroscope downward to view the posterior portion of the endometrial cavity.

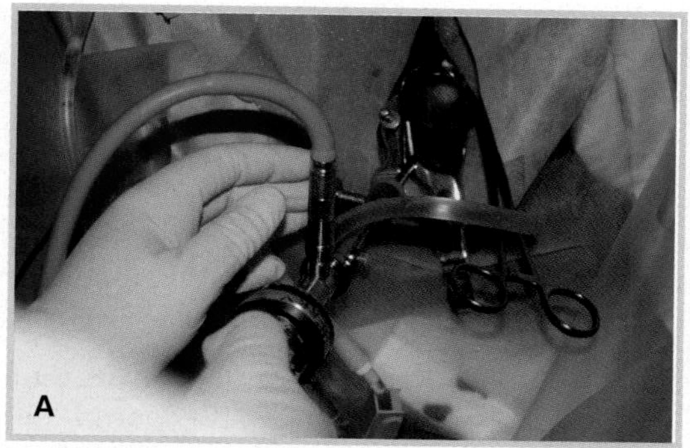

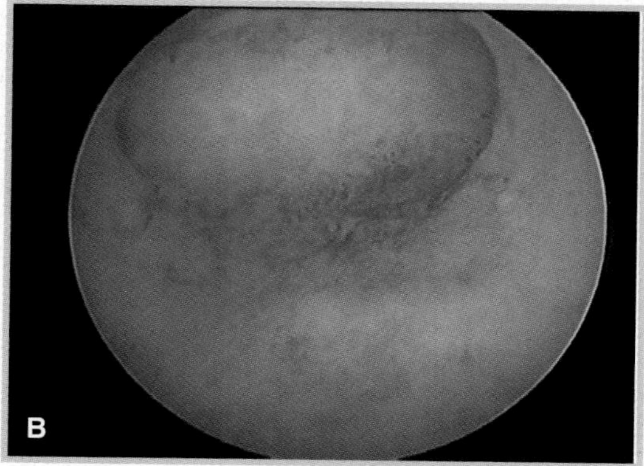

Step 9

Step 10. Rotate the hysteroscope to look upward as at the start.

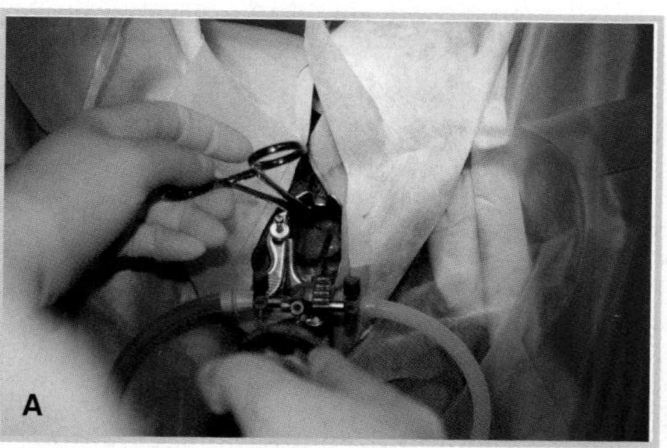

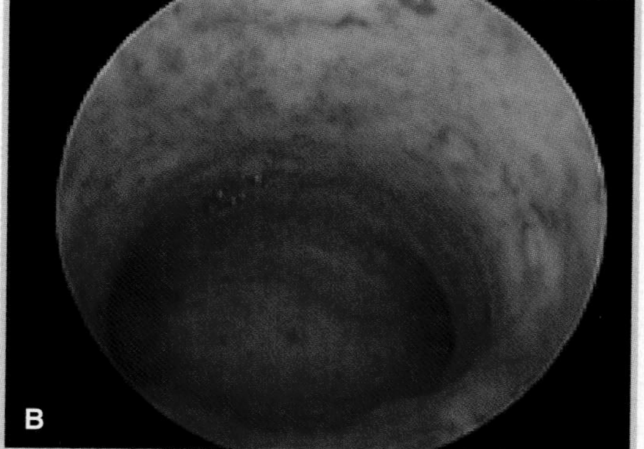

Step 10

Step 11. If a pressure bag has been used, reduce the pressure in the uterine cavity and repeat steps 8 to 12.

- **PEARL:** This is an important step in hysteroscopy. It allows the provider to gain as much information as possible from the procedure. Small polyps and fibroids may now become visible with the reduced pressure.
- **PEARL:** Use a combination of inflow and outflow changes to control distention. The provider will be amazed at how much information can be obtained.
- **PITFALL:** The endometrium will become edematous with prolonged procedures and multiple pressure changes. Most information is obtained in the first 5 minutes of the procedure.
- **PEARL:** Use the angle view to your advantage. Rotate the scope to view the tubal ostia and anterior and posterior walls. This limits manipulation of the hysteroscope in the cervix and vagina and decreases discomfort.

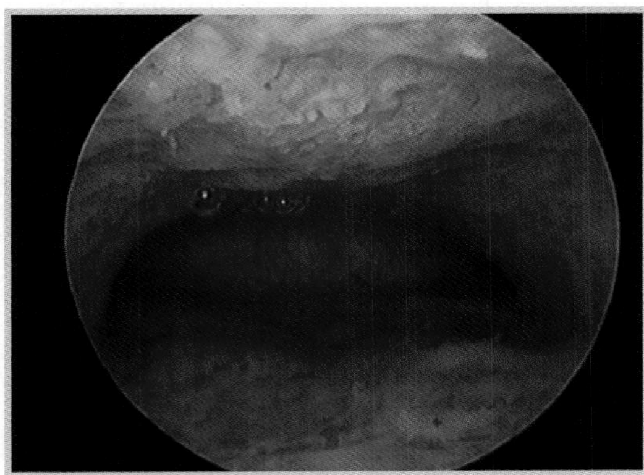

Step 11

Step 12. At this point, operative techniques may be employed, including targeted biopsy of suspicious lesions, polypectomy, and removal of small submucosal fibroids using scissors or grasping forceps passed down the operating channel. Intrauterine adhesions may be divided with scissors, and intrauterine devices or foreign bodies may be located and extracted with grasping forceps. Essure hysteroscopic sterilization may also be performed (refer to Chapter 75). At the completion of the procedure, all instrumentation is removed from the vagina.

- **PEARL:** A small amount of bleeding from the tenaculum site and cervix is expected. Thus, a sanitary napkin should be provided.

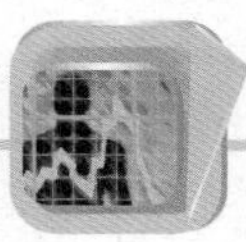

Complications

- Bleeding
- Infection
- Uterine perforation
- Cervical trauma
- Pain
- Cramps
- Anesthetic reactions (see Chapter 82)

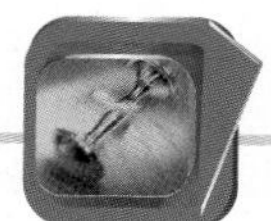

Pediatric Considerations

Office hysteroscopy should not be performed in the pediatric population. If hysteroscopy is necessary, the procedure should be performed in a hospital setting where appropriate anesthesia may be administered.

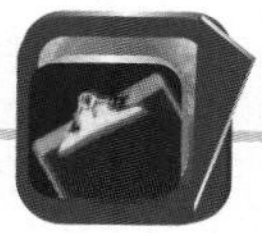

Postprocedure Instructions

Patients may experience vaginal bleeding and mild abdominal cramping after the procedure. Patients are advised to take ibuprofen (600 to 800 mg) every 6 to 8 hours as needed for pain. Pelvic rest for 1 week is advised. Patients should be instructed to notify their provider if they experience fevers, heavy vaginal bleeding, or severe cramping that is unrelieved by pain medication.

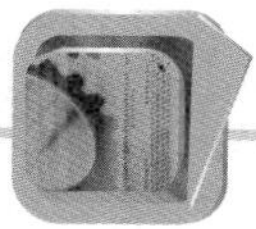

Coding Information and Supply Sources

Office hysteroscopes are available from Olympus, Karl Storz, Richard Wolf, ACMI, and many smaller makers. Most companies can arrange a compact mobile system with or without video systems. They also sell under-buttock drapes and pouches to capture excess fluid. There are also numerous leasing companies that will supply equipment long term or by the case.

The remainder of the equipment is available through general medical suppliers.

CPT Code	Description	2008 Average 50th Percentile Fee	Global Period
58555	Hysteroscopy, diagnostic (separate procedure)	$1,018.00	0
58558	Hysteroscopy, surgical; with sampling (biopsy) of endometrium and/or polypectomy, with or without D&C	$1,613.00	0
58559	Hysteroscopy, surgical; with lysis of intrauterine adhesions (any method)	$1,894.00	0
58560	Hysteroscopy, surgical; with division or resection of intrauterine septum (any method)	$2,146.00	0
58561	Hysteroscopy, surgical; with removal of leiomyomata	$2,831.00	0
58562	Hysteroscopy, surgical; with removal of impacted foreign body	$1,596.00	0
58563	Hysteroscopy, surgical; with endometrial ablation (e.g., endometrial resection, ' electrosurgical ablation, thermoablation)	$1,889.00	0
58565	Hysteroscopy, surgical; with bilateral fallopian tube cannulation to induce occlusion by placement of permanent implants	$2,319.50	90

CPT is a registered trademark of the American Medical Association.
2008 average 50th Percentile Fees are provided courtesy of 2008 MMH-SI's copyrighted Physicians' Fees and Coding Guide.
Note that paracervical block is not reimbursed by Medicare when used in conjunction with these codes.

Patient Education Handout

A patient education handout, "Office Hysteroscopy," can be found on the book's companion Web site.

Bibliography

Bakour SH, Jones SE, O'Donovan P. Ambulatory hysteroscopy: evidence-based guide to diagnosis and therapy. *Best Pract Res Clin Obstet Gynaecol.* 2006;20:953–975.

Campo R, Van Belle Y, Rombauts L, et al. Office mini-hysteroscopy. *Hum Reprod Update.* 1999;5:73–81.

Isaacson K. Office hysteroscopy: a valuable but under-utilized technique. *Curr Opin Obstet Gynecol.* 2002;14:381–385.

2008 MAG Mutual Healthcare Solutions, Inc.'s Physicians' Fee and Coding Guide. Duluth, Georgia. MAG Mutual Healthcare Solutions, Inc. 2007.

CHAPTER 82

Paracervical Block Anesthesia

Jay M. Berman, MD, FACOG
Assistant Professor, Department of Obstetrics and Gynecology, Wayne State University School of Medicine, Hutzel Women's Hospital, Detroit, MI

Samantha E. Montgomery, MD
Resident, Department of Obstetrics and Gynecology
Wayne State University School of Medicine, Detroit, MI

Paracervical block anesthesia has been used since 1925 and was originally refined for pain management during cervical dilation for voluntary termination of pregnancy. It was a popular method of analgesia for the first stage of labor, but has since fallen out of favor in North America due to the risk of fetal bradycardia and rare reports of fetal or neonatal death related to its use. Although paracervical blocks for labor remain popular throughout the rest of the world and the incidence of fetal bradycardia has greatly declined due to the standardization of injection methods, use in North America is now repopularized for ambulatory gynecologic procedures including office hysteroscopy, manual vacuum aspiration, treatment for incomplete abortion, and loop electrosurgical excision procedure (LEEP) and laser ablation procedures.

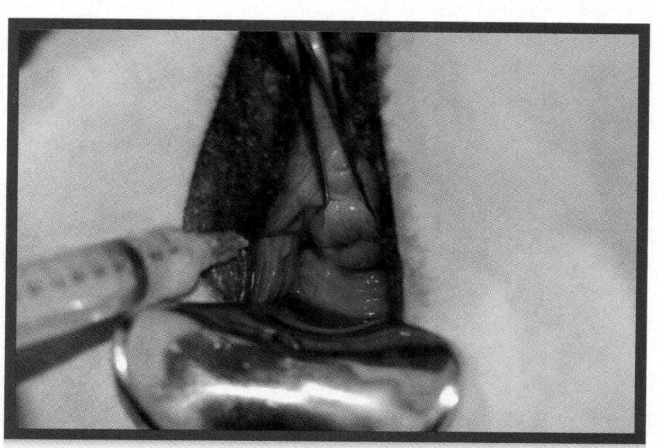

Because of the relative ease of administration, lack of special equipment and independence from the anesthesiologist, the paracervical block lends itself well to outpatient gynecologic surgery.

Innervation of the uterine cervix arises from the Lee-Frankenhäuser plexus, which is located lateral to the junction of the cervix and uterus at the base of the broad ligament. The Frankenhäuser ganglion houses the visceral afferent nerve fibers from the upper vagina, cervix and uterus. Sensory information is then carried to the spinal cord in T10–T12 and the L1 segmental nerves. Pain signals from cervical dilatation are transmitted primarily via this plexus and may be targeted for anesthesia by paracervical block.

Local anesthetics used for paracervical block are derived from the amide class of anesthetics. These agents are metabolized by N-dealkylation and hydroxylation by microsomal P-450 enzymes in the liver and are metabolized much more slowly than agents from the ester class. Possible anesthetic choices, their strength, onset of action, duration of action and maximal dosages are outlined in Table 82-1. Ten milliliters of 1%

TABLE 82-1. Anesthetic Choices for Cervical Blocks

Anesthetic	Strength	Onset	Duration of Action	Maximal Dose
Lidocaine (Xylocaine)	1%	Rapid	45–60 min	4.5 mg/kg
2-Chloroprocaine	2%	Rapid	30–45 min	10.0 mg/kg
Bupivacaine (Marcaine)	0.25%	Slow	46–80 min	2.0 mg/kg

lidocaine or 2% chloroprocaine without epinephrine may be used for paracervical block. Bupivacaine should be used in a 0.125% dilution by mixing 50/50 with normal saline.

The toxic effects of local anesthetics are generally manifested in the central nervous system (CNS) and the cardiovascular system. Early symptoms of CNS toxicity include circumoral numbness, tongue paresthesia, and dizziness at a plasma concentration of 4 mg/mL. Blurry vision results at a plasma concentration of 6 mg/mL. With exposure to increasingly toxic doses, excitatory symptoms develop, including restlessness, agitation, nervousness, and paranoia at 8 mg/mL. This period of excitation precedes CNS depression characterized by slurred speech, drowsiness, and unconsciousness. Muscle twitching precedes the onset of tonic–clonic seizures at 10 mg/mL, and finally, respiratory arrest occurs at 20 mg/mL. Cardiovascular toxicity develops at blood levels of local anesthetic that are almost three times that required to produce seizures—approximately 26 mg/mL. For this reason, cardiovascular toxicity is generally seen only in the setting of local blocks administered to patients under general anesthesia. Intravascular administration may produce hypotension, atrioventricular heart block, idioventricular rhythms, and life-threatening arrhythmias such as ventricular tachycardia and fibrillation. In general, amide anesthetics are used for paracervical blocks. Because these agents are metabolized in the liver, any condition which decreases hepatic blood flow (congestive heart failure, vasopressors) or function (cirrhosis) increases the risk of anesthetic toxicity. Many providers use lidocaine as 1% or 2% with 1:200,000 epinephrine, which prolongs the duration of action from ≤1 hour to 2 to 6 hours. This compares to the duration of action of bupivacaine 0.25% without epinephrine and maintains lidocaine's rapid onset of action.

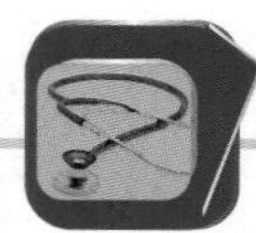

Equipment

- Gynecologic speculum of appropriate size
- Single tooth tenaculum
- Povidine-iodine solution
- Sterile cotton balls or gauze
- 10-cc syringe, control top preferred but not necessary
- 22-gauge spinal needle or needle and needle extender
- Local anesthetic of choice (see Table).
- Crash cart with appropriate medications.
- Intravenous supplies
- Automatic external defibrillator
- Pulse oximeter
- Portable or wall oxygen with mask and nasal prongs

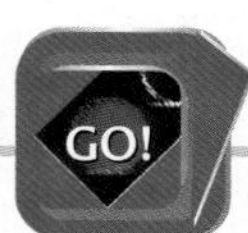

Indications

- Diagnostic hysteroscopy
- Endometrial ablation
- Hysteroscopic female sterilization

- Cervical biopsy
- LEEP. This procedure is most commonly done with intracervical block.

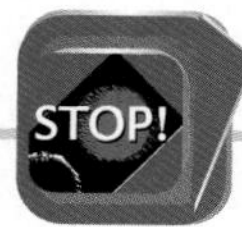

Contraindications

- Known hypersensitivity to any of the components of the anesthetic
- Hypersensitivity to the antiseptic agent
- Cardiac disease and hypertension are relative contraindications to anesthetic agents containing epinephrine.

The Procedure

Step 1. Prepare the tray of instruments including speculums, tenaculum, antiseptic, gauze.

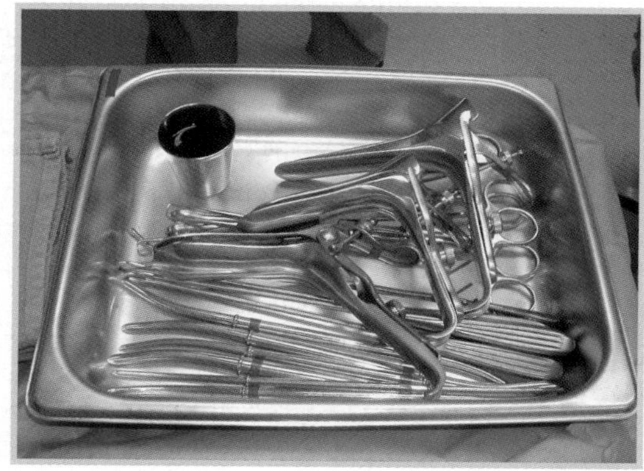

Step 1

Step 2. Fill the syringe with 10 mL of the appropriate local anesthetic (see Table 1).

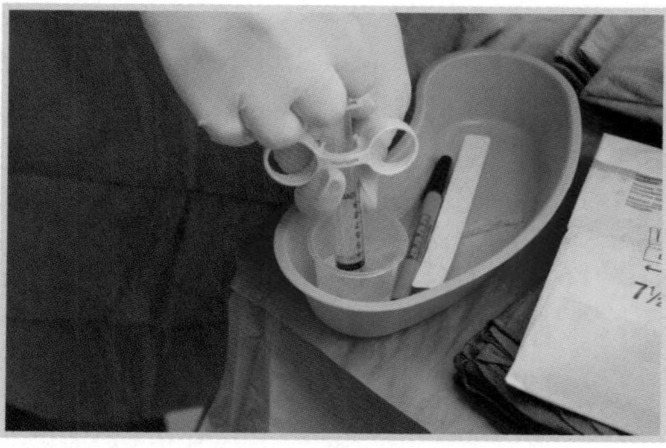

Step 2

Step 3. Attach the 22-gauge spinal needle or the 22-gauge needle with needle extender to the syringe.

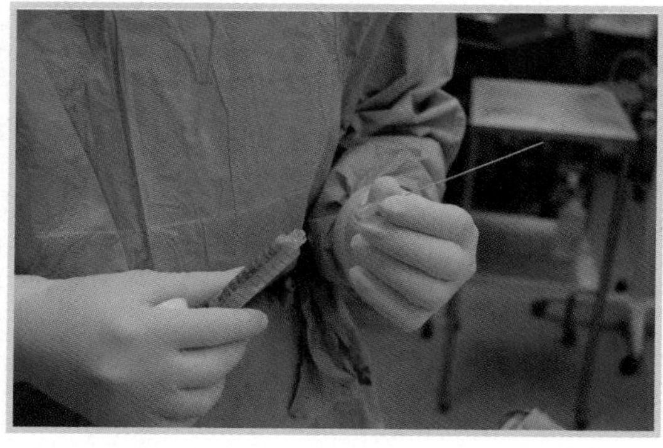

Step 3

Step 4. With the patient in the lithotomy position, the vagina and cervix are cleansed with Betadine. Exposure of the uterine cervix may then be achieved with a sterile speculum or with a weighted speculum and vaginal retractor. The sites for local anesthetic infiltration are selected. The aim is to avoid the uterine vessels and ureters that are located bilaterally at the 3- and 9-o'clock positions. Generally, injections of anesthetic at the 4- or 5- and 7- or 8-o'clock positions are sufficient.

- **PEARL:** Multiple injections at 4, 5, 7, and 8 o'clock have been shown to be no more efficacious than two injections in a randomized-controlled trial involving 82 women.

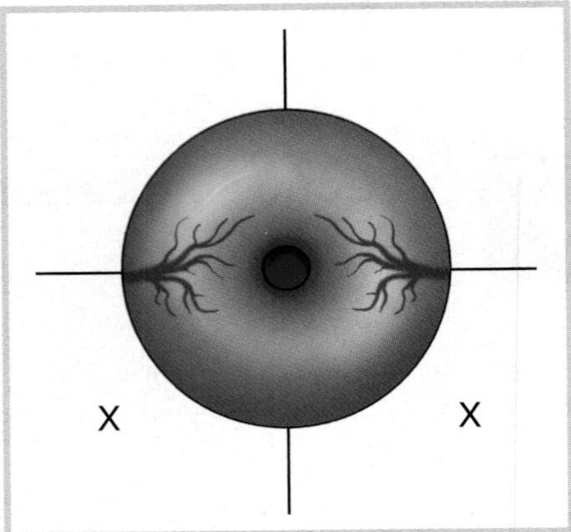

Step 4

Step 5. A 22-gauge spinal needle or 23-gauge needle with a needle extender is applied to the lateral edge of the cervix, taking care not to apply traction to the vaginal fornix as this may result in the uterine vessels being brought to a more superficial position. The needle is then advanced up to a depth of 0.5 cm, which allows infiltration of the uterosacral ligaments that carry the nerve bundles from the uterine corpus. One study found that less pain was experienced when local anesthetic was injected to a depth of 1.5 inches (3.81 cm); however, deeper injections carry the risk of intravascular injection. Most practitioners use a depth of 2 to 4 mm. This allows for palpable or visible mucosal swelling and slow intravascular absorption maximizing exposure of Frankenhäuser's plexus to the anesthetic agent.

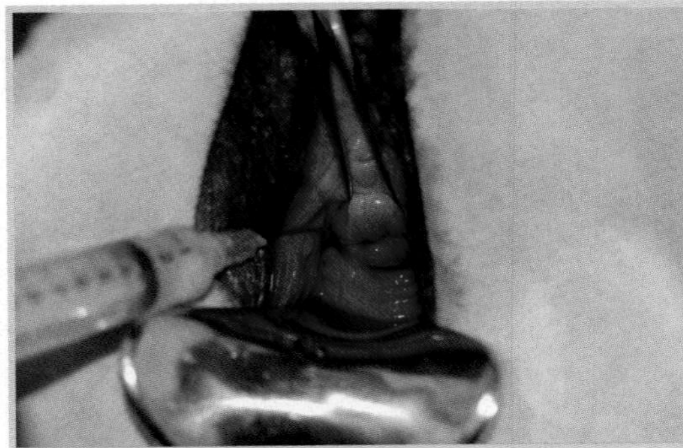

Step 5

Step 6. Aspirate prior to injection so as to avoid intravascular injection. Inject 3 to 5 mL of local anesthetic bilaterally. No more than 12 to 20 mL total should be used. Some authors support the theory that analgesia comes not from the anesthetic per se but from the volume-mediated distention of the tissues, which may exert enough pressure of the autonomic nerves to attenuate the conduction of pain fibers.

- **PITFALL:** Many failed anesthetics are due to impatience on the part of the provider. Think of your dentist giving local and then walking out of the room for 5 to 10 minutes. It is convenient to assemble all of the other procedural instruments (i.e., LEEP or Essure) only *after* the block is in place. This avoids provider impatience and starting too soon. Wait for the anesthetic to take effect before beginning the procedure.

- **PITFALL:** Inadvertent intravascular injection is the leading cause of adverse events.

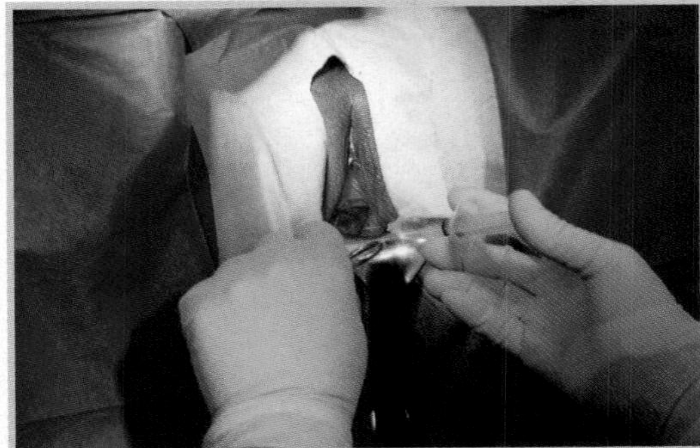

Step 6

In paracervical block, the location of the needle is close to the uterine arteries. Inadvertent vascular injections can cause CNS stimulation with seizures followed by CNS depression and possible respiratory arrest.

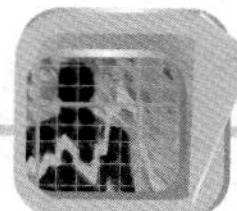

Complications

- Hypersensitivity: esters more likely than amides to elicit an allergic reaction as they are metabolized to p-aminobenzoic acid, which is a known allergen.
- If used in labor:
  - Bleeding from the vaginal fornices
  - Fetal scalp injection
  - Parametrial hematoma
  - Fetal bradycardia
  - Sacral plexus trauma
  - Fetal death
  - Infection and deep abscess formation
- CNS toxicity
- Respiratory arrest at doses of 20 mg/mL
- Cardiovascular toxicity
- Intravascular administration may produce hypotension, atrioventricular heart block, idioventricular rhythms, and life-threatening arrhythmias such as ventricular tachycardia and fibrillation

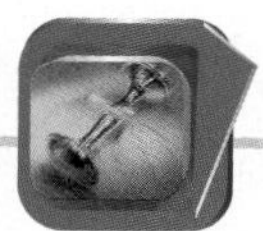

Pediatric Considerations

Paracervical block is not a useful technique in the pediatric population. Any extensive vaginal or cervical procedure in this population would require a general anesthetic.

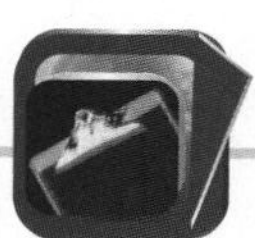

Postprocedure Instructions

Postprocedure counseling is generally not required except to state that the anesthetic effect may last for several hours after the procedure. Patients should be encouraged to start oral pain medication before the anesthetic wears off.

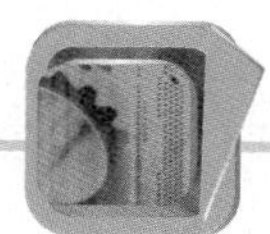

Coding Information and Supply Sources

CPT Code	Description	2008 Average 50th Percentile Fee	Global Period
64435-51	Paracervical block	$348.00	0

CPT is a registered trademark of the American Medical Association.
2008 average 50th Percentile Fees are provided courtesy of 2008 MMH-SI's copyrighted Physicians' Fees and Coding Guide.

The higher fee for in office procedures reflects the cost of the anesthetic agent and other disposables items including syringes, needles, gauze, instruments, sterilization and drapes

All of the items for this procedure are purchased from our office general medical supply such as Moore Medical or Henry Schein.

Patient Education Handout

A patient education handout, "Paracervical Block" can be found on the book's Web site.

Bibliography

Aimakhu VE, Ogunbode O. Paracervical block anesthesia for minor gynecologic surgery. *Int J Gynaecol Obstet.* 1972;10:66–71.

Glanta JC, Shomento S. Comparison of paracervical block techniques during first trimester pregnancy termination. *Int J Gynaecol Obstet.* 2001; 72:171–178.

Gomez PI, Gaitan H, Nova C, et al. Paracervical block in incomplete abortion using manual vacuum aspiration: randomized clinical trial. *Obstet Gynecol.* 2004;5:943–951.

Wiebe ER, Rawling M. Pain control in abortion. *Int J Gynaecol Obstet.* 1995;50:41–46.

Macarthur A. Other techniques for obstetric pain management. Caudal, paracervical, and pudendal blocks. *Tech Regional Anesth Pain Managt.* 2001;5:18–23.

Wiebe ER. Comparison of the efficacy of different local anesthetics and techniques of local anesthesia in therapeutic abortions. *Am J Obstet Gynecol.* 1992;167:131–140.

2008 MAG Mutual Healthcare Solutions, Inc.'s Physicians' Fee and Coding Guide. Duluth, Georgia. MAG Mutual Healthcare Solutions, Inc. 2007.

CHAPTER 83

Pessaries

Sandra M. Sulik MD, MS, FAAFP
Associate Professor Family Medicine
SUNY Upstate and St. Joseph's Family Medicine Residency, Fayetteville, NY

Amber Shaff, MD
Resident, St. Joseph's Family Medicine Residency, Syracuse, NY

Alessandra D'Avenzo, MD
Resident, St. Joseph's Family Medicine Residency, Syracuse, NY

Pessaries are effective tools in the managements of the pelvic floor prolapse (PFP) and stress urinary incontinence. PFP is more common with increasing age and is both uncomfortable and distressing for many women. It is estimated that PFP affects approximately 50% of women older than age 50, with a lifetime prevalence of 30% to 50%. Women with clinically significant PFP may complain of a sensation of a vaginal bulge that can be accompanied by symptoms of urinary, bowel, or sexual dysfunction. Nevertheless, most of these women do not seek medical advice because of the fear of cancer or simply because of embarrassment. The etiology of the PFP is complex and multifactorial. Risk factors include multiparity, childbirth, congenital or acquired connective tissue abnormalities, denervation or weakness of the pelvic floor, aging, menopause, and factors associated with chronically raised intra-abdominal pressure (i.e. constipation).

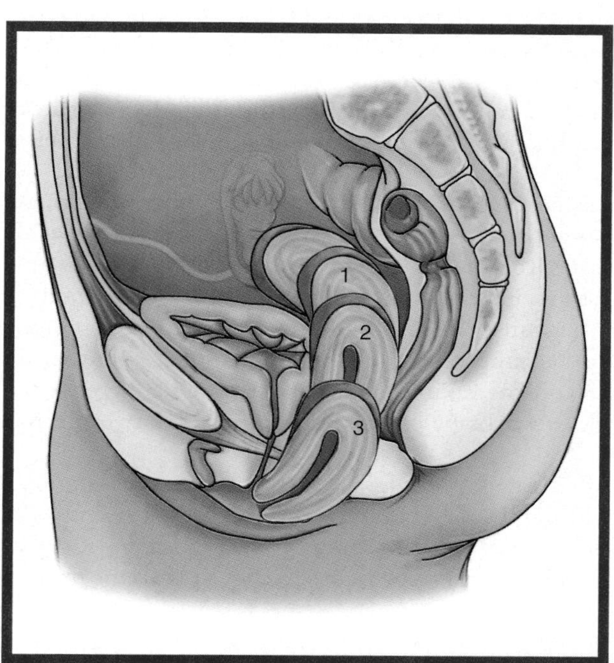

Treatment of PFP depends on the severity of the prolapse, its symptoms, and the woman's overall health. Options include conservative, mechanical, and surgical treatments. Generally, conservative or mechanical management is reserved for those women who cannot or are unwilling to have surgery or in women who have not completed child-bearing. An extensive range of mechanical devices have been described for prolapse. These consist mainly of silicone Pessaries that are inserted and left in the vagina to prevent PFP.

Uterine prolapse is classified as first degree when the cervix is visible when pushing down on the perineum, as second degree when the cervix is visible outside the vaginal introitus while the uterine fundus remains inside, and as third degree (procidentia) when the entire uterus is outside of the vaginal introitus. Uterine prolapse can lead to incontinence, vaginitis, cystitis, and possible uterine malignancy. Vaginal prolapse includes rectocele, where the rectum herniates into the posterior vaginal wall; cystocele, where the bladder herniates into the anterior vaginal wall; and vaginal vault prolapse, where any vaginal portion may prolapse.

Women who are considered poor surgical candidates because of severe co-morbidities, such as cardiovascular disease, osteoporosis with multiple compression fractures, and steroid-dependent chronic obstructive pulmonary disease are excellent candidates for pessary placement. In different surveys, 87% to 98% of practitioners reported the use pessaries in their practice and 77% as first line of treatment of PFP.

Most symptoms related to PFP, such as bulge and pressure, improve in 71% to 90% of patients with pessary use. Urgency and voiding difficulties have also been shown to improve in 40% of women. In 20% of patients, however, an occult incontinence can occur when the pessary is used. The pessary can also be used preoperatively to predict how a woman will respond to prolapse surgery. There is a risk that 4% to 6% of women will develop de novo urge incontinence or voiding difficulty when the pessary is placed. Approximately 50% of patients continued to use the pessary at 24 months. Previous hysterectomy and increasing parity were risk factors associated with pessary failure, whereas no difference has been found in age, ethnicity, or degree of PFP.

Patient evaluation starts with an accurate history of her daily activities, level of functioning, symptoms, and the impact of PFP or urinary incontinence on patient quality of life. Another important part of the history is the assessment of the patient's capacity to understand the pessary function, maintenance, and the importance of follow-up. It is important to assess degree of discomfort with sexual activity as well. Recent data demonstrate a substantial number of pessary patients have increased frequency of intercourse and improvement in the quality of sexual life.

Important in the physical exam is the evaluation of the pelvic floor strength, severity of prolapse, specific pelvic floor defects, and health of the vaginal epithelium. The exam should be performed while the patient is in a semirecumbent lithotomy position. Careful examination of the genitalia identifying excoriation, erythema of the vulva, and vaginal introitus is important. The genital hiatus, defined as the middle of the external urethral meatus to the posterior midline hymenal ring, is measured, and a size >5 cm decreases the likelihood of success for pessary fitting. A short vagina (<6 cm) also decreases the success of pessary fitting. Pelvic floor strength is important in retaining the pessary and is evaluated by placing two fingers in the patient's vagina while she is performing a Kegel maneuver. The use of vaginal estrogen cream is generally recommended if the epithelium is atrophic.

More than 200 types of pessaries have been developed in the past, of which approximately 20 types are still in use today, although not all pessary types are available in all countries. Pessaries are divided into two general categories: support pessaries and space-filling pessaries. Support pessaries, like the ring pessary, use a spring mechanism that rests in the posterior fornix and against the posterior aspect of the pubic symphysis. The space-filling pessaries, like the cube pessary or the donut, function either by creating suction between the device and the vaginal walls or just filling a larger space than the genital hiatus. The Gellhorn works by combining both of the two mechanisms.

Pessaries are currently made of silicone or, rarely, of latex. Rigid pessaries are no longer recommended, and if found during the pelvic exam, should be promptly removed. Generally speaking, a clinician should choose a pessary based on the type of pelvic organ prolapse (POP) found on the pelvic exam. Another approach is to choose the same pessary for all defects.

There are some basic rules that can aid in the choice of a pessary. Anterior vaginal wall defects, like a cystocele, as well as stage II apical compartment defects are best controlled with ring pessaries. Lever pessaries also seem to work well in controlling cystoceles. Gellhorns are best used for the management of stage III or IV uterine or vaginal vault prolapse or rectocele. The donut pessary can be useful in managing the uterine procidentia or vaginal vault eversion. Posterior vaginal wall defects, such as enterocele or rectocele, are better managed by using space occupying pessaries, such as the donut or the Gellhorn. A wide genital hiatus is generally caused by a damaged levator muscles and if the patient is unable to contract the pelvic floor, a space-filling device is recommended.

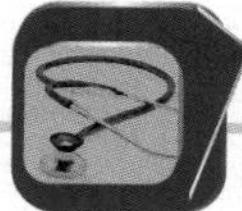

Equipment

- Pessary kit or various sizes of different pessaries
- Water-based lubricant
- Fluid absorbent pads
- Vaginal speculum
- Nonsterile gloves

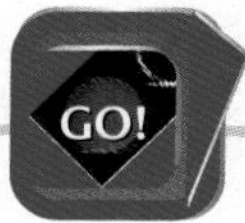

Indications

- Stress urinary incontinence
- Vaginal vault prolapse
- Cystocele
- Rectocele
- Enterocele
- Uterine prolapse
- Preoperative preparation/evaluation

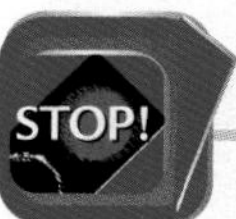

Contraindications

- Active vaginitis, atrophic changes, and vaginal ulcerations should be treated and fully resolved before the use of the pessary.
- Noncompliance
- Silicone or latex allergy (if using an Inflatoball)

The Procedure

Step 1. If fitting the patient for pelvic organ prolapse, fit with an empty bladder. If fitting for stress incontinence, fit with a full bladder. Place patient in the dorsal lithotomy position and perform bimanual exam. Examine the vulva and vaginal epithelium. Assess vaginal floor length in the same fashion as measuring for a diaphragm. During the bimanual examination, place the middle finger into the posterior cul-de-sac. Use the thumb to mark the point where the symphysis pubis abuts the index finger. Assess pelvic floor strength by having the patient tighten her muscles around your fingers. Identify the type of prolapse, cystocele, or rectocele.

- **PEARL:** If severely atrophic epithelium noted, the use of vaginal estrogen cream will help prevent erosions and aid in comfort.

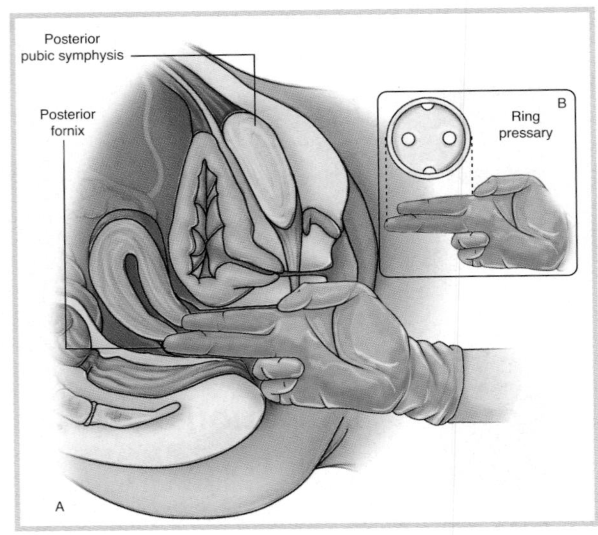

Step 1

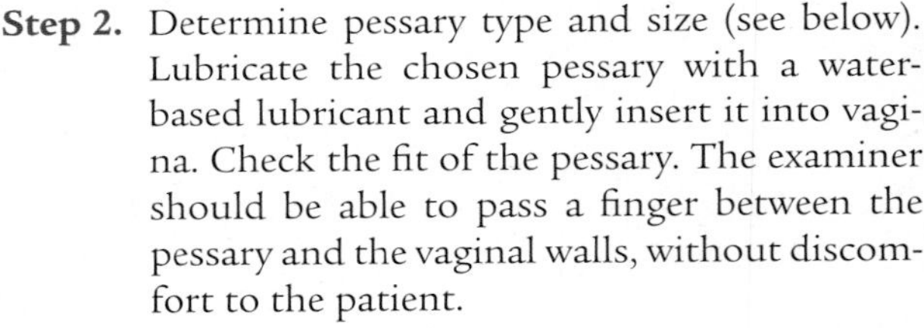

Step 2. Determine pessary type and size (see below). Lubricate the chosen pessary with a water-based lubricant and gently insert it into vagina. Check the fit of the pessary. The examiner should be able to pass a finger between the pessary and the vaginal walls, without discomfort to the patient.

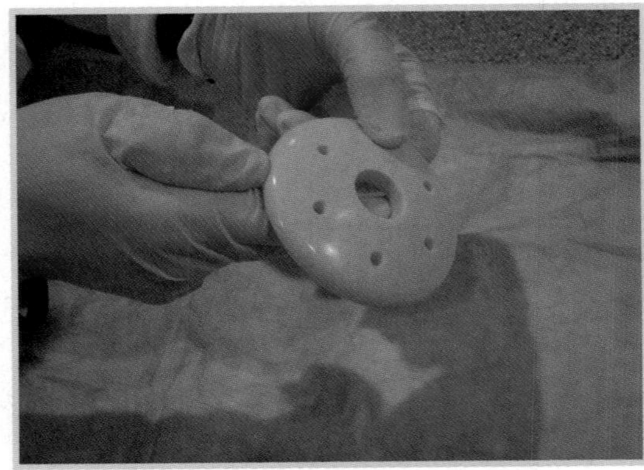

Step 2

Step 3. Have patient sit, stand, Valsalva, and cough to determine if pessary will dislodge or if prolapse or urine leakage occurs. If the pessary dislodges or there is leakage of urine, try the next larger size. If the pessary is uncomfortable, try the next smaller size. If there is correct placement, the patient should be unable to feel the pessary in place. Once the correct pessary is determined, have patient void.

- **PITFALL:** If the patient is unable to void, the pessary is too large and the next smaller size should be tried.

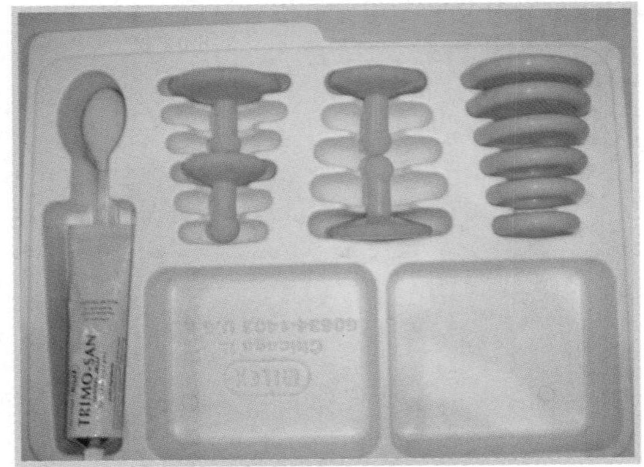

Step 3

Step 4. The patient should be instructed in how to insert and remove the pessary. Have the patient insert and remove the pessary before she leaves the office.

- **PITFALL:** Some patients are unable to remove the pessary on their own. In this case, the patient should return to the office every 6 to 8 weeks for removal, cleaning of the pessary, and inspection of the vaginal walls.
- **PEARL:** If the patient is unable to remove the pessary daily, she should insert one applicator of Trimo-San into the vagina three times per week to help decrease the amount and odor of the vaginal discharge.

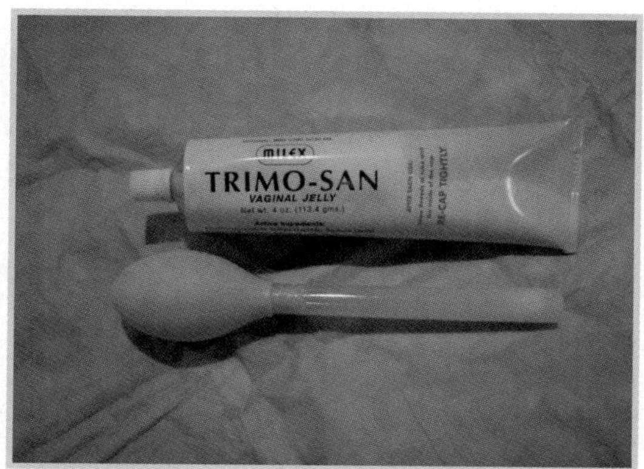

Step 4

Choosing and Using a Pessary

Ring Pessary

Step 5. There are two types of ring pessaries, without and with support. The ring is a support-type device and comes in sizes from 0 to 9. Special orders can be placed for sizes 10 to 15. Sizes 3 to 5 are the most commonly used. The ring pessary is excellent for mild uterine and vaginal prolapse, cystocele, and stress incontinence. It is acceptable for enterocele.

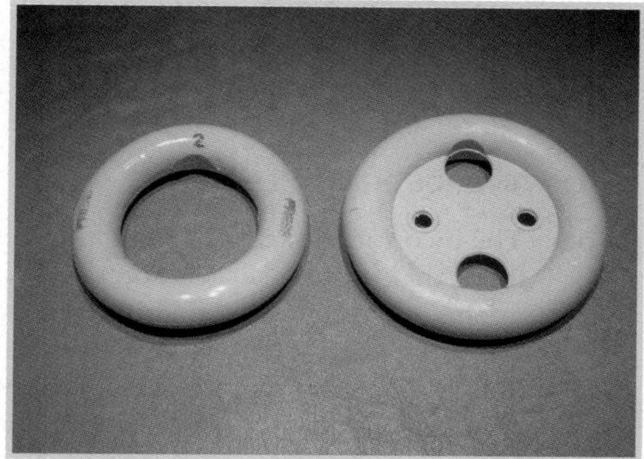

Step 5

Step 6. Ring pessaries are easy to insert, using the same folding technique as for fitting a diaphragm. Insert the pessary after applying a water-soluble lubricant on the rim of the device. Fold the device in half at the notch.

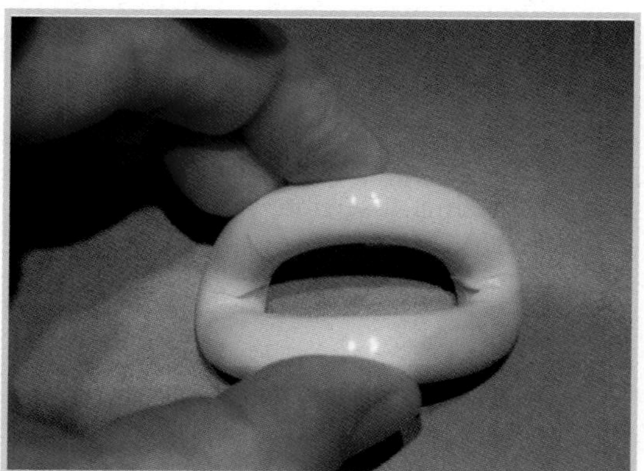

Step 6

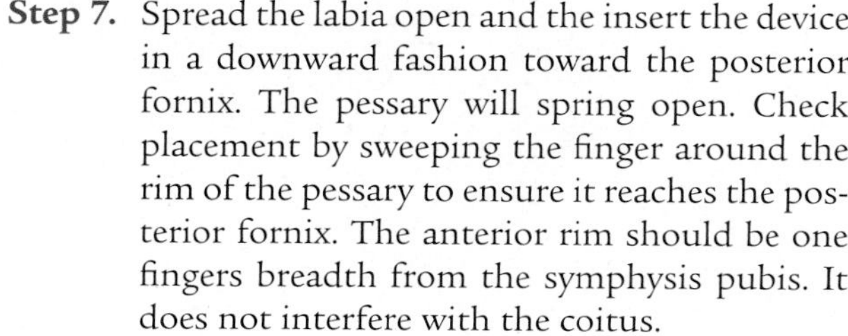

Step 7. Spread the labia open and the insert the device in a downward fashion toward the posterior fornix. The pessary will spring open. Check placement by sweeping the finger around the rim of the pessary to ensure it reaches the posterior fornix. The anterior rim should be one fingers breadth from the symphysis pubis. It does not interfere with the coitus.

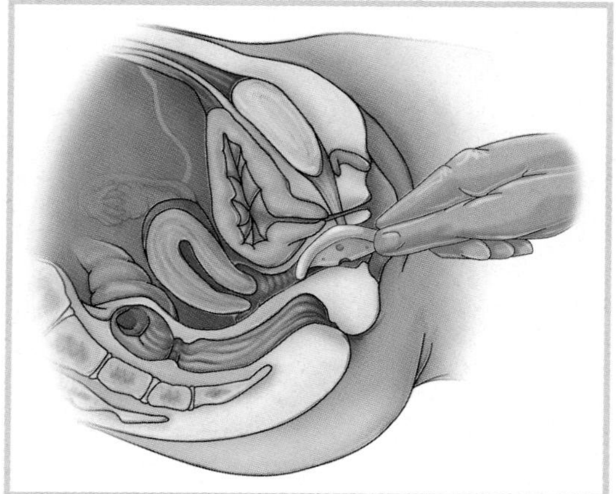

Step 7

Step 8. The pessary sits high in the vagina from the posterior fornix to just behind the symphysis pubis. Removal is achieved by turning the notch until it is anterior, then the pessary is pulled in a downward fashion and withdrawn.

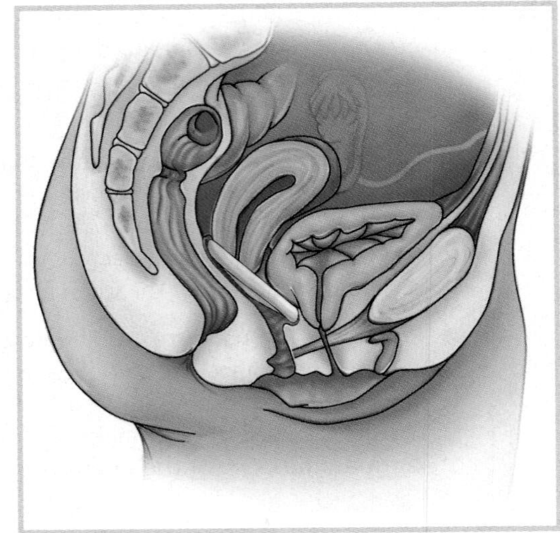

Step 8

Incontinence Ring Pessary

Step 9. The incontinence ring is a ring pessary with a knob that is placed at the anterior vagina just at the pubic notch. The knob provides additional support to the bladder neck during any increased abdominal pressure (i.e., Valsalva, cough, or laugh) to further prevent leakage of urine.

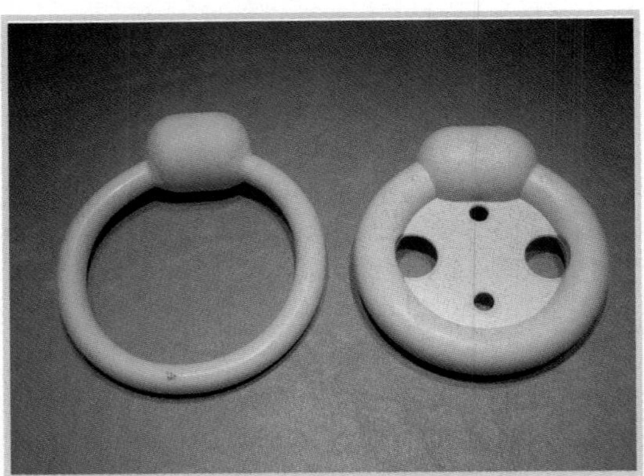

Step 9

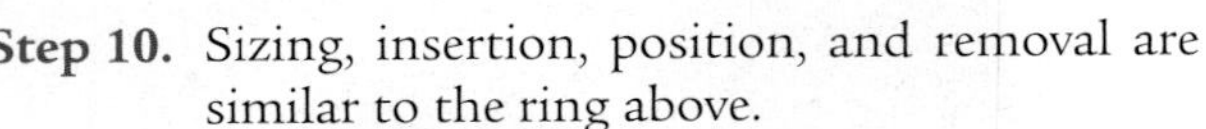

Step 10. Sizing, insertion, position, and removal are similar to the ring above.

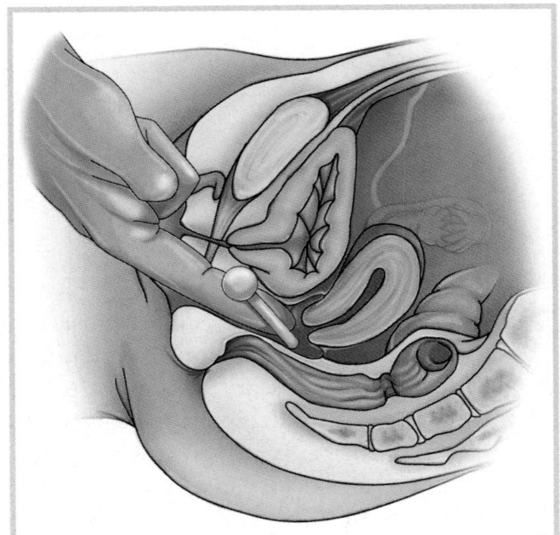

Step 10

Shaatz Pessary

Step 11. The Shaatz pessary lies in the supportive category and is best-suited for mild uterine prolapse, cystocele, and stress urinary incontinence. It is fit like the ring pessary. Most common used sizes are 3 to 6. This pessary can be used in cases where the ring does not provide enough support.

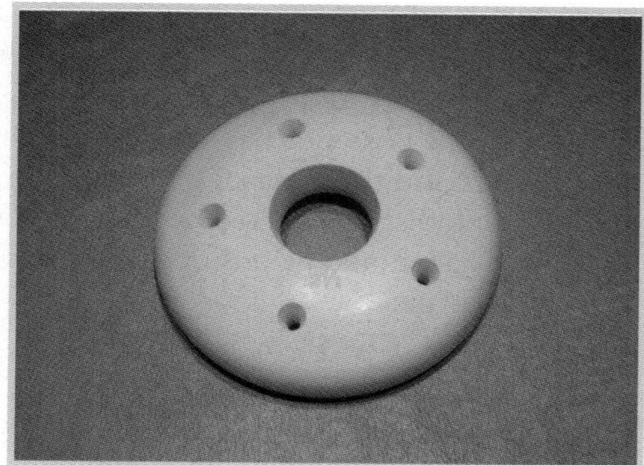

Step 11

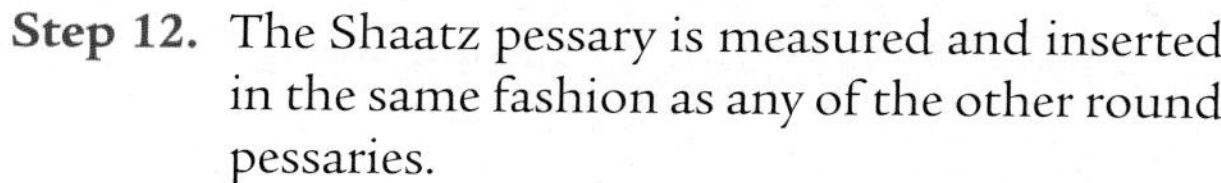

Step 12. The Shaatz pessary is measured and inserted in the same fashion as any of the other round pessaries.

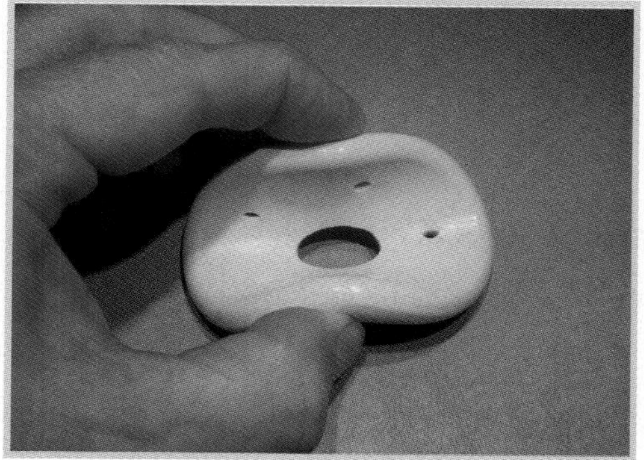

Step 12

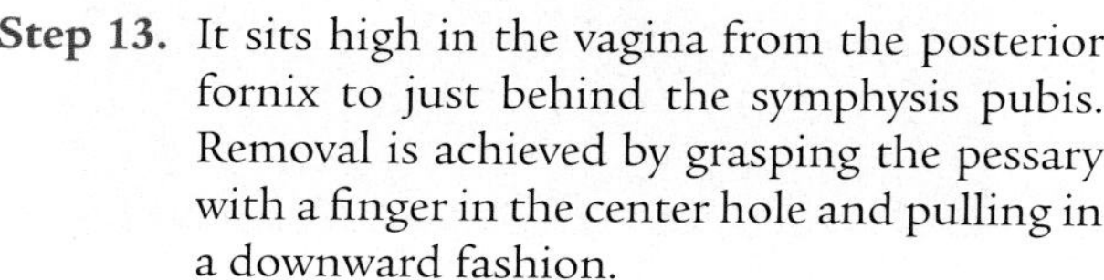

Step 13. It sits high in the vagina from the posterior fornix to just behind the symphysis pubis. Removal is achieved by grasping the pessary with a finger in the center hole and pulling in a downward fashion.

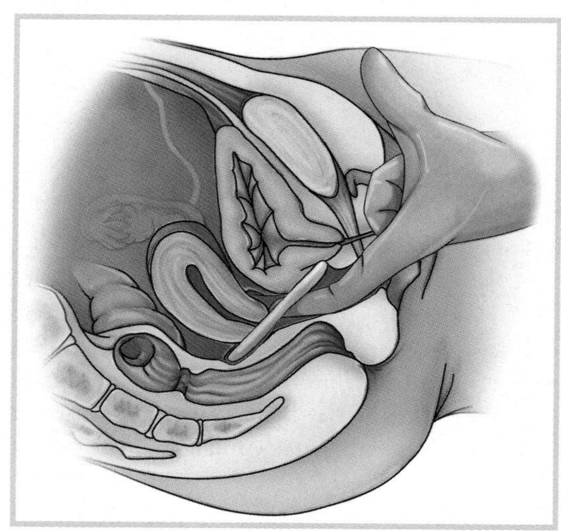

Step 13

Lever Pessary

Step 14. There are three types of lever pessaries (support pessary): the Hodge, Hodge-Smith and Risser. Any of the three are indicated in second-degree uterine and vaginal prolapse, or cystocele. The lever pessaries have also been used in pregnancy for cervical incompetence with or without cerclage. The Hodge pessaries are designed for patients with a shallow pubic arch and, without support, can be used for cervical incompetence in pregnancy. The Smith variant was modified to fit patients with a narrow pubic arch, whereas the Risser was further modified to accommodate patients with a flatter arch. They come in size 0 through 9. Generally, sizes 2 to 4 are the most commonly used.

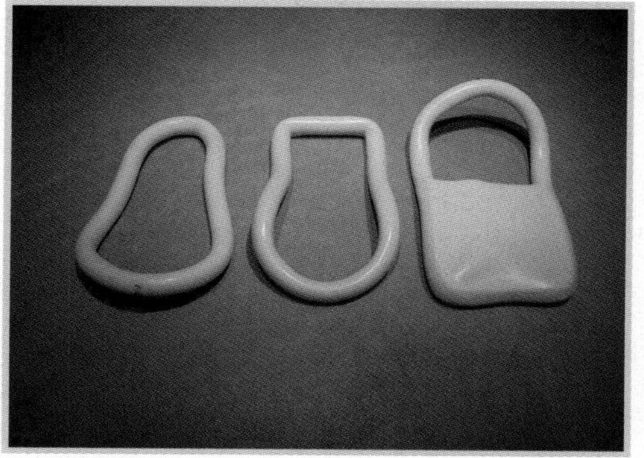

Step 14

Step 15. To insert the Lever pessary, the uterus should be manually anteverted, and the pessary folded along its axis is inserted into the vagina with the posterior bar positioned behind the cervix and the anterior bar behind the pubic symphysis. The curved portion of the posterior bar should be positioned into the posterior fornix.

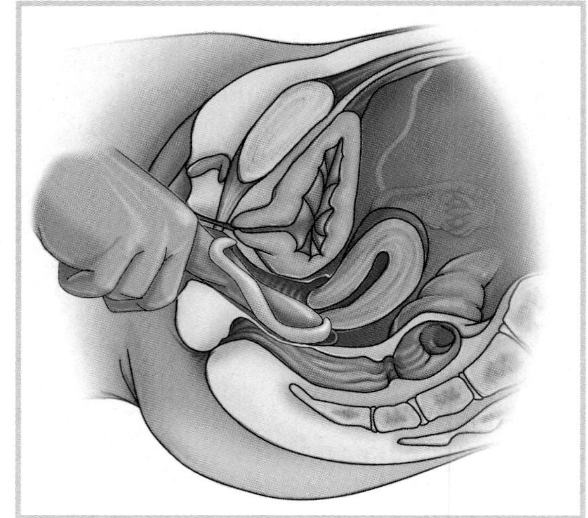

Step 15

Regula Pessary

Step 16. The Regula pessary is best-suited for first- and second-degree uterine prolapse. A number of different sizes of this pessary must be available to adequately fit the patient. Warn the patient that a number of different sizes are often needed to find the best fit to the vaginal vault while accommodating the degree of prolapse.

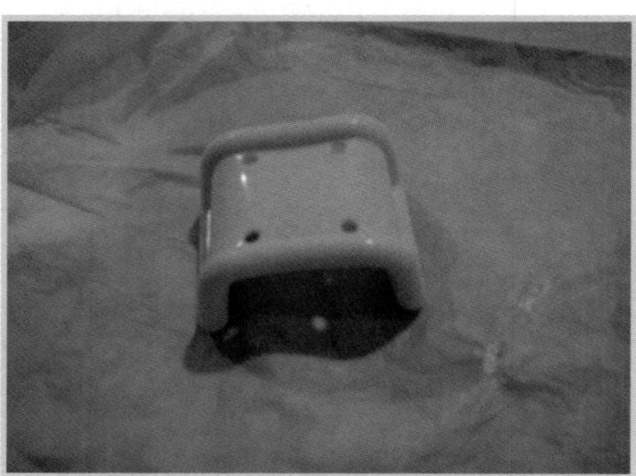

Step 16

Step 17. This pessary is shaped with a flexible bridge that abuts the cervix expanding horizontally when pressure in the pelvic cavity occurs. As the pressure is exerted by the cervix/uterus onto the arch of the pessary, it automatically spreads the heels outward. This mechanism helps prevent expulsion of the pessary.

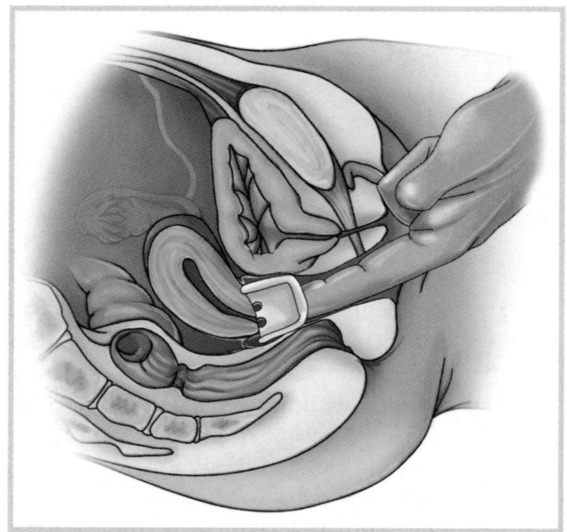

Step 17

Step 18. The pessary is folded in half lengthwise, inserted into the vagina, and then turned and pushed up towards the cervix. Removal is accomplished by grasping one of the sides of the pessary and pulling downward.

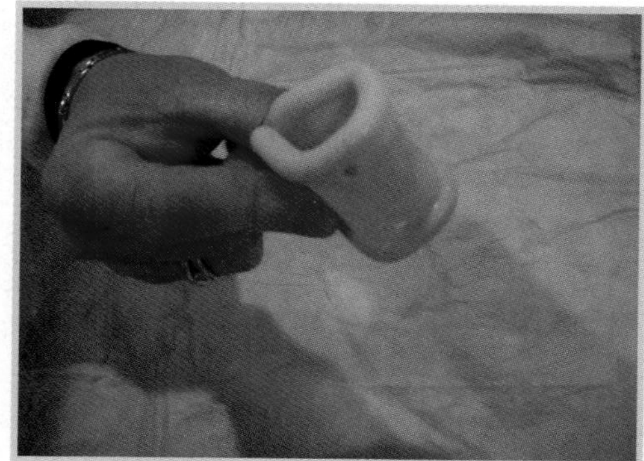

Step 18

Gellhorn Pessary

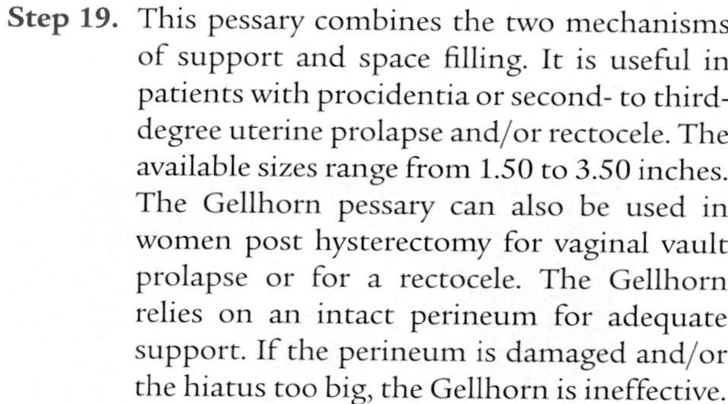

Step 19. This pessary combines the two mechanisms of support and space filling. It is useful in patients with procidentia or second- to third-degree uterine prolapse and/or rectocele. The available sizes range from 1.50 to 3.50 inches. The Gellhorn pessary can also be used in women post hysterectomy for vaginal vault prolapse or for a rectocele. The Gellhorn relies on an intact perineum for adequate support. If the perineum is damaged and/or the hiatus too big, the Gellhorn is ineffective.

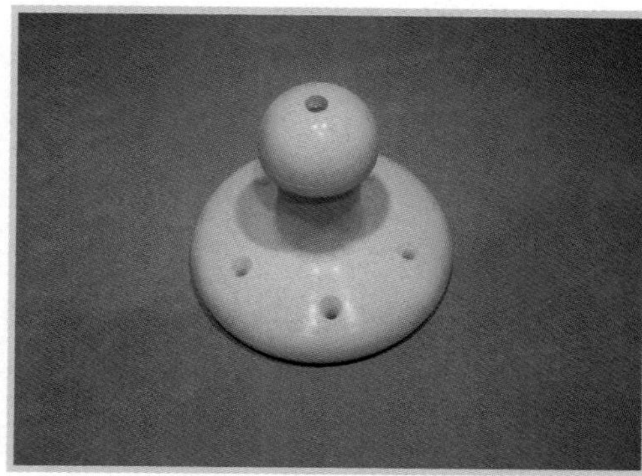

Step 19

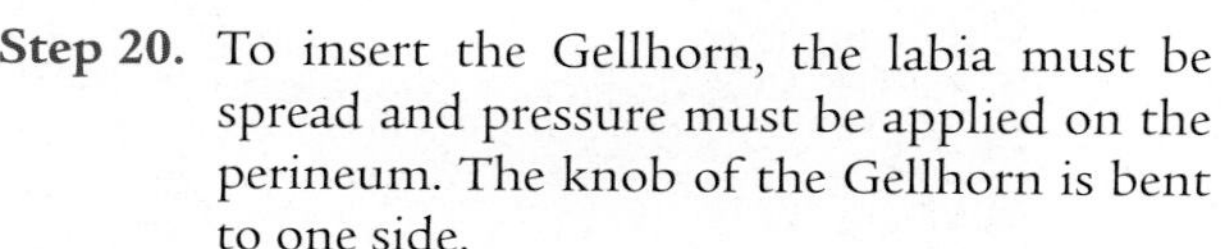

Step 20. To insert the Gellhorn, the labia must be spread and pressure must be applied on the perineum. The knob of the Gellhorn is bent to one side.

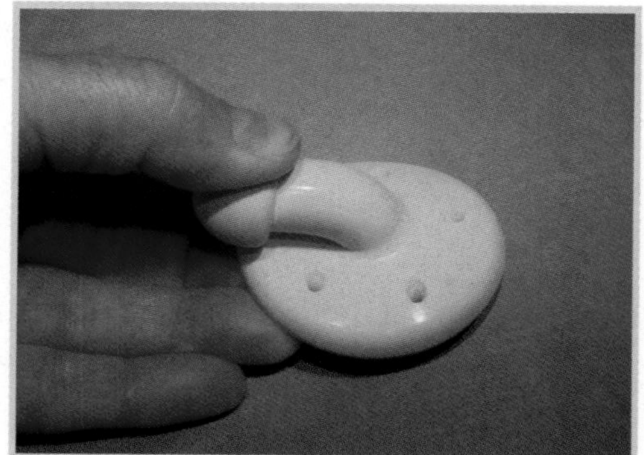

Step 20

Step 21. The Gellhorn is inserted obliquely through the introitus with the concave part directed toward the cervix, and the stem folded and oriented toward the introitus.

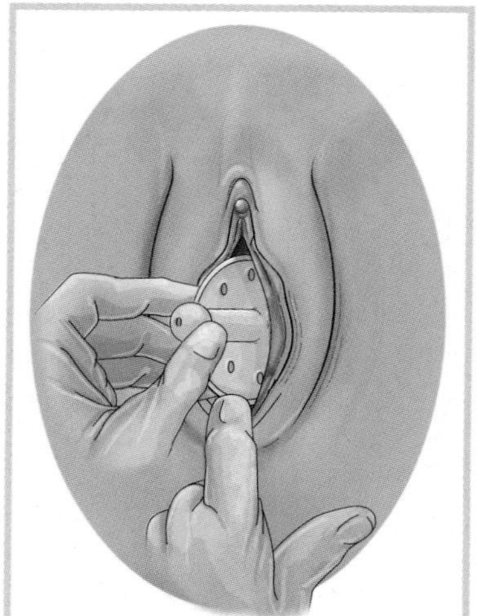

Step 21

Step 22. When in place, the dish part of the pessary lies over the cervix with the stem pointing outward. Coitus is contraindicated with the Gellhorn in place. Removal of this pessary is often difficult, as the suction must be broken before the pessary is pulled out. This is accomplished by wedging the tip of the index finger anywhere along the side of the pessary, then grasping the pessary or handle if necessary and pulling down and out. It can be difficult for some patients to insert and remove the pessary on their own.

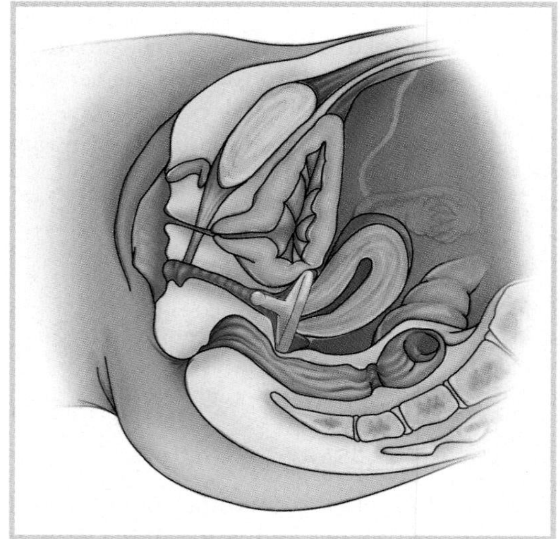

Step 22

Donut Pessary

Step 23. The donut is a space-filling type of device that works very well for all prolapse types, except for major posterior wall defects. It can be used in presence of decreased perineal support, but with good introital integrity. The pessary size is available from 0 to 7, and sizes 2 to 4 are generally most used.

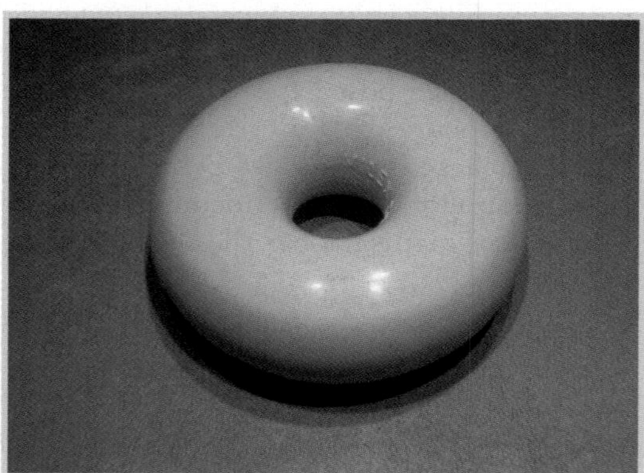

Step 23

Step 24. The donut is inserted similar to the ring, squeezing the sides to reduce its diameter.

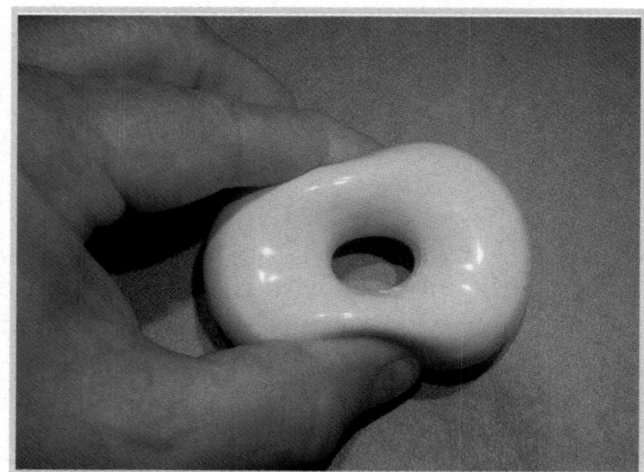

Step 24

Step 25. It is then inserted into position and allowed to resume its formed shape.

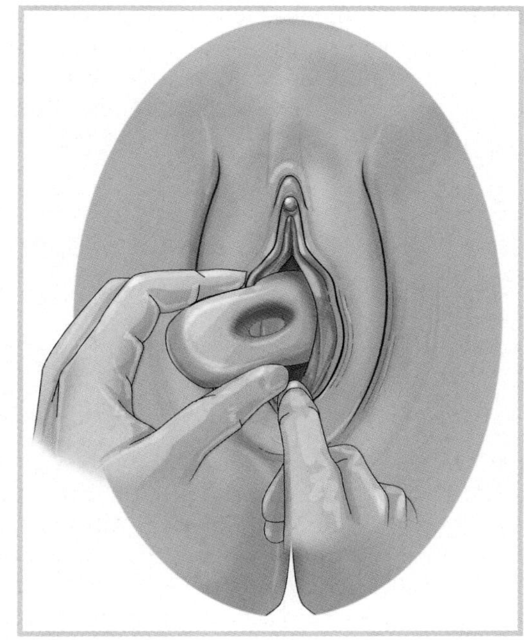

Step 25

Step 26. Once in the vagina, it should comfortably fit. Removal is accomplished by grasping the donut using the hole in the center and pulling downward. Although easy to insert and remove, because of its hard rubbery consistency, the donut can be difficult to manage for the older patients with arthritis.

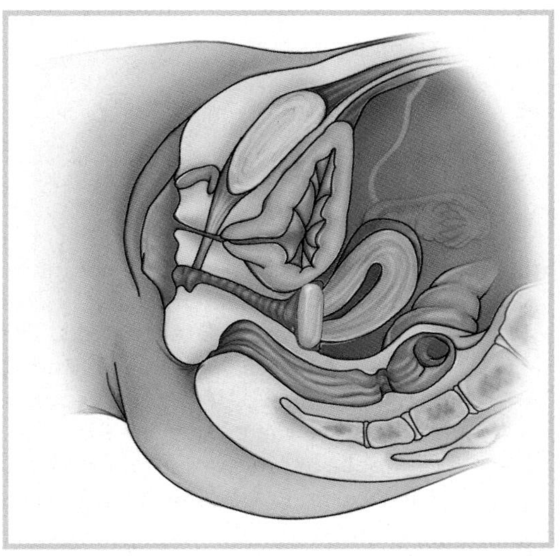

Step 26

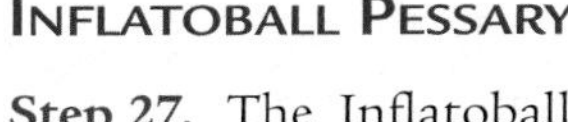

Inflatoball Pessary

Step 27. The Inflatoball is another donut-type pessary. This is the only latex rubber pessary available and, therefore, cannot be used in the latex-allergic patient.

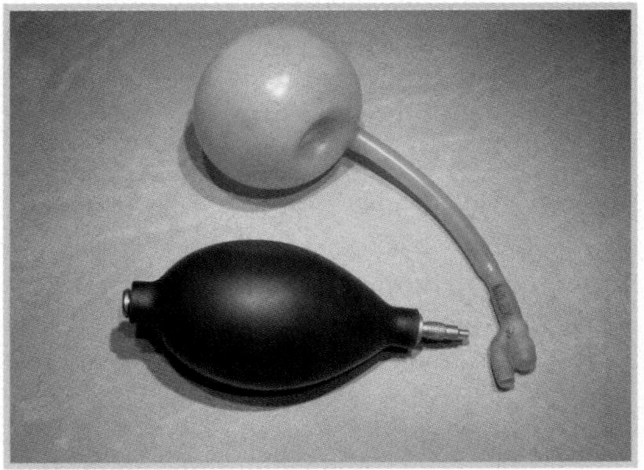

Step 27

Step 28. The Inflatoball comes in three sizes, and insertion and removal are easily taught to the patient. The pump is attached to the inflation tube and the ball stopper moved into the side tube.

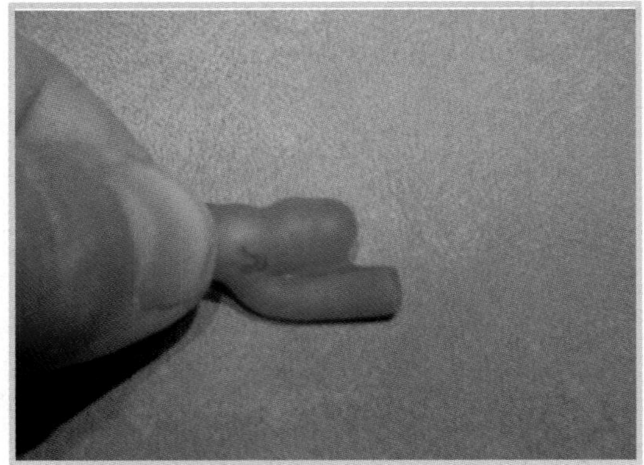

Step 28

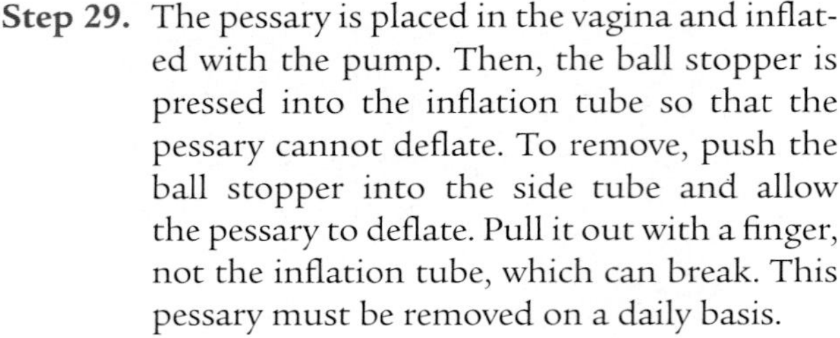

Step 29. The pessary is placed in the vagina and inflated with the pump. Then, the ball stopper is pressed into the inflation tube so that the pessary cannot deflate. To remove, push the ball stopper into the side tube and allow the pessary to deflate. Pull it out with a finger, not the inflation tube, which can break. This pessary must be removed on a daily basis.

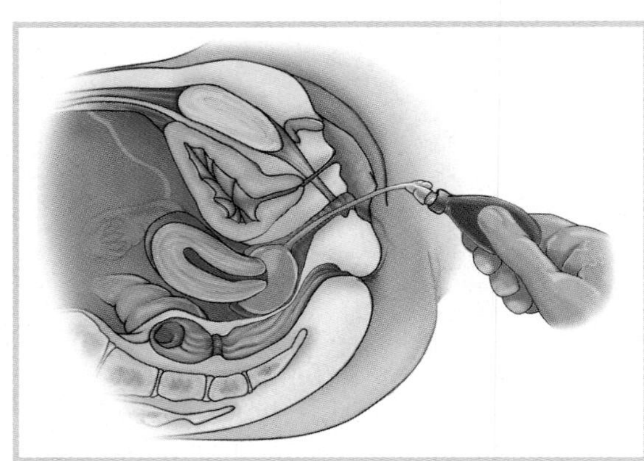

Step 29

Cube Pessary

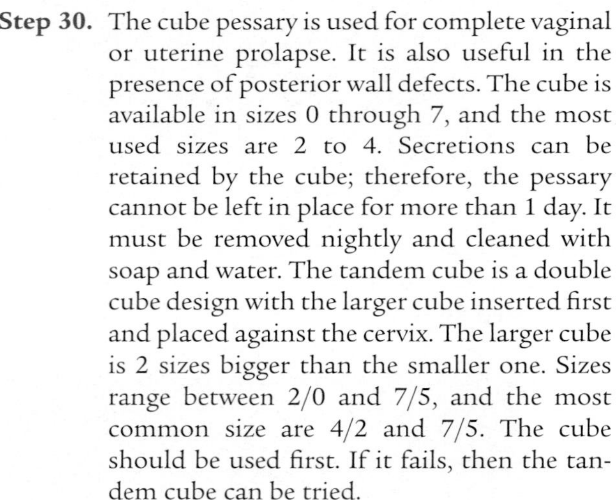

Step 30. The cube pessary is used for complete vaginal or uterine prolapse. It is also useful in the presence of posterior wall defects. The cube is available in sizes 0 through 7, and the most used sizes are 2 to 4. Secretions can be retained by the cube; therefore, the pessary cannot be left in place for more than 1 day. It must be removed nightly and cleaned with soap and water. The tandem cube is a double cube design with the larger cube inserted first and placed against the cervix. The larger cube is 2 sizes bigger than the smaller one. Sizes range between 2/0 and 7/5, and the most common size are 4/2 and 7/5. The cube should be used first. If it fails, then the tandem cube can be tried.

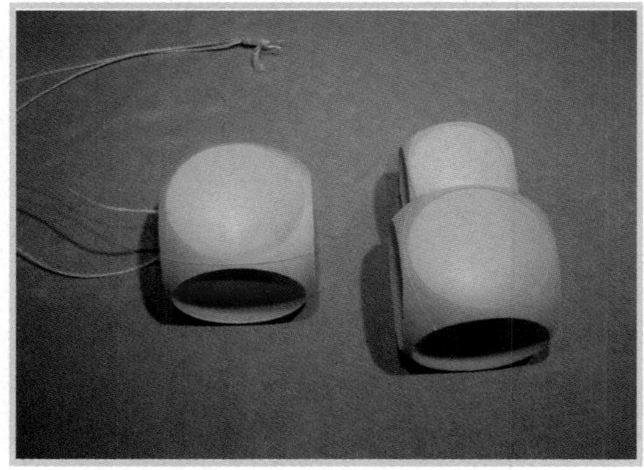

Step 30

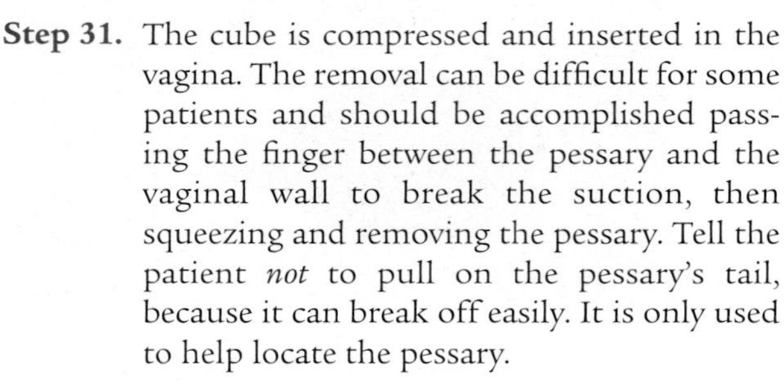

Step 31. The cube is compressed and inserted in the vagina. The removal can be difficult for some patients and should be accomplished passing the finger between the pessary and the vaginal wall to break the suction, then squeezing and removing the pessary. Tell the patient *not* to pull on the pessary's tail, because it can break off easily. It is only used to help locate the pessary.

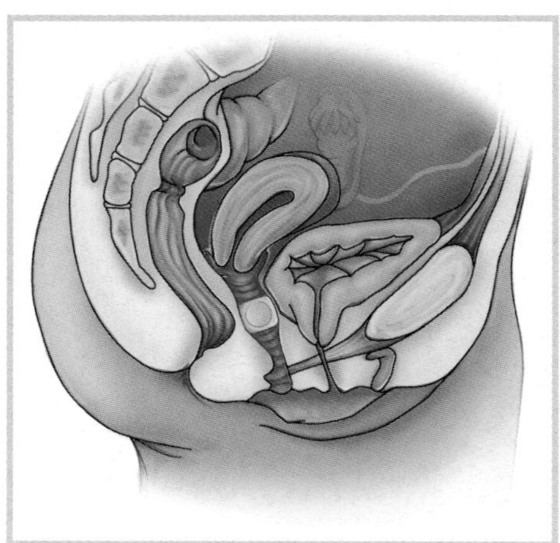

Step 31

Gehrung Pessary

Step 32. The Gehrung (saddle) pessary provides support for cystocele, rectocele, and some cases of procidentia. It is available in sizes 0 to 8, although the most used sizes are 2 to 5. The Gehrung with knob can be used for the same indications as the Gehrung but treats stress incontinence as well as cystocele/recotcele.

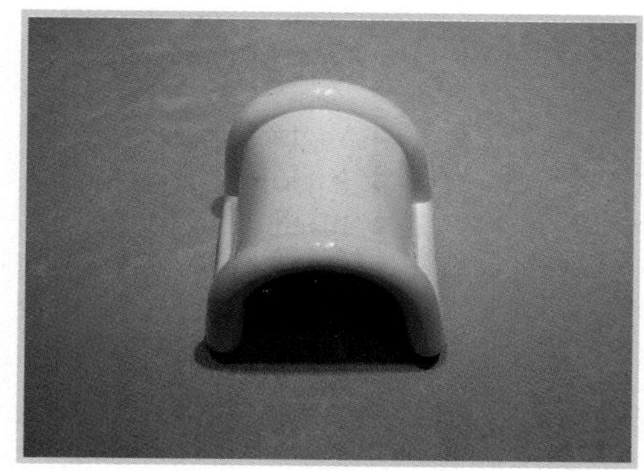

Step 32

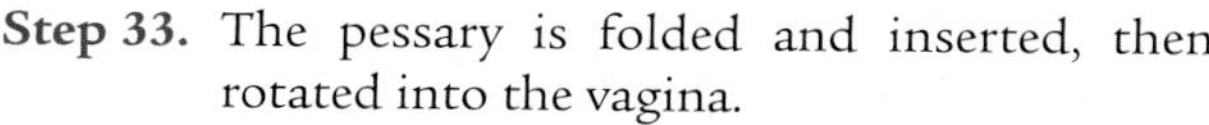

Step 33. The pessary is folded and inserted, then rotated into the vagina.

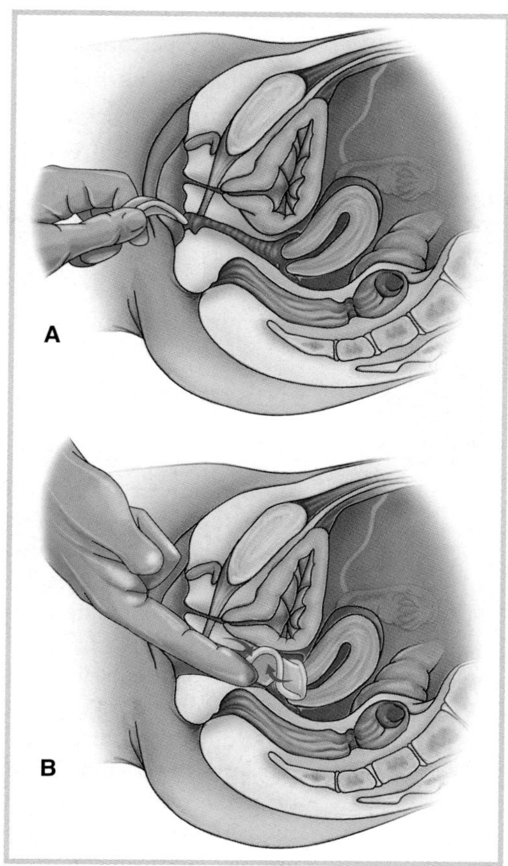

Step 33

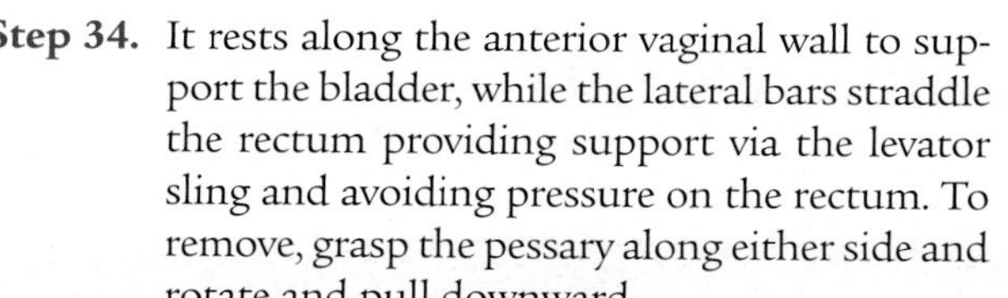

Step 34. It rests along the anterior vaginal wall to support the bladder, while the lateral bars straddle the rectum providing support via the levator sling and avoiding pressure on the rectum. To remove, grasp the pessary along either side and rotate and pull downward.

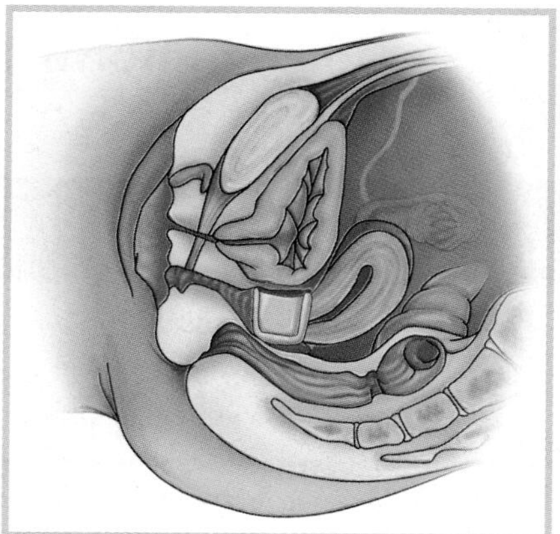

Step 34

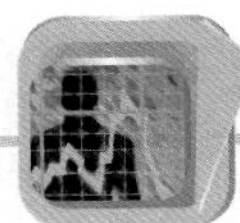

Complications

- Vaginal discharge
- Vaginitis
- Bleeding or spotting
- Vaginal erosion or ulceration

Rare Complications

- Pessary impaction
- Vesicovaginal fistula
- Urosepsis
- Bowel or bladder erosion
- Cervical perforation
- Urinary incontinence
- Urinary obstruction
- Pessary expulsion or shifting

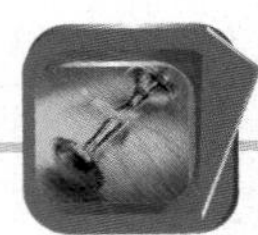

Pediatric Considerations

Pessaries can be used in female infants with uterine prolapse occurring in the first days of their life due to spinal cord defects.

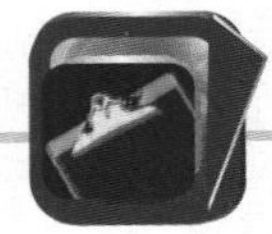

Postprocedure Instructions

There is no consensus or evidence regarding the management of pessaries, and most recommendations are based on expert opinion. Ideally, patients should remove their device nightly, clean with mild soap and water, and replace in the morning. Many patients find this practice cumbersome and, therefore, remove the pessary several times during the week but not on a daily basis. Ideally the patient should be seen within 24–48 hours after initial fitting and should be seen more frequently in the first year. It is recommended that during the first year, visits should be at 3 month intervals, and then increased to 6 month intervals. Patients who need more assistance or have decreased capacity should be seen more frequently. Pessaries should be removed and cleansed at every visit. A pelvic exam should also be performed at each visit to inspect for signs of vaginitis, vaginal atrophy, erosions, ulcerations or any other complications. If the patient experiences itching or irritation, a vaginal douche with dilute vinegar or hydrogen peroxide can be infrequently used. If the patient experiences vaginal ulceration, remove pessary until healing occurs, and use estrogen cream one-half of an applicator every night or a full applicator 3 times a week. Recheck the vaginal walls before reinsertion.

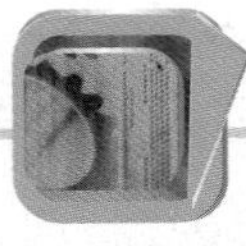

Coding Information and Supply Sources

CPT Code	Description	2008 Average 50th Percentile Fee	Global Period
57160	Pessary fitting	$158.00	0
A4561	Rubber pessaries	40–50 a piece	XXX
A4562	Nonrubber pessaries	***	XXX

*Medicare supply reimbursement is about $50 for nonrubber pessaries and $17 for rubber pessary.

CPT is a registered trademark of the American Medical Association.

2008 average 50th Percentile Fees are provided courtesy of 2008 MMH-SI's copyrighted Physicians' Fees and Coding Guide.

ICD9 DIAGNOSTIC CODES

618.0 Vaginal wall prolapse, rectocele, cystocele (female, without uterine prolapse)
618.1 Uterine prolapse without vaginal wall prolapsed
618.2 Uterovaginal prolapsed
618.4 Rectocele or cystocele with prolapsed, female
618.5 Posthysterectomy vault prolapsed
618.6 Enerocele, vaginal
618.8 Pelvic relaxation
621.6 Symptomatic retroflexed uterus
625.6 Stress incontinence
654.5 Cervical incompetence in pregnancy

Suppliers

- Milex Products, Inc., 311 N. Normandy, Chicago, IL 60634 (phone: 1-800-621-1278; Web site: http://www.milexproducts.com).
- Uromed, 1095 Windward Ridge Parkway, Suite 170, Alpharetta, GA 30005 (phone 1-888-987-6633; Web site: http://www.uromed.com).

Patient Education Handout

Patient education handouts, **"Vaginal Pessary"** and **"How to Use a Pessary"** can be found on the book's Web site.

Bibliography

Bash K. Review of vaginal pessaries. *Obstet Gynecol Surv.* 2000;55:455–460.
Clemons JL, Aguilar VC, Tillighast TA, et al. Patients satisfaction and changes in prolapse and urinary symptoms in women who were fitted successfully with pessary for pelvic organ prolapse. *Am J Obstet Gynecol.* 2004;190:1025–1029.
Cundiff GW, Weidner AC, Visco AG, et al. A Survery of pessary use by American Urogynecologist Society. *Obstet Gynecol.* 2000;95:931–935.
de Mola J, Carpenter S. Management of genital Prolapse in neonates and young women. *Obstet Gynecol Survey* 1996;51:253–260.
Fernando R, Thakar R, Sultan A, et al. Pessaries in symptomatic pelvic organ prolapse. *Is College Obstet Gynecol.* 2006;108:93–99.
Rodriguez-Trowbridge E, Fenner D. Practicalities and pitfalls of pessaries in older women. *Clin Obstet Gynecol.* 2007;50:709–719.
Subak LL, Waetjen LE, van den Eeden S, et al. Cost of pelvic organ prolapse surgery in the United States. *Obstet Gynecol.* 2001;98:646–651.
Trowbridge E, Fenner D. Practicalities and pitfalls of pessaries in older women. *Clin Obstet Gynecol.* 2007;50:709–719.
Trowbridge E, Fenner D. Conservative management of pelvic organ prolapse. *Clin Obstet Gynecol.* 2005;48:668–681.
Weber AM, Richter HE. Pelvic organ prolapse. *Obstet Gynecol.* 2005;106:615–634.
2008 MAG Mutual Healthcare Solutions, Inc.'s Physicians' Fee and Coding Guide. Duluth, Georgia. MAG Mutual Healthcare Solutions, Inc. 2007.

CHAPTER 84

No-Scalpel Vasectomy

Brian Elkins, MD, DABFM, FAAFP
Associate Professor of Clinical Family Medicine
Louisiana State University Health Sciences Center, Shreveport, LA

Vasectomy is a surgical procedure that accomplishes permanent sterilization for men. The procedure generally involves interrupting the flow of sperm through the vas deferens on each side. Semen production is unaffected (except for the absence of viable sperm) and sexual function does not change. Vasectomy may be performed in the office with anxiolysis and local anesthesia, making it a very cost-effective method of preventing pregnancy. Vasectomy is generally safer than permanent female sterilization via tubal ligation because it requires only local anesthesia and does not require entry into the peritoneal cavity.

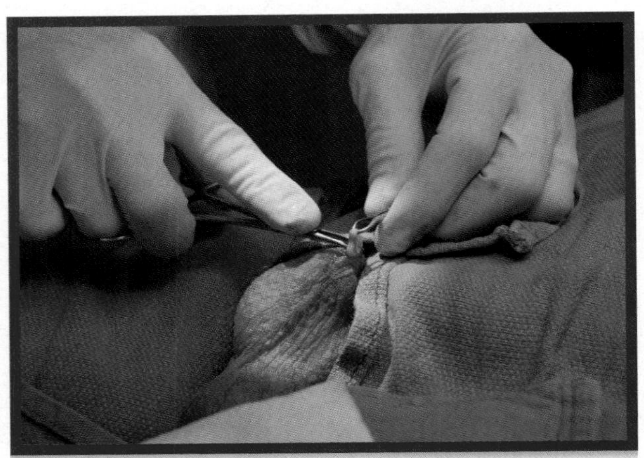

The procedure consists of three major portions: (a) accessing the vas, (b) disrupting the vas, and (c) closure. There are numerous variations of each portion of the procedure. Accessing the vas may be done through either one midline opening or two lateral openings, and may utilize either an open or a "no-scalpel" technique. The no-scalpel technique utilizes a specialized ring clamp to grasp the vas deferens percutaneously and a sharply pointed hemostat to create the opening and to dissect out and elevate the vas. The no-scalpel technique is somewhat more difficult to perform but has been shown to result in fewer complications, such as bleeding and infection.

Disruption of the vas usually involves excision of a portion of the vas on each side and is often followed by some type of occlusion, such as luminal cautery, clips, or suture ligation. Luminal cautery is superior to suture ligation; the interposition of a layer of fascia between the prostatic and testicular ends of vas deferens on each side has been shown to increase the success rate. Leaving the testicular end open has been shown in some studies to decrease the incidence of chronic testicular pain. The method described here utilizes luminal cautery of the prostatic vas, leaving the testicular end open and performing fascial interposition. The scrotal entry wound utilized in no-scalpel vasectomy heals spontaneously and does not require closure.

The excised portions of vas deferens can be sent for pathological examination if desired. Alternatively, they can be retained in formalin until sterilization is confirmed by semen analysis, at which time they can be discarded; or they can be sent for analysis at a later time if the procedure fails.

Because sperm remain in the vasa deferentia and seminal vesicles proximal to the site of surgery, vasectomy is not effective immediately. Patients must be cautioned to rely on another form of contraception until cleared with a semen analysis. Semen analysis is delayed until 3 months after the procedure because azoospermia may normally take this length of time to occur. The semen analysis consists of a single unspun specimen viewed on a slide under low magnification. Although complete azoospermia has traditionally been used as the criteria for successful sterilization, the presence of rare nonmotile sperm may persist in up to one third of men postvasectomy and is rarely associated with pregnancy.

Despite of the intent of the procedure to result in permanent sterilization, about 6% of men eventually seek a reversal. Unfortunately for these men, vasectomy reversal is difficult, expensive, and is not always successful. Change in marital status is the most commonly cited reason for seeking vasectomy reversal. Younger men should be counseled carefully regarding this risk, because age younger than 30 years at the time of the procedure has been shown to be a predictive desire for later reversal. Interestingly, patients with no children are less likely to seek later reversal.

Patients should be instructed to clip the hair on the anterior scrotum below the penis short (but not to shave as this increases risk of infection). Patients should bring an athletic supporter with them to wear home after the procedure. Patients also need to have someone to drive them home. Some providers recommend diazepam 10 mg orally prior to the procedure for anxiolysis; make sure to obtain informed consent before the patient is under the influence of the drug. Intravenous sedation can also be used if available.

The most common complication of vasectomy is bleeding or hematoma formation. In most cases, this can be managed conservatively with anti-inflammatory medications and will resolve spontaneously; rarely, surgical exploration may be required to locate and cauterize or ligate a bleeding vessel. Failure of the procedure may occur and has been divided into "early" versus "late" failure, depending on whether azoospermia was never achieved ("early failure"), or whether azoospermia was followed by a subsequent semen analysis demonstrating the presence of motile spermatozoa ("late failure," usually discovered after a pregnancy occurs). The technique described here has a 0.3% reported failure rate. Infection may occur but is uncommon. Sperm granuloma may occur with open-ended techniques but may often be asymptomatic and usually can be managed with anti-inflammatory medications. Congestive epididymitis may also occur but is less frequent with open-ended techniques than with clipping or ligation of the vas.

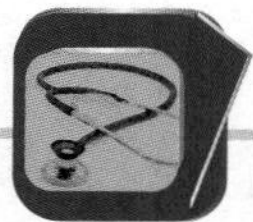

Equipment

- No-scalpel vasectomy ring clamp
  - Note: The Li forcep is the original no-scalpel vasectomy ring clamp. An alternative instrument, the Wilson forcep, is also available. The Wilson forcep is pictured in the procedure photographs in this chapter. The operator may choose either forcep depending on experience and preference.
- No-scalpel vasectomy hemostat
- Lidocaine 1%, 10 mL, with a 30-guage needle
- Lidocaine 1%/bupivicaine 0.5% 1:1, 10 mL, with a 1 ¼′ 27-guage needle
- Narrow-tipped thermal or electrical cautery
- Single-tooth Adson forcep
- Small hemostats ("mosquitoes")
- Iris scissor
- Needle driver

- 4-0 polyglycolic acid absorbable suture with an RB-1 tapered (atraumatic) needle
- Antibiotic ointment
- Nonadherent dressing
- Large pack of 4 × 4 gauze pads "fluffed"

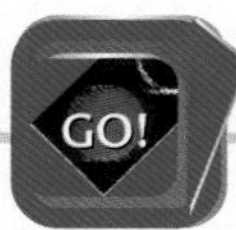

Indications

- A desire for permanent male sterilization

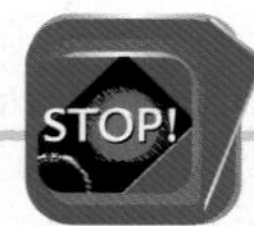

Contraindications

- Active local or nearby infection
- Varicocele
- Large inguinal hernia
- Coagulopathy
- Uncertainty about the procedure
- Desire for possible later reversal
- Current pregnancy (relative)
- Recent major life event affecting the decision (relative)

The Procedure

Step 1. The patient's penis can be taped so that it does not drape over the scrotum. The hair on the anterior scrotum is clipped short with clippers if not already done by the patient. The scrotum is prepped with chlorhexidine solution or other surgical prep and is draped with sterile drapes. Be sure to include the posterior scrotum and adjacent upper thighs in the prep. Some place a warmed bag of normal saline on the scrotum over a sterile towel for several minutes at this point to assist with relaxation of the cremasteric muscles. This is an ideal time to verify that the vas deferens can be palpated and easily isolated and elevated on both sides prior to the start of the procedure.

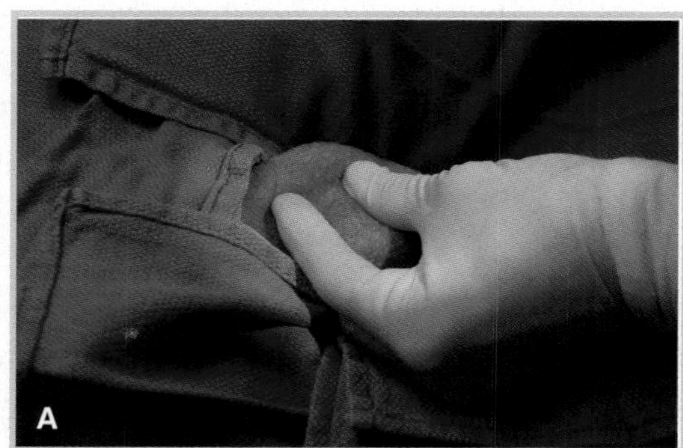

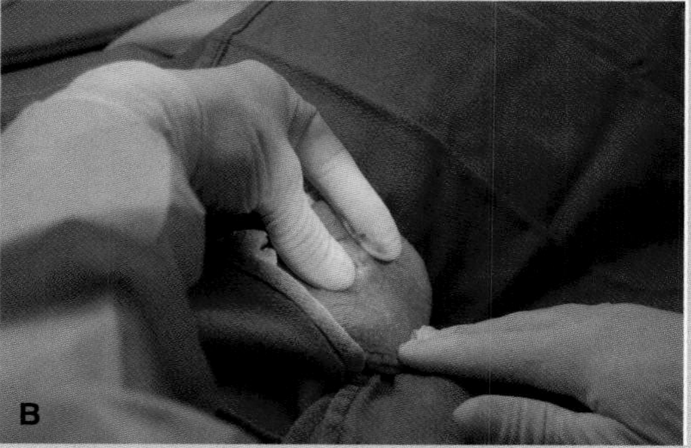

Step 1

Step 2. The skin of the anterior midline scrotum is infiltrated with 1% lidocaine. Alternatively, two separate lateral areas can be anesthetized if two lateral points will be used to access the vasa. Use the smallest amount possible, about 0.5 to 1 mL, to minimize distortion of the tissues. The anesthetized area can be circled with a surgical marking pen for later reference if needed. Perform a perivasal block on each side. First, grasp the vas with the three-point fixation technique: the thumb and forefinger stretch the vas on the anterior surface of the scrotum while the third finger is located posteriorly, pressing the vas forward between the thumb and forefinger.

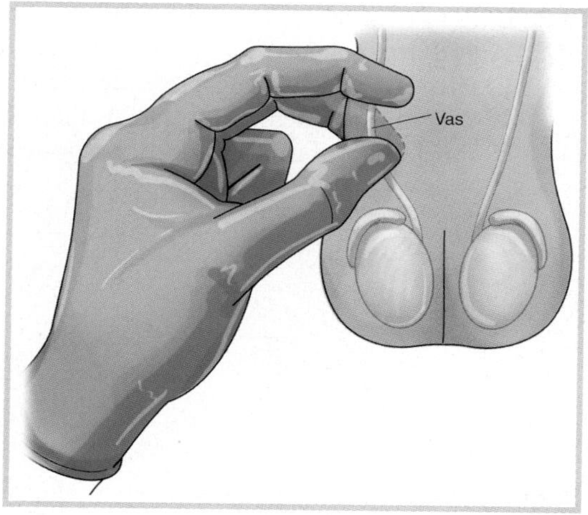

Step 2

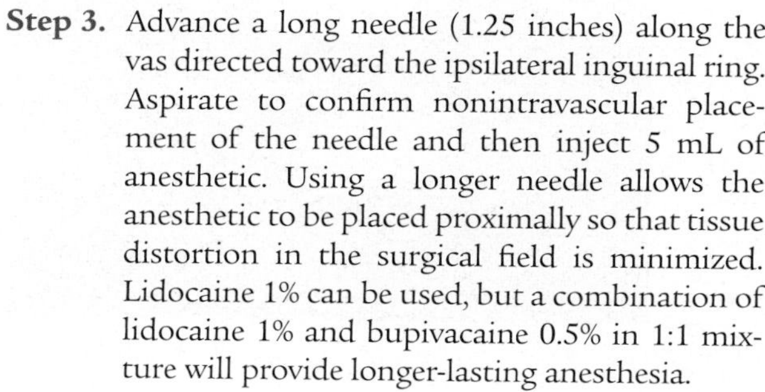

Step 3. Advance a long needle (1.25 inches) along the vas directed toward the ipsilateral inguinal ring. Aspirate to confirm nonintravascular placement of the needle and then inject 5 mL of anesthetic. Using a longer needle allows the anesthetic to be placed proximally so that tissue distortion in the surgical field is minimized. Lidocaine 1% can be used, but a combination of lidocaine 1% and bupivacaine 0.5% in 1:1 mixture will provide longer-lasting anesthesia.

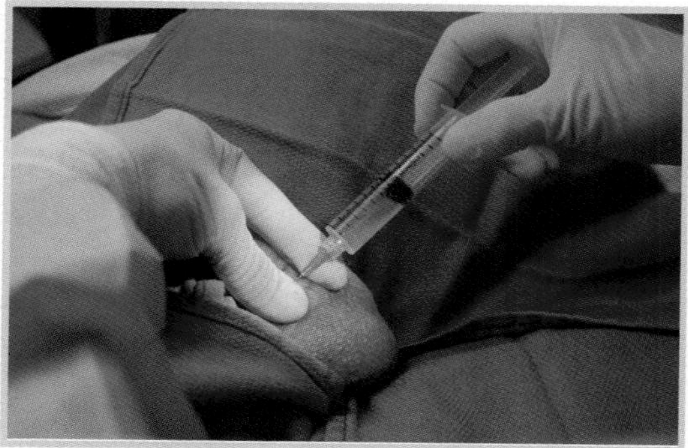

Step 3

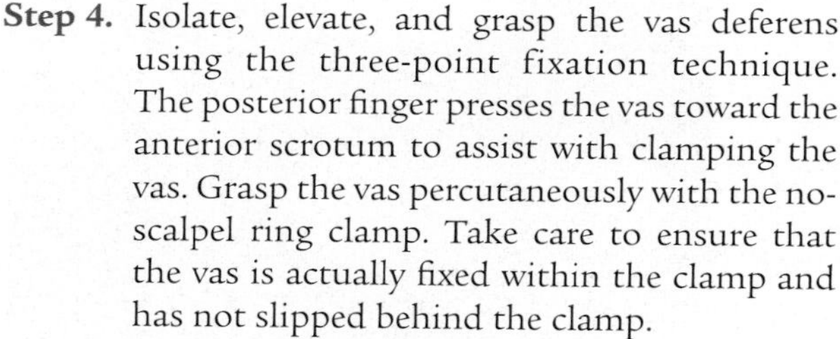

Step 4. Isolate, elevate, and grasp the vas deferens using the three-point fixation technique. The posterior finger presses the vas toward the anterior scrotum to assist with clamping the vas. Grasp the vas percutaneously with the no-scalpel ring clamp. Take care to ensure that the vas is actually fixed within the clamp and has not slipped behind the clamp.

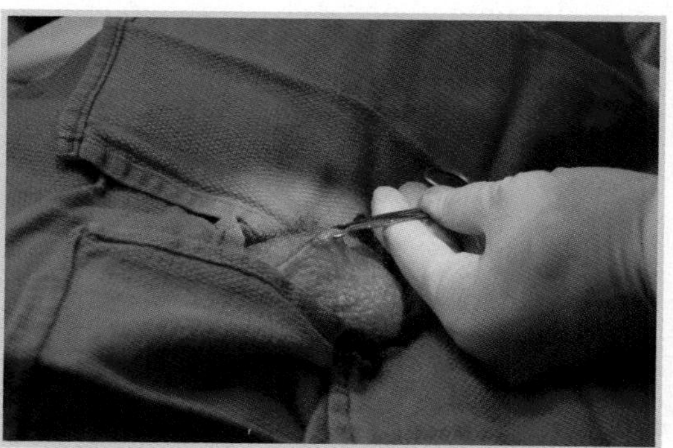

Step 4

Step 5. Open the no-scalpel hemostat and pierce the skin with one tip. Press firmly until you feel a slight "pop" sensation indicating the tip has pierced the vas.

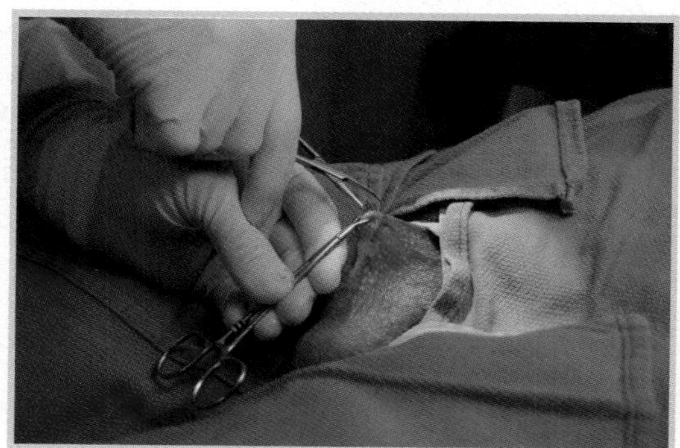

Step 5

Step 6. Remove the hemostat, close the tips, and insert both tips together in the hole created in step 5. Dissect to the vas by spreading the tips apart. You may need to reinsert the hemostat and spread several times until the vas is exposed.

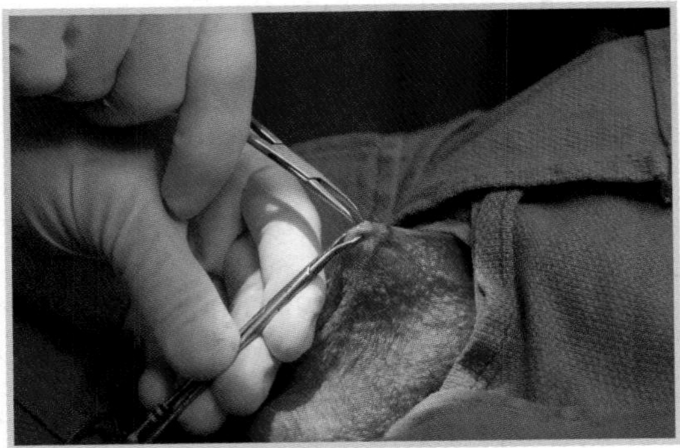

Step 6

Step 7. Once the vas is exposed, open the hemostat and insert one tip into the vas. Rotate your wrist to bring the tip upward. This should elevate a small portion of the vas essentially free of surrounding connective tissue.

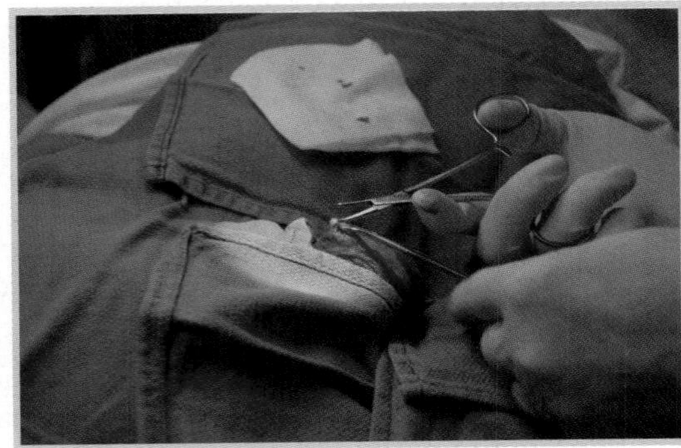

Step 7

Step 8. With the vas still elevated, using your other hand grasp through the vas with the ring clamp.

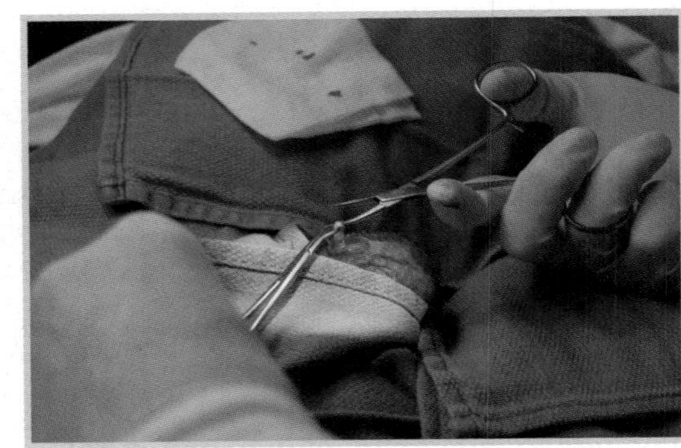

Step 8

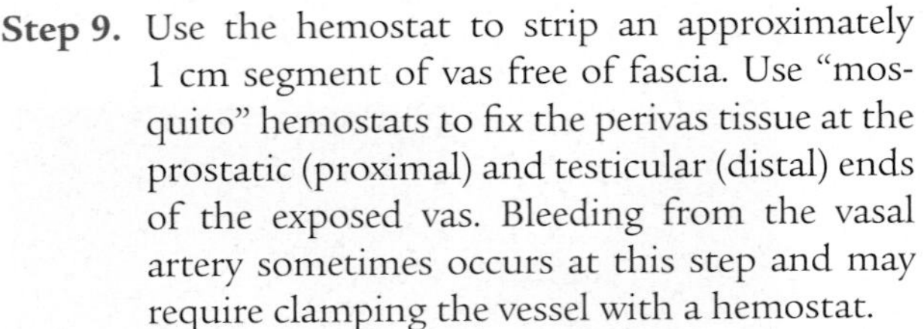

Step 9. Use the hemostat to strip an approximately 1 cm segment of vas free of fascia. Use "mosquito" hemostats to fix the perivas tissue at the prostatic (proximal) and testicular (distal) ends of the exposed vas. Bleeding from the vasal artery sometimes occurs at this step and may require clamping the vessel with a hemostat.

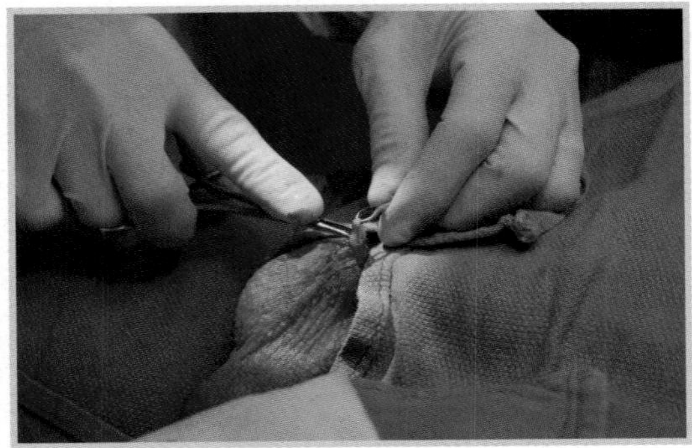

Step 9

Step 10. Using the ring clamp still clamped through the vas, elevate the vas and partially incise the prostatic end of the vas, exposing the lumen but leaving a portion of the wall intact for traction.

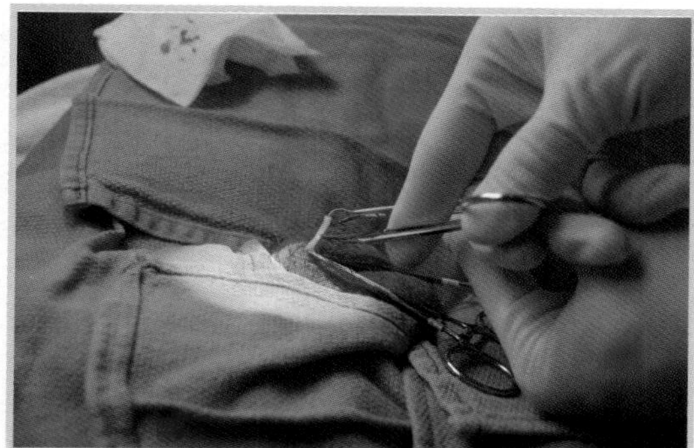

Step 10

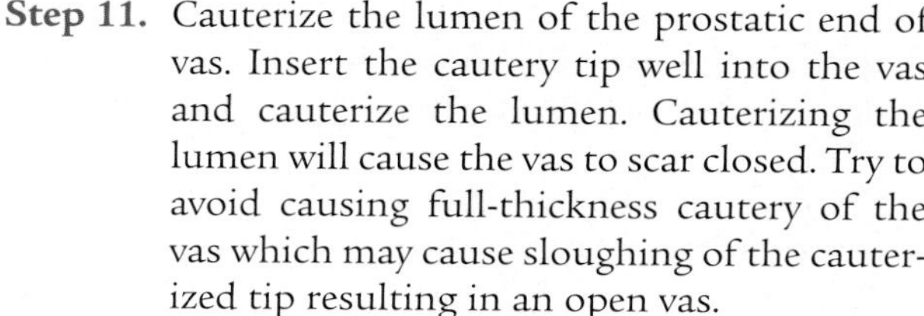

Step 11. Cauterize the lumen of the prostatic end of vas. Insert the cautery tip well into the vas and cauterize the lumen. Cauterizing the lumen will cause the vas to scar closed. Try to avoid causing full-thickness cautery of the vas which may cause sloughing of the cauterized tip resulting in an open vas.

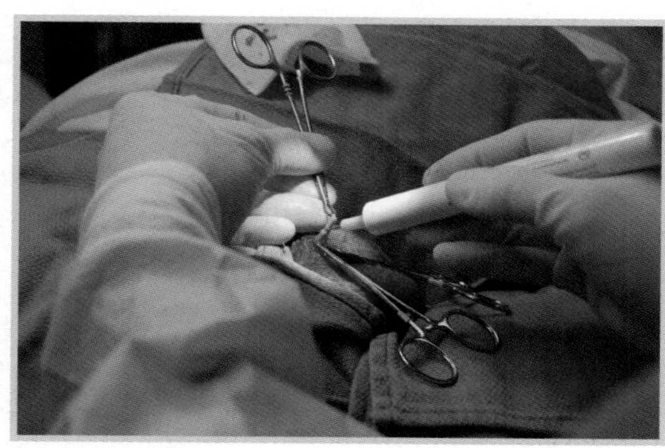

Step 11

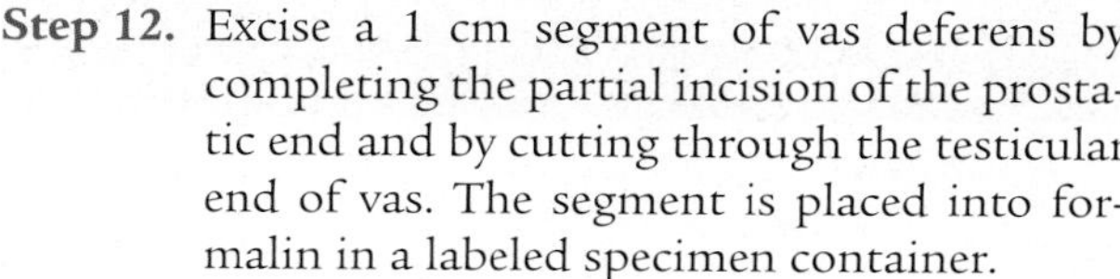

Step 12. Excise a 1 cm segment of vas deferens by completing the partial incision of the prostatic end and by cutting through the testicular end of vas. The segment is placed into formalin in a labeled specimen container.

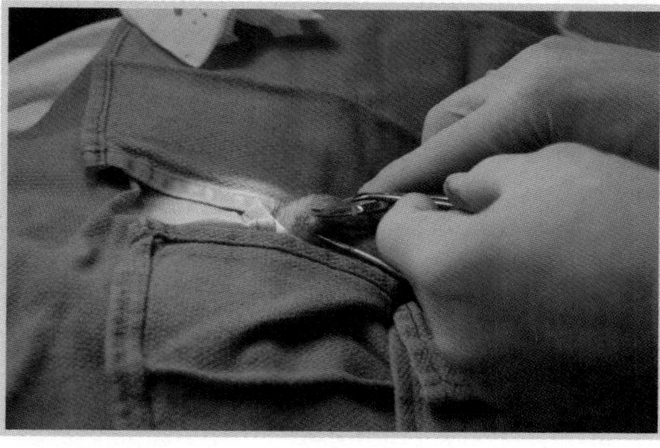

Step 12

Step 13. Place a purse string suture in the perivas fascia over the testicular end of vas using the 4-0 absorbable suture and tapered needle. (This can also be placed over the prostatic end of vas if desired. In some cases, the fascia is easier to bring up on one or the other side for the purse string suture.) When the purse string suture is tied, a layer of fascia should interpose between the two free ends of vas. Check the area for hemostasis, and when satisfactory, allow the fascia and remaining free end of vas to drop back into the scrotum. Repeat steps 4 through 13 for the opposite side. The entry wound can usually be left open. Apply antibiotic ointment and cover first with a small nonadherent gauze pad followed by several 4 × 4 gauze pads "fluffed" to provide cushioning. Assist the patient in putting on the athletic supporter so that the dressing remains in place.

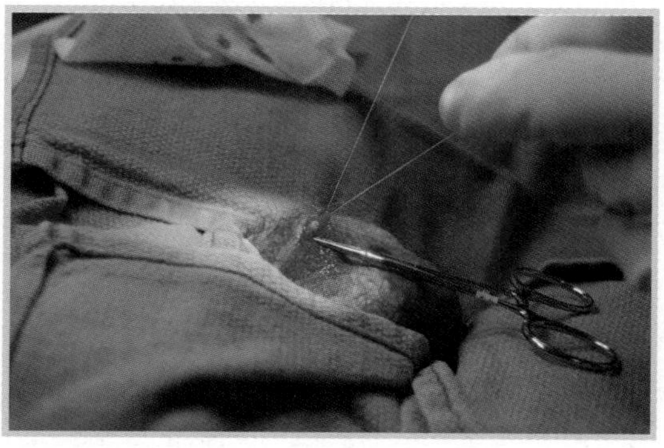

Step 13

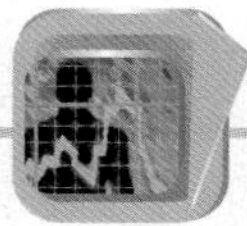

Complications

- Hematoma
- Pain, infection, and bleeding
- Congestive epididymitis
- Sperm granuloma
- Failure (about 0.3%)

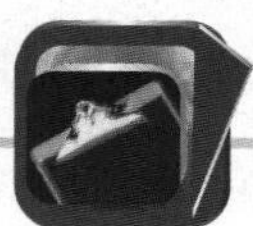

Postprocedure Instructions

Patients are instructed to rest and to intermittently place an ice pack on the groin on the day of the procedure. On the second day, the patient may ambulate to a limited degree. Activity may return to normal by the third day for most patients, although some prefer to avoid heavy lifting for 1 week. Patients should wear the athletic supporter for about 1 week for comfort.

Patients should be carefully counseled to obtain a semen analysis 3 months after the procedure to verify sterilization and to use another form of contraception until then.

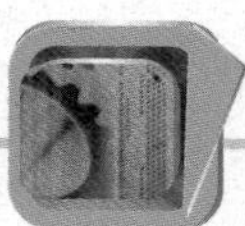

Coding Information

The following code may be reported for either bilateral vasectomy or for unilateral vasectomy (e.g., in the case of a patient who previously had an orchiectomy).

CPT Code	Description	2008 Average 50th Percentile Fee	Global Period
55250	Vasectomy, unilateral or bilateral, including postoperative semen examination(s)	$824.00	90

CPT is a registered trademark of the American Medical Association.
2008 average 50th Percentile Fees are provided courtesy of 2008 MMH-SI's copyrighted Physicians' Fees and Coding Guide.

Patient Education Handout

A patient education handout, "Postvasectomy Care for Adults" can be found on the book's Web site.

Bibliography

Alderman PM. Complications in a series of 1224 vasectomies. *J Fam Pract.* 1991;33:579–584.

Chawla A, Bowles B, Zini A. Vasectomy follow-up: clinical significance of rare nonmotile sperm in postoperative semen analysis. *Urology.* 2004;64:1212–1215.

Clenney TL, Higgins JC. Vasectomy techniques. *Am Fam Physician.* 1999;60:137–152.

Dassow P, Bennett JM. Vasectomy: an update. *Am Fam Physician.* 2006;74:2069–2074, 2076.

Labrecque M, Nazerali H, Mondor M, et al. Effectiveness and complications associated with 2 vasectomy occlusion techniques. *J Urol.* 2002;168:2495–2498.

Li SQ, Goldstein M, Zhu J, et al. No-scalpel vasectomy. *J Urol.* 1991;145:341–344.

Potts JM, Pasqualotto FF, Nelson D, et al. Patient characteristics associated with vasectomy reversal. *J Urol.* 1999;161:1835–1839.

2008 MAG Mutual Healthcare Solutions, Inc.'s Physicians' Fee and Coding Guide. Duluth, Georgia. MAG Mutual Healthcare Solutions, Inc. 2007.

CHAPTER 85

Laparoscopic Tubal Cauterization

Danielle Cooper, MD
Assistant Professor of Obstetrics and Gynecology
Louisiana State University Health Sciences Center, Shreveport, LA

The laparoscopic tubal cauterization is a procedure used to permanently surgically sterilize a woman. This is an elective procedure with virtually no absolute contraindications unless the patient is a poor surgical candidate. There are numerous methods for achieving permanent sterilization, but many women prefer the laparoscopic technique due to its effectiveness, rapid recovery, and outpatient basis. Bipolar coagulation is now the most commonly used laparoscopic occlusion method in the United States.

Even though this is considered a permanent form of contraception, reversal is possible. Informed consent is extremely important, with special attention given to the patient's most common complaint postoperatively, which is regret. All other contraceptive options must be reviewed and documented as well as consent for a possible laparotomy incision if unexpected anatomy or complications are incurred intraoperatively. The patient must also be made aware of the risk of tubal ligation failure resulting in either an intrauterine pregnancy or an ectopic pregnancy. The 5-year cumulative probability of pregnancy for women with three or more sites of bipolar coagulation is 3.2 per 1,000 procedures. The 10-year cumulative probability of ectopic pregnancy after bipolar coagulation is 17.1 per 1,000 procedures.

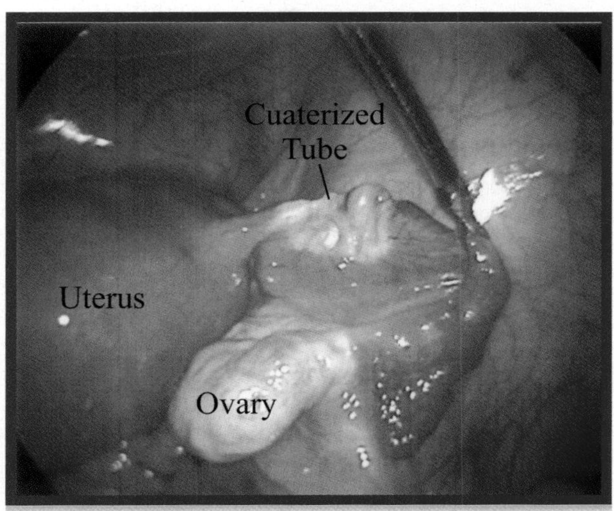

Another contraceptive method should be utilized for 1 month prior to the procedure, and a negative pregnancy test should be performed the day of surgery. Even though reversibility is an option, the patient must be made aware of the complications and expense associated with trying to reverse the tubal ligation. Even with reanastomosis, there is no guarantee of fertility. Younger age at the time of sterilization is a significant risk factor for developing future regret. There are nonsurgical, reversible, equally effective methods of contraception available to the patient, such as an intrauterine device or Depo-Provera, that should be discussed. The patient must be aware of the operative complications from both surgery and anesthesia. The option of male sterilization with vasectomy should be offered and explored with the patient prior to proceeding to the operating room.

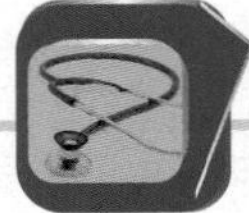

Equipment

- Anesthesiologist
- General endotracheal anesthesia
- Oral gastric tube
- Laparoscope with light source
- Bipolar operating forceps
- Ammeter
- Blunt probe
- Hulka uterine manipulator (optional)
- No. 11 blade
- Two trocars—10 mm and 5 mm
- Needle driver
- Veress needle
- Saline
- CO_2 gas
- Skin forceps
- 0 and 4.0 absorbable monofilament

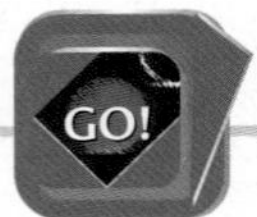

Indications

- Patient requests permanent surgical sterilization

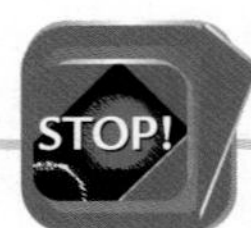

Contraindications

- Poor surgical candidate due to cardiac or pulmonary disease
- Morbidly obese, thus prohibiting laparoscopic use
- Severe pelvic adhesive disease distorting anatomy, making fallopian tubes unidentifiable
- History of previous tubal ligation failure—bilateral salpingectomy then indicated

The Procedure

Step 1. The patient is consented and taken to the operating room, where general endotracheal anesthesia is obtained and an oral gastric tube is inserted. She is placed in the dorsal lithotomy position utilizing Allen stirrups.

- **PEARL:** Positioning is very important to avoid unintentional injury. The arms of the patient may be tucked by her side to prevent brachial plexus injury; however, this may not be possible based on the patient's body habitus. If the patient's arms are perpendicular

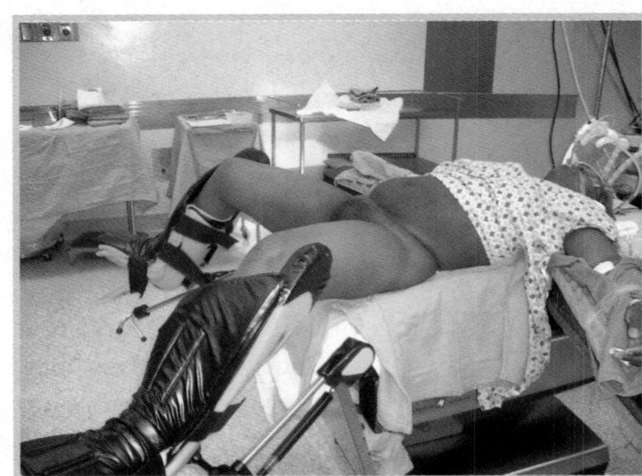

Step 1

to her body, take precautions to not lean against her arms during the procedure.

- **PEARL:** Some surgeons will utilize a shoulder harness because of the Trendelenburg positioning that will be necessary during the procedure. Others avoid these because of their high association with arm and neck injury.

Step 2. A bivalve speculum is inserted into the vagina. The cervix is cleaned with chlorhexidine cleanser. The anterior lip of the cervix is grasped, uterus sounded, and a Hulka uterine manipulator is inserted into the uterine cavity and attached to the anterior cervical lip. The initial tenaculum is removed. The speculum is removed from the vagina, and the bladder is drained. The nurse will then cleanse and drape the patient's abdomen.

- **PITFALL:** It is possible to perforate the uterus with the uterine sound or the Hulka uterine manipulator; therefore, respect for the tissue needs to be maintained.
- **PEARL:** The uterine manipulator is optional but will allow for better visualization and manipulation of the fallopian tubes. Some surgeons will just place a sponge stick in the vagina to raise the uterus into the visual field during the procedure.

Step 3. A 10-mm infraumbilical skin incision is made with the no. 11 blade. The abdominal cavity is lifted, and a Veress needle is inserted into the incision at a 45-degree angle until passing into the peritoneal cavity.

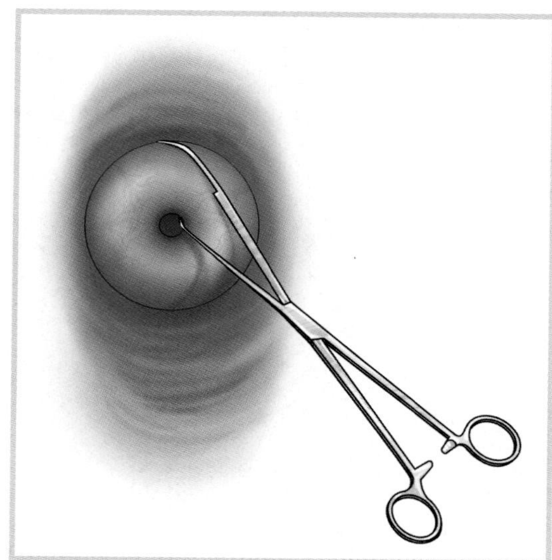

Step 2

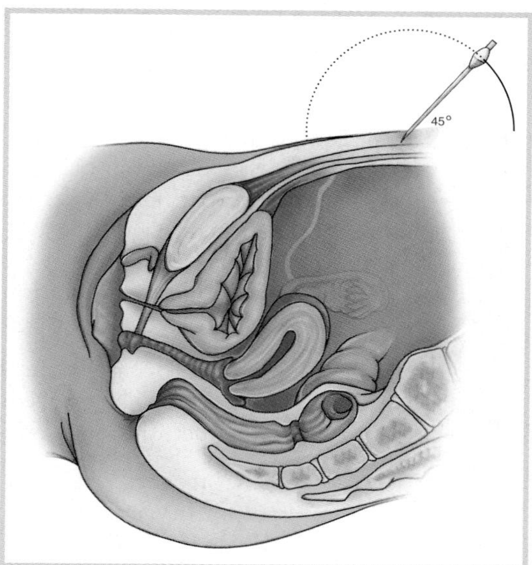

Step 3

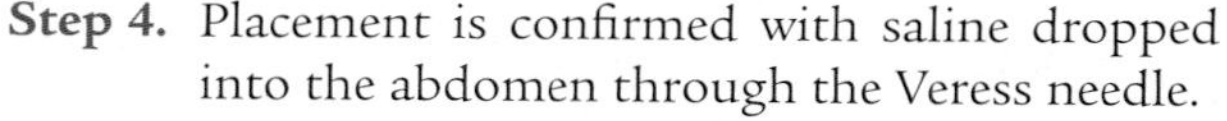

Step 4. Placement is confirmed with saline dropped into the abdomen through the Veress needle.

- **PITFALL:** Umbilical hernias or previous surgeries may prevent Veress needle use, and a cutdown procedure may be needed to avoid bowel injury.
- **PEARL:** In obese patients, the Veress needle is introduced directly into the abdomen at a 90-degree angle.
- **PEARL:** If you are unable to manually grasp the abdomen and lift, towel clamps may be placed lateral to the incision and used to lift the abdominal wall.

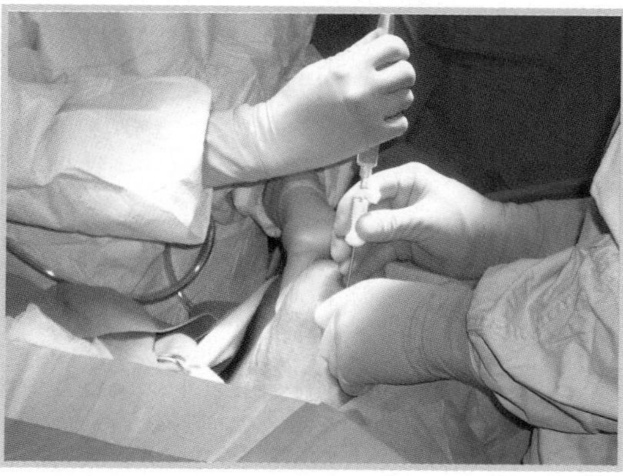

Step 4

Step 5. CO_2 gas is instilled into the peritoneal cavity until 15 to 18 mm Hg of intra-abdominal pressure is achieved; usually at least 3 L of CO_2 gas is needed for sufficient insufflation.

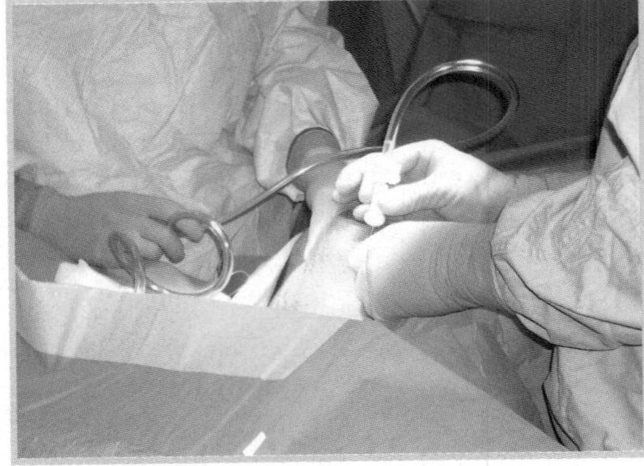

Step 5

Step 6. A 10-mm trocar is passed through the incision at a 45-degree angle, and a laparoscope is inserted to confirm intra-abdominal placement. The entire abdomen and pelvis are visually surveyed.

- **PITFALL:** In obese patients, the trocar is introduced directly into the abdomen at a 90-degree angle.

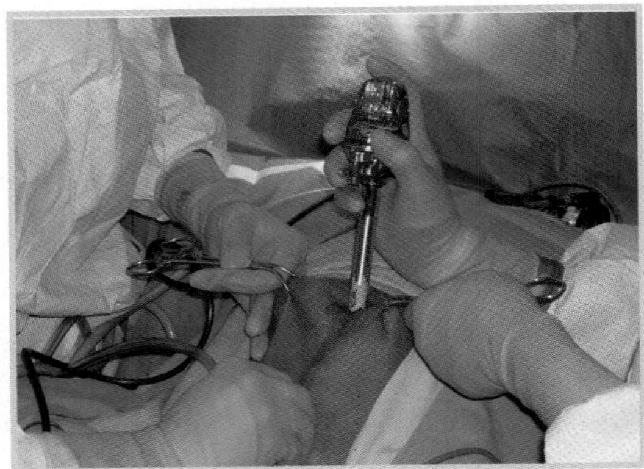

Step 6

Step 7. The patient is placed in the Trendelenburg position. The uterine manipulator lifts the uterus into the visual field. A second 5-mm midline incision is made with the no. 11 blade, 2 cm above the pubic symphysis. A 5-mm trocar is placed through this incision under direct visualization with the laparoscope.

- **PITFALL:** Failure to empty the bladder prior to the start of the procedure can result in bladder perforation.
- **PITFALL:** The trocar is aimed at the patient's sacrum in the midline, and too lateral of placement can result in significant injury and hemorrhage.
- **PEARL:** The uterus can be placed anterior to the bowel and protect both large and small bowel from injury with introduction of the second trocar.
- **PITFALL:** Aggressive manipulation of the uterus can result in uterine perforation.

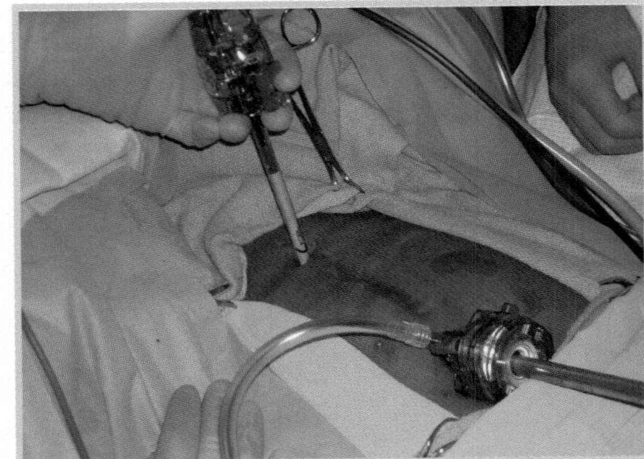

Step 7

Step 8. A blunt probe used to expose the entire fallopian tube and ovary on each side and maneuver the remainder of the bowel out of the pelvis.

- **PITFALL:** Severe pelvic adhesive disease may limit the ability to visualize the entire fallopian tube, but this must be achieved. If significant adhesive disease is encountered, it may be managed laparoscopically; alternatively, convert the case to an open procedure, and perform a laparotomy.

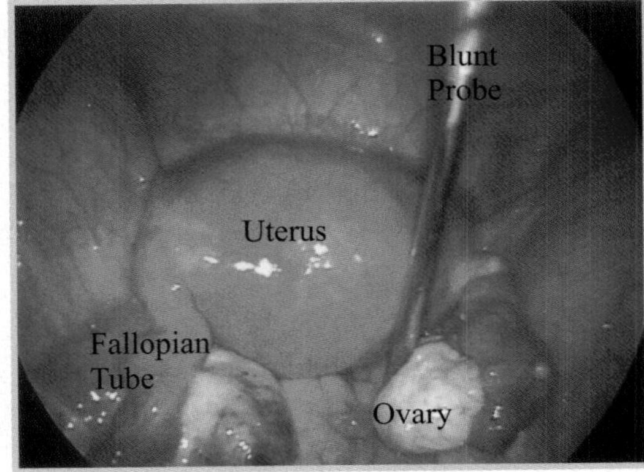

Step 8

Step 9. Bipolar operating forceps are used to grasp each tube in the ampullary region (approximately 2 to 3 cm from the cornu), placed on tension to ensure no contact with any other structures, and electrodessication is begun. Current is applied until an ammeter shows that tissue grasped has been completely desiccated.

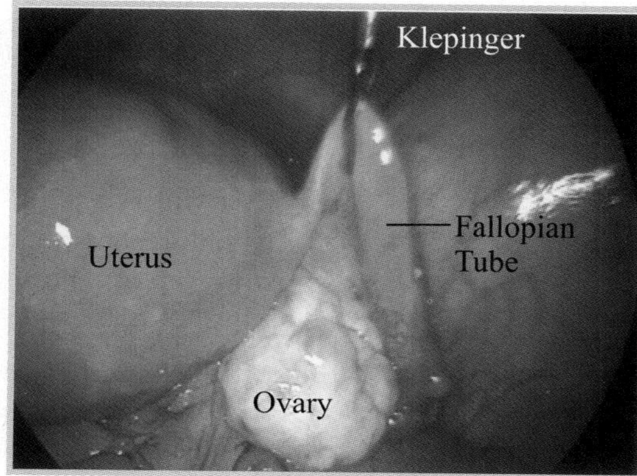

Step 9

Step 10. Regrasp the tube adjacent to this area, and begin desiccation. This is performed until at least 3 cm of contiguous tube is destroyed. Repeat on the opposite fallopian tube.

- PITFALL: Care must be taken to ensure that no other structures contact the desiccating forceps due to peripheral burn that occurs causing injury. The most common reason for failure of this method is related to incomplete desiccation of the endosalpinx.

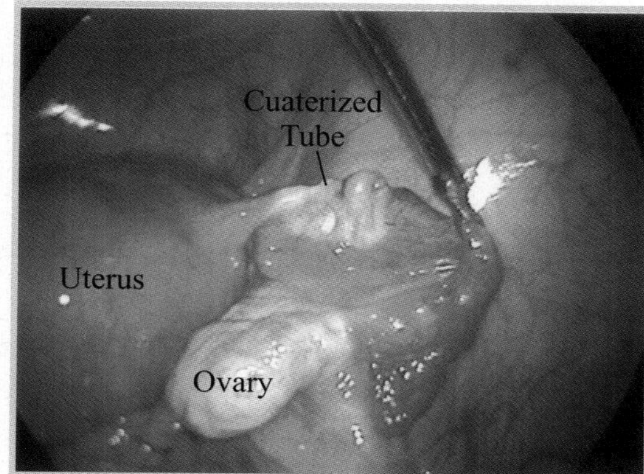

Step 10

Step 11. Remove all instruments from the abdomen and pelvis. A single 0 absorbable monofilament suture is used to close the fascial incision at the infraumbilical port site. Any other port sites >5 mm will also need to be closed in a similar fashion. The skin is reapproximated with a 4.0 absorbable monofilament in a running subcuticular fashion. Operative sites are bandaged. The Hulka uterine manipulator is removed. The patient is awakened and taken to recovery room. Once postoperative anesthesia protocols are met, the patient may be discharged home.

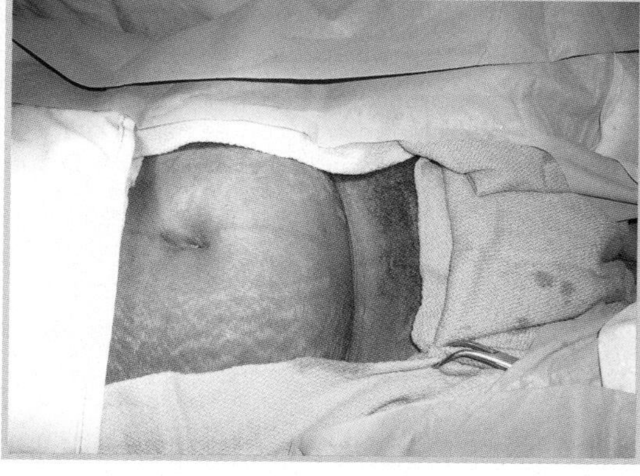

Step 11

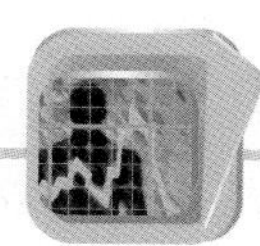

Complications

- Mortality: Risk of death from tubal sterilization is 1 to 2 cases per 100,000 procedures; most of these are complications of general anesthesia. Cardiopulmonary arrest and hypoventilation are reported as the leading cause of death. Sepsis as a cause of death is directly related to bowel perforations or electrical bowel burns.
- Unintended laparotomy occurs with 1% to 2% of laparoscopic procedures.
- Bowel injury can occur during the insertion of the insufflation needle or trocar or during electrocoagulation. Small injuries from the needle or trocar with no bleeding or leakage of enteric contents can be managed expectantly; all others require prompt laparotomy.

- Vascular injury can occur during insufflation needle or trocar insertion. Injury to a large vessel is life threatening, and immediate laparotomy with direct pressure to control bleeding until repair (usually by a vascular surgeon) can be performed.
- Pain: Chest and shoulder pain may be experienced postoperatively due to trapped CO_2 gas.
- Tubal failure: Surgical sterilization is highly effective and considered a definitive form of contraception; however, it has a failure rate of 0.1% to 0.8% in the first year. At least one third of these are ectopic pregnancies.
- Regret: Poststerilization regret is a complex condition caused by unpredictable life events. Young age, low parity, single-parent status, or being in an unstable relationship are risk factors for regret.

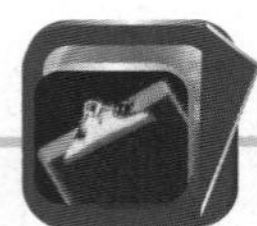

Postprocedure Instructions

The patient is advised to use over-the-counter nonsteroidal anti-inflammatory drugs for pain. A narcotic pain prescription may be given for any breakthrough pain she may be experiencing. If the patient experiences any fever (>100.4), heavy bleeding (> one pad per hour), abdominal pain (unrelieved by pain medication), and excessive nausea or vomiting, she should return to the hospital immediately. Follow up on an outpatient basis in 2 weeks to ensure proper healing of the incisions.

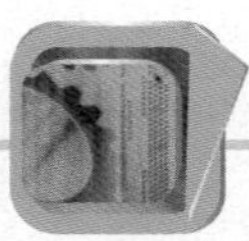

Coding Information and Supply Sources

CPT Code	Description	2008 Average 50th Percentile Fee	Global Period
58670	Laparoscopy, surgical; with fulguration of oviducts (with or without transaction)	$1,688.00	90

CPT is a registered trademark of the American Medical Association.
2008 average 50th Percentile Fees are provided courtesy of 2008 MMH-SI's copyrighted Physicians' Fees and Coding Guide.

ICD-9 Code

V25.2 Sterilization

Patient Education Handout

A patient education handout, "Tubal Sterilization," can be found on the book's Web site.

Bibliography

American College of Obstetricians and Gynecologists. *Benefits and Risks of Sterilization*. ACOG Practice Bulletin 46. Washington, DC: Author; 2003.

Peterson HB, Xia Z, Wilcox LS, et al. for the U.S. Collaborative Review of Sterilization Working Group. Pregnancy after tubal sterilization with bipolar electrocoagulation. *Obstet Gynecol.* 1999;94:163–167.

Stovall TG, Mann WJ. Surgical sterilization of women. Up to Date. Available at http://www.uptodate.com. Accessed July 1, 2008.

2008 MAG Mutual Healthcare Solutions, Inc.'s Physicians' Fee and Coding Guide. Duluth, Georgia. MAG Mutual Healthcare Solutions, Inc. 2007.

SECTION EIGHT

GASTROENTEROLOGY

CHAPTER 86

Abdominal Paracentesis

E. J. Mayeaux, Jr., MD, DABFP, FAAFP

Professor of Family Medicine, Professor of Obstetrics and Gynecology
Louisiana State University Health Sciences Center, Shreveport, LA

Abdominal paracentesis is a safe and effective diagnostic and therapeutic procedure used in the evaluation of a variety of abdominal problems, including ascites, abdominal injury, acute abdomen, and peritonitis. Ascites may be recognized on physical examination as abdominal distention and the presence of a fluid wave. Therapeutic paracentesis is employed to relieve respiratory difficulty due to increased intra-abdominal pressure caused by ascites.

Midline and lateral approaches can be used for paracentesis, with the left-lateral technique more commonly employed. The left-lateral approach avoids air-filled bowel that usually floats in the ascitic fluid. The patient is placed in the supine position and slightly rotated to the side of the procedure to further minimize the risk of perforation during paracentesis. Because the cecum is relatively fixed on the right side, the left-lateral approach is most commonly used.

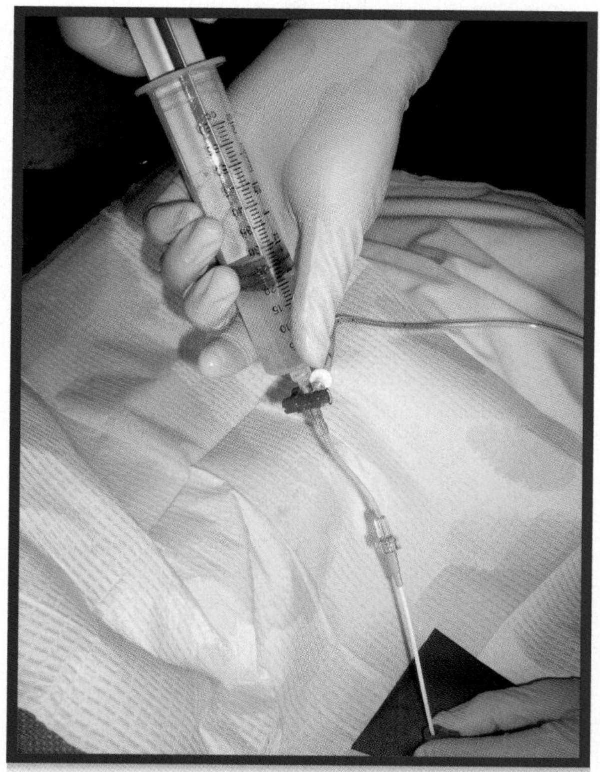

Most ascetic fluid reaccumulates rapidly. Some experts recommend that no more than 1.5 L of fluid be removed in any single procedure. Patients with severe hypoproteinemia may lose additional albumen into reaccumulations of ascites fluid and develop acute hypotension and heart failure. Cancer patients with malignant effusions may also need repetitive therapeutic paracentesis. Intravenous fluid and vascular volume support may be required in these patients if larger volumes are removed.

After diagnostic paracentesis, fluid should be sent to the laboratory for Gram stain; culture; cytology; protein, glucose, and lactate dehydrogenase levels; and blood cell count with a differential cell count. A polymorphonuclear cell count of >500 cells/mm^3 is highly suggestive of bacterial peritonitis. An elevated peritoneal fluid amylase level or a level greater than the serum amylase level is found in pancreatitis. Grossly bloody fluid in the abdomen (>100,000 red blood cells/mm^3) indicates more severe trauma or perforation of an abdominal organ. The classic positive test for hemoperitoneum is the inability to read newspaper type through the paracentesis lavage fluid.

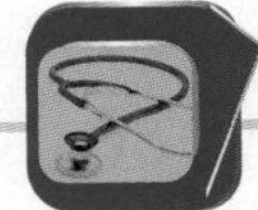

Equipment

Disposable paracentesis/thoracentesis kits usually include the following:

- Antiseptic swab sticks
- Fenestrated drape
- Lidocaine 1%, 5-mL ampule
- Syringe, 10 mL
- 2-inch-long injection needle
- No. 11 blade scalpel
- 14-gauge catheter over 17-gauge × 6-inch needle with three-way stopcock or one-way valve, self-sealing valve, and a 5-mL Luer Lock syringe
- Syringe, 60 mL
- Tubing set with roller clamp
- Drainage bag or vacuum container
- Specimen vials or collection bottles (3)
- Gauze, 4 inch × 4 inch
- Adhesive dressing

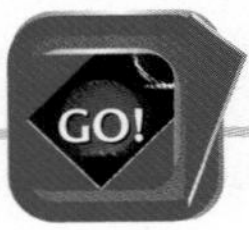

Indications

- Evaluation of ascites fluid to help determine etiology, to differentiate transudate versus exudate, to detect the presence of cancerous cells, or to address other considerations
- Evaluation of blunt or penetrating abdominal injury
- Relief of respiratory distress due to increased intra-abdominal pressure
- Evaluation of acute abdomen
- Evaluation of acute or spontaneous peritonitis
- Evaluation of acute pancreatitis

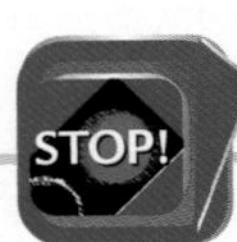

Contraindications

- Acute abdomen requiring immediate surgery (absolute contraindication)
- Severe thrombocytopenia (platelet count <20 × 103/μL)
- Coagulopathy (international normalized ratio [INR] >2.0)
- In patients without clinical evidence of active bleeding, routine labs such as prothrombin time (PT), activated partial thromboplastin time (aPTT), and platelet counts may not be needed prior to the procedure.
- Severe bowel distention (use extra caution)
- Multiple previous abdominal operations
- Pregnancy (absolute to midline procedure)
- Distended bladder that cannot be emptied with a Foley catheter (relative contraindication)
- Obvious infection at the intended site of insertion (relative contraindication)
- Severe hypoproteinemia (relative contraindication)
- Intra-abdominal adhesions

The Procedure

Step 1. The anatomy of the abdominal wall is shown. The insertion sites may be midline or through the oblique transversus muscle, which is lateral to the thicker rectus abdominus muscles.

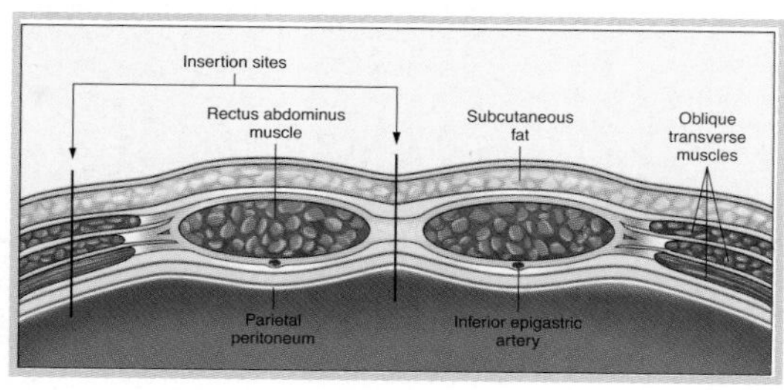

Step 1

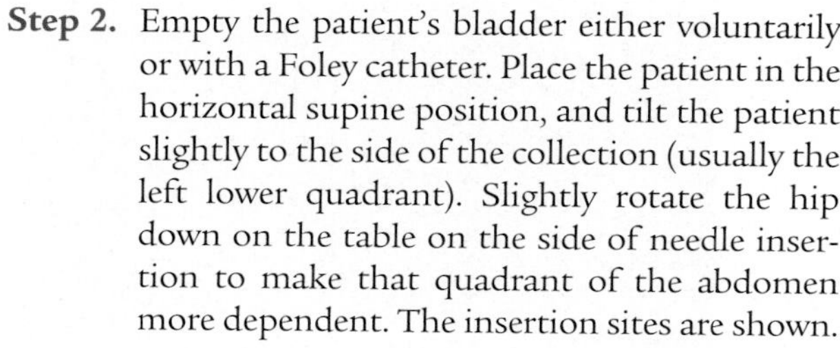

Step 2. Empty the patient's bladder either voluntarily or with a Foley catheter. Place the patient in the horizontal supine position, and tilt the patient slightly to the side of the collection (usually the left lower quadrant). Slightly rotate the hip down on the table on the side of needle insertion to make that quadrant of the abdomen more dependent. The insertion sites are shown.

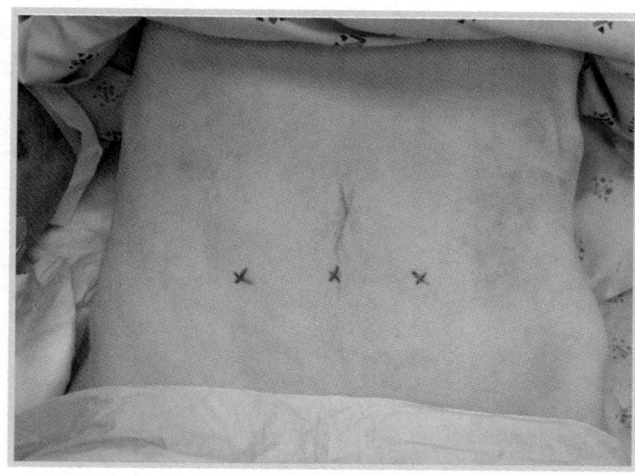

Step 2

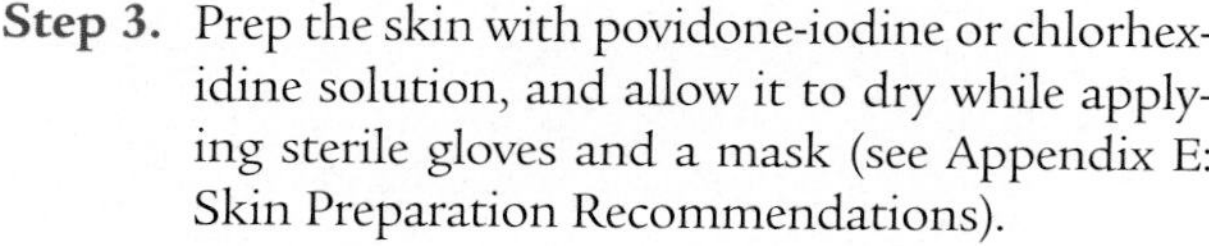

Step 3. Prep the skin with povidone-iodine or chlorhexidine solution, and allow it to dry while applying sterile gloves and a mask (see Appendix E: Skin Preparation Recommendations).

- **PEARL:** Prep a wide area so that an undraped area is not inadvertently exposed if the drape slides a little.

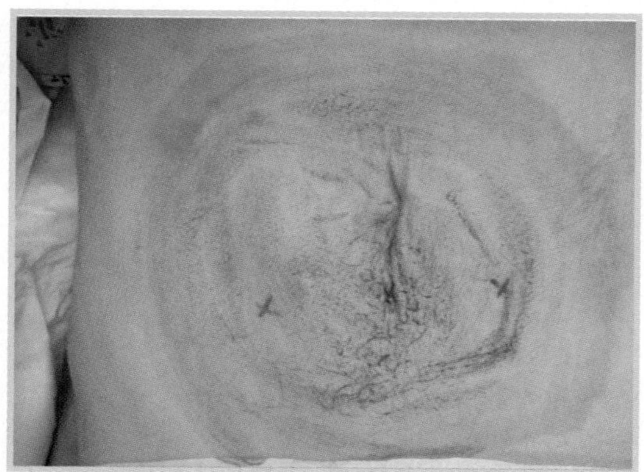

Step 3

Step 4. Center the sterile drape about one third of the distance from the umbilicus to the anterior iliac crest.

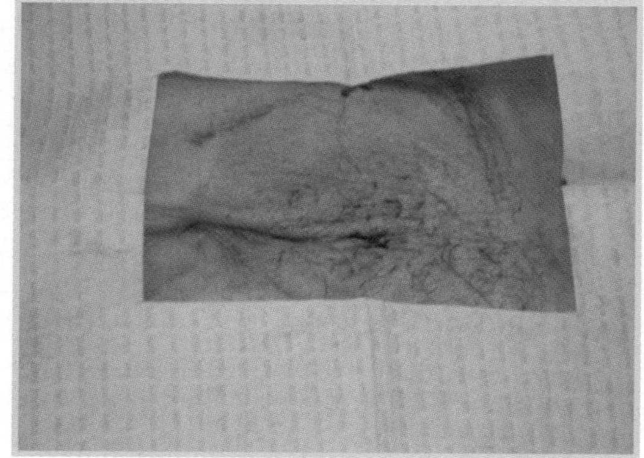

Step 4

Step 5. Infiltrate the skin and subcutaneous tissues with a 1% solution of lidocaine with epinephrine. A 2-inch needle is then inserted perpendicular to the skin to infiltrate the deeper tissues and peritoneum with anesthetic.

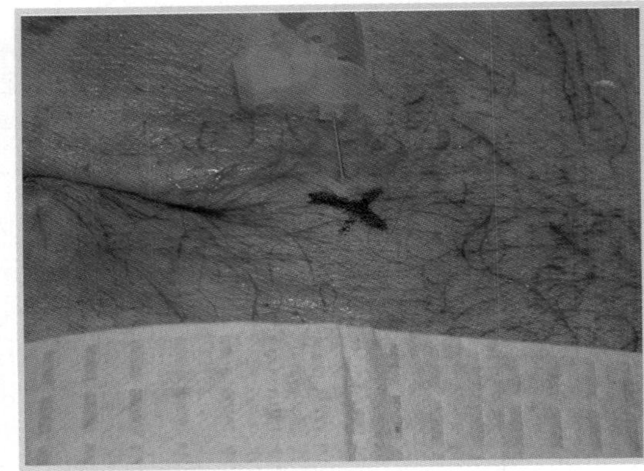

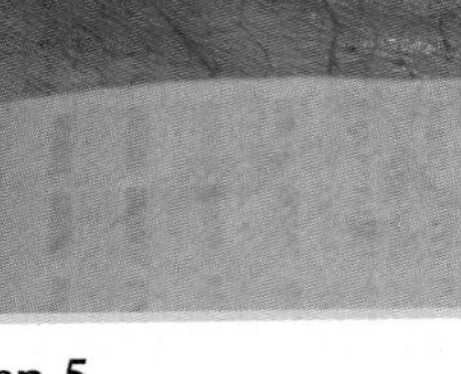

Step 5

Step 6. Insert the catheter/introducer through the skin. The nondominant hand then stretches the skin to one side of the puncture site, and the needle is further inserted to create a Z tract.

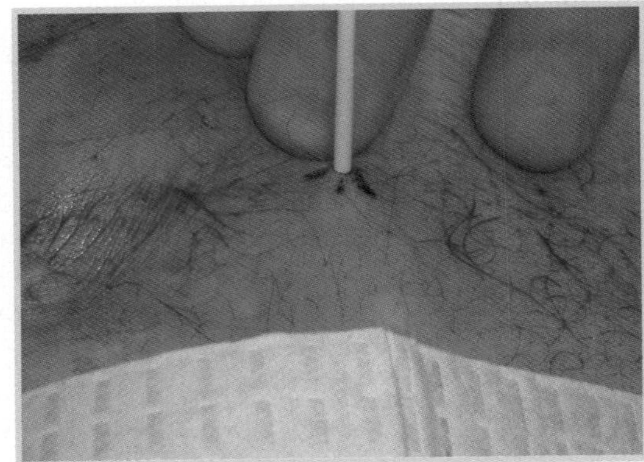

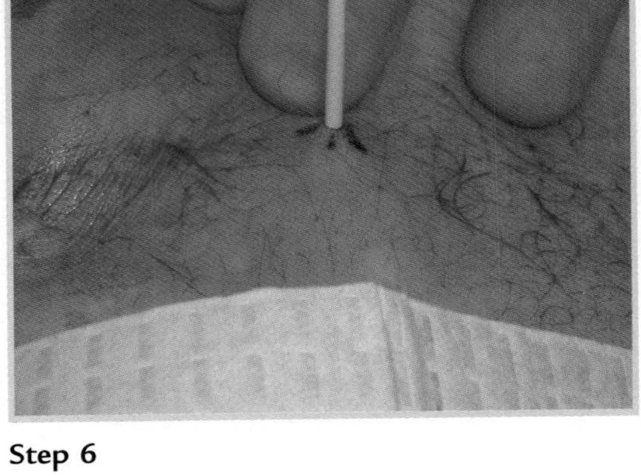

Step 6

Step 7. Advance the catheter until a "pop" is felt and the catheter penetrates the peritoneum. Release the pressure on the skin after the introducer enters the peritoneum. Advance the catheter into the abdominal cavity.

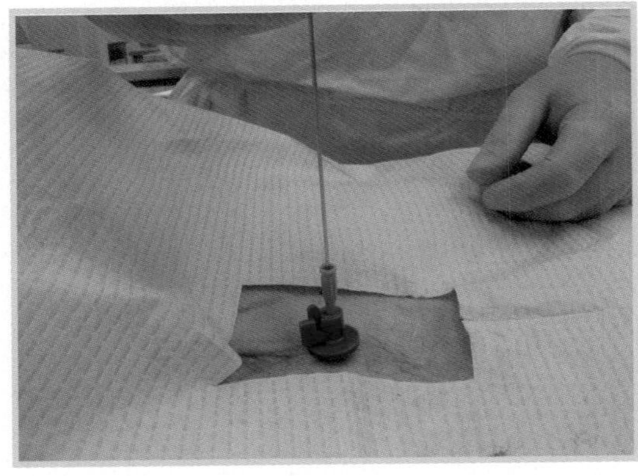

Step 7

Step 8. Remove the introducer, and attach the syringe. Draw the fluid into the syringe. If no fluid returns, rotate, slightly withdraw, or advance the catheter until fluid is obtained. If still no fluid returns, abort the procedure, and try an alternative site or method. Ascites fluid may be removed by attaching a three-way stopcock or one-way valve, a 60-cc syringe to one arm, and drainage tubing and bag to the other arm. If lavage is desired, such as for detecting hemoperitoneum after trauma, connect intravenous tubing to the three-way stopcock. Remove excess fluid and then infuse 700 to 1,000 mL of Ringer lactate or normal saline into the abdominal cavity. Gently roll the patient from side to side. Then, remove the fluid as described above or using a trap-suction arrangement.

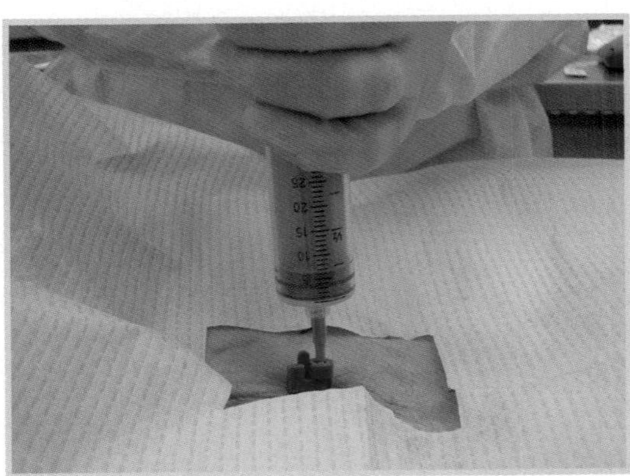

Step 8

Step 9. After the procedure, gently remove the catheter, and apply direct pressure to the wound. Observe the characteristics of the fluid, and send it for the appropriate studies. If the insertion site is still leaking fluid after 5 minutes of direct pressure, suture the site with a vertical mattress suture. Apply a pressure dressing.

- PITFALL: Gauze dressing should be applied when rare, persistent drainage occurs.

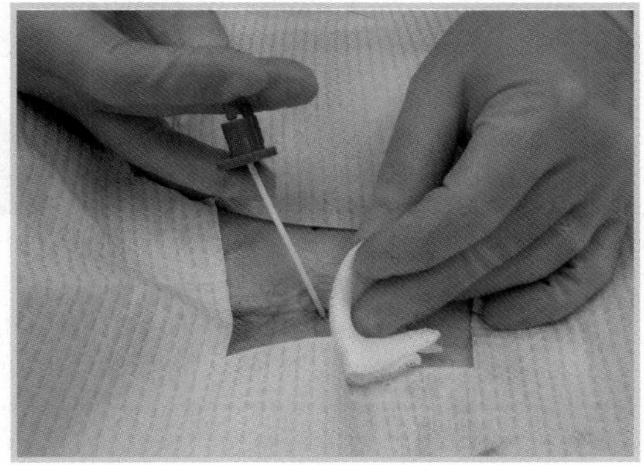

Step 9

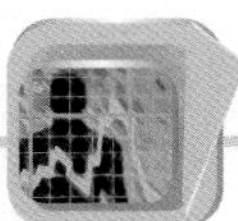

Complications

- Abdominal radiographs should be obtained before paracentesis, because air may be introduced during the procedure and may interfere with interpretation.
- Perforation of bladder and stomach (emptied prior to the procedure to decrease the risk)
- Bowel perforation
- Laceration of a major blood vessel
- Loss of catheter or guide wire in the peritoneal cavity
- Abdominal wall hematomas
- Pneumoperitoneum
- Bleeding
- Perforation of the pregnant uterus
- Infection
- Persistent leak from the puncture site
- Postparacentesis hypotension
- Dilutional hyponatremia
- Hepatorenal syndrome

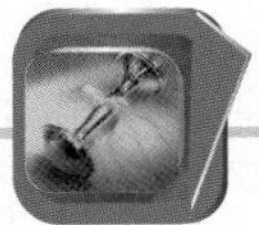

Pediatric Considerations

Pediatric patients may not cooperate with placement of catheter placement. Because of the risks of damage to vessels, nerves, and so forth, consider conscious sedation with intramuscular injections or oral administration of sedating medications such as Versed and Ketamine.

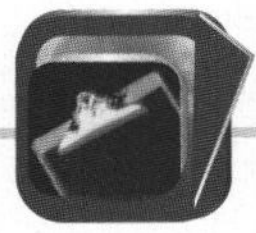

Postprocedure Instructions

The patient should be instructed to monitor the bleeding of the area and return if any abnormal bleeding is noted. The patient should also be educated to call with questions or concerns regarding pain, numbness, or discomfort in the area. The patient should also monitor for evidence of infection. Lastly, the patient should be advised to clean the area with warm soap and water and pat the area dry.

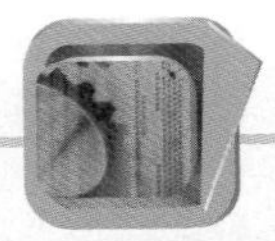

Coding Information and Supply Sources

CPT Code	Description	2008 Average 50th Percentile Fee	Global Period
49080	Peritoneocentesis, abdominal paracentesis, or peritoneal lavage, initial	$344.00	0
49081	Peritoneocentesis, abdominal paracentesis, or peritoneal lavage, subsequent.	$271.00	0

Paracentesis trays that include all instruments needed to perform the procedure can be ordered from the following manufacturers:

- Arrow Medical Products Ltd., 2400 Bernville Road, Reading, PA 19605 (phone: 1-800-233-3187; Web site: http://www.arrowintl.com/)
- Baxter, One Baxter Parkway, Deerfield, IL 60015-4625 (phone: 1-847-948-2000; fax: 847-948-3642; Web site: http://www.baxter.com)
- American Hospital Supply (phone: 1-407-475-1168; Web site: http://www.americanhospitalsupply.com/)
- Cardinal Health, Inc., 7000 Cardinal Place, Dublin, OH 43017 (phone: 1-800-234-8701; Web site: http://www.cardinal.com/)
- Owens and Minor, 4800 Cox Road, Glen Allen, VA 23060-6292 (phone: 1-804-747-9794; fax: 1-804-270-7281)
- Allegiance Healthcare Corp., McGraw Park, IL 60085 (phone: 1-847-689-8410; Web site: http://www.cardinal.com/mps/brands/specialprocedures/diagnostictrays.asp)

Patient Education Handout

A patient education handout, "Paracentesis," can be found on the book's Web site.

Bibliography

Cappell MS, Shetty V. A multicenter, case-controlled study of the clinical presentation and etiology of ascites and of the safety and clinical efficacy of diagnostic abdominal paracentesis in HIV seropositive patients. *Am J Gastroenterol.* 1994;89:2172–2177.

Guarner C, Soriano G. Spontaneous bacterial peritonitis. *Semin Liver Dis.* 1997;17:203–217.

Gupta S, Talwar S, Sharma RK, et al. Blunt trauma abdomen: a study of 63 cases. *Indian J Med Sci.* 1996;50:272–276.

Halpern NA, McElhinney AJ, Greenstein RJ. Postoperative sepsis: reexplore or observe? Accurate indication from diagnostic abdominal paracentesis. *Crit Care Med.* 1991;19:882–886.

Mansoor T, Zubari S, Masiullah M. Evaluation of peritoneal lavage and abdominal paracentesis in cases of blunt abdominal trauma—a study of fifty cases. *J Indian Med Assoc.* 2000;98:174–175.

Romney R, Mathurin P, Ganne-Carrié N, et al. Usefulness of routine analysis of ascitic fluid at the time of therapeutic paracentesis in asymptomatic outpatients. Results of a multicenter prospective study. *Gastroenterol Clin Biol.* 2005;29(3):275–279.

Runyon BA. Management of adult patients with ascites caused by cirrhosis. *Hepatology.* 1998;27:264–272.

Stephenson J, Gilbert J. The development of clinical guidelines on paracentesis for ascites related to malignancy. *Palliat Med.* 2002;16:213–218.

Thomson A, Cain P, Kerlin P, et al. Serious hemorrhage complicating diagnostic abdominal paracentesis. *J Clin Gastroenterol.* 1998;26:306–308.

Watanabe A. Management of ascites: a review. *J Med.* 1997;28:21–30.

Webster ST, Brown KL, Lucey MR, et al. Hemorrhagic complications of large volume abdominal paracentesis. *Am J Gastroenterol.* 1996;91:366–368.

2008 MAG Mutual Healthcare Solutions, Inc.'s Physicians' Fee and Coding Guide. Duluth, Georgia. MAG Mutual Healthcare Solutions, Inc. 2007.

CHAPTER 87

Anoscopy with or without Biopsy

Larry S. Sasaki, MD, FACS
Assistant Clinical Professor of Surgery
Louisiana State University Health Sciences Center, Shreveport, LA

Anoscopy is a diagnostic and therapeutic technique for the anal canal. Anoscopy is performed in the office without sedation. Office evaluation of common anorectal complaints such as "hemorrhoids" will necessitate a thorough examination. This is best accomplished by performing an anoscopy. Frequently, examiners will substitute a rigid or flexible sigmoidoscopy to visualize the anal canal. This is a suboptimal examination because anal canal lesions may easily be missed, for example, as can occur when a lesion is hidden between the hemorrhoidal columns. Additionally, barium enema examination has been used to substitute a for thorough anorectal examination. This also has resulted in many missed anal lesions. Anoscopy provides the best means of examining the anal canal for hemorrhoids, fissures, fistulas, neoplasms, or other lesions.

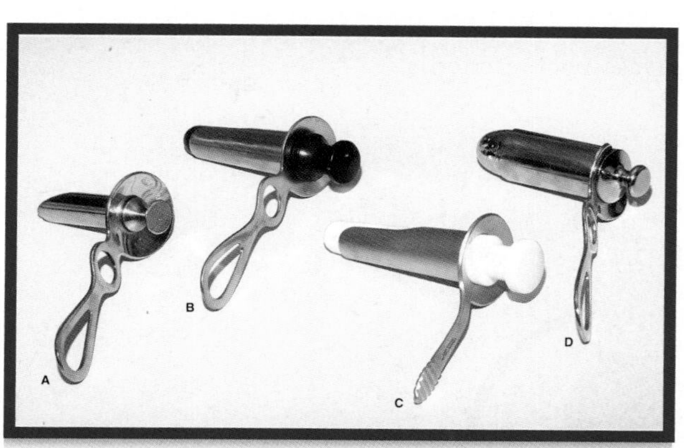

Anoscopy is accomplished by using one of several different instruments. There are several different nondisposable anoscopes available. Anoscopes shown include the (A) Hirschman, available in three sizes: 9/16 inch (1.43 cm), 11/16 inch (1.75 cm), and 7/8 inch (2.2 cm), (B) Pennington, (C) Fansler-Ives, and (D) Chelsea Eaton.

There is also a fiberoptic anoscope that has the convenience of a disposable sheath. It also allows the provider to work at a greater distance from the anus and often in a more comfortable position.

Biopsy can be performed by using rectal biopsy forceps. If a neoplastic lesion is identified, a biopsy may be performed. However, biopsy may not be necessary if surgical referral is planned.

No bowel preparation is needed for an anoscopic examination. A digital examination should precede an anoscopic examination to assess whether the patient will tolerate passage of an anoscope. Inspection and palpation alone can reveal the presence of some fissures, fistulas, perianal dermatitis, masses, thrombosed external hemorrhoids, condyloma, and other growths.

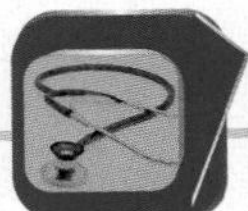

Equipment

Anoscopic Examination

- Surgical water-soluble lubricant
- Anoscope: disposable fiberoptic anoscope or metallic anoscopes
- Illumination instrument

Biopsy Equipment

- Biopsy forceps
- Anorectal pure anesthetic cream or combination with steroid (optional)
- 1% lidocaine with epinephrine
- Silver nitrate
- Cotton-tip applicators

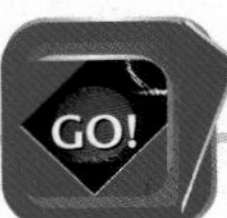

Indications

- Rectal symptoms: bleeding, itching, swelling, or pain
- Anal lesion or mass

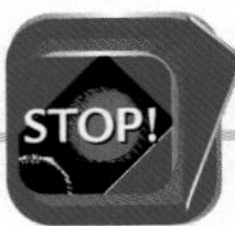

Contraindications

- Anal stricture or stenosis
- Severe pain
- Bleeding diathesis
- Acute cardiovascular conditions (vasovagal reaction)
- Acute abdominal conditions

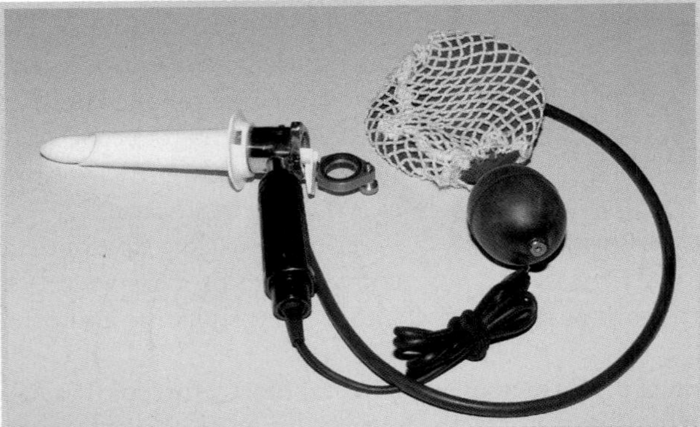

Figure 2

The Procedure

Anoscopic Examination

Step 1. Place the patient in the left lateral decubitus position. Inspect the perianal skin. A simple gooseneck lamp for illumination is ideal. Note the location of any lesions with respect to the patient's anterior, posterior, left lateral, and right lateral positions. This is frequently designated by the use of "o'clock" descriptions. With o'clock description, the "12 o'clock" position is the anterior midline of the anus (likewise, 3 o'clock is left lateral, 6 o'clock is posterior midline, and 9 o'clock is right lateral). The patient shown has a posterior anal fissure (6 o'clock) and a hypertrophic anal papilla on the right lateral aspect of anal canal (9 o'clock).

- **PITFALL:** Lesions such as an anal fissure may be too painful for anoscopy. Do not perform anoscopy in this setting.

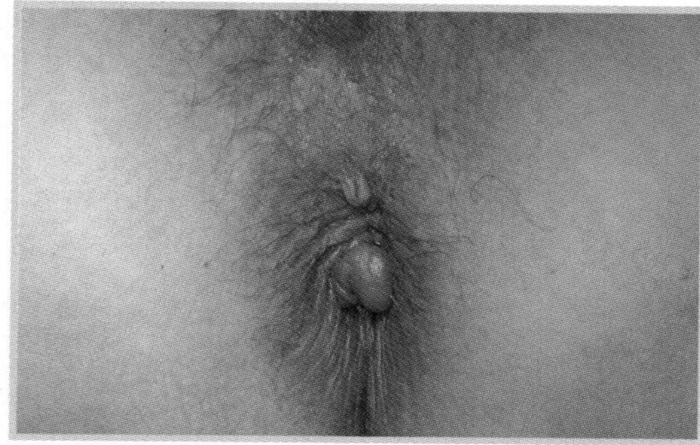

Step 1

Step 2. Anoscopy is not necessary for diagnosis of an anal fissure. Simply stretching the perianal skin can expose and diagnose an anal fissure. If symptoms are consistent with an anal fissure, then a trial of medical treatment may be warranted. Of course, referral to a surgeon may be also made at this time.

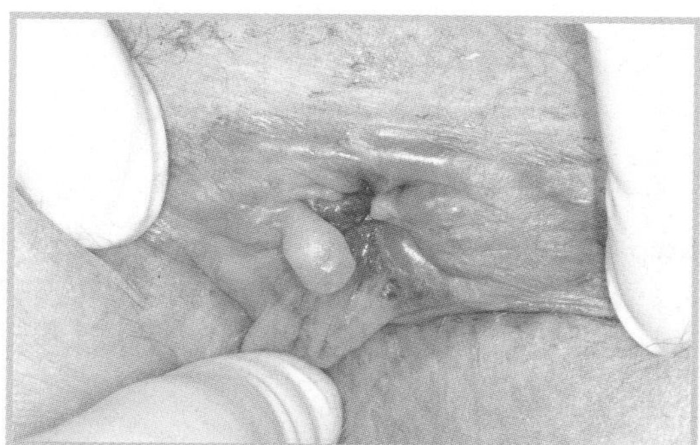

Step 2

Step 3. Palpate the perianal region to identify lesions such as a perirectal abscess, fistula, or mass. Digital examination is gently performed with careful assessment of the degree of discomfort.

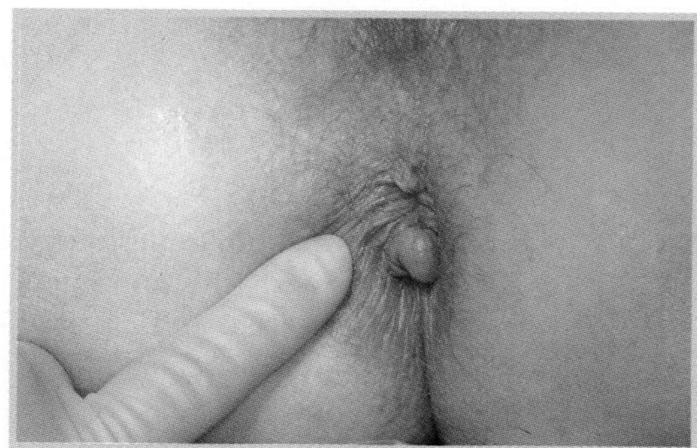

Step 3

Step 4. During digital examination, the anal canal should be palpated between the index finger and thumb, especially if an anal fistula or mass is suspected. If this can be accomplished without undue pain, then anoscopic examination can be performed.

- **PITFALL:** Painful anal lesions such as fissures may not be adequately anesthetized with anal creams. Do not perform anoscopy in this setting.
- **PEARL:** Some providers prefer a topical anesthetic such as 2.5% prilocaine and 2.5% lidocaine (EMLA) cream.

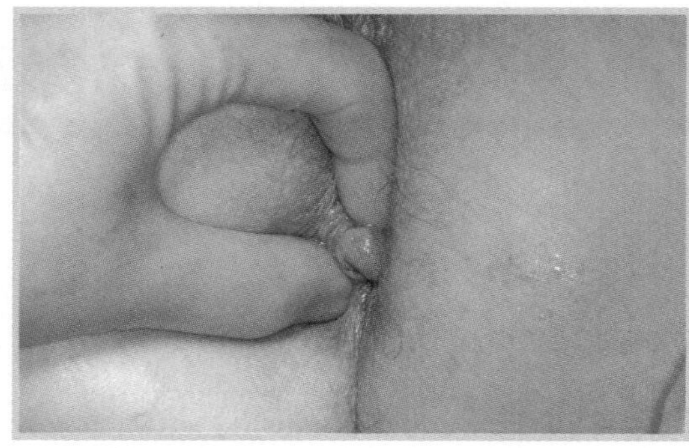

Step 4

Step 5. Gently insert the well-lubricated anoscope with obturator.

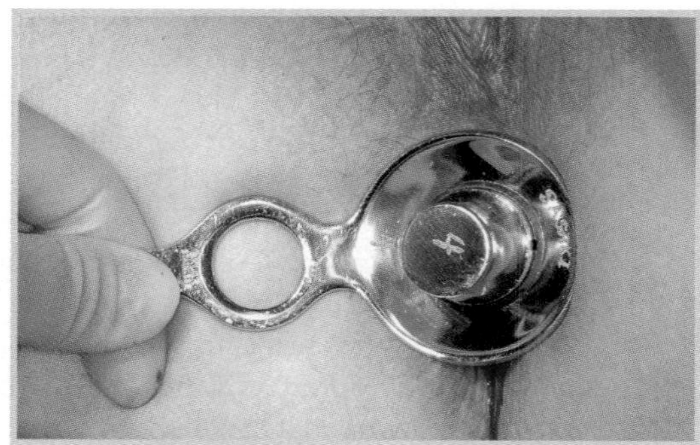

Step 5

Step 6. Remove the obturator to visualize the anal canal. Reinsert the obturator *prior* to rotating the anoscope to visualize another quadrant of the anal canal.

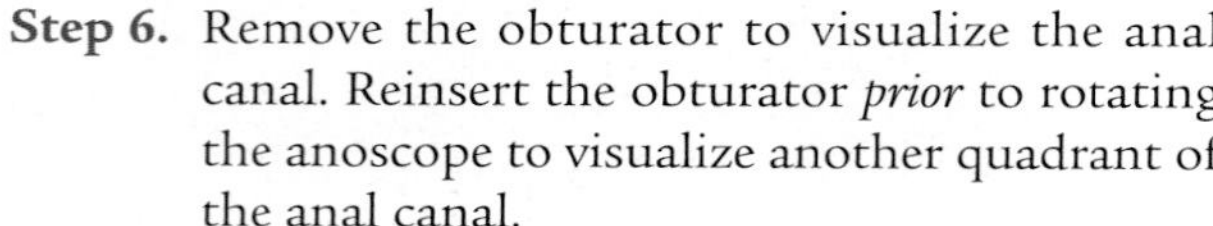

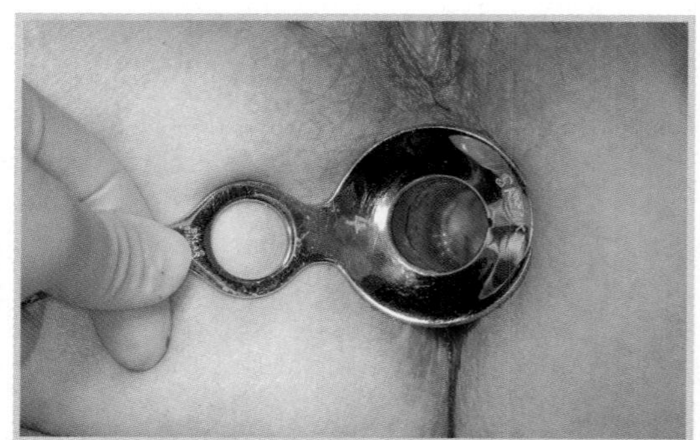

Step 6

Step 7. Examine the epithelium for lesions. Examples of lesions seen with the anoscope include (A) prominent internal and external hemorrhoid complex and (B) an anal fissure.

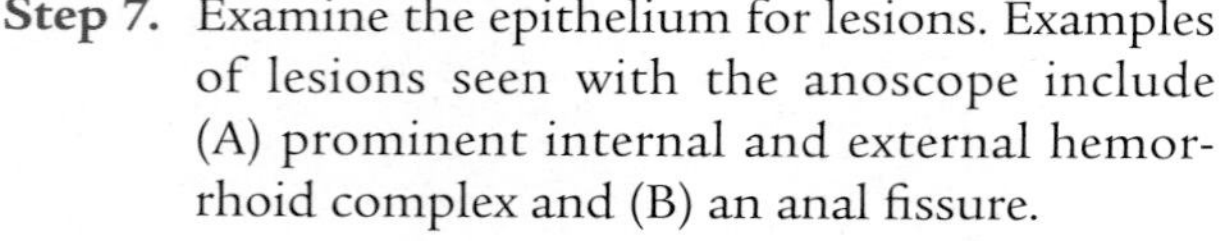

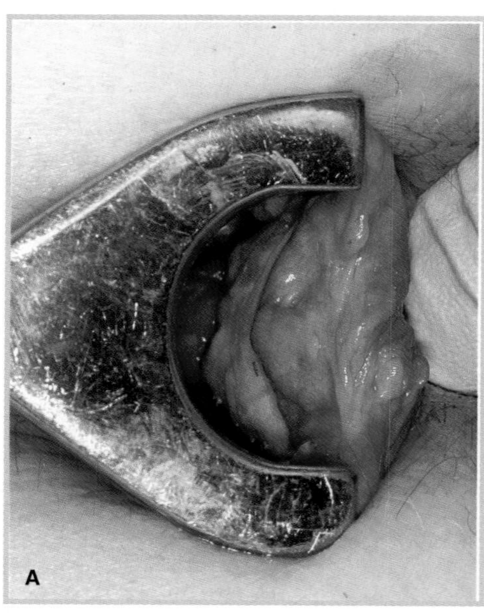

A

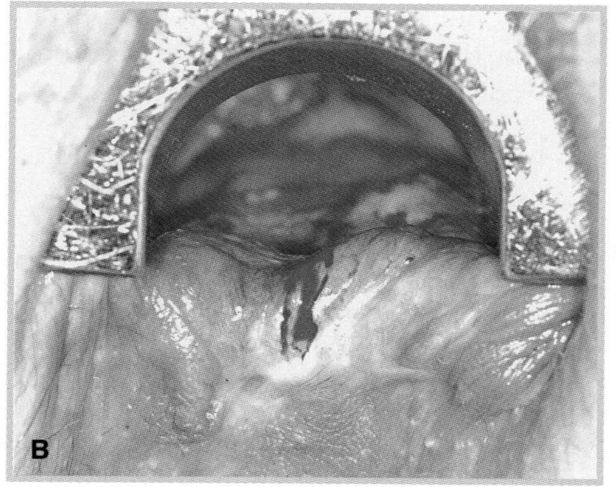
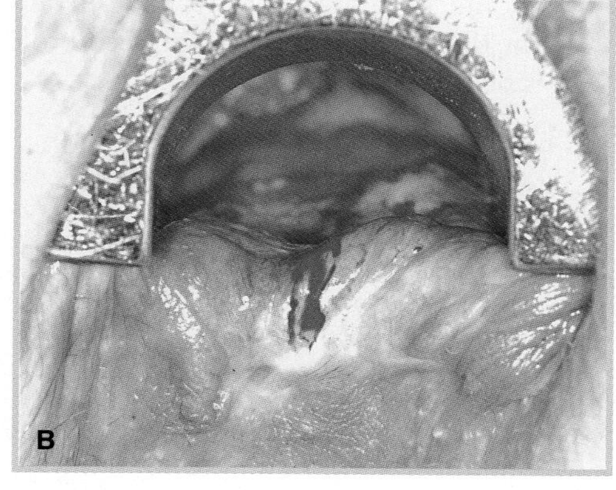

Step 7

Step 8. Other examples of lesions seen with the anoscope include (A) an anal fistula with the internal opening (marked by the probe) located at the posterior midline and dentate line and (B) an anal condyloma.

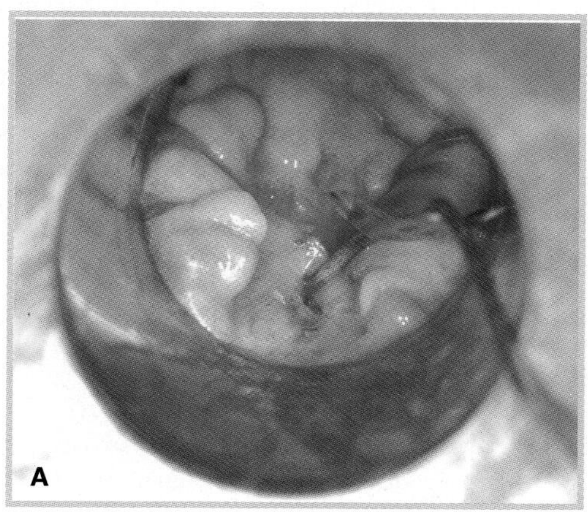

Step 8

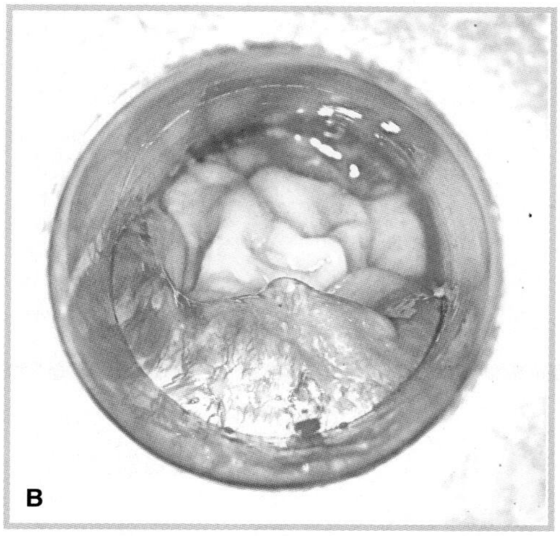

Anoscopic Biopsy

Step 9. Anoscopic biopsy can be performed with relative ease and safety. Bleeding is rarely a problem, so unelectrified biopsy forceps may be used. The biopsy is done under direct vision. Note the location of the biopsy site relative to the o'clock description and depth. The depth

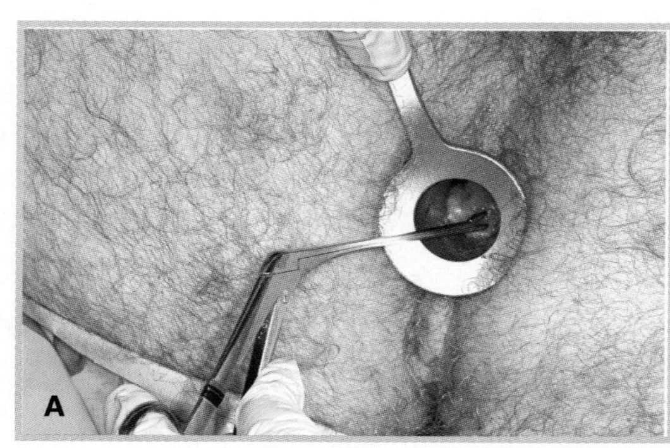

should be characterized by its distance from the dentate line (e.g., "3 mm distal to the dentate line").

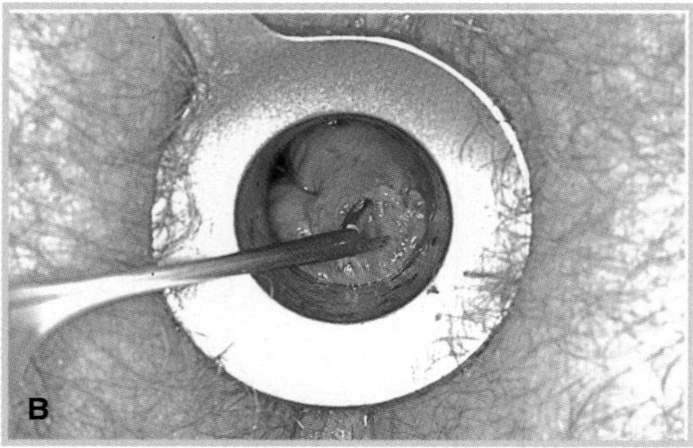

Step 9

Step 10. Biopsy of anal canal lesions may be painful. A single biopsy is well tolerated; however, multiple biopsies may require injection of local anesthetic (1% lidocaine with epinephrine).

- **PEARL:** Pathologic lesions such as an exophytic neoplasm are usually asensate, and thus a local anesthetic is usually unnecessary.

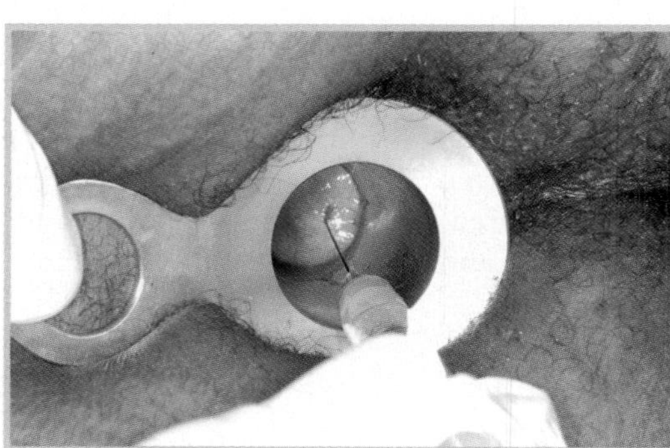

Step 10

Step 11. Bleeding is usually self-resolving and does not require further treatment. However, if the bleeding is pulsatile, then additional measures may be required. The biopsy site can be tamponaded with a cotton-tip applicator soaked with 1% lidocaine with epinephrine or cauterized using silver nitrate. Failed attempts to control bleeding mandate packing the anal canal with gauze and an immediate referral to surgery.

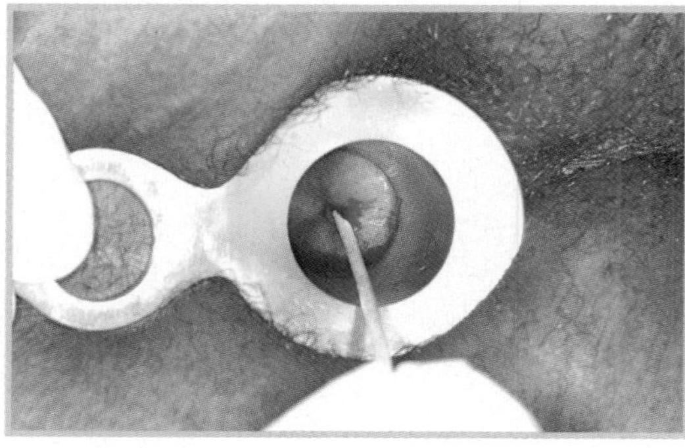

Step 11

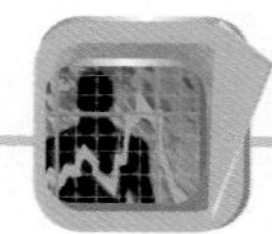

Complications

- Minor lacerations, abrasions, or tearing of hemorrhoids
- Bleeding occasionally occurs after biopsy
- Infection (rare)

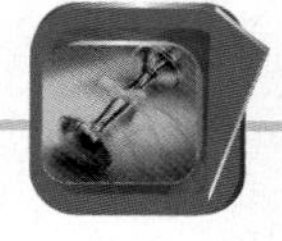

Pediatric Considerations

These conditions are rarely encountered in the pediatric population.

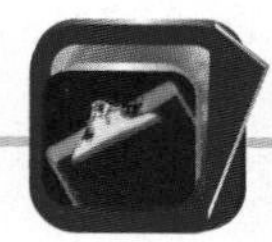

Postprocedure Instructions

Instruct the patient to bathe in a warm tub as needed for spasms or pain. Have the patient report excessive rectal bleeding (especially blood clots), fever ≥101°F, severe or worsening rectal pain, difficulties with urination, redness and swelling around the anus, or a yellow discharge from anus.

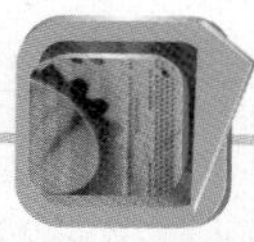

Coding Information and Supply Sources

CPT Code	Description	2008 Average 50th Percentile Fee	Global Period
46600	Anoscopy	$117.00	0
46606	Anoscopy with biopsy, single or multiple	$244.00	0

Suppliers

The Ives slotted anoscope ($160) is available from Redfield Corporation, 336 West Passaic Street, Rochelle Park, NJ. Phone: 1-800-678-4472. Web site: http://www.redfieldcorp.com.

A suggested anesthesia tray that can be used for this procedure is described in Appendix F.

Patient Education Handout

A patient education handout, "Anoscope with Biopsy," can be found on the book's companion Web site.

Bibliography

Corman ML. *Colon and Rectal Surgery*. 5th ed. Philadelphia: Lippincott; 2004:55–60.

Indinnimeo M, Cicchini C, Stazi A, et al. Analysis of a follow-up program for anal canal carcinoma. *J Exp Clin Cancer Res.* 2001;20:199–203.

Kelly SM, Sanowski RA, Foutch PG, et al. A prospective comparison of anoscopy and fiber endoscopy in detecting anal lesions. *J Clin Gastroenterol.* 1986;8:658–660.

Korkis AM, McDougall CJ. Rectal bleeding in patients less than 50 years of age. *Dig Dis Sci.* 1995;40:1520–1523.

Lewis JD, Brown A, Localio AR, et al. Initial evaluation of rectal bleeding in young persons: a cost-effectiveness analysis. *Ann Intern Med.* 2002;136:99–110.

2008 MAG Mutual Healthcare Solutions, Inc.'s Physicians' Fee and Coding Guide. Duluth, Georgia. MAG Mutual Healthcare Solutions, Inc. 2007.

CHAPTER 88

Anal Cytology and High-Resolution Anoscopy

Naomi Jay, RN, NP, PhD

Co-Director HPV Research Studies,
Department of Medicine, University of California San Francisco, San Francisco, CA

Mary M. Rubin, RNC, PhD, CRNP

Associate Clinical Professor, Department of Nursing, Coordinator, Gyn Oncology and Dysplasia Research, Department of OB/GYN and Medicine, University of California, San Francisco, San Francisco, CA

The cervix is used as a model for anal human papilloma virus (HPV)-associated disease based on similar anatomy and pathophysiology. Both the cervix and anus consist of squamous epithelium, which abuts columnar epithelium inducing squamous metaplasia. These areas undergoing squamous metaplasia are most susceptible to abnormal changes caused by HPV. The same strains of HPV found in the female genital tract are found in the anal canal of women and men. They induce the same range of disease in the anus as in the cervix, vagina, and vulva.

Anal disease is classified with similar cytology and histology taxonomies as the cervix, although in the anus, squamous intraepithelial lesions (SIL) is often called anal intraepithelial neoplasia (AIN) grades I, II, and III. High-grade AIN (HGAIN) is considered to be the precursor lesion to anal squamous cell cancer (SCC), and as such, screening procedures used for the cervix including cytology and colposcopy have been adapted for screening of anal HPV-associated disease. Sensitivity and specificity of anal cytology

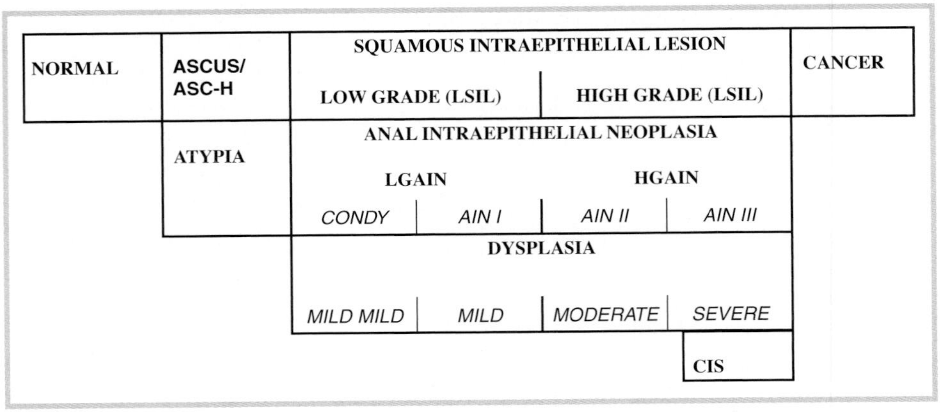

NORMAL	ASCUS/ ASC-H	SQUAMOUS INTRAEPITHELIAL LESION				CANCER
		LOW GRADE (LSIL)		HIGH GRADE (LSIL)		
	ATYPIA	ANAL INTRAEPITHELIAL NEOPLASIA				
		LGAIN		HGAIN		
		CONDY	*AIN I*	*AIN II*	*AIN III*	
		DYSPLASIA				
		MILD MILD	*MILD*	*MODERATE*	*SEVERE*	
					CIS	

Figure 1

are similar to cervical cytology, and liquid-based cytology has been shown to improve quality of samples. As a screening test for anal cancer, anal cytology has been shown to be cost-effective. In the anal canal, colposcopy is called high-resolution anoscopy (HRA). Colposcopy techniques and terminology have been validated for anal canal disease.

There are several principles of screening when using anal cytology and HRA. Anal cytology is used for identification of populations and individuals with HPV-associated diseases through cytology screening programs. HRA is used for detection of lesions, histologic diagnosis of disease, and treatment of disease, specifically HGAIN and prevention of cancer development. It is also used for early detection of nonsymptomatic cancer.

Before an anal cytology exam or HRA, instruct the patient to avoid douching, enemas, or insertion of anything per rectum 24 hours prior to the procedure. Obtain relevant history, including current anal symptoms such as pruritus, bleeding, and pain. Determine prior history of anal or perianal condyloma and whether treatments were surgical or office based. Also determine prior history of any anal abnormalities such as fissures, fistula, abscesses, or hemorrhoids requiring intervention. Ask about any prior treatments that may have caused scarring or other alterations in the normal anal mucosa such as abscess lancing, fistula repairs, or hemorrhoidectomies. Obtain informed consent with explanation of the procedures to be performed.

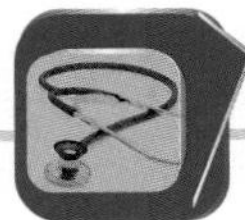

Equipment

Much of the equipment is similar to that used for cervical examinations. Most gynecology or dysplasia practices have these supplies without significant additional cost

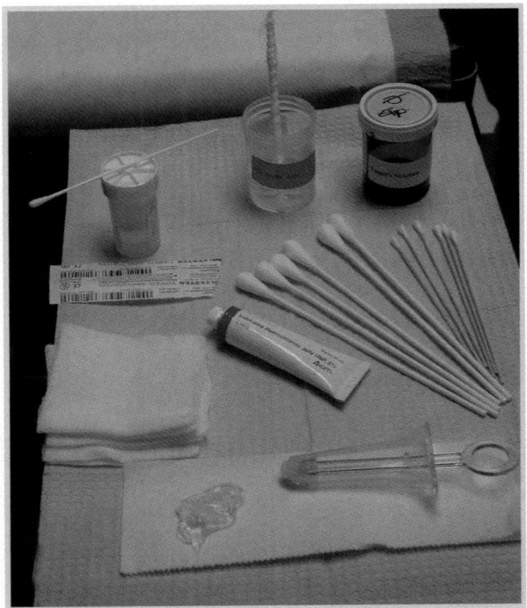

Figure 2

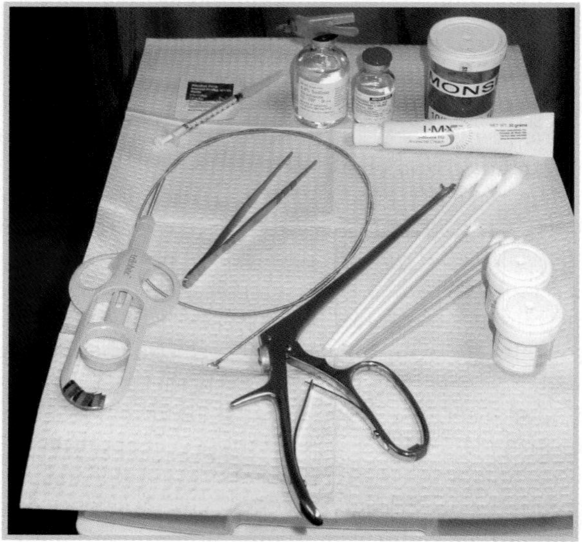

Figure 3

for performing these procedures. A procedure tray for examination includes the following:

- Cytology liquid medium (or conventional slide with fixative solution)
- Dacron swab
- Anoscope (disposable or sterilized metal)
- 3% acetic Acid
- Nonsterile cotton swabs
- Nonsterile Scopettes
- Nonsterile 4 × 4 gauze pads
- Lugol solution
- K-Y Jelly mixed with 1% to 5% lidocaine gel

For intra-anal biopsies, the following additional equipment is needed:

- Monsel solution or silver nitrate sticks
- Formalin
- Baby-Tischler punch biopsy or endoscopy forceps

For perianal biopsies the following additional equipment is needed:

- 1% to 5% lidocaine gel/cream
- 1% lidocaine with epinephrine and sodium bicarbonate (2 mL per 10 cc of lidocaine)
- Small pick-up forceps
- 30-gauge needle
- 22-gauge needle
- 1-cc syringe

Colposcope

The following specifications are recommended for colposcopes intended for HRA:

- Double objective lens with magnification up to 25 to 40×
- Oculars that magnify 10 to 20×
- Angled eye pieces, as the straight-on view is ergonomically difficult for HRA
- Side-swing arm to brace clinician's arm while holding the anoscope for long periods
- Green filter for evaluation of vascular changes

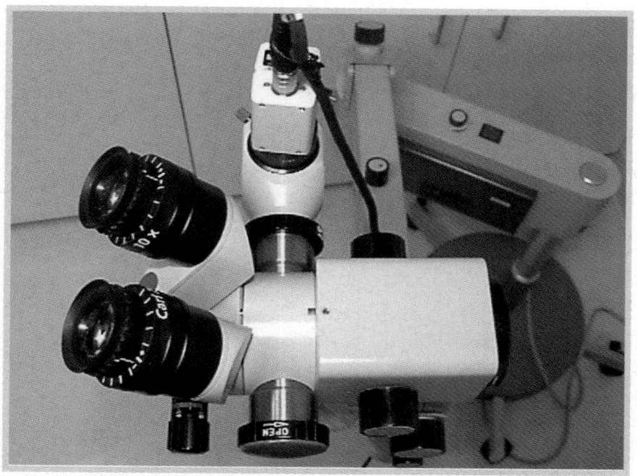

Figure 4

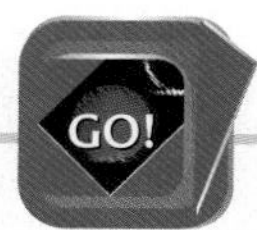

Indications

Populations to screen include the following:

- HIV-seropositive individuals
- Immune-compromised individuals (organ transplant recipients, autoimmune diseases)
- HIV-seronegative women with a history of anal or perianal warts, genital high-grade SIL (HSIL), or cancer
- HIV-seronegative men who have sex with men with a history of anal or perianal warts or prior receptive anal intercourse

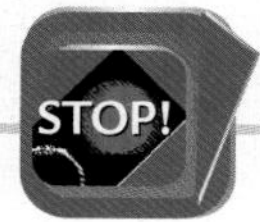

Contraindications

- There is no contraindication for cytology screening or HRA, although patients who have recently undergone anal procedures such as hemorrhoidectomy, fistula repair, or fulguration of anal warts should defer examination until healed.
- Biopsy should be deferred in patients with platelets <65,000 or in patients who are neutropenic or who are on anticoagulant therapies.

The Procedure

Step 1. The anatomy of the anus is depicted.

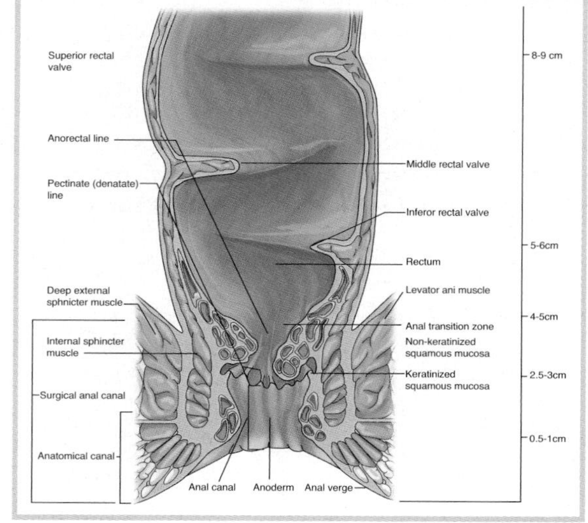

Step 1

Step 2. The anus is composed of squamous epithelium. The rectum or colon is columnar epithelium. The anal canal is mucosa lined, and the anal margin is epidermal. The proximal end of the anal canal begins at the junction of the ani muscle and external anal sphincter and extends to the anal verge. It is 2 to 4 cm in length and is shorter in women compared with that found in men. The distal end of the anal canal is the dentate line, which is approximately equivalent to the original squamocolumnar junction (SCJ) in colposcopic terminology. The dentate line is considered to be a "fixed" anatomic zone, whereas the anal transformation zone (AnTZ) is dynamic and undergoing squamous metaplasia. The AnTZ is the current SCJ. The anal margin begins at the verge and represents the transition from mucosal to epidermal epithelium and extends to the perianal skin.

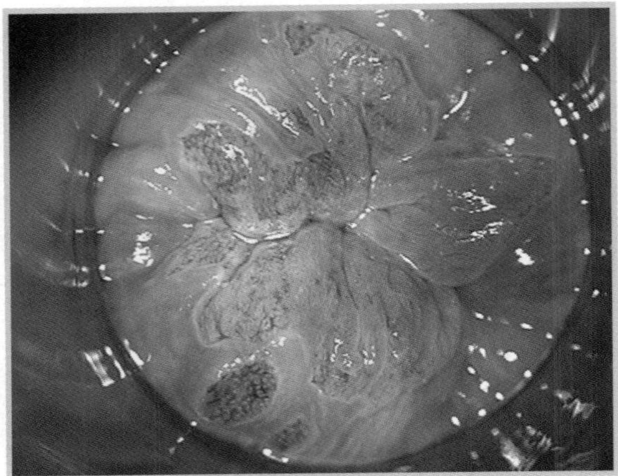

Step 2

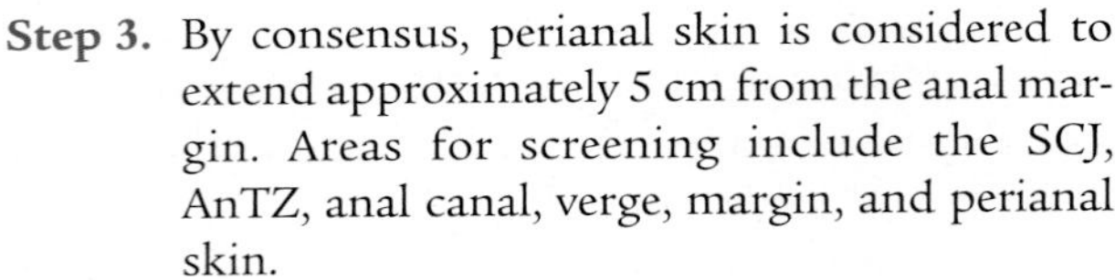

Step 3. By consensus, perianal skin is considered to extend approximately 5 cm from the anal margin. Areas for screening include the SCJ, AnTZ, anal canal, verge, margin, and perianal skin.

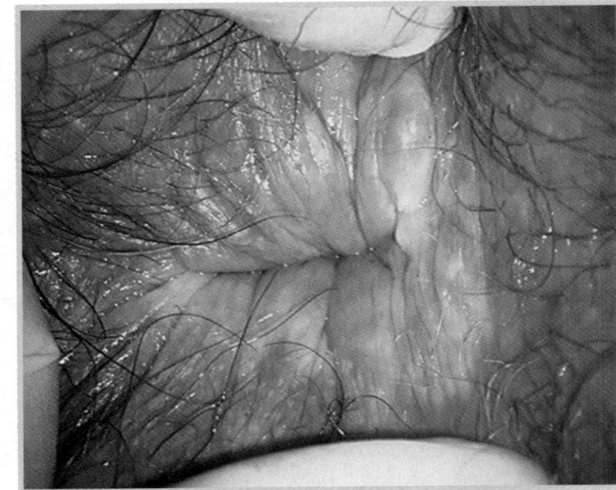

Step 3

Performing Anal Cytology

Step 1. The anal cytology specimen should be performed first to provide the highest yield of cells. Gently separate the buttocks. The patient can hold his or her right cheek to facilitate the view.

- PITFALL: There must be no lubrication prior to obtaining a cytology sample, as the lubricant may interfere with the processing and interpretation of the sample.

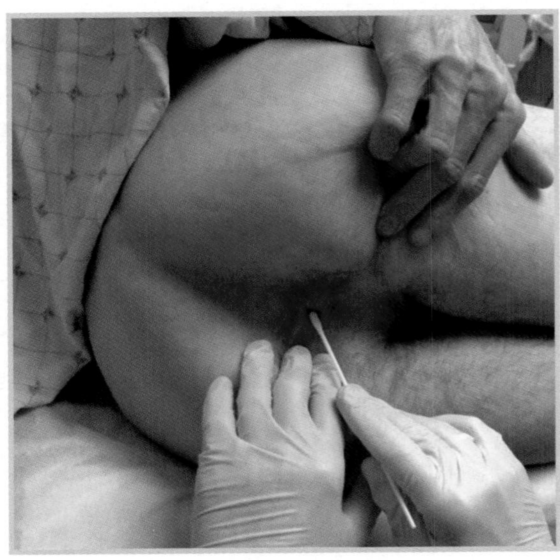

Step 1

Step 2. Insert a moistened Dacron swab approximately 3 to 4 cm into the anus to assure sampling of cells from the AnTZ. If initial resistance is encountered, change the position of the swab and reinsert.

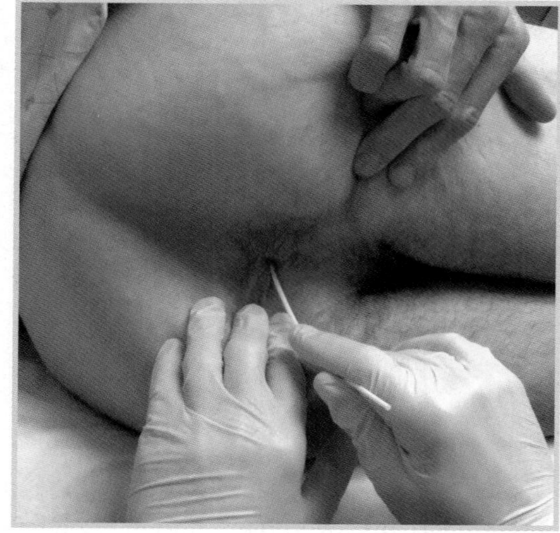

Step 2

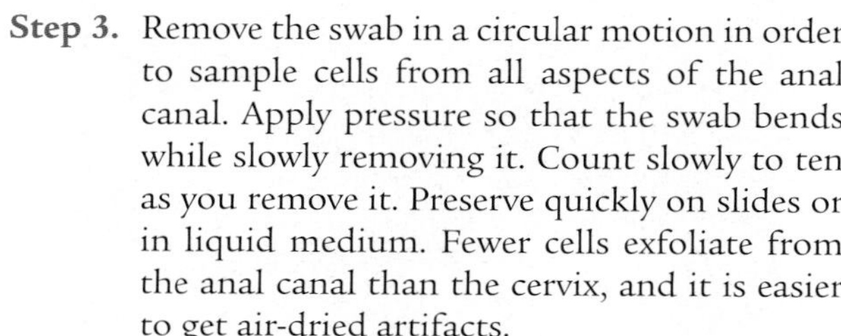

Step 3. Remove the swab in a circular motion in order to sample cells from all aspects of the anal canal. Apply pressure so that the swab bends while slowly removing it. Count slowly to ten as you remove it. Preserve quickly on slides or in liquid medium. Fewer cells exfoliate from the anal canal than the cervix, and it is easier to get air-dried artifacts.

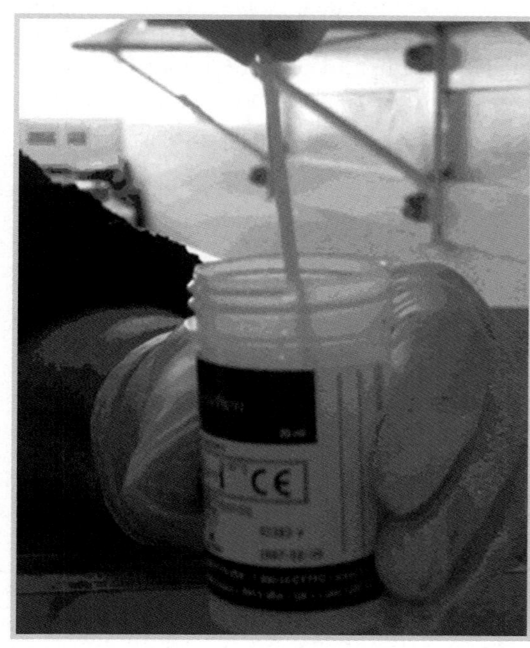

Step 3

Performing High-Resolution Anoscopy

Step 1. Assist the patient into one of the following positions: left lateral, lithotomy if also performing cervical exam (but most women prefer to switch to left lateral for the HRA), or prone (if overhead colposcope is available). In the left lateral and prone positions, the patient should be as close to the bottom edge of the table as possible to facilitate focusing the colposcope.

Step 2. Be clear and consistent in describing location of lesions and the position used. The "anal clock" is different from the "gynecologic clock." In the prone position, posterior is 12:00, while in the lithotomy position, it is 6:00. When referring patients for follow-up to anal surgeons, it is helpful to use anatomic descriptors (posterior, anterior, left or right lateral) in place of or in addition to the "clock" positions.

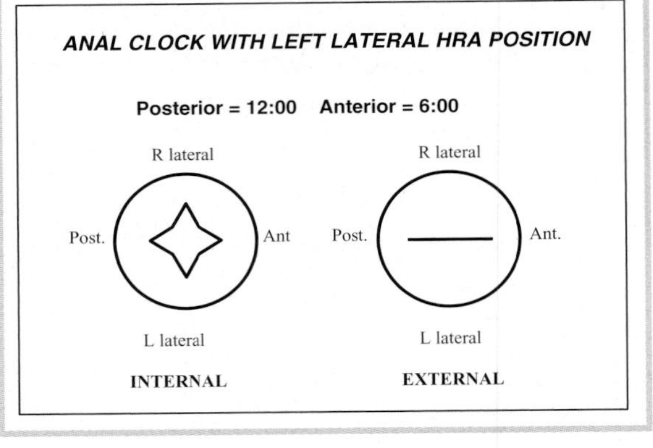

Step 2

Step 3. Obtain a cytology specimen if needed (new patients or those referred with abnormal cytology specimens >3 months old). Lubricate the anal canal with K-Y Jelly mixed with 1% to 5% lidocaine. Perform a digital rectal exam, and palpate for warts, masses, ulcerations, fissures, and focal areas of discomfort or pain. The presence of hard and fixed lesions should increase your index of suspicion for cancer, since these are not the usual presentation of hemorrhoids and warts.

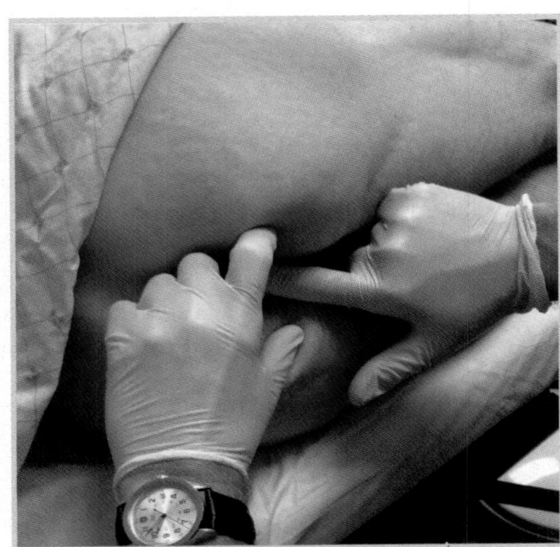

Step 3

Step 4. Insert the anoscope, and remove the obturator.

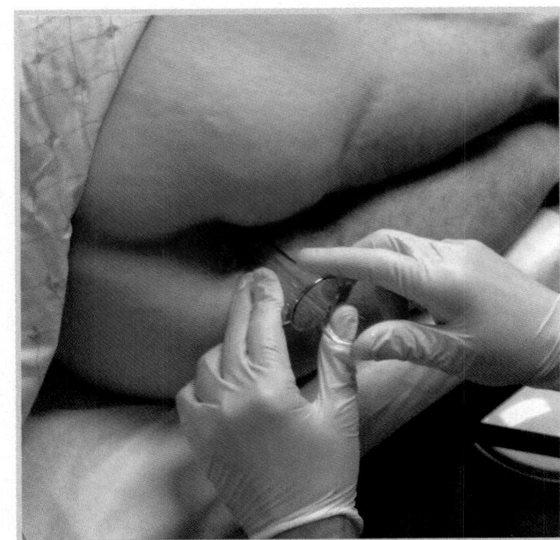

Step 4

Step 5. Insert a cotton swab wrapped in gauze that has been soaked in acetic acid.

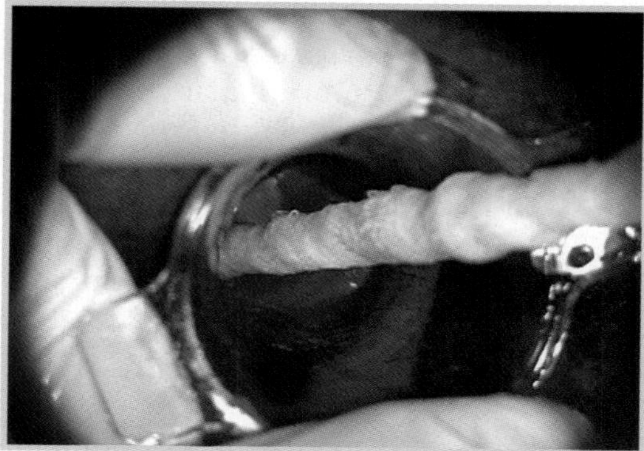

Step 5

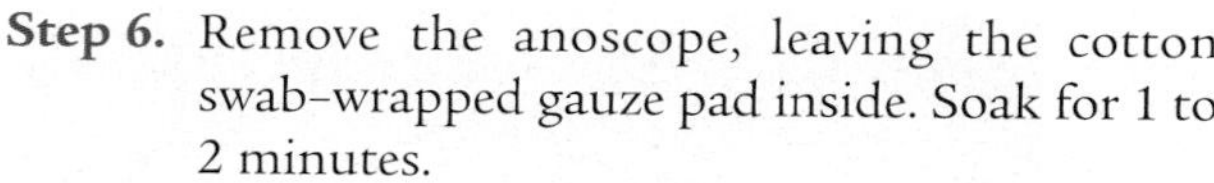

Step 6. Remove the anoscope, leaving the cotton swab-wrapped gauze pad inside. Soak for 1 to 2 minutes.

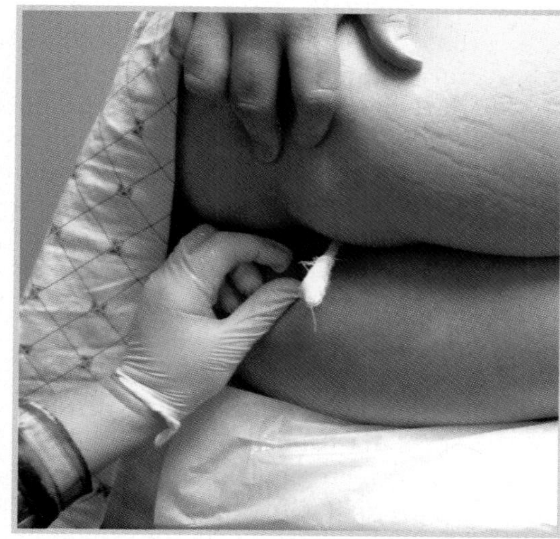

Step 6

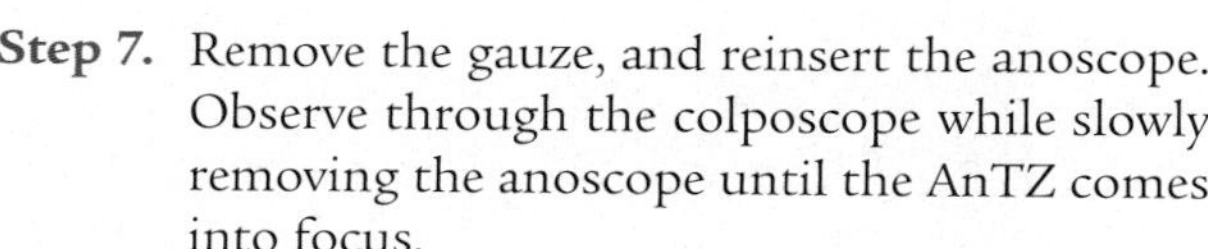

Step 7. Remove the gauze, and reinsert the anoscope. Observe through the colposcope while slowly removing the anoscope until the AnTZ comes into focus.

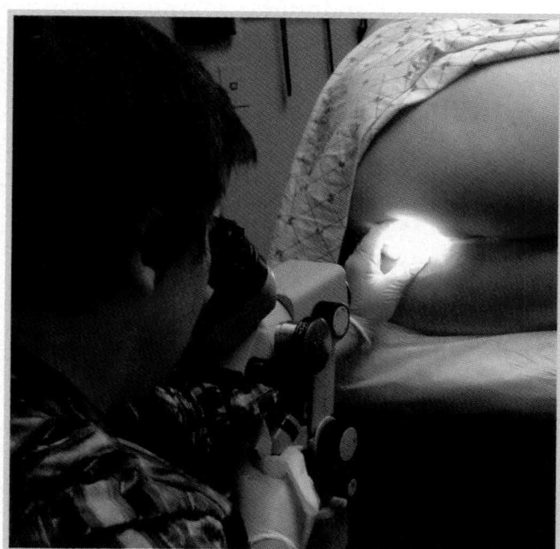

Step 7

Step 8. Continue to apply acetic acid with Scopettes or cotton swabs during the exam. Using cotton swabs to manipulate the folds, hemorrhoids, or prolapsing mucosa as well as adjusting the anoscope will help to view all aspects of the AnTZ. In most cases, the entire AnTZ should be seen, and the exam will be considered satisfactory. Continue withdrawing the anoscope until the entire canal has been observed.

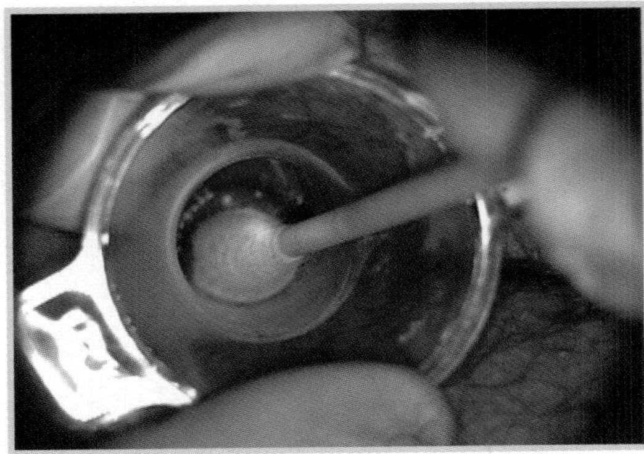

Step 8

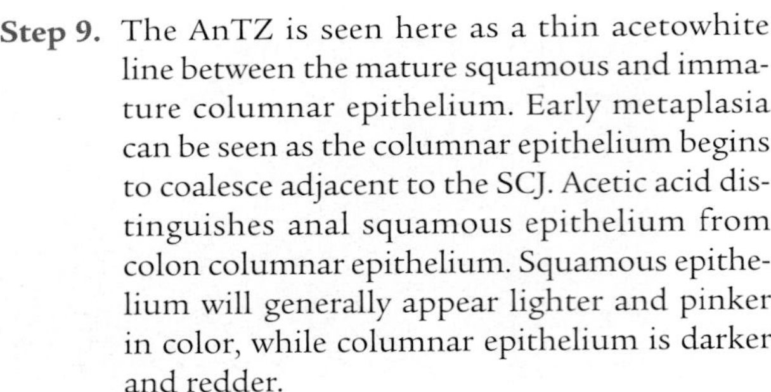

Step 9. The AnTZ is seen here as a thin acetowhite line between the mature squamous and immature columnar epithelium. Early metaplasia can be seen as the columnar epithelium begins to coalesce adjacent to the SCJ. Acetic acid distinguishes anal squamous epithelium from colon columnar epithelium. Squamous epithelium will generally appear lighter and pinker in color, while columnar epithelium is darker and redder.

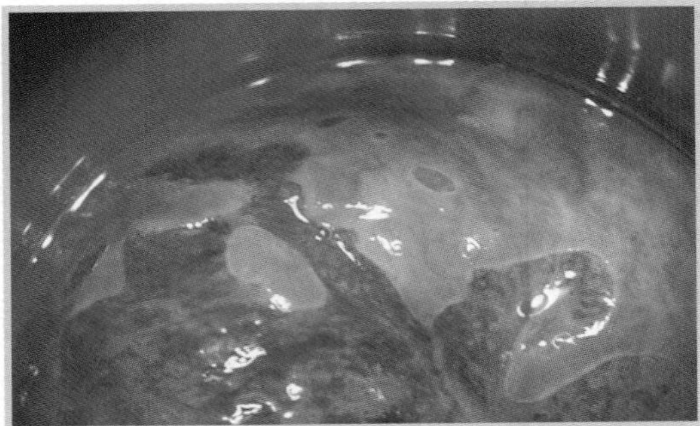

Step 9

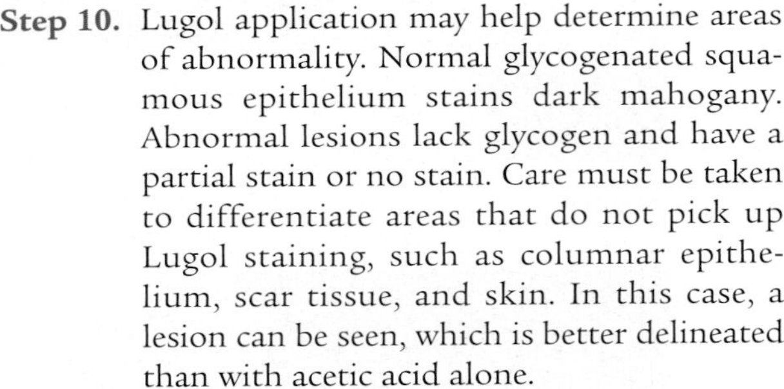

Step 10. Lugol application may help determine areas of abnormality. Normal glycogenated squamous epithelium stains dark mahogany. Abnormal lesions lack glycogen and have a partial stain or no stain. Care must be taken to differentiate areas that do not pick up Lugol staining, such as columnar epithelium, scar tissue, and skin. In this case, a lesion can be seen, which is better delineated than with acetic acid alone.

- PITFALL: Review allergy to iodine during history taking. If patient has an allergic reaction to shellfish or has known allergy to iodine from prior procedures, do not use during the examination.

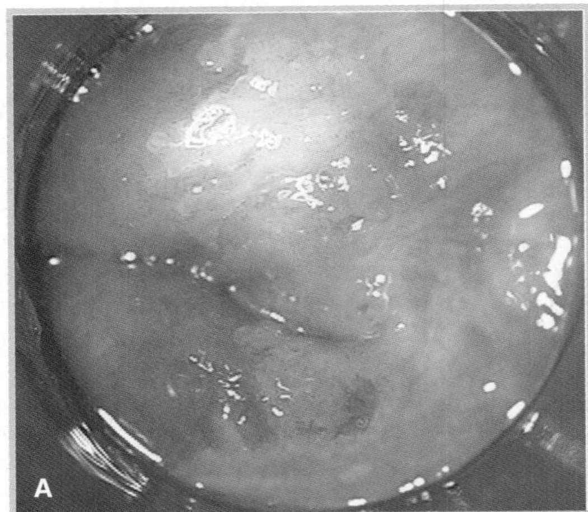

A

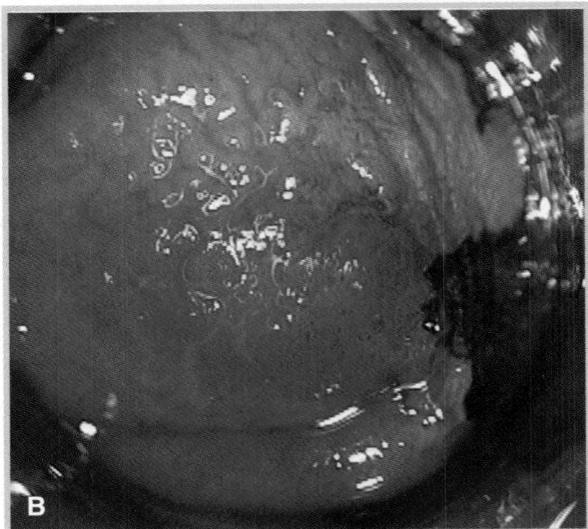

B

Step 10

Step 11. Commonly recognized cervical lesion characteristics that help distinguish cervical low-grade SIL (LSIL) and HSIL are also seen in anal lesions and help guide the clinician in choosing areas for biopsy. A typical raised low-grade AIN (LGAIN) is shown in part A and a typical flat high-grade AIN (HGAIN) is shown in part B.

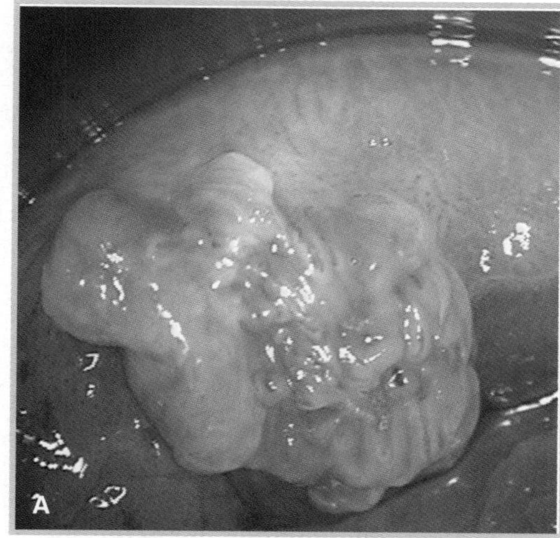

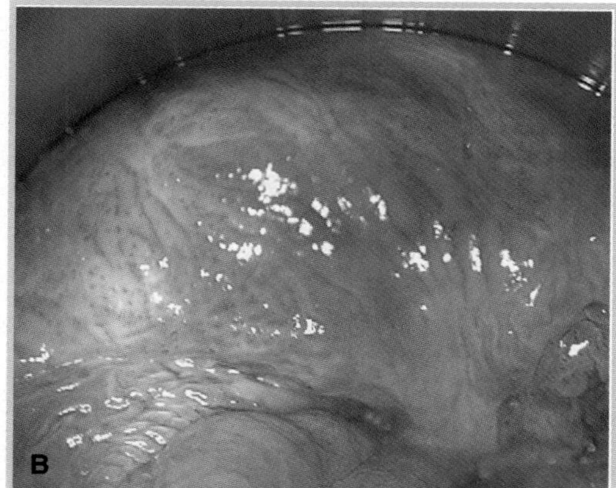

Step 11

Step 12. Biopsies are directed at areas thought to represent the highest grade of abnormality. Anal biopsies should be smaller than those typically taken of the cervix using forceps no larger than 2 to 3 mm. Internal biopsies do not require anesthesia. External biopsies require injecting a small amount of 1% lidocaine with epinephrine buffered with sodium bicarbonate (2 cc NaHC03: 10 cc lidocaine), similar to biopsies of the vulva. The injection can be preceded by numbing medication topically with lidocaine gel or spray. Monsel solution or silver nitrate is used for hemostasis, although the pressure of the anal walls will generally stop bleeding for internal biopsies.

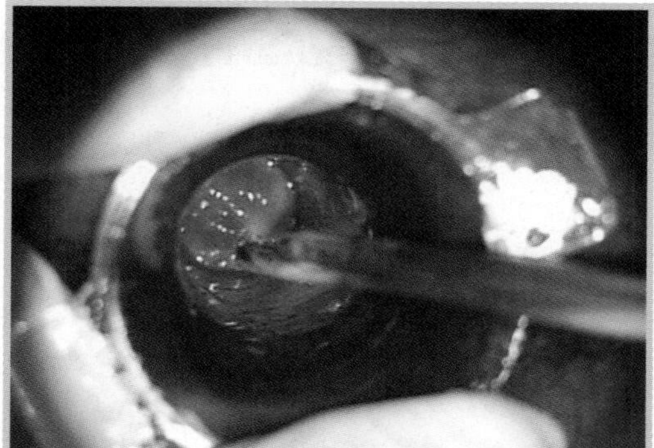

Step 13

Step 13. Insert closed forceps through the anoscope while looking through the colposcope.

- **PEARL:** Closing the forceps will prevent unintentional injury.

Step 14. Once the forceps is adjacent to the lesion, open in the direction that allows for the forceps to grab the tissue. For some lesions, the forceps will need to be positioned upside down.

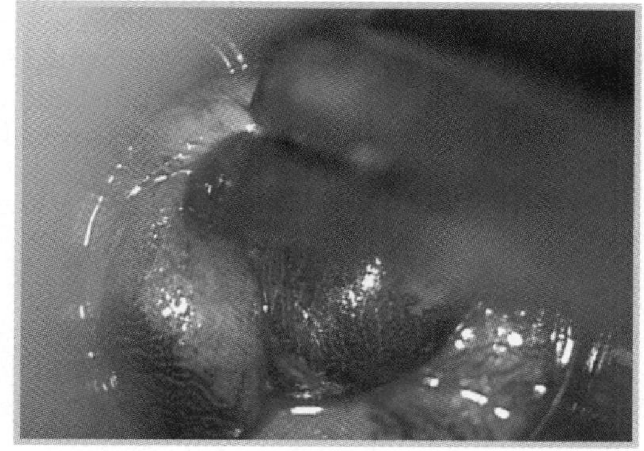

Step 14

- PITFALL: Patients on warfarin (Coumadin) or daily aspirin may have increased bleeding with biopsy. If the platelet count is <65,000, approach the biopsy with caution or postpone until count improves. It is no longer considered necessary to provide antibiotic prophylaxis prior to biopsy in patients with history of endocarditis or otherwise at risk for heart valve disease.

Step 15. To obtain a small sample, the forceps should not be opened the entire width but rather should be partially closed before closing and grabbing the tissue. Monsel solution can be applied to the biopsy site for hemostasis, although most small biopsy samples will coagulate spontaneously once the anoscope is removed.

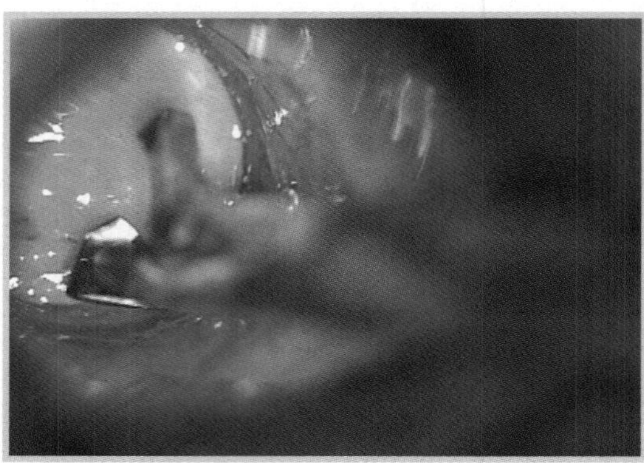

Step 15

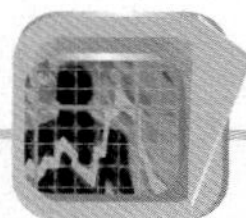

Complications

- Bleeding with bowel movements for several days post biopsy
- Infection (rare)
- Problematic bleeding (rare)

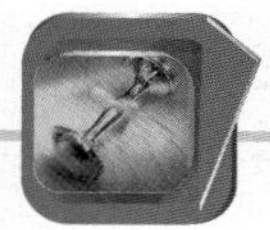

Pediatric Considerations

Since cytology screening is not usually done until a patient has been sexually active, this procedure is not routinely done in a pediatric population.

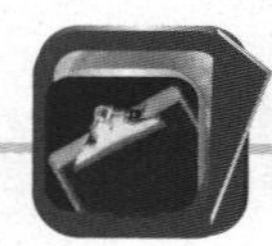

Postprocedure Instructions

Patients should be told to expect slight bleeding with bowel movements for several days post biopsy. There may be mild postprocedure pain associated with biopsy of lesions in and around the anal canal. Rarely, a patient may require medication such as hydrocodone.

Comfort measures include avoiding constipation by increasing fiber in the diet during a few days following biopsy. If the patient requires pain medications, stool softeners may be necessary, depending on their routine bowel habits. Avoid hot and spicy foods. Soaking in warm water will facilitate faster healing and relieve any pain associated with biopsy. Lidocaine 1% to 5% gel/cream can be applied to perianal tissue when biopsies have been performed.

Follow-up will depend on the results of the cytology, histology, and the clinical indications for the referral. See Figure 5.

Triage for Anal Cytology and High-Resolution Anoscopy

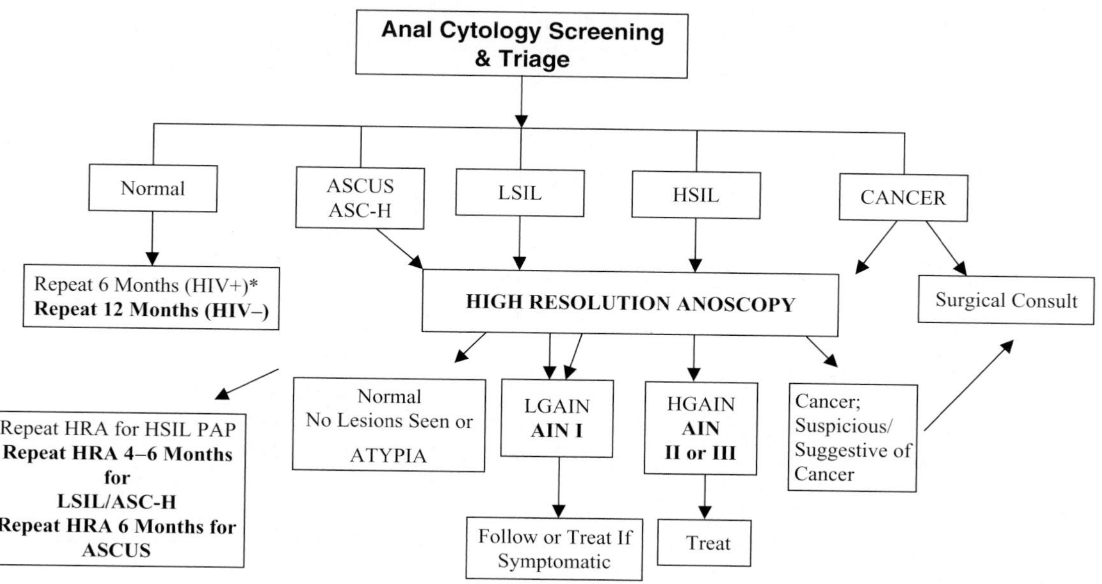

Figure 5

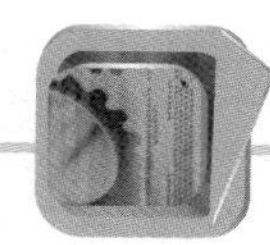

Coding Information and Supply Sources

CPT Code	Description	2007 Average 50th Percentile Fee	Global Period
46600	Anoscopy	$117.00	0
46606	Anoscopy with biopsy, single or multiple	$244.00	0
46900	Destruct lesion(s) anus simple, chemical (e.g., trichloroacetic acid)	$400.00	10
46916	Destruct lesion(s) anus simple, cryosurgery	$424.00	10

Use a -22 modifier for use of microscope with any of above.
CPT is a registered trademark of the American Medical Association.
2008 average 50th Percentile Fees are provided courtesy of 2008 MMH-SI's copyrighted Physicians' Fees and Coding Guide.

ICD-9 Codes

078.11	Anal condyloma
211.4	Benign neoplasms of the anus (AIN I or AIN II)
230.5	HGAIN (AIN III) or carcinoma in situ of the anus
239.2	Anal dysplasia (nonspecific)
154.2	Anal cancer
042	HIV

Supplies for HRA needed in addition to standard colposcopy supplies include the following:

Item	Manufacturer	Contact information
Anoscopes	Cardinal Healthcare	800-477-3800
Endoscopic forceps	Fibertech Forceps	714-522-7112
Endoscopic forceps	ESCO Medical Instruments	631-689-9153
Infrared coagulator	Redfield Corporation	http://www.redfieldcorp.com

Patient Education Handout

A patient education handout, "Anal Cancer Screening," can be found on the book's Web site.

Bibliography

Darragh T, Jay N, Tupkelewicz B, et al. Comparison of conventional cytologic smears and ThinPrep preparations from the anal canal. *Acta Cytol.* 1997;41,4:1167–1170.

Frisch M, Biggar RJ, Goedert JJJ. HPV associated cancers in patients with HIV infection and AIDS. *JNCI.* 2000;92(18):1500–1510.

Goldie S, Kuntz K, Weinstein M, et al. The clinical effectiveness and cost-effectiveness of screening for ASIL in homosexual and bisexual HIV-positive men. *JAMA.* 1999;281:1822–1829.

Jay N, Berry JM, Hogeboom C, et al. Colposcopic appearance of ASIL; relationship to histopathology. *Dis Colon Rectum.* 1997;40:919–928.

O'Connor JJ. The study of anorectal disease by colposcopy. *Dis Colon Rectum.* 1977;20(7):570–572.

Palefsky J, Holly E, Hogeboom C, et al. Anal cytology as a screening tool for ASIL. *JAIDS.* 1997;14:415–422.

Scholefield JH, Ogunbiyi OA, Smith JH, et al. Anal colposcopy and the diagnosis of AIN in high-risk gynecologic patients. *Int J Gyn Cancer.* 1994;4:119–426.

2008 MAG Mutual Healthcare Solutions, Inc.'s Physicians' Fee and Coding Guide. Duluth, Georgia. MAG Mutual Healthcare Solutions, Inc. 2007.

CHAPTER 89

Colonoscopy

Jeffrey A. German, MD

Associate Professor, Department of Family Medicine
Louisiana State University Health Sciences Center, Shreveport, LA

Clint N. Wilson, MD

Chief Resident, Family Medicine Residency
Louisiana State University Health Sciences Center, Shreveport, LA

Colonoscopy refers to the endoscopic examination of the entire colon and rectum and often includes the terminal ileum. Common activities performed during colonoscopy include inspection, biopsy, photography, and video recording. The procedure is technically challenging and requires considerable training and experience. High-quality examinations require good clinical judgment, anatomy and pathology recognition, technical skill in manipulating the scope and performing biopsies, appropriate patient monitoring, and well-maintained and clean equipment to ensure patient safety. Video colonoscopes enable complete examinations of the entire colon in more than 90% of examinations.

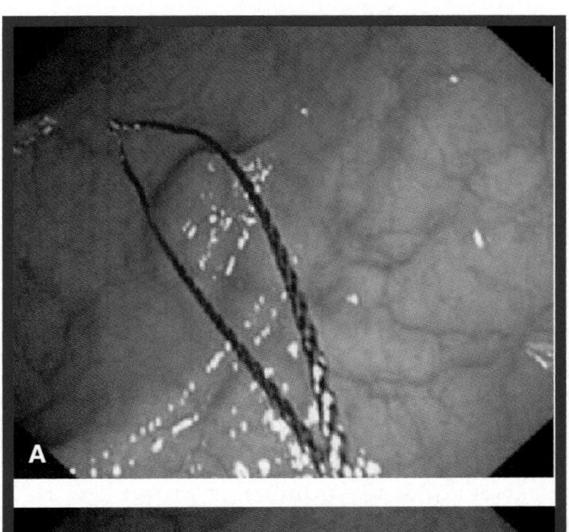

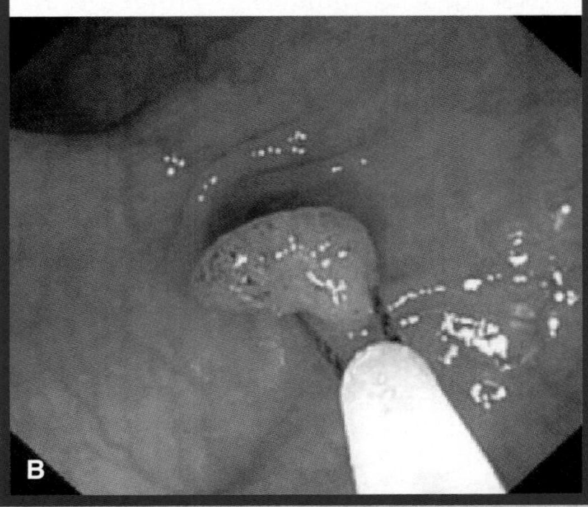

Most colorectal cancers appear to develop from benign neoplastic (adenomatous) lesions. Americans of average risk have a 6% lifetime risk of developing colon cancer. Adenomas occur in about 30% of individuals at age 50 years and 55% at age 80 years. Several screening modalities are advocated to detect early adenomas and cancer, including colonoscopy every 10 years after age 50. Colonoscopy has sensitivities of 75% to 85% for polyps <1 cm in diameter and 95% for larger polyps and cancers. The specificity for the examination approaches 100%.

A single screening colonoscopy in asymptomatic individuals at age 65 has been advocated for reducing mortality from colorectal cancer. Several analyses have suggested that a single screening or repeated screenings every 10 years after age 50 may be a cost-effective strategy. Despite increased insurance coverage for colonoscopy screening, the feasibility of screening an entire population has yet to be established.

Colonoscopy is the diagnostic procedure of choice for patients with a positive fecal occult blood test (FOBT). Approximately 50% of individuals with a positive FOBT have a neoplastic lesion (adenomas, 38%; cancer, 12%) at endoscopy. Patients with long-standing ulcerative colitis should undergo colonoscopy with biopsy to examine for dysplasia beginning 8 years after the development of pancolitis or 15 years after the development of distal disease.

Colonoscopy is indicated for villous adenomas of any size that are discovered during flexible sigmoidoscopy. Distal tubular adenomas are not associated with an increase in proximal adenomas, and some clinicians do not believe that colonoscopy is required after removal of a small, distal tubular adenoma. Historically, adenomas >1 cm in diameter have been referred for colonoscopy. Larger colonic lesions are more often villous or tubulovillous, necessitating colonoscopic removal of the lesion and examination for synchronous lesions. Some studies suggest that purely tubular lesions >1 cm in diameter can be followed without immediate colonoscopy. This strategy may be problematic, because a biopsy sample from within a large lesion may fail to recognize the most significant pathology (i.e., missed villous or cancerous elements). Despite some contrary opinions, colonoscopy is generally not indicated after the diagnosis of a hyperplastic distal polyp.

Average procedure times for experienced endoscopists are about 10 minutes to reach the cecum and 30 minutes to complete the entire procedure. Inadequate preparation is the most common reason for prolonged or incomplete examinations. Most individuals in the United States receive 3 to 4 L of a polyethylene glycol–based electrolyte solution the day before the examination. Some studies have suggested that longer procedures and greater discomfort occur in women undergoing the procedure, possibly because of their anatomically longer colons and greater sigmoid mobility. Older individuals may present greater difficulty in reaching the cecum.

Colonoscopy routinely is performed after the administration of conscious sedation. Intravenous midazolam and meperidine have been the drugs most commonly employed. Unfortunately, 15% of individuals receiving these two medications are dissatisfied with their sedation. Propofol is an intravenous, short-acting sedative used for the induction of general anesthesia. Propofol may provide superior sedation and more rapid recovery, but its safety in office situations has not been demonstrated. Studies have shown that the procedure can be performed in selected individuals without sedation, with relatively high (70% to 85%) rates of patients willing to undergo a similar procedure again without sedation. Many physicians feel more comfortable with routine administration of sedation to improve procedure acceptance among patients. Chapter 4 contains guidelines for monitoring the patient receiving conscious sedation at endoscopy.

Polypectomy is the most commonly performed therapeutic procedure during colonoscopy. With regard to polyps found at the time of endoscopy, 85% to 90% can be removed with the endoscope, but patients can experience considerable morbidity from bleeding or colon perforation due to polypectomy. There is a strong relationship between complication rates of diagnostic and therapeutic colonoscopy and the experience of the endoscopist. The highest rates of these complications appear in the first 500 procedures.

Colonoscopy can be safely learned only with direct, one-on-one supervision by an experienced proctor or preceptor. Debate exists about the number of procedures that trainees need to perform to become competent in colonoscopy, and no scientific data currently exists correlating the volume of colonoscopies performed with acquisition of competence. Individual practitioners have varying levels of manual dexterity and experience with flexible sigmoidoscopy and can acquire skills at differing rates. Studies show that when observable factors are used to determine technical competency in colonoscopy (reach-the-cecum rate, time to complete procedure, and rate of complications), family physicians, gastroenterologists, and general surgeons are all comparable.

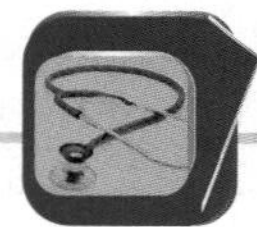

Equipment

- Conscious sedation drugs and equipment
- Colonoscope and video monitoring equipment
- Biopsy forceps, snare, electrosurgical generator

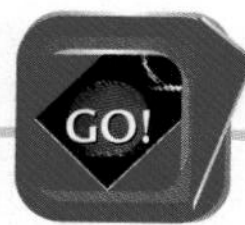

Indications

- Evaluation of a radiographic abnormality
- Screening of asymptomatic individuals for colon neoplasia or cancer
- Evaluation of unexplained gastrointestinal bleeding
- Positive FOBT
- Unexplained iron-deficiency anemia
- Examination for a synchronous colon neoplastic lesion when a lesion is found in the rectosigmoid
- Surveillance or follow-up study after removal of a prior neoplastic lesion
- Suspected inflammatory bowel disease or surveillance for previously diagnosed inflammatory bowel disease
- Evaluation of symptoms suggestive of significant colon disease (e.g., chronic diarrhea, weight loss, abdominal or pelvic pain)
- Therapeutic procedures (e.g., polyp removal, foreign body removal)

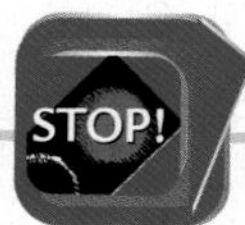

Contraindications (Relative)

- Fulminant colitis
- Acute diverticulitis
- Hemodynamically unstable patient
- Recent (<3 months) myocardial infarction
- Recent (<1 week) bowel surgery
- Uncooperative patient
- Coagulopathy or bleeding diathesis
- Known or suspected perforation
- When the procedure results will not produce a change in management

The Procedure

Step 1. The patient is placed on the examination table in the left lateral position. Intravenous access is obtained, and sedation is administered. Appropriate patient monitoring includes frequent vital signs, oximetry, and heart rhythm (electrocardiographic) evaluation throughout the procedure. Chapter 91 provides instruction for scope insertion and examination techniques in the rectosigmoid during colonoscopy.

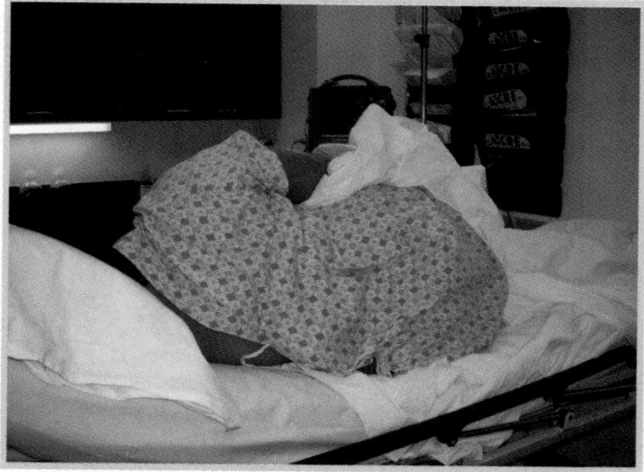

Step 1

Step 2. Traversing the rectosigmoid junction is the one of the most difficult aspects of the procedure. Prior pelvic surgery may produce extensive adhesions in this area (see Chapter 91 for techniques to pass through this area). Insert the scope only through visible lumen. The wall of the descending (left) colon has a characteristic circular appearance with encircling folds.

- **PITFALL:** Sliding the scope along the colon wall (i.e., slide-by technique) is not advocated, as this technique may result in perforation at the rectosigmoid junction.

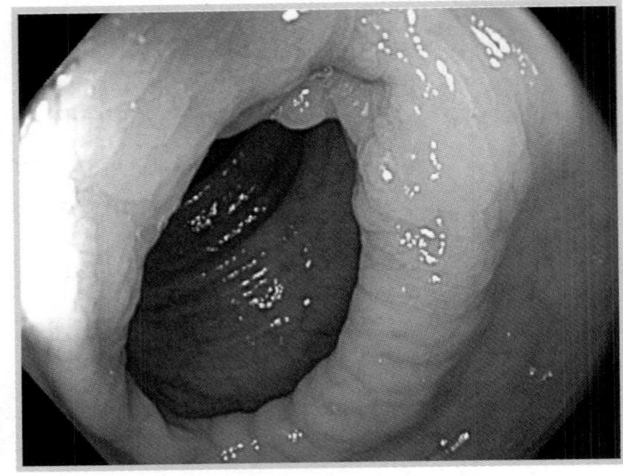

Step 2

Step 3. A sharp turn appears at the splenic flexure. A bluish color of the vascular spleen may be visible through the colon wall.

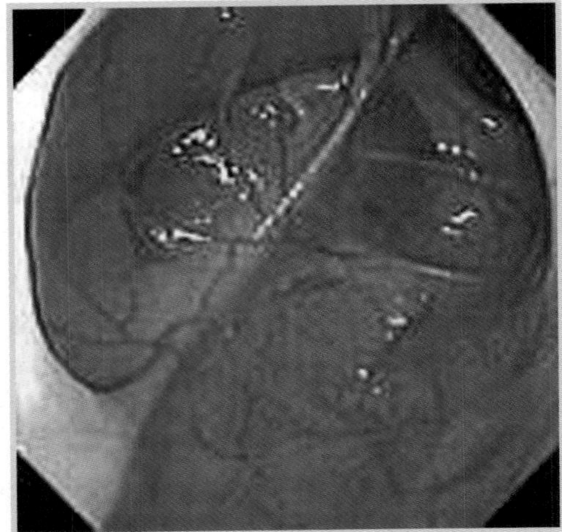

Step 3

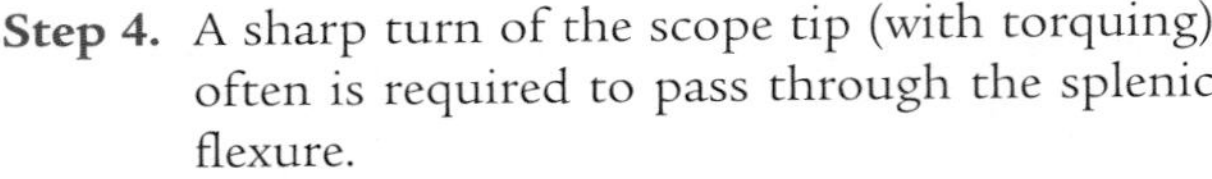

Step 4. A sharp turn of the scope tip (with torquing) often is required to pass through the splenic flexure.

The lumen of the transverse colon has a characteristic triangular appearance.

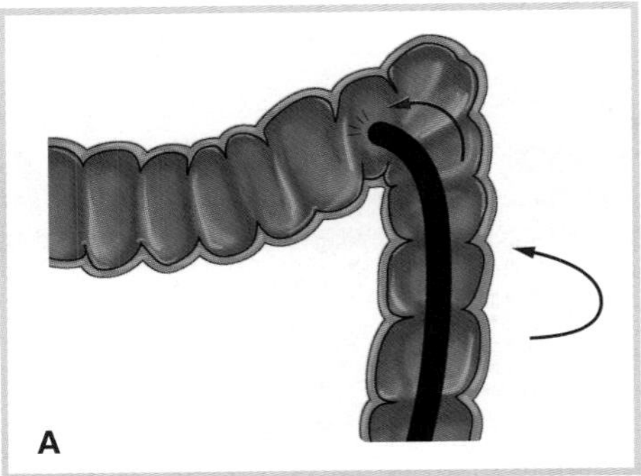

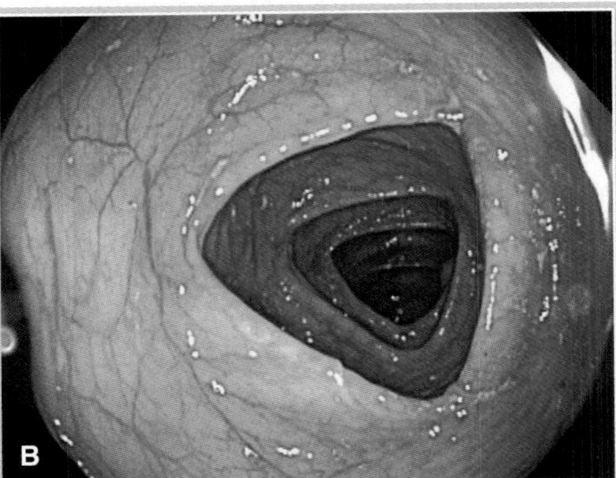

Step 4

Step 5. The passage through the transverse colon is relatively straight. Another sharp angle exists at the hepatic flexure. The hepatic flexure can be identified by the bluish brown shadow of the liver seen through the colon wall.

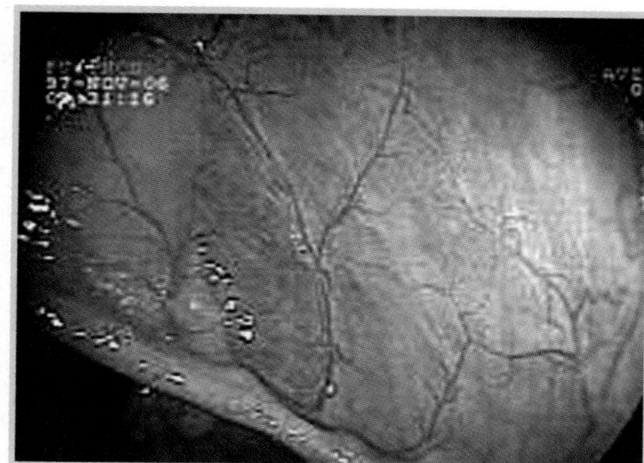

Step 5

Step 6. The examiner may notice transillumination through the left upper abdominal wall from the endoscope light. The assistant can press down on the patient's right upper abdomen to facilitate the downward deflection of the scope tip into the ascending (left) colon. The ascending colon has a characteristic pattern of mucosal folds that do not encircle the lumen completely.

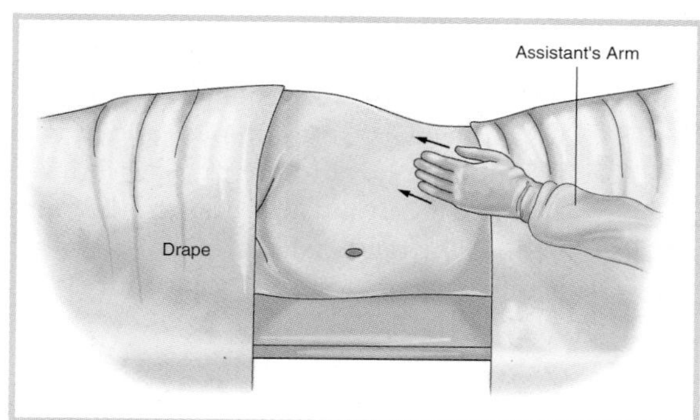

Step 6

Step 7. Avoid the creation of loops within the colon, which can increase discomfort and risk of complications. Keep the instrument as straight (short) as possible. Repeated short insertions and withdrawals and aspiration of air at the flexures can pleat the colon wall onto the instrument. Abdominal pressure by the assistant can eliminate loops in the transverse or sigmoid colon and facilitate more rapid insertion.

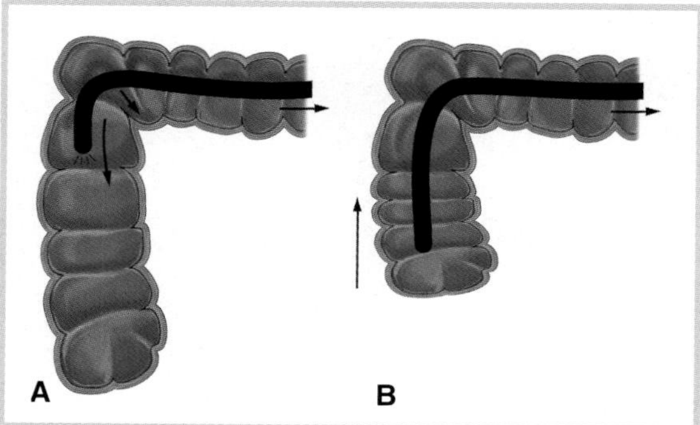

Step 7

Step 8. Traversing the left colon can be challenging. The scope tip is advanced by pulling back on the endoscope, causing paradoxical insertion. The scope tip is centered in the lumen, and suction is applied to further advance the scope through the colon. The ileocecal and appendiceal orifices may be recognized when the cecum is reached. The appendiceal orifice (shown) often appears on a "crow's foot," and the three taeniae form a confluent fold leading to the orifice. In many examinations, the appendiceal orifice may not be seen. Feeling the scope tip in the patient's right lower quadrant through the abdominal wall or seeing the light transilluminating through abdominal wall can help to assure the endoscopist that the cecum has been reached, but seeing landmarks such as the appendiceal orifice, "crow's foot," and ileocecal valve are necessary to confirm the scope's location within the colon.

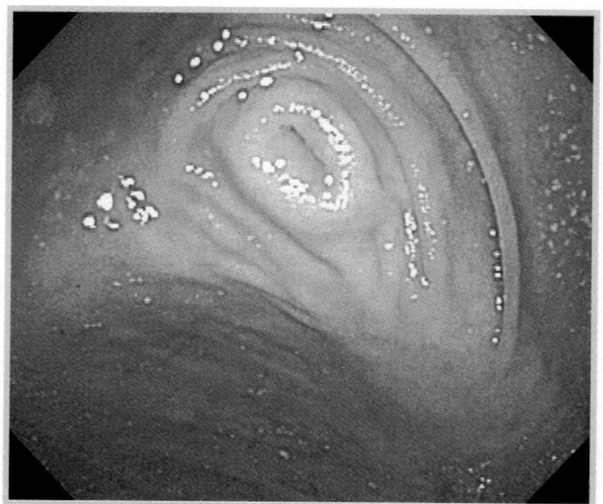

Step 8

Step 9. Attempt to intubate the ileocecal orifice, which often appears as a slit on the medial wall 3 cm above the pole (i.e., most proximal portion) of the ascending colon. First, aspirate the fluid from the cecal pole. The ileocecal orifice often is angled downward, and several attempts may be required for intubation. Angle the scope tip toward the orifice, and position the tip just past the orifice. Gently withdraw the scope until the angled tip flattens the D-shaped mucosal fold.

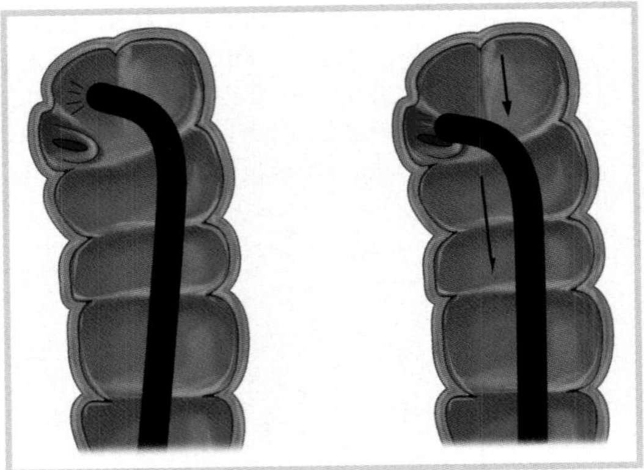

Step 9

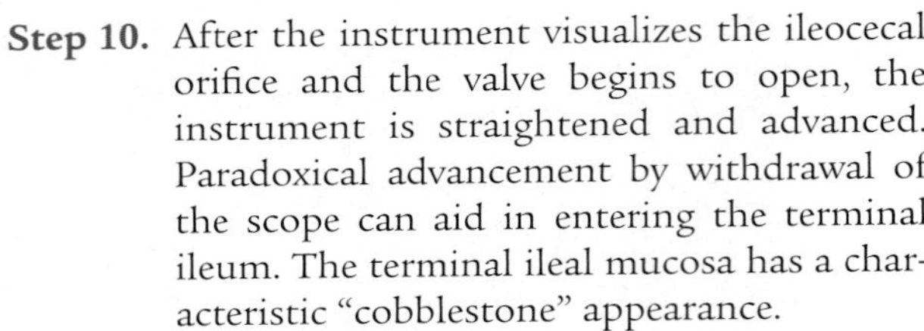

Step 10. After the instrument visualizes the ileocecal orifice and the valve begins to open, the instrument is straightened and advanced. Paradoxical advancement by withdrawal of the scope can aid in entering the terminal ileum. The terminal ileal mucosa has a characteristic "cobblestone" appearance.

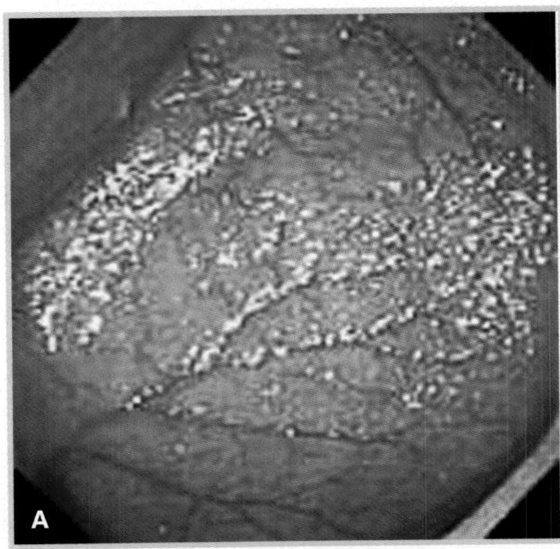

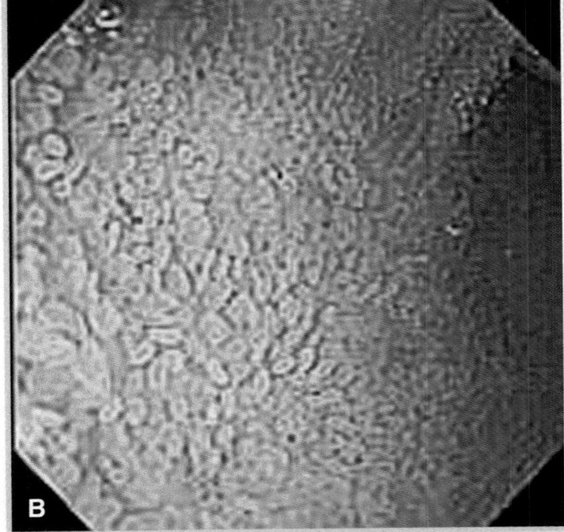

Step 10

Step 11. Visualization is performed on withdrawal of the scope. Withdrawal must be slow, with careful inspection of the entire circumferential wall before the scope is moved. Inspect behind every fold to ensure that hidden lesions are not missed. After a polyp is discovered, the scope is positioned a few centimeters away. The electrocautery snare is inserted through the biopsy channel. The snare sheath is positioned next to the polyp, the wire loop is advanced over the polyp, and the wire loop is slowly secured over the base of the polyp or pedicle. In order to reduce the risk of performation, the scope tip is maneuvered so that the snare loop is not touching the colon wall. Apply the electrocautery current.

- PITFALL: Colonic explosion has occurred in individuals undergoing electrosurgical polypectomy. Explosion of intraluminal methane gas is unlikely if the colon has been adequately prepped.

Step 12. Small polyps can be retrieved through the scope using the snare or grasping forceps. Larger polyps can be removed by suctioning the polyp against the scope and withdrawing the scope.

- PITFALL: Reinsertion of the scope may be needed if the scope has to be withdrawn to remove a large polyp. The polyp may obscure the scope tip, making adequate visualization of the colon wall during withdrawal difficult.
- PITFALL: Occasionally, polyps fall away or are mishandled, or a large number must be removed. Unretrieved polyps can be recovered after the procedure. Patients may strain to move them out of the colon, or added bowel prep solution (i.e., polyethylene glycol solution or phosphate enema) can be administered through the scope to induce evacuation. The fluid is filtered so that the polyps can be recovered for histologic examination.
- PITFALL: Suspected perforation after polypectomy necessitates hospital observation and evaluation.

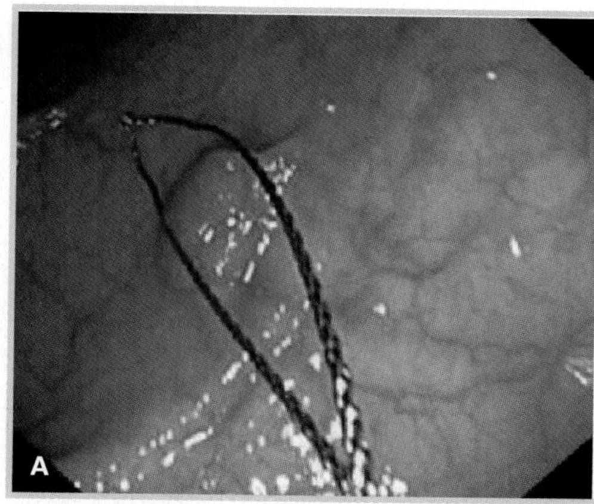

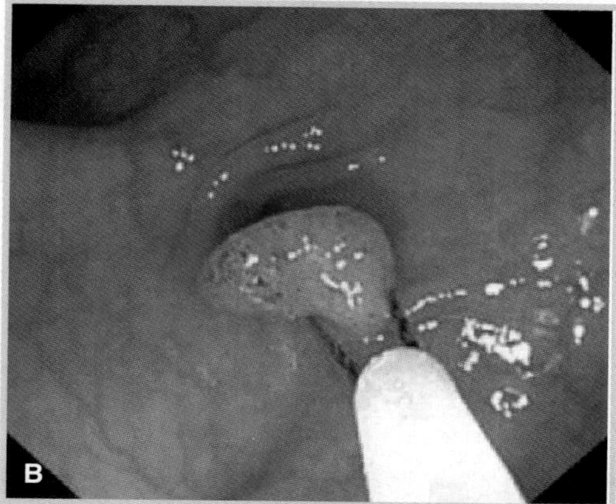

Step 11

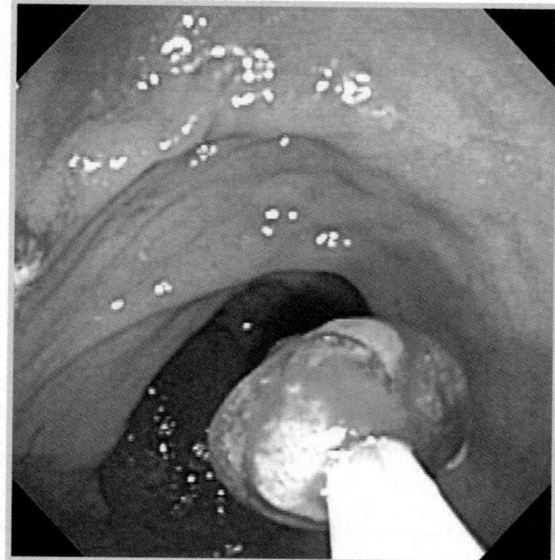

Step 12

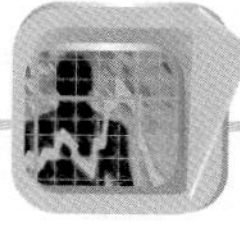

Complications

- Perforation: 1 to 2 per 1,000 procedures (studies from diagnostic colonoscopies only, however)
- Bleeding following polypectomy
- Adverse reaction from sedatives such as respiratory depression, allergic reaction, or cardiac dysrhythmia

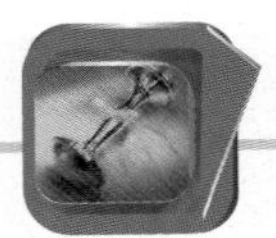

Pediatric Considerations

Pediatric endoscopes are available, which have a narrower diameter than adult endoscopes.

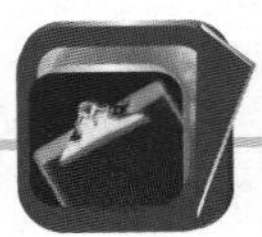

Postprocedure Instructions

Patients are usually monitored for 30 minutes after the procedure to make sure that they have recovered completely from sedation. Someone must drive them home, but they can resume a regular diet right away. They should be warned to contact their provider immediately if they experience severe abdominal pain (not just gas cramps); a firm, distended abdomen; vomiting; fever; or bleeding greater than a few tablespoons.

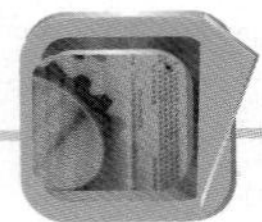

Coding Information and Supply Sources

Current Procedural Terminology (CPT) codes listed here include the terminology "proximal to the splenic flexure" in the code descriptor. However, for reporting purposes, colonoscopy is the examination of the entire colon from the rectum to the cecum and may include examination of the terminal ileum. For an incomplete colonoscopy, with full preparation administered with the intent to perform a full colonoscopy, use the colonoscopy codes above with a -52 modifier to signify reduced services. In the office setting, a tray charge can be billed (99070 or A4550) to help cover procedure costs.

CPT Code	Description	2008 Average 50th Percentile Fee	Global Period
45378	Flexible colonoscopy with brushing, washing	$1,041.00	0
45379	Flexible colonoscopy with removal of foreign body	$1,238.00	0
45380	Flexible colonoscopy with one or more biopsies	$1,143.00	0
45382	Flexible colonoscopy with bleeding control by coagulator	$1,371.00	0
45383	Flexible colonoscopy with ablation of tumors or polyps	$1,389.00	0
45384	Flexible colonoscopy with tumor or polyp removal by hot biopsy forceps	$1,358.00	0
45385	Flexible colonoscopy with tumor or polyp removal by snare technique	$1,491.00	0

CPT is a registered trademark of the American Medical Association.
2008 average 50th Percentile Fees are provided courtesy of 2008 MMH-SI's copyrighted Physicians' Fees and Coding Guide.

Common ICD-9 Codes

Abdominal mass	789.3
Anemia, unexplained	280.9
Iron deficiency anemia secondary to blood loss, anemia	280.0
GI bleeding, acute	578.9
GI bleeding, occult	578.1
X-ray abnormality	793.4

Weight loss, severe	783.2
Benign neoplasm colon	211.3
Constipation, slow transit	564.01
Constipation, outlet dysfunction	564.02
Diverticulosis with blood	562.12
Rectal bleeding	569.3
Personal Hx CRCa	V10.05
Family Hx CRCa	V16.0
Ulcerative colitis	556.9
Rectal pain	569.42
Change in bowel habits	787.99
Personal Hx colon polyps	V12.72
Abdominal mass	789.3
Anemia, unexplained	280.9
GI bleeding, acute	578.9
GI bleeding, occult	578.1
X-ray abnormality	793.4
Weight loss, severe	783.2

Instrument and Materials Ordering

- Recommendations for endoscope cleaning appear in Appendix K: Recommendations for Endoscope Disinfection
- Complete endoscopy equipment such as endoscopes, light sources, video endoscopy monitors, cleaning and disinfection aids, and mouthpieces are available from the following manufacturers:

  Olympus Corporation, Center Valley, PA (http://www.olympusamerica.com)

  Pentax Precision Instrument Corporation, Montvale, NJ (http://www.pentaxmedical.com)
- Intravenous materials (e.g., intracaths, normal saline solution, intravenous tubing) can be obtained from local hospitals or surgical supply houses.
- Propofol (1% Diprivan) injection is available from AstraZeneca, Wilmington, DE (http://www.astrazeneca-us.com). Meperidine (Demerol) injection is available from Wyeth-Lederle (http://www.wyeth.com). Midazolam (Versed) injection is available from Roche, Nutley, NJ (http://www.roche.com).
- Guidelines for monitoring patients receiving conscious sedation appear in Chapter 4.

Patient Education Handout

A patient education handout, "Colonoscopy," can be found on the book's Web site.

Bibliography

Akerkar GA, Yee J, Hung R, et al. Patient experience and preferences toward colon cancer screening: a comparison of virtual colonoscopy and conventional colonoscopy. *Gastrointest Endosc.* 2001;54:310–315.

American Academy of Family Physicians. AAFP Colonoscopy position paper. Available at http://www.aafp.org. Accessed February 1, 2008.

American Academy of Family Physicians. AAFP policies: colonoscopy privileging. Available at http://www.aafp.org. Accessed January 1, 2008.

American Society for Gastrointestinal Endoscopy. Appropriate use of gastrointestinal endoscopy. Consensus statement of the ASGE. *Gastrointest Endosc.* 2000;52:831–837.

American Society for Gastrointestinal Endoscopy. Statement on role of short courses in endoscopic training. Guidelines for clinical application. *Gastrointest Endosc.* 1999;50: 913–914.

American Society for Gastrointestinal Endoscopy. The role of colonoscopy in the management of patients with colonic polyps neoplasia. Guidelines for clinical application. *Gastrointest Endosc.* 1999;50:921–924.

Anderson JC, Messina CR, Cohn W, et al. Factors predictive of difficult colonoscopy. *Gastrointest Endosc.* 2001;54:558–562.

Arezzo A. Prospective randomized trial comparing bowel cleaning preparations for colonoscopy. *Surg Laparosc Endosc Percutan Tech.* 2000;10:215–217.

Bond JH, Frakes JT. Who should perform colonoscopy? How much training is needed? *Gastrointest Endosc.* 1999;49:657–659.

Charles RJ, Chak A, Cooper GS, et al. Use of open access in GI endoscopy at an academic medical center. *Gastrointest Endosc.* 1999;50:480–485.

Hoffman MS, Butler TW, Shaver T. Colonoscopy without sedation. *J Clin Gastroenterol.* 1998;26:279–282.

Imperiale TF, Wagner DR, Lin CY, et al. Risk of advanced proximal neoplasms in asymptomatic adults according to the distal colorectal findings. *N Engl J Med.* 2000;343:169–174.

Kim WH, Cho YJ, Park JY, et al. Factors affecting insertion time and patient discomfort during colonoscopy. *Gastrointest Endosc.* 2000;52:600–605.

Lee JG, Leung JW. Colonoscopic diagnosis of unsuspected diverticulosis. *Gastrointest Endosc.* 2002;55:746–748.

Lieberman DA, Rex DA. Feasibility of colonoscopy screening: discussion of issues and recommendations regarding implementation [Editorial]. *Gastrointest Endosc.* 2001;54:662–667.

Marshall JB, Perez RA, Madsen RW. Usefulness of a pediatric colonoscope for routine colonoscopy in women who have undergone hysterectomy. *Gastrointest Endosc.* 2002;55:838–841.

Nelson DB, McQuaid KR, Bond JH, et al. Procedural success and complications of large-scale screening colonoscopy. *Gastrointest Endosc.* 2002;55:307–314.

Noble J, Greene HL, Levinson W, et al. Tumors of the large bowel. In: Noble J, Greene HL, Levinson W, et al., eds. *Textbook of Primary Care Medicine.* St. Louis: Mosby; 2001:953–959.

Patel K, Hoffman NE. The anatomical distribution of colorectal polyps at colonoscopy. *J Clin Gastroenterol.* 2001;33:222–225.

Rex DK. Colonoscopic withdrawal technique is associated with adenoma miss rates. *Gastrointest Endosc.* 2000;51:33–36.

Simon JB. Screening colonoscopy: is it time [Commentary]? *Can Med Assoc J.* 2000;163:1277–1278.

Sipe BW, Rex DK, Latinovich D, et al. Propofol versus midazolam/meperidine for outpatient colonoscopy: administration by nurses supervised by endoscopists. *Gastrointest Endosc.* 2002;55:815–825.

Sonnenberg A, Delco F. Cost-effectiveness of a single colonoscopy in screening for colorectal cancer. *Arch Intern Med.* 2002;162:163–168.

Wexner SD, Litwin D, Cohen J, et al. Principles of privileging and credentialing for endoscopy and colonoscopy. *Gastrointest Endosc.* 2002;55:367–369.

Worthington DV. Colonoscopy: procedural skills. AAFP position paper. *Am Fam Physician.* 2000;62:1177–1182.

2008 MAG Mutual Healthcare Solutions, Inc.'s Physicians' Fee and Coding Guide. Duluth, Georgia. MAG Mutual Healthcare Solutions, Inc. 2007.

CHAPTER 90

Esophagogastroduodenoscopy

Michael B. Harper, MD, DABFM
Professor of Clinical Family Medicine
Louisiana State University Health Sciences Center, Shreveport, LA
Albert L. Smith, III, MD
Chief Resident Family Medicine
Louisiana State University Health Sciences Center, Shreveport, LA

Esophagogastroduodenoscopy (EGD) is an endoscopic procedure that allows clinicians to diagnose and treat multiple problems in the upper gastrointestinal tract. EGD is indicated for the evaluation of a variety of abdominal and chest symptoms. It can be safely performed in an office setting. When compared to radiographic procedures, EGD has greater sensitivity and specificity for diagnosis of mucosal abnormalities and allows biopsies for histology and testing for *Helicobacter pylori* infection. Radiographic studies are superior to EGD in evaluating motility of the esophagus and stomach.

There are several potential benefits when primary care providers perform EGD, especially if it is done in the office setting. These benefits include rapid assessment of patients' complaints, improved access to the procedure, increased patient comfort, reduced costs, improved provider understanding of the involved pathology, and improved health-care quality for the patient.

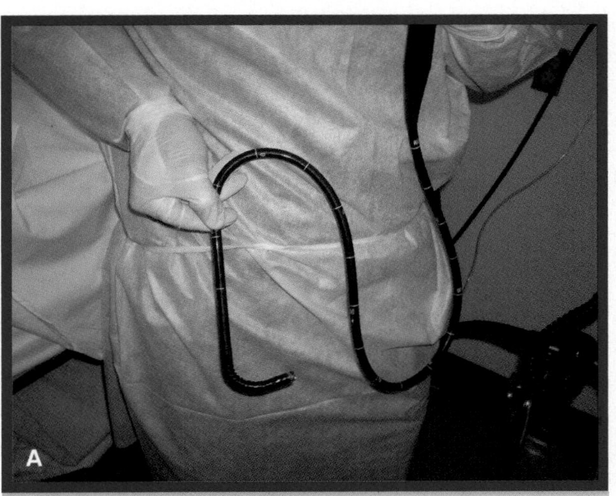

In the United States, procedural (conscious) sedation is typically used during EGD. Intravenous benzodiazepine, diazepam or midazolam, is often combined with an intravenous narcotic, meperidine or fentanyl, to improve patient comfort. Midazolam causes amnesia in most patients. Guidelines for monitoring the patient receiving conscious sedation for gastrointestinal endoscopy are included in Chapter 4. Topical anesthesia of the oral cavity can be achieved by gargling with a viscous 2% lidocaine solution or by spraying the posterior pharynx with 20% benzocaine (Hurricaine spray), but this latter method can cause methemoglobinemia. A public health advisory warning of this complication has been issued by the U.S. Food and Drug Administration. Patients who smoke and patients who have asthma, bronchitis, or chronic obstructive pulmonary disease (COPD) are at higher risk of methemoglobinemia.

Nonintravenous methods of sedation have been used successfully for EGD. Practitioners may be more comfortable with administering similar medications by nonintravenous routes in an office setting. Patients can take the benzodiazepine triazolam (Halcion, 0.25 or 0.5 mg) orally 1 hour before the procedure. Butorphanol tartrate nasal spray (Stadol) can be administered (one or two sprays) immediately before the procedure if additional anesthesia is required. Good results from this regimen were reported in a pilot study, but this regimen has not been compared with intravenous regimens. Patients undergoing nonintravenous sedation are monitored similarly to those undergoing intravenous sedation. Cost savings can be achieved by avoiding the placement of an intravenous line for the procedure. Consent must be obtained before any anesthesia is administered.

In many countries (Asia and Europe), patients commonly do not receive sedation for EGD. Smaller diameter endoscopes make this approach more feasible. Pediatric endoscopes (7.9 or 9.0 mm outer diameter) and ultrathin endoscopes (<6 mm) are available. The later can be inserted intranasally.

EGD is most commonly performed to evaluate patients with signs or symptoms of acid-peptic disorders who do not respond to appropriate medical therapy. Patients >50 years of age, as well as those with signs or symptoms of serious organic disease, should be evaluated promptly. Alarm features for serious disease include weight loss, refractory vomiting, early satiety, dysphagia, and gastrointestinal bleeding. If active bleeding is suspected, the patient should be evaluated in the controlled environment of a hospital endoscopy suite. Good patient outcomes often follow proper patient selection, and specialty referral of medically unstable or high-risk patients appears prudent.

Testing for *H. pylori*, the bacteria highly associated with antral gastritis and peptic ulcer disease, is an important component of the EGD examination. *H. pylori* produce urease, the enzyme involved in breakdown of urea to ammonia. Ammonia can be evaluated colorimetrically, and a red color change is seen in the gel testing medium when urease activity is present in the biopsy specimen. If patients are treated with antibiotics or proton pump inhibitors prior to the EGD, the test is less sensitive because of the suppression of the bacteria. To maximize sensitivity, take four biopsy specimens. Two biopsies should be from the antrum, one from the lesser curvature (at or near the incisura), and the other from the greater curvature. Take two additional biopsies from the body of the stomach, one along the greater curvature and the other near the cardia. This approach yields nearly 100% sensitivity for the infection in patients who have not been on antibiotics or a proton pump inhibitor for the previous 3 to 4 weeks.

Correct identification of pathology is a major challenge in learning EGD. Experience helps, but even seasoned endoscopists consult books and atlases to review their visual observations. Photographic or videotape recordings of procedures can help with documentation and learning. When nonvascular abnormalities are seen, biopsy is particularly useful to help identify the pathology. Although referral may be required for unusual or uncertain pathology, EGD is appropriately performed in primary care practices.

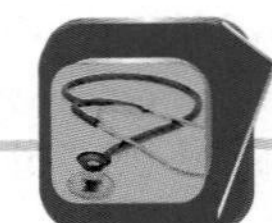

Equipment

- Video endoscopes are available in a variety of pediatric to adult sizes.
- Supporting equipment includes the instrument stack containing a light source, insufflator, suction, and video recorder/photo printer.
- Instruments include biopsy forceps, snares, and injecting needles.

Recommended Atlases

- Keeffe EB, Jeffrey RB, Lee RG. *Atlas of Gastrointestinal Endoscopy*. Philadelphia: Appleton & Lange; 1998.
- Martin DM, Lyons RC. *The Atlas of Gastrointestinal Endoscopy*. http://www.endoatlas.com/atlas_1.html

■ Murra-Saca J. *El Salvador Atlas of Gastrointestinal Videoendoscopy*. http://www.gastrointestinalatlas.com
■ Owen DA, Kelly JK. *Atlas of Gastrointestinal Pathology*. Philadelphia: WB Saunders; 1994.
■ Schiller KF, Cockel R, Hunt RH, et al. *A Colour Atlas of Gastrointestinal Endoscopy*. Philadelphia: WB Saunders; 1987.
■ Silverstein FE, Tytgat Guido NJ. *Atlas of Gastrointestinal Endoscopy*. St. Louis: Mosby; 1997.
■ Tadataka Y. *Atlas of Gastroenterology*. Philadelphia: Lippincott Williams & Wilkins; 2004.

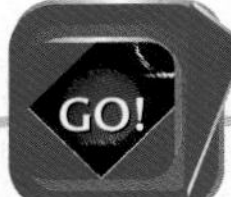

Indications

- Dyspepsia unresponsive to medical therapy
- Periodic surveillance of patients with biopsy-proven Barrett esophagus
- Dysphagia or odynophagia
- Persistent vomiting of unknown origin
- Documentation of *H. pylori*
- Persistent regurgitation of undigested food
- Suspected malabsorption
- Periodic monitoring of patients with gastric polyps or Gardner syndrome
- Documentation of clearance of gastric ulcers
- Iron-deficiency anemia
- Atypical chest pain with negative cardiac workup
- Esophageal reflux symptoms unresponsive to medical therapy
- Evaluation of upper gastrointestinal bleeding
- Suspected bezoar
- Suspected Zenker diverticulum
- Suspected upper intestinal or gastric obstruction
- Dyspepsia associated with serious signs such as weight loss
- Evaluation of abnormal radiographic findings
- Screening for gastric cancer (especially in high-risk populations such as the Japanese)

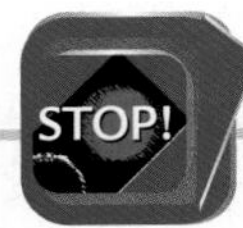

Contraindications (Relative)

- Known or suspected perforated viscus
- Acute, severe, or unstable cardiopulmonary disease
- Uncooperative patient
- Coagulopathy or bleeding diathesis
- Severe or active upper gastrointestinal bleeding
- Patients requiring therapeutic EGD that cannot be performed by the practitioner in that setting
- Hemodynamically unstable patient

The Procedure

Step 1. The first step in any endoscopic procedure is to determine that all functions of the endoscope are working properly. Turn on the light source, and confirm the image is clear. If using a videoendoscope, perform the white balance maneuver.

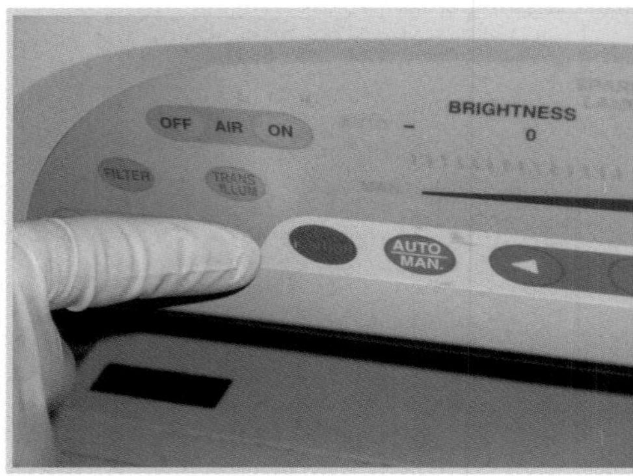

Step 1

Step 2. Covering the air/water button introduces air and can be checked by placing the tip into water and watching for bubbles to be produced.

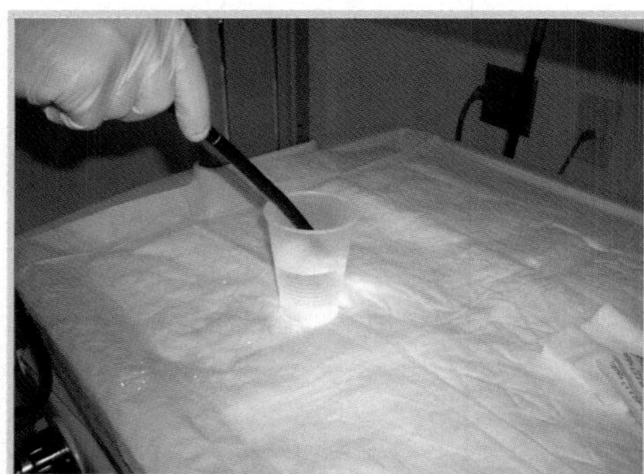

Step 2

Step 3. Pushing this button all the way down ejects a small amount of water to clean the lens. Check suction by suctioning a small amount of water through the endoscope.

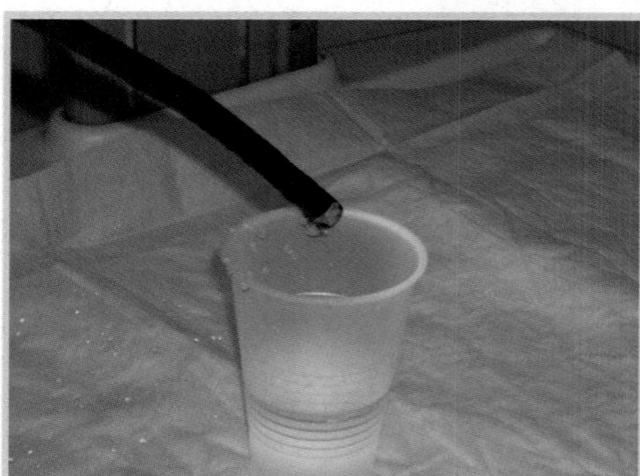

Step 3

Step 4. Be sure the tip will fully deflect by rotating both control wheels fully in both directions while observing and feeling for free movement. Remember the tip will deflect upward 170 degrees and deflect only 90 degrees in the other directions.

The tip of the endoscope is shown with the components labeled.

The head of the endoscope is depicted in the figure.

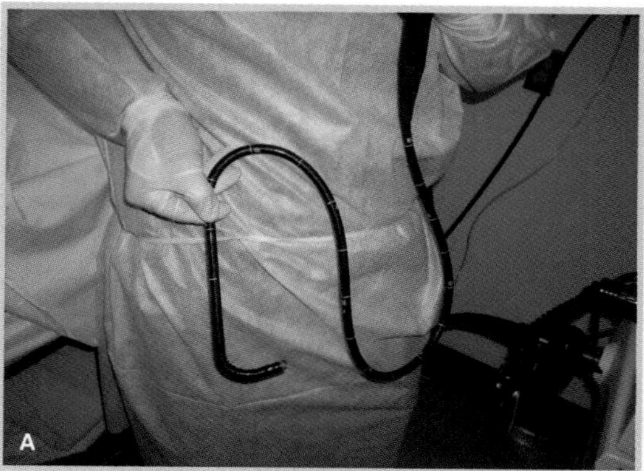

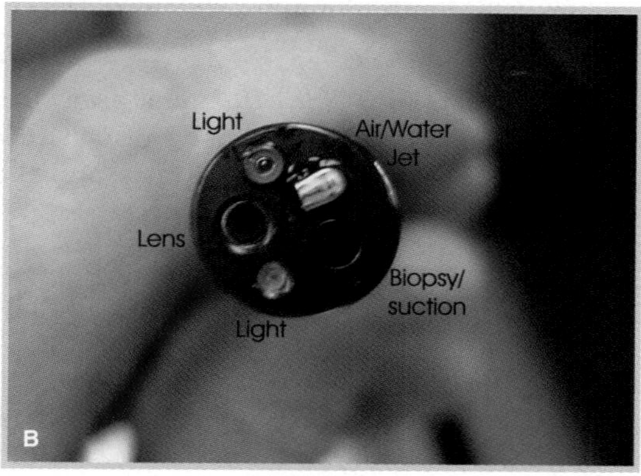

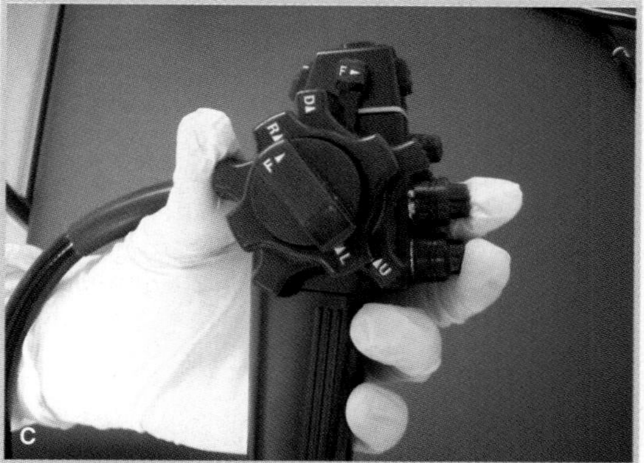

Step 4

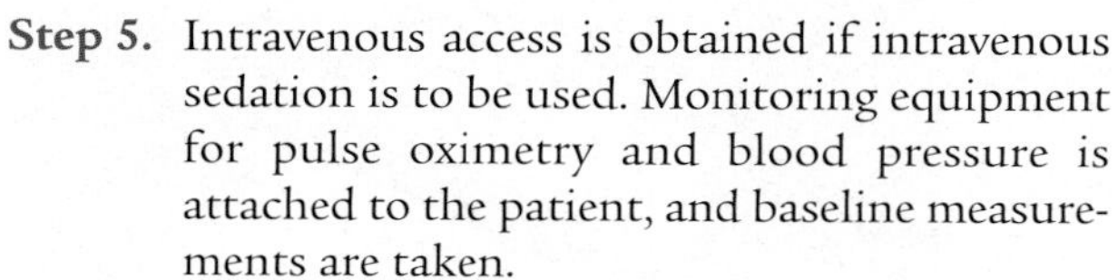

Step 5. Intravenous access is obtained if intravenous sedation is to be used. Monitoring equipment for pulse oximetry and blood pressure is attached to the patient, and baseline measurements are taken.

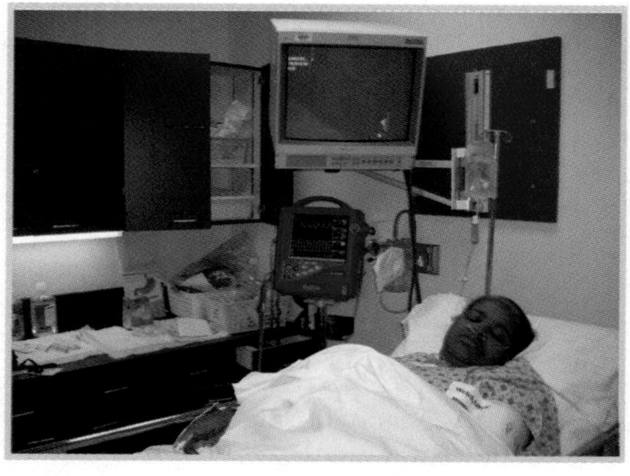

Step 5

Step 6. Dentures are removed, and oral topical anesthesia is administered. The patient can swish, gargle, and swallow 5 to 10 mL of 2% viscous lidocaine. Benzocaine spray is then applied to the posterior pharyngeal wall to blunt the gag reflex. The examiner's gloved left index finger or tongue depressor is used to depress the tongue, exposing the pharynx for two 2- to 5-second sprays. Avoid touching the patient's tissues, which would contaminate the extension spray tubing from the multiuse spray bottle, or use replacement tubing with each procedure. Some endoscopists do not use topical anesthesia and rely solely on conscious sedation for the procedure.

- **PITFALL:** The benzocaine spray has a pungent taste, even with flavoring added. Warn the patient about the taste, and allow time for a brief respite before the second spray.

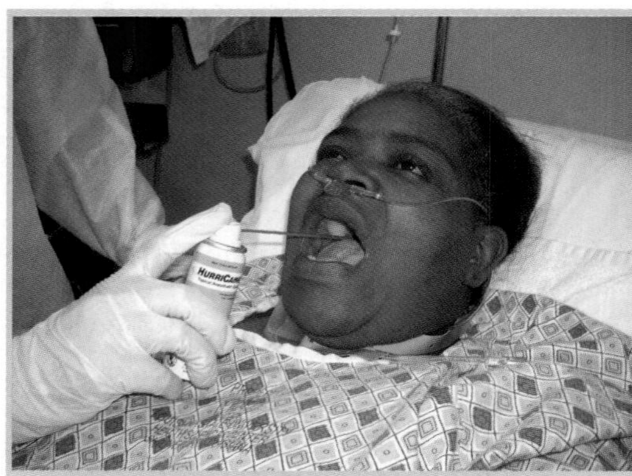

Step 6

Step 7. The patient is positioned in the left lateral decubitus position. A pillow is placed beneath the patient's head, and the head is tilted with the chin to the chest. Disposable absorbent pads are placed beneath the patient's head and neck for secretions that may drain during the procedure. The assistant may need to hold the head during insertion of the endoscope and should have suction readily available throughout the procedure. The mouthpiece is placed, and the patient is asked to gently but firmly place the teeth around the mouthpiece.

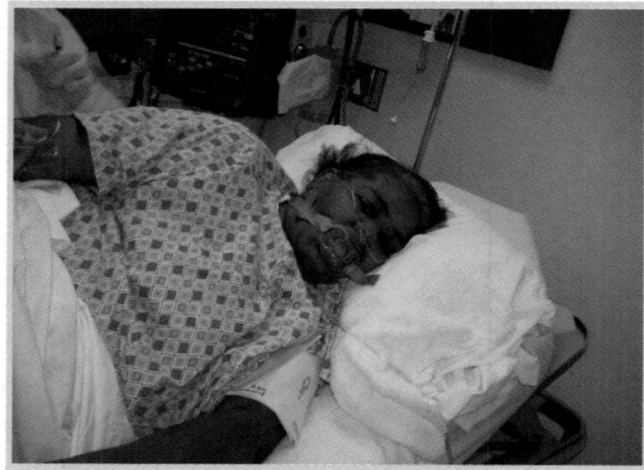

Step 7

Step 8. Anesthesia is then administered. Intravenous fentanyl (50 to 100 μg) or meperidine (25 to 75 mg) along with midazolam (1 to 2 mg) or diazepam (1 to 5 mg) is administered to achieve sedation. The proper level of sedation is recognized when the patient has slurred speech and dozes off but is still able to respond to questions and commands. Additional sedation may be used during the procedure to keep the patient comfortable as long as oxygen saturation and blood pressure are satisfactory. This step can be replaced with oral triazolam 1 hour before the procedure and intranasal butorphanol tartrate immediately prior to the procedure as described previously. Lubricate the distal end of the endoscope.

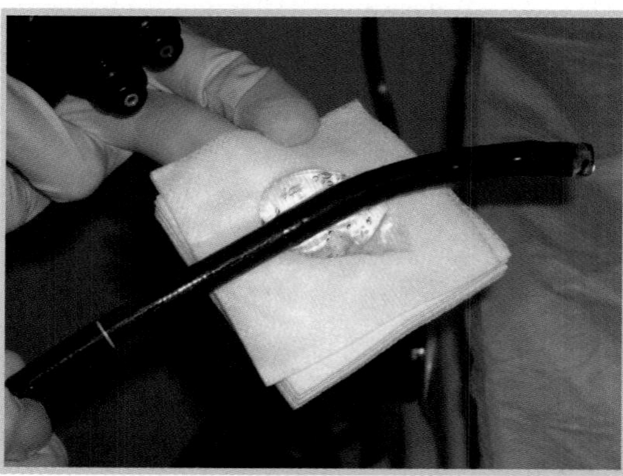

Step 8

Step 9. Insert the endoscope through the mouthpiece. The endoscope should slide easily over the posterior tongue. At about 8 cm from the incisors, deflect the tip downward to view the larynx. The scope is inserted slowly and kept off the side walls of the hypopharynx to limit gagging.

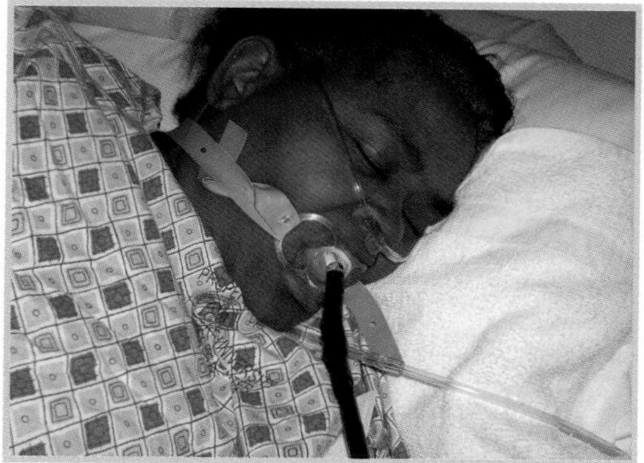

Step 9

Step 10. The scope tip is inserted to the posterior larynx, away from the vocal cords, just proximal to the closed cricopharyngeus muscle (scope inserted 15 to 18 cm from the incisors). This photo shows the view with an upward deflection in the endoscope tip.

Alternatively, this photo shows the view with a downward deflection in the endoscope tip.

- **PEARL:** The advantage of using a downward deflection is the tip cannot be overly deflected (it will bend only 90 degrees downward).

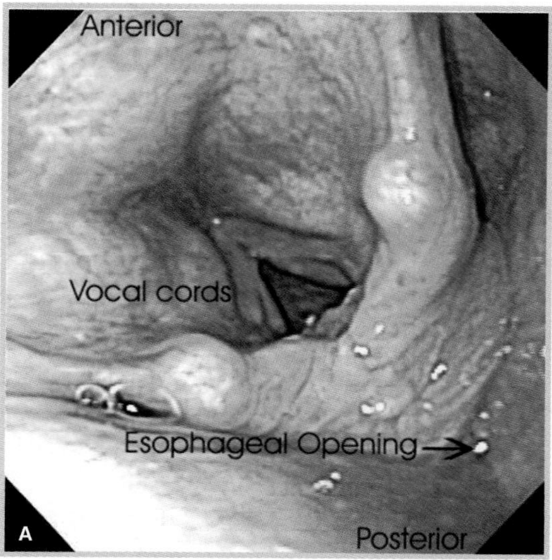

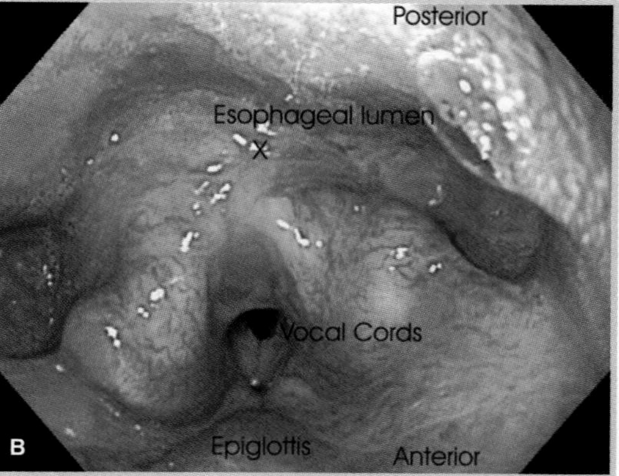

Step 10

Step 11. Ask the patient to swallow, which opens the muscle and allows access to the esophagus. The scope tip is inserted as the patient swallows, and if the esophagus is intubated, the characteristic appearance of the upper esophagus can be seen.

- **PITFALL:** The patient often gags when the scope is inserted. As soon as intubation is accomplished, stop and prevent movement of the scope tip. This allows the patient to resume normal respiratory pattern and become accustomed to the sensation created by the tube. Calm verbal encouragement should be used to assist the patient through this most difficult aspect of the procedure.
- **PITFALL:** Tracheal intubation can happen if the tube is forcibly inserted with the scope tip positioned over the vocal cords. The endoscope usually produces gagging and distress from the inability to breath and possibly from laryngospasm. The scope should be completely withdrawn if tracheal intubation is suspected or occurs (i.e., tracheal rings are visualized).

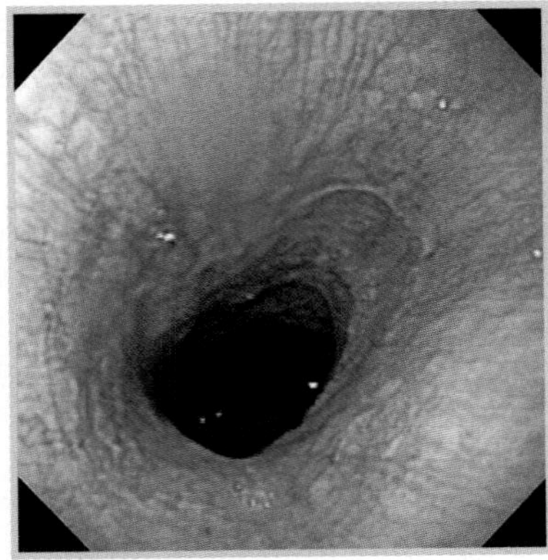

Step 11

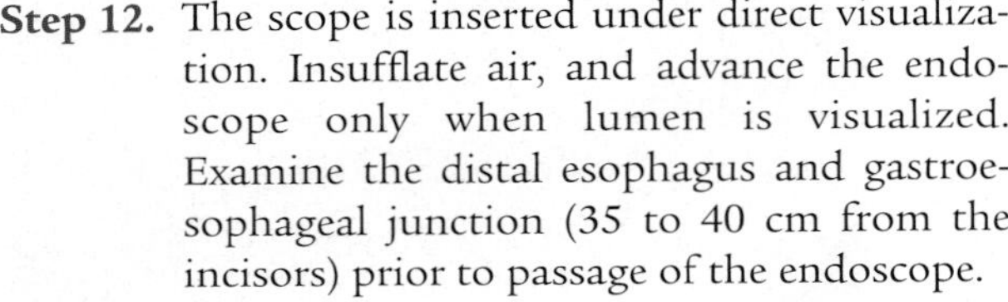

Step 12. The scope is inserted under direct visualization. Insufflate air, and advance the endoscope only when lumen is visualized. Examine the distal esophagus and gastroesophageal junction (35 to 40 cm from the incisors) prior to passage of the endoscope.

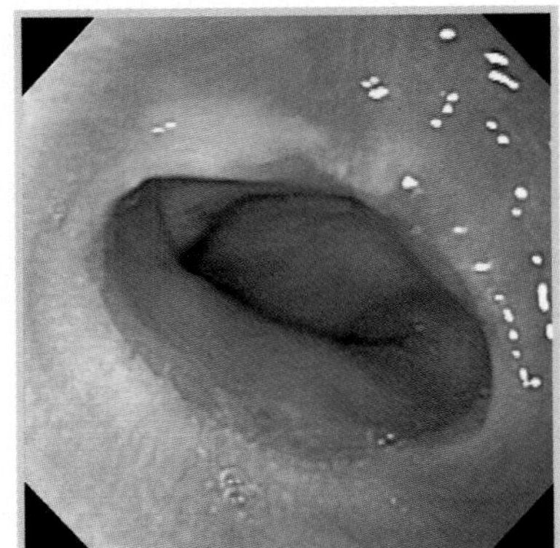

Step 12

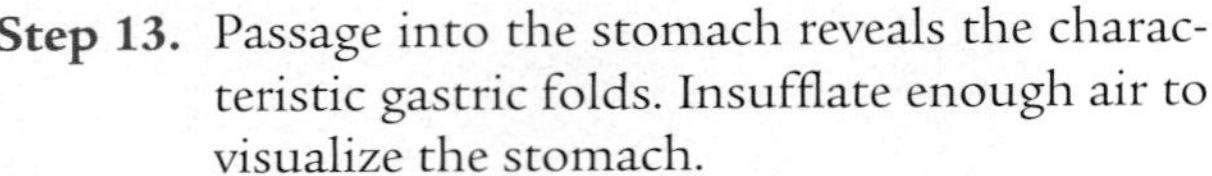

Step 13. Passage into the stomach reveals the characteristic gastric folds. Insufflate enough air to visualize the stomach.

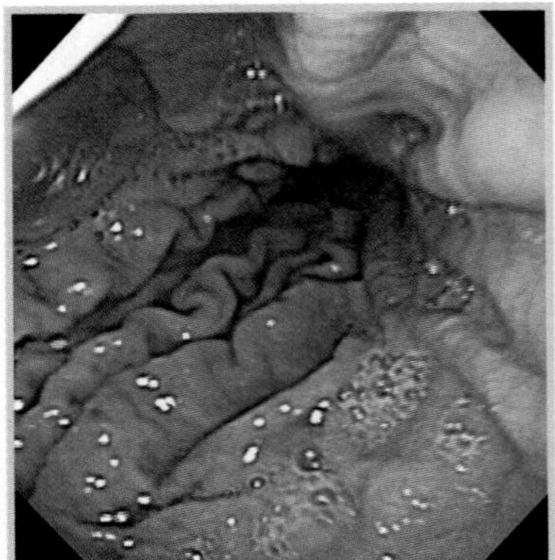

Step 13

Step 14. Pass the endoscope to the antrum. The longitudinal folds of the body can be used to determine the long axis and assist in finding the antrum and pylorus. Angulation of the scope tip may be required. Position the scope tip just proximal to the pylorus, and insert the scope as the pylorus opens after a contraction. You may need to insufflate more air during this step, but do not use excessive amounts.

- PITFALL: The longer the scope is in the stomach, the greater is the degree of pylorospasm. Rapid intubation of the duodenum is advocated to reduce difficulty in passing through the pylorus.
- PITFALL: Often, the scope tip slips back into the stomach, and the scope must be reinserted into the duodenum.

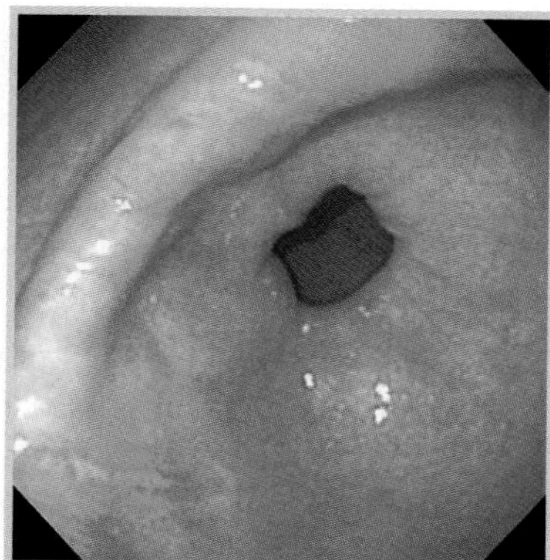

Step 14

Step 15. As the endoscope enters the duodenum, examine the mucosa for duodenitis before scope passage. The lumen will typically be seen down and right. By moving the scope tip up, examine the anterior wall, down to examine the posterior wall, left for the inferior wall, and right to see the superior wall.

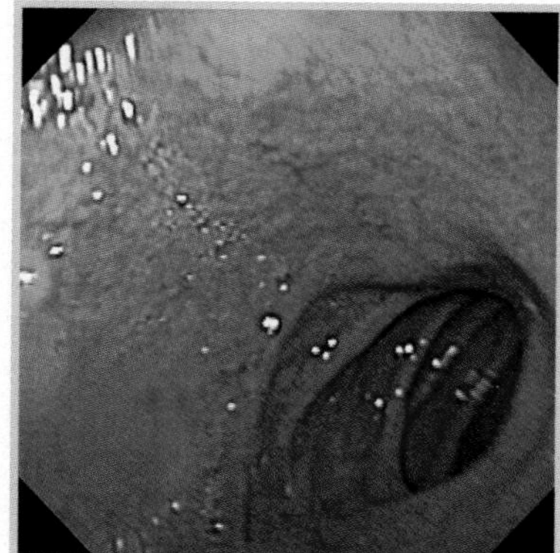

Step 15

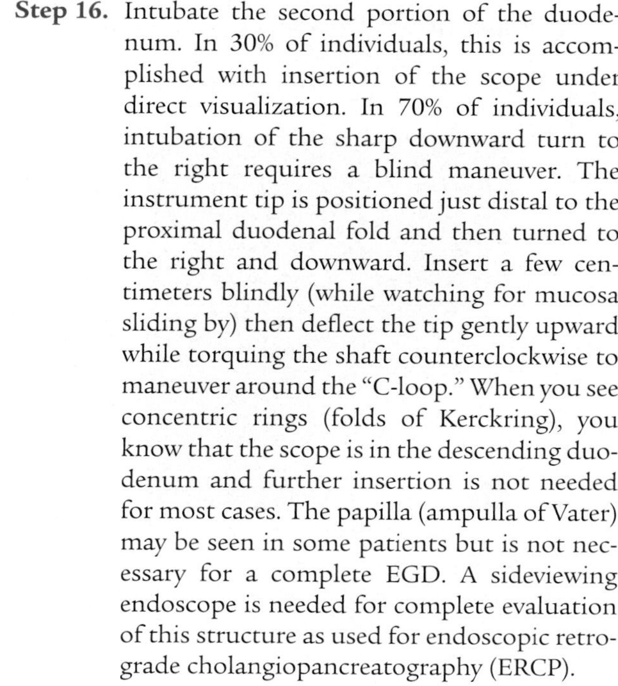

Step 16. Intubate the second portion of the duodenum. In 30% of individuals, this is accomplished with insertion of the scope under direct visualization. In 70% of individuals, intubation of the sharp downward turn to the right requires a blind maneuver. The instrument tip is positioned just distal to the proximal duodenal fold and then turned to the right and downward. Insert a few centimeters blindly (while watching for mucosa sliding by) then deflect the tip gently upward while torquing the shaft counterclockwise to maneuver around the "C-loop." When you see concentric rings (folds of Kerckring), you know that the scope is in the descending duodenum and further insertion is not needed for most cases. The papilla (ampulla of Vater) may be seen in some patients but is not necessary for a complete EGD. A sideviewing endoscope is needed for complete evaluation of this structure as used for endoscopic retrograde cholangiopancreatography (ERCP).

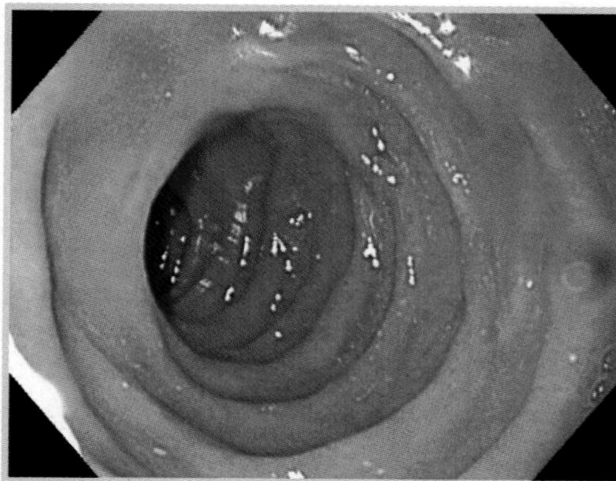

Step 16

Step 17. Withdraw the scope slowly to allow examination of the duodenal bulb if it was not thoroughly seen upon insertion. Often the endoscope comes out of the pylorus and must be reinserted to fully evaluate the duodenal bulb. After thorough examination of the duodenum, the scope is brought back into the stomach.

- **PITFALL:** Do not biopsy pulsatile or vascular lesions, because the resulting bleeding can be extensive and difficult to control.
- **PITFALL:** Esophageal ulcerations or erosions may be better assessed by brushing or washing. The esophagus is much thinner than the stomach, and risk of perforation from biopsy is greater at this location. Beware of biopsying the base of a deep gastric ulcer, because perforation can occur in this situation.

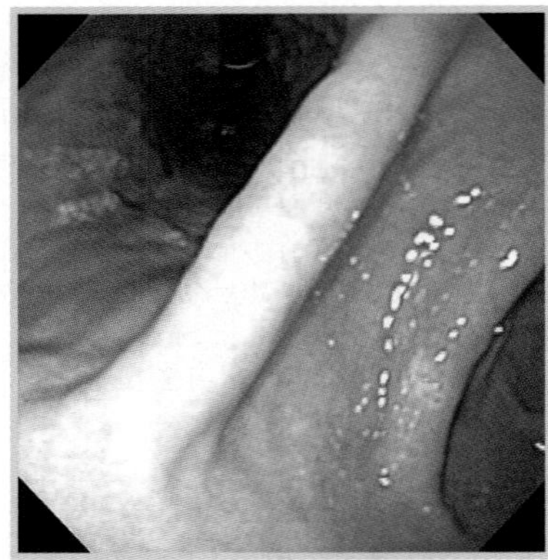

Step 17

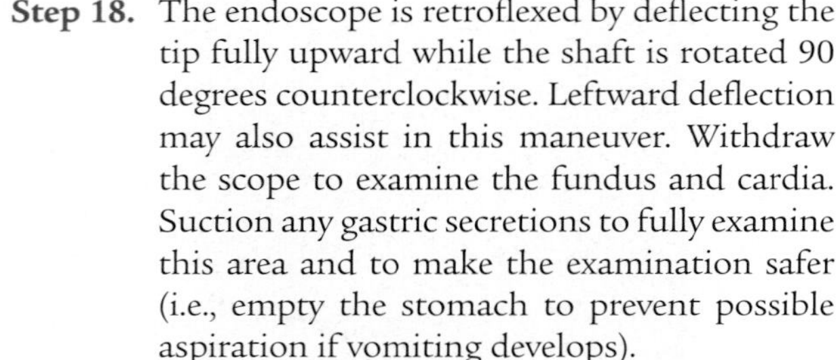

Step 18. The endoscope is retroflexed by deflecting the tip fully upward while the shaft is rotated 90 degrees counterclockwise. Leftward deflection may also assist in this maneuver. Withdraw the scope to examine the fundus and cardia. Suction any gastric secretions to fully examine this area and to make the examination safer (i.e., empty the stomach to prevent possible aspiration if vomiting develops).

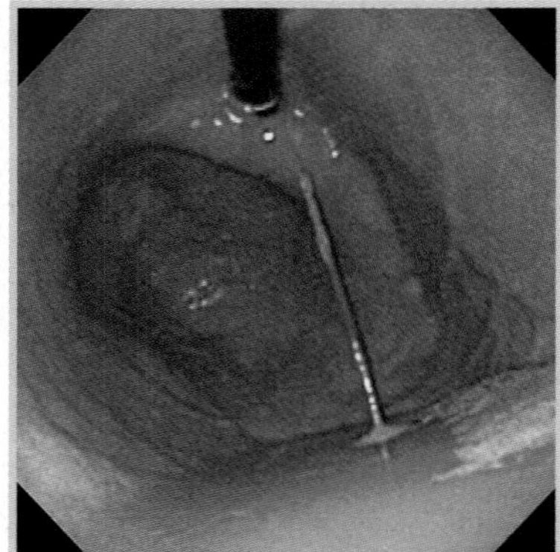

Step 18

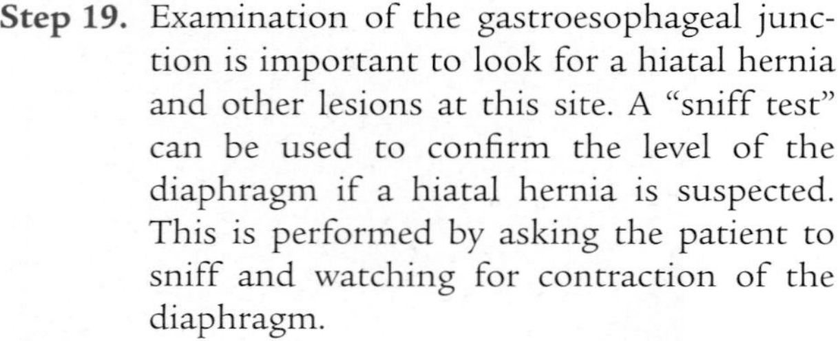

Step 19. Examination of the gastroesophageal junction is important to look for a hiatal hernia and other lesions at this site. A "sniff test" can be used to confirm the level of the diaphragm if a hiatal hernia is suspected. This is performed by asking the patient to sniff and watching for contraction of the diaphragm.

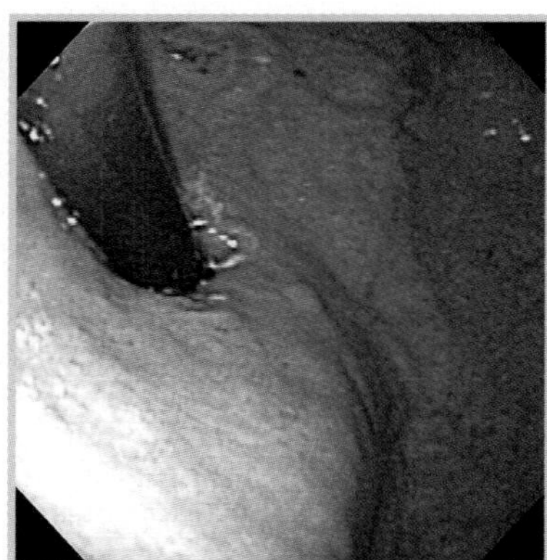

Step 19

Step 20. Biopsies are then obtained for *H. pylori* testing (CLOtest). Because of the risk of malignancy, multiple biopsies are performed on all gastric ulcers along the raised edges. In contrast, duodenal ulcers do not require biopsy. Biopsy also is performed on abnormal growths, polyps, or other nonvascular pathologic changes.

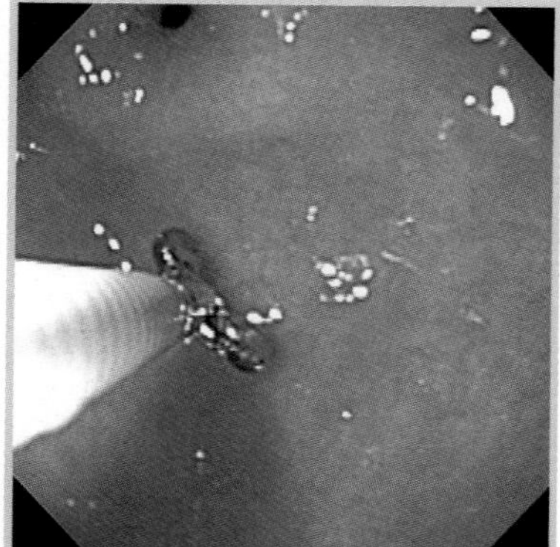

Step 20

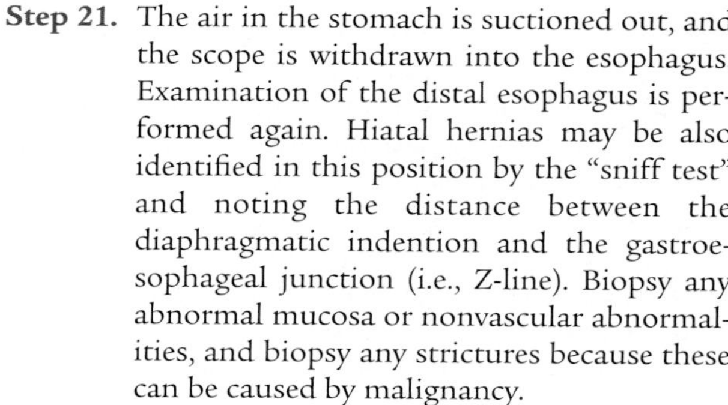

Step 21. The air in the stomach is suctioned out, and the scope is withdrawn into the esophagus. Examination of the distal esophagus is performed again. Hiatal hernias may be also identified in this position by the "sniff test" and noting the distance between the diaphragmatic indention and the gastroesophageal junction (i.e., Z-line). Biopsy any abnormal mucosa or nonvascular abnormalities, and biopsy any strictures because these can be caused by malignancy.

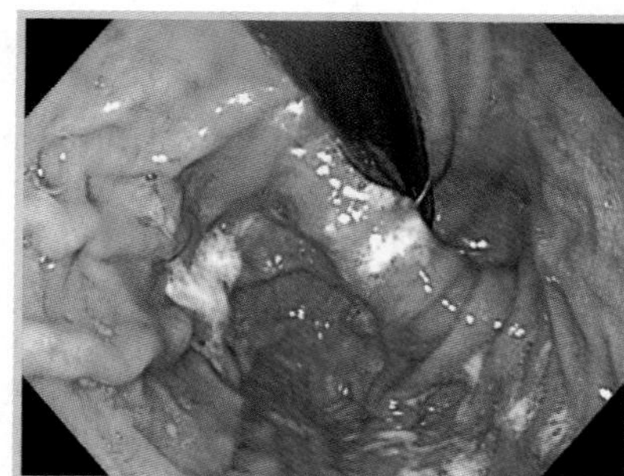

Step 21

Step 22. Withdraw the scope, examining the esophagus and larynx on removal. Pay special attention to the proximal esophagus because this may have been passed blindly upon initial insertion of the scope. Remove the mouthpiece. Wipe off any oral secretions that have drained from the mouth. Observe the patient until the sedation wears off or the patient is stable for discharge with a family member or caregiver.

- PITFALL: Lesions in the proximal esophagus may be missed upon initial insertion of the endoscope. Examine this area carefully.

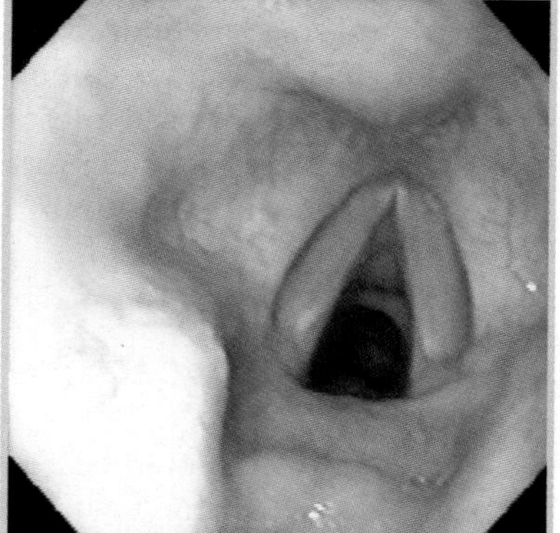

Step 22

Step 23. Immediately following the procedure, begin the cleaning process by suctioning an enzyme solution through the endoscope, and follow manufacturer's recommendations for disinfection. Recommendations for endoscope disinfection are included in Appendix K: Recommendations for Endoscope Disinfection.

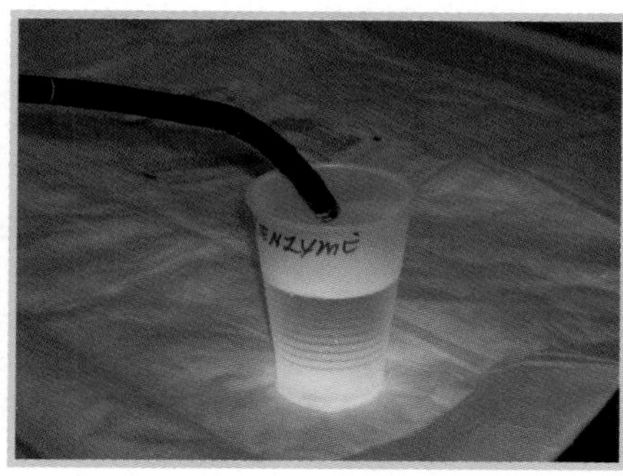

Step 23

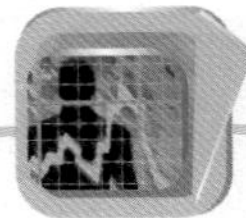

Complications

- Perforation of stomach, esophagus, or duodenum
- Bleeding at biopsy site
- Adverse reaction to anesthesia or medication, including
  - Respiratory depression
  - Apnea
  - Hypotension
  - Excessive sweating
  - Bradycardia
  - Laryngospasm

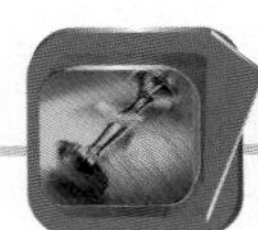

Pediatric Considerations

Pediatric indications for EGD are similar to adult indications. Ingestions of foreign objects and caustic materials are more common in the pediatric population. Caustic items such as watch batteries should be retrieved from the esophagus urgently. Oral mucosa damage should be useful in determining the need for further evaluation of questionable liquid ingestion. Most coins will advance to the stomach within 24 hours, but a foreign body impacted in the esophagus should be removed within 24 hours. Size and shape of a foreign object is another important consideration. Objects >3 cm in length young children and 5 cm in length in ages up to adolescence should be promptly removed. Sharp or pointed objects should be urgently recovered.

A standard adult gastroscope (≥9.7 mm) is appropriate for most children weighing >25 kg. A smaller gastroscope (7.9 or 9.0 mm outer diameter) is recommended for infants and smaller children. Also, pediatric endoscopes have correspondingly smaller biopsy forceps with a reduced bite appropriate for thinner small bowel.

Refer to the anesthesia chapter for pediatric anesthesia (see Chapter 122). Some important considerations involve airway safety and anesthesia selection. The necessary equipment and training for definitive airway protection should be readily available.

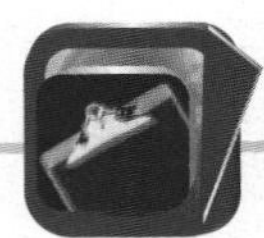

Postprocedure Instructions

Someone should be available to take the patient home after the procedure and stay with the patient for a while. Patients should not be allowed to drive themselves because of the sedation.

Patients should call their health-care provider if any of these conditions arise after endoscopy: chest pain, severe abdominal pain, fever, black stools, or hematemesis. Patients might find relief from a transitory sore throat with warm saltwater gargling or throat lozenges.

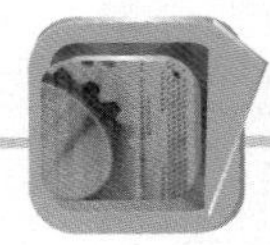

Coding Information and Supply Sources

For comprehensive upper gastrointestinal (GI) endoscopic procedures, 43239 is the code most commonly reported. In the office setting, a surgery tray charge may be billed in addition (99070 or A4550) to cover some of the administrative costs.

CPT Code	Description	2008 Average 50th Percentile Fee	Global Period
43200	Esophagoscopy with or without brushings	$729.00	0
43202	Esophagoscopy with biopsies	$772.00	0
43234	Simple primary upper GI endoscopy	$720.00	0
43235	Upper GI endoscopy, including duodenum with brushings	$779.00	0
43239	Upper GI endoscopy, including duodenum with biopsies	$879.00	0

ICD-9 Codes

Abdominal mass	789.3
Anemia, unexplained	280.9
GI bleeding, acute	578.9
GI bleeding, occult	578.1
X-ray abnormality	793.4
Dyspepsia, severe	536.8
Dysphagia/odynophagia	787.2
Early satiety	789.0
Epigastric pain	789.0
Food slicking	787.2
Heartburn, meal related	787.1
Indigestion, severe	787.3
Nausea, chronic (vomiting)	787.0
Pain (substernal/paraxiphold)	786.5
Reflux of food (regurgitation)	787.0
Weight loss, severe	783.2
Cancer surveillance in high risk patients	V 67.9
Esophageal stricture	564.2
Gastric retention	782.0
History of duodenitis	535.6
History of esophagitis	530.1
History of gastritis	535.4
History of hiatal hernia	553.3
Monitoring a gastric ulcer	531.9
Peptic ulcer disease	533.0
Pyloroduodenal stenosis	537.0
Varices	456.0

Suppliers

Complete endoscopy equipment such as endoscopes, light sources, video endoscopy monitors, cleaning and disinfection aids, and mouthpieces are available from these suppliers:

- Olympus Corporation, Center Valley, PA. Web site: http://www.olympusamerica.com.
- Pentax Precision Instrument Corporation, Montvale, NJ. Web site: http://www.pentaxmedical.com
- A viscous 2% lidocaine topical solution is available from Alpharma USPD, Bridgewater, NJ. Web site: http://www.alpharma.com.
- Benzocaine 20% spray (Hurricaine topical anesthetic) is available in several flavors from Beutlich Pharmaceuticals, Waukegan, IL. Web site: http://www.beutlich.com
- CLOtest kits can be obtained from Tri-Med Specialties, Roswell, GA. Web site: http://www.kchealthcare.com/global/index.asp.

- Butorphanol tartrate (Stadol) nasal spray is available from Bristol-Myers Squibb. Web site: http://www.bms.com.

Intravenous materials (e.g., Intracaths, normal saline solution, intravenous tubing) can be obtained from local hospitals or surgical supply houses.

Recommendations for endoscope cleaning appear in Appendix K.

Patient Education Handout

A patient education handout, "Esophagogastroduodenoscopy (EGD)," can be found on the book's companion Web site.

Bibliography

Ackerman RJ. Performance of gastrointestinal tract endoscopy by primary care providers. *Arch Fam Med.* 1997;6:52–58.

American Academy of Family Providers. *Esophagogastroduodenoscopy: A Short Course in Basic Skills and Cognitive Knowledge.* Kansas City: American Academy of Family Providers; 1992.

American Society for Gastrointestinal Endoscopy. *Appropriate Use of Gastrointestinal Endoscopy: A Consensus Statement from the American Society for Gastrointestinal Endoscopy.* Manchester, MA: American Society for Gastrointestinal Endoscopy; 1989.

Axon AT. Working party report to the World Congresses. Disinfection and endoscopy: summary and recommendations. *J Gastroenterol Hepatol.* 1991;6:23–24.

Bytzer P, Hansen JM, Schaffalitzky DE, et al. Empirical H2-blocker therapy or prompt endoscopy in management of dyspepsia. *Lancet.* 1994;343:811–816.

Cass OW, Freeman ML, Peine CJ, et al. Objective evaluation of endoscopy skills during training. *Ann Intern Med.* 1993;118:40–44.

Coleman WH. Gastroscopy: a primary diagnostic procedure. *Prim Care.* 1988;15:1–11.

Fleisher D. Monitoring the patient receiving conscious sedation for gastrointestinal endoscopy: issues and guidelines. *Gastrointest Endosc.* 1989;35:262–266.

Genta RM, Graham DY. Comparison of biopsy sites for the histopathologic diagnosis of *Helicobacter pylori*: a topographic study of *H. pylori* density and distribution. *Gastrointest Endosc.* 1994;40:342–345.

Health and Public Policy Committee, American College of Providers. Endoscopy in the evaluation of dyspepsia. *Ann Intern Med.* 1985;102:266–269.

Health and Public Policy Committee, American College of Providers. Clinical competence in diagnostic esophagogastroduodenoscopy. *Ann Intern Med.* 1987;107:937–939.

Hocutt JE, Rodney WM, Zurad EG, et al. Esophagogastroduodenoscopy for the family provider. *Am Fam Provider.* 1994;49:109–116, 121–122.

LaLuna L, Allen ML, DiMarino AJ. The comparison of midazolam and topical lidocaine spray versus the combination of midazolam, meperidine, and topical lidocaine spray to sedate patients for upper endoscopy. *Gastrointest Endosc.* 2001;53:289–293.

Lieberman DA, Wuerker CK, Katon RM. Cardiopulmonary risk of esophagogastroduodenoscopy: role of endoscope diameter and systemic sedation. *Gastroenterology.* 1985;88:468–472.

Nelson DB, Block KP, Bosco JJ, et al. Technology status evaluation report: ultrathin endoscopes. *Gastrointest Endosc.* 2000;51:786–789.

Rodney WM, Weber JR, Swedberg JA, et al. Esophagogastroduodenoscopy by family providers phase a national multisite study of 2500 procedures. *Fam Pract Res J.* 1993;13:121–131.

Sgammato J. Should you be doing EGD? *Fam Pract Manag.* 1994;1:63–77.

Silverstein MD, Petterson T, Talley NJ. Initial endoscopy or empirical therapy with or without testing for *Helicobacter pylori* for dyspepsia: a decision analysis. *Gastroenterology.* 1996;110:72–83.

Spach DH, Silverstein FE, Stamm WE. Transmission of infection by gastrointestinal endoscopy and bronchoscopy. *Ann Intern Med.* 1993;118:117–128.

Susman J, Rodney WM. Numbers, procedural skills and science: do the three mix? [Editorial] *Am Fam Provider.* 1994;49:1591–1592.

Swedberg JA. Sedation for office esophagogastroduodenoscopy [Editorial]. *Arch Fam Med.* 1995;4:583–584.

Woodliff DM. The role of upper gastrointestinal endoscopy in primary care. *J Fam Pract.* 1979;8:715–719.

Zuber TJ. A pilot project in office-based diagnostic esophagogastroduodenoscopy comparing two nonintravenous methods of sedation and anesthesia. *Arch Fam Med.* 1995;4:601–607.

Zuber TJ. *Office Procedures.* Kansas City: American Academy of Family Providers; 1998:23–33.

2008 MAG Mutual Healthcare Solutions, Inc.'s Physicians' Fee and Coding Guide. Duluth, Georgia. MAG Mutual Healthcare Solutions, Inc. 2007.

CHAPTER 91

Flexible Sigmoidoscopy

Jeffrey A. German, MD

Associate Professor, Department of Family Medicine
Louisiana State University Health Sciences Center, Shreveport, LA

Clint N. Wilson, MD

Chief Resident, Family Medicine Residency
Louisiana State University Health Sciences Center, Shreveport, LA

Flexible sigmoidoscopy is a commonly performed technique for examination of the rectum and distal colon. Sigmoidoscopy has been advocated every 3 to 5 years for individuals older than 50 years of age as a screening strategy to detect adenomas and colon cancer. The technique is safe, easily performed in an office setting, and produces a 30% to 40% reduction in colon cancer mortality. Training in endoscopic maneuvering and in anatomy and pathology recognition is required for the performance of sigmoidoscopy. Experienced practitioners often perform the procedure in less than 10 minutes. Most physicians report comfort with performing the procedure unsupervised after completing 10 to 25 preceptor-guided sessions.

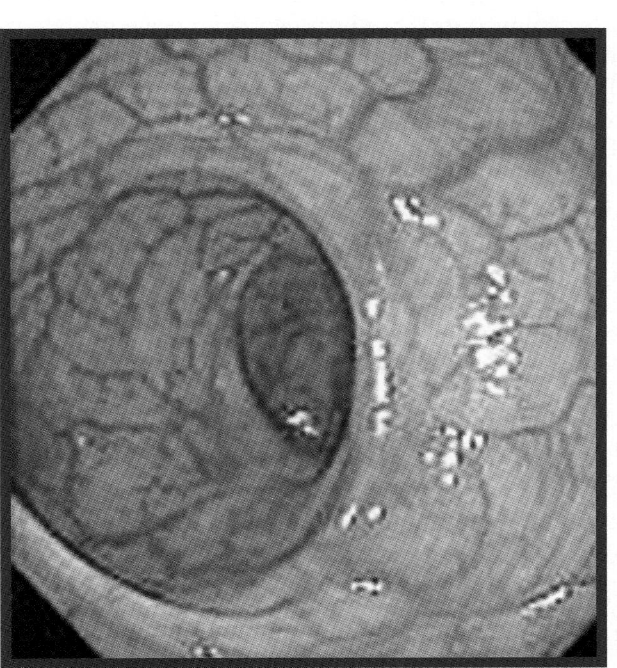

About 60% of all colorectal cancers are within reach of the sigmoidoscope. Rectal bleeding in individuals older than 50 years should be evaluated by full colonoscopy because of the risk for isolated proximal neoplasms beyond the view of the sigmoidoscope. Multiple options exist when evaluating a younger individual with rectal bleeding. For persons between the ages of 30 and 39 years, the incidence of colon cancer is only three cases per 1,000 people, but differentiating the few with serious pathology from those with anal disease can be difficult. Because proximal lesions also peak in individuals before the age of 40 years, full colonoscopy and flexible sigmoidoscopy with barium enema are appropriate strategies for individuals between the ages of 30 and 49 years. Most bleeding in individuals younger than 30 years is caused by benign anal disease. Flexible sigmoidoscopy is a reasonable option in that age group if anoscopic findings are normal.

About 7% to 10% of flexible sigmoidoscopies reveal the presence of adenomas. Historically, the presence of an adenoma necessitated referral for colonoscopy to look for proximal neoplasia. Some physicians have recommended colonoscopy only for larger (>1 cm) adenomas, because larger lesions were more likely to have higher-risk villous features. However, the major benefit of universal biopsy of polyps discovered at sigmoidoscopy may be to distinguish tubular adenomas from villous adenomas. Persons with tubular adenomas of any size appear to have the same rate of proximal neoplasia as individuals with no adenomas at sigmoidoscopy (about 5.5%). A distal tubulovillous or villous adenoma has a higher rate of proximal neoplasia (about 12%), and this finding should incur referral for colonoscopy.

Diminutive (<5 mm) polyps found at sigmoidoscopy often are hyperplastic. Although hyperplastic polyps generally are not thought to be associated with proximal adenomas, this opinion is not universally accepted in the literature. Many practices offer barium enema, and others recommend no further screening when hyperplastic polyps are found on sigmoidoscopic biopsy.

Many physicians recommend full colonoscopy for colon cancer screening every 10 years for all individuals older than 50 years. Individuals at higher risk (i.e., those with a family history of colon cancer) may benefit from this strategy. Significant feasibility issues continue to prevent this approach from being recommended for population screening. A more feasible strategy is to perform screening sigmoidoscopy at age 50 for average-risk individuals. Only a small proportion of screened individuals with an occult proximal neoplasm will have the lesion progress to symptomatic colon cancer, and those that do progress take many years. Periodic sigmoidoscopy followed by a single screening colonoscopy at age 65 may be a more appropriate, cost-effective population strategy.

The average procedure time for sigmoidoscopy without biopsy is about 17 minutes. Performance of a biopsy adds about 10 minutes to the procedure. Although it is desirable to insert the entire scope length (60 to 70 cm), the average depth of insertion is about 52 cm. Both procedure time and the depth of insertion appear to be operator dependent. Women have a more acute angle at the rectosigmoid junction, making endoscope passage more difficult. Studies in women also demonstrate that a history of prior pelvic or abdominal surgery increases the discomfort and decreases the depth of endoscope insertion. Sigmoidoscopy in women averages insertion depths of only 40 cm.

In a large series in England, about 80% of individuals rated the discomfort of sigmoidoscopy as "no or mild pain." The remainder rated their discomfort as moderate to severe, with women reporting significantly more discomfort. About 16% stated that their discomfort was greater than what they expected. Most procedures can be performed without sedation or analgesia, but if patients insist, premedication options include oral diazepam (10 mg) or triazolam (0.5 mg) taken 1 hour before the procedure, intranasal butorphanol (two squirts) immediately before the procedure, or intramuscular ketorolac (60 mg) administered 30 minutes before the procedure.

Adequate preparation of the left colon is essential for flexible sigmoidoscopy. Eating after midnight is highly associated with stool in the sigmoid, and patients must be instructed to consume only clear liquids the morning of the procedure. Most practices recommend the administration of one or two enemas before the procedure. Home administration of the enemas may reduce patient embarrassment and time demands on office nursing staffs. However, many patients refuse to administer home enemas, feeling unable to perform the task or fearing a mess. Proper education of enema administration and offering an alternate, orally administered bowel preparation may reduce noncompliance with home bowel cleansing.

Individuals often choose not to undergo sigmoidoscopy. Offering fecal occult blood testing simultaneously with sigmoidoscopy can cause some patients to avoid the invasive procedure. Increased acceptance of sigmoidoscopy can be achieved by sending a letter describing the significance of colon cancer and inviting individuals to participate in colon screening. Other factors that may favorably increase the uptake of the procedure include enthusiasm of the primary care physician and staff for the procedure, telephone reminders before the procedure, higher levels of general education in the target population, and skill of the practitioner performing endoscopy (especially for repeated screening).

About one half of primary care physicians who are trained to perform flexible sigmoidoscopy do not continue the procedure in practice. One study documented that the main deterrents to continuing to offer the service included the time required to perform the procedure, the availability of the procedure from other physicians in their locale, and the availability of adequately trained staff. Low reimbursement for the time involved in the procedure, especially from the Medicare program, is often cited as a reason for discontinuing sigmoidoscopy screening.

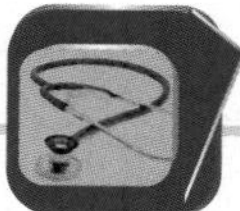

Equipment

- Sigmoidoscope and video monitoring equipment

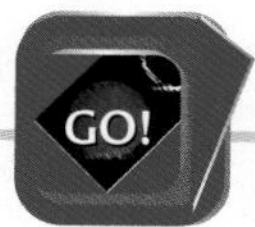

Indications

- Colorectal cancer screening
- Evaluation of bright red rectal bleeding, especially in younger patients
- Evaluation of an abnormal finding on rectal examination (e.g., palpable mass, polyp)
- Evaluation of a woman with prior gynecologic malignancy
- Evaluation of an abnormality identified radiographically
- Investigation of abdominal pain
- Suspected foreign body
- Evaluation of symptoms that could be attributable to the colon (e.g., weight loss, iron-deficiency anemia, persistent diarrhea, change in bowel habits, painful defecation)
- Surveillance of colon pathology (e.g., inflammatory bowel disease, prior polypectomy)
- Follow-up after colectomy

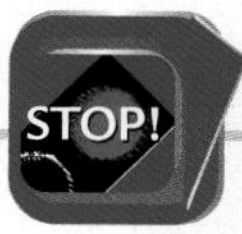

Contraindications (Relative)

- Acute peritonitis
- Uncooperative patient
- Coagulopathy or bleeding diathesis
- Acute diverticulitis (do not insert the scope past a newly discovered inflamed diverticulum)
- Acute fulminant colitis
- Suspected ischemic bowel necrosis
- Inadequate bowel preparation
- Extensive pelvic adhesions
- Severe cardiac or pulmonary disease
- Pelvic adhesions (especially women with a prior hysterectomy), which can increase the procedure's discomfort
- Toxic megacolon
- Anticoagulant or aspirin use at time of the procedure (discontinue aspirin at least 10 days before and coumadin at least 2 days before the procedure)
- Paralytic ileus
- Large (>5 cm) abdominal aneurysm
- Suspected perforation of the bowel

The Procedure

Step 1. The patient is positioned in the Sims or left lateral decubitus position, with the left side of the body down on the table. The right hip and knee are both flexed, and the left leg remains fairly straight. A rectal examination is performed with the lubricated, gloved index finger. The nondominant hand lifts the right buttock. The anal canal and distal rectum are examined for pathology and to exclude any obstruction, foreign body, or stool that may prevent endoscope insertion. Use of 5% lidocaine ointment may decrease discomfort from the subsequent endoscopic procedure.

- **PITFALL:** Overly aggressive performance of a digital examination will make the patient uncomfortable and possibly reduce patient tolerance of the ensuing endoscopy. Perform the examination gently, and talk to the patient (i.e., verbal anesthesia) from the very beginning.
- **PEARL:** Because the endoscope does not visualize the anal canal well, many authorities recommend performance of anoscopy before sigmoidoscopy (see Chapter 87).

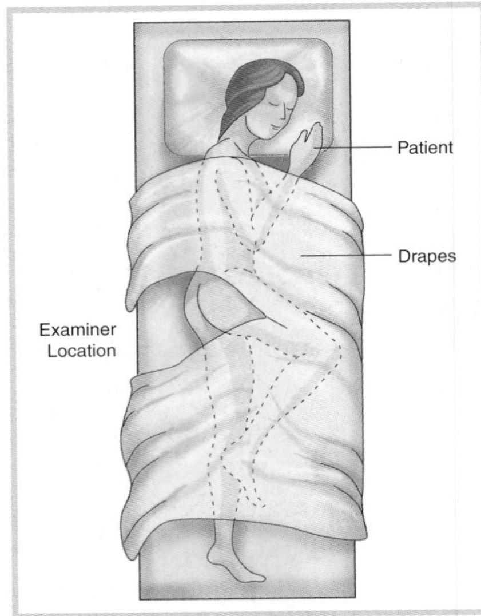

Step 1

Step 2. The endoscope is held in the left hand. The umbilical cord to the light source sits over the thumb web space and travels across the wrist. The endoscope head sits in the palm of the hand. The left thumb operates the inner (up and down) and outer (right and left) control knobs. The index finger and middle finger depress the air or water and suction valves. The left fourth and fifth fingers grasp and support the endoscope.

- **PITFALL:** Many individuals with small hands complain about the difficulty of holding the endoscope. It may be difficult for the thumb to reach the outer knob if the operator's hand is small. Most operators can learn to manipulate the wheels with the left hand only; however, in rare cases, individuals with small hands must learn to operate the wheels using the right hand.

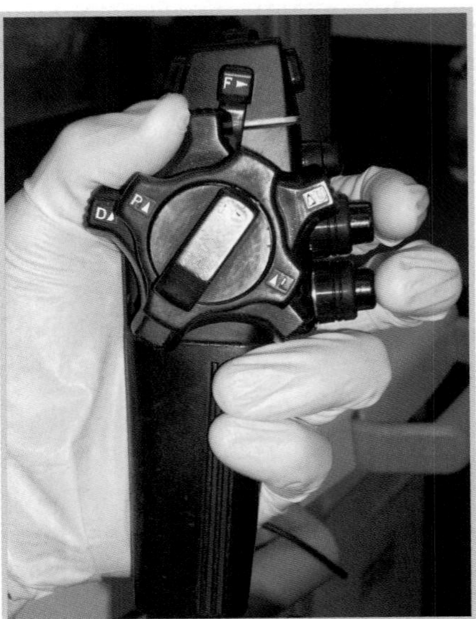

Step 2

Step 3. The right hand is used to grasp the scope and to twist the scope (A). This helps with the insertion techniques described later. As the left thumb moves the scope tip up and down (B), the right hand can torque the curled scope tip to move it right or left (C). Alternately, some practitioners prefer to have a nurse assistant perform the scope insertion and withdrawal and to use the right hand to work the outer (right or left) knob. Insertion by a second person limits the ability to feel tension on the colon wall and to perform torquing maneuvers.

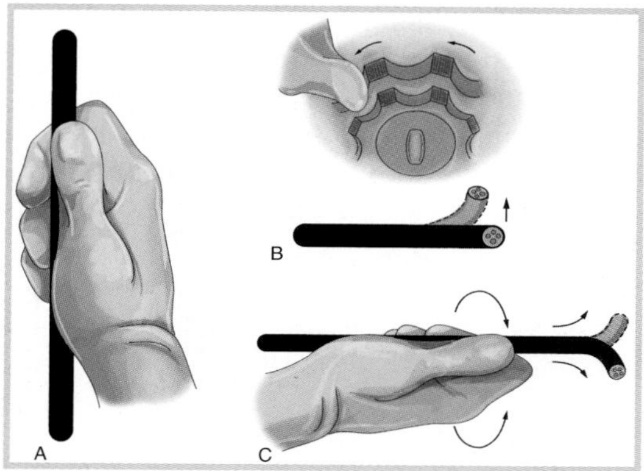

Step 3

Step 4. The scope is lubricated with water-soluble jelly, and insertion is performed by direct insertion of the scope tip into the anus or by pushing the scope tip inside with the index finger behind the scope. Some practitioners press tangentially on the anal verge to facilitate insertion.

- PITFALL: Do not apply lubricating jelly on the tip of the scope, as it will smear the lens and distort the image.
- PITFALL: Care must be taken when inserting the scope in women to avoid an embarrassing and potentially injurious intravaginal insertion.

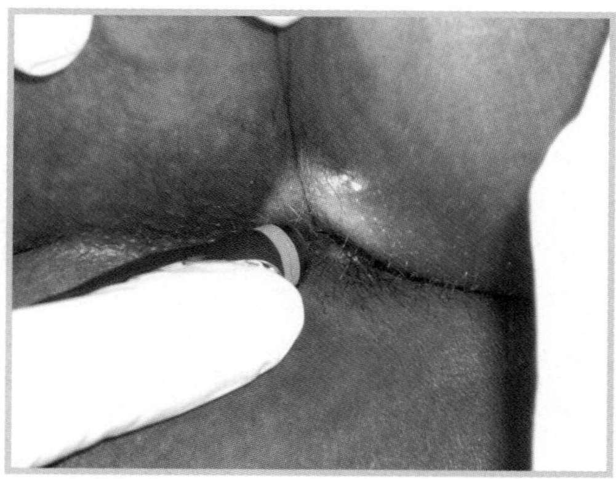

Step 4

Step 5. The scope is inserted into the rectum (7 to 17 cm), and air is insufflated to reveal the lumen. Some practitioners suction fluid from the rectum. The lumen is used as a guide for insertion, thereby reducing patient discomfort and risk of perforation. Air can be continuously or intermittently inserted to open the inside of the colon for passage and viewing.

- PITFALL: Avoid suctioning any solid stool (shown), because this can rapidly dry and clog the suction channel, necessitating costly repairs to the endoscope. Even fluid in the rectum may have stool, and suctioning should be performed only when needed.

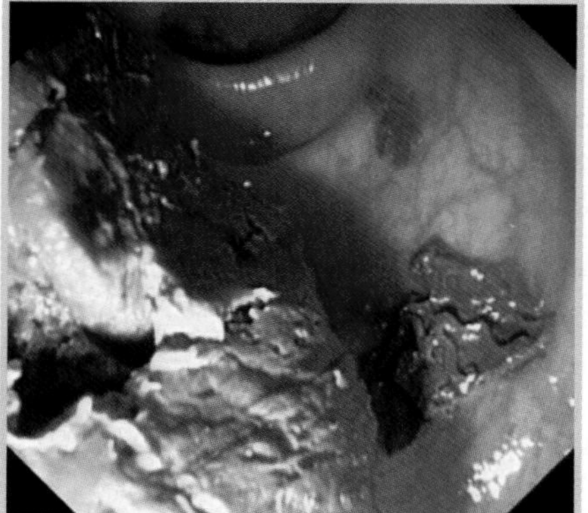

Step 5

Step 6. Insert the scope as rapidly as possible to limit patient discomfort and spasm, which can make insertion more difficult. Three transverse folds of mucosa are seen in the rectum, and these are passed to enter the rectosigmoid.

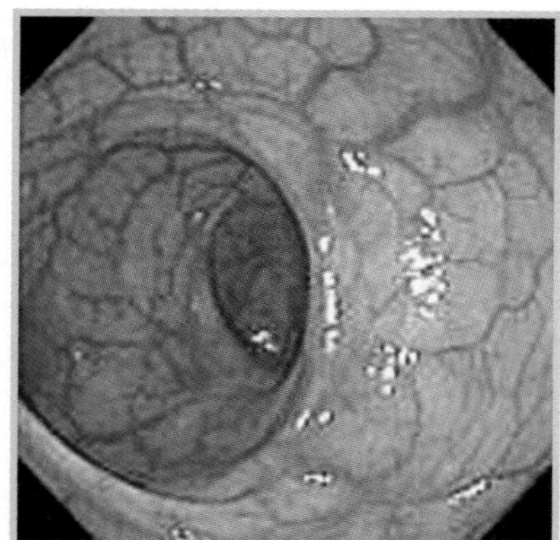

Step 6

Step 7. When maneuvering around folds or bends, torquing the endoscope with the right hand allows passage through turns. Dithering is the rapid back-and-forth motion that sometimes facilitates finding the lumen and passing the scope.

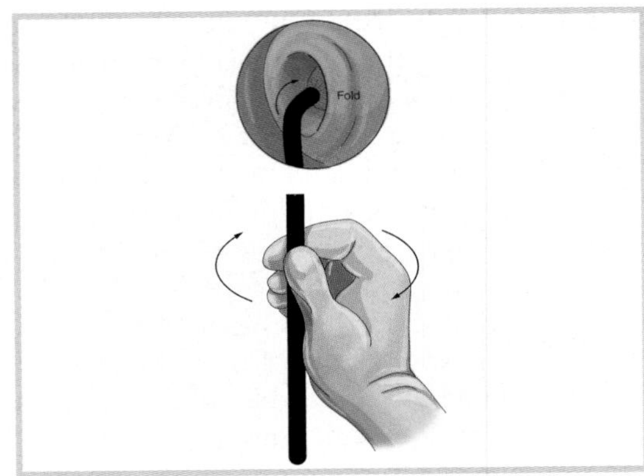

Step 7

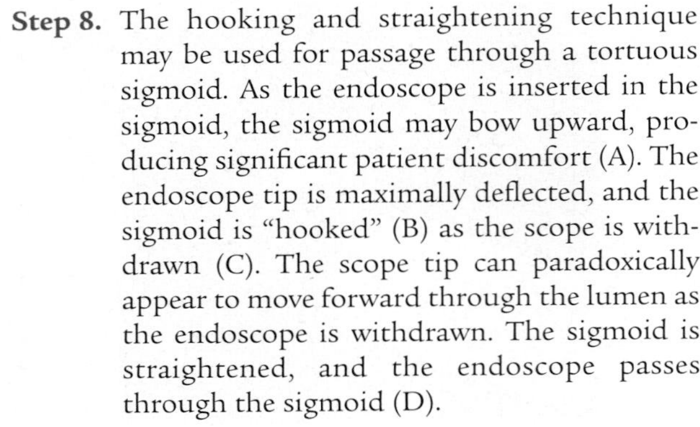

Step 8. The hooking and straightening technique may be used for passage through a tortuous sigmoid. As the endoscope is inserted in the sigmoid, the sigmoid may bow upward, producing significant patient discomfort (A). The endoscope tip is maximally deflected, and the sigmoid is "hooked" (B) as the scope is withdrawn (C). The scope tip can paradoxically appear to move forward through the lumen as the endoscope is withdrawn. The sigmoid is straightened, and the endoscope passes through the sigmoid (D).

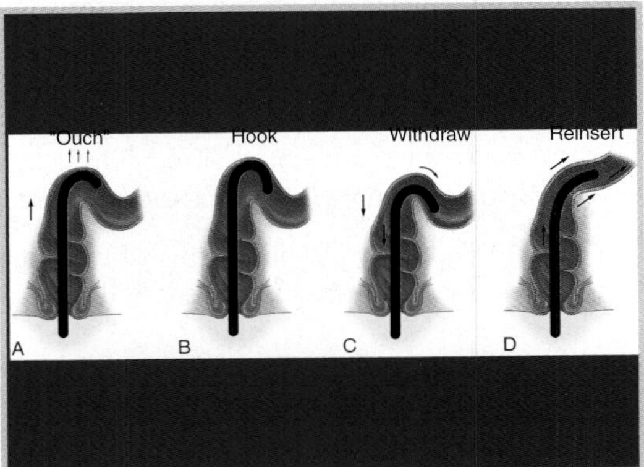

Step 8

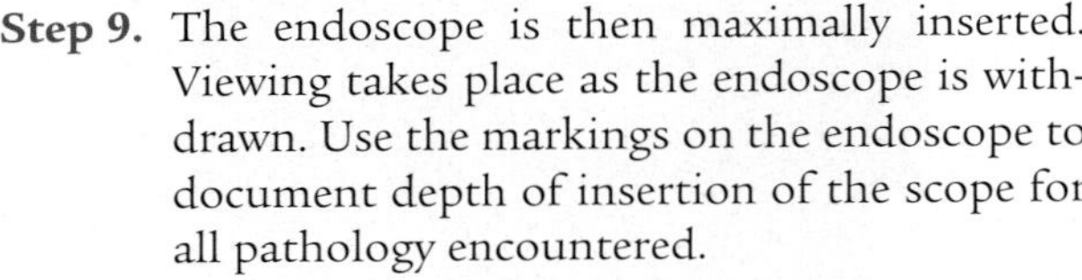

Step 9. The endoscope is then maximally inserted. Viewing takes place as the endoscope is withdrawn. Use the markings on the endoscope to document depth of insertion of the scope for all pathology encountered.

- **PITFALL:** Do not mistake a large diverticular orifice for the lumen. The posterior walls of diverticular sacs can be quite thin, and perforation is easily accomplished by inadvertent entry into a diverticular sac.

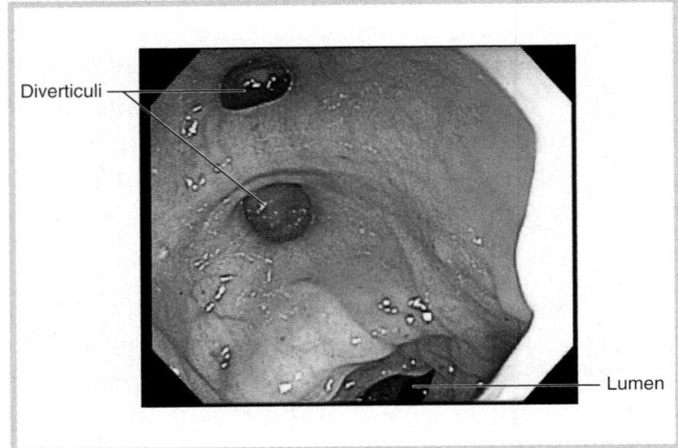

Step 9

Step 10. Biopsy is performed by threading the metal biopsy instrument through the biopsy channel. The open biopsy forceps can serve as a guide to the size of lesions, measuring approximately 5 mm when opened. A syringe-like plunger on the end of the biopsy forceps is used to open and close the forceps.

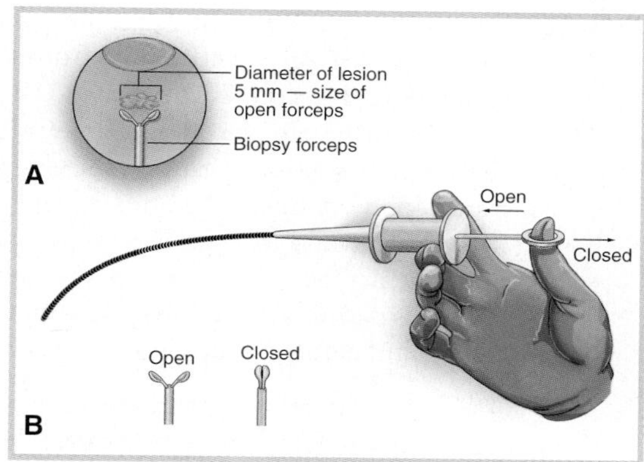

Step 10

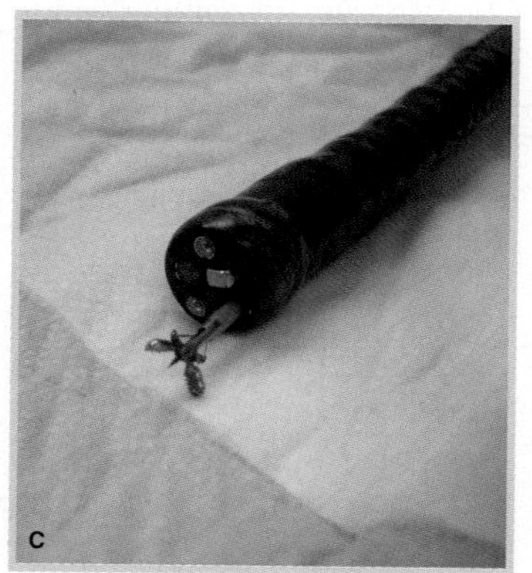

Step 11. After the endoscope is withdrawn to the rectum (i.e., 10 to 15 cm inserted), the scope tip is retroverted to examine the distal rectal vault. This area is not well visualized by the forward-directed scope as it passes the area. Retroversion is achieved by maximally deflecting both the inner and outer knobs with the left thumb while simultaneously inserting the scope with the right hand.

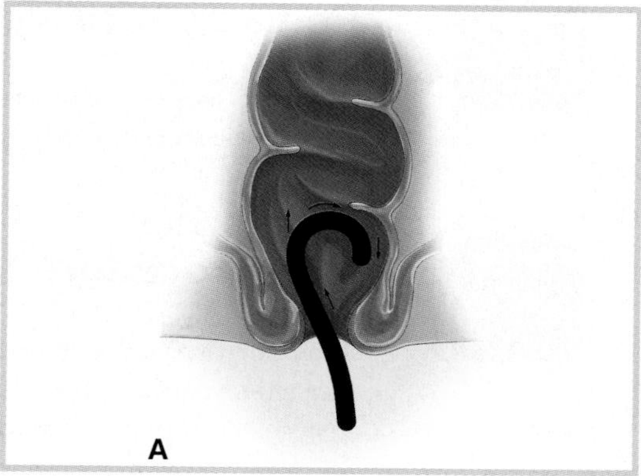

Step 11

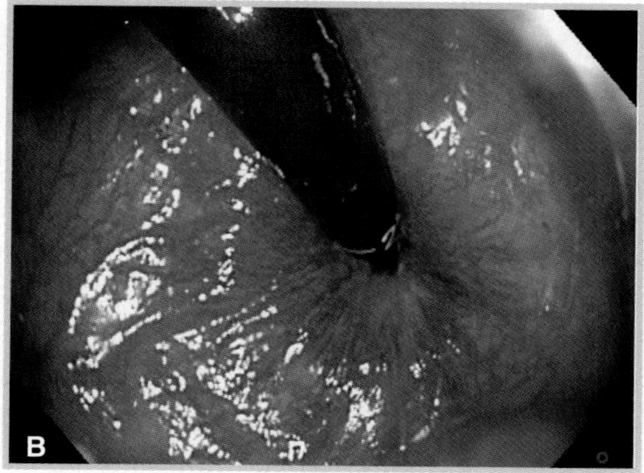

Step 12. Finally, the scope is straightened and the lumen viewed. Air is withdrawn from the rectum before the scope is withdrawn. The scope tip is immediately placed in soapy water, and the water is suctioned to prevent clogging of the suction channel. The anus is wiped clean with gauze, and the patient is offered the opportunity to go to the bathroom. The patient is permitted to get dressed after the procedure and before the findings are discussed.

- **PITFALL:** Vasovagal responses are possible during or after the procedure. Patients should be allowed to sit for a minute with the legs dangling off the table before being allowed to get off the examination table.

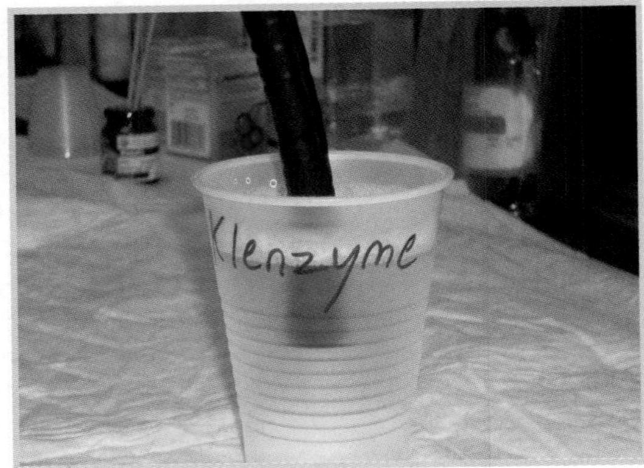

Step 12

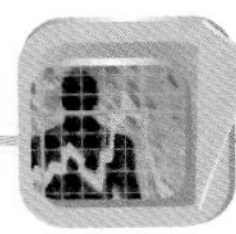

Complications

- Perforation
- Bleeding following polypectomy

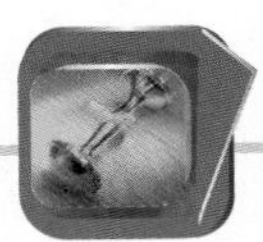

Pediatric Considerations

Pediatric scopes are available that are of a smaller diameter than adult scopes. Alternatively, a gastroscope can be used.

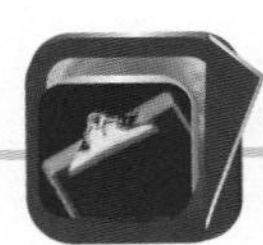

Postprocedure Instructions

After the procedure, patients may resume their regular diet and activity. They should be warned to contact their doctor immediately if they experience severe abdominal pain (not just gas cramps); a firm, distended abdomen; vomiting; fever; or bleeding greater than a few tablespoons.

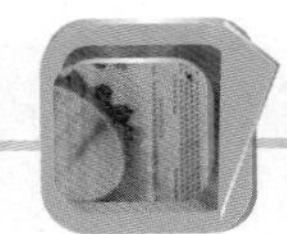

Coding Information and Supply Sources

For coding purposes, sigmoidoscopy involves examination of the entire rectum and sigmoid colon and may include a portion of the descending colon.

CPT Code	Description	2008 Average 50th Percentile Fee	Global Period
45330	Flexible sigmoidoscopy with or without brushings or washings	$300.00	0
45331	Flexible sigmoidoscopy with single or multiple biopsies	$413.00	0
45332	Flexible sigmoidoscopy with foreign body removal	$537.00	0
45333	Flexible sigmoidoscopy with tumor, polyp, lesion removal (hot biopsy forceps)	$631.00	0
45334	Flexible sigmoidoscopy with control of bleeding (cautery, coagulator)	$610.00	0

Common ICD-9 Codes

Abdominal mass	789.3
Anemia, unexplained	280.9
Iron deficiency anemia secondary to blood loss	280.0
GI bleeding, acute	578.9
GI bleeding, occult	578.1
X-ray abnormality	793.4
Weight loss, severe	783.2
Benign neoplasm colon	211.3
Constipation, slow transit	564.01
Constipation, outlet dysfunction	564.02
Diverticulosis with blood	562.12
Rectal bleeding	569.3
Personal Hx CRCa	V10.05
Family Hx CRCa	V16.0
Ulcerative colitis	556.9
Rectal pain	569.42
Change in bowel habits	787.99

Instrument and Materials Ordering

- The Ives slotted anoscope is available from Redfield Corporation, 336 West Passaic Street, Rochelle Park, NJ (phone: 800-678-4472; http://www.redfieldcorp.com)
- Recommendations for endoscope cleaning appear in Chapter 4.
- Complete endoscopy equipment such as endoscopes, light sources, video endoscopy monitors, cleaning and disinfection aids, and mouthpieces are available from the following manufacturers:
  - Olympus Corporation, Center Valley, PA (http://www.olympusamerica.com)
  - Pentax Precision Instrument Corporation, Montvale, NJ (http://www.pentaxmedical. com)
- A viscous 2% lidocaine topical solution is available from Alpharma USPD, Bridgewater, NJ (http://www.alpharma.com)
- Butorphanol tartrate (Stadol) nasal spray is available from Bristol-Myers Squibb (http://www.bms.com)
- Intravenous materials (e.g., intracaths, normal saline solution, intravenous tubing) can be obtained from local hospitals or surgical supply houses.

Patient Education Handout

A patient education handout, "Flexible Sigmoidoscopy," can be found on the book's website.

Bibliography

American Academy of Family Physicians. *Flexible Sigmoidoscopy Preceptorial Training Program: A Syllabus for the Physician Starting to Perform Flexible Sigmoidoscopy in the Office*. Kansas City, MO: Author; 1985.

Atkin WS, Hart A, Edwards R, et al. Uptake, yield of neoplasia, and adverse effects of flexible sigmoidoscopy screening. *Gut*. 1998;42:560–565.

Cohen LB. A new illustrated "how to" guide to flexible sigmoidoscopy. *Prim Care Cancer*. 1989;9:13–20.

Davis PW, Stanfield CB. Flexible sigmoidoscopy: illuminating the pearls for passage. *Postgrad Med*. 1999;105:51–62.

Esber EJ, Yang P. Retroflexion of the sigmoidoscope for the detection of rectal cancer. *Am Fam Physician*. 1995;51:1709–1711.

Herman M, Shaw M, Loewen B. Comparison of three forms of bowel preparations for screening flexible sigmoidoscopy. *Gastroenterol Nurs*. 2001;24:178–181.

Holman JR, Marshall RC, Jordan B, et al. Technical competence in flexible sigmoidoscopy. *J Am Board Fam Pract*. 2001;14:424–429.

Levin TR, Palitz A, Grossman S, et al. Predicting advanced proximal colonic neoplasia with screening sigmoidoscopy. *JAMA*. 1999;281:1611–1617.

Lewis JD, Asch DA. Barriers to office-based screening sigmoidoscopy: does reimbursement cover costs? *Ann Intern Med*. 1999;130:525–530.

Lewis JD, Asch DA, Ginsberg GG, et al. Primary care physicians' decisions to perform flexible sigmoidoscopy. *J Gen Intern Med*. 1999;14:297–302.

Lund JN, Buckley D, Bennett D, et al. A randomized trial of hospital versus home administered enemas for flexible sigmoidoscopy. *Br Med J*. 1998;317:1201.

Mayberry MK, Mayberry JF. Towards better informed consent in endoscopy: a study of information and consent processes in gastroscopy and flexible sigmoidoscopy. *Eur J Gastroenterol Hepatol*. 2001;13:1467–1476.

McCallion K, Mitchell RM, Wilson RH, et al. Flexible sigmoidoscopy and the changing distribution of colorectal cancer: implications for screening. *Gut*. 2001;48:522–525.

Ransohoff DF, Lang CA. Sigmoidoscopic screening in the 1990s. *JAMA*. 1993;269:1278–1281.

Rees MK. We should all be performing flexible sigmoidoscopy. *Mod Med*. 1987;55:3, 12.

Sanowski RA. *Flexible Fiberoptic Sigmoidoscopy*. Research Triangle Park, NC: Glaxo, 1992.

Verne JE, Aubrey R, Love SB, et al. Population based randomized study of uptake and yield of screening by flexible sigmoidoscopy compared with screening by faecal occult blood testing. *Br Med J*. 1998;317:182–185.

Wallace MB, Kemp JA, Trnka YM, et al. Is colonoscopy indicated for small adenomas found by screening flexible sigmoidoscopy? *Ann Intern Med*. 1998;129:273–278.

Williams JJ. Why family physicians should perform sigmoidoscopy [Editorial]. *Am Fam Physician*. 1990;4:1722, 1724.

Winawer SJ. Office screening for colorectal cancer. *Prim Care Cancer*. 1993;13:37–46.

Zuber TJ. Flexible sigmoidoscopy. *Am Fam Physician*. 2001;63:1375–1380, 1383–1388.

Zuber TJ. *Office Procedures. The Academy Collection Quick Reference Guides for Family Physicians*. Baltimore: Williams & Wilkins; 1999:35–42.

2008 MAG Mutual Healthcare Solutions, Inc.'s Physicians' Fee and Coding Guide. Duluth, Georgia. MAG Mutual Healthcare Solutions, Inc. 2007.

CHAPTER 92

Treatment of Internal Hemorrhoids

Larry S. Sasaki, MD, FACS
Assistant Clinical Professor of Surgery
Louisiana State University Health Sciences Center, Shreveport, LA

Hemorrhoidal disease affects more than a million Americans each year. Most sufferers will avoid medical attention and self-medicate with over-the-counter treatments. This accounts for the lucrative business of nonprescriptive hemorrhoidal treatments.

Hemorrhoids are vascular cushions of the anus. These vascular cushions are a normal anatomic part of the anus; thus, hemorrhoids are not pathologic. However, the term *hemorrhoids* is most commonly meant to describe symptoms due to enlargement of these vascular cushions. They are also considered varicose veins of the anus and rectum. Symptoms range from painless swelling to painful thrombosis.

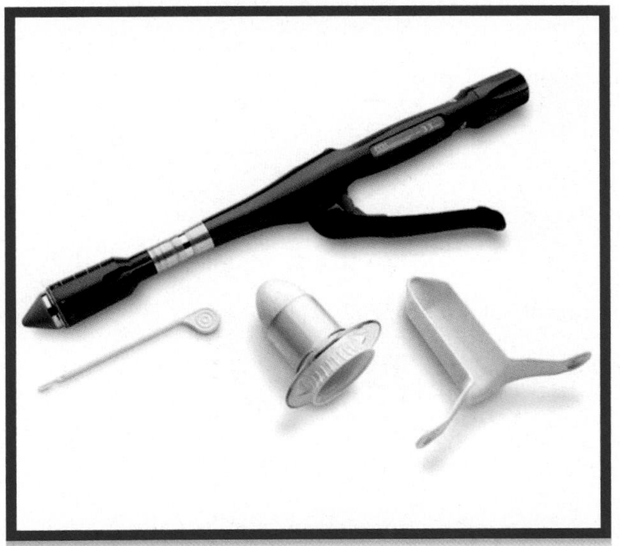

The probable pathogenesis of symptomatic hemorrhoids is the abnormal dilatation of the internal hemorrhoidal venous plexus and destruction of the suspensory ligaments of the internal hemorrhoids (corrugator cutis ani). The suspensory ligaments and connective tissue deteriorate with age, usually after the third decade of life. Subsequently, hemorrhoidal dilatation and prolapse may occur, resulting in swelling, erosion, bleeding, thrombosis, and pain.

Medical treatment of internal hemorrhoids are primarily used to alleviate the symptoms. A wide variety of anal creams and suppositories are composed of a combination of topical steroids and anesthetics. Any of the prescription-strength combinations should suffice. Warm tub or sitz baths should be taken at least four times daily and after bowel movements. Fiber supplementation should be taken to prevent constipation and straining.

Persistent internal hemorrhoidal symptoms such as bleeding, swelling, and prolapse that are unresponsive to medical treatment warrant additional treatment options. Common office treatments include infrared coagulation and rubber band ligation, which will be outlined later. Other less utilized office treatments include cryosurgery, sclerotherapy, and bipolar diathermy.

Hemorrhoids that are unresponsive or refractory to medical and office treatments are candidates for surgery. A new less invasive procedure with dramatically less pain and morbidity is the procedure for prolapsed hemorrhoids (PPH). PPH is preferable over the conventional hemorrhoidectomy for these reasons. It is performed on an outpatient basis. The PPH removes a circumferential band of anorectal mucosa and submucosa above the dentate line with a circular stapler. This effectively treats hemorrhoids that are bleeding and prolapsing by reducing the blood flow to the internal hemorrhoids and repositions the anal canal tissue resulting in "lifting up" the hemorrhoidal tissue. Ultimately, patients experience less pain and recover faster than patients who are treated with conventional hemorrhoidectomy procedures.

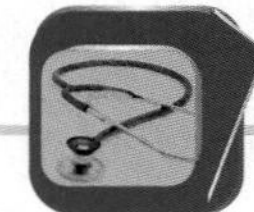

Equipment

- Surgical water-soluble lubricant
- Anoscopes: disposable fiber optic or metallic
- Illumination instrument
- Preferred treatment devices:
  - Redfield infrared coagulator (Model #IRC 2100)
  - McGivney hemorrhoid rubber band ligator

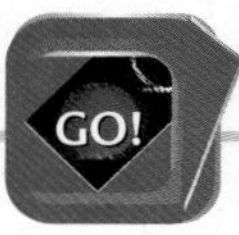

Indications

- Rectal symptoms: bleeding, itching, swelling, pain
- Prolapse

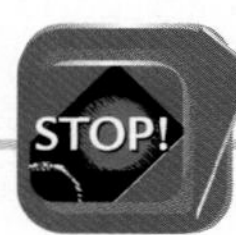

Contraindications

- Bleeding diathesis
- Anal stenosis (relative due to discomfort of anoscope)

The Procedure

Step 1. Internal hemorrhoids are defined by their anatomic position in the anus, which is above the dentate line. External hemorrhoids develop below the dentate line.

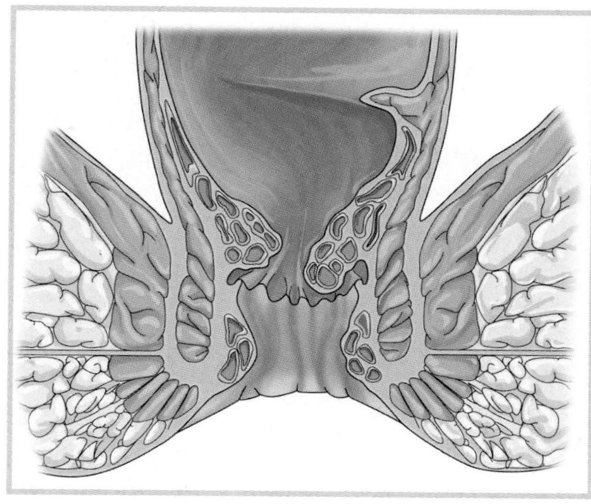

Step 1

Step 2. The most common presenting complaint of hemorrhoids is bleeding. Other common symptoms include itching, pain, swelling, and mucous discharge. Anoscopy is the optimal diagnostic examination for the anal canal. Thus, the initial physical examination should include anoscopy. Later, either rigid or flexible proctosigmoidoscopy should be performed. Those patients with occult blood in stool, or those 50 years of age or older, should undergo a colonoscopy.

- **PITFALL:** A diagnosis of "hemorrhoids" may conceal a colorectal cancer.
- **PEARL:** All rectal bleeding must have a thorough colorectal examination. All occult blood in stool must have a colonoscopy.

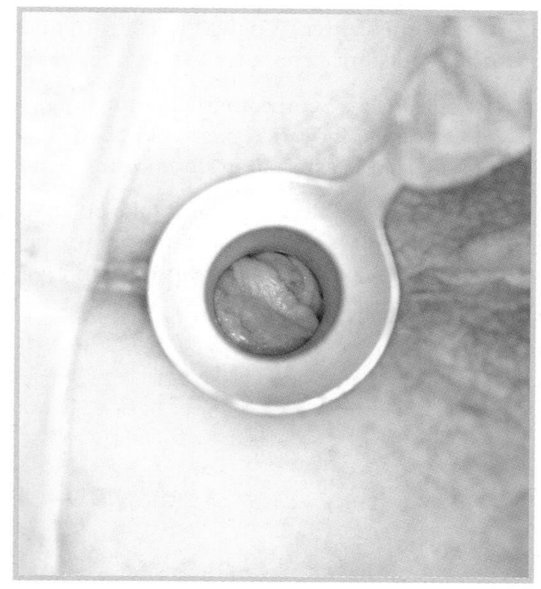

Step 2

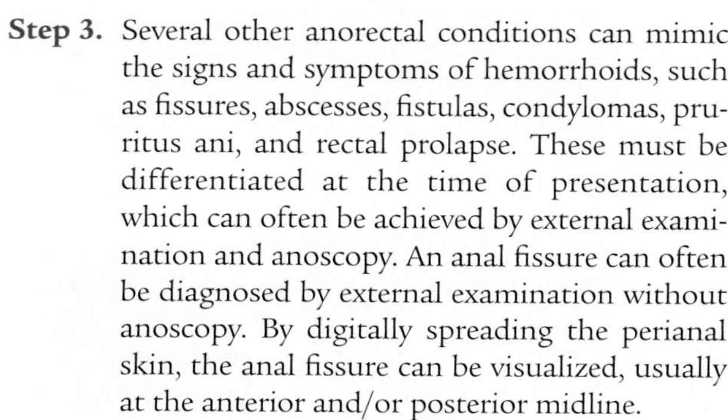

Step 3. Several other anorectal conditions can mimic the signs and symptoms of hemorrhoids, such as fissures, abscesses, fistulas, condylomas, pruritus ani, and rectal prolapse. These must be differentiated at the time of presentation, which can often be achieved by external examination and anoscopy. An anal fissure can often be diagnosed by external examination without anoscopy. By digitally spreading the perianal skin, the anal fissure can be visualized, usually at the anterior and/or posterior midline.

- **PITFALL:** Anoscopy performed for an anal fissure may cause excessive discomfort and is unnecessary.

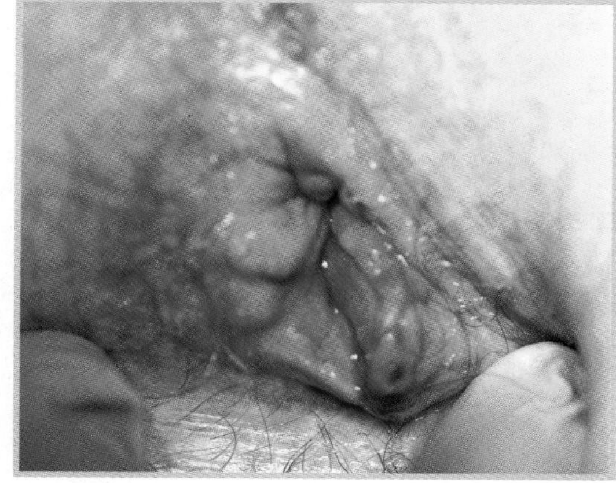

Step 3

- **PEARL:** Anal fissures are most commonly located at the anterior and/or posterior midline. Look for the frequently associated anal skin tag.

Step 4. Perirectal abscesses and anal fistulas can be diagnosed by external examination. Anoscopy is helpful in identifying the internal opening of an anal fistula. The internal opening is identified with the fistula probe.

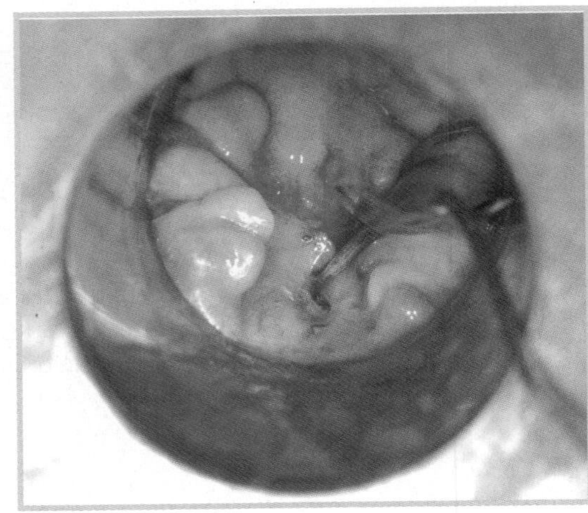

Step 4

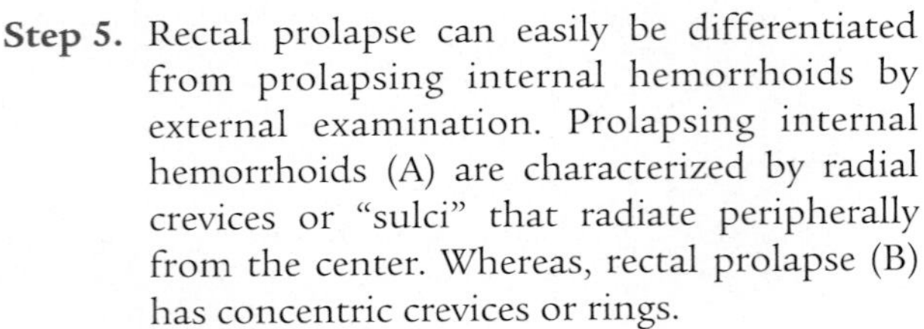

Step 5. Rectal prolapse can easily be differentiated from prolapsing internal hemorrhoids by external examination. Prolapsing internal hemorrhoids (A) are characterized by radial crevices or "sulci" that radiate peripherally from the center. Whereas, rectal prolapse (B) has concentric crevices or rings.

- **PITFALL:** Symptomatic hemorrhoids, even prolapsing, can regress and have an unremarkable external examination.
- **PEARL:** Have the patient take an enema in the office to allow for symptomatic hemorrhoids and rectal prolapse to enlarge and prolapse.

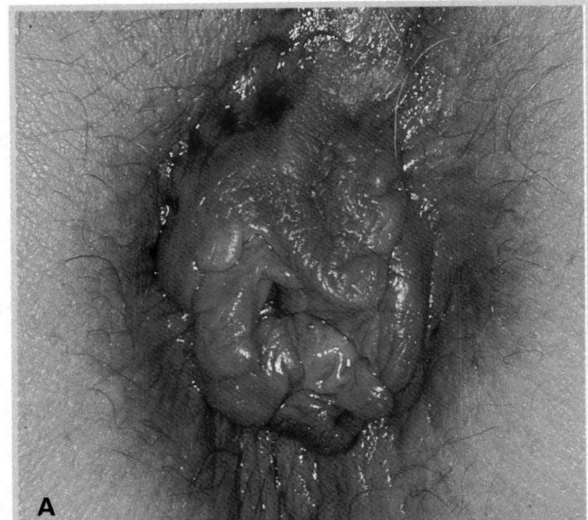

A

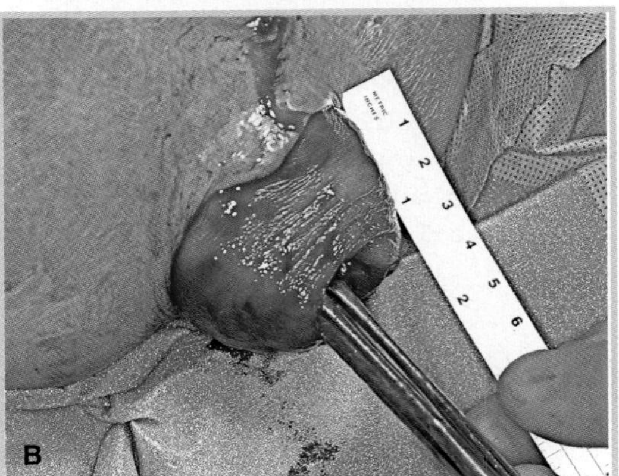

B

Step 5

Infrared Coagulation

Step 1. An infrared coagulation is applied directly with a probe through an anoscope. An assistant holds the anoscope in place.

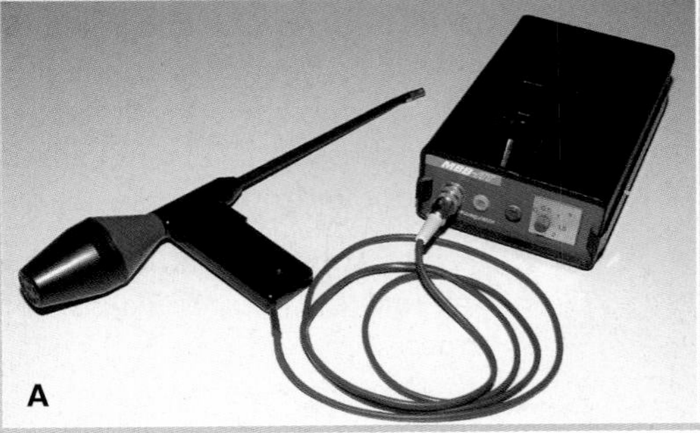

A

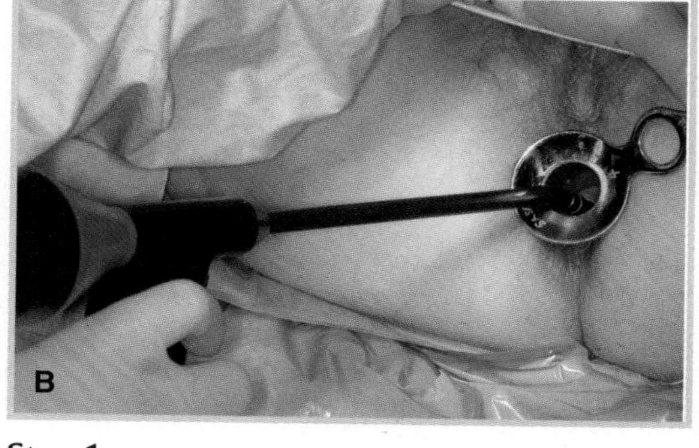

Step 1

Step 2. Three to five pulses are applied to the normal mucosa above the hemorrhoidal column. Try to avoid applying the pulse directly on the hemorrhoid. Pulses are 1 to 1.5 seconds in duration. Treatments may be repeated every 2 weeks.

- **PEARL:** Any patient with bleeding is a candidate. Prolapse is not as effectively treated with this method.

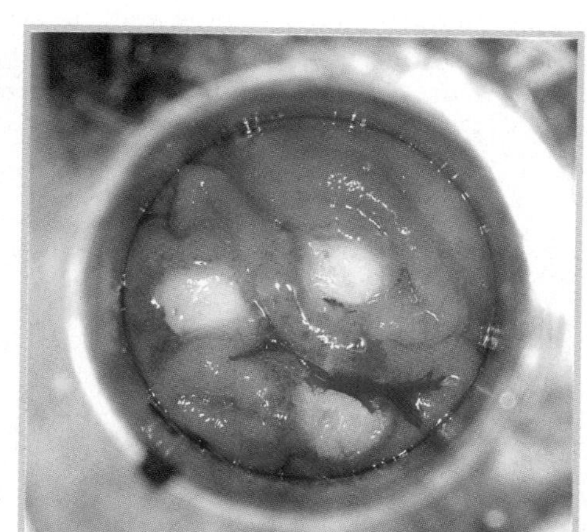
Step 2

Rubber Band Ligation

Step 1. The McGivney hemorrhoid rubber band ligator is used to ligate internal hemorrhoids. Placement of the rubber band above the dentate line should be painless. The mucosa at the proximal apex of the hemorrhoidal column is grasped with the forceps while the patient is asked whether "pain" or "pressure" are felt. If pain is ilicited, then the forceps should be repositioned more proximally (i.e., away from the dentate line). Once an area of "pressure" is reported, then the rubber band is deployed. If despite grasping a more proximal area the patient still reports "pain," then the procedure should be abandoned, and surgical treatment may be indicated. Usually, there are three major hemorrhoidal columns that will require ligation: (1) left lateral, (2) right anterior, and (3) right posterior. The first session of rubber banding should be performed only once. If the patient tolerates this well, then the other areas can be treated 3 to 4 weeks later.

- **PEARL:** Any patient with bleeding, prolapse, or both is a candidate.

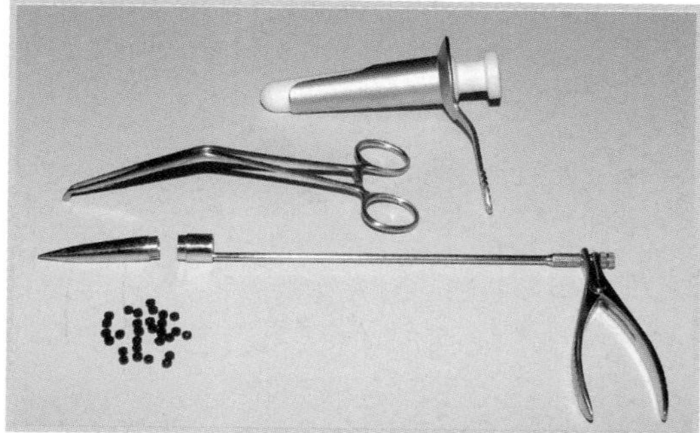
Step 1

Step 2. Prepare rubber band ligator by placing *two* bands on the end of the device.

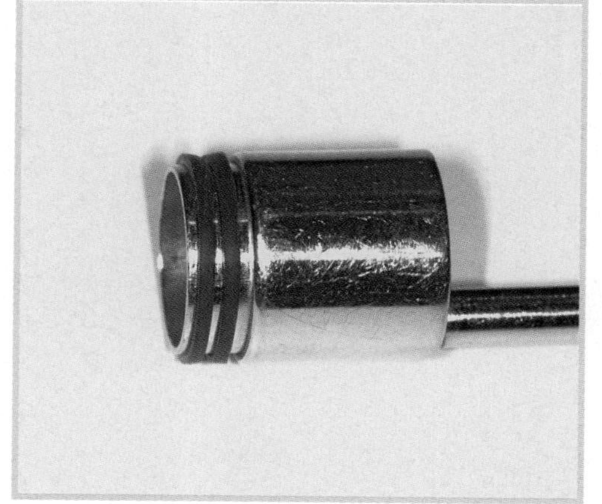
Step 2

Step 3. Insert an anoscope, and examine the canal circumferentially to identify the largest hemorrhoidal columns.

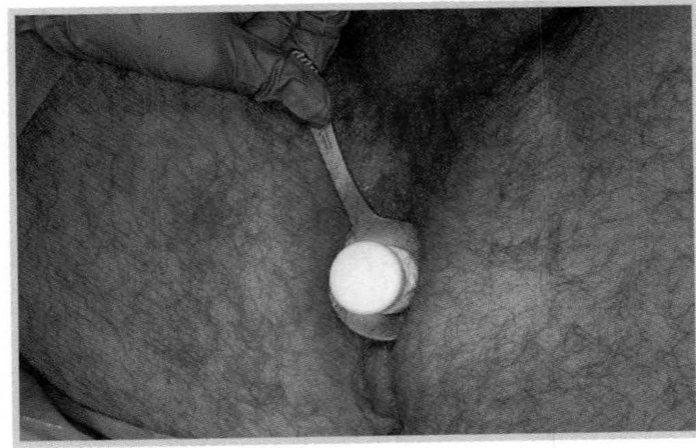

Step 3

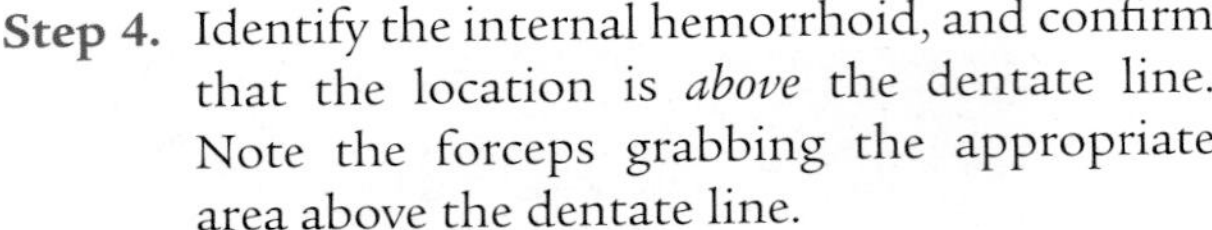

Step 4. Identify the internal hemorrhoid, and confirm that the location is *above* the dentate line. Note the forceps grabbing the appropriate area above the dentate line.

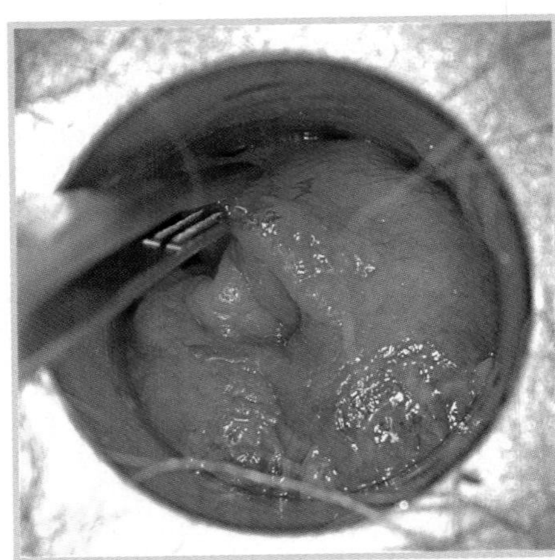

Step 4

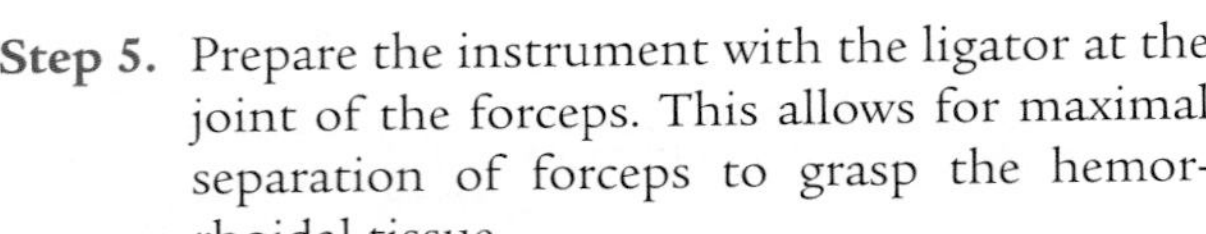

Step 5. Prepare the instrument with the ligator at the joint of the forceps. This allows for maximal separation of forceps to grasp the hemorrhoidal tissue.

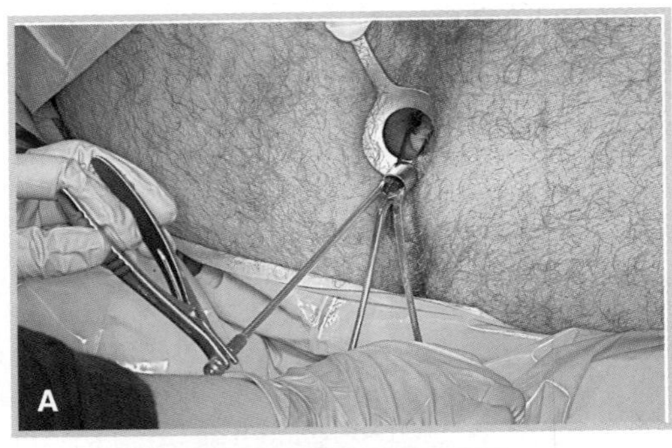

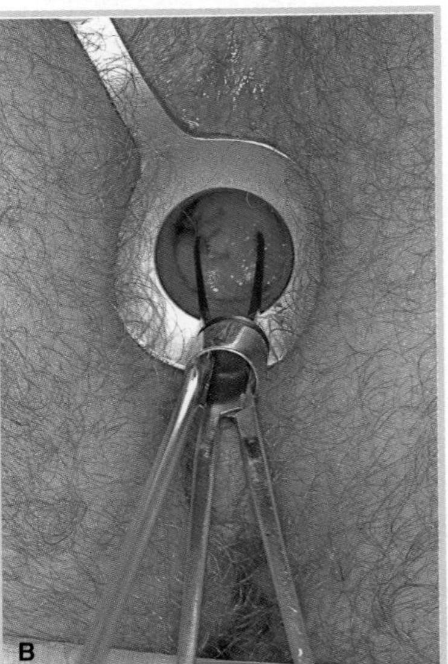

Step 5

Step 6. Grasp the internal hemorrhoidal tissue to be ligated above the dentate line. The patient should report "pressure" but not "pain." Gently advance the ligator against the rectal wall while applying traction on the forceps to optimize correct deployment of rubber bands at the *base* of the redundant internal hemorrhoidal tissue.

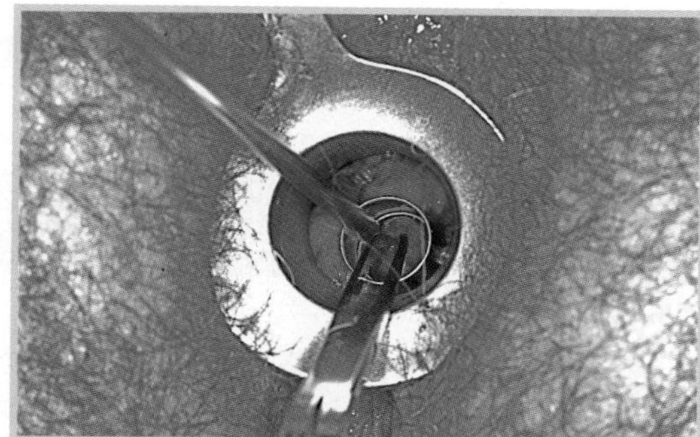

Step 6

Step 7. Examine the rubber band. The patient should *not* report "pain." If painful, then the rubber band should be removed by using suture scissors.

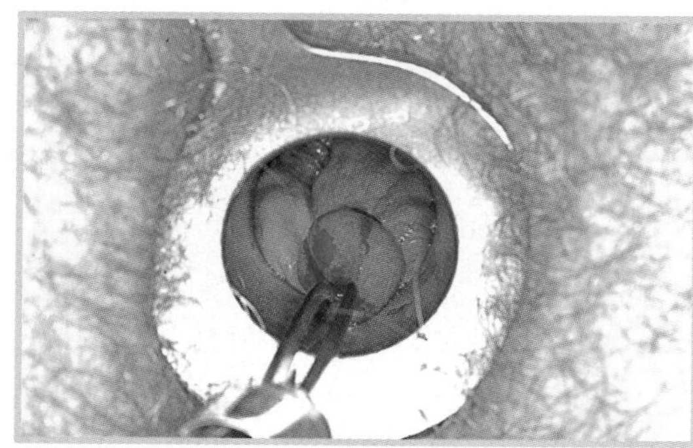

Step 7

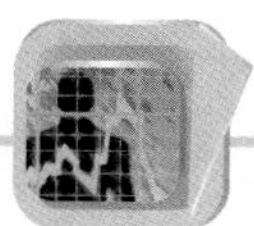

Complications

- Bleeding
- Pain
- Infection, such as pelvic sepsis
- Urinary retention (mandates examination to identify possible infection)

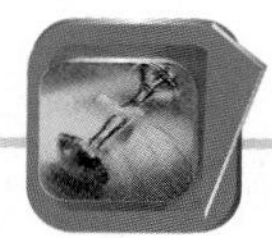

Pediatric Considerations

Hemorrhoids are rare in the pediatric population.

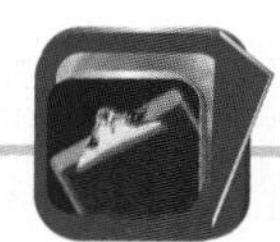

Postprocedure Instructions

Instruct patients to bathe in a warm tub as needed for spasm or pain. Have them report excessive rectal bleeding, especially blood clots, or any signs of infection. Narcotics should be avoided after hemorrhoid treatment, as they can produce further constipation, straining, and bleeding.

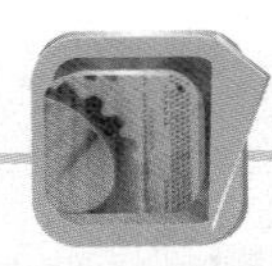

Coding Information and Supply Sources

CPT Code	Description	2008 Average 50th Percentile Fee	Global Period
46600	Anoscopy	\$117.00	0
46606	Anoscopy with biopsy, single or multiple	\$244.00	0
46934	Destruction of internal hemorrhoids, any method (such as infrared coagulation)	\$606.00	90
46945	Ligation of internal hemorrhoid, Rubber band, single procedure	\$449.00	90
43946	Ligation of internal hemorrhoid, rubber band, multiple procedure	\$537.00	90

Add CPT -78 modifier to 46934 for repeated procedures.
CPT is a registered trademark of the American Medical Association.
2008 average 50th Percentile Fees are provided courtesy of 2008 MMH-SI's copyrighted Physicians' Fees and Coding Guide.

Common ICD-9 Codes

Hemorrhoid uncomplicated	455.6
Hemorrhoid bleeding or prolapsed	455.8
Hemorrhoid external	455.3
Hemorrhoid external thrombosed	455.4
Hemorrhoid bleeding or prolapsed external	455.5
Hemorrhoid internal	455.0
Hemorrhoid internal thrombosed	455.1
Hemorrhoid bleeding or prolapsed internal	455.2

Equipment Sources

- The infrared coagulator and the metal, slotted Ives anoscope are available from Redfield Corporation, 336 West Passaic Street, Rochelle Park, NJ (phone: 800-678-4472; http://www.redfieldcorp.com).
- The McGivney hemorrhoidal ligator (including loading cone), latex O-rings (i.e., rubber bands), and McGivney hemorrhoid grasping forceps are available from Miltex Inc., 589 Davies Dr., York, PA 17402 (phone: 800-645-8000; http://www.ssrsurgical.com).

Patient Education Handout

A patient education handout, "Hemorrhoid Treatment," can be found on the book's Web site.

Bibliography

Ambrose NS, Morris D, Alexander-Williams J, et al. A randomized trial of photocoagulation or injection sclerotherapy for the treatment of first- and second-degree hemorrhoids. *Dis Colon Rectum*. 1985;28:238–240.

Corman, ML. *Colon and Rectal Surgery* (5th ed.). Baltimore: Lippincott; 2004:165–180.

Johanson JF, Rimm A. Optimal nonsurgical treatment of hemorrhoids: a comparative analysis of infrared coagulation, rubber band ligation, and injection sclerotherapy. *Am J Gastroenterol*. 1992;87:1601–1606.

Ganio E, Altomare F, Gabrielli F, et al. Prospective randomized multicenter trial comparing stapled with open hemorrhoidectomy. *British J Surg*. 2001;88:669–674.

Walker AJ, Leicester RJ, Nicholls RJ, et al. A prospective study of infrared coagulation, injection and rubber band ligation in the treatment of haemorrhoids. *Int J Colorectal Dis*. 1990;5:113–116.

2008 MAG Mutual Healthcare Solutions, Inc.'s Physicians' Fee and Coding Guide. Duluth, Georgia. MAG Mutual Healthcare Solutions, Inc. 2007.

CHAPTER 93

Pilonidal Cyst or Abscess Management

Robert W. Smith, MD, MBA, FAAFP

Vice Chair for Education, Department of Family Medicine
University of Pittsburgh School of Medicine, Pittsburgh, PA

Pilonidal cysts will most often require immediate intervention by the clinician when they have become infected. The cause of such cysts has been long debated in the literature. While approximately 40% of patients have a family history of pilonidal disease, and patients with midline hair accumulations (between the eyebrows and in the umbilical and sacrococcygeal regions) seem to have an increased risk of disease, the congenital nature of the disease has never been conclusively proven.

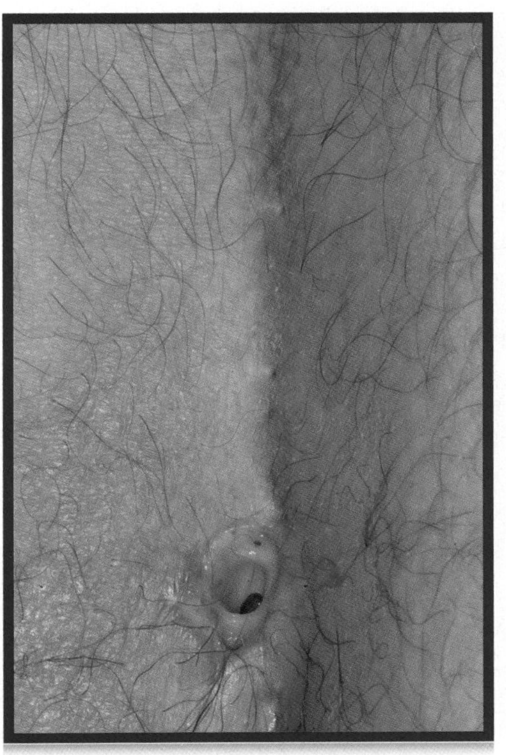

Pilonidal (literally "hair location") disease occurs in asymptomatic, subclinical, and acute abscess stages. The management at each stage requires a different approach. As the traditional name implies, hair has been traditionally implicated in the etiology of disease. Reports have demonstrated, however, that hair is only found in about one half of the cases on surgical incisions. Present theories include repetitive trauma to tense skin that is felt to have a predilection for sinus tracts into which hair, skin debris, or other material is introduced over time, forming microabscesses that predominately are anaerobic, although *Staphylococcus aureus* is also common. This trauma often occurs in areas of pressure, most commonly the sacrococcygeal region. Patients with obesity, family history, deep clefts, pre-existing sinuses, stretched skin, and repeated microtrauma are felt to be at increased risk of developing abscesses in the sacrococcygeal region. It should be recalled, however, that pilonidal sinuses can occur anywhere on the skin surface, although with much lower frequency. While adult men are more commonly affected than women, the reverse ratio is true in children.

Asymptomatic sinus tracts may be discovered by patients serendipitously or by clinicians on routine physical examination. These sinuses can often be quite extensive and require referral to a surgeon for further evaluation and management. Management by the surgeon in the asymptomatic phase may include cautery, crystallized phenol, or more commonly complete extensive excision, often including flaps. Subclinical disease usually occurs in patients after the resolution of an acute abscess, whether spontaneously resolving or managed by the clinician by incision and drainage during the acute phase. Again, subacute or recurrent disease requires extensive debridement and therefore referral to a surgeon for management.

Acute pilonidal abscess, however, is a common presenting problem for the clinician in the primary care or emergency room setting. Pain in the midline of the cleft of the buttocks is the most common presenting feature. Diagnosis of abscess is made by clinical examination. While ultrasound and other imaging techniques have been tried for asymptomatic and subclinical disease, they have not proved valuable in an acute abscess. Careful attention should be paid to distinguish pilonidal abscesses from perirectal or perianal abscesses, which may need more extensive initial intervention. The latter are more commonly located outside the midline and have direct extensions into the mucosa of the anal canal. Pilonidal abscess is more commonly midline and superior to the anal verge by several centimeters. While pain is the most common presenting symptom, fever may occur with deeper abscesses prior to the onset of pain. Erythema, thin overlying skin, induration, tenderness, and edema in the proper location lead to the diagnosis.

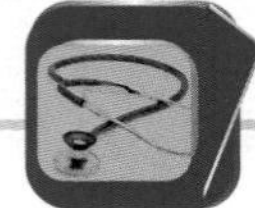

Equipment

- The standard skin tray supplies shown in Appendix G may be used for this procedure.
- The suggested anesthesia tray shown in Appendix F may be used for this procedure.
- Skin preparation recommendations shown in Appendix E may be used for this procedure.
- Iodoform gauze will be needed unless the patient is allergic to iodine, in which case petroleum gauze will be sufficient.
- Other than proper personal protective gear (mask, eye shield, gown), no special equipment is necessary for this procedure.
- Appropriate culture transport medium for both aerobes and anaerobes should be available.
- A specimen container should be available for any foreign body (e.g., hair) that may be found in the event that pathological analysis is considered.

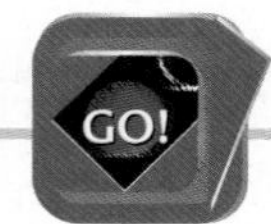

Indications

- Nonresolved abscess that is edematous, fluctuant, and tender to touch

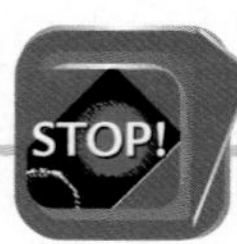

Contraindications (Relative)

- Immunocompromised patients (require referral and perhaps hospitalization)
- Recurrent disease (consider for referral for definitive resection)
- Patients with a question of perianal or perirectal abscess or sinus (refer)
- Large abscess that cannot be properly anesthetized in the office setting
- Children under the age of 10 years or adults incapable of remaining still for the procedure

The Procedure

Step 1. The procedure, its complications, alternatives, and expected course should be discussed with the patient. A proper consent should be obtained. Place the patient in the prone position on a variable-height table.

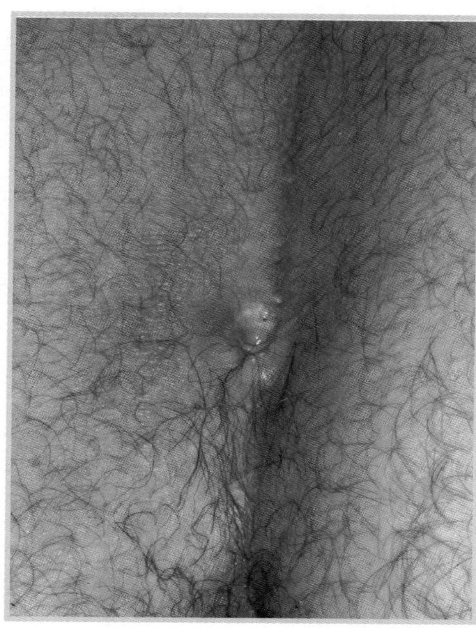

Step 1

Step 2. Prep the skin with povidone iodine or chlorhexadine solution (see Appendix E), and drape the patient in a sterile manner. Administer a local field block to the surrounding skin, including infiltration of the deeper subcutaneous tissues. In adults, this may require up to 10 cc of 2% lidocaine (with or without epinephrine). Refer to Chapter 2 for the technique.

- **PITFALL:** While heat and time may lead to a more fluctuant abscess, additional risk is incurred. No more than 48 hours of expectant treatment should be required to intervene in an unresolved abscess.
- **PITFALL:** Patients unable to tolerate the prone position (e.g., chronic obstructive pulmonary disease) can be placed in the lateral decubitus position.
- **PITFALL:** Do not inject the abscess itself. The lidocaine will not be effective in relieving the pain, and the possibility of spontaneous, uncontrolled rupture may prolong the procedure.
- **PEARL:** Lidocaine-prilocaine (EMLA) cream or cryo topical anesthetic may be utilized prior to injection of the tender area.
- **PEARL:** It is important to wait for 10 minutes to assure adequate deep anesthesia. If anesthesia is inadequate, wait an additional 10 minutes and test again prior to further injection.

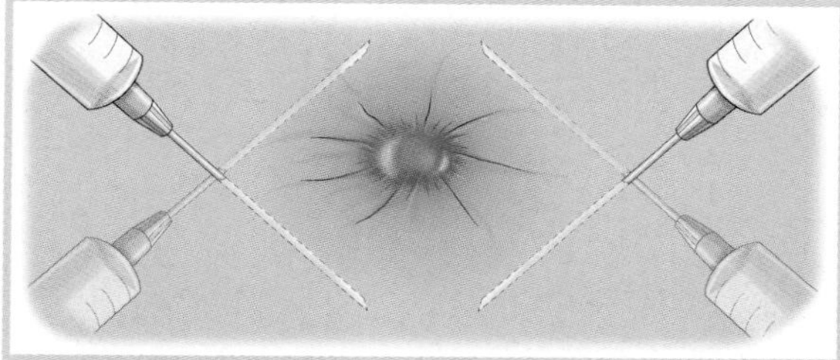

Step 2

Step 3. An incision is made with a no. 11 blade in the cephalocaudal orientation 1 cm lateral to the midline of the abscess. Ensure that an adequate incision is made, as these abscesses are often larger than they appear, both in width and in depth. Immediate spontaneous expulsion of purulent material and debris should be expected.

- **PITFALL:** An inadequate incision can result in incomplete drainage and recurrence.
- **PITFALL:** Explosive results may be a hazard to the clinician and assistant, and appropriate protective gear should be required. Expect the abscess to be foul smelling due to the high likelihood of anaerobes.

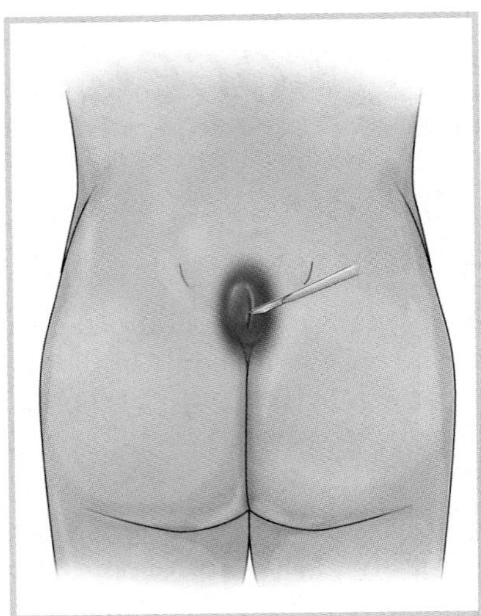

Step 3

Step 4. In larger abscesses, an elliptical incision of overlying skin may be required for larger abscesses in order to allow for adequate drainage.

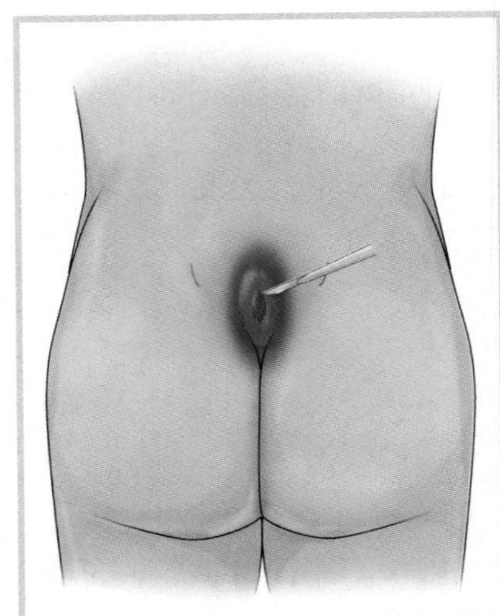

Step 4

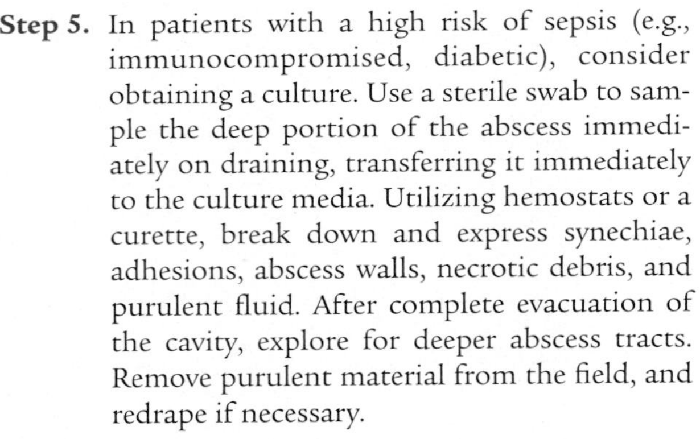

Step 5. In patients with a high risk of sepsis (e.g., immunocompromised, diabetic), consider obtaining a culture. Use a sterile swab to sample the deep portion of the abscess immediately on draining, transferring it immediately to the culture media. Utilizing hemostats or a curette, break down and express synechiae, adhesions, abscess walls, necrotic debris, and purulent fluid. After complete evacuation of the cavity, explore for deeper abscess tracts. Remove purulent material from the field, and redrape if necessary.

- **PITFALL:** Inadequate agitation may leave behind microabscesses that will lead to recurrence.
- **PITFALL:** Large quantities of purulent material are often obtained, creating an exposure risk to the clinician and staff. Proper redraping reduces likelihood of cross contamination.

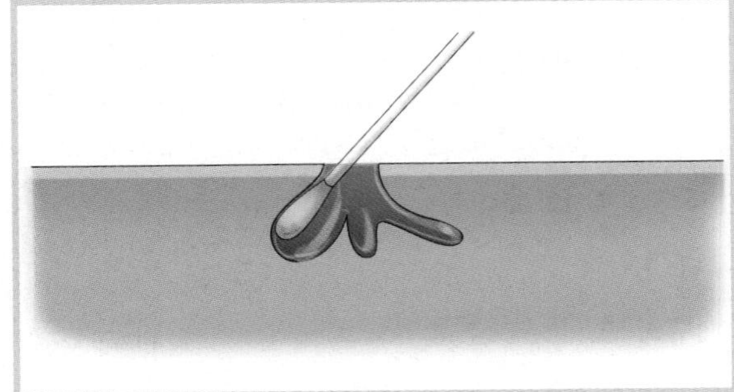

Step 5

Step 6. Utilizing Adson forceps, pack with the largest appropriate iodoform gauze in ample quantity to fill the abscess cavity by grabbing the ribbon and progressively layering the gauze into the open wound. Leave 2 cm of gauze to protrude from the open wound. Cover with a sterile dressing.

- **PITFALL:** Do not use iodoform in patients with iodine allergy. Utilize petroleum or plain gauze instead.

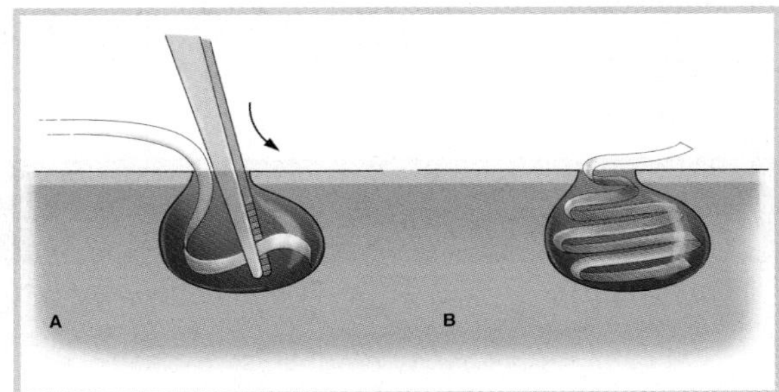

Step 6

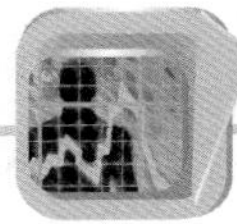

Complications

- Systemic infection
- Extension of abscess
- Recurrence
- Missed diagnosis of squamous cell carcinoma
- Inadvertent entry into perirectal abscess tract
- Anesthesia reaction
- Hemorrhage

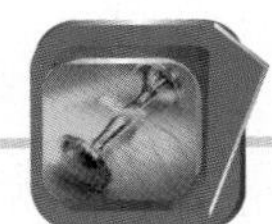

Pediatric Considerations

Conscious sedation may be required for preadolescent children, those with disabilities who are unable to maintain the prone position, or those whose behaviors would preclude management under local anesthesia.

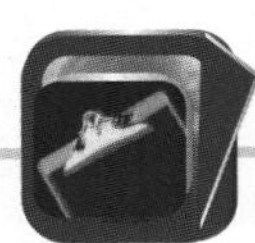

Postprocedure Instructions

- Pain relief is usually instantaneous and nearly complete on drainage of the abscess. However, providing adequate pain medication and a follow-up phone call is suggested.
- Schedule a wound check for 24 hours, and pull out about 2 cm at that time, leaving the remainder for the future.
- Complete packing removal can usually occur within 3 to 7 days.
- Referral to a surgeon after resolution may be indicated if there is concern for incomplete resolution and in order to perform more extensive excision.
- Immediate referral and/or hospitalization should be considered if the patient develops signs of sepsis.
- Antibiotics are usually not required in immunocompetent patients who do not have coexisting cellulitis.

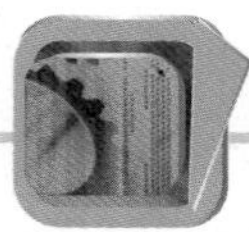

Coding Information and Supply Sources

CPT Code	Description	2008 Average 50th Percentile Fee	Global Period
10080	I & D of pilonidal abscess, simple (not requiring excision of skin or deep exploration)	$191.00	10
10081	I & D of pilonidal abscess, complicated	$350.00	10

CPT is a registered trademark of the American Medical Association.
2008 average 50th Percentile Fees are provided courtesy of 2008 MMH-SI's copyrighted Physicians' Fees and Coding Guide.

Supply Sources

Moore Medical LLC
PO Box 1500
New Britain, CT 06050-1500

Medical Supply Group
2101 NW 33rd Street
Suite 600A
Pompano Beach, FL 33069

The Physician's Resource for Medical Equipment, Inc.
306 Country Club Drive
Mountaintop, PA 18707

Bibliography

Brook I, Anderson KD, Controni G, et al. Aerobic and anaerobic bacteriology of pilonidal cyst abscess in children. *Am J Dis Child.* 1980;134(7):679–680.

DaSilva JH. Pilonidal cyst, cause and treatment. *Dis Colon Rectum.* 2000;42:1146–1156.

Hosseini SV, Bananzadeh AM, Rivaz M, et al. The comparison between drainage, delayed excision and primary closure with excision and secondary healing in management of pilonidal abscess. *Int J Surg.* 2006;4(4):228–231.

Hull TL, Wu J. Pilonidal disease. *Surg Clin North Am.* 2002;82(6):1169–1185.

Jensen SL, Harling H. Prognosis after simple incision and drainage for a first-episode acute pilonidal abscess. *Br J Surg.* 1988;75(1):60–61.

2008 MAG Mutual Healthcare Solutions, Inc.'s Physicians' Fee and Coding Guide. Duluth, Georgia. MAG Mutual Healthcare Solutions, Inc. 2007.

CHAPTER 94

Excision of Thrombosed External Hemorrhoids

E. J. Mayeaux Jr., MD, DABFP, FAAFP
Professor of Family Medicine, Professor of Obstetrics and Gynecology
Louisiana State University Health Sciences Center, Shreveport, LA
Larry S. Sasaki, MD, FACS
Assistant Clinical Professor of Surgery
Louisiana State University Health Sciences Center, Shreveport, LA

Acute thrombosis of external hemorrhoids can cause extreme discomfort and disability. The condition frequently manifests in younger individuals, and up to one third of women experience the condition immediately postpartum. Straining with defecation is believed to be causative, and individuals often report pain after severe bouts of diarrhea or constipation. Examination often reveals a tender, enlarged, perianal mass, with the blue clot seen through the skin. Drainage or mild bleeding can occur if the clot ruptures through the skin.

External hemorrhoids are composed of the dilated tributaries of the inferior rectal vein, and they appear below the dentate line. Because the specialized anoderm in the anal canal below the dentate line is heavily innervated, thrombosed external hemorrhoids can produce excruciating discomfort. Acutely thrombosed hemorrhoids benefit from surgical intervention, and many physicians still consider this the treatment of choice. Thrombosis that has been present more than 72 hours generally should be treated conservatively, because the pain from the surgery often exceeds the pain experienced from slow resolution of the lesion. Conservative management includes sitz baths, oral analgesics, stool softeners, nonsteroidal anti-inflammatory drugs (NSAIDs), and topical anesthetics such as lidocaine. Topical nifedipine and topical nitroglycerin appear to be promising interventions for more rapid symptom resolution in patients not surgically treated.

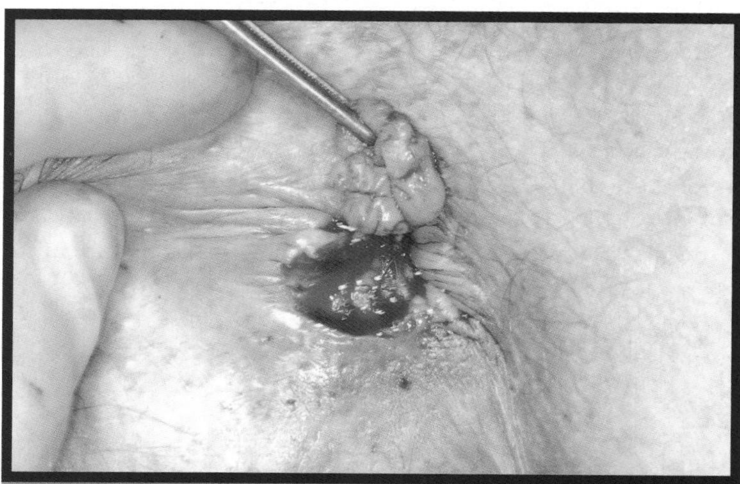

Primary care physicians historically have performed incision and drainage procedures on thrombosed hemorrhoids. This procedure can remove large clots, but reports of high recurrence rates within 24 hours have led many physicians to advocate more extensive surgical intervention. A fusiform excision is recommended, with removal of the clot adherent to the overlying skin. Many physicians advocate removal of the entire underlying hemorrhoidal complex. Some have reported increased discomfort in individuals whose wounds are closed with sutures, but subcutaneous closure provides the benefit of more rapid healing and less drainage from the surgical site. Arterioles in the hemorrhoidal complex may experience spasm when cut. Sutured wounds are less likely to experience brisk bleeding from the surgery site several hours after the procedure once the spasm is relieved.

The natural history of thrombosed hemorrhoids is slow resolution over 1 to 2 weeks. The swollen tissue diminishes to form an external skin tag. Tags are almost always asymptomatic, and surgical removal usually is not indicated.

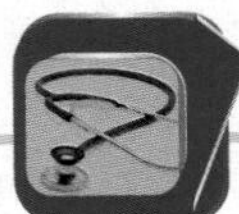

Equipment

- The recommended surgical tray for office surgery is listed in Appendix G. Suggested suture removal times are listed in Appendix J.
- A suggested anesthesia tray that can be used for this procedure is listed in Appendix F.
- Skin preparation accommodations appear in Appendix E.
- One inch of 2% lidocaine jelly (Xylocaine) placed on the corner of the drape.
- Ive's anoscope.
- Surgical scissors.
- Surgical forceps.
- Electrocautery.

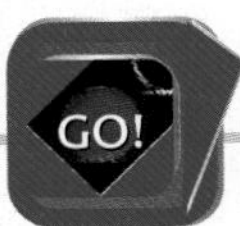

Indications

- Severe symptoms (e.g., pain, itching) requiring surgical intervention
- Ulcerated or ruptured external thrombosed hemorrhoids
- Recurrent thrombosis after incision procedure

Contraindications (Relative)

- Uncooperative patient
- Coagulopathy or bleeding diathesis
- Presence of symptoms for more than 72 hours (may still consider surgery, but pain of surgery may exceed pain of conservative management)
- Presence of complicating disease (e.g., fissures, fistulas, cancer) that require more extensive surgery

The Procedure

Step 1. The patient is placed in the left lateral decubitus position on an absorbent pad. A gloved assistant should be available. Inspect the area. Flex the right hip and knee, and place a drape over the patient's waist and legs.

- **PEARL:** If solid tumors or unusual tissue characteristics are discovered at the time of surgery, histologic analysis of the tissue is warranted.

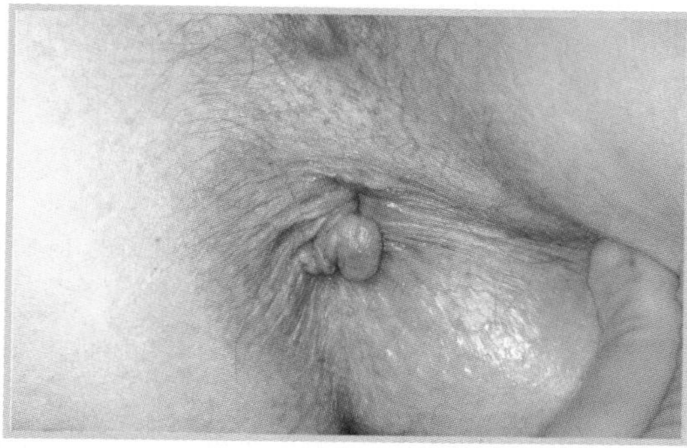

Step 1

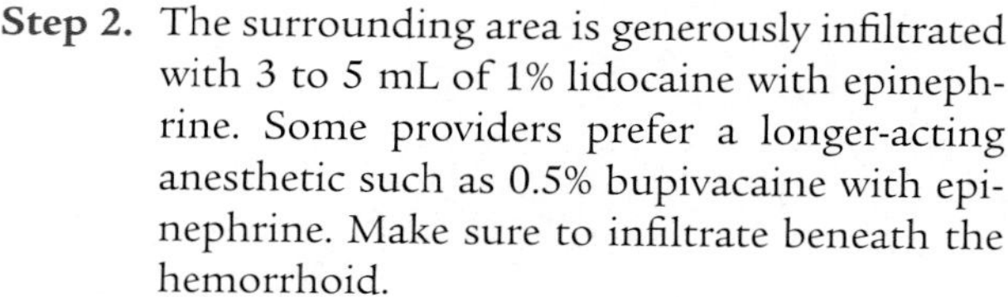

Step 2. The surrounding area is generously infiltrated with 3 to 5 mL of 1% lidocaine with epinephrine. Some providers prefer a longer-acting anesthetic such as 0.5% bupivacaine with epinephrine. Make sure to infiltrate beneath the hemorrhoid.

- **PITFALL:** The perianal tissues are highly vascular. Avoid intravascular injection of the anesthetic when injecting into these tissues.

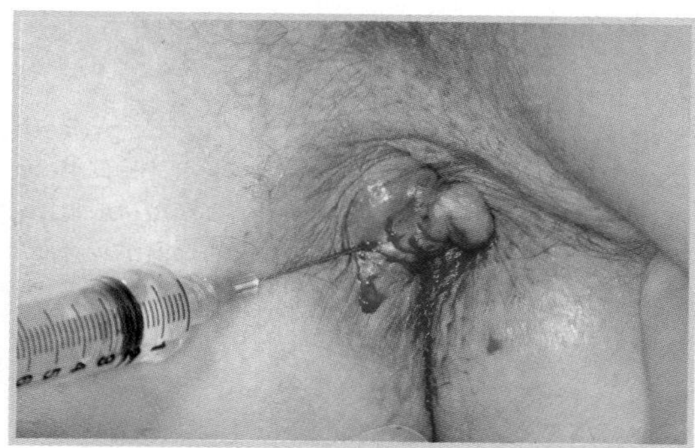

Step 2

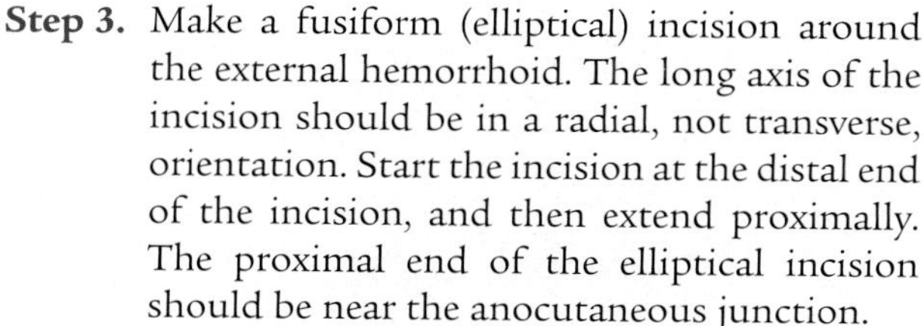

Step 3. Make a fusiform (elliptical) incision around the external hemorrhoid. The long axis of the incision should be in a radial, not transverse, orientation. Start the incision at the distal end of the incision, and then extend proximally. The proximal end of the elliptical incision should be near the anocutaneous junction.

- **PITFALL:** Do not extend the proximal end of the incision too proximally (i.e., dentate line or above). This may result in a proximal end that is difficult to expose and control bleeding.
- **PEARL:** You can use scalpel for the initial incision; however, many providers find that they have better control of both making the incision and subsequently removing the hemorrhoid with the scissors. Scissors also save some time because you do not have to switch instruments.

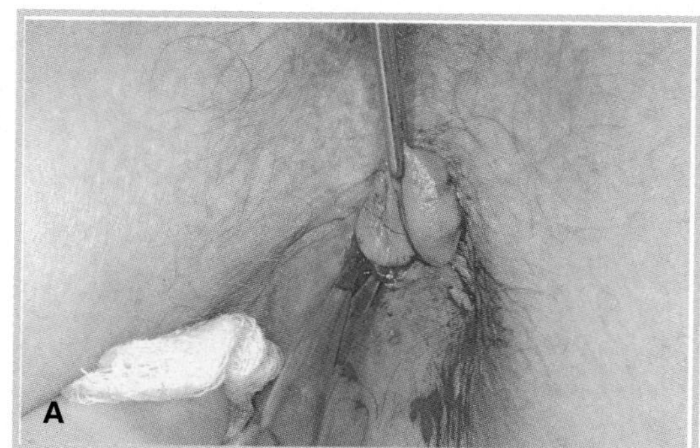

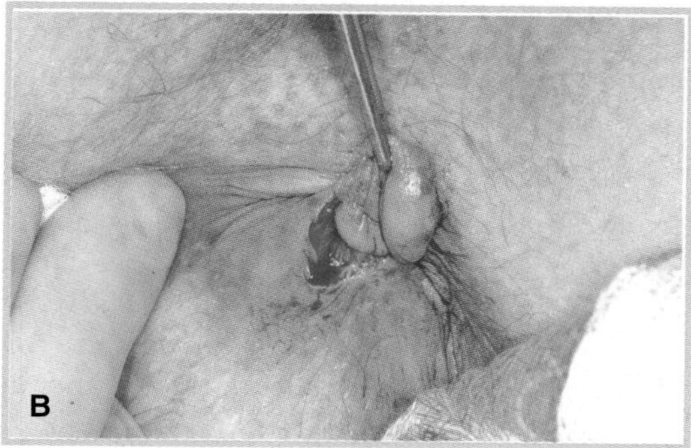

Step 3

Step 4. After the skin incision, grasp the central island of skin. Undermine this central island of skin with scissors, cutting deeply enough to maintain attachment of the thrombosed hemorrhoid to the overlying skin. If additional hemorrhoidal complexes (veins) are seen beneath the clot, these can be excised with tissue scissors.

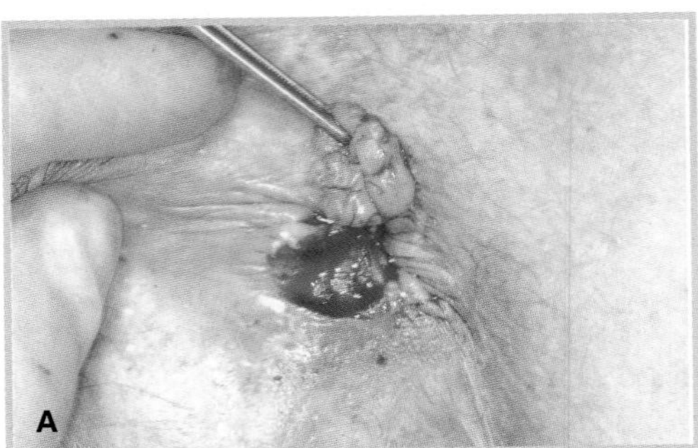

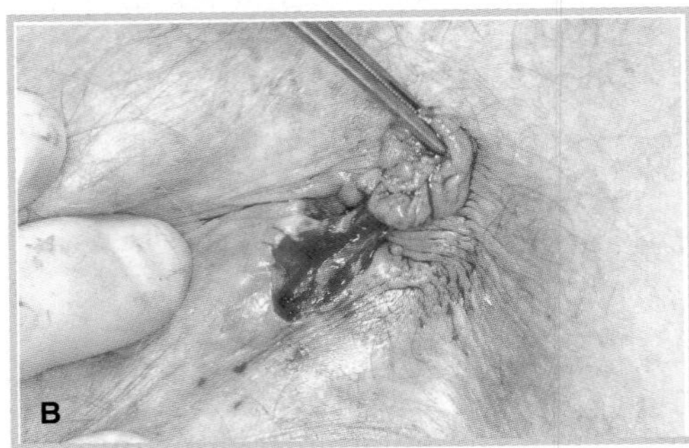

Step 4

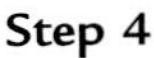

Step 5. Bleeding can occur during the procedure. The electrocautery is used for hemostasis. Clamping a hemostat on a bleeding vessel inside the wound also often provides effective control. The instrument can be removed after a minute.

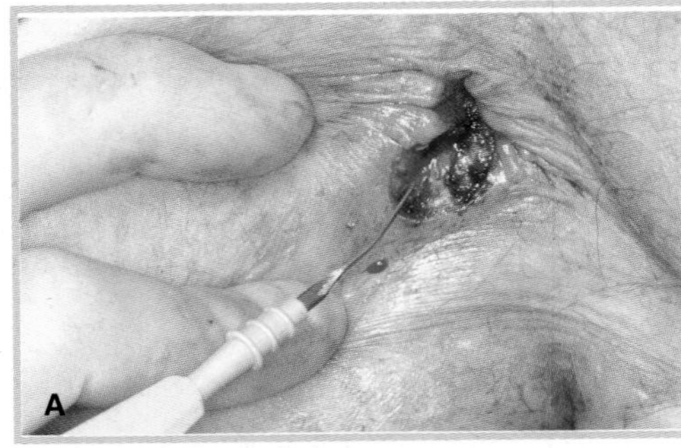

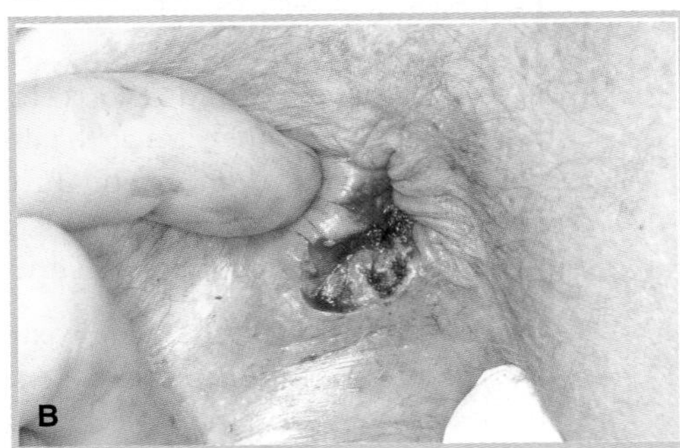

Step 5

Step 6. Leave the area open, with healing accomplished by secondary intention. The final appearance after hemorrhoidectomy is shown.

- **PEARL:** Most providers do not close the defect because the wound heals nicely without suturing and time is saved without suturing. Also, the wound frequently dehisces with suture closure anyway.

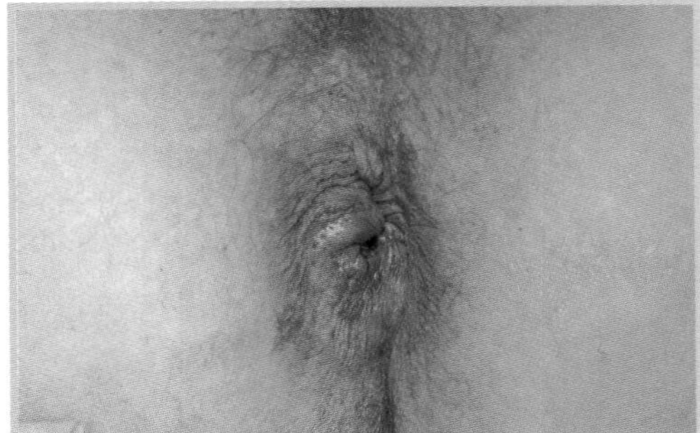

Step 6

Step 7. Apply bulky gauze dressing over the defect (not in the anus), which may be changed as needed.

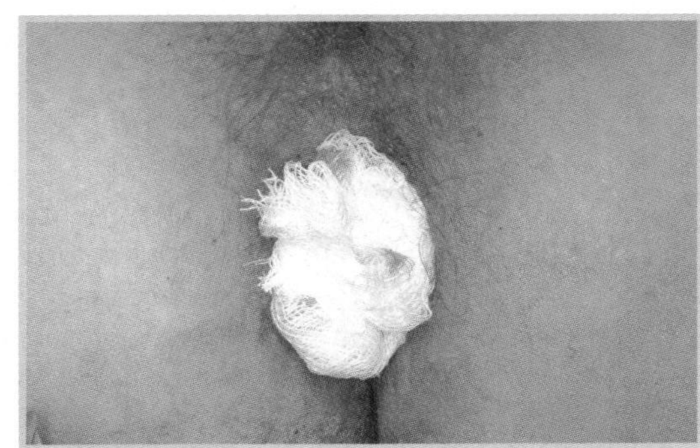

Step 7

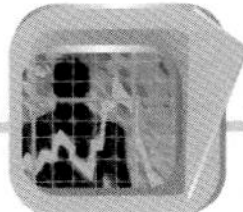

Complications

- Bleeding
- Scarring
- Anal stenosis
- Infection
- Pain

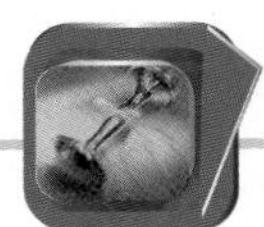

Pediatric Considerations

This condition is very rare in the pediatric population.

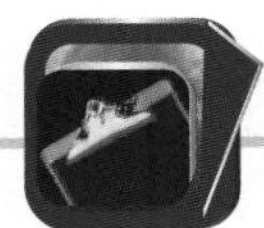

Postprocedure Instructions

Arrange for the patient to have a follow-up visit at 4 to 6 weeks postprocedure. If coexisting internal hemorrhoids are found during the procedure, they can be treated at this visit. Emphasize to the patient the need for soft stools. Use multiple modalities to soften the stools, such as stool softeners, stool-bulking agents, fiber-rich foods, and increased daily consumption of fluids.

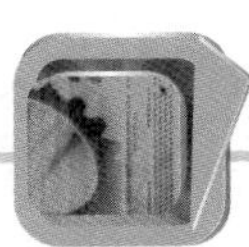

Coding Information and Supply Sources

CPT Code	Description	2008 Average 50th Percentile Fee	Global Period
46083	Incision of thrombosed external hemorrhoid	$353.00	10
46221	Hemorrhoidectomy by rubber band ligation	$360.00	0
46250	External hemorrhoidectomy, complete	$1,045.00	90
46320	Enucleation or excision of external thrombotic hemorrhoid	$371.00	10

CPT is a registered trademark of the American Medical Association.
2008 average 50th Percentile Fees are provided courtesy of 2008 MMH-SI's copyrighted Physicians' Fees and Coding Guide.

ICD-9 Codes

Hemorrhoid uncomplicated	455.6
Hemorrhoid bleeding or prolapsed	455.8
Hemorrhoid external	455.3
Hemorrhoid external thrombosed	455.4
Hemorrhoid bleeding or prolapsed external	455.5
Hemorrhoid internal	455.0
Hemorrhoid internal thrombosed	455.1
Hemorrhoid bleeding or prolapsed internal	455.2

Instrument and Materials Ordering

The instruments on the office surgical tray (see Appendix G) are appropriate for hemorrhoidal surgery. The addition of two straight hemostats may be beneficial. Some physicians prefer to grasp and elevate the clot and hemorrhoidal complex using an Allis clamp. All instruments are available from surgical supply houses or instrument dealers. A suggested anesthesia tray that can be used for this procedure is listed in Appendix F.

Patient Education Handout

A patient education handout, "Hemorrhoids," can be found on the book's companion Web site.

Bibliography

Abramowitz L, Sobhani I, Benifla JL, et al. Anal fissure and thrombosed external hemorrhoids before and after delivery. *Dis Colon Rectum.* 2002;45:650–655.

Buls JG. Excision of thrombosed external hemorrhoids. *Hosp Med.* 1994;30:39–42.

Friend WG. External hemorrhoids. *Med Times.* 1988;116:108–109.

Grosz CR. A surgical treatment of thrombosed external hemorrhoids. *Dis Colon Rectum.* 1990;33:249–250.

Hulme-Moir M, Bartolo DC. Hemorrhoids. *Gastroenterol Clin.* 2001;30:183–197.

Hussain JN. Office management of common anorectal problems. *Prim Care Clin Office Pract.* 1999;26:35–51.

Janicke DM, Pundt MR. Anorectal disorders. *Emerg Med Clin North Am.* 1996;14:757–788.

Leibach JR, Cerda JJ. Hemorrhoids: modern treatment methods. *Hosp Med.* 1991;27:53–68.

Medich DS, Fazio VW. Hemorrhoids, anal fissure, and carcinoma of the colon, rectum, and anus during pregnancy. *Surg Clin North Am.* 1995;75:77–88.

Nagle D, Rolandelli RH. Primary care office management of perianal and anal disease. *Gastroenterology.* 1996;23:609–620.

Orkin BA, Schwartz AM, Orkin M. Hemorrhoids: what the dermatologist should know. *J Am Acad Dermatol.* 1999;41:449–456.

Perrotti P. Conservative treatment of acute thrombosed external hemorrhoids with topical nifedipine. *Dis Colon Rectum.* 2001;44:405–409.

Schussman LC, Lutz LJ. Outpatient management of hemorrhoids. *Prim Care.* 1986;13:527–541.

Zuber TJ. Diseases of the rectum and anus. In: Taylor RB, David AK, Johnson TA, et al., eds. *Family Medicine Principles and Practice.* 5th ed. New York: Springer-Verlag; 1998:788–794.

Zuber TJ. Hemorrhoidectomy for thrombosed external hemorrhoids. *Am Fam Physician.* 2002;65:1629–1632, 1635–1636, 1639.

2008 MAG Mutual Healthcare Solutions, Inc.'s Physicians' Fee and Coding Guide. Duluth, Georgia. MAG Mutual Healthcare Solutions, Inc. 2007.

SECTION NINE

Eye, Ear, Nose, and Throat Procedures

CHAPTER 95

Anterior Epistaxis Treatment

Stacy Kanayama, MD, ATC
Assistant Professor of Family Medicine
Louisiana State University Health Sciences Center, Shreveport, LA

E. J. Mayeaux, Jr., MD, DABFP, FAAFP
Professor of Family Medicine, Professor of Obstetrics and Gynecology
Louisiana State University Health Sciences Center, Shreveport, LA

Epistaxis (i.e., nosebleed) is a condition commonly seen in the primary care setting. Because the blood supply to the nasal cavity originates in the carotid arteries, epistaxis may produce profuse bleeding. This chapter focuses on the more common anterior bleeds. Around 80% to 90% of nosebleeds originate in the anterior part of the nasal septum known as the Kiesselbach plexus. The Kiesselbach plexus is readily accessible to objects inserted into the nose. The presence of nasal trauma, recent use of intranasal agents, presence of a foreign body, recent infection, nasal allergy, and absence of sensation of blood flowing down the back of the throat all suggest an anterior site of bleeding.

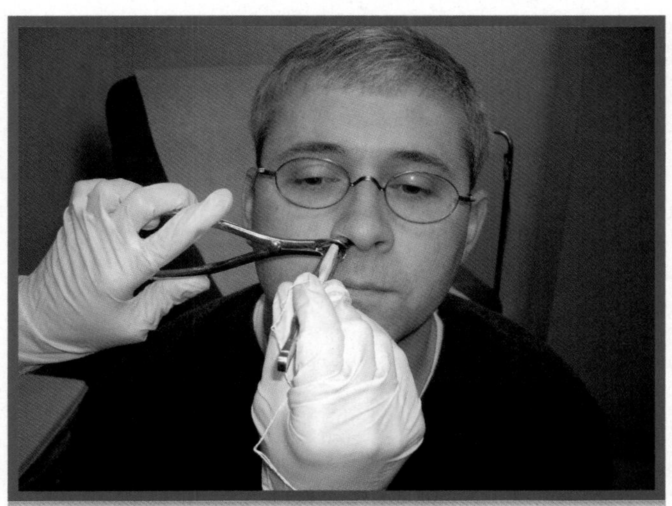

Local and systemic disorders may cause nosebleeds (Table 95-1). In a patient older than 40 years of age, bleeding is often posterior and may be associated with systemic disease. The site of bleeding should be identified in all patients, even those in whom the bleeding has stopped, because the severity of the problem and the treatment options vary by site. If serious bleeding exists, the highest priority is to secure the patient's airway, breathing, and circulation. One third of children presenting with recurrent epistaxis have a diagnosable coagulopathy.

When a patient presents with epistaxis, obtain a brief history to determine the duration and severity of bleeding and the presence of any contributing factors. Patients who present with epistaxis typically have a history of intermittent bleeding that may be either active or temporarily controlled at the time of presentation. If bleeding is severe, consider getting a complete blood cell count (CBC) and clotting studies. Determine if the bleeding originates in the anterior or posterior part of the nasal cavity. It may be difficult to determine the source of the bleeding, because clots may be present and blood can reflux into the unaffected side. Have the patient blow his or her nose to dislodge clots. Suction with a Fraser tip may be helpful. Adequate lighting and suction are essential to a good

TABLE 95-1. Common Causes of Epistaxis

- Infections such as rhinitis, nasopharyngitis, and sinusitis
- Trauma, inflicted (e.g., facial bone fractures) and self-induced (e.g., nose picking)
- Nasal foreign body
- Mucosal atrophy from chronic steroid nasal sprays
- Nasal surgery
- Local irritants such as nasal sprays and cocaine abuse
- Dry nasal mucosa
- Allergic and atrophic rhinitis
- Hypertension and atherosclerotic cardiovascular disease
- Tumors and polyps, benign or malignant
- Nasal defects, congenital or acquired
- Bleeding disorders, including hemophilia A, hemophilia B, von Willebrand disease, thrombocytopenia, and hypoprothrombinemia
- Liver disease
- Renal failure or uremia
- Disseminated intravascular coagulation
- Drug induced, including nonsteroidal anti-inflammatory drugs (especially salicylates), heparin, warfarin, thrombolytics, and heavy metals

physical examination. The physical examination should include vital signs, evaluation for orthostasis, and inspection of the oral cavity and nasopharynx.

Anterior epistaxis usually can be stopped by direct pressure, use of vasoconstrictors, simple cautery, and packing. The first therapy is usually direct pressure, accomplished by grasping the alae distally using the closed hand technique. This provides firm compression and makes it easier for the patient to maintain his or her grip. Time the nasal compression (5 to 10 minutes), because patients usually underestimate the elapsed time. If direct pressure is unsuccessful, apply a combined vasoconstrictive agent and anesthetic (Table 95-2) using a spray bottle, atomizer, or pledget. A moistened pledget provides better contact with the nasal mucosa while also providing a local tamponade effect.

Chemical cautery with silver nitrate sticks is effective treatment for minor anterior nasal bleeding. First, control bleeding using vasoconstrictors, direct pressure, or both, as it is difficult to cauterize an actively bleeding area by chemical means alone. Electrical and thermal cautery also may be used, but these are no better at hemorrhage control than chemical cautery. Battery-powered, disposable, heat cautery devices are difficult to control for the depth of cautery, and significant injury can occur.

Anterior nasal packing should be considered when the previous methods fail after three attempts. Prepare the nasal cavity with a combined vasoconstrictor and anesthetic agent (Table 95-2). The nasal cavity is packed using strips of petrolatum- or iodoform-impregnated gauze or an appropriate commercial device. If nasal packing does not control

TABLE 95-2. Vasoconstrictive and Anesthetic Agents for Epistaxis

- 0.5%–1.0% phenylephrine (Neo-Synephrine) mixed 2:1 with 4% lidocaine up to a total dosage of 4 mg/kg of lidocaine
- 0.05% oxymetozaline (Afrin) mixed with 4% lidocaine up to a total dosage of 4 mg/kg of lidocaine
- 0.25 mL of 1% (1:1,000 concentration) epinephrine mixed with 20 mL of 4% lidocaine up to a total dosage of 4 mg/kg of lidocaine

isolated anterior bleeding, the anterior pack should be reinserted to ensure proper placement. Leave anterior packs in place for 48 hours. Ask the patient to report any fever or recurrent bleeding and to return immediately if bleeding recurs or if there is a sensation of blood trickling down the back of the throat.

Commercial products have been developed specifically to make the insertion of an anterior nasal pack easier and more comfortable for the patient. Polyvinyl alcohol (PVA) compressed foam sponges are made of dehydrated, spongelike material that expands on contact with moisture. They may be more comfortable than a balloon or gauze packing. It has been reported that the efficacy of this device is comparable to other methods. Gelfoam packs also can be used.

Posterior packing may be required for uncontrolled posterior bleeding. Posterior padding requires skill and practice in the face of vigorous bleeding and is best performed in emergency departments or hospital settings by physicians experienced in such insertion.

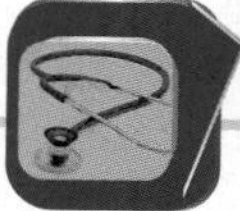

Equipment

- Handsfree light source (can be an overhead surgical lamp, battery-operated headlamp, or light held by an assistant)
- Nasal speculum
- Cotton-tipped applicators
- Frazier tip suction tip connected to continuous wall suction
- Bayonnet forceps
- Material to tamponade the site of bleeding, potentially including cotton pledgets, gelfoam packs, and Merocel nasal sponges
- Chemical cautery agent
- Topical antibiotic ointment (e.g., Bacitracin or Neosporin) if using Merocel
- Local medication for vasoconstriction: either 0.5% to 1.0% phenylephrine (Neo-Synephrine) or 0.05% oxymetozaline (Afrin) nasal spray
- Local medication for anesthesia: 4% lidocaine (up to 4 mg/kg total dose)
- Personal protective equipment including eyewear, mask, gown, and gloves

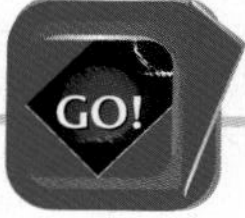

Indications

- Epistaxis that persists despite adequate external pressure

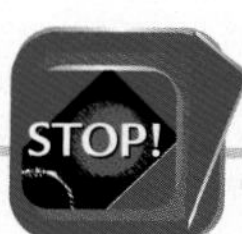

Contraindications

- No current epistaxis
- Clotting abnormalities, as aggressive packing may cause further bleeding (normalize clotting mechanisms before removing nasal packs if possible)
- Chronic obstructive pulmonary disease (monitor for a drop in oxygen partial pressure)
- Trauma, especially facial trauma (consider referral)
- Known or suspected cerebrospinal fluid leak
- Drug abuse (e.g., cocaine)
- Allergy to anesthetics or vasoconstrictors

The Procedure

Step 1. Arterial anatomy of the nasal septum. The Kiesselbach plexus is a complex anastomosis of arterioles in the superficial region of the nasal mucosa on the nasal septum. It is fed by the septal branches of the anterior ethmoid (AE), posterior ethmoid (PE), sphenopalatine (S), superior labial (SL), and greater palatine (GP) arteries.

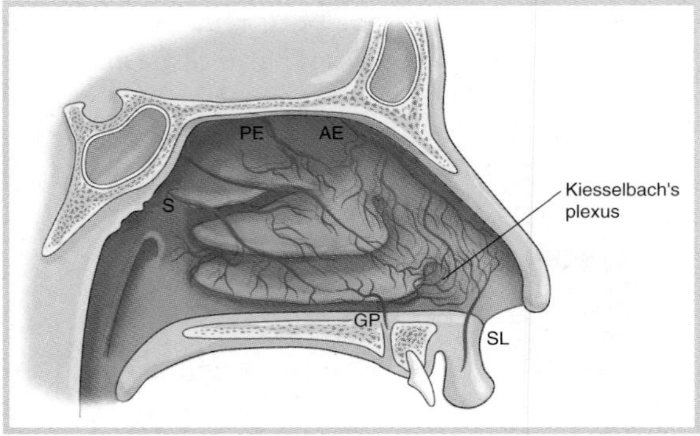

Step 1

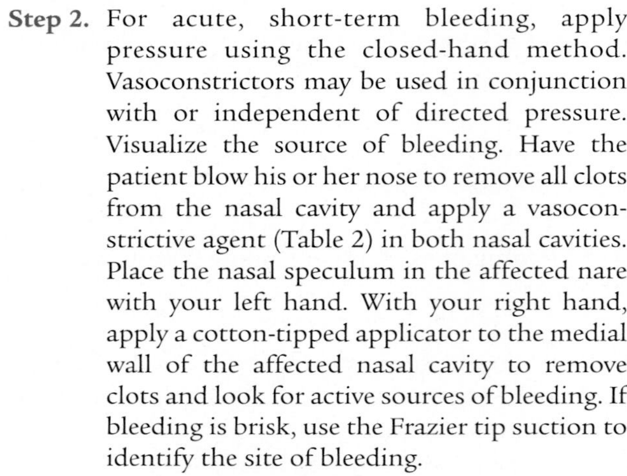

Step 2. For acute, short-term bleeding, apply pressure using the closed-hand method. Vasoconstrictors may be used in conjunction with or independent of directed pressure. Visualize the source of bleeding. Have the patient blow his or her nose to remove all clots from the nasal cavity and apply a vasoconstrictive agent (Table 2) in both nasal cavities. Place the nasal speculum in the affected nare with your left hand. With your right hand, apply a cotton-tipped applicator to the medial wall of the affected nasal cavity to remove clots and look for active sources of bleeding. If bleeding is brisk, use the Frazier tip suction to identify the site of bleeding.

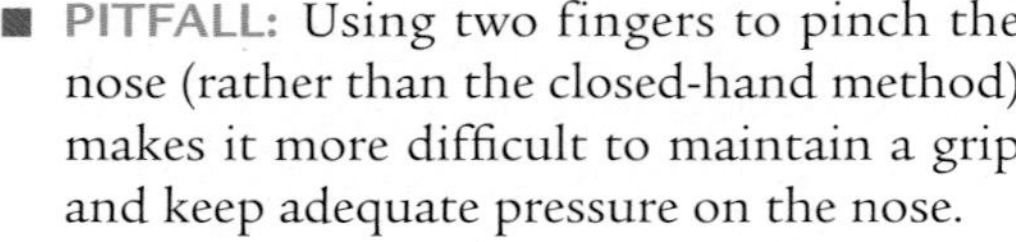

- PITFALL: Using two fingers to pinch the nose (rather than the closed-hand method) makes it more difficult to maintain a grip and keep adequate pressure on the nose.
- PITFALL: Bleeding will sometimes stop after application of a vasoconstictive agent and subsequent direct pressure. Wait at least 1 hour to make certain that bleeding is controlled before putting away your equipment and releasing the patient.
- PITFALL: If you cannot visualize the site of active bleeding by utilizing a nasal speculum and Frazier tip suction, the bleeding is likely to be from a posterior source and will require referral for posterior packing. In this instance, the anterior nares will need to be packed by utilizing Merocel as described below to slow down the bleeding.

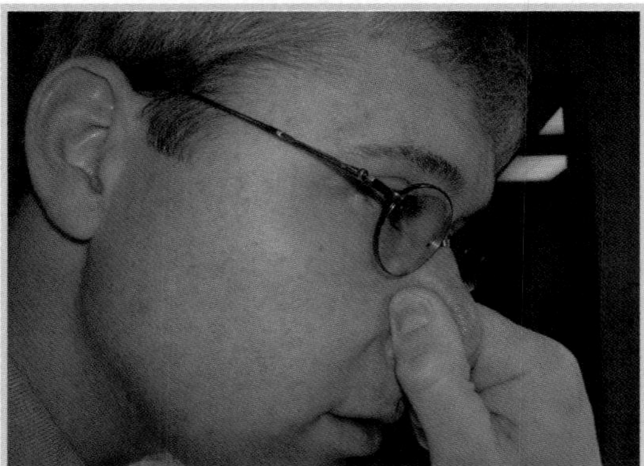

Step 2

Step 3. Chemical cautery or gelfoam can be used if anterior epistaxis cannot be controlled with vasoconstrictors, direct pressure, or both. Prepare the nasal cavity with combined vasoconstrictor and anesthetic agent. After the

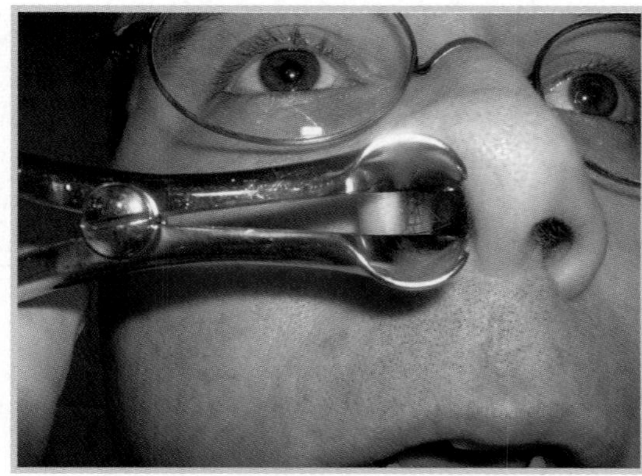

Step 3

bleeding has stopped, dry the mucosa. Visualize the nasal cavity using a nasal speculum to ensure proper gauze placement. Cauterize the mucosa by touching the bleeding source with the tip of a silver nitrate stick for 10 to 15 seconds. Wipe away any residual silver nitrate, and apply antibiotic ointment if desired. Alternatively, gently place a piece of gelfoam against the site of bleeding. The blood at the site will adhere it to the surface of the nasal cavity. Carefully remove the nasal speculum, and observe for any further bleeding.

- PITFALL: Tissue necrosis may occur if both sides of the septum are cauterized in the same session.

Step 4. Next, apply gauze packing for resistant anterior epistaxis. Using bayonet forceps, grasp one end of a long strip of ¼-inch petrolatum, iodoform, or plain gauze saturated with antibiotic ointment approximately 2 to 3 cm from its end. Allow the end to double over so that the first pass applies two layers of gauze.

- PITFALL: Blind packing often results in loose placement of the gauze and inadequate compression. Inadequate packing is probably the most common cause of treatment failure.

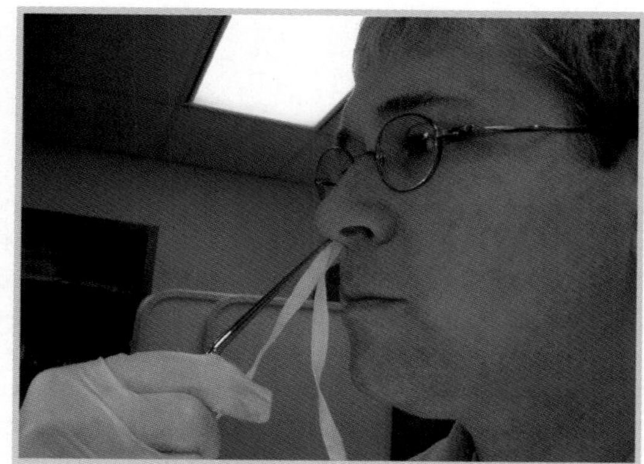

Step 4

Step 5. Insert the gauze through the nasal speculum to the posterior limit of the floor of the nose.

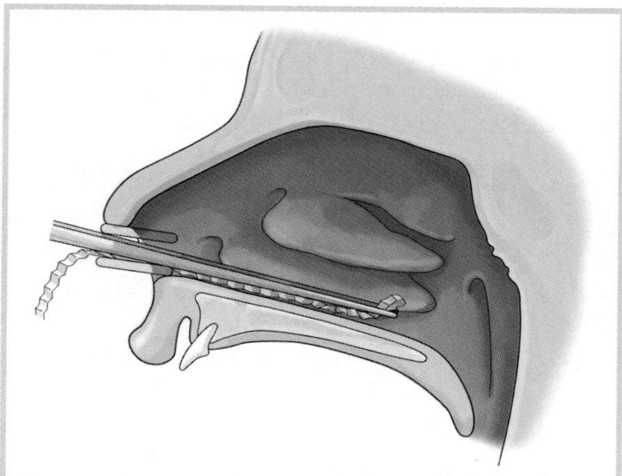

Step 5

Step 6. Withdraw the bayonet forceps and nasal speculum. Reintroduce the nasal speculum on top of the first layer of packing. Grasp another loop of gauze with the bayonet forceps. Insert the gauze on top of the previous course using an "accordion" technique so that part of each layer lies anterior to the previous layer, preventing the gauze from falling posteriorly into the nasopharynx. With each layer, use the forceps to gently push the underlying strip downward.

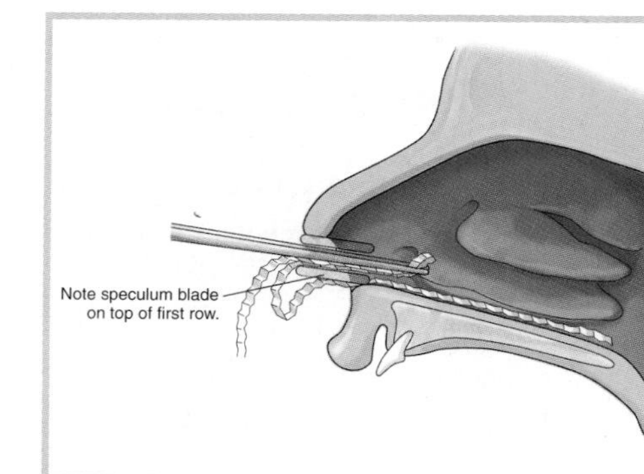
Note speculum blade
on top of first row.

Step 6

Step 7. Repeat until the entire nasal cavity is filled with layers of packing material. Observe the patient for 30 minutes to make sure that adequate hemostasis has been achieved.

- **PEARL:** If the patient complains of choking or a foreign body sensation in the back of the throat, look for layers of an anterior nasal pack that have fallen backward into the nasopharynx.

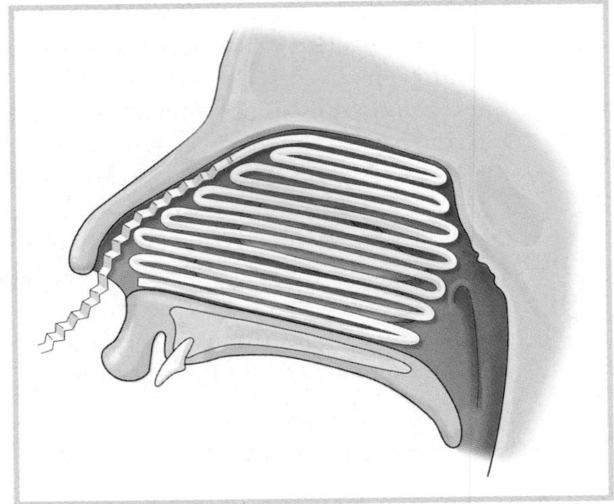

Step 7

Step 8. Alternatively, the PVA compressed foam sponge may be used for anterior packing. PVA sponges absorb blood and secretions from the nasal cavity, quickly expanding to fill the cavity and tamponade the bleeding. Before insertion into the bleeding nasal cavity, cover the sponge with antibiotic ointment. Insert the sponge directly into the nare, placing it posteriorly until resistance is felt. The proximal end of the sponge should be flush with the nasal opening. Repeat this procedure for the nonbleeding nasal cavity. Packing both sides prevents deviation of the nasal septum, allowing the site of bleeding to be effectively tamponaded by the packing.

- **PEARL:** Drops of the vasoconstrictive agent can be added to the PVA sponge if further expansion is needed.
- **PEARL:** Some sponges have a suture attached to one end to facilitate future removal. The suture needs to be left outside the nasal cavity and can be taped to the cheek to keep it out of the way.

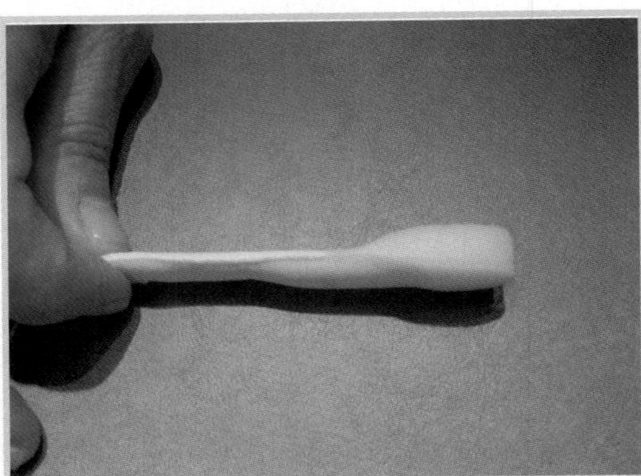

Step 8

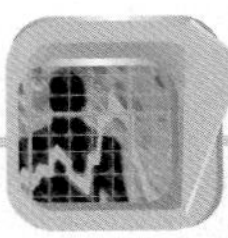

Complications

- Continued bleeding
- Rebleeding with removal of pledget/gelfoam or packing
- Sinusitis
- Pain
- Toxic shock syndrome (very rare)
- Septal perforations (very rare)

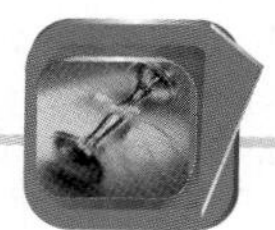

Pediatric Considerations

Anterior nosebleed management may be managed as in the adult population. However, referral to a specialist may be necessary for an uncooperative patient.

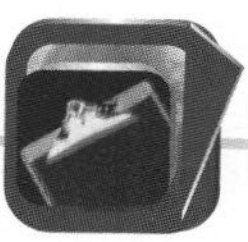

Postprocedure Instructions

All patients with anterior epistaxis should refrain from blowing the nose, avoid digital trauma, and use a room humidifier. Saline nasal spray can be used to maintain the moisture of nasal mucosal membranes. Patients with any type of nasal packing should be prescribed both analgesic medication and prophylactic oral antibiotics (amoxicillin-clavulanate, fluoroquinolones) to prevent development of sinusitis and toxic shock syndrome. Patients should be instructed to pinch their nares for 15 to 20 minutes prior to seeking medical care if bleeding recurs. If this stops the bleeding, there is no immediate need for them to seek medical attention for the epistaxis. The nasal packing should remain in place for 24 to 48 hours, and the patient should come in for follow-up at that time.

If the bleeding is controlled, instruct the patient not to manipulate the external nares or insert foreign objects or fingers into the nasal cavity. Petrolatum or triple antibiotic ointment may be applied to dry nasal mucosa with a cotton-tipped applicator once or twice each day for several days. Have patients avoid aspirin or nonsteroidal anti-inflammatory drugs for 3 or 4 days. If bleeding recurs, the patient should use home measures such as over-the-counter nasal sprays or direct pressure for 5 to 10 minutes before returning for medical care. If bleeding continues after repeating compression twice more, have the patient seek immediate medical help.

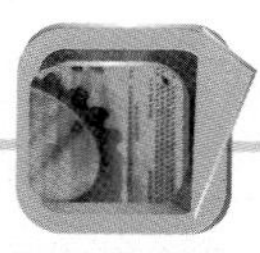

Coding Information and Supply Sources

CPT Code	Description	2008 Average 50th Percentile Fee	Global Period
30901	Control nasal hemorrhage, anterior, simple (limited cautery and nasal packing), any method	$221.00	0
30903	Control nasal hemorrhage, anterior, complex (extensive cautery and nasal packing), any method	$327.00	0

Patient Education Handout

A patient education handout, "Nosebleeds," can be found on the book's Web site.

Bibliography

Chopra R. Epistaxis: a review. *J R Soc Health.* 2000;120:31–33.

Frazee TA, Hauser MS. Nonsurgical management of epistaxis. *J Oral Maxillofac Surg.* 2000;58:419–424.

Kotecha B, Fowler S, Harkness P, et al. Management of epistaxis: a national survey. *Ann R Coll Surg Engl.* 1996;78:444–446.

Murthy P, Laing MR. An unusual, severe adverse reaction to silver nitrate cautery for epistaxis in an immunocompromised patient. *Rhinology.* 1996;34:186–187.
O'Donnell M, Robertson G, McGarry GW. A new bipolar diathermy probe for the outpatient management of adult acute epistaxis. *Clin Otolaryngol.* 1999;24:537–541.
Pond F, Sizeland A. Epistaxis: strategies for management. *Aust Fam Physician.* 2000;29:933–938.
Pope LER, Hobbs CGL. Epistaxis: an update on current management. *Postgrad Med J.* 2005;81:309–314.
Pothula V, Alderson D. Nothing new under the sun: the management of epistaxis. *J Laryngol Otol.* 1998;112:331–334.
Randall DA. Epistaxis packing. Practical pointers for nosebleed control. *Postgrad Med.* 2006;119:77–82.
Randall DA, Freeman SB. Management of anterior and posterior epistaxis. *Am Fam Physician.* 1991;43:2007–2014.
Sandoval C, Dong S, Visintainer P, et al. Clinical and laboratory features of 178 children with recurrent epistaxis. *J Pediatr Hematol Oncol.* 2002;24:47–49.
Srinivasan V, Sherman IW, O'Sullivan G. Surgical management of intractable epistaxis: audit of results. *J Laryngol Otol.* 2000;114:697–700.
Swoboda TK. Epistaxis. In: Meldon S, Ma OJ, Woolard R, eds. *Geriatric Emergency Medicine*. New York: McGraw-Hill; 2003:475–478.
Tan LK, Calhoun KH. Epistaxis. *Med Clin North Am.* 1999;83:43–56.
2008 MAG Mutual Healthcare Solutions, Inc.'s Physicians' Fee and Coding Guide. Duluth, Georgia. MAG Mutual Healthcare Solutions, Inc. 2007.

CHAPTER 96

Cerumen Impaction Removal

Michael G. Lamb, MD
Clinical Associate Professor of Medicine
University of Pittsburgh Medical Center, Pittsburgh, PA

Jeannette E. South-Paul, MD
Andrew W. Mathieson Professor and Chair, Department of Family Medicine
University of Pittsburgh School of Medicine, Pittsburgh, PA

Cerumen impaction is one of the most common problems one encounters in primary care medicine. It is estimated that 150,000 ear irrigations are done each day in the United States and 25,000 each day in the United Kingdom. One study reported that the average family doctor sees 108 patients a year with cerumen impactions. The incidence of cerumen impaction is nearly 28% in mentally retarded adults (i.e., patients with Down syndrome often have narrow ear canals). Almost 40% of nursing home residents have been shown to have cerumen impaction. Elderly adults with intellectual deterioration and those who wear hearing aids also get this problem more frequently.

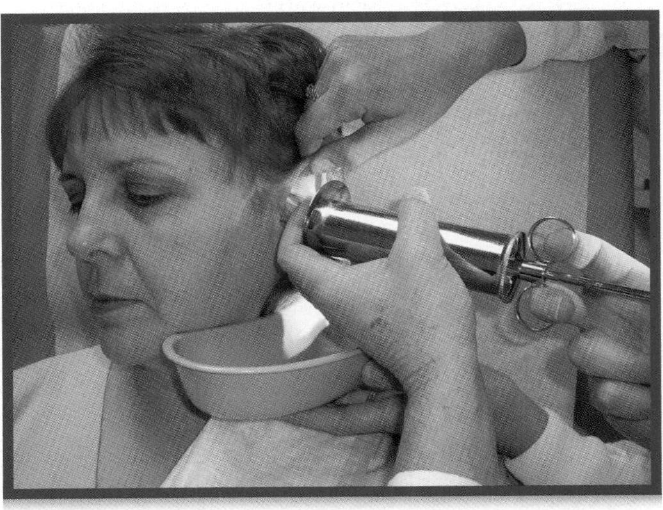

This problem is not only common but is also a cause of significant morbidity (i.e., otic pruritus, ear discomfort, recurrent external otitis, dizziness, vertigo, tinnitus, decreased hearing, hearing loss, social withdrawal, decreased cognition, poor work performance, and poor school performance). One study reported 80% improvement in hearing after the removal of impacted cerumen. Resolution of dizziness, vertigo, and tinnitus has been reported as well. Improvement in cognitive function has also been documented with successful treatment of cerumen impaction in selected groups. Overall, however, there have been few evidence-based studies in relation to outcomes data and the treatment of cerumen impaction.

There are two major types of cerumen: wet and dry. The dry type of ear wax is gray-yellow, tan, or brown-yellow in color. It is difficult to remove by curettage but is easily flushed out with gentle irrigation. Wet cerumen is dark brown and sticky and has a higher concentration of lipids. It is relatively impervious to water and hence is best removed by manual curettage. Therefore, the type of ear wax involved in the impaction will determine the general approach to treatment (irrigation vs. curettage). There are a number of proprietary solvents that are touted as being effective in dissolving ear wax. For the most part, controlled studies do not show them to be any more effective than plain water.

There is some controversy in regards to what is the best type of irrigation syringe to use. The "old-fashioned" metal syringe has been used for more than 2,000 years. Recently aural jet irrigation devices have become somewhat popular. Normal tympanic membranes in cadavers rupture at an overpressure between 0.5 and 2.0 atm. Atrophic tympanic membranes rupture between 0.3 and 0.8 atm. The tensile strength of the tympanum declines with advanced age. The standard metal syringe used in ear canal irrigation generates a maximum overpressure of 0.3 atm. When used gently, the pressure generated by this device is thus clearly less than the threshold for rupturing both normal and atrophic tympanic membranes. The authors of this chapter have performed more than 1,000 such irrigations without causing a perforation of the tympanum. The literature quotes a perforation rate of 1 in 1,000 patients when the standard metal syringe is used. In contrast, one study reported a perforation rate in cadavers of 6% with aural jet irrigation. It would seem that the standard metal syringe, when used properly, is safer than the aural jet devices.

The patient must be informed of the potential complications of cerumen removal, especially bleeding, which is relatively common with curettage. Mild dizziness and a full feeling in the ear are somewhat common after irrigation. A tympanic membrane perforation should never occur in a cooperative patient, because the curette should not come anywhere close to the tympanic membrane. A good general rule is to never advance the curette greater than half the length of the external otic canal. There are several types of ear curettes. They can be composed of metal or plastic. A curette with a wirelike loop on the end is useful for removing dry cerumen. Hard cerumen plugs are best removed with a firm metal spoon-type curette with a slightly angled probe on the end.

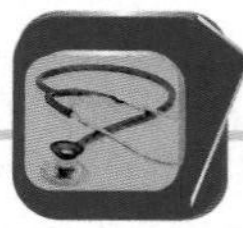

Equipment

- Cerumen curettes: metal loop type, metal spoon type, metal angulated spoon type, or plastic loop type
- Metal syringe with a piston-type mechanism (plastic types are also available)
- Kidney-shaped metal or plastic basin (to catch irrigation water)
- Standing gooseneck lamp (to illuminate the ear canal opening)
- Protective drape (to cover the patient's neck and shoulder)
- Otoscope

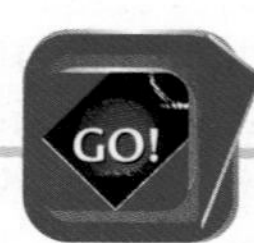

Indications

- Cerumen impaction. Because of the associated morbidity (especially in relation to decreased hearing), cerumen impaction should always be corrected if 50% or greater of the ear canal is occluded, providing that the patient can hold still or is able to be held still.

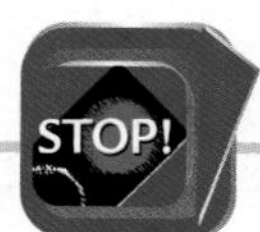

Contraindications

Curettage

- Inability to cooperate, hold still, or be held still
- Excessive cough reflex
- Anticoagulation with warfarin (Coumadin)
- Thrombocytopenia

- Coagulopathy
- Otitis externa
- Otic bleeding
- Suspected tympanic membrane perforation
- Otic furuncle or pustule
- Inability to adequately visualize (excess inner ear hair and unusual ear canal anatomy)

Irrigation

- Prior ruptured tympanum
- History of tympanostomy tubes
- Acute otitis media
- Acute, chronic, or recurrent otitis externa
- Recurrent or chronic otitis media
- Diabetes
- Other immunosuppressed hosts
- Inability to cooperate
- Hemotympanum
- Bloody discharge from the ear
- Recent ear pain
- Failure after five irrigation attempts to remove any significant amounts of cerumen
- Recurrent vertigo

The Procedure

Irrigation for the Removal of Cerumen

Step 1. Several papers have been written recommending a specific protocol for cerumen removal. Although there are some common general considerations, there is no evidence-based consensus. Have an assistant bring kidney-shaped basins, curettes, and an irrigation syringe into the examination room.

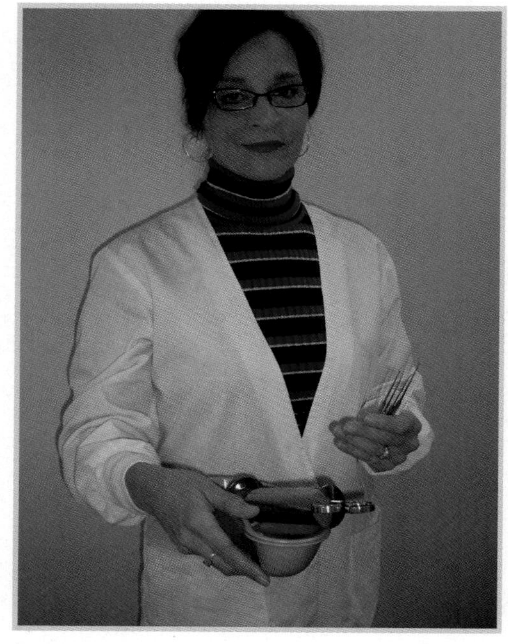

Step 1

Step 2. Inspect the irrigation syringe and be sure that the piston mechanism moves smoothly.

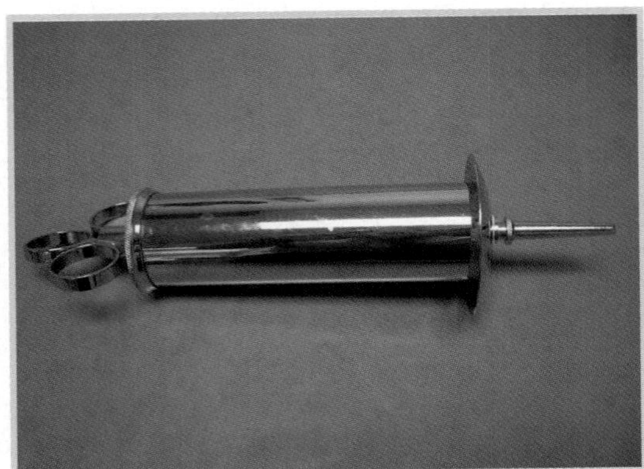

Step 2

Step 3. Carefully examine the ears before irrigation. (If possible, check for intact tympanic membrane, look for any evidence of otitis media or otitis externa, and check for tragal tenderness, blood in the ear canal, and the type of cerumen.)

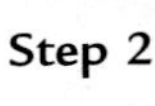

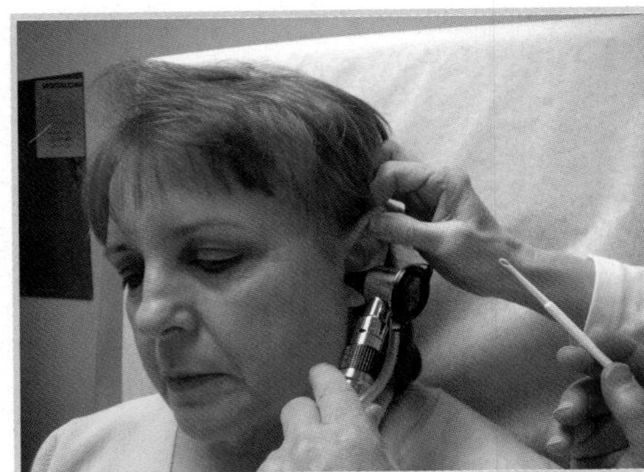

Step 3

Step 4. Check to be sure all fittings on the irrigation syringe are tight.

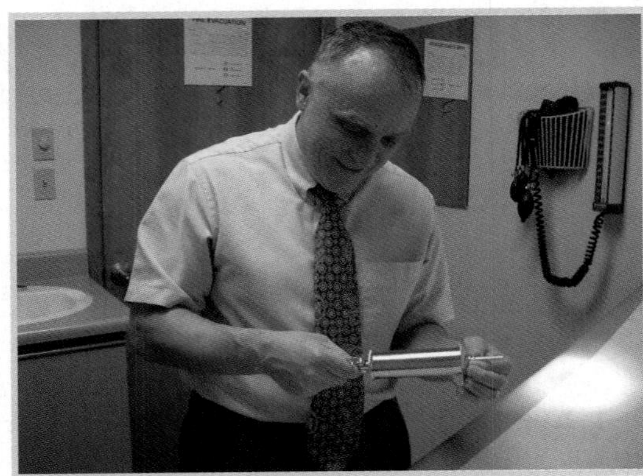

Step 4

Step 5. Fill a kidney-shaped basin with lukewarm water.

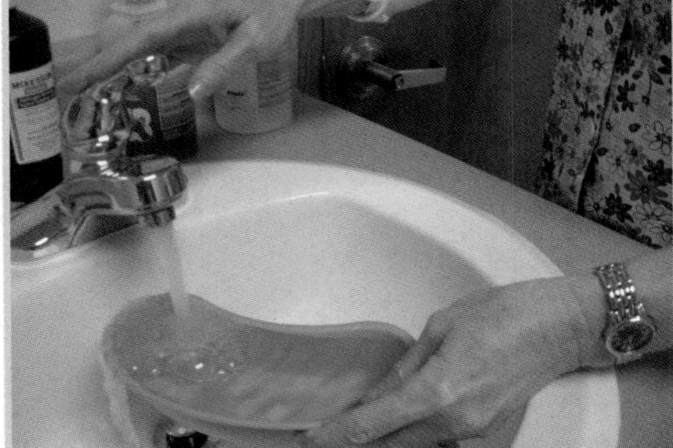

Step 5

Step 6. Fill the ear syringe with lukewarm water

- **PITFALL:** Using water that is too warm or too cold increases the risk of stimulation of the vestibular reflex and associated nystagmus and nausea.

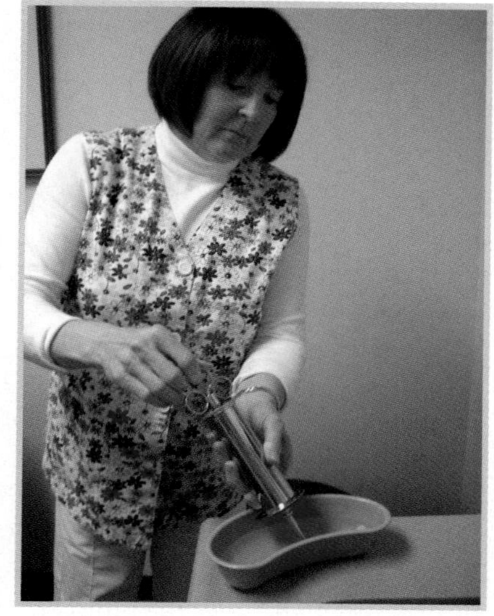

Step 6

Step 7. Express any air from the syringe and refill by aspirating more water into the syringe (this prevents a loud gurgling noise from occurring, which is obviously not pleasant for the patient).

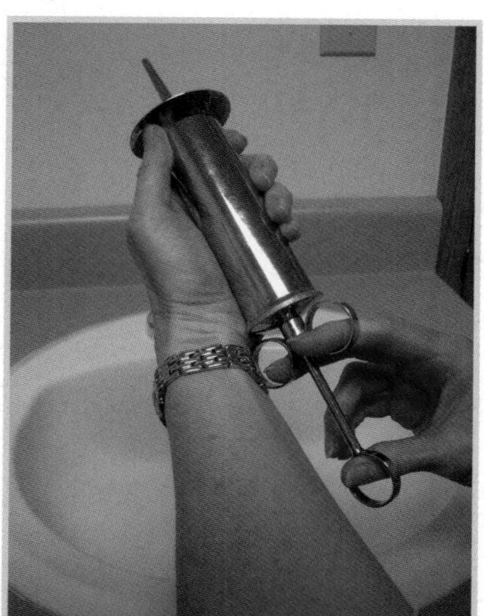
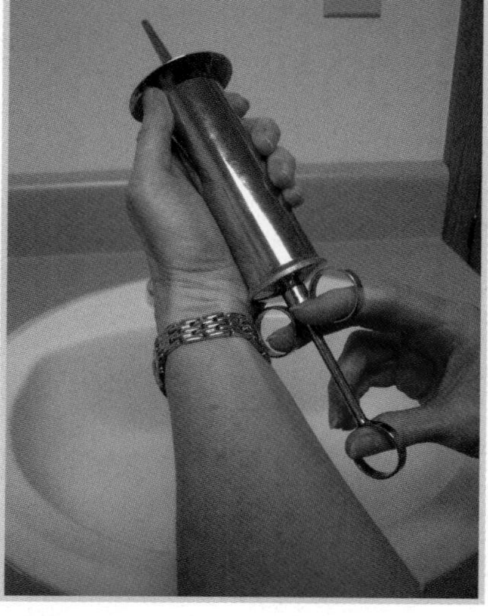

Step 7

Step 8. Drape the patient's shoulder and lateral neck with a protective barrier and direct the light from a standing gooseneck lamp onto the patient's ear.

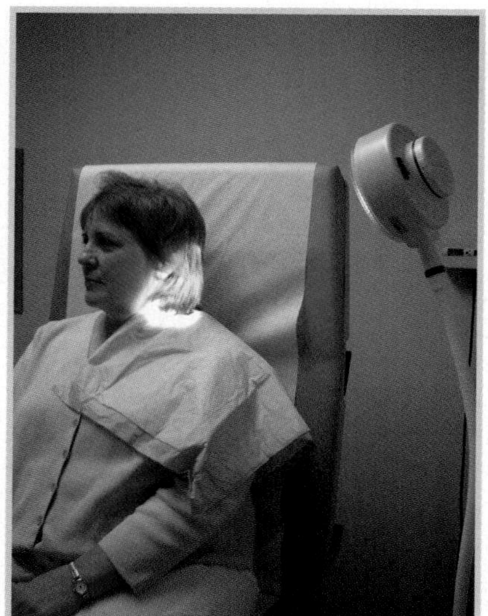

Step 8

Step 9. Have your assistant gently retract the pinnae to open the ear canal.

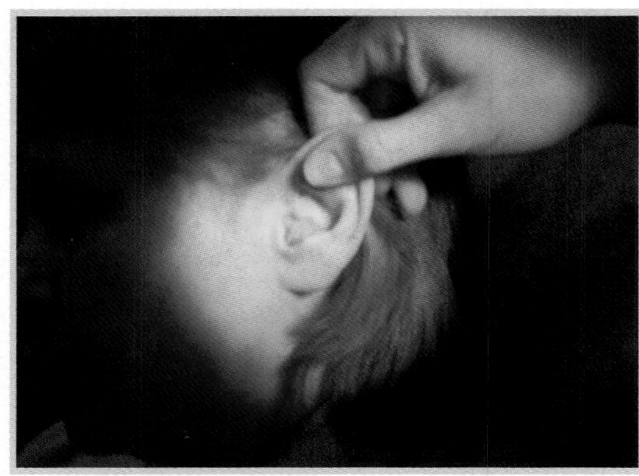

Step 9

Step 10. Grasp the nipple of the syringe between the second and third fingers. Place the thumb of the opposite hand over the plunger.

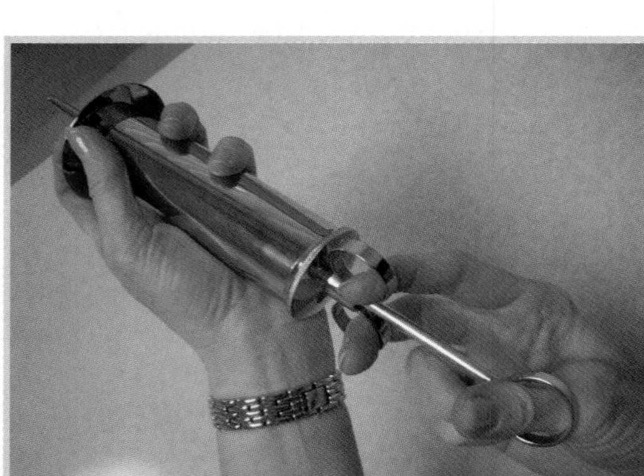

Step 10

Step 11. Place only the tip of the syringe in the canal.

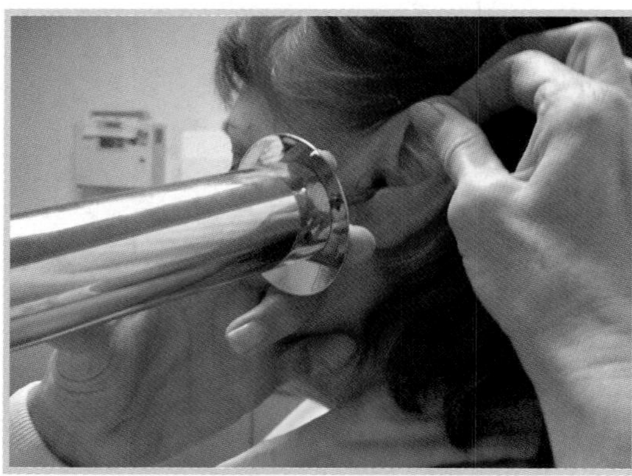

Step 11

Step 12. Have an assistant hold the kidney-shaped basin under the ear to catch the irrigation water.

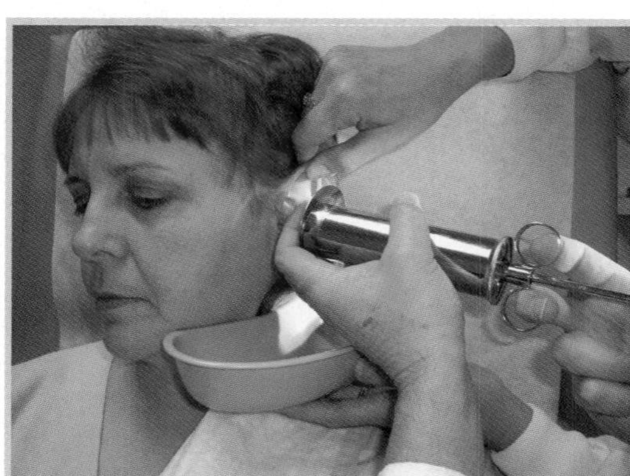

Step 12

Step 13. Gently irrigate the ear by pressing with only mild force on the irrigation piston. If significant resistance is encountered, re-evaluate the ear canal. Re-examine the ear with an otoscope to ascertain progress, and repeat the irrigation procedure until the cerumen is removed.

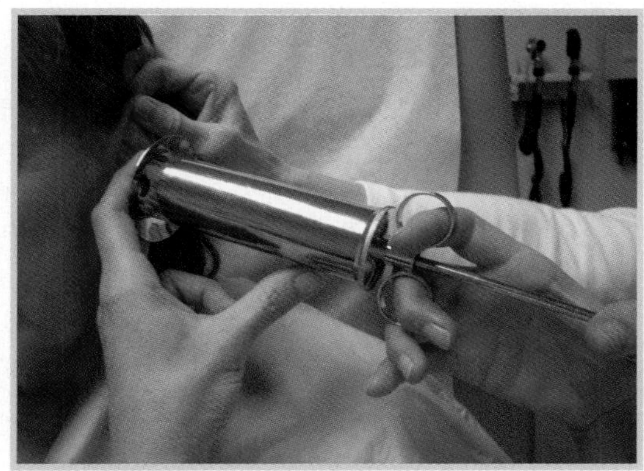

Step 13

Cerumen Removal by Curette

Step 1. A bright light should be shined on the ear while an assistant gently retracts the earlobe to open the canal as much as possible. The patient should be sitting and should be informed that this is an uncomfortable but not painful procedure. He or she must be told to be very still. Putting up the back of the exam table may help the patient hold still. The patient need only to say "stop" to halt the procedure. This should be the case if any pain is being produced. Choose the type of curette to be used.

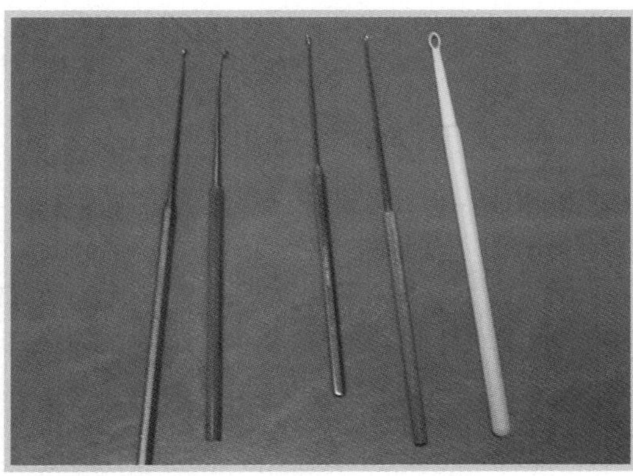

Step 1

Step 2. The angled curette usually works best in most adult cerumen impactions.

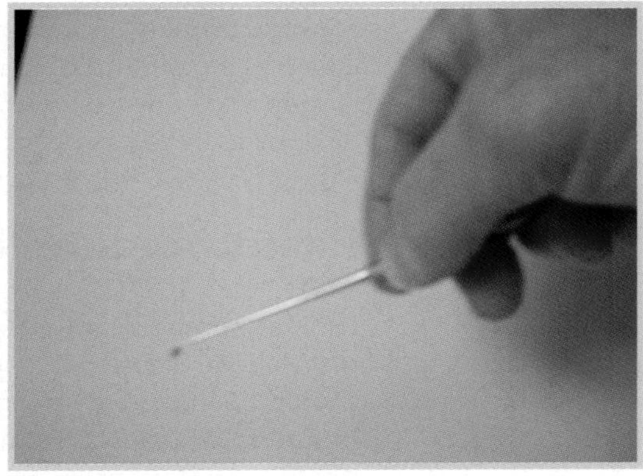

Step 2

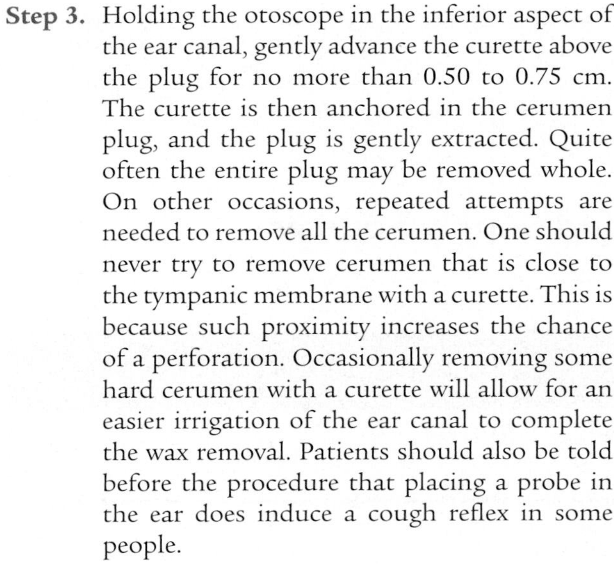

Step 3. Holding the otoscope in the inferior aspect of the ear canal, gently advance the curette above the plug for no more than 0.50 to 0.75 cm. The curette is then anchored in the cerumen plug, and the plug is gently extracted. Quite often the entire plug may be removed whole. On other occasions, repeated attempts are needed to remove all the cerumen. One should never try to remove cerumen that is close to the tympanic membrane with a curette. This is because such proximity increases the chance of a perforation. Occasionally removing some hard cerumen with a curette will allow for an easier irrigation of the ear canal to complete the wax removal. Patients should also be told before the procedure that placing a probe in the ear does induce a cough reflex in some people.

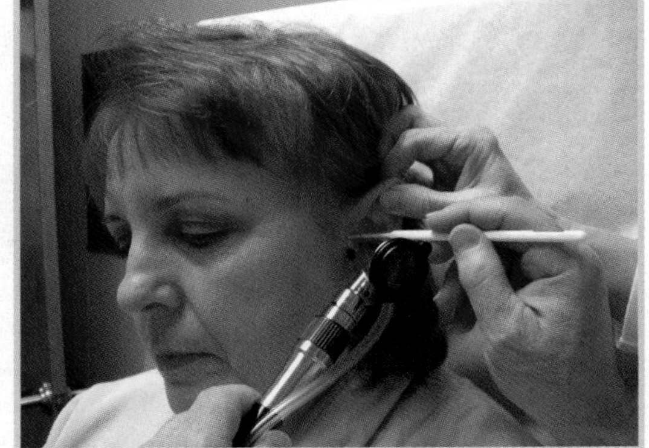

Step 3

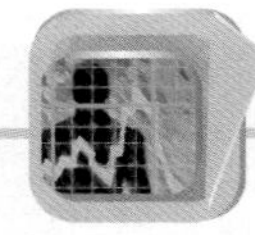

Complications

Irrigation Technique

- Perforated tympanic membrane (1 in 1,000 incidence)
- Minor bleeding from the ear canal
- Ear canal laceration
- Otitis media
- External otitis
- Vertigo
- Tinnitus
- Hemotympanum
- Malignant external otitis (in diabetics)

Curettage Technique

- Perforated tympanic membrane
- Minor bleeding from the ear canal
- Ear canal laceration

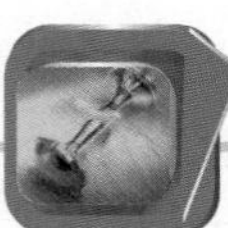

Pediatric Considerations

Adolescents are usually able to cooperate well with either ear cleaning procedure. This is usually not the case with infants and children. These patients often must be held in a "fetal position" by an assistant while the cerumen is removed with a curette. Because cerumen in infants and children is usually of the dry type, a plastic loop curette is recommended. This curette also is less likely to scratch or abrade the ear canal (an important consideration in a potentially uncooperative patient). A trained assistant is preferred over enlisting a parent to hold the child. Irrigation is difficult in infants and small children. It is probably done best with a 3- to 5-cc non-Luer-tip plastic syringe. Obviously this must be done as gently as possible.

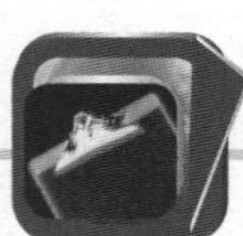

Postprocedure Instructions

Patients should be informed that a full or stuffy feeling in the ear is common after irrigation. The presence of ear pain, tinnitus, fever, vertigo, or bloody drainage from the ear should be immediately reported because these can be signs of significant complications. In general, if one is careful and follows the appropriate guidelines, complications related to cerumen impaction treatment are quite rare.

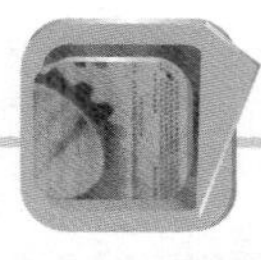

Coding Information and Supply Sources

CPT Code	Description	2008 Average 50th Percentile Fee	Global Period
69210	Removal impacted cerumen (separate procedure), one or both ears	$101.00	0

CPT is a registered trademark of the American Medical Association.
2008 average 50th Percentile Fees are provided courtesy of 2008 MMH-SI's copyrighted Physicians' Fees and Coding Guide.

- Otoscopes, ear curettes, emesis or ear basins, gooseneck lamps, and ear syringes can be obtained from medical supply houses.
- Cerumen-softening agents such as mineral oil, triethanolamine (Cerumenex), carbamide peroxide (Debrox), or cresyl acetate (Cresylate) may be obtained from pharmacies.

Patient Education Handout

A patient education handout, "Ear Wax Removal," can be found on the book's companion Web site.

Bibliography

Bird S. The potential pitfalls of ear syringing: minimizing the risks. *Aust Fam Physician.* 2003;(March):150–151.

Eckhof J. A quasi randomized trial of water as a softening agent of persistent ear wax. *Br J Gen Pract.* 2001;51:635–637.

Guest J, Greenier M, Robinson A, et al. Impacted cerumen: composition, production, epidemiology and management. *Q JM.* 2004;97(8):477–488.

Hedgard-Jansen J, Bonding P. Experimental pressure induced rupture of the tympanic membrane in man. *Acta Otolaryng.* 1993;109:62–67.

Memel D, Langley C, Watkins C. Effectiveness of ear syringing in general practice. *Br J Gen Pract.* 2002;(Nov.): 906–911.

Sharp J, Wilson J. Ear wax removal: a survey of current practice. *Br Med J.* 1990;301:1251–1253.

Sorensen VZ, Bonding P. Can ear irrigation cause rupture of the normal tympanic membrane? *J Laryngol Otol.* 1991;101:75–78.

Zikk D, Lane B, Birchall M, et al. Invasive external otitis after removal of impacted cerumen by irrigation. *N Engl J Med.* 1991;325(13):969–970.

2008 MAG Mutual Healthcare Solutions, Inc.'s Physicians' Fee and Coding Guide. Duluth, Georgia. MAG Mutual Healthcare Solutions, Inc. 2007.

CHAPTER 97

Chalazia Removal

Thomas B. Redens, MD

Director, Cornea/External Disease/Refractive Surgery LSUHSC-Shreveport
Program Director, LSUHSC Dept Ophthalmology-Shreveport, Shreveport, LA

Chalazia appear as chronic subcutaneous nodules of the eyelid. Chalazia develop from obstruction of the meibomian gland duct at the eyelid margin and almost always have a radial orientation to the lid margin. Leaking sebaceous material from an engorged, obstructed gland induces lipogranulomatous inflammation. Chalazia usually are sterile, although lesions frequently become secondarily infected.

Chalazia are often confused with hordeolums or styes. Hordeolums are associated with infection of a meibomian gland (or other accessory eyelid gland) and manifest as suddenly appearing, erythematous, tender lumps in the eyelids that usually form abscesses and drain spontaneously. Although hordeolums usually are self-limited, they can evolve into chalazia with chronicity.

Keeping in mind two important differentiators between chalazia and hordeola will minimize diagnostic confusion: (1) Hordeola are quite painful, while chalazia are usually painless, and (2) Chalazia are chronic, while hordeola are usually acute. Chalazia often appear in individuals with skin disorders such as seborrheic dermatitis or rosacea and are highly associated with blepharitis.

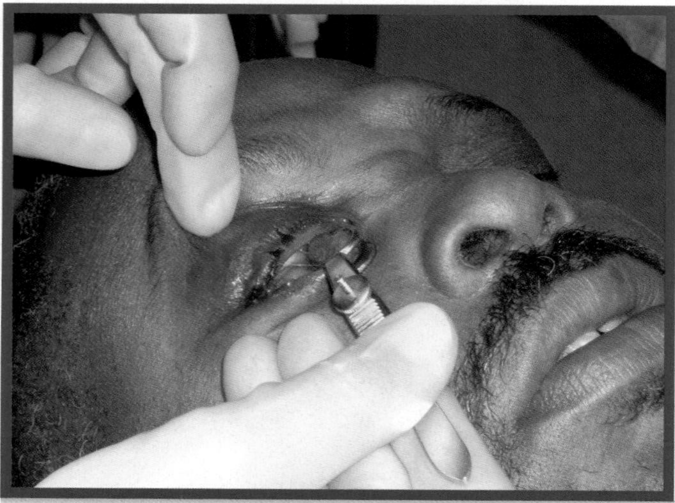

Conservative care is frequently all that is needed for successful treatment of chalazia, as opening of the duct will often result in resolution of the inflammation. The application of warm moist compresses four times daily should be the initial therapy. Patients are instructed to use a clean washcloth soaked in hot water (emphasize—not scalding!) and to hold this washcloth against their closed eyes. When the water cools, the patient is to reheat the washcloth and repeat the compress. This should be done for several minutes. Along with the compresses, basic lid hygiene is essential. The patient should use baby shampoo for lid scrubs by placing a drop of the shampoo on their fingertip and gently massages the lid margin/lash line while the eye is closed. More than one third of lesions will resolve over 3 months with this therapy, although usually 1 month of warm compress therapy is usually sufficient to identify those who will respond to conservative management.

The second tier of conservative therapy is antibiotic therapy. The most commonly used agents are tetracycline (250 mg BID) or doxycycline (100 mg qd). Usually, results are seen within 1 to 2 months after starting this therapy. Antibiotic therapy is quite useful in preventing recurrence, and the patient must continue the regimen of warm compresses and lid hygiene. Importantly, prior to initiation of either warm compresses/lid hygiene with or without antibiotic therapy, the clinician should physically palpate the chalazia—if the nodule is hard, more aggressive measures are needed.

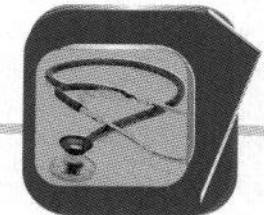

Equipment

For intralesional steroid injections:

- Tuberculin syringe with a 30-gauge needle
- 0.05 to 0.2 mL triamcinolone (5 mg/dL)
- Proparacaine 1% or tetracaine 0.5%

For incision and curettage:

- 1% lidocaine without epinephrine
- Proparacaine 1% or tetracaine 0.5%
- Plastic corneal shield
- Ophthalmic ointment
- Chalazion forceps
- No. 11 blade
- Chalazion currette

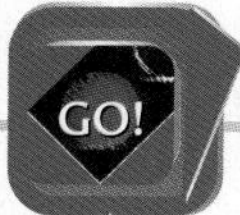

Indications

- Chronic internal eyelid nodules, often with recurrent nature
- Cosmetic deformity from chalazia
- Chronic irritation from chalazia
- Visual disturbance (induction of astigmatism) from chalazia

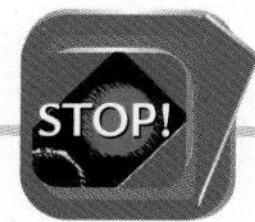

Contraindications

- Hordeolums (self-limited)
- Chalazia that have not undergone conservative management
- Chalazia associated with chronic unilateral blepharitis or loss of eyelashes due to the possibility of malignancy—especially sebaceous cell carcinoma
- Chalazia associated with cicatrizing eye disorders (i.e., ocular cicatricial pemphigoid, Stevens-Johnson syndrome)
- Darkly pigmented patients (depigmentation associated with intralesional steroid)

The Procedure

Intralesional Triamcinolone

Step 1. Stabilize the patient's head. The patient should be in the supine position, and an assistant may be needed to immobilize the patient's head. Inject 0.05 to 0.2 mL of the triamcinolone solution into the chalazion. If using the external approach, position the needle obliquely to avoid possible injury to the globe.

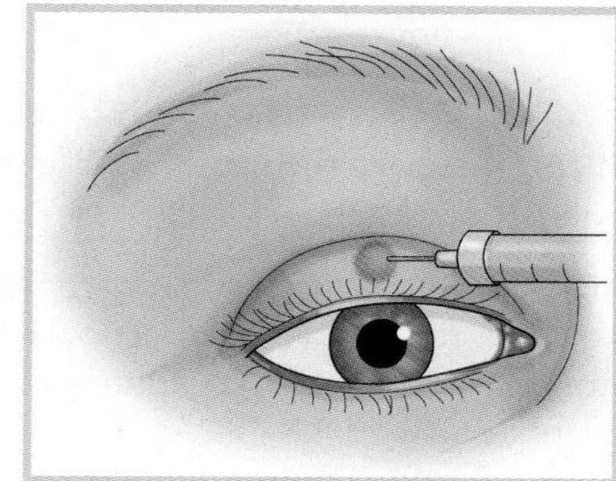

Step 1

Step 2. If approaching internally, administer 1 drop of anesthetic (proparacaine or tetracaine), and stabilize the lid. Instilling gel lidocaine (2% to 4%) into the inferior cul-de-sac and having the patient keep the eyes closed for several minutes prior to the injection allows good conjunctival anesthesia and substantially decreases patient discomfort. Use gentle pressure over the injection site to minimize bleeding.

- **PEARL:** Remember to include skin depigmentation and ocular injury in the consent.

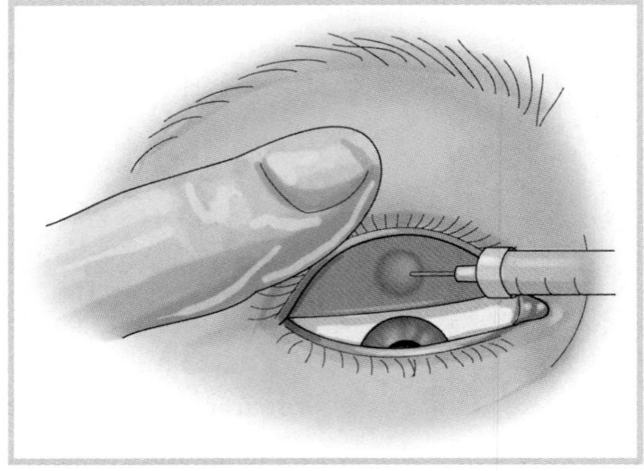

Step 2

Incision and Curettage

Step 1. Stabilize the patient's head. The patient should be in the supine position, and an assistant may be needed to immobilize the patient's head. The use of gel lidocaine is strongly encouraged. The figure shows a patient with a large inferonasal chalazion (with a small external component that has been partially expressed). Place a plastic corneal shield following the topical anesthesia. The shield is placed by having the patient look down while the clinician gently elevates the upper lid and then slides the shield under the upper lid. A suction cup device is also available for placement and removal of the corneal shield.

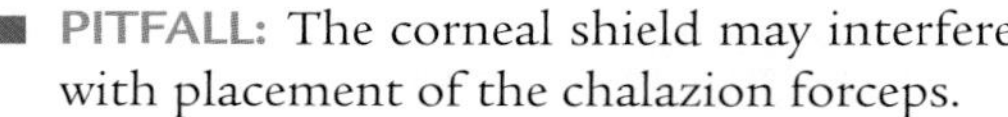

- **PITFALL:** The corneal shield may interfere with placement of the chalazion forceps.

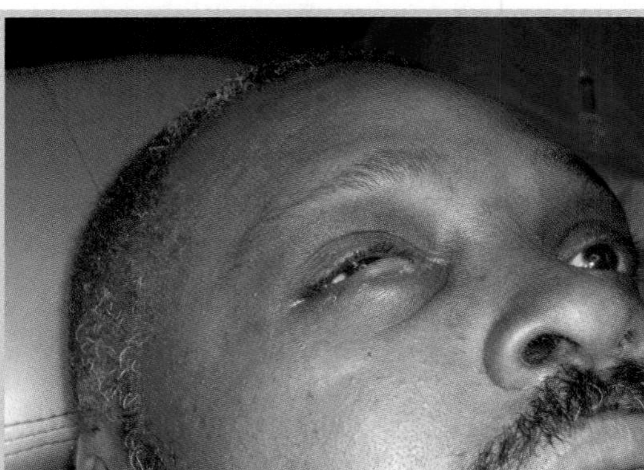

Step 1

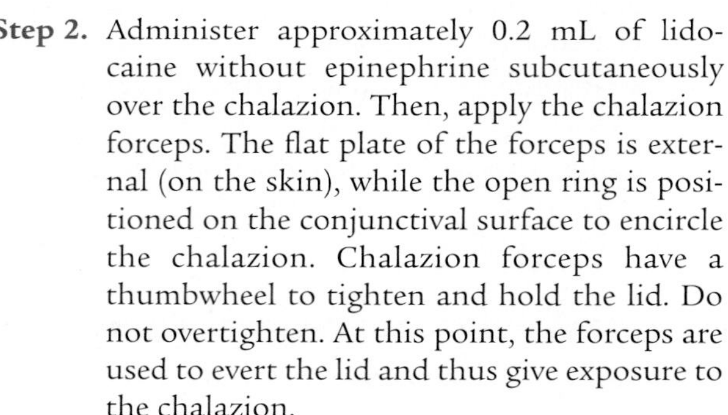

Step 2. Administer approximately 0.2 mL of lidocaine without epinephrine subcutaneously over the chalazion. Then, apply the chalazion forceps. The flat plate of the forceps is external (on the skin), while the open ring is positioned on the conjunctival surface to encircle the chalazion. Chalazion forceps have a thumbwheel to tighten and hold the lid. Do not overtighten. At this point, the forceps are used to evert the lid and thus give exposure to the chalazion.

- **PITFALL:** This step usually gives incomplete anesthesia, as the tarsus is difficult to completely anesthetize.
- **PEARL:** Use great care in everting the eyelid using these forceps, as disinsertion of the levator may occur with resultant permanent ptosis.

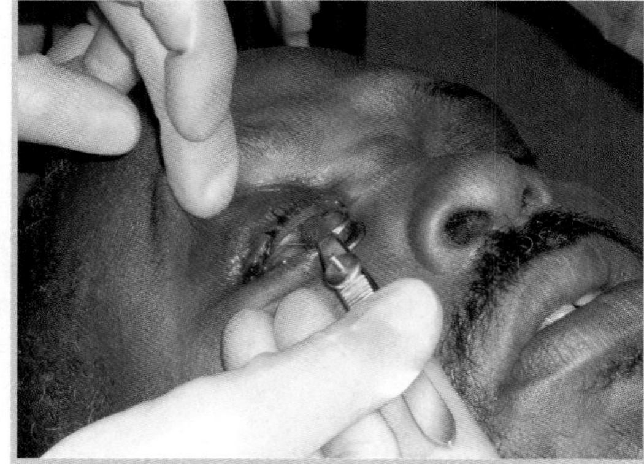

Step 2

Step 3. Using the no. 11 blade, carefully incise over the chalazion (3 mm usually is adequate). Do not make the incision full thickness (through to the skin) or through the lid margin.

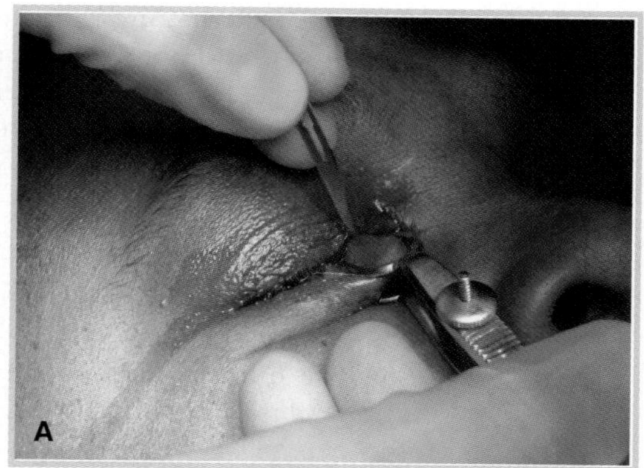

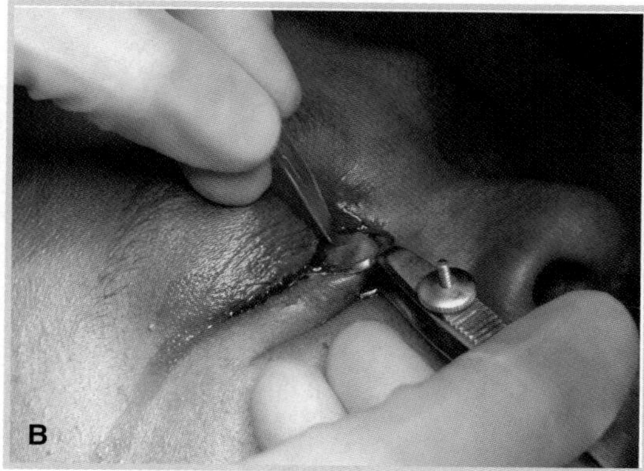

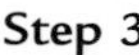

Step 3

Step 4. Using the chalazion curette, gently remove all the lipogranulomatous inflammatory material from the cavity, including scraping all walls.

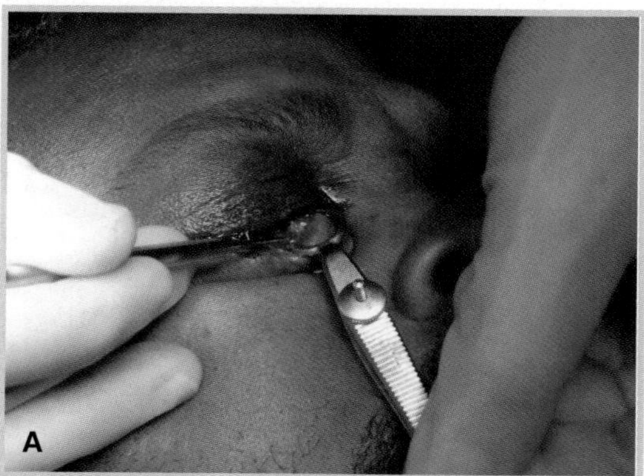

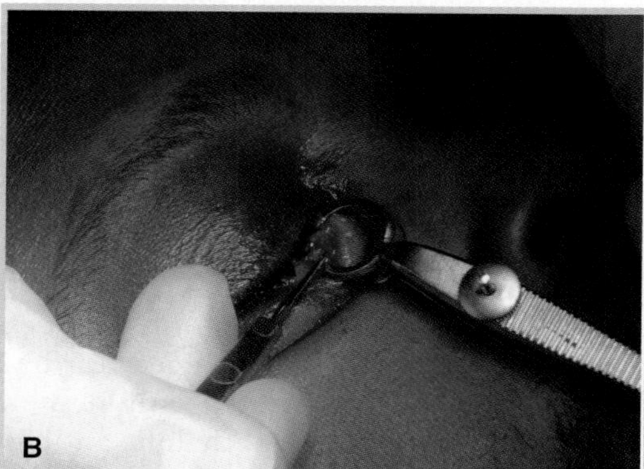

Step 4

Step 5. Carefully remove both the curette and the forceps from the lid, and apply gentle pressure with gauze. The figure shows the patient's lid after completion of the curettage, with gentle pressure being applied to the site with a cotton-tipped applicator.

- **PITFALL:** Note that with intralesional steroid injection or incision and curettage, have the patient sit up slowly. Vasovagal reactions are quite common with these procedures.

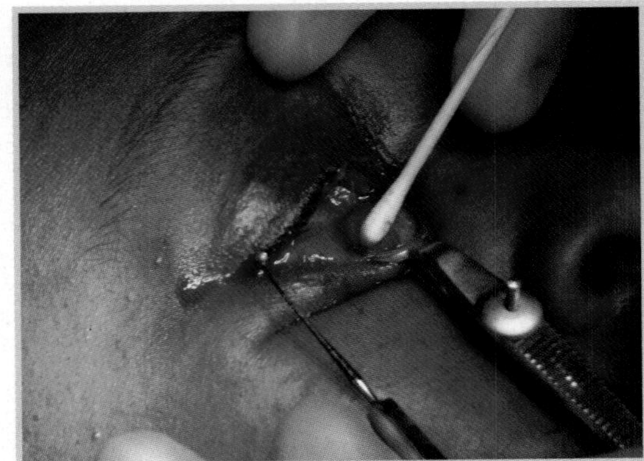

Step 5

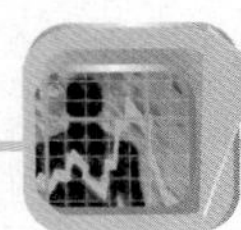

Complications

- Recurrence of chalazion
- Skin depigmentation (in darkly pigmented individuals)
- Infections (uncommon secondary to the rich vascular supply of the lids)
- Bleeding (ask the patient about anticoagulant medications or bleeding disorders)—also usually not a significant problem
- Ptosis (after use of chalazion forceps)—more common in the elderly
- Conjunctival scarring—rare, associated with large incisions and other ocular diseases (i.e., ocular cicatricial pemphigoid).
- Central retinal artery occlusion (rare)—associated with periocular steroid injections (including the lids)
- Ocular injury

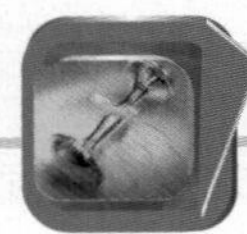

Pediatric Considerations

Generally, children (or the mentally challenged) with chalazia require general anesthesia for either injection or incision and curettage. The same procedures and complications apply.

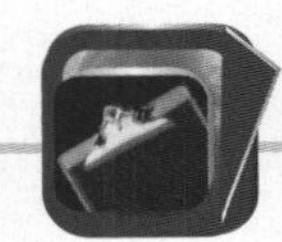

Postprocedure Instructions

Instruct patients to call or return immediately if any change in vision, significant swelling, purulence, or excessive bleeding occurs. Reassure patients that a small amount of blood-tinged tearing and a mild foreign body sensation with blinking is normal (associated with incision and curettage). Patients often are more comfortable with a TID ophthalmic antibiotic following incision and curettage, although its use is not mandated.

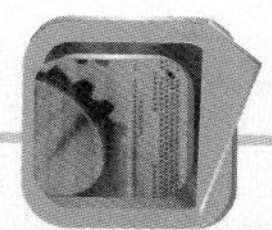

Coding Information and Supply Sources

CPT Code	Description	2008 Average 50th Percentile Fee	Global Period
67800	Excision of chalazion, single	$283.00	10
67801	Excision of chalazia, multiple, same lid	$450.00	10
67805	Excision of chalazia, multiple, different lids	$539.00	10
67808	Excision under general anesthesia or requiring hospitalization	$892.00	90

CPT is a registered trademark of the American Medical Association.
2008 average 50th Percentile Fees are provided courtesy of 2008 MMH-SI's copyrighted Physicians' Fees and Coding Guide.

Common ICD-9 Code

Chalazion 373.2

Supplies

- Chalazion forceps and curettes may be obtained from Katena Products, Inc., 4 Stewart Court, Denville, NJ 07834 USA (800-225-1195; http://www.katena.com).
- Other instruments and supplies may be found in Appendix G.

Patient Education Handout

A patient education handout, "Chalazion," can be found on the book's Web site.

Bibliography

Epstein GA, Putterman AM. Combined excision and drainage with intralesional corticosteroid injection in the treatment of chronic chalazia. *Arch Opthalmol.* 1988;106:514–516.

Mannis MJ, Macsai MS, Huntley AC. *Eye and Skin Disease*. Philadelphia: Lippincott-Raven Publishers; 1996:644–647.

Ostler HB, Maibach HI, Hoke AW, et al. *Diseases of the Eye and Skin—A Color Atlas*. Philadelphia: Lippincott Williams & Wilkins; 2004:183, 196–197.

Vidaurri LJ, Pe'er J. Intralesional corticosteroid treatment of chalazia. *Ann Ophthalmol.* 1986;18:339–340.

2008 MAG Mutual Healthcare Solutions, Inc.'s Physicians' Fee and Coding Guide. Duluth, Georgia. MAG Mutual Healthcare Solutions, Inc. 2007.

CHAPTER 98

Conjunctival and Corneal Foreign Object Removal

E. J. Mayeaux Jr., MD, DABFP, FAAFP

Professor of Family Medicine, Professor of Obstetrics and Gynecology
Louisiana State University Health Sciences Center, Shreveport, LA

Man T. Ton, MD

Third Year Family Medicine Resident
Louisiana State University Health Sciences Center, Shreveport, LA

Conjunctival and corneal foreign objects are commonly seen problems in the primary care office and in the emergency department. Removal of the foreign object is usually easy accomplished and can be performed in the outpatient setting. When a patient presents, document a thorough history including job type, the condition of the eye before injury, probable type of foreign body (especially if it may be iron based), mechanism of injury, and whether first aid was rendered. Always test and document the patient's vision before and after treatment. Use a Snellen chart or an equivalent visual acuity chart if possible.

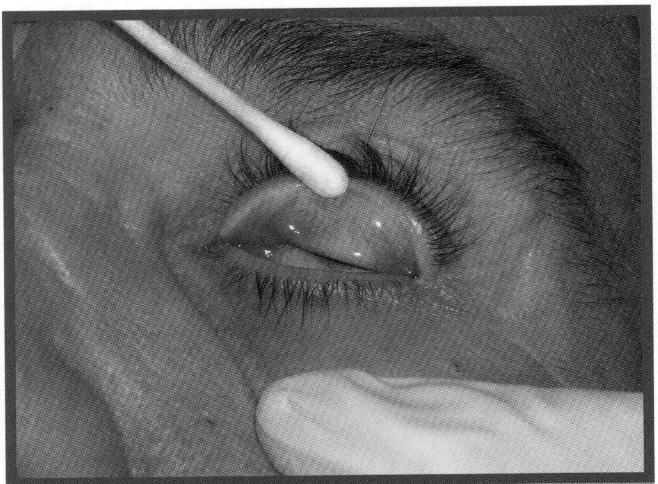

Because of the risk of complications, obtaining informed consent is a necessity prior to treatment. Possible complications of foreign body removal include infection, incomplete removal of a foreign body, perforation of the cornea, scarring, and permanent visual impairment. Special care must be taken with iron-based foreign objects, because rust is toxic to the cornea and may prevent it from healing.

The corneal and conjunctival epithelia are some of the fastest-healing areas of the body. If considerable progress toward healing has not been made within 24 hours of foreign body extraction, re-examine for additional foreign bodies or signs of infection. Pain may be an important indicator of developing corneal ulceration or the presence of an additional foreign body. Therefore, local anesthetic drops and topical steroids should not be prescribed for outpatient use. The other reasons to avoid local anesthetic drops are because they may retard corneal healing and might lead to corneal perforation. They are often used during mechanical removal of foreign objects in the clinical setting only.

If the patient has significant pain, consider using a cycloplegic agent to decrease spasm of the iris. Apply antibiotic drops or ointment for prophylaxis. An ointment may be better than drops because of its lubricant effect and ability to help reduce disruption of the newly generated epithelium. Oral pain medication should be prescribed as indicated. Instruct the patient not to rub the eye, because it may disrupt the new epithelial layers of the cornea.

Traditionally, eye patches were applied, on the theory that they decreased photophobia, tearing, foreign body sensation, pain, and healing time. However, studies indicate that patching does not improve pain scores, healing times, or treatment outcomes. It may also decrease patient compliance with treatment plans.

Clinicians must use extreme caution when attempting to remove foreign objects by mechanical means such as cotton-tipped applicators or needles. Object removal is most successful in cases of recent, superficial foreign bodies. Any downward pressure on the object may result in more damage to the epithelium or deeper layers. If clinicians are unsure of their ability to remove an object without exerting downward pressure on it, the patient should be referred to an ophthalmologist for removal.

Re-epithelialization is complete in 3 to 4 days for more than 90% of patients, but it can take weeks. Re-examine every 24 hours until the eye is healed. Perform and document a visual acuity test on the last visit. Continue antibiotic drops or ointment for an additional 3 days after the eye is free of symptoms. The patient may be unusually receptive at this time to education about eye safety measures such as protective eyewear. If the pain increases at any time during the follow-up or signs of conjunctival or orbital infection are seen, immediately refer the patient to an ophthalmologist.

It is important to know when to refer patients to an ophthalmologist to decrease the risk of impaired vision or blindness. Indications for immediate referral include an intraocular presence of an object, a large corneal epithelial defect, a corneal infiltrate or white spot, corneal opacity, or a purulent discharge. The patient should also be referred to an ophthalmologist immediately for any chemical injury, or if pain or functional impairment persists after irrigation. Possible acid or alkali contamination of the eye is a true ophthalmologic emergency.

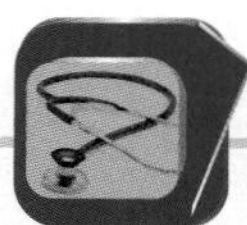

Equipment

- A Snellen chart or equivalent visual acuity chart can be obtained from Premier Medical, P. O. Box 4132, Kent, WA 98032. Phone: 1-800-955-2774. Web site: http://premieremedical.safeshopper.com
- Medications: topical ophthalmic anesthetic (e.g., tetracaine [Pontocaine] or proparacaine [Opthetic]), cycloplegic drops, topical antibiotics ointment (e.g., erythromycin [Ilotycin], bacitracin, or sulfacetamide).
- Magnification devices, loupes, and Wood's lights may be ordered from medical supply companies. Fluorescein strips may be ordered from pharmacies.
- Other materials: cotton-tipped swabs, hypodermic needle (26 gauge), sterile water, bag of normal saline with IV drip tubing, ophthalmoscope.

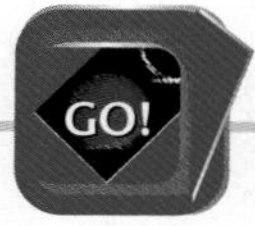

Indications

- Small, conjunctival, or corneal foreign bodies embedded <24 hours

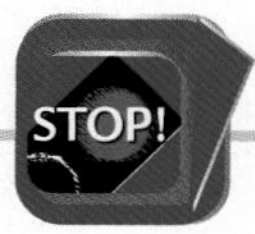

Contraindications

- Foreign bodies embedded in the cornea for >24 hours (i.e., risk of infection)
- Iron-based foreign bodies, which may cause a rust ring (relative contraindication)
- Uncooperative patient
- Deeply or centrally embedded foreign bodies (i.e., ophthalmologic referral)

- Possible acid or alkali contamination of the eye (i.e., ophthalmologic emergency)
- Ruptured globe (i.e., ophthalmologic emergency)
- Hyphema, lens opacification, abnormal anterior chamber examination, or irregularity of the pupil (i.e., possible ruptured globe, which is an ophthalmologic emergency)
- Signs or symptoms of infection (i.e., ophthalmologic referral)

The Procedure

Step 1. Check and record the patient's visual acuity using a Snellen chart.

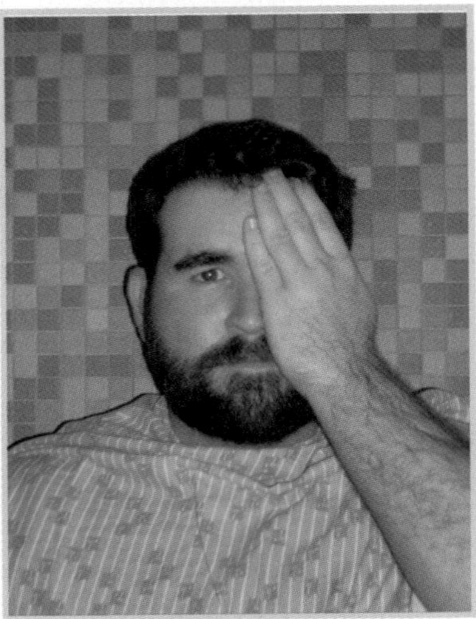

Step 1

Step 2. Position the patient in the supine position. For corneal foreign bodies, position the patient's head so that the foreign body and the eye are in the most elevated position. For conjunctival foreign bodies, position the head to give the examiner maximal access to the affected area.

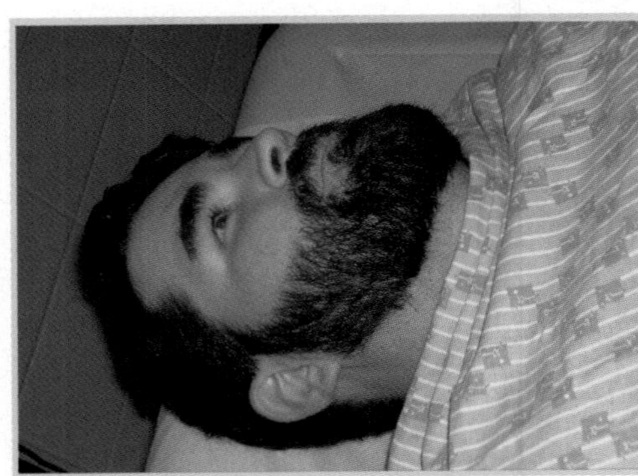

Step 2

Step 3. Hold the patient's eyelids apart with your thumb and index finger of the nondominant hand. Ask the patient to fix and maintain his or her gaze on a distant object and to hold the head as motionless as possible throughout the procedure.

- **PEARL:** A wire eye speculum may be used but usually is not available in primary care offices.

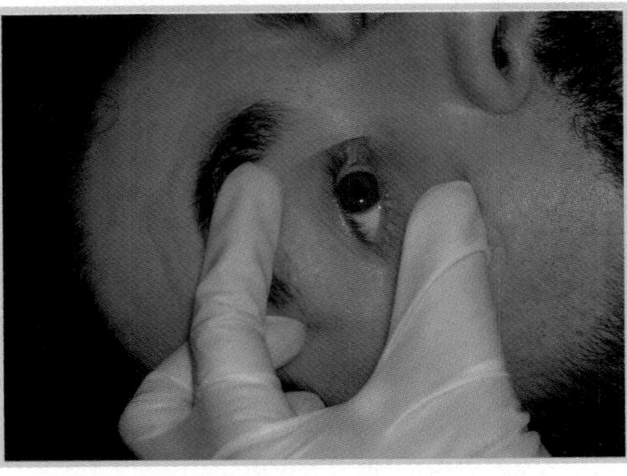

Step 3

Step 4. If a foreign body under the lid is suspected, evert the eyelid by placing the cotton-tipped swab on top of the lid and roll the lid over the swab.

- **PITFALL:** Vertical scratches on the cornea may indicate a foreign body embedded in the upper lid, necessitating eyelid eversion and examination with a cotton-tipped applicator.

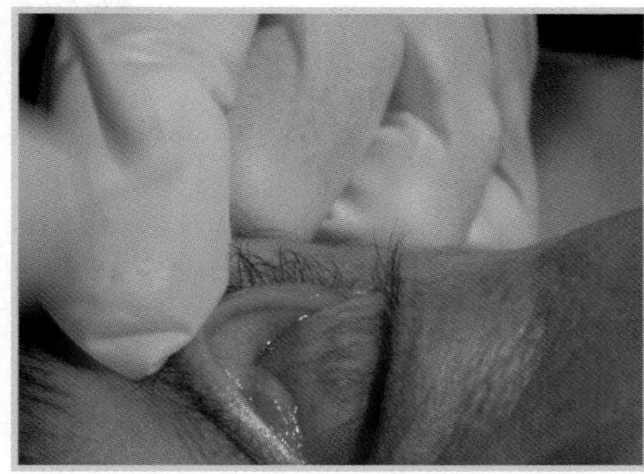

Step 4

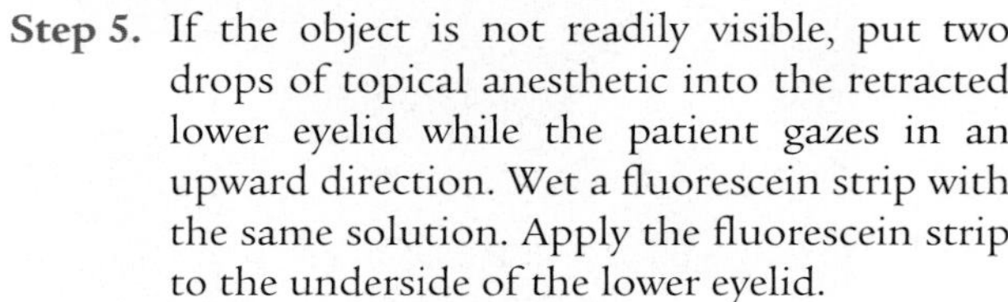

Step 5. If the object is not readily visible, put two drops of topical anesthetic into the retracted lower eyelid while the patient gazes in an upward direction. Wet a fluorescein strip with the same solution. Apply the fluorescein strip to the underside of the lower eyelid.

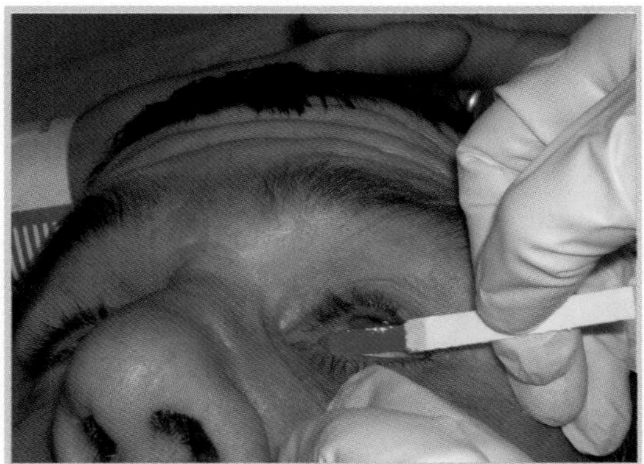

Step 5

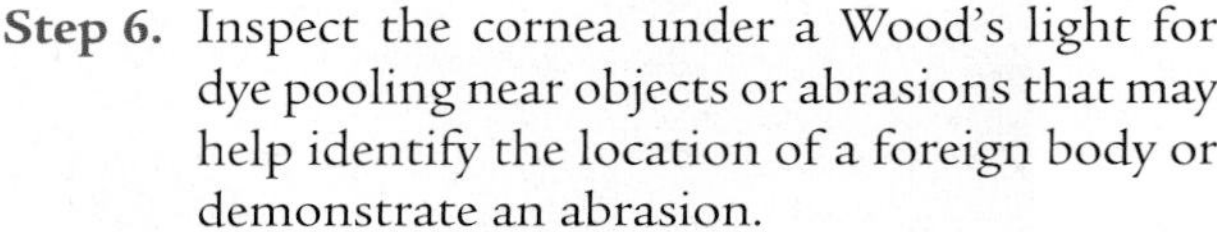

Step 6. Inspect the cornea under a Wood's light for dye pooling near objects or abrasions that may help identify the location of a foreign body or demonstrate an abrasion.

- **PITFALL:** Putting drops directly on a scratched cornea can be very painful.

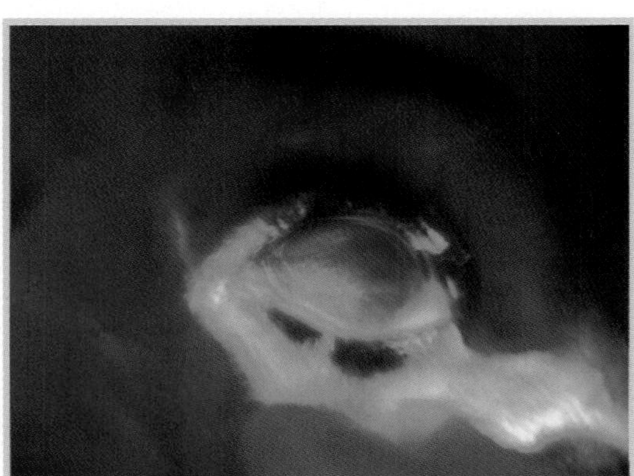

Step 6

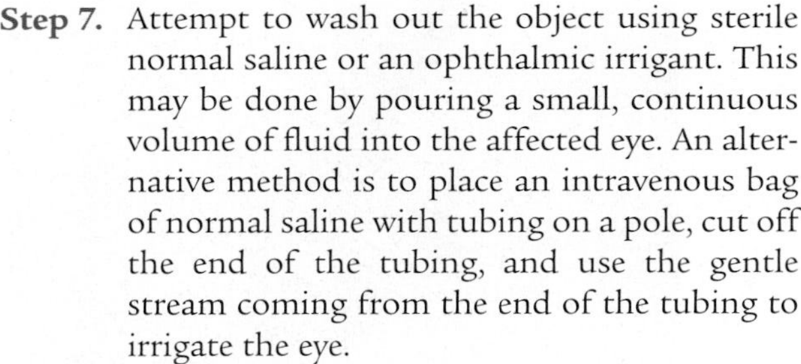

Step 7. Attempt to wash out the object using sterile normal saline or an ophthalmic irrigant. This may be done by pouring a small, continuous volume of fluid into the affected eye. An alternative method is to place an intravenous bag of normal saline with tubing on a pole, cut off the end of the tubing, and use the gentle stream coming from the end of the tubing to irrigate the eye.

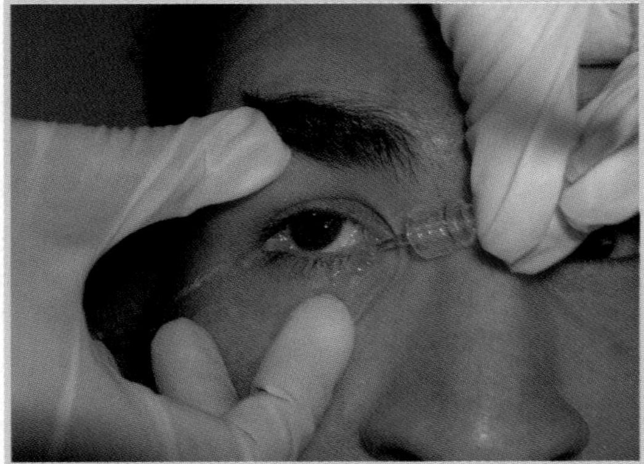

Step 7

Step 8. If this is unsuccessful, attempt to dislodge the object using a cotton-tipped applicator or corner of a soft cotton gauze. Moisten the cotton with local anesthetic, and gently lift the object by lightly touching it.

- PITFALL: Never use force or rub the cornea because this can produce pain, damage the epithelium, and cause deeper corneal injuries.

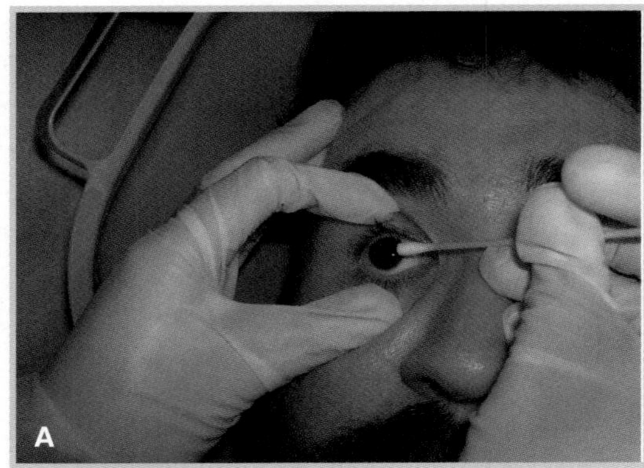

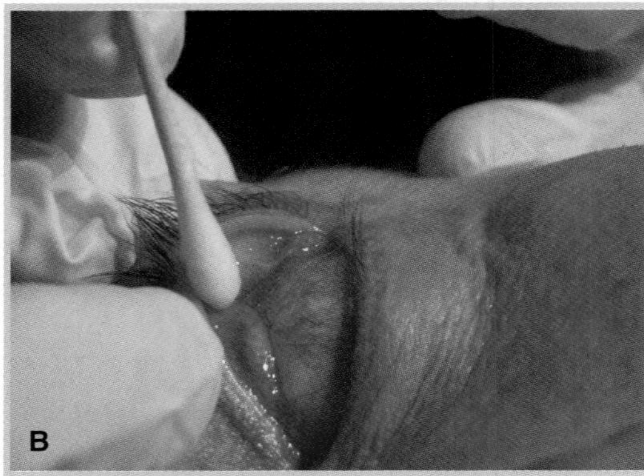

Step 8

Step 9. If the object is still lodged, a sterile needle may be used to remove the object. Place a 26-gauge needle on a tuberculin syringe and hold it in with a pencil grip. Stabilize your operating hand on the patient's brow or zygomatic arch. Approach the object with the needle bevel upward from a tangential direction.

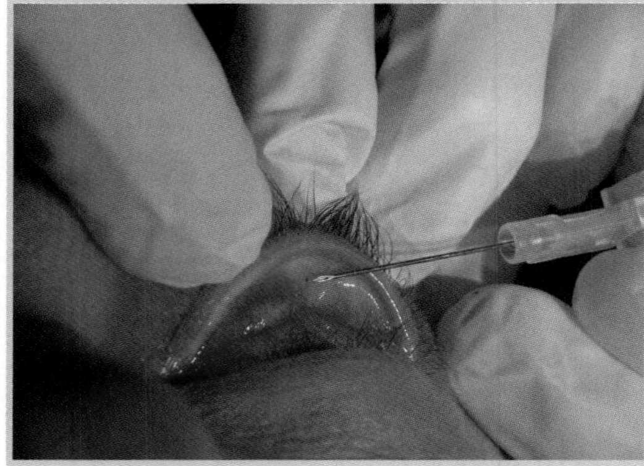

Step 9

Step 10. Use the needle tip to gently lift the object. Turn the patient's head laterally, and copiously irrigate the eye. Retest and record the patient's visual acuity.

- PITFALL: If the object cannot be readily removed, refer the patient for removal under slit lamp by an ophthalmologist.
- PITFALL: If any residual corneal rust is found, immediately refer the patient to an ophthalmologist because rust is toxic to the corneal epithelium.

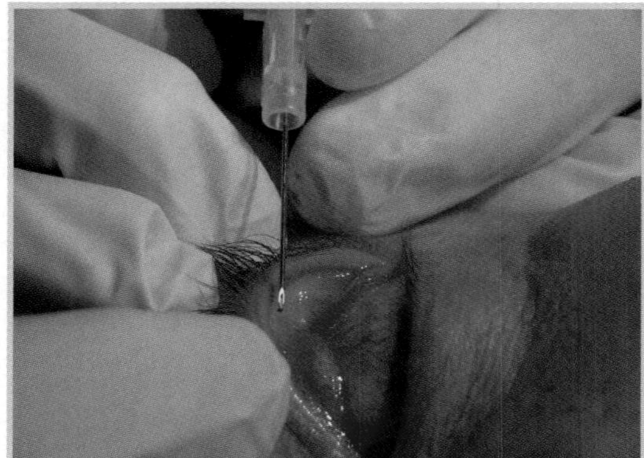

Step 10

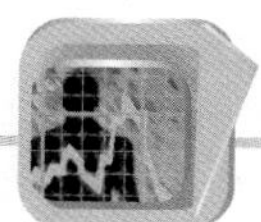

Complications

- Infection
- Perforation of the cornea
- Scarring
- Visual impairment
- Corneal ulceration

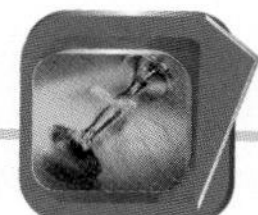

Pediatric Considerations

The history is less specific, because the child might not be able to describe the symptoms or the mechanism of the injury. Any time a child cannot or refuses to open an eye, penetrating trauma must be ruled out. After that, an attempt to measure visual acuity with an age-appropriate technique is recommended. Topical ophthalmic anesthetic can be used to facilitate the examination, which is similar to that in an adult. Warn the child and the parents that the anesthetic will cause a burning sensation at first.

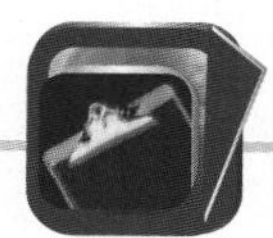

Postprocedure Instructions

For small abrasions (<3 mm), no follow-up is necessary if the patient's vision is good. Contact-lens-related abrasions required daily follow-up until the abrasion is healed to avoid ulceration. Large abrasions (>3 mm) with a symptom of decreasing vision require close follow-up.

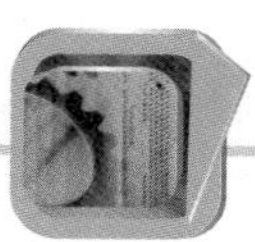

Coding Information and Supply Sources

CPT Code	Description	2008 Average 50th Percentile Fee	Global Period
65205	Removal of foreign body, external eye, conjunctivally superficial	$161.00	0
65210	Removal of foreign body, external eye, conjunctivally embedded	$207.00	0
65220	Removal of foreign body, external eye, corneal without slit lamp	$196.00	0
65222	Removal of foreign body, corneal with slit lamp	$248.00	0

CPT is a registered trademark of the American Medical Association.
2008 average 50th Percentile Fees are provided courtesy of 2008 MMH-SI's copyrighted Physicians' Fees and Coding Guide.

All of the necessary supplies can be obtained from hospital supply houses or pharmacies.

Patient Education Handout

A patient education handout, "Conjunctival and Corneal Foreign Object Removal," can be found on the book's companion Web site.

Bibliography

Appen RE, Hutson CE. Traumatic injuries: office treatment of eye injury, 1: injury due to foreign materials. *Postgrad Med.* 1976;60:223–225, 237.

Gumus K, Karakucuks, Mirza E. Corneal injury from a metallic foreign body—an occupational hazard. *Eye Contact Lens.* 2007;33(5):259–260.

Holt GR, Holt JE. Management of orbital trauma and foreign bodies. *Otolaryngol Clin North Am.* 1988;21:35–52.

Kaiser PK. A comparison of pressure patching versus no patching for corneal abrasions due to trauma or foreign body removal: Corneal Abrasion Patching Study Group. *Ophthalmology.* 1995;102:1936–1942.

Le Sage N, Verreault R, Rochette L. Efficacy of eye patching for traumatic corneal abrasions: a controlled clinical trial. *Ann Emerg Med.* 2001;38:129–134.

Nayeen N, Stansfield D. Management of corneal foreign bodies in A&E departments. *Arch Emerg Med.* 1992;9:257.

Newell SW. Management of corneal foreign bodies. *Am Fam Physician.* 1985;31:149–156.

Owens JK, Scibilia J, Hezoucky N. Corneal foreign bodies—first aid, treatment, and outcomes: skills review for an occupational health setting. *AAOHN J.* 2001;49:226–230.

Peate WF. Work related eye injuries and illnesses. *Am Fam Physician.* 2007;75:7.

Reich JA. Removal of corneal foreign bodies. *Aust Fam Physician.* 1990;19:719–721.

Stout A. Corneal abrasion. *Pediatric Rev.* 2006;27:11.

2008 MAG Mutual Healthcare Solutions, Inc.'s Physicians' Fee and Coding Guide. Duluth, Georgia. MAG Mutual Healthcare Solutions, Inc. 2007.

CHAPTER 99

Flexible Fiber-Optic Nasolaryngoscopy

T. S. Lian, MD FACS
Associate Professor of Otolaryngology-Head and Neck Surgery
Louisiana State University Health Sciences Center, Shreveport, LA

Flexible fiber-optic nasolaryngoscopy is useful technique to allow for a thorough examination of the hypopharynx and larynx. As the fiber-optic endoscope is passed through the nasal cavity and the nasopharynx, these areas are easily examined as well. Direct examination of the areas can provide for a more thorough examination as opposed to indirect techniques such as mirror examination as well as more limited examination using a nasal speculum.

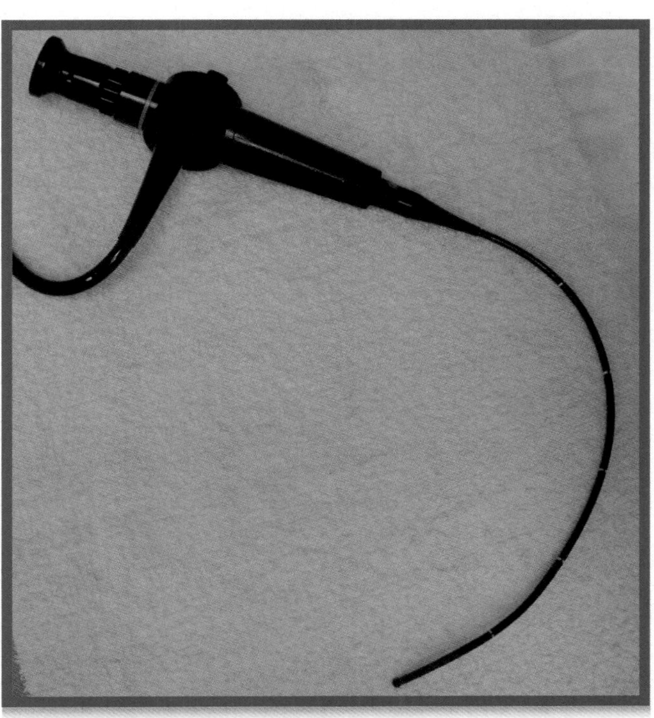

A thorough understanding of the anatomy of the nasal cavity, nasopharynx, hypopharynx, and larynx is necessary in order to completely realize the utility of flexible fiber-optic nasolaryngoscopy. Anatomical structures that can be identified and used as landmarks for orientation when passing the scope via the nasal cavity include the floor of the nose, nasal septum, and inferior turbinate. Similarly, familiarity with the nasopharyngeal opening of the eustachian tubes and posterior nasopharyngeal wall as well as the nasal side of the soft palate is necessary when advancing the scope.

Flexible fiber-optic nasolaryngoscopy is not only useful in the identification of pathology such as masses, but it is also a dynamic examination, as the movement of the soft palate and the vocal cords can be assessed. Another useful feature of flexible fiber-optic nasolaryngoscopy is that a recording of the exam can be made when the scope is attached to a camera. This documentation is useful, as previous examinations can be reviewed and compared.

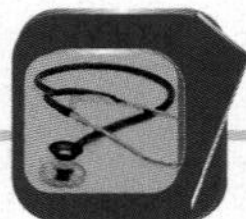

Equipment

- Numerous flexible fiber-optic laryngoscopes are available; however, they all have basic common features, including a monocular eye piece for viewing; hand piece with controls to flex the tip of the scope; and the fiber-optic bundle, which is inserted during examination. The diameter of most fiber-optic bundles range from 3 to 4 mm, with the working length typically being up to 300 mm. A light source is also required.

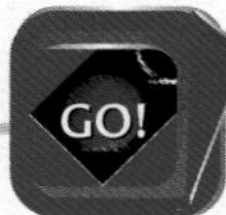

Indications

- Odynophagia
- Dysphagia
- Hemoptysis
- Dysphonia (hoarseness)
- Dyspnea
- Stridor
- Epistaxis
- Chronic nasal airway obstruction
- Foreign body
- Unilateral serous otitis media in an adult

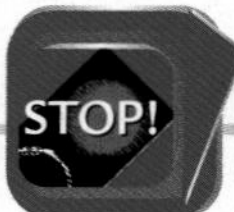

Contraindications

- Uncooperative patient
- Intractable bleeding
- Impeding airway collapse
- Suspected epiglottitis/supraglottitis in a child

The Procedure

Step 1. Obtain informed consented. Ask the patient if breathing is better through one side of the nose relative to the other. If there is a perceived difference, one should plan on introducing and passing the scope through the side of the nose that is easier to breathe through. Topical decongestant spray such as phenylephrine (Neo-Synephrine) or oxymetazoline (Afrin) as well as an anesthetic such as 4% topical lidocaine is insufflated into the nasal cavity. Benzocaine spray can also be sprayed into the oral cavity and oropharynx for further anesthetic effect.

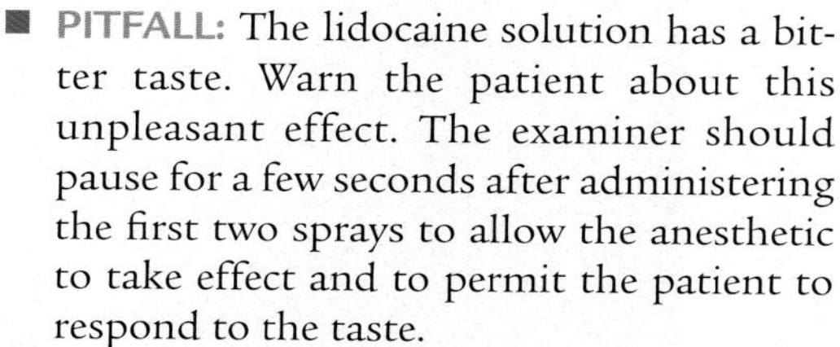

- PITFALL: The lidocaine solution has a bitter taste. Warn the patient about this unpleasant effect. The examiner should pause for a few seconds after administering the first two sprays to allow the anesthetic to take effect and to permit the patient to respond to the taste.

Step 2. The scope is typically held with the dominant hand guiding the fiber-optic bundle and the nondominant hand holding the eyepiece end of the scope and operating the flexion/extension control.

Step 3. The thumb is used to slide the deflection control to cause the tip of the scope to deflect up or down. Strong twisting action of the right first and second fingers torque the scope tip from its vertical motion to the right and left, and continued up-and-down movement of the left thumb facilitates right and left turning.

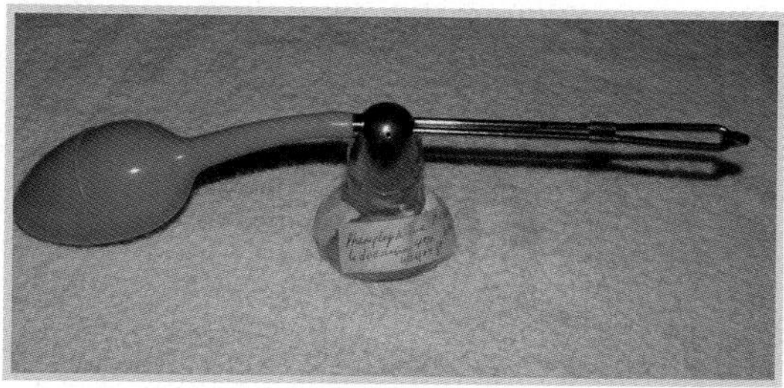

Step 1

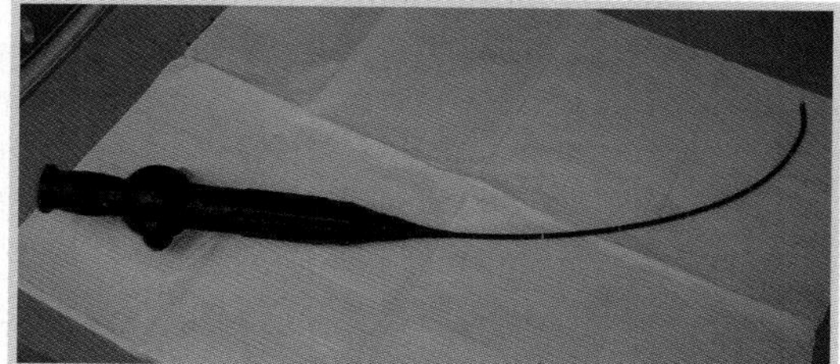

Step 2

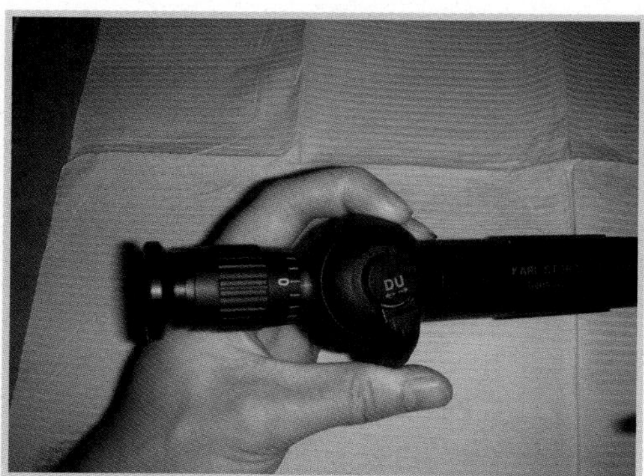

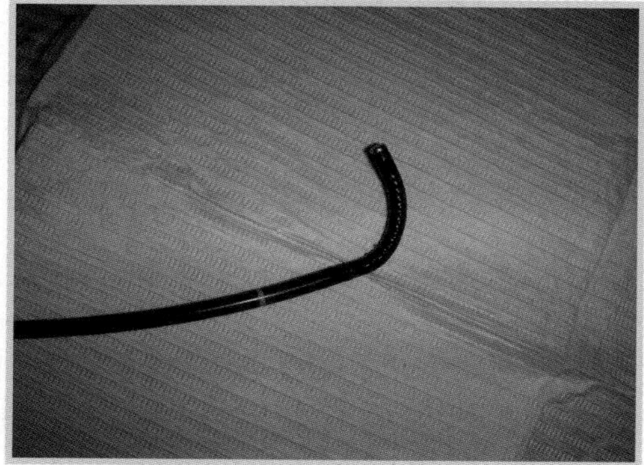

Step 3

Step 4. The patient assumes and maintains a sitting, upright "sniffing" position with the neck slightly extending, allowing for the chin to be slightly elevated.

- **PITFALL:** A patient's glasses can interfere with anchoring the hand to the patient's face or be hit during the procedure. Consider asking the patient to remove glasses before the procedure.

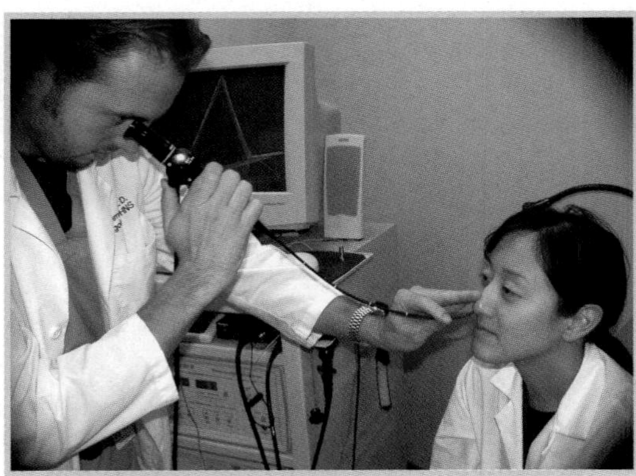

Step 4

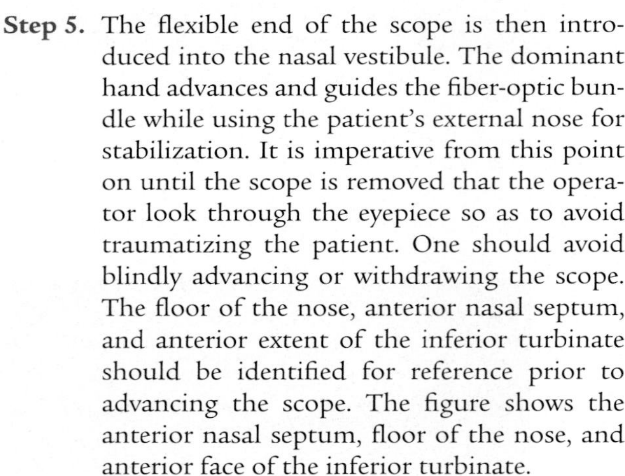

Step 5. The flexible end of the scope is then introduced into the nasal vestibule. The dominant hand advances and guides the fiber-optic bundle while using the patient's external nose for stabilization. It is imperative from this point on until the scope is removed that the operator look through the eyepiece so as to avoid traumatizing the patient. One should avoid blindly advancing or withdrawing the scope. The floor of the nose, anterior nasal septum, and anterior extent of the inferior turbinate should be identified for reference prior to advancing the scope. The figure shows the anterior nasal septum, floor of the nose, and anterior face of the inferior turbinate.

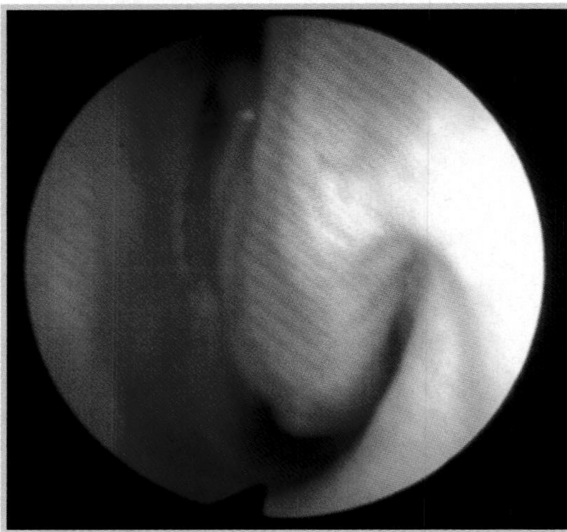

Step 5

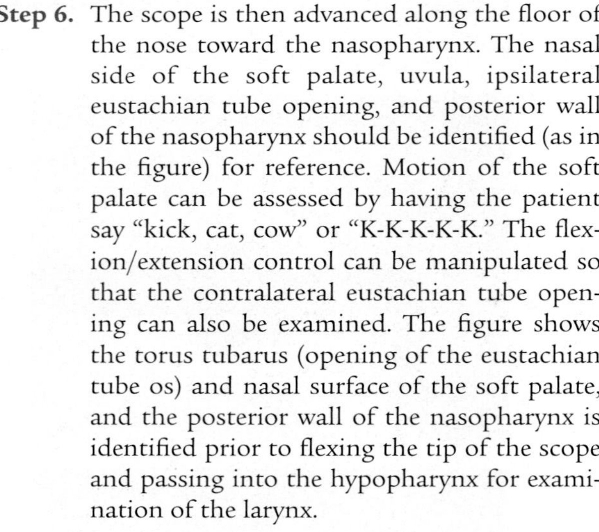

Step 6. The scope is then advanced along the floor of the nose toward the nasopharynx. The nasal side of the soft palate, uvula, ipsilateral eustachian tube opening, and posterior wall of the nasopharynx should be identified (as in the figure) for reference. Motion of the soft palate can be assessed by having the patient say "kick, cat, cow" or "K-K-K-K-K." The flexion/extension control can be manipulated so that the contralateral eustachian tube opening can also be examined. The figure shows the torus tubarus (opening of the eustachian tube os) and nasal surface of the soft palate, and the posterior wall of the nasopharynx is identified prior to flexing the tip of the scope and passing into the hypopharynx for examination of the larynx.

- **PITFALL:** During insertion of the endoscope, mucus can adhere and obscure the view through the scope. Gently tap the tip of the scope against the wall of the nasopharynx to clean the view on the scope. If the view becomes obscured while examining the larynx, have the patient swallow to clear the tip of the scope. It is almost never necessary to completely withdraw the scope to clear the lens.

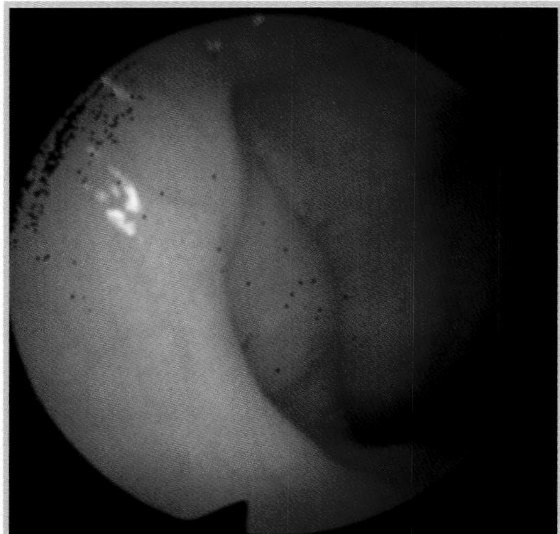

Step 6

Step 7. With the posterior wall of the nasopharynx in view, the tip of the scope is flexed down, and the scope is advanced into the oropharynx and hypopharynx. In this position, numerous anatomical structures can be examined to include the base of tongue, vallecula, lateral and posterior pharyngeal walls, epiglottis, aryepiglottic folds, arytenoids, true and false vocal folds, and the glottic aperture (and to a certain extent, the pyriform sinuses and subglottis). The vallecula and base of tongue may be better seen by having the patient stick out the tongue. Normal true vocal cords should appear white relative to the other more pink mucosal surfaces. The free edge of the true vocal cords are smooth and linear in the normal situation. Any irregularity in this area, such as a mass, would be expected to affect the normal vibratory nature of the true vocal cords and result in hoarseness. Assessment of true vocal cord motion can be made by having the patient say "eeee." In the normal circumstance, the true vocal cords approximate to the midline on phonation. Acute unilateral true vocal cord paresis or paralysis/immobility can result in incomplete approximation of the true vocal cords with a resultant weak and breathy voice. Frank aspiration of secretions may also be observed in the setting of unilateral vocal cord paralysis. Further assessment of true vocal cord abduction can be made by having the patient sniff in through the nose. In the absence of bilateral true vocal cord abduction, the patient may experience an element of stridor and/or dyspnea, which may require urgent securing of the airway, particularly in the acute setting of bilateral vocal cord paralysis. The posterior glottis should also be examined, as this area commonly appears thickened and relatively pale in cases of chronic laryngopharyngeal reflux or relatively erythematous in the acute situation. The procedure is completed by withdrawing the scope while looking through the eyepiece until the end of the scope has exited the nose.

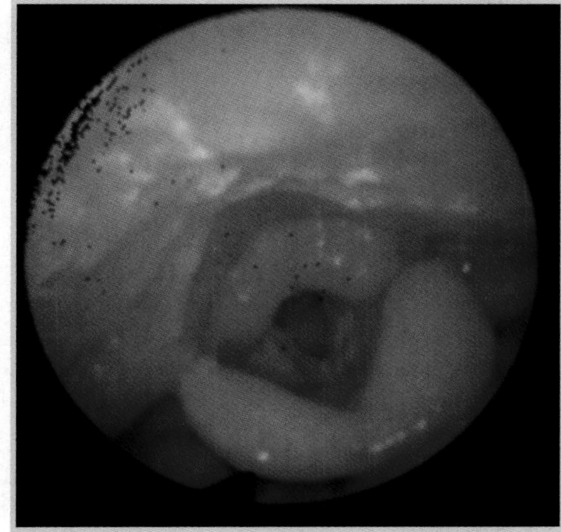

Step 7

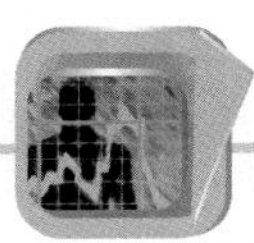

Complications

- Mucosal abrasion
- Bleeding
- Laryngospasm

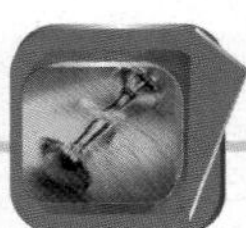

Pediatric Considerations

Flexible fiber-optic nasolaryngoscopy can be performed in children depending on cooperativity and availability of pediatric/neonatal flexible laryngoscopes. Such scopes have a relatively small fiber bundle diameter.

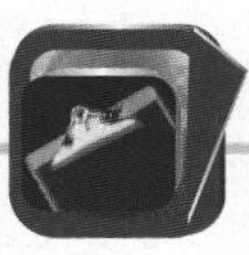

Postprocedure Instructions

Patients are instructed to refrain from eating and drinking for at least 45 minutes subsequent to the application of the anesthetics so as to avoid aspiration.

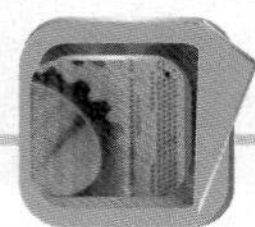

Coding Information and Supply Sources

CPT Code	Description	2008 Average 50th Percentile Fee	Global Period
31575	Laryngoscopy, flexible fiber optic; diagnostic	$352.00	0
92511	Nasopharyngoscopy with endoscope	$230.00	0
31231	Nasal endoscopy, diagnostic (unilateral or bilateral)	$327.00	0

CPT is a registered trademark of the American Medical Association.
2008 average 50th Percentile Fees are provided courtesy of 2008 MMH-SI's copyrighted Physicians' Fees and Coding Guide.

ICD-9 Codes

Odynophagia	786.1
Dysphagia	787.20
Hemoptysis	786.3
Hoarseness/dysphonia	784.49
Vocal cord polyp	784.4
Dyspnea	786.05
Stridor	786.1
Epistaxis	784.7
Chronic nasal airway obstruction	478.19
Foreign body	933.0

Supplies

Nasolaryngoscopes may be ordered from the following suppliers:

- Olympus USA, 2 Corporate Center Drive, Melville, NY 11747 (www.olympusamerica.com)
- WelchAllyn, 4341 State Street Road, Skaneateles Falls, NY 13153 (phone: 800-535-6663; www.welchallyn.com/medical)
- Endosheath Technology, Vision Sciences, 9 Strathmore Road, Natick, MA 01760 (phone: 800-874-9975; http://www.visionsciences.com/)
- Pentax, 30 Ramtand Road, Orangeburg, NY 10962 (phone: 800-431-5880; www.pentax-endoscopy.com)

Additional supplies can be obtained as follows:

- Lidocaine hydrochloride (4% solution or 2% jelly) is available from Astra Pharmaceuticals, Westborough, MA (phone: 508-366-1100) or through a local pharmacy.

Oxymetazoline hydrochloride (0.05%) (Afrin spray) is produced by Schering-Plough, Kenilworth, NJ (phone: 908-298-4000) and is available through a local pharmacy.

Patient Education Handout

A patient education handout, "Flexible Fiberoptic Nasolaryngoscopy," can be found on the book's Web site.

Bibliography

Bent J. Pediatric laryngotracheal obstruction: current perspectives on stridor. *Laryngoscope.* 2006;116(7):1059.

Couch ME, Blaugrund J, Kunar D. History, physical examination and the preoperative evaluation. In: Cummings CW, Haughey BH, Thomas, JR, et al., eds. *Cummings Otolaryngology: Head and Neck Surgery* (4th ed.). Philadephia: Elsevier Mosby; 2005:3–24.

Plant RL, Samlan RA. Visual documentation of the larynx. In: Cummings CW, Haughey BH, Thomas, JR, et al., eds. *Cummings Otolaryngology: Head and Neck Surgery* (4th ed.). Philadephia: Elsevier Mosby; 2005:1989–2007.

Zarnitz P. Guidelines for performing fiberoptic flexible nasal endoscopy and nasopharyngolaryngoscopy on adults. *ORL Head Neck Nurs.* 2005;23(2):13–18.

2008 MAG Mutual Healthcare Solutions, Inc.'s Physicians' Fee and Coding Guide. Duluth, Georgia. MAG Mutual Healthcare Solutions, Inc. 2007.

CHAPTER 100

Foreign Body Removal from the Nose and the Ear

T. S. Lian, MD, FACS

Associate Professor of Otolaryngology–Head and Neck Surgery
Louisiana State University Health Sciences Center, Shreveport, LA

Foreign bodies in the nose or ear are more commonly found in the pediatric population but also present in the mentally challenged adult. The placement of the foreign body is frequently not witnessed. The foreign body may therefore be present for a relatively long period of time with associated soft tissue edema, erythema, or even frank purulence, reflecting the presence of infection. Expansion or swelling of the foreign body may also have occurred if the foreign body is of vegetable or organic material.

Foreign bodies typically consist of small household items such as plastic beads or organic material including beans or peas. Small batteries deserve special mention because if left in place, a corrosive injury may result. If the foreign body remains relatively proximal to the respective opening, such as in the nasal vestibule anterior to the inferior turbinate or in the external auditory canal lateral to the bony cartilaginous junction, then foreign body removal can usually be accomplished easily in the clinic setting. Typically, the further away the foreign body is from the external meatus of the ear canal or the nares, the more challenging the removal becomes, and otolaryngology consultation should be considered. Because the nasal mucosa and the cutaneous lining of the ear are relatively fragile, one must exercise caution in instrumenting these areas because problematic bleeding can result. Use of irrigation to extract a foreign body from the ear canal is not recommended, particularly if the integrity of the tympanic membrane is not known.

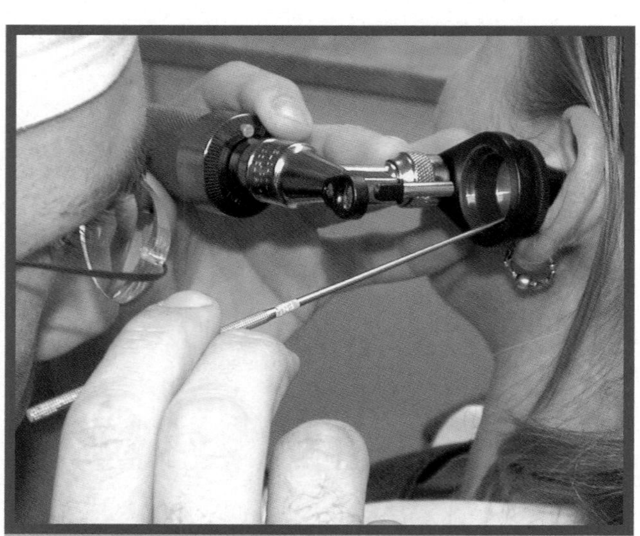

If local anesthesia is needed for removal of an object from the auditory canal, place the affected ear in the nondependent position, and instill 2% lidocaine or 20% benzocaine into the canal, allowing it to remain for 10 minutes. This is especially useful with an insect in the ear. Many insects, especially cockroaches, grasp the lining of the canal to resist extraction. Local anesthetic provides anesthesia, and it kills the insect, making it easier to remove. Do not use local anesthesia if the tympanic membrane may be disrupted. Use of suction with an appropriate suction tip can rapidly remove most insects without the need to use an anesthetic to kill the insect. Oral, intravenous, or general anesthesia may be necessary in individuals who cannot tolerate instrumentation.

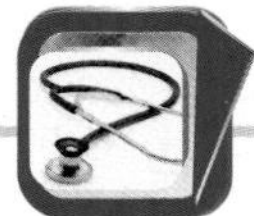

Equipment

- Otoscope
- Day hook
- Nasal speculum
- Suction and suction tips
- Head light
- Alligator forceps
- Bayonet forceps

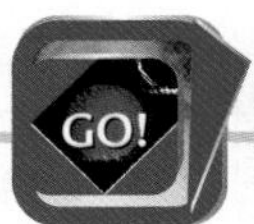

Indications

- Foreign body in the nasal cavity or external auditory canal

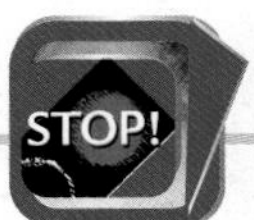

Contraindications (Relative)

- An uncooperative patient or infant who cannot be restrained
- Marked bleeding
- Limited visualization
- Distal location or displacement of the foreign body
- Trauma-induced distortion of the normal anatomy
- Previous ear surgery (because of increased risk of perforation)
- Known or suspected cholesteatoma

The Procedure

Step 1. Assemble the tools for removal of the foreign object. Blunt hooks, forceps, speculums, and suction are the primary instruments used to remove foreign bodies.

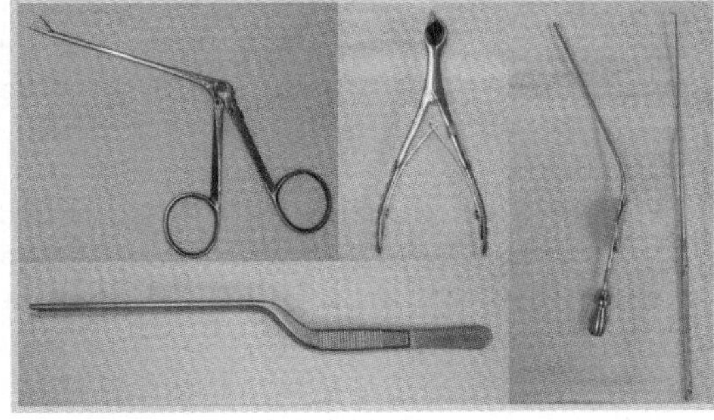

Step 1

Step 2. Depending on the cooperativity of the patient, the patient can be placed in either a sitting or supine position. To facilitate a traumatic removal, children should be secured so as to avoid movement. With use of an otoscope, the ear canals should be examined to identify the foreign body, including its shape and position. Similarly, the nasal cavity is inspected with use of a nasal speculum and head light. It is important to examine both ears or both sides of the anterior nasal cavity as a contralateral foreign body may be found.

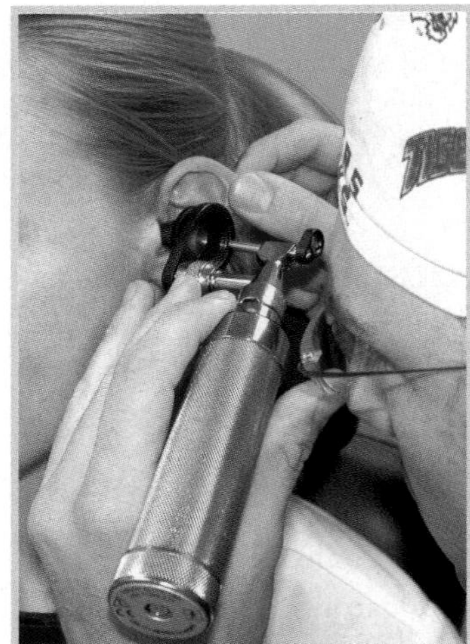

Step 2

Step 3. Once the foreign body has been identified and a decision has been made to attempt removal, the appropriate instrument is selected based on the shape of the presenting aspect of the foreign body. For a foreign body in the ear, use an otoscope and blunt-tip hook. The nondominant hand holds the scope while the dominant hand uses the hook. Note how the nondominant hand stabilizes the scope with the patient's cheek.

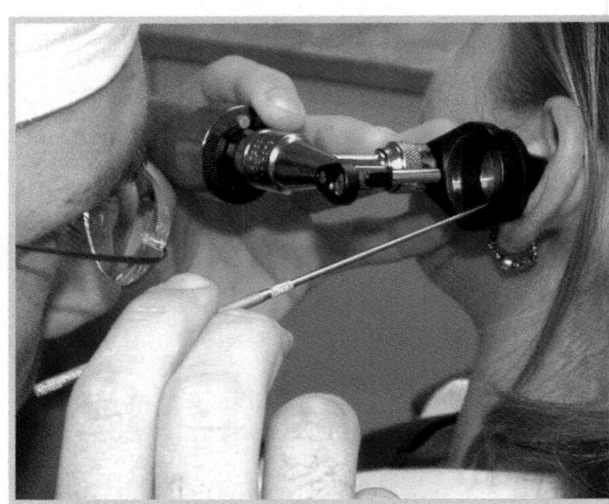

Step 3

Step 4. Use a nasal speculum and blunt-tip hook to remove a foreign body.

- **PEARL:** Note how using a headlight frees up both hands so that they can be used for instrumentation.

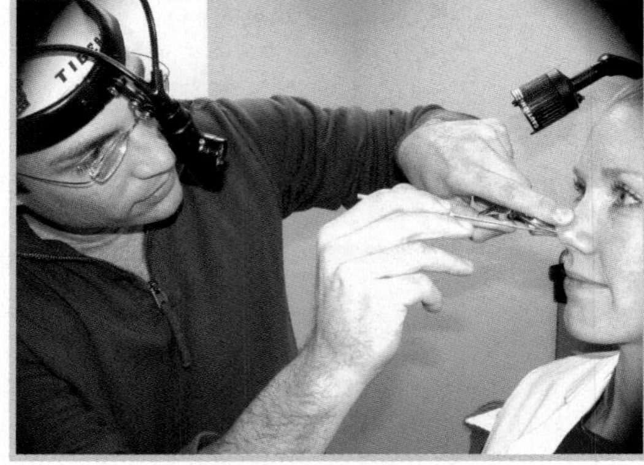

Step 4

Step 5. Smooth or rounded objects are best removed with use of a right-angled blunt hook such as a Day hook. The hook is introduced such that the hook remains relatively flush to the soft tissues, allowing the end of the instrument to pass distal to the foreign body. The hook is then rotated 90 degrees and withdrawn along with the foreign body. If the foreign body has a broad flat edge, the object may be grasped with forceps and removed. If the foreign body is an insect, suction can be introduced to rapidly suction the insect out. Similarly if the foreign body is particulate, or falls apart when manipulated with forceps or hooks, use of suction maybe most appropriate.

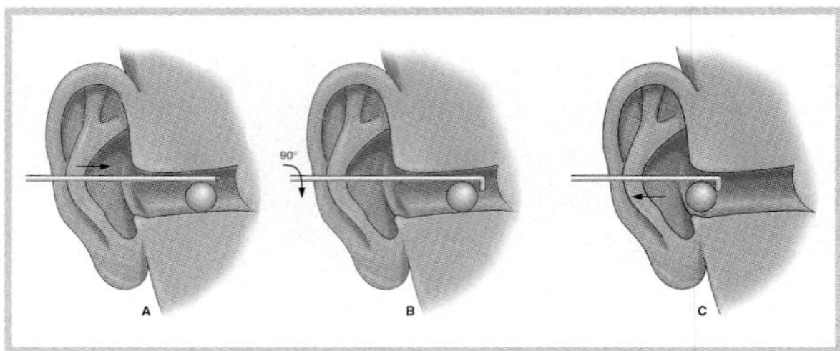

Step 5

- **PITFALL:** Regardless of which instrument is being used for removal, if manipulation results in displacement of the foreign body further back in the nasal cavity or further down the external auditory canal, attempts at removal should cease and otolaryngology consultation should be considered.
- **PITFALL:** If bleeding occurs such that visualization of the object is obscured, attempts at removal should be stopped and otolaryngology consultation should be initiated.

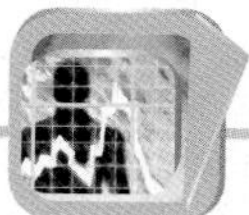

Complications

- Bleeding
- Abrasion
- Infection
- Perforation
- Aspiration
- Nausea or vomiting with removal of an object in the ear

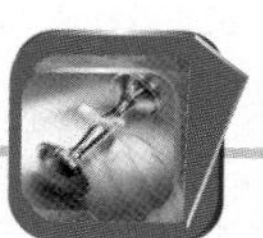

Pediatric Considerations

In some cases, limited cooperation of the pediatric patient may be such that it is safer to perform foreign body removal in an operating room setting under anesthesia to facilitate an atraumatic removal.

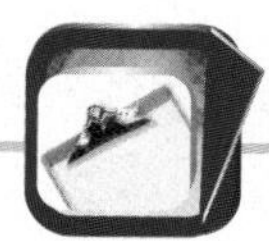

Postprocedure Instructions

After removal of the foreign body, the nasal cavity or ear canal should be examined again for any further foreign bodies as well as to identify any associated injury.

Removal of Nasal Foreign Body

After the procedure, instruct the patient to watch for signs of infection. If mucous membrane injury occurs, have the patient return for a follow-up visit in 1 or 2 days. Recommend saline irrigations three times each day for 1 week if mucosal injury has occurred. Obtain an otolaryngology consultation for severe injuries such as septal and turbinate mucosal injuries in apposition to each other.

Removal of Ear Foreign Body

Instill three drops of antibiotic drops to the ear three times each day for 7 days if ear canal trauma or tympanic membrane perforation is present. Obtain an otolaryngology consultation for persistent perforations. Audiometry and tympanometry testing need to be done if tympanic membrane injury or perforation is present, with otolaryngology consultation as necessary.

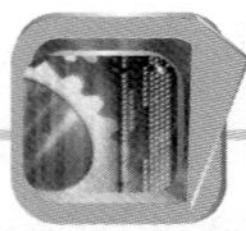

Coding Information and Supply Sources

CPT Code	Description	2008 Average 50th Percentile Fee	Global Period
30300	Removal intranasal foreign body, without general anesthesia	$275.00	10
69200	Removal foreign body from external auditory canal, without general anesthesia	$197.00	0

CPT is a registered trademark of the American Medical Association.
2008 average 50th Percentile Fees are provided courtesy of 2008 MMH-SI's copyrighted Physicians' Fees and Coding Guide.

ICD-9 Codes

Foreign body ear	931
Foreign body nose	932
Foreign body upper air passage	933.0

Supplies

Instruments such as suction tips, alligator forceps, ear curettes, attic hooks, ear speculums, or nasal speculums may be obtained from most national supply houses, such as AllHeart.com-Professional Appearances, Inc., 431 Calle San Pablo, Camarillo, CA 93012 (fax: 805-445-8816; Web site: http://store.yahoo.com/allheart/index.html) or Atlantic Medical Supply, 65-14 Brook Avenue, Deer Park, NY 11729 (phone: 516-249-0191; Web site: http://www.atlanticmedsupply.com).

Patient Education Handout

A patient education handout, "Foreign Bodies in the Ears or Nose," can be found on the book's companion Web site.

Bibliography

Antonelli PJ, Ahmadi A, Prevatt A. Insecticidal activity of common reagents for insect foreign bodies of the ear. *Laryngoscope*. 2001;111:15–20.

Couch ME, Blaugrund J, Kunar D. History, physical examination and the preoperative evaluation. In: *Cummings Otolaryngology-Head and Neck Surgery*. (4th ed.) Philadephia: Elsevier Mosby; 2005:3–24.

D'Cruz O, Lakshman R. A solution for the foreign body in nose problem. *Pediatrics*. 1988;81:174.

Heim SW, Maughan KL. Foreign bodies in the ear, nose, and throat. *Am Fam Physician*. 2007;76:1185–1189.

Jensen JH. Technique for removing a spherical foreign body from the nose or ear. *Ear Nose Throat J*. 1976;55:46.

Mishra A, Shukla GK, Bhatia N. Aural foreign bodies. *Indian J Pediatr*. 2000;67:267–269.

Reddy IS. Foreign bodies in the nose and ear. *Emerg Med J*. 2001;18:523.

Schulze SL, Kerschner J, Beste D. Pediatric external auditory canal foreign bodies: a review of 698 cases. *Otolaryngol Head Neck Surg*. 2002;127(1):73–78.

Thompson SK, Wein RO, Dutcher PO. External auditory canal foreign body removal: management practices and outcomes. *Laryngoscope*. 2003;113(11):1912–1915.

2008 MAG Mutual Healthcare Solutions, Inc.'s Physicians' Fee and Coding Guide. Duluth, Georgia. MAG Mutual Healthcare Solutions, Inc. 2007.

CHAPTER 101

Tympanometry

T. S. Lian, MD, FACS
Associate Professor of Otolaryngology–Head and Neck Surgery
Louisiana State University Health Sciences Center, Shreveport, LA

Tympanometry is essentially a measure of aural immittance. Immittance [im(pedance) + (ad)mittance] can be described as how energy travels through a system. In terms of the ear, immittance reflects the relative ease of the passage of sound energy through the hearing mechanism, and impedance is the opposition of the passage of sound energy. Tympanometry measures aural immittance with the use of air pressure. In normal situations, the air pressure is equal on both sides of the tympanic membrane, and thus aural immittance is optimal because the tympanic membrane moves most effectively under these pressure conditions. During tympanometry, the pressure in the external auditory canal is varied with application of negative and positive pressure. The movement of the tympanic membrane in terms of compliance is plotted against the variation of pressure, resulting in a graphic representation of immittance called a tympanogram. Because the eustachian tube is involved in pressure equalization of the middle ear space, a relative negative pressure peak seen in a tympanogram would reflect inadequate ventilation by the eustachian tube. This eustachian tube dysfunction can be related to inflammation/infection, masses, and neuromuscular disorders. Tympanometry can also be used to measure the volume of the external auditory canal. A relatively high volume is evidence of a tympanic membrane perforation. Normal volumes in adults range from 0.5 to 2.0 mL and in children range from 0.3 to 1.0 mL.

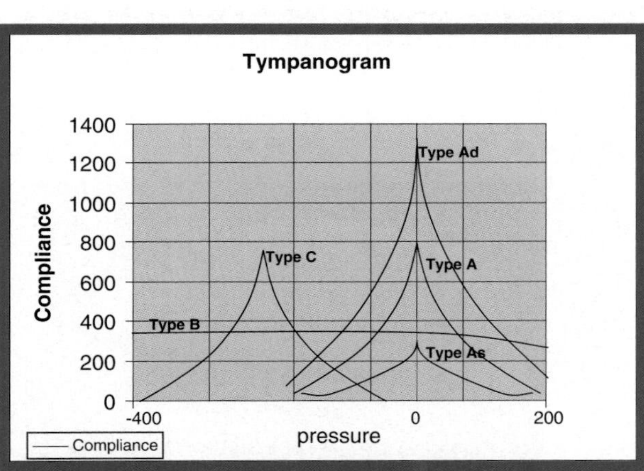

A common method for describing tympanograms was popularized by Jerger. This description involves three basic types of tympanograms: types A, B, and C. Type A is a normal tympanogram. Type Ad describes a highly compliant tympanic membrane where there is little impedance. This situation may occur in the face of ossicular discontinuity or scarring of the tympanic membrane in the absence of hearing loss. The type As pattern suggests decreased compliance and can be found in cases of ossicular fixations such as otosclerosis. A type B tympanogram describes a flat tympanogram where there is no peak in compliance and little if any change in compliance with changes of pressure. A Type B tympanogram would be found in cases of middle ear effusions as in serous otitis media; however, a flat tympanogram associated with a relatively high volume would suggest a tympanic membrane perforation. A type C tympanogram has a compliance peak in the negative pressure range beyond an air pressure of −100 mm H_2O as occurs when there is inadequate ventilation of the middle ear space, which is reflective of eustachian tube dysfunction.

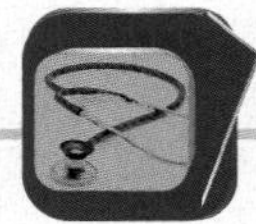

Equipment

- Portable tympanometer

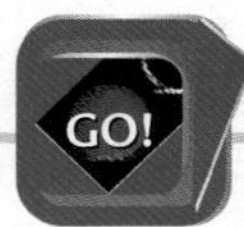

Indications

- Decreased hearing
- Hearing loss
- Possible ear infection or perforation

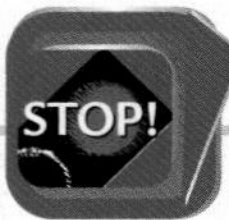

Contraindications

- Bleeding
- Otorrhea
- External otitis
- Acute external auditory canal trauma
- Occlusion of the external auditory canal

The Procedure

Tympanometry is relatively easy to perform and typically lasts only a few seconds. A portable tympanometer is shown.

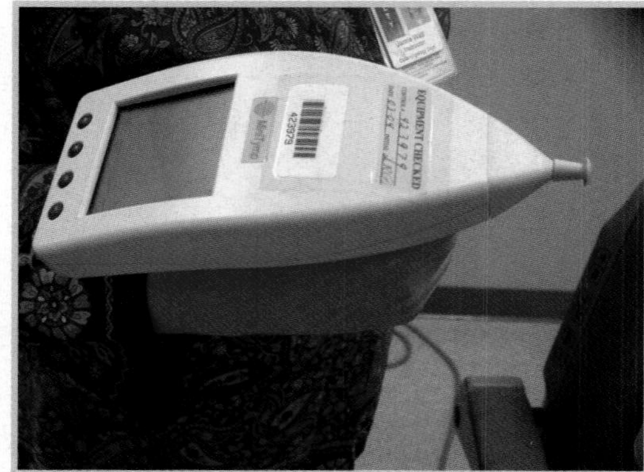

Figure 2

Step 1. Prior to performing the procedure, otoscopy should be performed to assess for any relative contraindications for tympanometry as well as the patency of the external auditory structures. An obstructed or impacted cerumen should be removed prior to tympanometry.

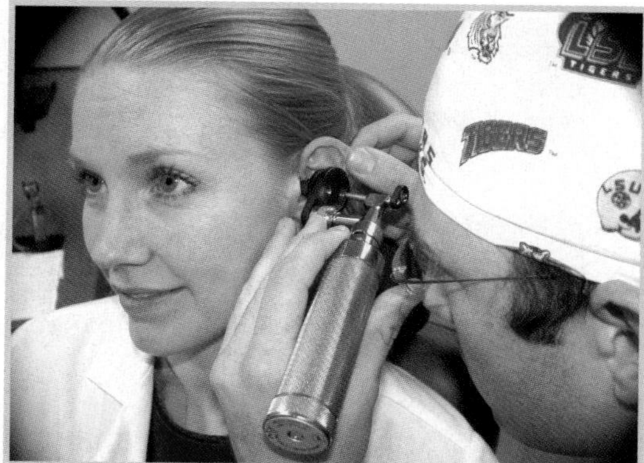

Step 1

Step 2. With the patient in the sitting position, the helix is gently grasped and pulled in a superior posterior direction.

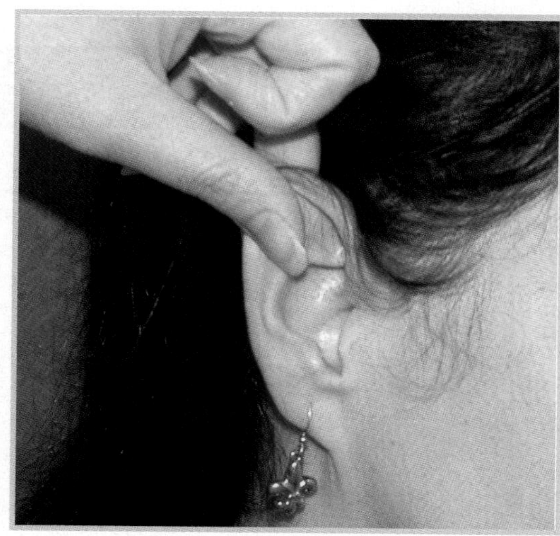

Step 2

Step 3. The tympanometry probe is then inserted into the external auditory canal meatus, forming an airtight seal. Pressure readings are then taken, and the tympanogram and associated volume are displayed by the tympanometer. The probe is then removed.

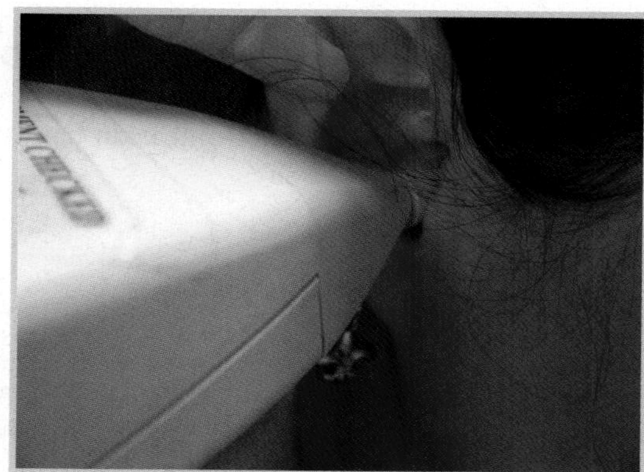

Step 3

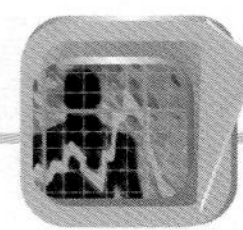

Complications

- Abrasion of the external auditory meatus

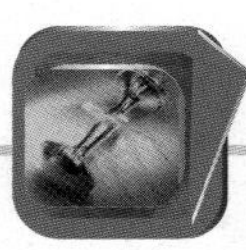

Pediatric Considerations

In the infant, tympanometry can also be performed in the supine position.

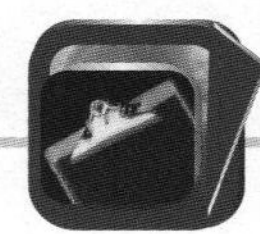

Postprocedure Instructions

General ear care instructions and any disease-specific instructions should be given.

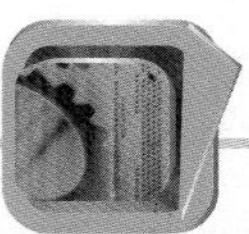

Coding Information and Supply Sources

CPT Code	Description	2008 Average 50th Percentile Fee	Global Period
92567	Tympanometry	$49.00	XXX

XXX, global concept does not apply.

2008 average 50th Percentile Fees are provided courtesy of 2008 MMH-SI's copyrighted Physicians' Fees and Coding Guide.

ICD-9 Codes

Conductive hearing loss	389.06
Serous otis media	381.10
Tympanic perforation	384.20
Tympanosclerosis	385.00
Cerumen impaction	380.4

Suppliers

Tympanometers can be obtained from most medical supply houses.

Patient Education Handout

A patient education handout, "Tympanometry," can be found on the book's companion Web site.

Bibliography

Hall JW, Antonelli PJ. Assessment of peripheral and central auditory function. In: *Head and Neck Surgery—Otolaryngology*. (3rd ed.). Philadephia: Lippincott Williams & Wilkins; 2001:1663–1664.

Jerger JF. Clinical experience with impedance audiometry. *Arch Otolaryngol.* 1970;92:11–24.

Koike KJ. *Everyday Audiology: A Practical Guide for Health Care Professionals*. San Diego: Plural Publishing; 2006.

2008 MAG Mutual Healthcare Solutions, Inc.'s Physicians' Fee and Coding Guide. Duluth, Georgia. MAG Mutual Healthcare Solutions, Inc. 2007.

SECTION TEN

MUSCULOSKELETAL PROCEDURES

CHAPTER 102

Carpal Tunnel Syndrome Injection

Edward A. Jackson, MD, DABFM, FABFM

Chair and Program Director, Synergy Medical Education Alliance

Professor, Department of Family Medicine, Michigan State College of Human Medicine

East Lansing, MI

Carpal tunnel syndrome is among the most frequent clinically presenting nerve entrapments. It is caused by the compression of the median nerve within the carpal canal. This canal is a space that is created by the carpal bones below and the transverse carpal ligament above. Any condition that either enlarges structures within the canal or decreases the size of the canal can produce compression on the median nerve. Things such as tumors, ganglia, or tenosynovitis of the flexor tendons of the wrist will reduce the canal space. Conditions such as pregnancy, amyloidosis, or thyroid dysfunctions may create edema that also can compress the canal.

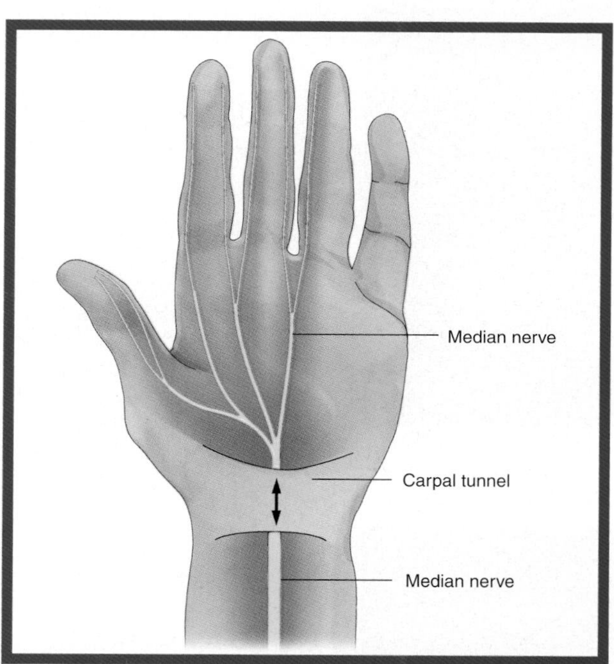

Carpal tunnel is more common in women (3:1 female-to-male ratio). Underlying causes for tenosynovitis such as repetitive injuries due to work activities such as typing or overuse should be corrected first. Control of illnesses such as thyroid conditions and diabetes should also be beneficial in the treatment.

Patients will usually complain of paresthesias (numbness) and pain in the median nerve distribution. The median nerve supplies sensation to the first three digits and the radial half of the fourth digit. Most patients complain of increased problems at nighttime, especially when they sleep on the wrist or maintain the wrist in a flexed position. As the syndrome persists, there may be pain radiating to the wrist and forearm with atrophy of the thenar muscles, especially the thumb abductors.

Testing for this syndrome often involves the Tinel and Phalen tests. The Tinel test creates a paresthesia by tapping upon the median nerve at the wrist (Figure 2). The Phalen test is performed by having the patient flex the wrists together for 30 to 60 seconds to reproduce paresthesias and numbness (Figure 3).

Both of these tests are poorly sensitive (20% and 46% respectively). Nerve conduction studies may provide more objective data and reveal a delay in the conduction of an electrical impulse across the carpal canal.

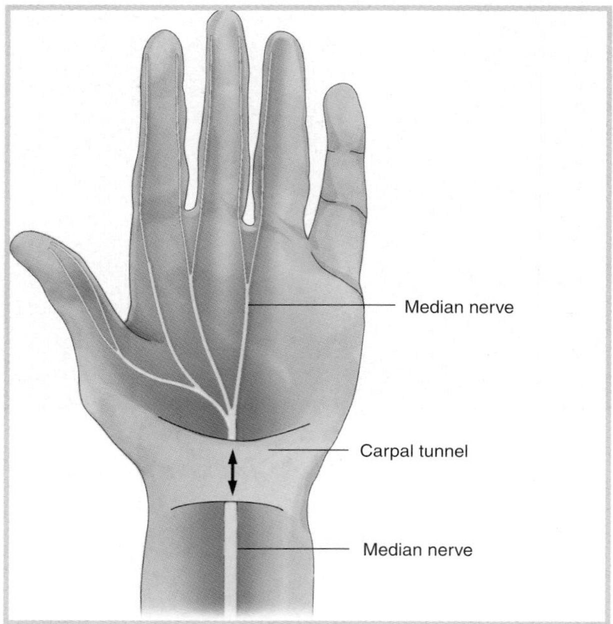

Figure 1

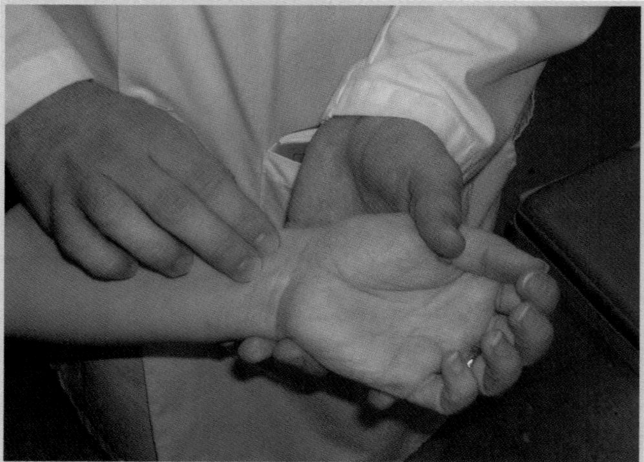

Figure 2

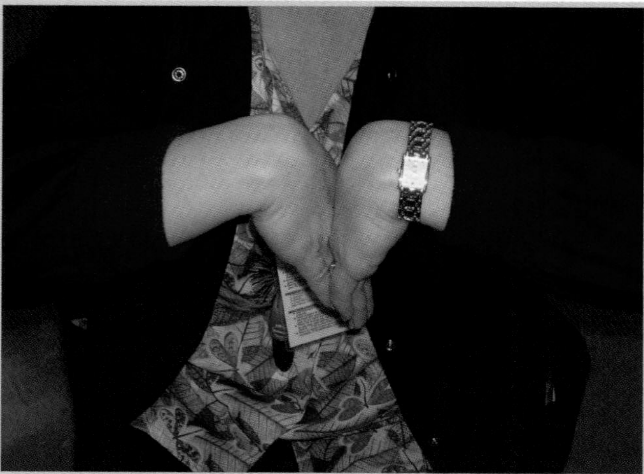

Figure 3

Conservative treatment may include rest, ice, the use of wrist splinting to limit flexion, and the use of nonsteroidal anti-inflammatory drugs (NSAIDS). Use of injected corticosteroids has been shown to improve the condition. Most studies can document at least a 70% short-term benefit with an injection of steroids. A repeat injection may be performed if symptoms recur but should be limited to two or three injections to limit crystalline deposition into the canal. If repeated injections fail, surgery should be considered.

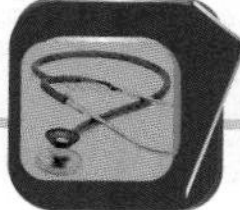

Equipment

- Povidone-iodine (or equivalent skin antiseptic)
- Alcohol pads
- Syringe, 5 cc
- Lidocaine 1% without epinephrine
- Steroid (0.5 cc) such as betamethasone (Celestone) or triamcinolone
- Adhesive bandages

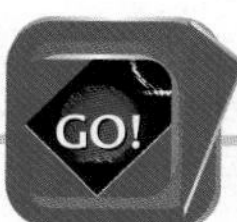

Indications

- Signs and symptoms suggesting median nerve compression in the carpal canal with the absence of severe symptoms or pain and absence of severe signs such as thenar muscle wasting

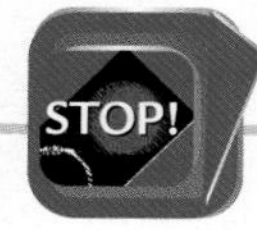

Contraindications

- Usually not done in pediatric populations
- Avoid during third trimester of pregnancy
- Overlying skin with signs and symptoms of cellulitis or infection
- A mass in the canal
- History of bleeding disorders or coagulopathy
- Uncooperative patient (relative)

The Procedure

Step 1. Place patient supine with affected arm fully extended. Face the patient's feet alongside the affected arm.

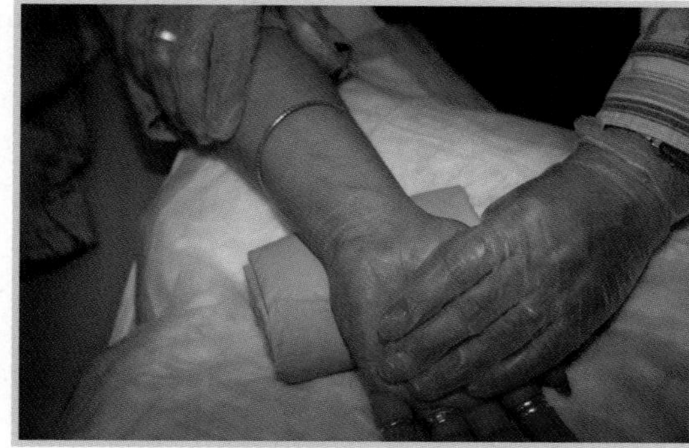

Step 1

Step 2. Have the patient make a fist against some resistance to locate the palmaris longus tendon. The needle can be inserted on either side of the palmaris longus tendon.

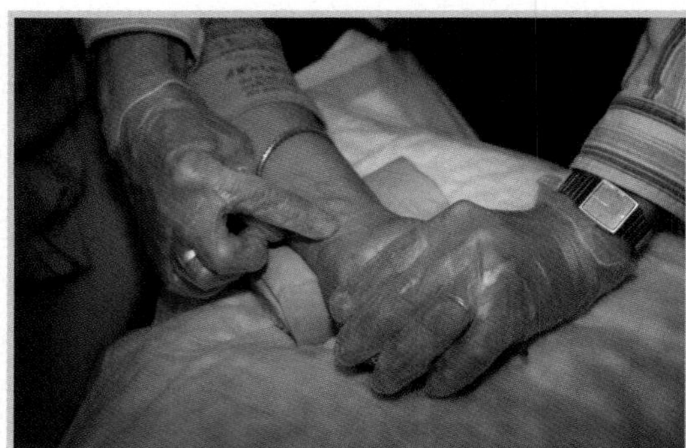

Step 2

Step 3. Locate the second wrist crease on the volar side of the wrist.

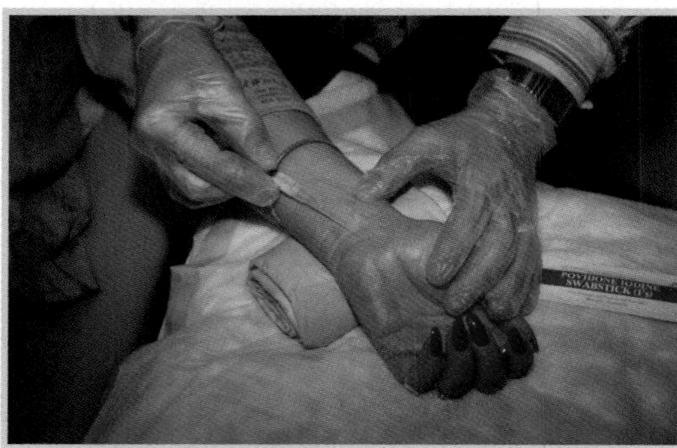

Step 3

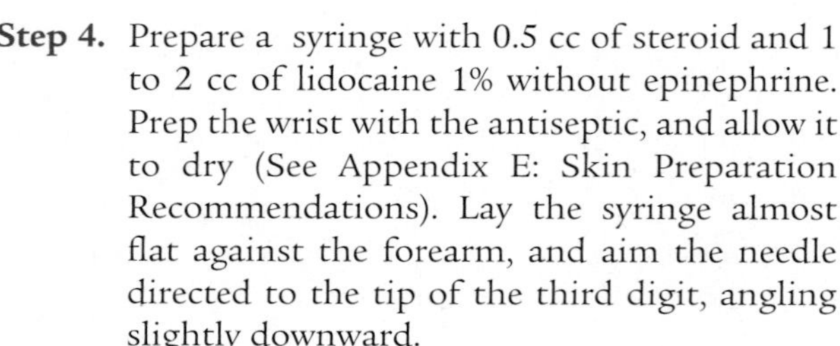

Step 4. Prepare a syringe with 0.5 cc of steroid and 1 to 2 cc of lidocaine 1% without epinephrine. Prep the wrist with the antiseptic, and allow it to dry (See Appendix E: Skin Preparation Recommendations). Lay the syringe almost flat against the forearm, and aim the needle directed to the tip of the third digit, angling slightly downward.

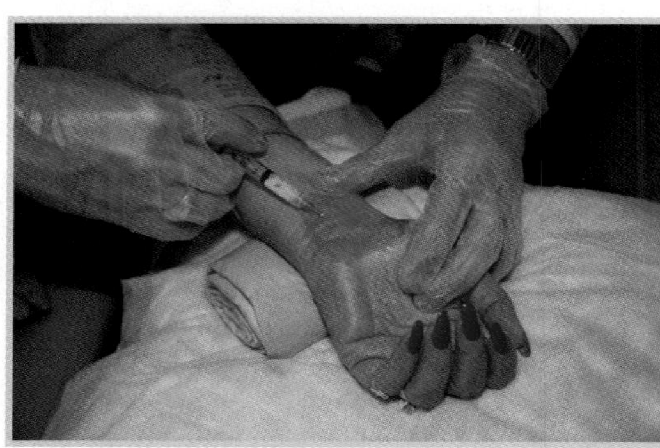

Step 4

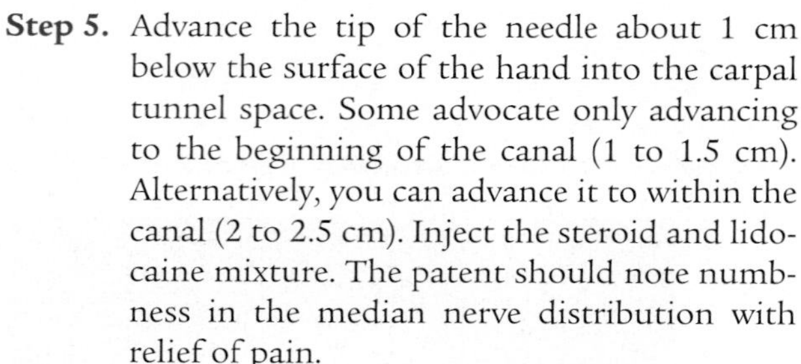

Step 5. Advance the tip of the needle about 1 cm below the surface of the hand into the carpal tunnel space. Some advocate only advancing to the beginning of the canal (1 to 1.5 cm). Alternatively, you can advance it to within the canal (2 to 2.5 cm). Inject the steroid and lidocaine mixture. The patent should note numbness in the median nerve distribution with relief of pain.

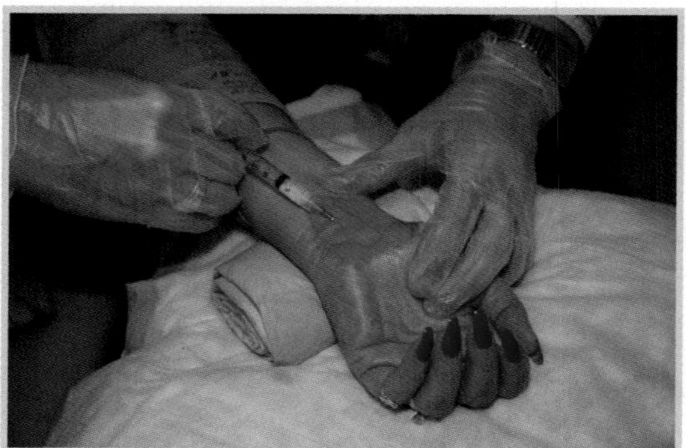

Step 5

Step 6. The needle is withdrawn, and an adhesive bandage is placed over the injection site. Consider using a splint and NSAIDs after the injection, and have the patient rest the wrist.

- PITFALL: The needle should pass easily into the canal. With resistance, withdraw and redirect the needle, still aiming for the tip of the third digit.
- PITFALL: If the needle touches or penetrates the nerve itself, the patient may experience pain and numbness in the median nerve distribution. Ask the patient to report if this happens. If the needle tip touches the nerve, withdraw and redirect the needle slightly upward but still aiming for the tip of the third digit.

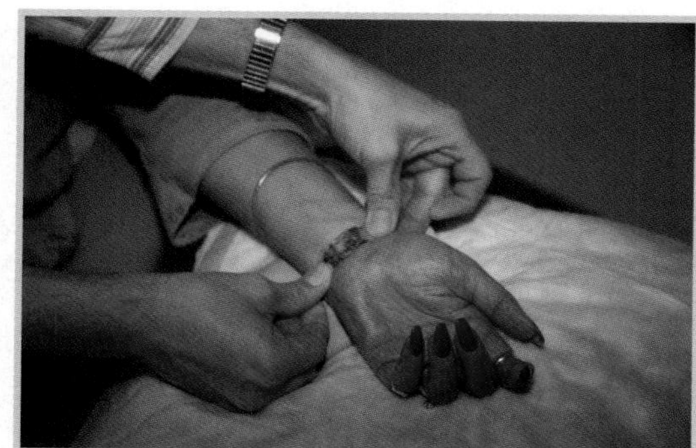

Step 6

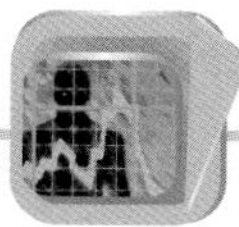

Complications

- Increased pain after steroid injection (temporary and usually resolves in 48 hours)
- Accidental injection into the median nerve
- Bruising of the skin

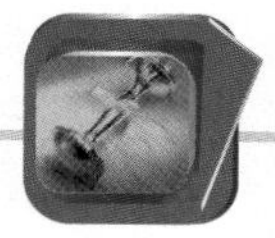

Pediatric Considerations

This syndrome is rarely found in children, and the procedure is usually not performed in this population.

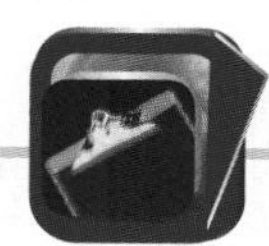

Postprocedure Instructions

Advise the patient to rest the wrist after the procedure. Encourage the patient to wear the splint if prescribed, which may improve the outcome. Also advise the patient to use ice and/or NSAIDS for pain relief if needed.

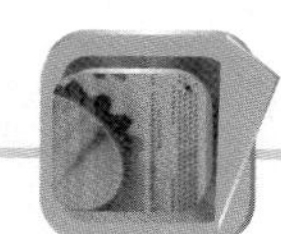

Coding Information and Supply Sources

CPT Code	Description	2008 Average 50th Percentile Fee	Global Period
20526	Injection, therapeutic (e.g.. local anesthetic, corticosteroid), carpal tunnel	$165.00	0

CPT is a registered trademark of the American Medical Association.
2008 average 50th Percentile Fees are provided courtesy of 2008 MMH-SI's copyrighted Physicians' Fees and Coding Guide.

Consult the ordering information that appears in Appendix G. Needles, syringes, and splints are available from local surgical supply houses. A suggested tray for performing soft tissue aspirations and injections is listed in Appendix I. Skin preparation recommendations appear in Appendix E.

Patient Education Handout

A patient education handout, "Carpal Tunnel," can be found on the book's companion Web site.

Bibliography

Biundo JJ. Regional rheumatic pain syndromes. In: Klippel JH, Weyand CM, Wortmann RL, eds. *Primer on the Rheumatic Diseases*. (11th ed.). Atlanta: Arthritis Foundation; 1997:136–148.

Buttaravoli P, Stair T. *Minor Emergencies: Splinters to Fractures*. St. Louis: Mosby; 2000:267–270.

Carpal tunnel syndrome. MayoClinic.com. Available at http://www.mayoclinic.com/health/carpal-tunnerl-syndrome/DS00326. Accessed February 6, 2007.

Carpal tunnel syndrome: pain in your hands and wrists. Familydoctor.org. http://familydoctor.org/023.xml?printxml. Updated August 2006. Accessed February 2, 2007.

Dammers JW, Veering MM, Vermeulen M. Injection with methylprednisolone proximal to the carpal tunnel: randomized double blind trial. *BMJ*. 1999;319:884–886.

Kasten SJ, Louis DS. Carpal tunnel syndrome: a case of median nerve injection injury and a safe and effective method for injecting the carpal tunnel. *J Fam Pract*. 1996;43:79–82.

Katz RT. Carpal tunnel syndrome: a practical review. *Am Fam Physician*. 1994;49:1371–1379.

Lee D, van Holsbeeck MT, Janevski PK, et al. Diagnosis of carpal tunnel syndrome: ultrasound versus electromyography. *Radiol Clin North Am*. 1999;37:859–872.

Mercier LR, Pettid FJ, Tamisiea DF, et al. *Practical Orthopedics*. (4th ed.). St. Louis: Mosby; 1991: 101–103.

Miller RS, Iverson DC, Fried RA, et al. Carpal tunnel syndrome in primary care: a report from ASPN. *J Fam Pract*. 1994;38:337–344.

Murphy MS, Amadio PC. Carpal tunnel syndrome: evaluation and treatment. *Fam Pract Recert*. 1992;14:23–40.

Olney RK. Carpal tunnel syndrome: complex issues with a "simple" condition [Editorial]. *Neurology*. 2001;56:1431–1432.

Seiler JG. Carpal tunnel syndrome: update on diagnostic testing and treatment options. *Consultant*. 1997;37:1233–1242.

Szabo RM. A management guide to carpal tunnel syndrome. *Hosp Med*. 1994;30:26–33.

von Schroeder HP. Review finds limited evidence for electrodiagnosis to predict surgical outcomes in people with carpal tunnel syndrome. *Evid Based Healthcare Sci Appr Health Pol*. 2000;4:92.

Wilson FC, Lin PP. *General Orthopedics*. New York: McGraw-Hill; 1997:259–260.

Wong SM, Hui AC, Tang A, et al. Local vs. systemic corticosteroids in the treatment of carpal tunnel syndrome. *Neurology*. 2001;56:1565–1567.

2008 MAG Mutual Healthcare Solutions, Inc.'s Physicians' Fee and Coding Guide. Duluth, Georgia. MAG Mutual Healthcare Solutions, Inc. 2007.

CHAPTER 103

De Quervain's Injection

Doug Aukerman, MD, FAAFP

Assistant Professor, Department of Orthopaedics, Rehabilitation and Sports Medicine
Assistant Professor, Department of Family and Community Medicine
Penn State Milton S. Hershey Medical Center
Hershey, PA
Team Physician, Penn State University
State College, PA

Stenosing tenosynovitis of the short and long thumb abductor tendons (i.e., abductor pollicis longus and extensor pollicis brevis) is a common cause of dorsal wrist pain near the radial styloid. Commonly known as de Quervain's tenosynovitis or Quervain's disease, the condition is usually related to overuse and chronic microtrauma to the first and second dorsal compartment tendons as they pass through a fibroosseous tunnel. This region is predisposed to stenosing tendosynovitis because of the confined space in the tunnel. Jobs requiring repetitive hand and wrist motion, especially those with frequent thumb extension and extreme lateral wrist deviations, increase the risk of this disorder. Certain sports (e.g., golf, racquet sports, fishing) have also been commonly associated with the condition. Additionally, pregnancy and care of a new born infant is associated with this tenosynovitis. Gonococcal infection historically was a cause of de Quervain's disease, but this is a very uncommon cause today.

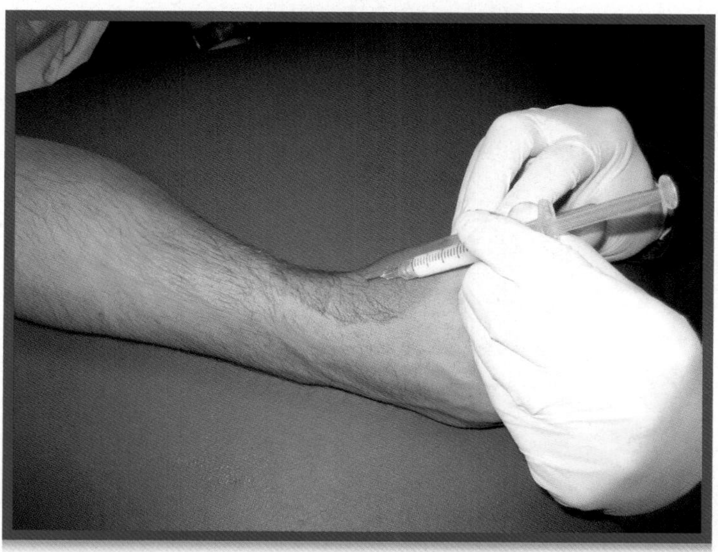

De Quervain's disease produces marked discomfort on gripping. Ulnar deviation, as reproduced with Finkelstein's test, causes marked pain. Visible swelling can often be observed over the abductor and extensor tendons, and palpable crepitus may be observed. Pain, tenderness, swelling, and warmth over the dorsal wrist on the radial side are common features on examination. Finkelstein's test is the classic diagnostic maneuver for De Quervain's. The differential diagnosis includes wrist arthritis, radial nerve compression at the wrist (Wartenberg's syndrome), and intersection syndrome (i.e., tendonitis and associated bursitis of the dorsal wrist extensors). Corticosteroid injection can resolve or cure the condition, especially if given early in the course of the disease. Some physicians believe that injection therapy offers the best prognosis for improvement in symptoms. Many physicians prefer to postpone injections until a trial of physical therapy, anti-inflammatory medication, and rest (with or without splinting or casting) have been prescribed. Up to three injections, given at monthly intervals, can be tried before surgical referral for release of the dorsal compartment.

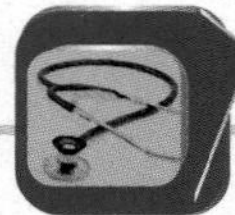

Equipment

- Povidone iodine (or equivalent skin antiseptic) (see Appendix E)
- Alcohol pads
- 3-cc syringe with 25- or 27-gauge needle
- Lidocaine 1% without epinephrine
- 0.5 cc of steroid such as Celestone or Triamcinolone
- Adhesive bandage

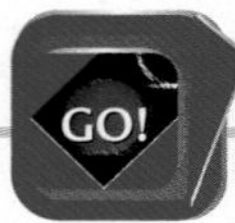

Indications

- DeQuevain's tenosynovitis not improved with rest, anti-inflammatory medication, stretching, and ice

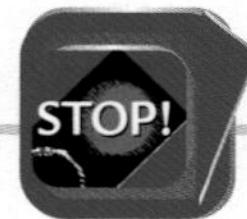

Contraindications

- Infection of overlying or nearby skin
- Bleeding disorders
- Allergic reaction to similar drug

The Procedure

Step 1. Finkelstein's test can help reproduce the symptom of DeQuevain's tenosynovitis. The test is performed by flexing the fingers around a flexed thumb and then passive ulnar deviation maximally at the wrist. The pain is experienced at the first and/or second dorsal compartments and radiates cephalad.

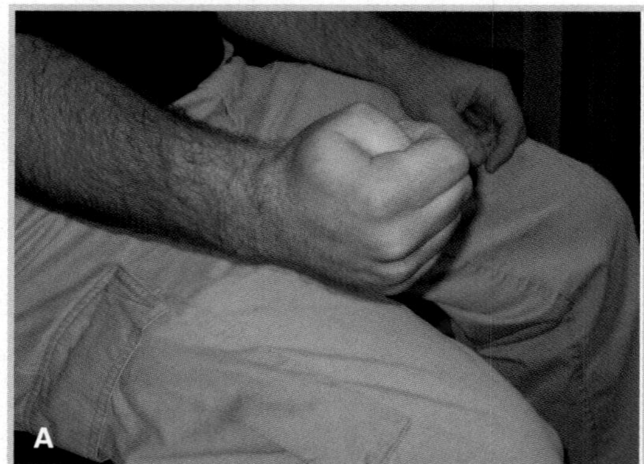

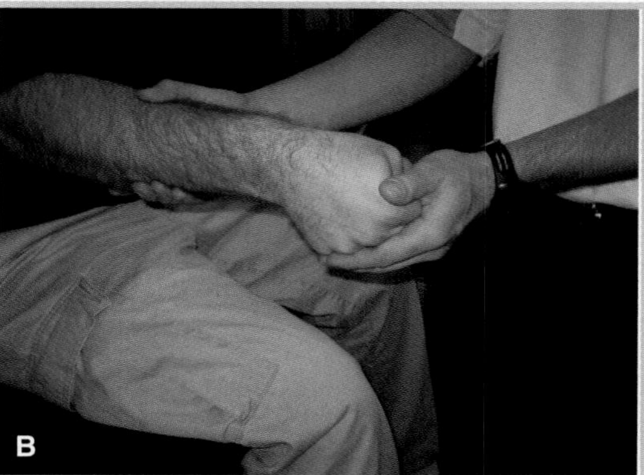

Step 1

Step 2. To perform the injection, maximally abduct thumb (accentuates abductor tendon) to help identify the first and second dorsal tendon and its sheath. Determine which dorsal tendon is affected.

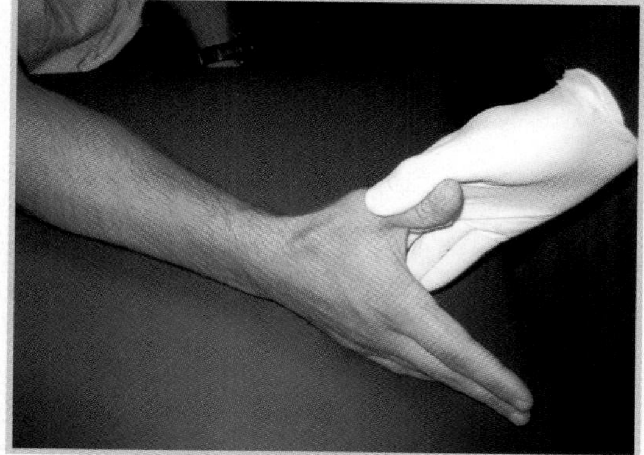

Step 2

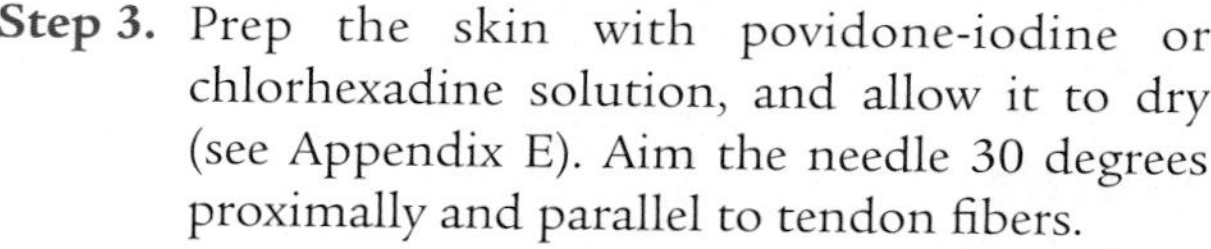

Step 3. Prep the skin with povidone-iodine or chlorhexadine solution, and allow it to dry (see Appendix E). Aim the needle 30 degrees proximally and parallel to tendon fibers.

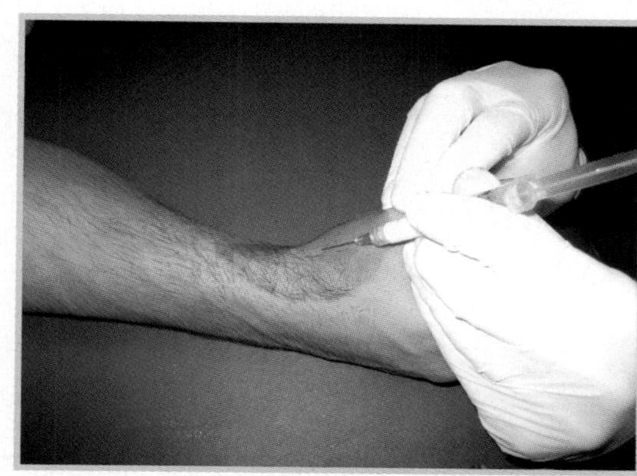

Step 3

Step 4. Have patient gently flex and extend involved finger. Insert the needle distally toward proximal direction to avoid intra tendinous injection. The needle should be entered with the tendon flexed and then extended before injection, which will release the tendon from the needle if the tendon is accidentally entered.

- **PEARL:** Insert the needle until patient experiences scratchy sensation, which indicates you are juxtaposed to the tendon and the tendon sheath. Have the patient actively move the thumb prior to injection, if the needle moves it indicates that you are within the tendon. DO NOT INJECT. Withdraw a few millimeters and have the patient move the thumb again. Never inject against resistance.

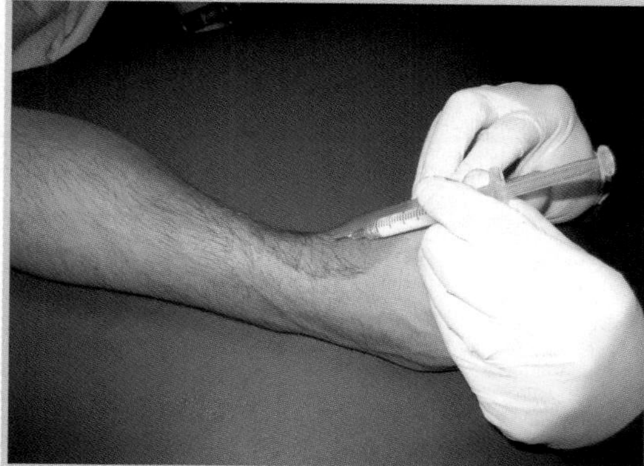

Step 4

Step 5. The injection can also be performed by entering the skin in the opposite direction.

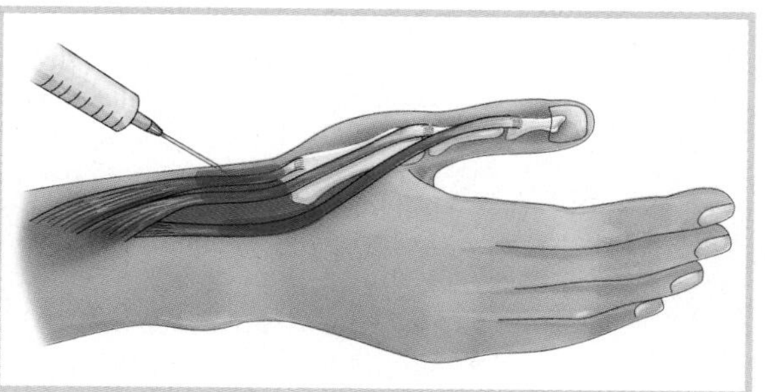

Step 5

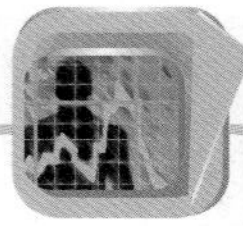

Complications

- Infection
- Tendon rupture
- Elevations of blood sugar in diabetics
- Misplaced injection causing excessive pain
- Post injection flare (corticosteroid induced crystal synovitis)
- Skin atrophy
- Skin hypopigmentation or hyperpigmentation

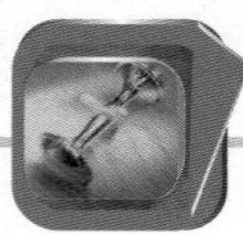

Pediatric Considerations

This syndrome is rarely found in children and the procedure is usually not performed in this population.

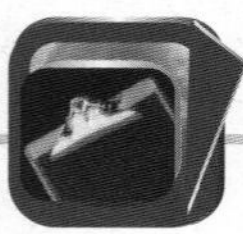

Postprocedure Instructions

Advise the patient to rest the wrist after the procedure. Encourage the patient to wear their splint, if prescribed, which may improve the outcome. Also advise the patient that they may use ice and/or nonsteroidal anti-inflammatory drugs for pain relief if needed.

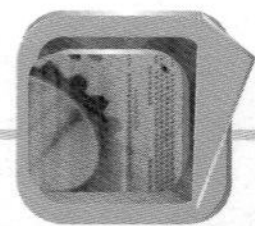

Coding Information and Supply Sources

CPT Code	Description	2008 Average 50th Percentile Fee	Global Period
20550	Injection(s); single tendon sheath, or ligament, aponeurosis (e.g., plantar "fascia")	$140.00	0

CPT is a registered trademark of the American Medical Association.

2008 average 50th Percentile Fees are provided courtesy of 2008 MMH-SI's copyrighted Physicians' Fees and Coding Guide.

Bibliography

Anderson LG. Aspirating and injecting the acutely painful joint. *Emerg Med.* 1991;23:77–94.

Brown JS. *Minor Surgery: A Text and Atlas.* London: Chapman & Hall Medical; 1997:165.

Hanlon DP. Intersection syndrome: a case report and review of the literature. *J Emerg Med.* 1999;17:969–971.

Kay NR. De Quervain's disease: changing pathology or changing perception? *J Hand Surg Br.* 2000;25:65–69.

Leversee JH. Aspiration of joints and soft tissue injections. *Prim Care.* 1986;13:579–599.

Mani L, Gerr F Work-related upper extremity musculoskeletal disorders. *Prim Care Clin Office Pract.* 2000;27:845–864.

Marx RG, Sperling JW, Cordasco FA. Overuse injuries of the upper extremity in tennis players. *Clin Sports Med.* 2001;20:439–451.

Owen DS, Irby R. Intra-articular and soft-tissue aspiration and injection. *Clin Rheumatol Pract.* 1986;Mar–May:52–63.

Rettig AC. Wrist and hand overuse syndromes. *Clin Sports Med.* 2001;20:591–611.

Ritchie JV, Munter DW. Emergency department evaluation and treatment of wrist injuries. *Emerg Med Clin North Am.* 1999;17:823–842.

Tallia AF, Cardone DA. Diagnostic and therapeutic injection of the wrist and hand region. *Am Fam Physician.* 2003;67(4):745–750.

Weiss AP, Akelman E, Tabatabai M. Treatment of DeQuervain's disease. *J Hand Surg Am.* 1994;19:595–598.

2008 MAG Mutual Healthcare Solutions, Inc.'s Physicians' Fee and Coding Guide. Duluth, Georgia. MAG Mutual Healthcare Solutions, Inc. 2007.

CHAPTER 104

Extensor Tendon Injury Repair

Doug Aukerman, MD, FAAFP
Assistant Professor, Department of Orthopaedics, Rehabilitation and Sports Medicine
Assistant Professor, Department of Family and Community Medicine
Penn State Milton S. Hershey Medical Center
Hershey, PA
Team Physician, Penn State University
State College, PA

Wayne Sebastianelli, MD
Professor, Department of Orthopaedics and Rehabilitation
Pennsylvania State University
Assistant Chief of Staff, Mount Nittany Medical Center
State College, PA

All lacerations to the hands or feet must be carefully examined for underlying tendon injury. To find such injuries, examine the patient for a functional deficit of the anatomic part. Flexor tendon injuries of the hand require complex specialized repairs and should be promptly referred to a surgical hand specialist. Although many extensor tendon injuries may also require specialized repair, extensor injuries to the dorsum of the hand (Verdan classification zone VI) may often be treated in the office or emergency department.

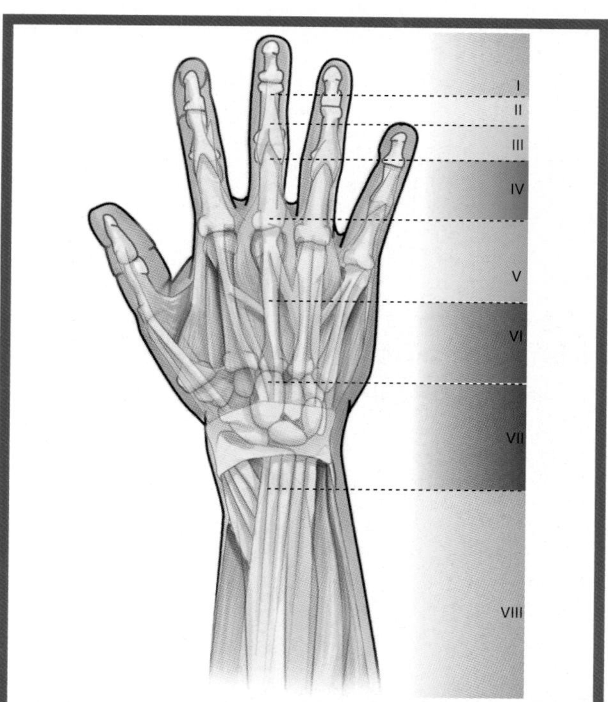

Even with normal function on finger examination, a tendon may be partially lacerated. Unrepaired partial tendon lacerations can result in delayed rupture 1 to 2 days after the initial injury. Repair any tendon that is >50% transected. If only a minimal laceration is discovered, apply a splint for 3 weeks, followed by passive motion exercises for 2 to 3 weeks.

A tendon that angles around curves, pulleys, or joints is surrounded by a thin tendon sheath. A lacerated tendon within an intact sheath often will not heal. If the sheath is absent or severed, the proximal part of the tendon will grow in an attempt to reattach to the distal portion, often resulting in adherence to surrounding structures. Adhesions are part of the repair process, and they may occasionally interfere with function. Patients who are compliant with instructions and motivated toward rehabilitation usually have a greater chance of a good outcome after tendon repair.

When the tendon is cut completely through, the ends may retract a significant distance from the site of trauma. Careful examination and extension of the incision may be necessary to identify both ends. However, extensor tendons on the dorsum of the hand are crosslinked and usually do not retract to the same degree as flexor tendons. During the first 2 weeks of healing, a repaired tendon develops a fibroblastic bulbous connection. Organized tendon collagen usually does not begin to form until the third week. By the end of the fourth week, swelling and vascularity markedly decrease. After the swelling has abated and the junction becomes strong, the tendon can fully perform its gliding motion. For tendon repairs to be successful, the tendons must be covered with healthy skin. Skin grafting should be performed when there is a significant area of skin avulsion or necrosis. Tendon injuries that are complicated by tissue maceration, contamination, or passage of more than 8 hours should be treated in the operating room.

Uncontrolled motion of the hand during the first 3 weeks after repair often results in rupture or attenuation of the repair. Classically, the repaired tendons are immobilized for 1 week to prevent rupture and to promote healing. Place a plaster splint on the palmar surface from the forearm to the fingertips. Place the wrist in 30 degrees of extension, the metacarpophalangeal joints in 20 degrees of flexion, and the fingers in slight flexion. Keep the fingers from flexing during splint changes. Active motion is started after 5 to 14 days to improve the final strength of the repair. Physical and occupational therapy consultation is usually helpful.

Strong healing can be observed as early as 6 weeks after the tendon repair. Some centers have shown that early, limited, controlled motion using specialized orthotics may improve outcomes (see Chow et al., 1989).

Extensor tendon injuries over fingers (Verdan classification zones I through IV) involve complex structures and often result in poor healing with office repair. Because these tendons lie close to the joint capsule, any complete tendon laceration over a joint should raise the suspicion of joint capsule injury and should be treated in the operating room. Lacerations directly over the metacarpophalangeal joints (zone V) may be successfully repaired in the office by skilled surgeons. Zone VI repairs are the most commonly performed repairs by primary care physicians. Possible complications of tendon repair include local infection, finger contracture, delayed tendon rupture, or local adhesions. Patients with associated digital fractures or with ragged lacerations tend to have poorer results.

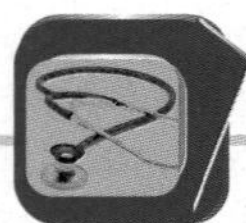

Equipment

- Sterile field
- Suture material (4-0 Ethibond or 4-0 Ticron)
- Lidocaine 1% plain

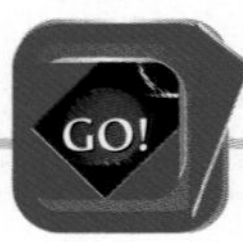

Indications

- Partially lacerated extensor tendon in the dorsum of the hand
- Transected extensor tendon in the dorsum of the hand

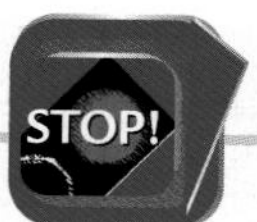

Contraindications

- Tendon injuries associated with tissue maceration
- Tendon injuries associated with contamination
- Tendon injuries more than 8 hours old
- Extensor tendon injuries over the dorsum of the fingers, flexor tendon injuries, or joint involvement should be referred to hand surgeon.

The Procedure

Step 1. Examine the hand laceration and identify the ends of the tendon. If the ends of the tendon have retracted from the skin incision, extend the fingers to push the tendon ends back to the incision site. Extensor tendon injuries may be repaired by direct end to end approximation using the Kessler or modified Bunnell technique.

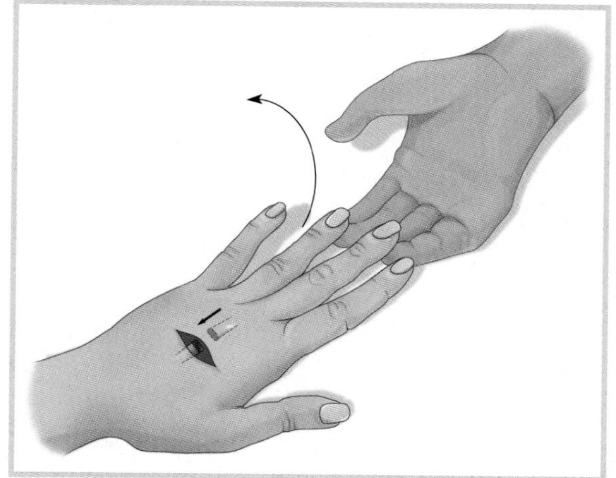

Step 1

The Kessler Technique

Step 2. Begin by passing suture in the proximal portion of the tendon and exiting through the cut end.

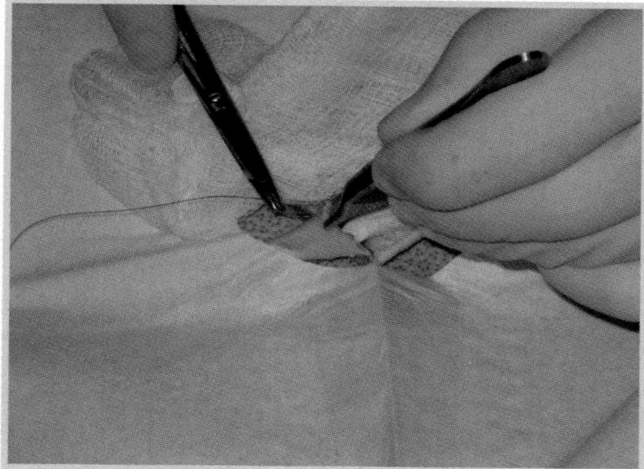

Step 2

Step 3. Then, pass the suture into the distal piece of tendon through the cut end and exit on the same side distally.

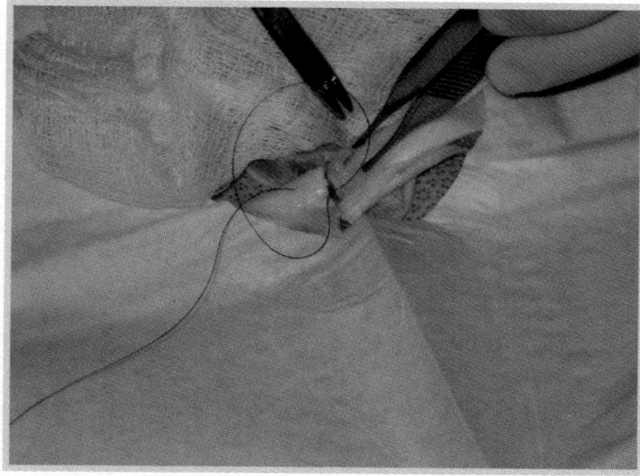

Step 3

Step 4. Leaving an external suture loop, a pass is then made through the substance of the tendon.

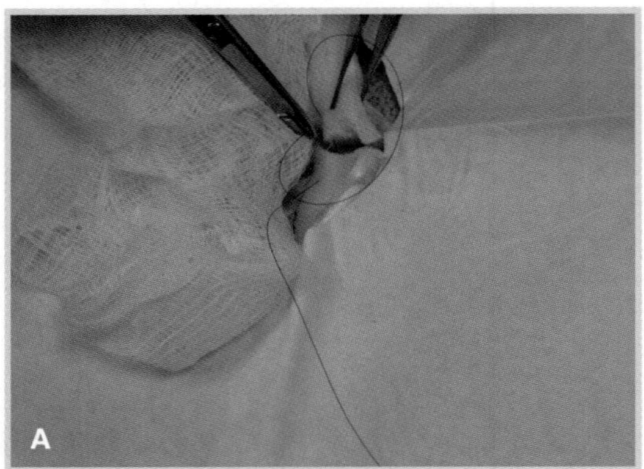

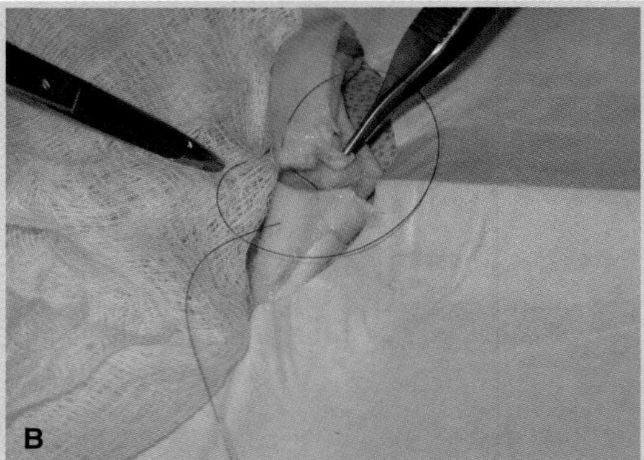

Step 4

Step 5. Leaving another external loop on the other side of the tendon, the suture is then passed from the outside portion of the distal tendon and out the cut end.

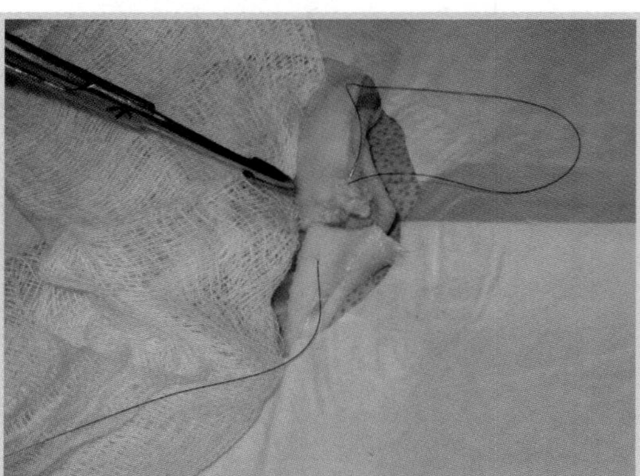

Step 5

Step 6. The suture then enters the proximal cut end of the tendon through the cut end and tension applied to bring the ends of the tendon together.

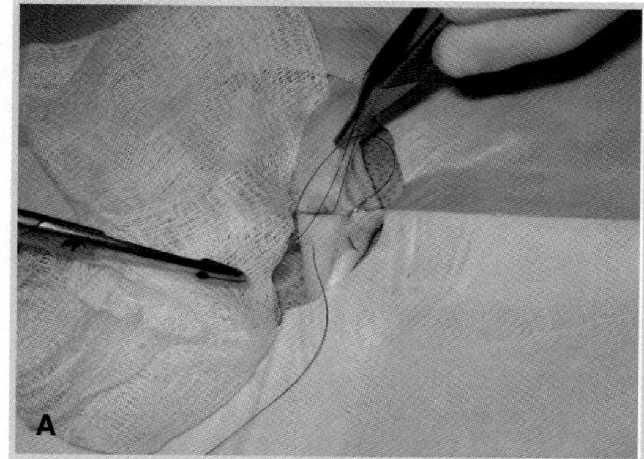

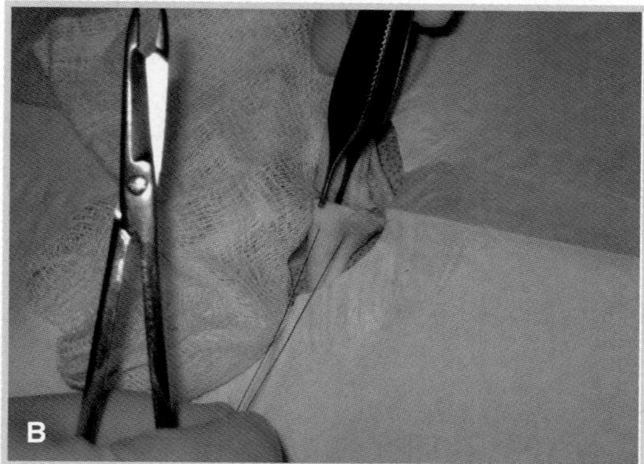

Step 6

Step 7. The suture ends can then be tied. (Note: The suture loop may also be tied to have the knot placed between the injured portion of the tendon).

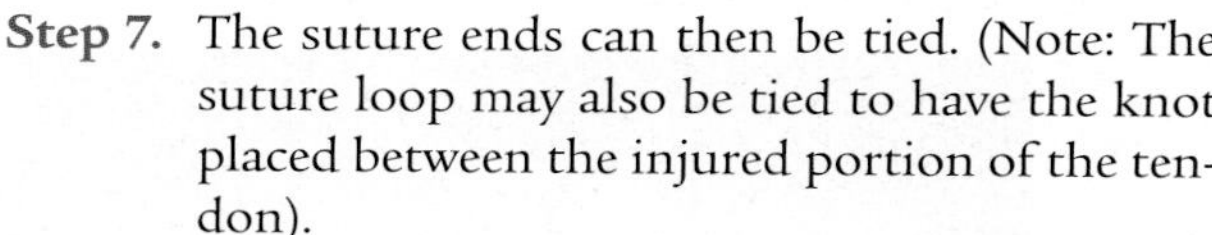

- **PITFALL:** Do not over tighten. If the tendon repair is under to much tension it will limit flexion after it heals.
- **PEARL:** Knot location placed dorsally allows for easier removal if the permanent suture knot becomes symptomatic.

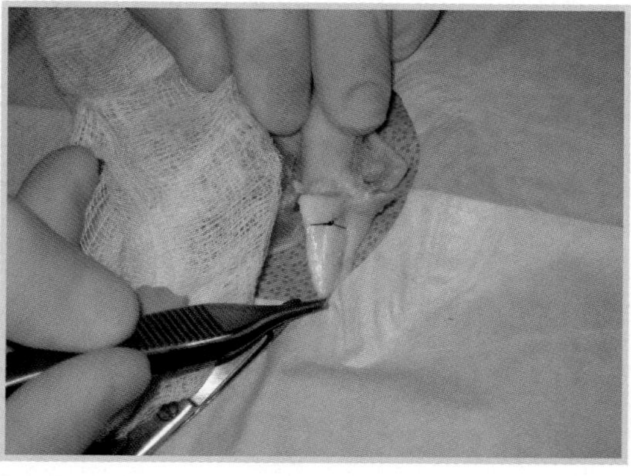

Step 7

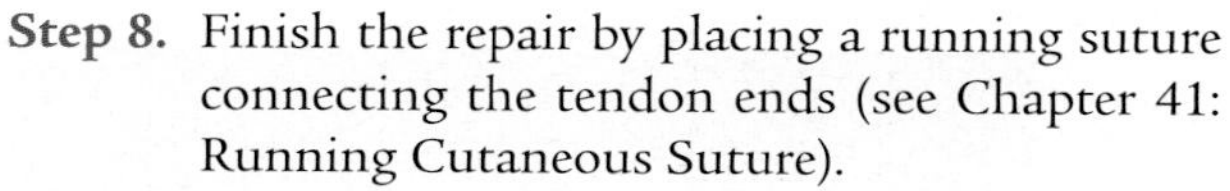

Step 8. Finish the repair by placing a running suture connecting the tendon ends (see Chapter 41: Running Cutaneous Suture).

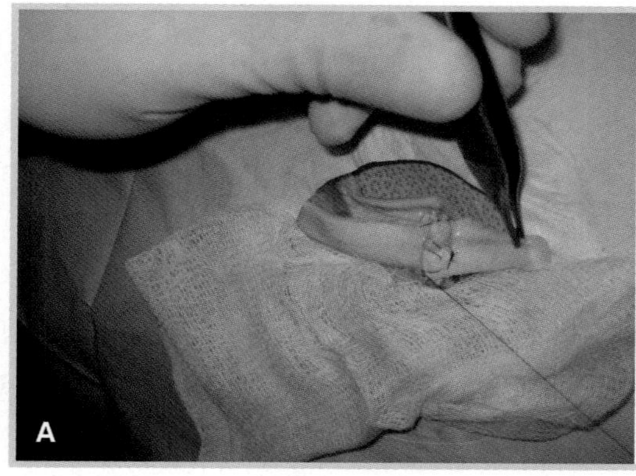

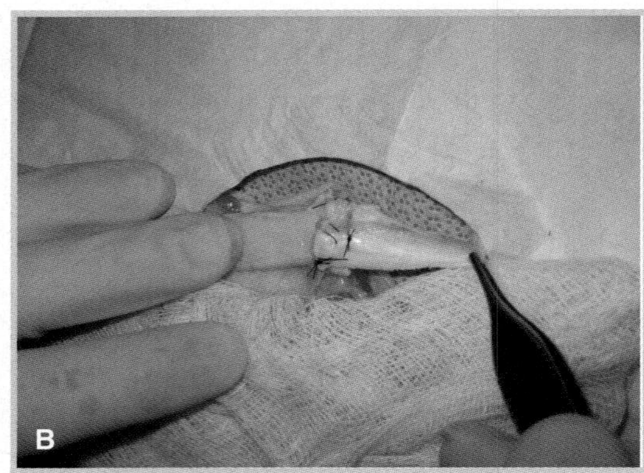

Step 8

End-to-end Repair with Simple Interrupted or Horizontal Mattress Sutures

Step 1. Begin by placing a simple interrupted suture at one edge of the tendon so as to close the defect (see Chapter 38).

- **CLINICAL PEARL:** Make sure to match the ends of tendons as anatomically as possible to ease repair and promote healing.

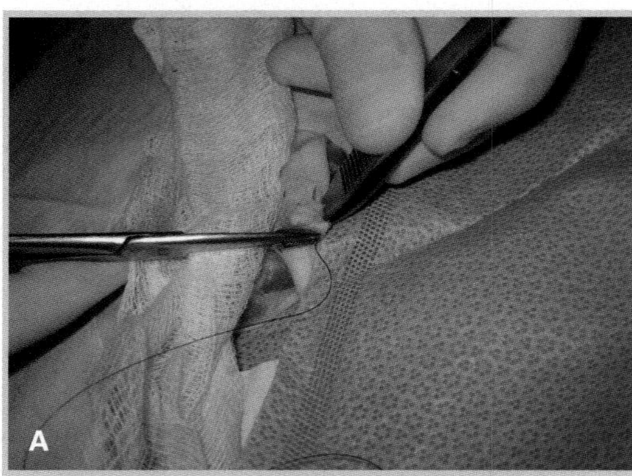

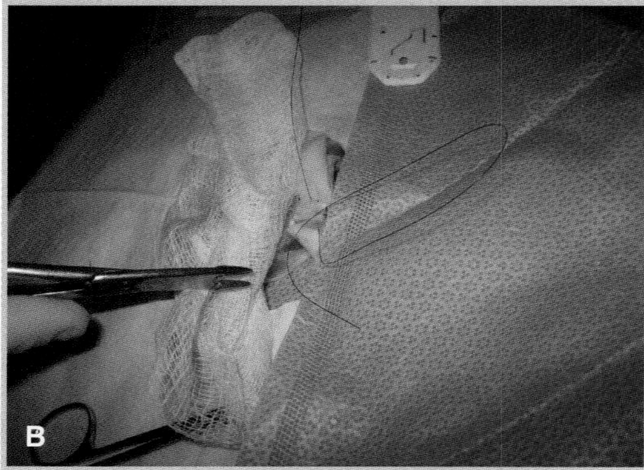

Step 1

Step 2. Tie the simple interrupted suture snugly but not so tight as to cause the ends to bulge.

- **CLINICAL PEARL:** Try to handle the tendon as little as possible and with as little compression from the forceps to minimize iatrogenic injury.

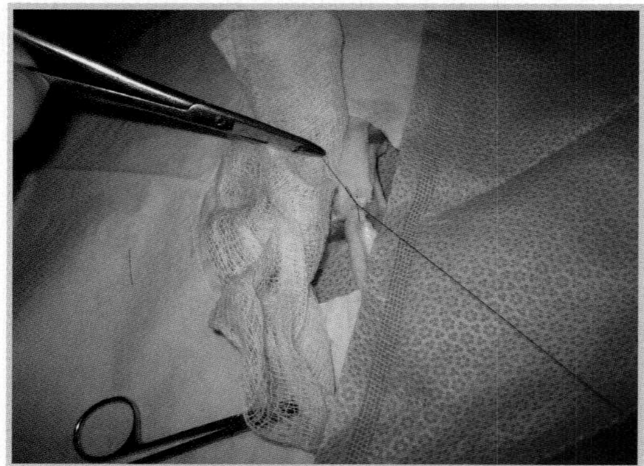

Step 2

Step 3. Continue placing interrupted sutures across the tendon to the opposite side.

- **PEARL:** This technique may also be accomplished using interrupted sutures (see Chapter 40).

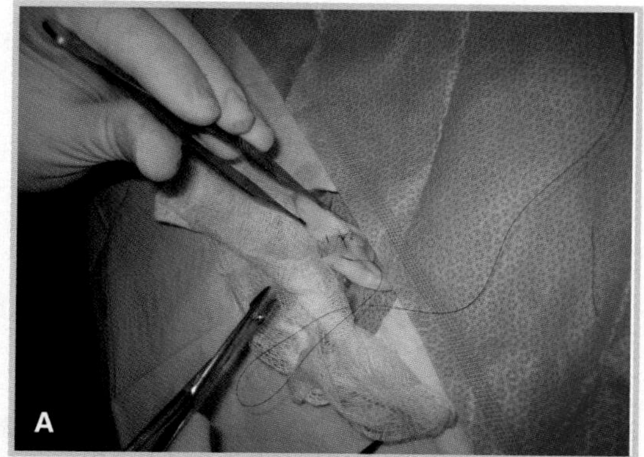

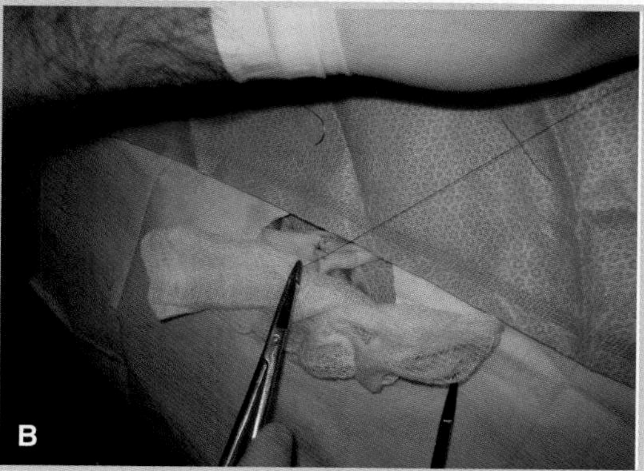

Step 3

Step 4. Continue placing interrupted sutures until the laceration is completely closed and tie off.

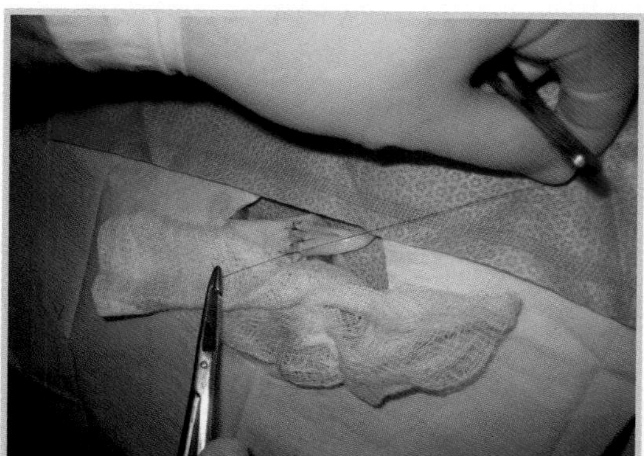

Step 4

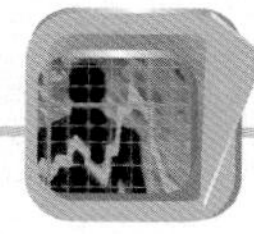

Complications

- Loss of flexion and stiffness from over tightening repair
- Infection
- Rerupture of tendon repair
- Adhesions
- Stiffness

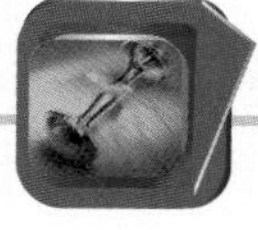

Pediatric Considerations

Pediatric patients often require sedation until the patient is splinted to reduce noncompliance with the procedure. Excessive motion during or immediately after the repair will weaken or place the repair at risk of re-rupture.

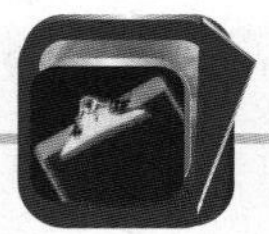

Postprocedure instructions

Splint the extremity in extension for 3 weeks. Begin active flexion and passive extension from 3 weeks to 6 weeks after injury. Instruct the patient to avoid aggressive use of hand and fingers for 10 to 12 weeks postinjury.

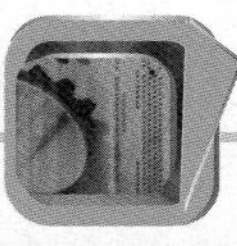

Coding Information and Supply Sources

CPT Code	Description	2008 Average 50th Percentile Fee	Global Period
26410	Extensor tendon repair, dorsum of hand, single; primary or secondary, each tendon	$1,559.00	90

For suture supply sources, see Appendix G.

Patient Education Handout

A patient education handout, "Extensor Tendon Injury Repair" can be found on the book's Web site.

Bibliography

Calabro JJ, Hoidal CR, Susini LM. Extensor tendon repair in the emergency department. *J Emerg Med.* 1986;4:217–225.

Chow JA, Dovelle S, Thomes LJ, et al. A comparison of results of extensor tendon repair followed by early controlled mobilisation versus static immobilisation. *J Hand Surg Br.* 1989;14:18–20.

Evans JD, Wignakumar V, Davis TR, et al. Results of extensor tendon repair performed by junior accident and emergency staff. *Injury.* 1995;26:107–109.

Ip WY, Chow SP. Results of dynamic splintage following extensor tendon repair. *J Hand Surg Br.* 1997;22:283–287.

Kerr CD, Burczak JR. Dynamic traction after extensor tendon repair in zones 6, 7, and 8: a retrospective study. *J Hand Surg Br.* 1989;14:21–22.

Kinninmonth AWG. A complication of the buried suture. *J Hand Surg Am.* 1990;15:959.

Kleinert HE. Report of the committee on tendon injuries. *J Hand Surg Am.* 1989;14:381.

Lee H. Double loop locking suture: a technique of tendon repair for early active mobilization, parts I and II. *J Hand Sung Am.* 1990;15:945.

Newport ML, Blair WF, Steyers CM. Long-term results of extensor tendon repair. *J Hand Surg Am.* 1990;15:961.

Purcell T, Eadie PA, Murugan S, et al. Static splinting of extensor tendon repairs. *J Hand Surg Br.* 2000;25:180–182.

Thomas D, Moutet F, Guinard D. Postoperative management of extensor tendon repairs in zones V, VI, and VII. *J Hand Ther.* 1996;9:309–314.

Wolock BS, Moore JR, Weiland AJ. Extensor tendon repair: a reconstructive technique. *Orthopedics.* 1987;10:1387–1389.

2008 MAG Mutual Healthcare Solutions, Inc.'s Physicians' Fee and Coding Guide. Duluth, Georgia. MAG Mutual Healthcare Solutions, Inc. 2007.

CHAPTER 105

Greater Trochanteric Bursa Injection

Anne Boyd, MD
Assistant Professor, Department of Family Medicine
University of Pittsburgh School of Medicine
Director, Primary Care Sports Medicine Fellowship Program
UPMC
Pittsburgh, PA

Scott Wissink, MD
Assistant Professor, Department of Orthopaedic Surgery
University of Pittsburgh
Monroeville, PA

Several bursae surround the greater trochanter of the femur. Two bursae that lie between the gluteus maximus muscle and the greater trochanter are thought to be of greatest clinical significance. The superficial bursa is immediately beneath the gluteus maximus over the lateral surface of the greater trochanter. Beneath the superficial bursa, is the appropriately named *deep bursa*. The deep bursa is larger and blankets the "cuff" of tissue around the greater trochanter formed by the attachment of the gluteus medius (posteriorly), gluteus minimus (anterolaterally), and vastus lateralis (anteriorly).

Although the term *bursitis* suggests that the primary pathology is inflammation at one or more of the peritrochanteric bursae, recent magnetic resonance imaging (MRI) evidence indicates that the majority of patients with clinical findings consistent with the diagnosis of trochanteric bursitis have tendinosis, or a partial or complete tear of the gluteus medius or minimus as their primary pathology, not trochanteric bursae inflammation. Current theory holds that gluteal tendinosis induces muscle atrophy, femoral head subluxation, and bursitis in the contiguous bursae and that subsequent impingement of the distended bursae results in painful range of motion. Regardless of the associated pathology, injection at the trochanter is often successful in treating symptoms. Most (61%) patients report improvement at 6 months following trochanteric bursa injection.

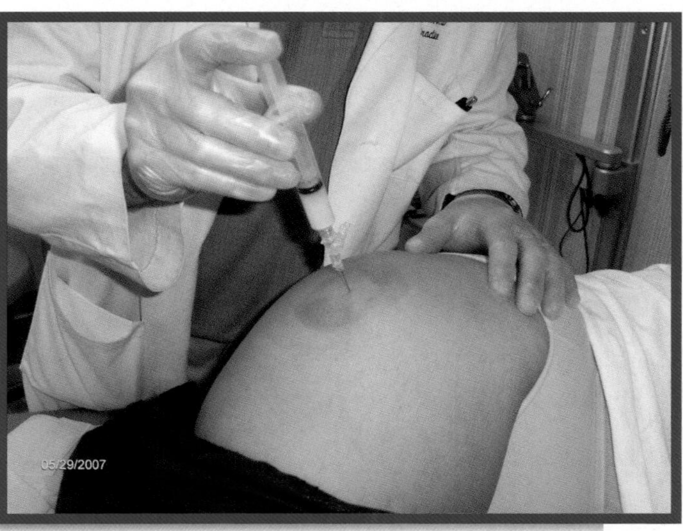

Leg length discrepancy, tight iliotibial band, arthritis of the hip, obesity, and lumbar spondylosis may be predisposing factors for the development of trochanteric bursitis. Once lumbar spine, hip, and other pathology have been excluded, the clinical presentation is usually sufficient to make a presumptive diagnosis. Patients complain of localized, lateral hip pain that is often worse when lying on the affected side at night. On examination, there is focal tenderness to palpation, and occasionally swelling, at the greater trochanter.

The differential diagnosis of hip pain includes osteoarthritis of the hip, iliotibial band syndrome, and adductor tendenopathy.

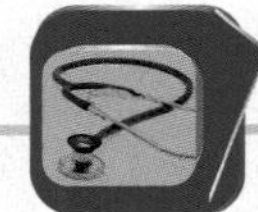

Equipment

- Syringe, 10 mL.
- Needle (22–25 gauge, 1.5 inches) on a 10-mL syringe (consider a longer needle for the obese patient).
- Methylprednisolone acetate (40 mg Depo-Medrol; 1 mL if 40 mg/mL). One mL of 40 mg/mL triamcinolone acetonide (Kenalog) is a reasonable alternative to Depo-Medrol but may carry a higher risk of atrophy than Depo-Medrol.
- 1% lidocaine (5 mL) without epinephrine.
- Consult the ordering information that appears in Appendix I. Needles, syringes, and corticosteroid preparations may be ordered from surgical supply houses or local pharmacies. A suggested tray for performing soft tissue aspirations and injections is listed in Appendix I. Skin preparation recommendations appear in Appendix E.

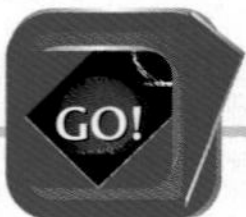

Indications

- Symptomatic discomfort at the greater trochanter of the hip

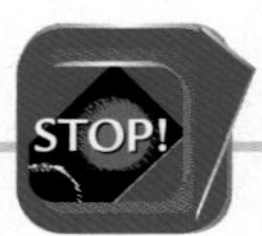

Contraindications

- Drug allergy to injectable materials
- Infection: septic arthritis, bacteremia, or cellulitis at the injection site
- Minimal relief after prior injections (relative)
- Underlying coagulopathy or uncontrolled anticoagulation (relative)
- Uncontrolled diabetes (relative)
- Joint prosthesis (scarring changes anatomy; foreign body increases risk for infectious complications) (relative)

The Procedure

Step 1. After informed consent is obtained, hands are washed, materials are prepared, and gloves are applied. Position the patient in the lateral recumbent position with the affected side up.

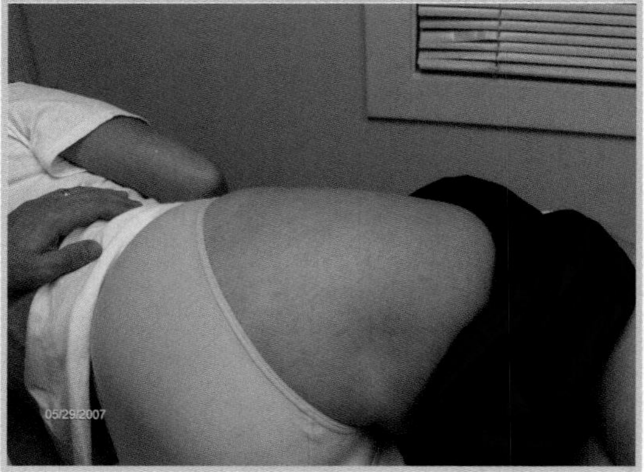

Step 1

Step 2. Identify the point of maximal tenderness, and mark the site with a pressure mark from a needle cap, pen, or fingernail.

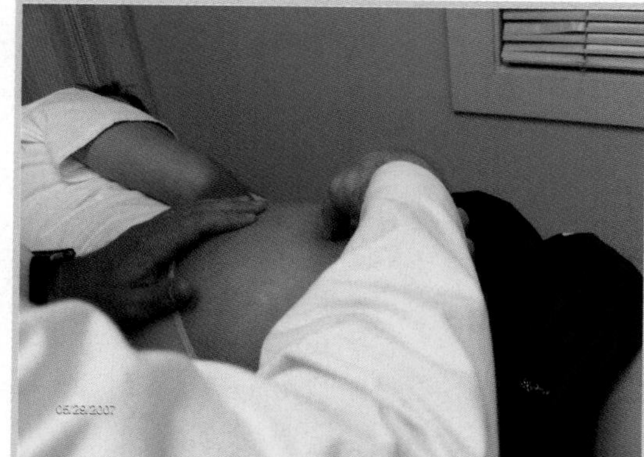

Step 2

Step 3. Swab the patient's skin with povidone-iodine, chlorhexidine solution, or 70% ethanol. (See Appendix E.) Do not touch the injection site after swabbing.

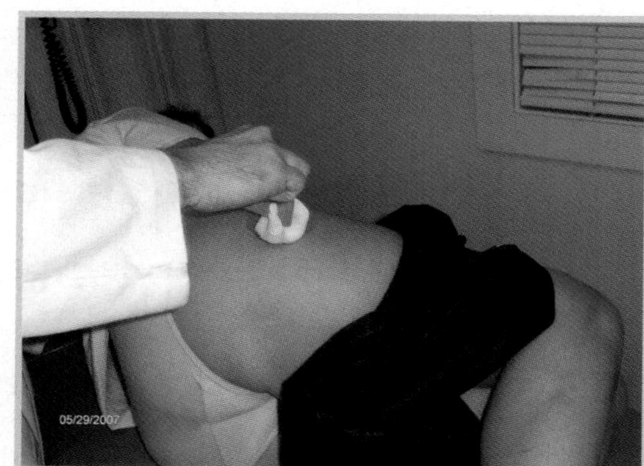

Step 3

Step 4. Insert the needle perpendicular to the skin and advance until the needle tip touches the bone. Withdraw the needle 2 to 3 mm, then aspirate and inject the steroid and lidocaine mixture. Have patient rest in the office for 20 to 30 minutes postinjection to ensure the patient tolerates the procedure and to review postprocedure instructions.

- **PEARL:** Maximal tenderness is often found at the muscle insertions along the superior and posterior borders of the greater trochanter. This may require larger injection volumes and/or a fanned technique to disperse the medication to the deep bursae, which superficially blankets the tendons described previously.
- **PITFALL:** Long-acting, low-solubility, fluorinated glucocorticoids (such as triamcinolone hexacetonide [Aristospan]) are considered inappropriate for soft tissue injections by some authors because of a higher risk of tissue atrophy. Triamcinolone acetonide (Kenalog) is a fluorinated triamcinolone, but solubility is intermediate to high. This makes Kenalog a reasonable alternative for this procedure but it may carry a higher risk of tissue atrophy than methylprednisolone.

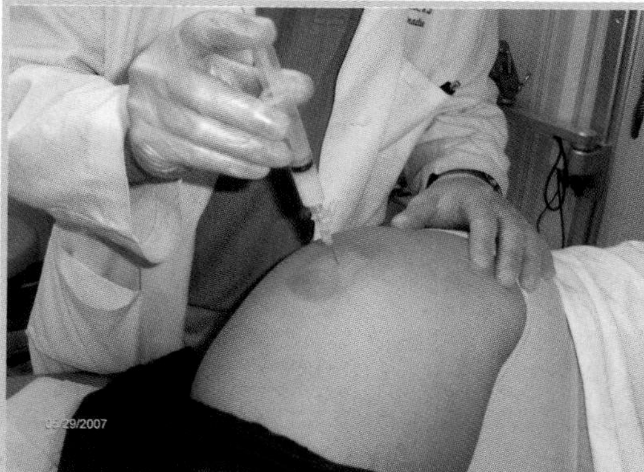

Step 4

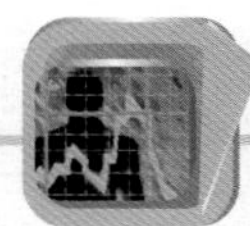

Complications

Local Effects

- Local infection (reported incidence range 1:3,000 to 1:50,000).
- Local reactions (swelling, tenderness, and warmth for up to 2 days).
- Steroid flare (1% to 10%; crystal-induced synovitis within 24 to 48 hours).
- Fat atrophy (especially at superficial soft tissue sites; worse with triamcinolone because it is less soluble and is fluorinated).
- Damage to local cartilage or nerves.

Systemic Effects

- Facial flushing (<15% of patients; within hours; lasts <3 or 4 days; women)
- Adrenal suppression (usually mild and transient; worse with stress)
- Transient increase in glucose

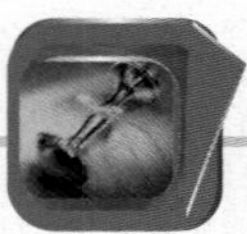

Pediatric Considerations

Trochanteric bursitis is rarely seen in children.

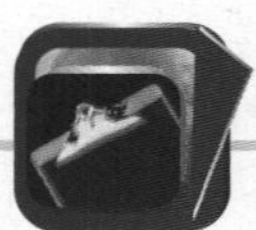

Postprocedure Instructions

Cover the injection site with a bandage. Ask the patient to gently move the area to spread the injected fluid. Advice about rest and timing between repeat injections is variable. Generally, avoiding aggravating activities for 24 hours is sufficient in this situation. Although evidence-based studies are lacking, general recommendations advise a respite of 6 weeks between injections and no more than three to four injections into the same region within a given year.

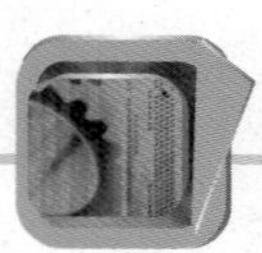

Coding Information and Supply Sources

CPT Code	Description	2008 Average 50th Percentile Fee	Global Period
20610	Arthrocentesis, aspiration, and/or injection of large joint or bursa	$ 176.00	0

ICD-9 Code

Trochanteric bursitis 726.5

Patient Education Handout

A patient education handout, "Trochanteric Bursitis," can be found on the book's companion Web site.

Bibliography

Alvarez-Nemegyei J, Canoso JJ. Evidence-based soft tissue rheumatology III: trochanteric bursitis. *J Clin Rheumatol.* 2004;10(3):123–124.

Bird PA, Oakley SP, Shnier R, et al. Prospective evaluation of MRI and physical examination findings in patients with greater trochanteric pain syndrome. *Arthritis Rheum.* 2001;44:2138–2145.

Cardone DA, Tallia AF. Diagnostic and therapeutic injection of the hip and knee. *Amer Fam Phys.* 2003;67(10):2147–2152.

Dunn T, Heller CA, McCarthy SW, et al. Anatomical study of the "trochanteric bursa." *Clinical Anat.* 2003;16:233–240.

Ines L. Soft tissue injections. *Best Pract Res Clin Rheum.* 2005;19(3):503–527.

Kingzett-Taylor A, Tirmal PF, Feller J, et al. Tendinosis and tears of gluteus medius and minimus muscles as a cause of hip pain: MR imaging findings. *Am J Roentgenol.* 1999;173:1123–1126.

Lievense A, Bierma-Zeinstra S, Schouten B, et al. Prognosis of trochanteric pain in primary care. *Br J Gen Pract.* March 2005:199–204.

Oakley SP, Bird P, Kirkham BW. Gluteus medius tears presenting as the clinical syndrome of trochanteric bursitis (abstract). *Arthritis Rheum.* 1999;42(Suppl 9):S340.

Shbeeb MI, Matteson EL. Trochanteric bursitis (greater trochanter pain syndrome). *Mayo Clin Proc.* 1996;71:565–569.

Walker P, Kannangara S, et al. Lateral hip pain. *Clin Orthop Relat Res.* 2007;Apr;457:144–149.

2008 MAG Mutual Healthcare Solutions, Inc.'s Physicians' Fee and Coding Guide. Duluth, Georgia. MAG Mutual Healthcare Solutions, Inc. 2007.

CHAPTER 106

Knee Joint Aspiration and Injection

Daniel L. Stulberg, MD, FAAFP
Associate Professor of Family and Community Medicine
University of New Mexico Health Sciences Center, Albuquerque, NM

Aspiration and/or injection of the knee joint are useful procedures for the office-based or hospital-based practitioner. Arthrocentesis may establish a diagnosis, relieve discomfort, detect hemarthrosis, drain off infected fluid, or instill medication. Even with the increased frequency of advanced imaging including magnetic resonance imaging (MRI), arthrocentesis can be very time and cost-efficient as well as therapeutic. This simple procedure can be a useful diagnostic and therapeutic tool for the practitioner.

Therapeutic injection of the knee joint may be performed without the presence of an effusion. Aspiration of fluid from a knee effusion can temporarily relieve pressure and reduce discomfort, but the fluid usually recollects unless the underlying process is self-limited or treated. Therefore, aspiration is more useful when the etiology of the effusion is unclear and analysis of the fluid will help the clinician treat the patient. The differential diagnosis includes osteoarthritis, injury, infection, rheumatic disorders, gout, and other less common disorders, so cell counts, Gram stains, cultures, and analysis for crystals are often performed based on the clinical situation.

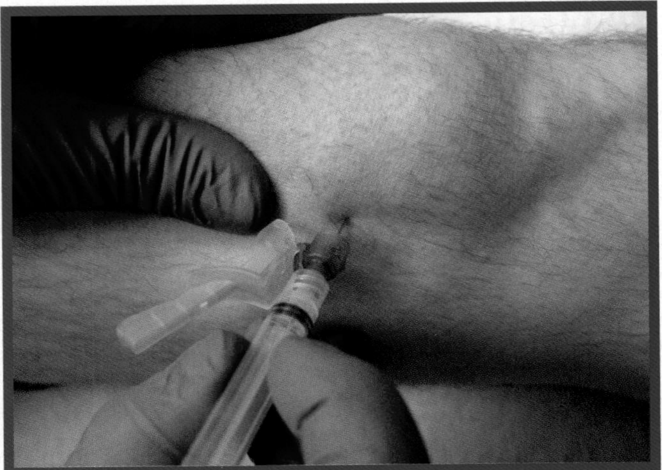

Effusion of the knee initially causes a rounder, full appearance to the knee with a loss of the "hollows" medially and laterally at the inferior portion of the patella. Larger effusions will cause swelling seen superiorly. With compression of one or two of these areas, the fluid will shift to the other areas and appear more prominent. The patella may even be ballottable (having a bouncing or floating feel) when compressed posteriorly. A variety of needle entry techniques have been described for the knee joint, and almost all are successful when large effusions are present. Common approaches are the superolateral or the medial from a supine position or the inferolateral from the sitting position with the knee flexed to 90 degrees.

As with any invasive procedure and the injection of medications, the clinician should weigh the risks and benefits of the procedure with the patient prior to proceeding. Corticosteroids can temporarily help with the pain and inflammation of osteoarthritis (Table 106-1) or help with a flare of gout. Viscosupplementation with

TABLE 106-1. Criteria for the Classification of Osteoarthritis of the Knee using Clinical and Laboratory Findings

The patient should complain of knee pain and have at least 5 of the following **9** features:
Age >50 yr
Stiffness <30 min
Crepitus
Bony tenderness
Bony enlargement
No palpable warmth
Erythrocyte sedimentation rate <40 mm/hr
Rheumatoid factor <1:40
Synovial fluid signs of osteoarthritis (clear to straw colored, high viscosity, 1,000–7,500 white blood cells/μL, 2.9–5.5 g of protein/dL)

Adapted from Blackburn WD. Approach to the patient with a musculoskeletal disorder. *Professional Commun.* 1st ed. New York; 2000:126.

hylan or hyaluronan (Synvisc and Orthovisc respectively) is approved for the treatment of osteoarthritis with longer-lasting reduction in pain versus corticosteroids based on a Cochrane database analysis. They are given as a series of three weekly injections. Intra-articular administration is thought to maximize local medication benefits while reducing systemic effects, but patients should be counseled regarding the risks of viscosupplementation and the risks of steroids as appropriate, including the risk of aseptic necrosis of the femoral or humeral head with the latter.

Steroids should not be injected into a joint if infection is suspected or confirmed. The total synovial white blood cell count (SWBC) can help classify the type of effusion. Typically, a SWBC of <2,500/mm^3 is found in noninflammatory fluid, and a SWBC between 2,500 and 25,000/mm^3 is found in inflammatory fluid. A 2007 systematic review of the literature by Margaretten et al. showed that a SWBC differential of 90% or higher segmented neutrophils has an increased likelihood ratio of 3.4 versus a likelihood ration of only 0.34 if the differential was <90% segmented neutrophils. The review also found increasing likelihood rations of 7.7 and 28 for SWBC >50,000/mm^3 and >100,000/mm^3 respectively.

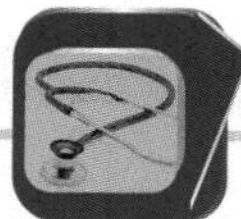

Equipment

- Sterile gloves are preferred by some; others use nonsterile gloves and a "no touch" sterile technique.
- Skin preparation agent: 70% isopropyl alcohol, povidone-iodine (Betadine), or chlorhexidine gluconate with 70% isopropyl alcohol (ChloraPrep) pads or applicator.
- Viscosupplementation agent or steroid for injection as indicated, most commonly 40 to 80 mg of methylprednisolone acetate (Solu-Medrol), 10 to 40 mg of triamcinolone hexacetonide (Aristospan), or 10 to 40 mg of triamcinolone acetonide (Kenalog).
- Syringe (3 to 10 mL, for administering medication).
- Syringe (20 to 60 mL, for aspirating effusion).
- One or two 21- to 22- gauge, 1.25-inch needles (to draw up injecting solutions, with the option of a second needle for performing arthrocentesis).
- Straight hemostat for stabilizing the needle if planning to aspirate first and then exchange the medication syringe for the aspiration syringe to inject without entering the joint a second time.

- 1% lidocaine for use as a local anesthetic as needed and for injection with corticosteroids.
- Red-top tube or vial for laboratory analysis and culture swab with medium for testing as indicated.
- Postprocedure bandage.

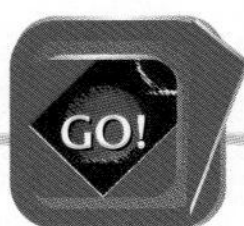

Indications

- Diagnostic evaluation of the cause of an effusion or an unexplained monoarthritis
- To limit joint damage from infected or inflamed joint fluid by serial removal of fluid
- Symptomatic relief by removing a large effusion or treatment of joint pain or inflammation (usually temporary)
- Diagnosis or treatment of a crystal-induced arthropathy
- Administration of viscous agents for symptomatic improvement of osteoarthritis
- Administration of glucocorticoids for symptomatic improvement of osteoarthritis

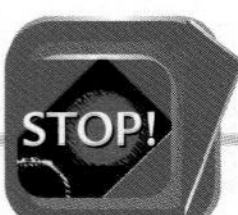

Contraindications

- Bacteremia or cellulitis overlying the joint
- Bleeding diathesis or coagulopathy
- Uncooperative patient
- Injection of steroids if septic arthritis is suspected or present
- Clinician is unfamiliar with the correct approach to the joint
- Presence of a joint prosthesis
- Lack of response to previous injections or aspirations
- Steroid injections should usually be limited to three to four times per year
- Poorly controlled diabetes or systemic illness (diabetes or illness may be more difficult to control with injection of steroids)
- Therapeutic injection for children and conditions other than those listed previously warrant consideration of a specialty evaluation or recommendation

The Procedure

Step 1. In skilled hands, injection into the knee joint can be completed in only a few seconds, so a local anesthetic is not usually used. For aspiration, for the patient with difficult anatomy, or for the less experienced clinician, a local anesthetic of 1% lidocaine plain injected subcutaneously at the injection site and toward the joint may be useful. See Appendix F. Some practitioners believe that a larger volume gives greater distribution of the medication and will use up to 10 mL or more of local anesthetic injected into the joint with the corticosteroid, and some studies have shown that injection of a volume of anesthetic alone can reduce symptoms.

- **PITFALL:** Limit the use of local infiltration to 1 to 2 mL to avoid causing swelling that would distort the usual landmarks and the ability to palpate the joint.
- **PEARL:** Marcaine can be mixed with the lidocaine to extend the anesthetic effect from approximately 1 hour to between 3 and 4 hours.
- **PITFALL:** Some experts recommend a new needle for each multidose vial and for the actual injection as well as using single-dose vials of unpreserved anesthetic to avoid possible precipitation of the steroid due to the preservative.

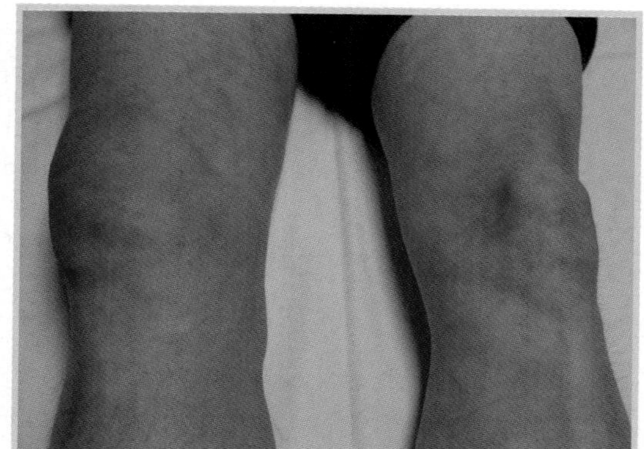

Step 1

Step 2. If aspiration and then injection is planned, draw the medication into a syringe, remove the needle, and place where the tip will remain sterile (optimally have an assistant hold it). Attach a 21- or 22-gauge needle to a 10- to 60-mL Luer lock syringe based on anticipated volume. Have a straight hemostat available to grasp and stabilize the needle after the aspiration.

- **PITFALL:** This can be done without an assistant, but make sure that sterility is maintained and that the needles are securely on the syringes with a Luer lock to prevent leakage or dislodgement but not so tight that they are difficult to remove during the procedure.

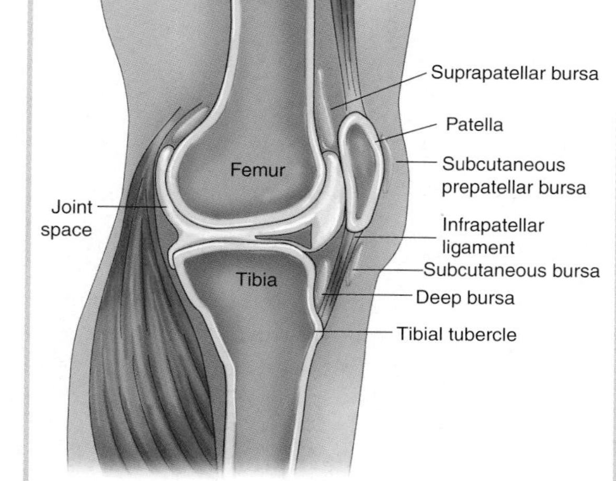

Step 2

Medial Approach (Supine Position with the Knee Slightly Flexed)

Step 3. Place a gloved hand around the patella with the thumb on the medial aspect and the fingers on the lateral edge of the patella.

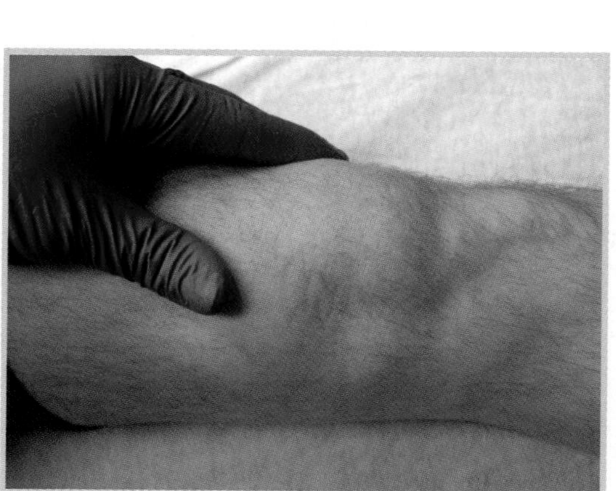

Step 3

Step 4. Pull the patella medially with the fingers at the same time as the thumb is used to slightly elevate the patella on the medial aspect, opening up a space under the patella and palpating the injection site at the midpoint of the medial aspect of the patella.

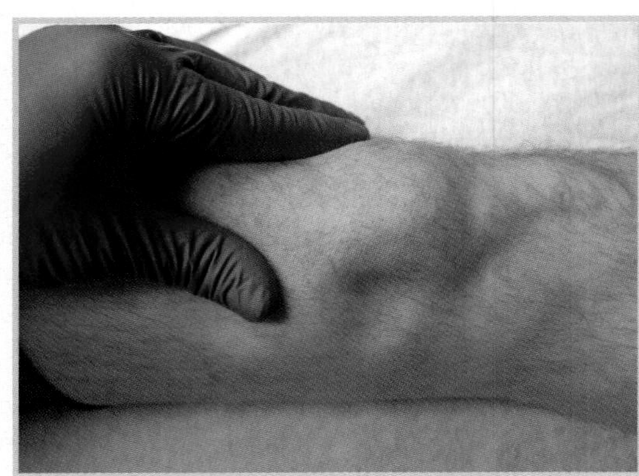

Step 4

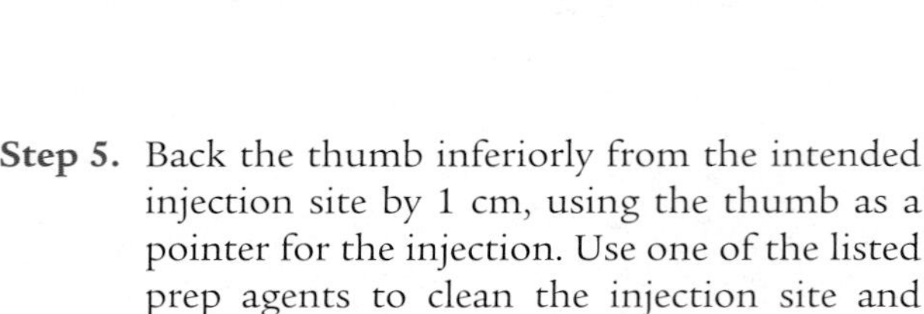

Step 5. Back the thumb inferiorly from the intended injection site by 1 cm, using the thumb as a pointer for the injection. Use one of the listed prep agents to clean the injection site and allow it to dry.

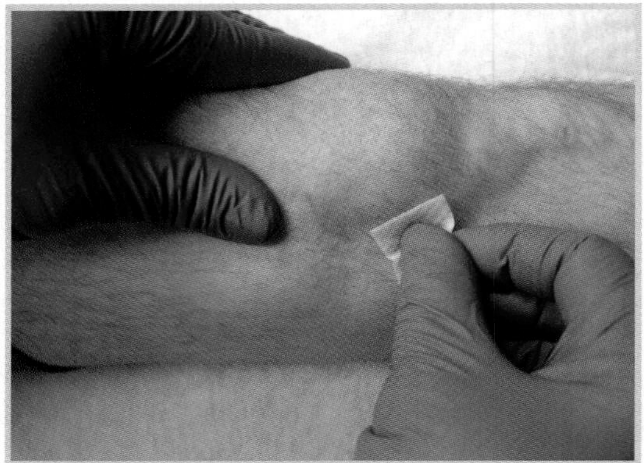

Step 5

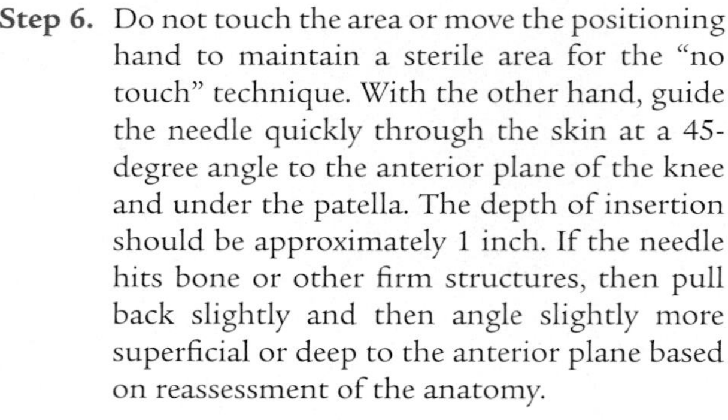

Step 6. Do not touch the area or move the positioning hand to maintain a sterile area for the "no touch" technique. With the other hand, guide the needle quickly through the skin at a 45-degree angle to the anterior plane of the knee and under the patella. The depth of insertion should be approximately 1 inch. If the needle hits bone or other firm structures, then pull back slightly and then angle slightly more superficial or deep to the anterior plane based on reassessment of the anatomy.

- **PITFALL:** The needle tip should pass easily and not touch nearby structures. Touching the needle to any structures within the joint can cause significant discomfort.

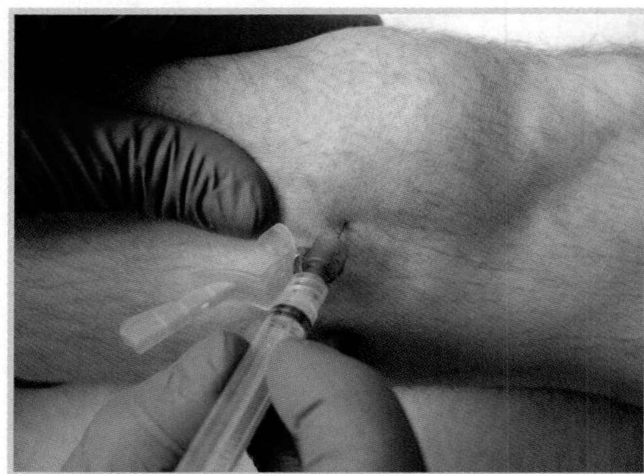

Step 6

Step 7. For aspiration, withdraw the desired amount of fluid. If the effusion is small, pressure applied by an assistant at the inferior and superior aspects of the patella at its medial and lateral margins can displace the fluid toward the aspirating needle. To avoid a second puncture and inject at the same time, grasp the hub of the needle with a straight hemostat, rest that hand against the patient, and stabilize the needle while unscrewing the syringe and then screwing on the medication syringe. Maintain the sterile condition of the

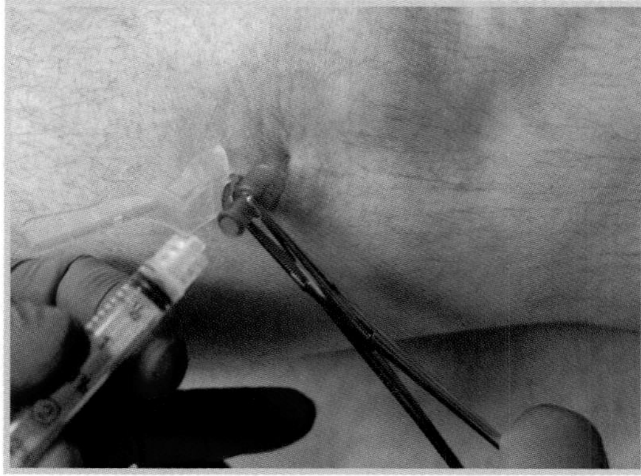

Step 7

connections by not allowing them to touch any other surfaces.

To inject the medication, push the plunger. There should be no resistance. If there is any resistance, then the needle is not in the joint space and should be repositioned. When there is no resistance, the medication can be injected in less then a second, and the needle removed very quickly to the relief of the patient, who is usually nervous but then pleased that the procedure was brief. Place a gauze pad or cotton ball over the site for any skin bleeding, and then apply an adhesive bandage. If lidocaine is used, the patient will usually note a reduction in pain in a matter of only a few minutes.

- PITFALL: Avoid movement of the needle when removing or reapplying a syringe. Movement of the needle is very painful.

Superolateral Technique

Step 8. In the same "no touch" sterile technique and setup as described previously, palpate the superolateral aspect of the patella. Insert the needle quickly through the skin 1 cm (approximately one fingerbreadth) superiorly and laterally to the patella. Then gently guide the needle beneath the patella at a 45-degree angle to the axis of the extremity, aiming the needle to the center of the joint toward the inferior portion of the patella.

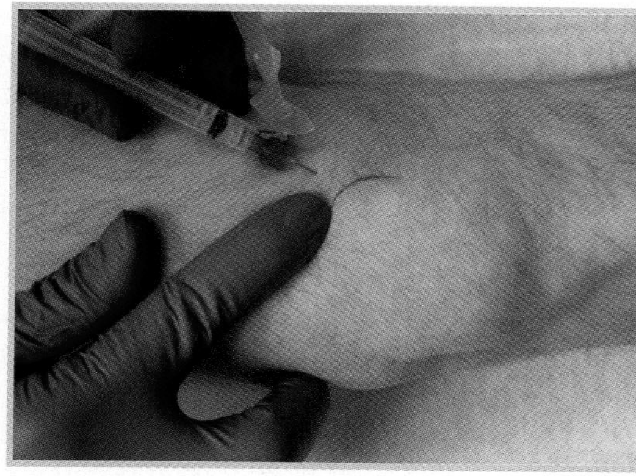

Step 8

Anterior (Sitting Flexed Knee) Technique

Step 9. With the patient sitting, the foot facing forward, and the knee flexed at 90 degrees, insert the needle slightly medially or laterally to the palpable infrapatellar tendon at its insertion on the inferior portion of the patella. Advance the needle posteriorly and slightly toward the midline.

- PITFALL: This technique is discouraged, because the needle tip may cause damage to the articular surfaces or the menisci. This direct approach may be acceptable when administering therapeutic viscous solutions (e.g., hyaluronic acid), because the knee cartilage has previously received significant wear.

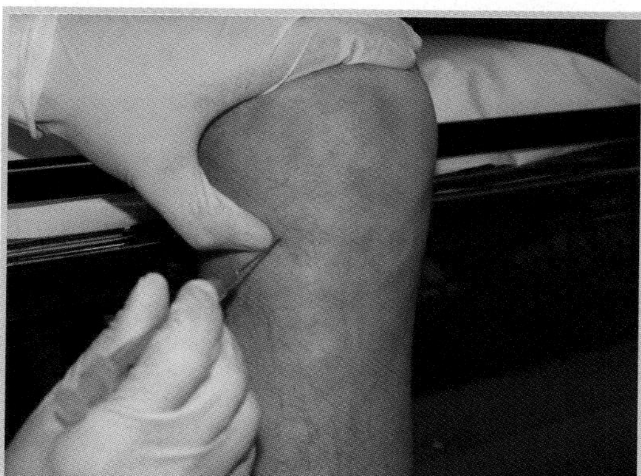

Step 9

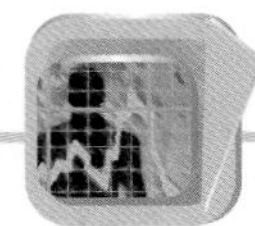

Complications

- Infection from arthrocentesis is rare and is believed to occur in <1 in 10,000 procedures.
- The knee is vulnerable to injury, and strenuous activity should be avoided in the first 24 hours after injection.
- Postinjection flare is a worsening of joint pain 12 to 72 hours after a steroid injection; nonsteroidal drugs may help.
- Theoretically, steroids may cause degeneration of the articular surface; limit them to three to four injections per year.

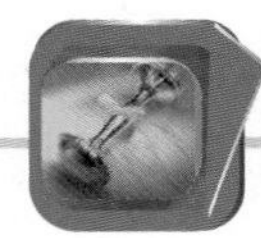

Pediatric Considerations

This is rarely used in pediatrics patients.

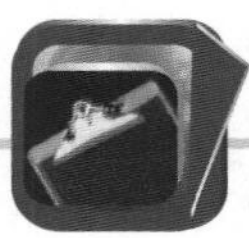

Postprocedure Instructions

Cautions regarding the risks and benefits of the procedure should have been discussed prior to the procedure but may be reinforced after the procedure. Even though the patient will likely feel better, the patient should rest for 1 to 2 days and avoid overusing the knee. The patient should watch for signs of infection, which could include fevers, increasing pain, warmth, or redness of the knee. The knee will usually feel much better for one to a few hours after the injection if an anesthetic was injected. This will wear off, and it will take 1 to 2 days before the steroid or viscosupplementation effects start. With steroids or viscosupplementation, there can be a flare and increased pain initially. This can be helped by icing the knee and taking a nonsteroidal anti-inflammatory drug (NSAID) if the patient can tolerate one. Flexible gel ice packs are commercially available, or a bag of frozen peas or corn can be molded over the knee (but should be discarded instead of consumed if used as an ice pack). Steroids and viscosupplementation will not help all patients, and the improvement in symptoms is useful, but only temporary, especially with steroids. If an effusion was tapped, there is a high likelihood that it will at least partially return.

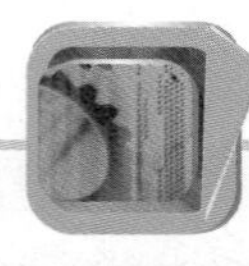

Coding Information and Supply Sources

CPT Code	Description	2008 Average 50th Percentile Fee	Global Period
20610	Aspiration or injection of major joint or bursa (knee)	$176.00	0

CPT is a registered trademark of the American Medical Association.
2008 average 50th Percentile Fees are provided courtesy of 2008 MMH-SI's copyrighted Physicians' Fees and Coding Guide.

All materials can be ordered through local medical supply companies. Lidocaine solution, injectable steroid solution (e.g., Celestone), and injectable viscous agents (e.g., Hyalgan) are available from local pharmacies or medical supply companies. A suggested tray for performing soft tissue aspirations and injections is listed in Appendix I: Suggested Tray for Soft Tissue Aspiration and Injection Procedures. Skin preparation recommendations appear in Appendix E.

Patient Education Handout

A patient education handout, "Knee Joint Aspiration and Injection," can be found on the book's companion Web site.

The author would like to acknowledge Chris McGrew, MD, for his review of the manuscript.

Bibliography

Blackburn WD. *Approach to the Patient with a Musculoskeletal Disorder*. Caddo (OK): Professional Communications; 1999.

Bellamy N, Campbell J, Robinson V, et al. Intra-articular corticosteroid for treatment of osteoarthritis of the knee. Cochrane Database of Systematic Reviews 2006:2. University of Queensland, Centre of National Research on Disability and Rehabilitation Medicine, Brisbane, Queensland, Australia. Cochrane Database of Systematic Reviews 2006, Issue 2. Art No.: CD005328. DOI: 10.1002/14651858. CD005328.pub 2.

Bellamy N, Campbell J, Robinson V, et al. Viscosupplementation for the treatment of osteoarthritis of the knee. Cochrane Database of Systematic Reviews 2006:2. University of Queensland, Centre of National Research on Disability and Rehabilitation Medicine, Brisbane, Queensland, Australia. Cochrane Database of Systematic Reviews 2006, Issue 2. Art No.: CD005321. DOI: 10.1002/14651858. CD005321.pub 2.

Margaretten ME, Kohlwes J, Moore D, et al. Does this adult patient have septic arthritis? *JAMA*. 2007;297:1478–1488.

Schumacher HR, Chen LX. Injectable corticosteroids in treatment of arthritis of the knee. *Am J Med*. November 2005;118(11).

2008 MAG Mutual Healthcare Solutions, Inc.'s Physicians' Fee and Coding Guide. Duluth, Georgia. MAG Mutual Healthcare Solutions, Inc. 2007.

CHAPTER 107

Olecranon Bursa Aspiration and Injection

Anne Boyd, MD
Assistant Professor, Department of Family Medicine
University of Pittsburgh School of Medicine
Director, Primary Care Sports Medicine Fellowship Program
UPMC
Pittsburgh, PA

Scott Wissink, MD
Assistant Professor, Department of Orthopaedic Surgery
University of Pittsburgh
Monroeville, PA

The olecranon bursa is situated between the tip of the olecranon and the skin. Its function is to prevent tissue damage by providing a mechanism for the skin to glide freely over this bony process. Because of its superficial location, this bursa is susceptible to inflammation from either acute or repetitive (cumulative) trauma. Nontraumatic inflammatory olecranon bursitis may result from gout, rheumatoid arthritis, calcium pyrophosphate deposition disease, or infection.

After an acute injury, the bursa can fill with blood or clear fluid to produce a tender, painful swelling over the elbow. Elbow pain that worsens during active or passive range of motion (ROM) should increase the clinician's suspicion of a fracture of the olecranon process and prompt him or her to obtain radiographs.

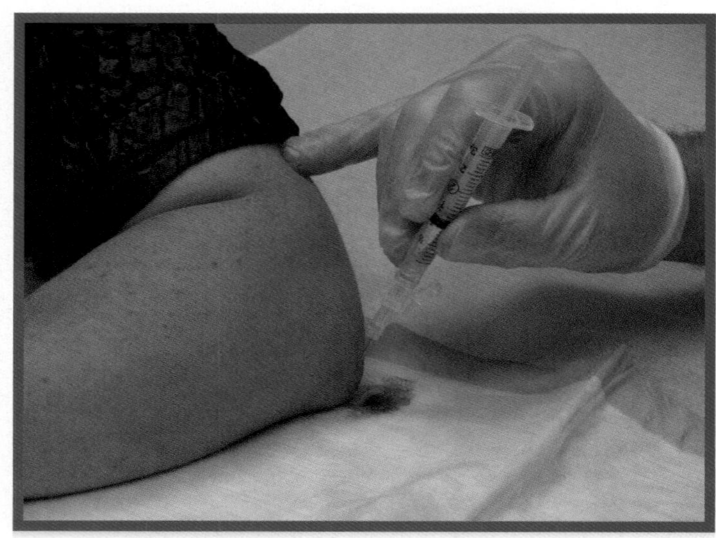

Nontraumatic inflammatory olecranon bursitis is diagnosed by the appearance of a fluctuant swelling over the elbow. The presence of erythema, warmth, and tenderness should alert the practitioner to the possibility of septic bursitis. However, positive cultures have also been obtained from distended bursae that do not exhibit the classic physical findings of infection. Therefore, testing to exclude infection before considering a corticosteroid injection is recommended, even if the clinical exam is atypical or fluid is not turbid on aspiration.

The leukocyte count can help determine whether joint fluid is infectious versus inflammatory. Within synovial aspirates, white blood cell (WBC) counts are assessed as follows:

- WBC count $<200/\mu L$ is considered normal.
- WBC count is considered noninflammatory at 200 to $2{,}000/\mu L$.
- WBC count in the range 2,000 to $100{,}000/\mu L$ is considered an indication of inflammation.
- WBC count $>100{,}000/\mu L$ is considered an indication of a septic condition.

Gram stain also is helpful in determining quickly whether bacterial infection appears to be present. If the Gram stain is positive, antibiotics should be started immediately and bursal corticosteroid injection must be avoided. Even if the Gram stain is negative or initially unavailable, antibiotics may seem indicated based on the mechanism of injury (e.g., abrasion or puncture), physical examination findings suggestive of infection (e.g., fever, significant local redness, and warmth), or the gross appearance of the aspirate (e.g., turbid, purulent). Gram stain should be followed by culture and sensitivity testing. The culture and sensitivity results should guide the use of antibiotics in cases of bacterial infection (usually cephalosporins or penicillinase-resistant penicillins). Crystal analysis may reveal monosodium urate crystals in a patient with gout, calcium pyrophosphate crystals in a patient with pseudogout, or hydroxyapatite crystals.

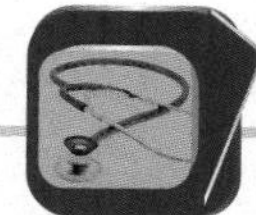

Equipment

- Needle (25 gauge, 1 inch long) on a 3-mL syringe loaded with 2 mL of 1% lidocaine with epinephrine (for anesthesia)
- Needle (18 gauge, 1.5 inches long) on a 10-mL syringe (for aspiration)
- Needle (22 to 25 gauge, 1.5 inches long) on a 3-mL syringe loaded with 0.5 mL (20 mg) of methylprednisolone acetate (Depo-Medrol) and 2 mL of 1% lidocaine without epinephrine (for steroid injection)

Consult the ordering information that appears in Appendix I. Needles, syringes, and corticosteroid preparations may be ordered from surgical supply houses or local pharmacies. A suggested tray for performing soft tissue aspirations and injections is listed in Appendix I. Skin preparation recommendations appear in Appendix E.

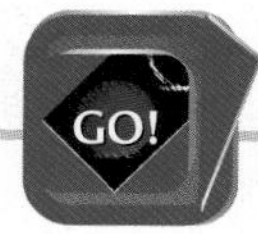

Indications

- Symptomatic or cosmetic concerns over distention of the olecranon bursa
- Suspicion of septic or crystalloid bursitis of the olecranon bursa

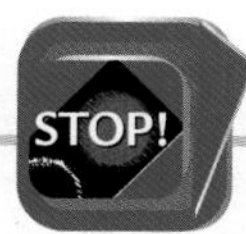

Contraindications (Relative)

- Uncooperative patient
- Coagulopathy or bleeding diathesis

The Procedure

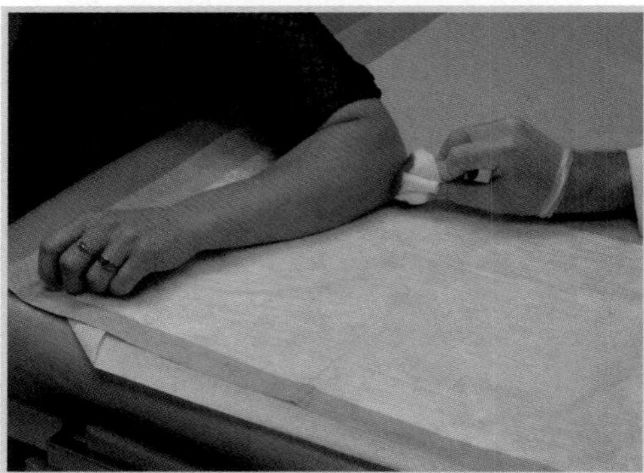
Step 1

Step 1. After informed consent is obtained, hands are washed, materials are prepared, and gloves are applied. With the patient seated, the elbow is flexed to 90 degrees and supported. Most practitioners prefer a lateral approach to avoid the ulnar nerve. Swab the patient's skin with povidone-iodine, chlorhexidine solution, or 70% ethanol (see Appendix E). Do not touch the injection site after swabbing.

- **PEARL:** When aspiration/injection is performed, use aseptic techniques to minimize the chance of causing iatrogenic infection.

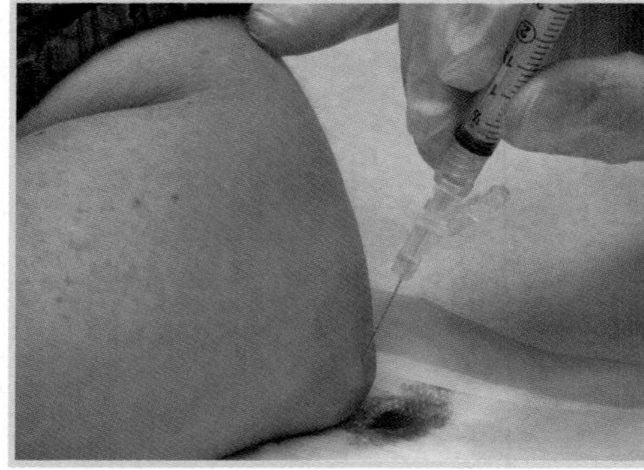
Step 2

Step 2. Insert a 25-gauge, 1-inch-long needle on a 3-mL syringe perpendicular to the skin, and inject approximately 2 mL of 1% lidocaine with epinephrine subcutaneously to create a small, raised wheal over the area you are going to insert the 18-gauge needle.

Step 3. Enter the bursa from the side (parallel to the plane of the forearm) and aspirate using an 18-gauge, 1.5-inch-long needle on a 10-mL syringe. Aspirated fluid should be sent for Gram stain, culture and sensitivity, white blood cell count and differential, and crystal analysis if there is any diagnostic uncertainty or if the clinician is considering injection of steroid at a later date. Apply pressure with a 4 × 4-inch gauze pad, clean the area with 70% ethanol, and apply a sterile bandage. Have patient rest in the office for 20 to 30 minutes postinjection to ensure patient tolerability of the procedure and to review postprocedure instructions.

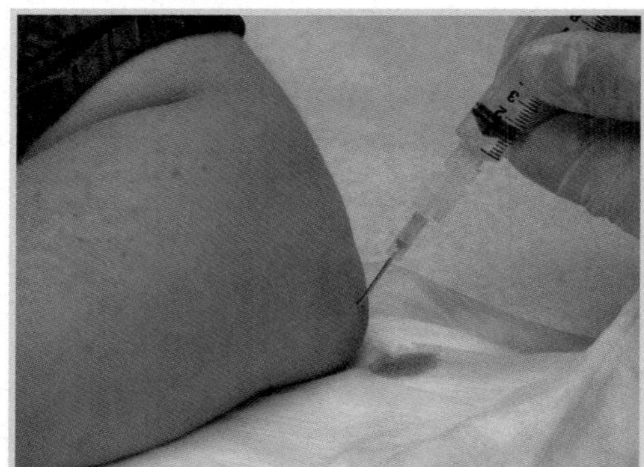
Step 3

Step 4. If aspirate from the initial procedure returns and indicates an inflammatory process alone (noninfectious process), a corticosteroid may be considered at a later date. To administer a steroid, repeat the preparation described and pictured in Step 1, then use a 22- to 25-gauge, 1.5-inch-long needle on a 3-mL syringe to inject 0.5 mL (20 mg) of methylprednisolone acetate (Depo-Medrol) and 2 mL of 1% lidocaine without epinephrine.

- **PITFALL:** Two procedures generally are needed if a steroid is to be used. The first is to perform the bacteriologic studies after aspiration. The second introduces the corticosteroid.
- **PITFALL:** Avoid injecting a steroid into a bursa with a subacute infection of the bursa or overlying skin.

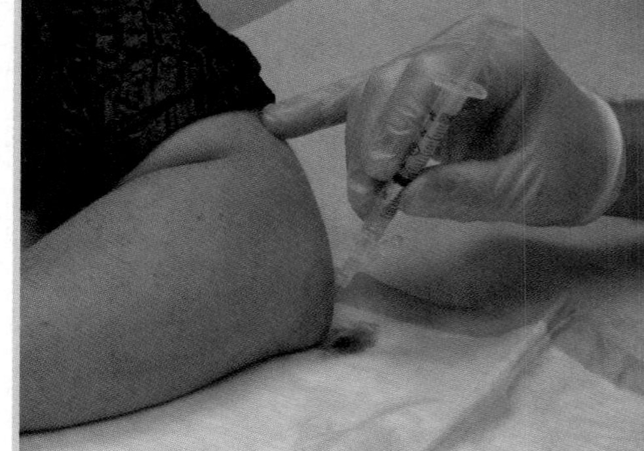
Step 4

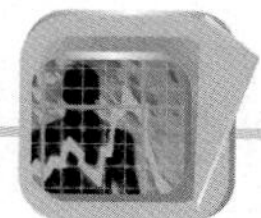

Complications

- Swelling: This may recur, particularly if the etiology is infectious or if pressure or icing at the site is not utilized after the procedure.
- Infection, which may be iatrogenic or a pre-existing, subacute infection that becomes acute.
- Persistent drainage through the injection tract.
- If a medial approach is used for the aspiration/injection, ulnar nerve injury is possible.
- Skin and fat atrophy and thinning, as well as hypopigmentation, are possible because of the superficial position of the bursa.

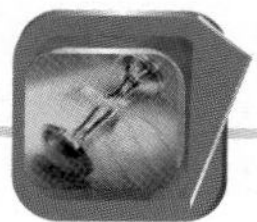

Postprocedure Instructions

After the injection, the patient may utilize nonsteroidal anti-inflammatory drugs (NSAIDs) and a compression dressing. For cases with repeated recurrence, consider the use of a posterior splint to limit elbow motion for 1 to 2 weeks following aspiration. The patient should return for re-evaluation within 1 week. At that time, assess for re-accumulation of the fluid, any persistent drainage, or any signs of infection. The decision whether to treat with empiric antibiotics depends upon the perceived likelihood of infection based on the history, physical examination, and analysis of the bursal aspirate.

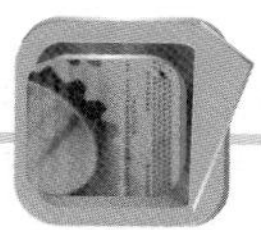

Coding Information and Supply Sources

CPT Code	Description	2008 Average 50th Percentile Fee	Global Period
20605	Arthrocentesis, aspiration, and/or injection of intermediate joint or bursa	$137.00	0

CPT is a registered trademark of the American Medical Association.
2008 average 50th Percentile Fees are provided courtesy of 2008 MMH-SI's copyrighted Physicians' Fees and Coding Guide.

ICD-9 Code

Olecranon bursitis 726.33

Patient Education Handout

A patient education handout, "Olecranon Bursitis," can be found on the book's companion Web site.

Bibliography

Griffin YG, Green W. *Essentials of Musculoskeletal Care.* (3rd ed.). Rosemont, IL: AAOS; 2005:269–273.

Pfenninger JL, Fowler GC. *Procedures for Primary Care.* (2nd ed.). St. Louis: Mosby; 2003:1479–1499.

Rouzier P. *The Sports Medicine Patient Advisor, Elbow (Olecranon) Bursitis.* (1st ed.). Amherst, MA: HBO & Company; 1999:206–207.

Saunders S, Longworth S. *Injection Techniques in Orthopaedic and Sports Medicine.* (2nd ed.). Philadelphia: WB Saunders; 2002:48–49.

Schumacher HR. Arthrocentesis, synovial fluid analysis, and synovial biopsy. In: *Primer on Rheumatic Diseases.* (10th ed.). Richmond: Arthritis Foundation; 1993:67–72.

2008 MAG Mutual Healthcare Solutions, Inc.'s Physicians' Fee and Coding Guide. Duluth, Georgia. MAG Mutual Healthcare Solutions, Inc. 2007.

CHAPTER 108

Plantar Fascia Injection

Doug Aukerman, MD, FAAFP

Assistant Professor, Department of Orthopaedics, Rehabilitation and Sports Medicine
Assistant Professor, Department of Family and Community Medicine
Penn State Milton S. Hershey Medical Center
Hershey, PA
Team Physician, Penn State University
State College, PA

Proximal plantar fasciitis is a common cause of heel pain in adults. The plantar fascia is a fibrous aponeurosis that originates from the medial tubercle of the calcaneus and provides dynamic shock absorption and static support to the longitudinal arch.

Individuals with pes planus (i.e., flat feet) or pes cavus (i.e., high arches) are at increased risk for developing plantar fasciitis. In athletes, overuse and improper footwear are the most common cause of plantar fasciitis. The pain of proximal plantar fasciitis is usually caused by collagen degeneration at the medial tubercle of the calcaneus (i.e., origin of the plantar fascia). It is caused by repetitive microtears of the plantar fascia that overcome the body's ability to repair itself.

The classic symptom of plantar fasciitis is that the worst pain occurs with the first few steps in the morning, lessening as activity continues. Pain may also be associated with prolonged standing, in which case it can worsen toward the end of the day. Often the pain may begin insidiously and become progressively worse over weeks to months. A history of an increase in weight-bearing activities is common, especially those involving running, due to repetitive microtrauma to the plantar fascia. On examination, the patient is maximally tender at the anteromedial region of the calcaneus. The tender area may extend distally from the insertion point along the proximal plantar fascia. The pain is often exacerbated by passive dorsiflexion of the toes or by having the patient stand on the tips of the toes. Diagnostic testing is usually not indicated. Plantar fasciitis is often called heel spurs because of the commonly associated x-ray findings, but 15% to 25% of the asymptomatic population has heel spurs, and many symptomatic individuals do not. The spurring on radiographs reflects the calcification resulting from the chronic nature or the microtrauma of the tight fascial tissue. Diagnostic testing is indicated in atypical cases of heel pain (Table 108-1) or in patients who are not responding to appropriate treatment.

TABLE 108-1. Differential Diagnosis of Heel Pain

Problem	Differentiating Clinical Features
Entrapment syndromes	Radiating burning pain, or numbness and tingling, mainly at night on the plantar surface of the foot
Calcaneal stress fracture	Pain with weight bearing; worsens with prolonged weight bearing
Paget's disease	Bowed tibias, kyphosis, headaches
Bone tumor	Deep bone pain; constitutional symptoms late in the course
Calcaneal apophysitis (Sever's disease)	Posterior heel pain in adolescents
Fat pad syndrome	Atrophy of heel pad
Heel bruise	History of acute impact injury
Bursitis	Usually retrocalcaneal; swelling, pain, and erythema of posterior heel
Plantar fascia rupture	Sudden, acute, knifelike pain, ecchymosis
Tendonitis	Pain mainly with resisted motions

Plantar fasciitis is usually a self-limiting condition, yet it may take 6 to 18 months to resolve with expectant management. Nonoperative treatment results in a 90% success rate. Rest alone is an effective treatment, but it is poorly accepted as a treatment modality by athletes, active adults, and persons whose occupations require extensive walking. Often, a planned period of "relative rest" that decreases the strain to the area can decrease the discomfort. Identifying and correcting the problems that place individuals at increased risk for plantar fasciitis, such as increased weight-bearing activity, high intensity of activity, hard walking or running surfaces, and worn-out shoes is important for long-term treatment success. The most common conservative treatment for plantar fasciitis is stretching and strengthening programs to correct functional risk factors such as tightness of the gastrocsoleus complex and weakness of the intrinsic foot muscles. Other commonly used treatments include use of orthotics, nonsteroidal anti-inflammatory drugs (NSAIDs), iontophoresis, ice, heat, heel cups, night splints, extracorporeal shock wave therapy, and plantar strapping. For individuals with flat feet, shoes with better longitudinal arch support may help.

Corticosteroid injections work best when administered early in the course of plantar fasciitis but are often reserved for recalcitrant cases. A foot radiograph is recommended before injecting steroids to rule out other causes of heel pain, such as stress fracture or tumor. Steroids can be injected through plantar or medial approaches with or without ultrasound guidance. Studies have found that steroid treatments have a success rate of at least 70%.

Rupture of the plantar fascia is a treatment risk found in up to 10% of patients after injection. Long-term plantar fascia rupture may be common. However, most individuals with rupture of the plantar fascia have resolution of symptoms with rest and rehabilitation. Other possible risks include fat pad atrophy, ecchymosis, and infection.

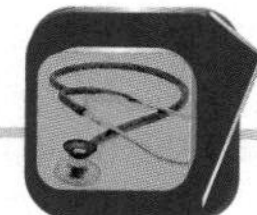

Equipment

- Iodine or chlorhexidine swabs
- Alcohol swabs
- Sterile syringe, 5 cc
- Lidocaine 1% without epinephrine
- Steroid (1 cc) such as betamethasone (Celestone) or triamcinolone
- Adhesive bandage

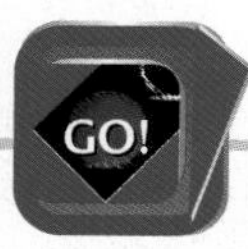

Indications

- Plantar fasciitis that is not improving or that is being treated with aggressive nonsurgical treatment

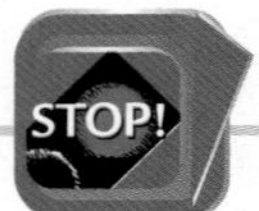

Contraindications

Absolute

- Local cellulitis
- Septic arthritis
- Acute fracture
- Bacteremia
- Joint prosthesis
- Achilles or patella tendinopathies
- Tumor
- History of allergy to the medications

Relative

- Minimal relief after two previous corticosteroid injections
- Coagulopathy or anticoagulation therapy
- Evidence of surrounding joint osteoporosis
- Uncontrolled diabetes mellitus
- Entrapment of posterior tibial nerve or its branches
- Fat pad atrophy

The Procedure

Medial Approach

Step 1. Place the patient in a comfortable position, sitting or lying on an examination table. Find the point of maximal tenderness, which is usually at or near the plantar fascia insertion on the calcaneus. Mark the area with the end of a sterile swab stick. Approach the injection using a medial approach, which improves patient comfort.

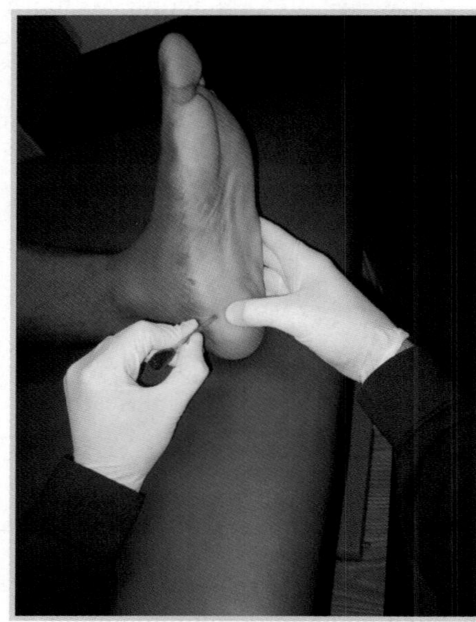

Step 1

Step 2. Clean the injection area with povidone-iodine, chlorhexidine, or alcohol (see Appendix E). Choose a 25-gauge needle that is 1 to 1.5 inches long.

- **PITFALL:** Use of a short, smaller-diameter needle may cause less discomfort, but it may fail to reach the intended area at the fascia insertion.

Step 3. Using sterile technique, insert the needle 1 to 2 cm above the sole, just past the end of the plantar fascia insertion on the calcaneus, aiming for the end of the bone. The needle is directed parallel to the surface of the sole, toward the area of maximal tenderness. The needle should be just cephalad to the plantar fascia and just distal to the insertion of the fascia to the calcaneus. Infiltrate the area with the diluted corticosteroid (1 cc of triamcinolone [40 mg mL] and 2 to 3 cc of 1% lidocaine). The needle may be drawn back and the medication infiltrated to bathe the aponeurosis in a fan shape just distal to the insertion.

- **PITFALL:** Do not inject against resistance. The medication should flow easily into the potential space around the fascia.
- **PITFALL:** Do not allow any steroid to leak into the fat pads on the plantar aspect of the foot, because this may cause fat atrophy or necrosis. If the specialized plantar fat pad atrophies, it is gone forever. Some authorities recommend against the direct plantar approach to avoid injury to this specialized cushioning fat beneath the heel.

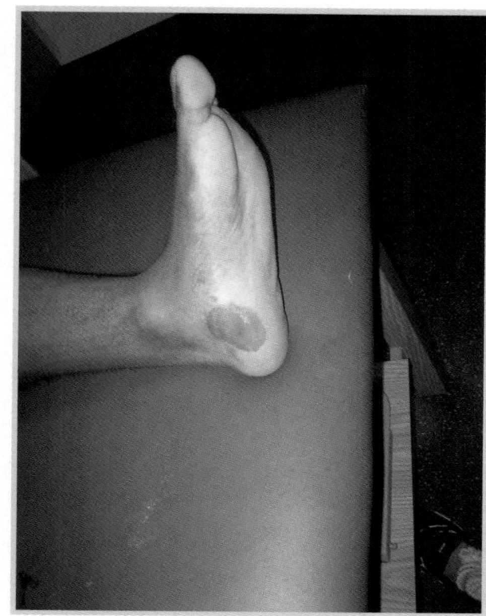

Step 2

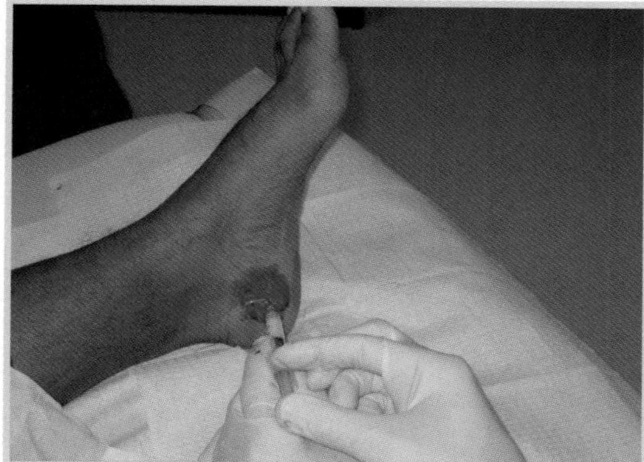

Step 3

Plantar Approach

Step 1. Find area on plantar surface of maximal tenderness. Mark with end of the swab.

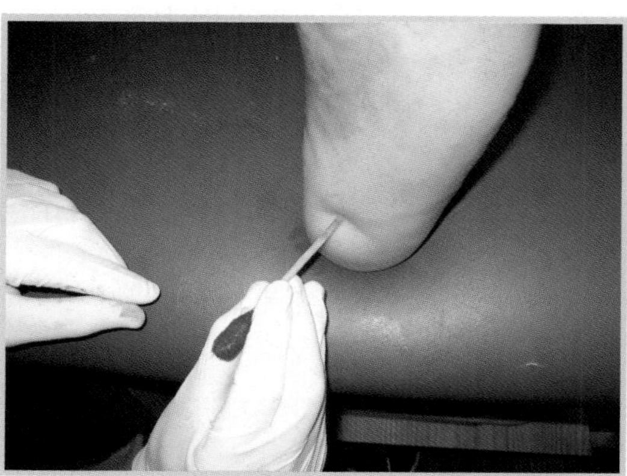

Step 1

Step 2. Clean skin with povidone-iodine or chlorhexidine. See Appendix E: Skin Preparation Recommendations.

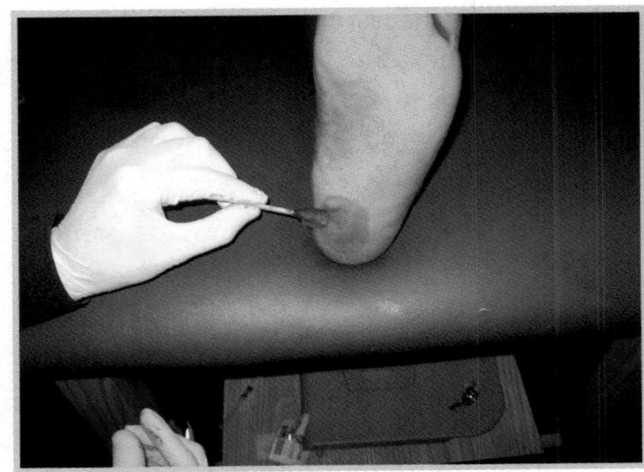

Step 2

Step 3. Infiltrate area with steroid and lidocaine mixture. Be sure not to allow mixture to leak into fat pad or to dermal layer.

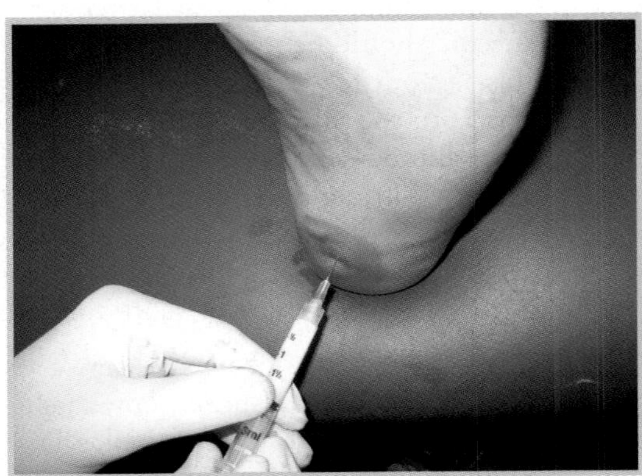

Step 3

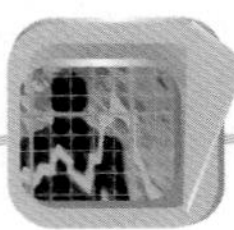

Complications

- Infection
- Bleeding
- Pain
- Fascia rupture
- Fat pad atrophy
- Skin hypopigmentation and atrophy

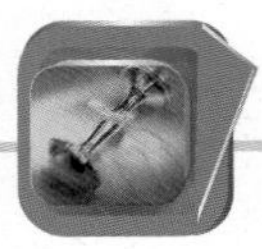

Pediatric Considerations

This procedure is not performed on a pediatric patient.

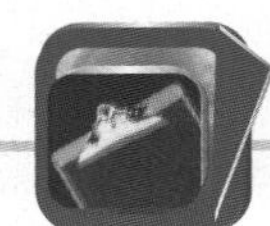

Postprocedure Instructions

Following the injection, apply slight pressure to the injection site to reduce the chance of steroid deposition into the dermal area. Ice may be applied to the area for patient comfort if the patient desires. Instruct the patient in ice and stretching for home treatment. A gel heel cup and arch support may be considered as adjunctive care.

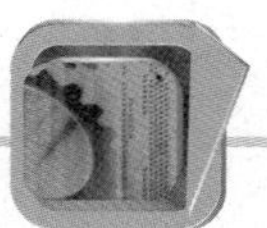

Coding Information and Supply Sources

CPT Code	Description	2008 Average 50th Percentile Fee	Global Period
20550	Injection(s); single tendon sheath, or ligament, aponeurosis (e.g., plantar "fascia")	$140.00	0

Note that this code and description has changed.

2008 average 50th Percentile Fees are provided courtesy of 2008 MMH-SI's copyrighted Physicians' Fees and Coding Guide.

Common materials for plantar fasciitis injection include a 3- or 5-mL syringe, 1% lidocaine without epinephrine, or 1% procaine, and 22-, 25-, or 27-gauge needles of various lengths. Injectable steroids can be found in local pharmacies.

Patient Education Handout

A patient education handout, "Plantar Fasciitis," can be found on the book's companion Web site.

Bibliography

Acevedo JI, Beskin JL. Complications of plantar fascia rupture associated with corticosteroid injection. *Foot Ankle Int.* 1998;19:91–97.

Furey JG. Plantar fasciitis: the painful heel syndrome. *J Bone Joint Surg.* 1975;57:672–673.

Gill LH, Kiebzak GM. Outcome of nonsurgical treatment for plantar fasciitis. *Foot Ankle Int.* 1996;17:527–532.

Kane D, Greaney T, Bresnihan B, et al. Ultrasound guided injection of recalcitrant plantar fasciitis. *Ann Rheum Dis.* 1998;57:383–384.

Khan KM, Cook JL, Taunton JE, et al. Overuse tendinosis, not tendinitis: a new paradigm for a difficult clinical problem (part 1). *Phys Sports Med.* 2000;28:38–48.

Kwong PK, Kay D, Voner RT, et al. Plantar fasciitis: mechanics and pathomechanics of treatment. *Clin Sports Med.* 1988;7:119–126.

Martin RL, Irrgang JJ, Conti SF. Outcome study of subjects with insertional plantar fasciitis. *Foot Ankle Int.* 1998;19:803–811.

Porter MD, Shadbolt B. Intralesional corticosteroid injection versus extracorporeal shock wave therapy for plantar fasciopathy. *Clin J Sport Med.* 2005;15(3):119–124.

Sellman JR. Plantar fascia rupture associated with corticosteroid injection. *Foot Ankle Int.* 1994;15:376–381.

Singh D, Angel J, Bentley G, et al. Plantar fasciitis. *BMJ.* 1997;315:172–175.

Stanley KL, Weaver JE. Pharmacologic management of pain and inflammation in athletes. *Clin Sports Med.* 1998;17:375–392.

Tallia AF, Cardone DA. Diagnostic and therapeutic injection of the ankle and foot. *Am Fam Physician.* 2003;68(7):1356–1362.

Taunton JE, Ryan MB, Clement DB, et al. A retrospective case-control analysis of 2002 running injuries. *Br J Sports Med.* 2002;36:95–101.

Tsai WC, Hsu CC, Chen CP, et al. Plantar fasciitis treated with local steroid injection: comparison between sonographic and palpation guidance. *J Clin Ultrasound.* 2006;34(1):12–16.

Wolgin M, Cook C, Graham C, et al. Conservative treatment of plantar heel pain: long-term follow-up. *Foot Ankle Int.* 1994;15:97–102.

Young CC, Rutherford DS, Niedfeldt MW. Treatment of plantar fasciitis. *Am Fam Physician.* 2001;63:467–474, 477–478.

2008 MAG Mutual Healthcare Solutions, Inc.'s Physicians' Fee and Coding Guide. Duluth, Georgia. MAG Mutual Healthcare Solutions, Inc. 2007.

CHAPTER 109

Shoulder Injection

Jeffrey A. German, MD, DABFM
Associate Professor, Department of Family Medicine
Louisiana State University Health Sciences Center, Shreveport, LA

Steven Kitchings, MD
Chief Resident, Family Medicine
Louisiana State University Health Sciences Center, Shreveport, LA

The shoulder comprises a series of joints and musculoskeletal tissues that afford extraordinary range of motion, making the shoulder the most mobile joint in the body. The glenohumeral, acromioclavicular, sternoclavicular, and scapulothoracic joints are all accessible for injection but can be difficult to enter and may be best injected by experienced physicians. However, the subacromial bursa is usually easily accessed and is the most commonly injected area in the shoulder. This chapter describes an injection technique into the subacromial bursa, commonly called a "shoulder injection." This procedure generally does not involve entering the shoulder joint.

Shoulder injections are easy to perform and often provide benefit for a number of painful shoulder conditions. Some shoulder disorders that may benefit from this technique include rotator cuff impingement syndrome, calcific tendonitis, subacromial/subdeltoid bursitis, and adhesive capsulitis. Anatomic proximity of the rotator cuff tendons and the bursa creates overlap among these conditions, allowing for a similar injection technique for these conditions.

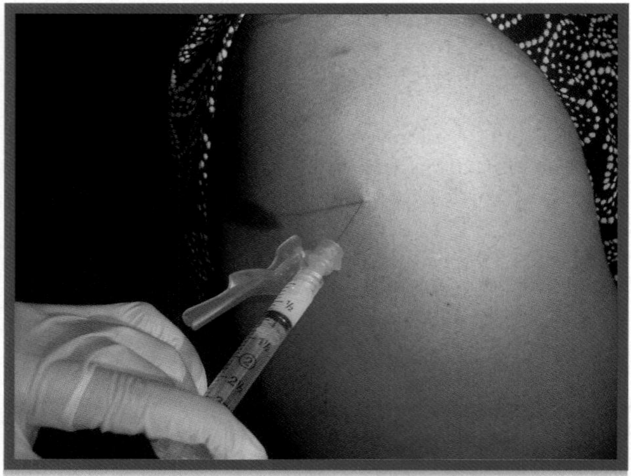

Impingement Syndrome

Impingement syndrome is one of the most common causes of pain in the adult shoulder. Impingement syndrome describes mechanical compression of the rotator cuff between the humeral head and the overlying acromion. Narrowing in this region is often attributed to spur formation on the anteroinferior acromion and may be related to excessive overhead use of the limb in certain sports and occupations. The symptoms of impingement can vary in severity and can reflect a spectrum of pathology ranging from mild changes of edema and hemorrhage, to more significant findings such as tendonitis and fibrosis, to actual tendon rupture and bony changes.

Patients with impingement commonly complain early of chronic aching in the shoulder. Acute onset of symptoms is much more suggestive of calcific tendonitis. The discomfort of impingement is frequently experienced at night when reaching over the head to grasp the pillow and when abducting the shoulder between 60 and 120 degrees. A test for impingement (Neer test) is considered positive when the patient experiences pain just distal to the anterior acromion when the examiner passively abducts the shoulder while preventing shoulder shrugging with the shoulder internally rotated. Pain at 90 degrees is considered mild impingement, pain at 60 to 70 degrees is moderate impingement, and pain at 45 degrees or below is considered severe impingement. Another test for rotator cuff pain is the flexion with internal rotation (Hawkins test). This test is performed by internally rotating the shoulder while the arm is flexed 90 degrees with the elbow bent to 90 degrees. Pain with internal rotation is a positive test.

Impingement syndrome generally is treated with exercises to restore flexibility and strength. Avoidance of painful activities is important early in the course of this disorder, and nonsteroidal anti-inflammatory drugs (NSAIDs) and ice therapy can be added to rest and physical therapy. Steroid injection may also provide symptom relief.

Calcific Tendinitis

Calcific tendonitis is irritation and inflammation caused by calcium deposits in the shoulder, most commonly in the supraspinatus tendon. It is estimated that 2% to 3% of the U.S. adult population suffers from this disorder, although many with the disorder are asymptomatic. The disorder is more common in middle-aged men in the dominant shoulder, and it may be connected to use and activity. More than 25% of individuals have bilateral shoulder involvement. Calcific tendonitis usually is characterized by an acute onset of intense shoulder pain that is not related to position or activity.

Because the subacromial bursa is adjacent to the supraspinatus tendon, most of the pain from calcific tendonitis is related to bursal inflammation. Point tenderness is identified over the lateral shoulder, and pain can be produced with active abduction from 60 to 120 degrees. Calcium can be detected on x-ray films (in external rotation); acute deposits are sharply delineated, whereas chronic calcium deposits are hazy and ill defined as they are being resorbed. Greater degrees of inflammation (i.e., greater pain) tend to result from rupture of the calcium deposit into the overlying bursa, causing a chemical bursitis. This typically precedes resolution of symptoms. Persistently large deposits may lead to disuse and eventually to frozen shoulder. Because the pain from calcific tendonitis can be severe, NSAIDs and injection with a local anesthetic and steroid are usually considered early in the course of therapy.

Supraspinatus Tendonitis and Subacromial Bursitis

Rotator cuff tendonitis unrelated to calcium deposition can occur. The supraspinatous tendon in particular can develop tendonitis as a result of repetitive activity, generally at or above shoulder height. Inflammation and/or a partial tear of the tendon lead to irritation of the subacromial bursa, and as a result, supraspinatus tendonitis and subacromial bursitis usually coexist. Patients often complain of shoulder pain aggravated by reaching, pushing, pulling, lifting, positioning the arm above the shoulder level, or lying on the affected side. Many physicians believe that these disorders almost always occur as part of the two previously discussed conditions.

The point of the shoulder (just under the acromion) is the location of maximal tenderness from supraspinatus tendonitis. Soft tissue disorders of the shoulder are difficult to differentiate clinically, because these conditions produce remarkably similar signs and symptoms. Injection therapy often is a valuable adjunct, unless there is evidence of complete rotator cuff tear or loss of motor function.

Frozen Shoulder (Adhesive Capsulitis)

Adhesive capsulitis (commonly referred to as *frozen shoulder*) refers to a stiffened glenohumeral joint that has lost significant range of motion. Patients with this disorder commonly complain of stiffness, although they may have pain and always have a global decreased range of motion of the shoulder. The decreased range of motion is both active and passive and is due to a contraction of the joint capsule. The etiology can be due to any condition, with the most common cause being rotator cuff tendonitis that leads to disuse of the shoulder, or it can be idiopathic.

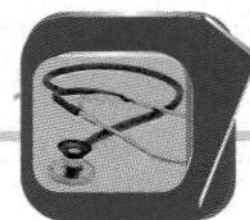

Equipment

- See Appendix I: Suggested Tray for Soft Tissue Aspiration and Injection Procedures.
- See Appendix E: Skin Preparation Recommendations.

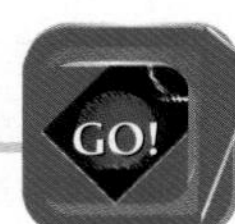

Indications

- Impingement syndrome
- Calcific tendonitis
- Supraspinatous tendonitis
- Subacromial bursitis
- Adhesive capsulitis (frozen shoulder)

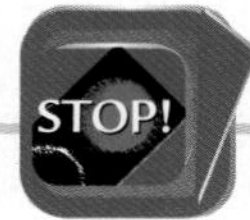

Contraindications

- Uncooperative patient
- Bleeding diathesis or coagulopathy
- Bacteremia or cellulitis overlying the lateral shoulder
- Evidence of complete rotator cuff tear

The Procedure

Lateral Approach

Step 1. The patient is positioned sitting up, with the hand of the affected side resting in the lap. Ask the patient to relax the shoulder and neck muscles. Downward traction on the elbow may be necessary to open the subacromial space.

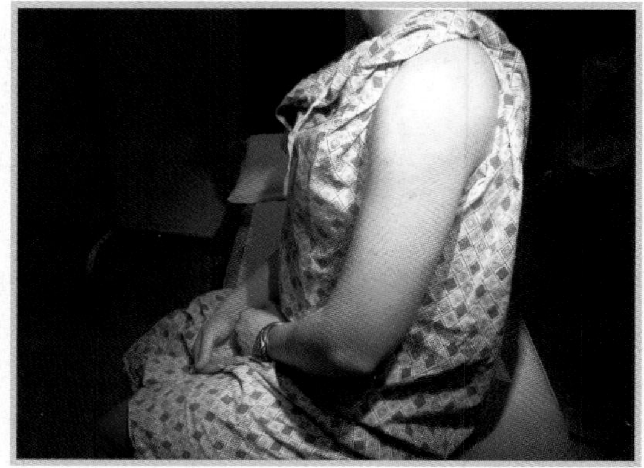

Step 1

Step 2. The anterior, lateral, and posterior border of the acromion is marked with a pen. The needle insertion site is approximately 1 to 1.5 inches below the midpoint of the lateral acromion.

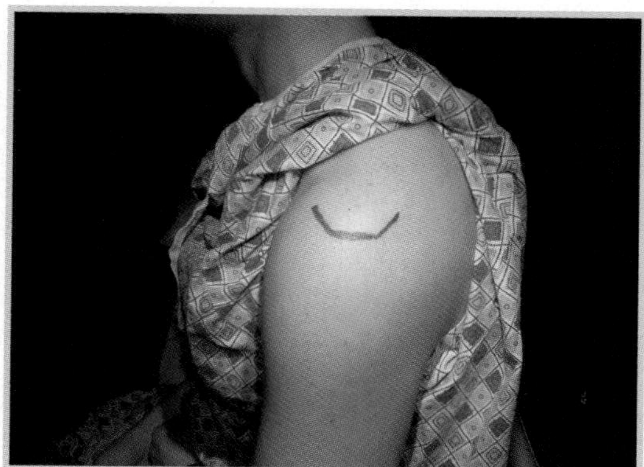

Step 2

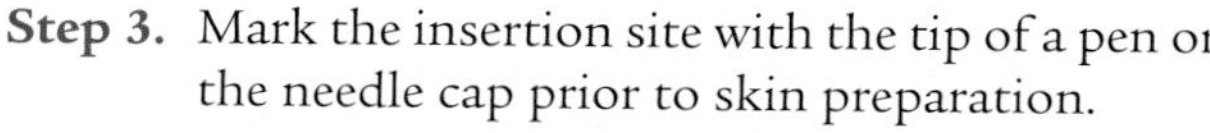

Step 3. Mark the insertion site with the tip of a pen or the needle cap prior to skin preparation.

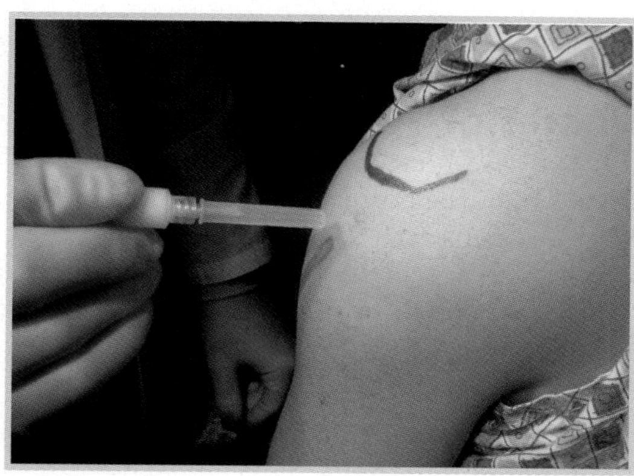

Step 3

Step 4. Prep the skin with povidone-iodine or chlorhexidine solution, and allow it to dry (see Appendix E: Skin Preparation Recommendations).

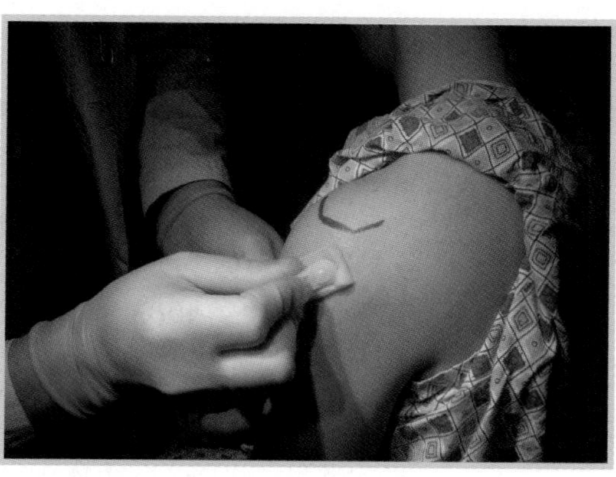

Step 4

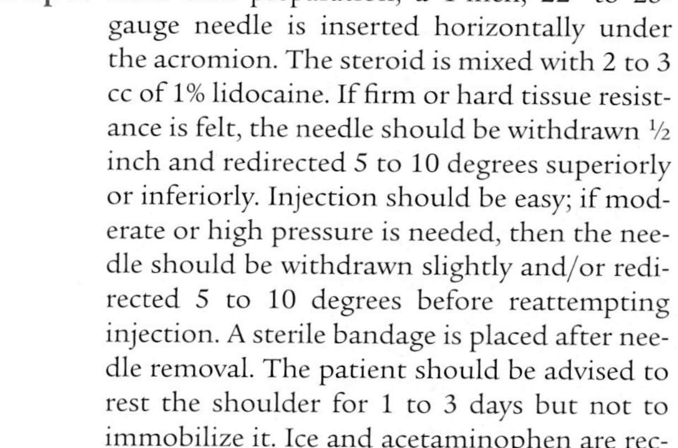

Step 5. After skin preparation, a 1-inch, 22- to 25-gauge needle is inserted horizontally under the acromion. The steroid is mixed with 2 to 3 cc of 1% lidocaine. If firm or hard tissue resistance is felt, the needle should be withdrawn ½ inch and redirected 5 to 10 degrees superiorly or inferiorly. Injection should be easy; if moderate or high pressure is needed, then the needle should be withdrawn slightly and/or redirected 5 to 10 degrees before reattempting injection. A sterile bandage is placed after needle removal. The patient should be advised to rest the shoulder for 1 to 3 days but not to immobilize it. Ice and acetaminophen are recommended for soreness.

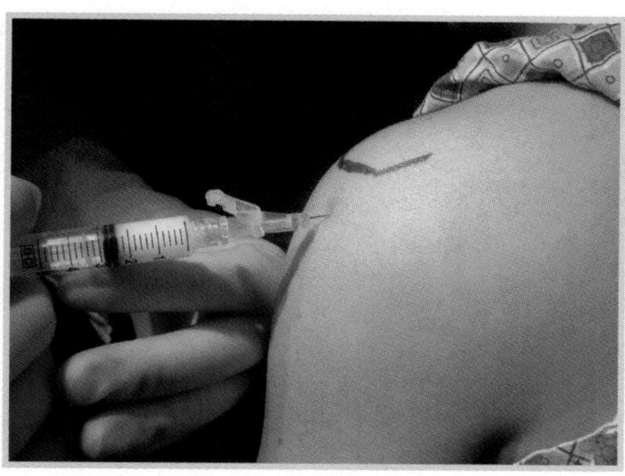

Step 5

Anterior Approach

Step 1. For the anterior approach, the needle should be placed below the acromion process, 1 cm lateral to the coracoid process and immediately medial to the head of the humerus. The needle is directed posteriorly and slightly superiorly and laterally. If the needle hits bone, it should be pulled back and redirected at a slightly different angle.

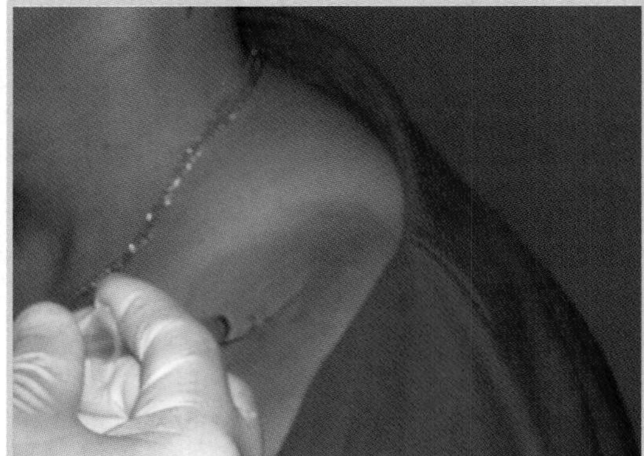

Step 1

Posterior Approach

Step 1. For the posterior approach, the needle should be inserted 2 to 3 cm inferior to the posterolateral corner of the acromion and directed anteriorly toward the coracoid process.

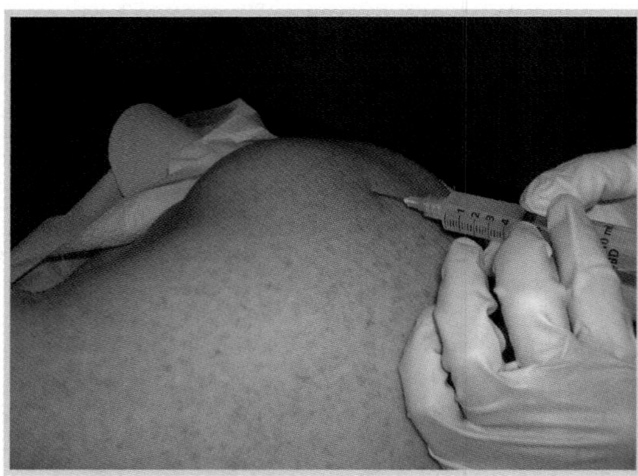

Step 1

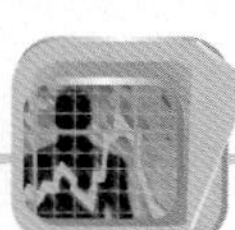

Complications

- Skin atrophy
- Vitiligo around injection site
- Dystrophic calcification around joint capsule
- Increase in blood glucose for up to 4 days
- Tendon rupture
- Postinjection flare
- Iatrogenic infection (very low incidence)
- Cushings syndrome (if frequency greater than one per month)
- Cataracts
- Facial erythema

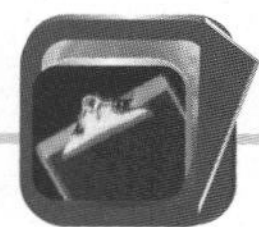

Postprocedure Instructions

The patient should remain seated or placed in supine position for several minutes after the injection. To ascertain whether the pharmaceuticals have been delivered to the appropriate location, the joint area may be put through a passive range of motion. The patient should remain in the office to be monitored for 30 minutes after the injection.

The patient should avoid strenuous activity involving the injected region for at least 48 hours. Patients should be cautioned that they may experience worsening symptoms during the first 24 to 48 hours, related to possible steroid flare, which can be treated with

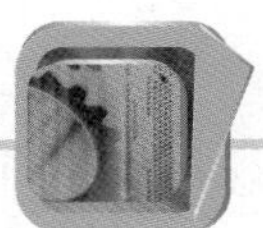

Coding Information and Supply Sources

CPT Code	Description	2008 Average 50th Percentile Fee	Global Period
20550	Injection(s); single tendon sheath, or ligament, aponeurosis (e.g., plantar "fascia")	$140.00	0
20605	Injection of intermediate joint (acromioclavicular) or bursa	$137.00	0
20610	Injection of major joint or bursa (shoulder)	$176.00	0

All materials can be ordered through local medical supply companies. Lidocaine solution, injectable steroid solutions are available from local pharmacies or medical supply companies. A suggested tray for performing soft tissue aspirations and injections is listed in Appendix I. Skin preparation recommendations appear in Appendix E.

Patient Education Handout

A patient education handout, "Shoulder Injection," can be found on the book's companion Web site.

Bibliography

Anderson BC. Frozen shoulder. UpToDate Web site. http://www.utdol.com. Accessed December 2007.

Anderson BC. Rotator cuff tendonitis. UpToDate Web site.http:// www.utdol.com. Accessed December 2007.

Anderson LG. Aspirating and injecting the acutely painful joint. *Emerg Med.* 1991;23:77–94.

Bell AD, Conaway, D. Corticosteroid injections for painful shoulders. *Int J Clin Pract.* 2005;59(10):1178–1186.

Blake R, Hoffman J. Emergency department evaluation and treatment of the shoulder and humerus. *Emerg Med Clin North Am.* 1999;17:859–876.

Brown JS. *Minor Surgery: A Text and Atlas.* (3rd ed.). London: Chapman & Hall; 1997.

Ike RW. Therapeutic injection of joints and soft tissues. In: Klippel JH, Weyand CM, Wortmann RL, eds. *Primer on the Rheumatic Diseases.* (11th ed.). Atlanta: Arthritis Foundation; 1997:419–421.

Jacobs LG, Barton MA, Wallace WA, et al. Intra-articulr distension and steroids in the management of capsulitis of the shoulder. *BMJ.* 1991;302:1498–1501.

Leversee JH. Aspiration of joints and soft tissue injections. *Prim Care.* 1986;13:579–599.

Mani L, Gerr E. Work-related upper extremity musculoskeletal disorders. *Prim Care Clin Office Pract.* 2000;27:845–864.

Mercier LR, Pettid FJ, Tamisiea DF, et al. *Practical Orthopedics.* (4th ed.). St. Louis: Mosby; 1995.

Owen DS, Irby R. Intra-articular and soft-tissue aspiration and injection. *Clin Rheum Pract.* March–May 1986;52–63.

Pando JA, Klippel JH. Arthrocentesis and corticosteroid injection: an illustrated guide to technique. *Consultant.* 1996;36:2137–2148.

Pronchik D, Heller MB. Local injection therapy: rapid, effective treatment of tendonitis/bursitis syndromes. *Consultant.* 1997;37:1377–1389.

Rowe CR. Injection technique for the shoulder and elbow. *Orthop Clin North Am.* 1988;19:773–777.

Wilson FC, Lin PP. *General Orthopedics.* New York: McGraw-Hill; 1997.

Wolf WB. Calcific tendonitis of the shoulder: diagnosis and simple, effective treatment. *Phys Sportsmed.* 1999;27:27–33.

Woodward TW, Best TM. The painful shoulder, part II: acute and chronic disorders. *Am Fam Physician.* 2000;61:3291–3300.

2008 MAG Mutual Healthcare Solutions, Inc.'s Physicians' Fee and Coding Guide. Duluth, Georgia. MAG Mutual Healthcare Solutions, Inc. 2007.

CHAPTER 110

The Short Arm Cast

Daniel L. Stulberg, MD, FAAFP

Associate Professor of Family and Community Medicine
University of New Mexico Health Sciences Center, Albuquerque, NM

Patients with orthopedic injuries commonly present to primary care offices or are referred there if the practitioner is skilled in their management. Knowing how to apply basic casts can expand one's practice of medicine and assist in the management and satisfaction of one's patients. Although most displaced fractures are managed with orthopedic consultation, primary care physicians manage many uncomplicated or nondisplaced fractures. Properly trained generalists may also perform some reductions.

The objective of early fracture management is immobilization of the fracture fragments. Internal fixation accomplishes this goal, but the costs and risks of internal fixation may be unnecessary for fractures that can be effectively treated with external devices such as casts. Casts are circumferential, rigid, molded to fit a body part, and do not accommodate swelling. Typically, they should be applied only after a period of splinting, usually 2 to 14 days, to allow resolution of swelling. Casts can be applied immediately for a clinical situation in which swelling is insignificant, such as with a suspected scaphoid fracture. A cast never completely immobilizes a fracture, but a well-molded cast provides enough relative immobilization to allow a fracture to heal. Casts provide the additional benefits of pain relief, protection of surrounding tissues (e.g., vessels, nerves), and maintenance of position after reduction of fracture fragments.

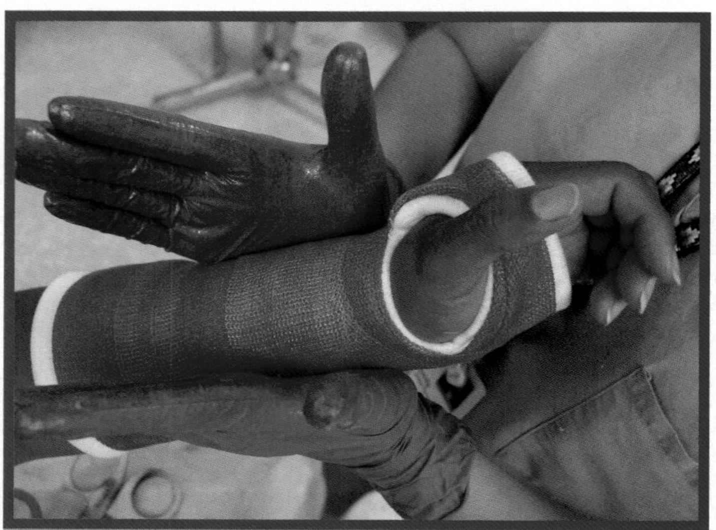

When applying a cast, place the injured part in a position of function, unless alternate positioning is required by the clinical situation. The position of function for the forearm is easily achieved by asking the patient to position the hand and wrist as if drinking a glass of water.

Plaster of Paris has been extremely popular as a cast material because of its ease of use, long shelf life, and low cost. Synthetic materials such as fiberglass provide the benefit of light weight and added strength, but at additional cost. The shelf life of some synthetic materials can be <6 months; the shelf life can be extended by turning over the packages every few months to prevent drying.

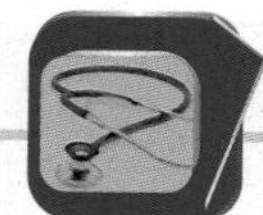

Equipment

- Cast material: fiberglass or plaster, two 2-, 3-, or 4-inch rolls based on patient size
- Stockinette: cotton or for waterproof casts—synthetic (3 M Synthetic Cast Stockinette)
- Cast padding: Cotton (BSN Specialist Cotton Cast Padding) or either synthetic cast padding (3M Scotchcast Wet or Dry Cast Padding or cast liner (Procel-Gore Cast Liner) for waterproof casts
- Nonsterile gloves
- Water basin
- Cast saw with vacuum attachment
- Cast spreader
- Bandage scissors
- A cut-resistant plastic strip (De-Flex Protective Strip) that provides protection from cuts and burns from cast saws during cast removal (optional if standard padding used)

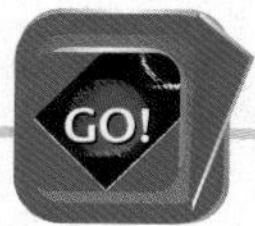

Indications

- Colles fracture (nondisplaced or after reduction)
- Nondisplaced metacarpal fractures
- Torus (buckle) or greenstick fracture of the distal radius
- Nondisplaced or suspected scaphoid fracture (refer if more than 1 mm of displacement)
- Clinically suspected scaphoid fracture with negative initial x-ray

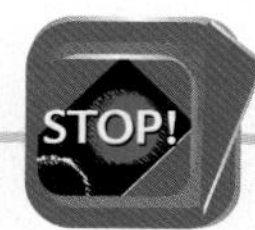

Relative Contraindications

- Unfamiliarity with appropriate methods or techniques
- Fractures best managed by specialty referral or surgical reduction or intervention
- Improperly functioning equipment (e.g., cast saw)
- Infection in tissues to be covered by a cast
- Open fractures

The Procedure

Step 1. A single layer of stockinette is applied, typically 3 inches. Cut the stockinette long enough so that it goes from the elbow to the distal interphalangeal joint of the third finger.

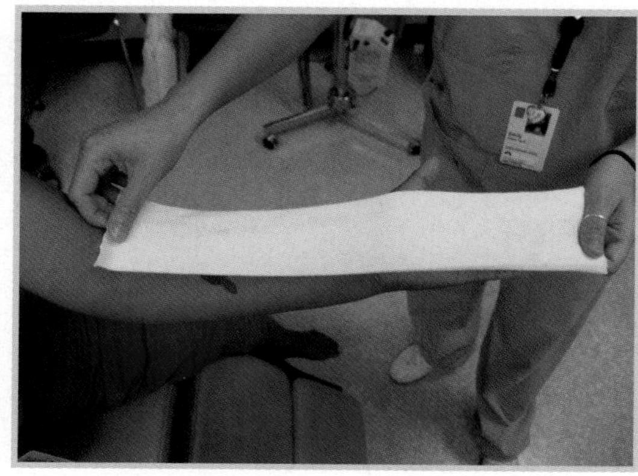

Step 1

Step 2. Cut a hole for the thumb. For scaphoid fractures, a thumb extension (spica) is added with 1-inch stockinette split at the base to overlap onto the radial aspect of the 3-inch stockinette and covering to the end of the thumb.

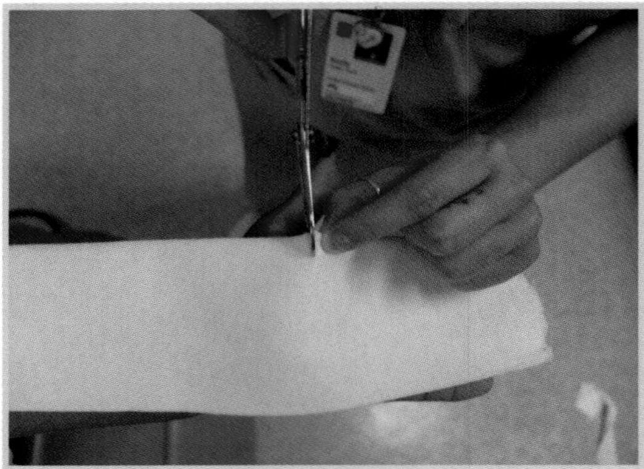
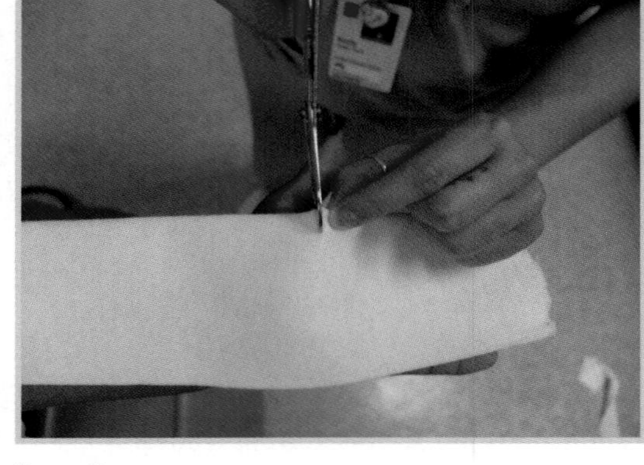

Step 2

Step 3. Apply the stockinette. The extra length on each end helps to create smooth edges on the cast.

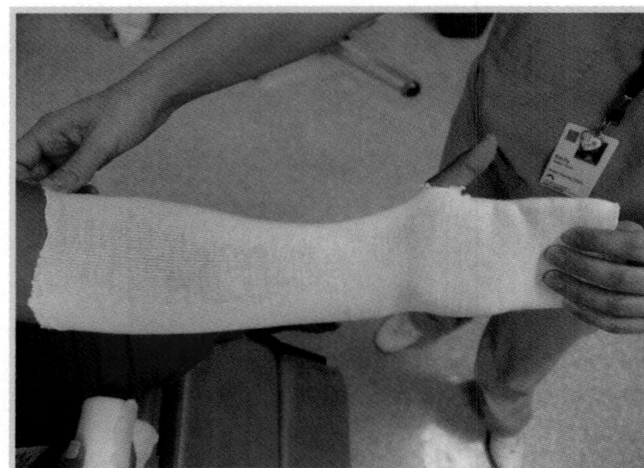

Step 3

Step 4. Apply the cast padding (starting either proximal or distal) covering from approximately 1 to 1.5 inches from the flexed elbow to the flexural crease of the palm to allow for adequate range of motion of the unaffected joints. The cast padding is applied to a double thickness by overlapping the roll 50% each turn.

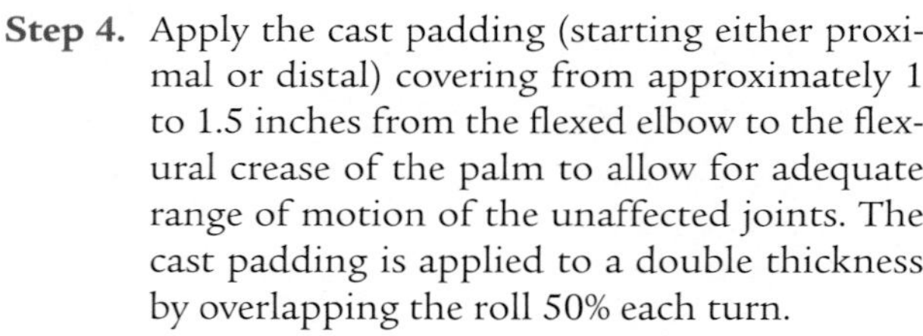

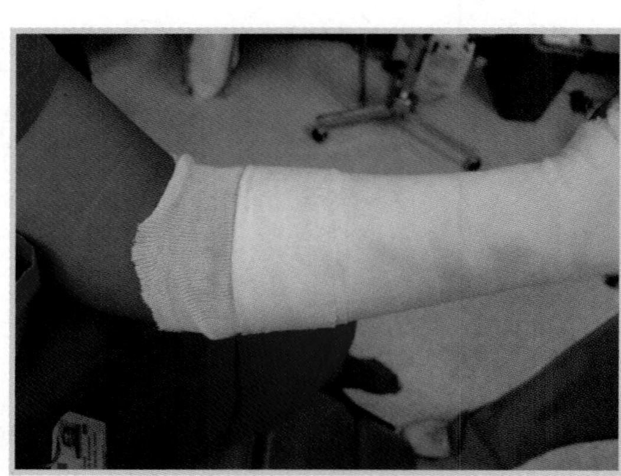

Step 4

Step 5. An extra roll of padding at the elbow as shown or a folded piece of padding at the palmar end of the cast help to reduce chafing and make the cast more comfortable at the cast ends.

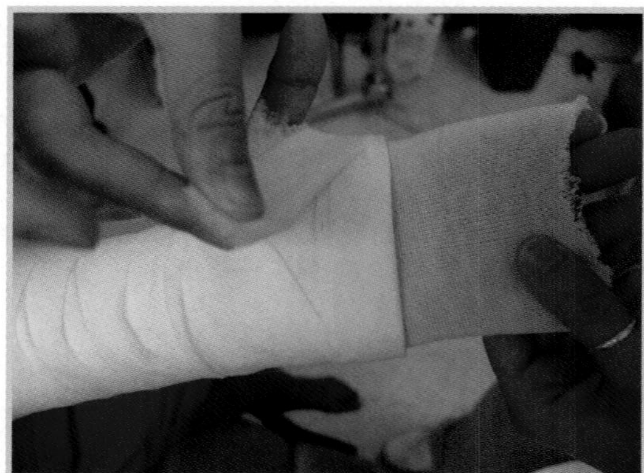

Step 5

Step 6. Partially tear the padding to slip the padding next to and around the base of the thumb.

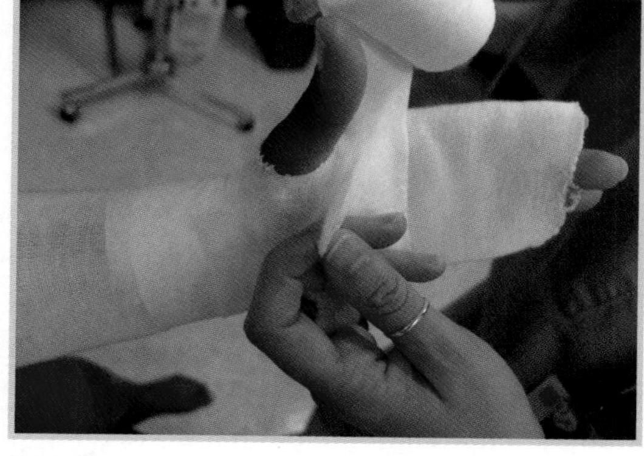

Step 6

Step 7. Apply cast padding and cast material while keeping the roll flat against the patient. This is like unrolling carpet with the bulk of the padding away from the patient. Doing the reverse would necessitate shifting the roll more from hand to hand. This allows the pad to roll on straight and not under too much tension.

- PITFALL: Do not use too much padding, because this makes the cast loose.
- PITFALL: Do not stretch the padding, because it will cause the padding and subsequent cast to be too tight.
- PITFALL: Some extra padding should be applied over bony prominences to avoid injury under the cast. An extra roll over the ulnar styloid can avoid problems at this site.

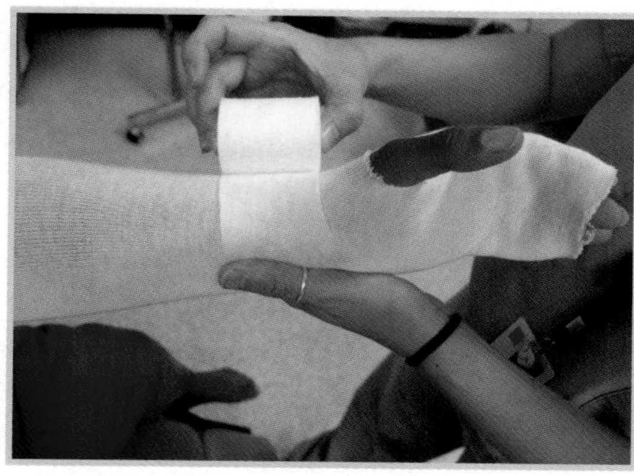

Step 7

Step 8. Place the plaster or fiberglass roll in lukewarm or room temperature water. For plaster, allow the plaster to sit in the water a few seconds, until the bubbling ceases. Remove the roll, and gently twist or gently squeeze the roll to remove excess water. Fiberglass can be applied without wetting if the clinician would like extra time for rolling it on or molding. The resin will react with ambient moisture in the air and harden in approximately 5 to 10 minutes.

- PITFALL: Never use hot water, which can cause an excess thermochemical reaction and extremely rapid setting of the cast material. The cast material should never be wrung out.

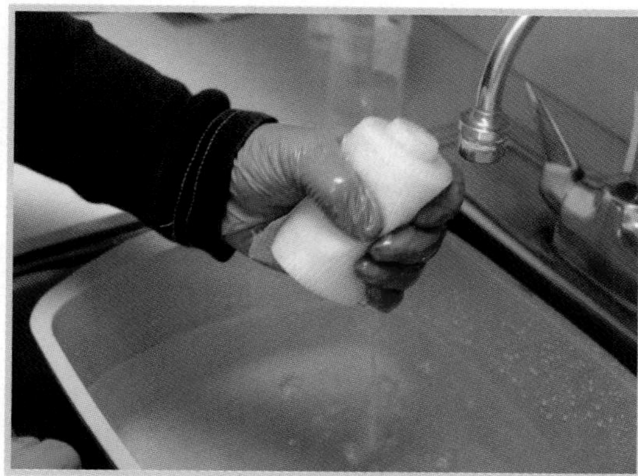

Step 8

Step 9. Start rolling either proximally or distally. Apply the cast material with only mild tension, applying it in the same manner as the cast padding, from one end to the other and overlapping 50% of the prior turn. When applying plaster over tapered parts, tucks or pleats may be needed to avoid ridges or creases. After the cast tape is anchored at the wrist, cut the fiberglass three quarters of the way across the strip at the thumb and fold the free corners under. This allows coverage of the hand without constricting the thumb. Alternatively, the cast tape can be folded accordion style or twisted 360 degrees around its lengthwise axis at the thumb web space. These latter techniques may cause a thicker cast at the web space, which can cause more rubbing at the base of the thumb.

- **PITFALL:** Apply the cast material while keeping the roll flat against the patient. This is like unrolling carpet with the bulk of the cast roll in your palm away from the patient. Reversing this necessitates shifting the roll more from hand to hand and also tends to cause too much tension as the roll is unwound by pulling away from the patient.

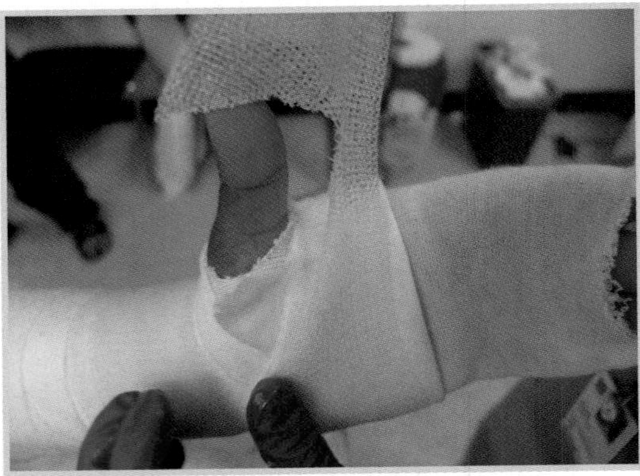

Step 9

Step 10. The stockinette and the underlying padding are folded over the edge of rolled cast material at the thumb, proximal, and distal aspects of the cast to form clean padded edges.

- **PITFALL:** If the cast material creates a sharp edge at the base of the thumb, trim the edge with bandage scissors or the cast saw.

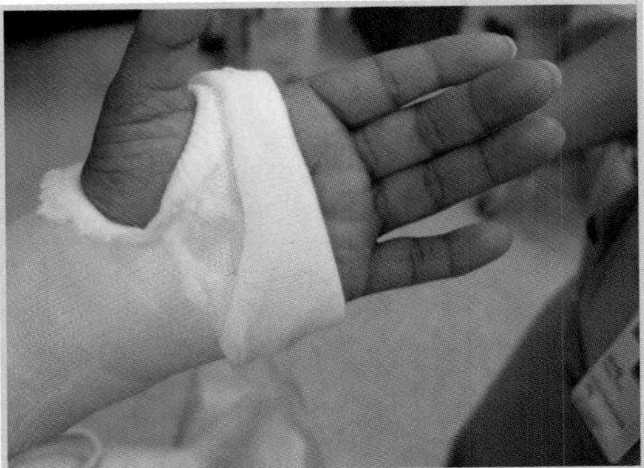

Step 10

Step 11. The folded-over stockinette is incorporated into the cast by rolling the casting tape back over the folded edge, either with the first roll or with a second roll if desired or if the arm is large and requires a second roll. For scaphoid fractures, the thumb is casted in a thumb extension (spica) position and the padding is folded back over the cast material to expose the distal aspect of the distal phalanx.

- **PITFALL:** The most common mistake made by novice physicians is to apply the cast to the metacarpophalangeal joints. All fingers need to be able to flex 90 degrees, and this means that the cast should end well short of the metacarpophalangeal joints.

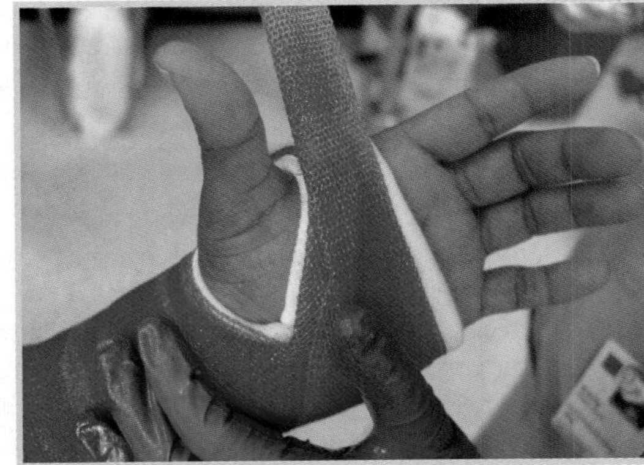

Step 11

Step 12. With wet gloved hands or using cast cream or hand lotion, smooth out any rough edges of the cast tape and mold the palm of the cast with an arm-wrestling-type handshake in a neutral position, unless a different position is required (i.e., for reduction of a Colles fracture).

- **PITFALL:** A poorly molded cast will not immobilize the area appropriately and can apply undue pressure at the wrong areas.

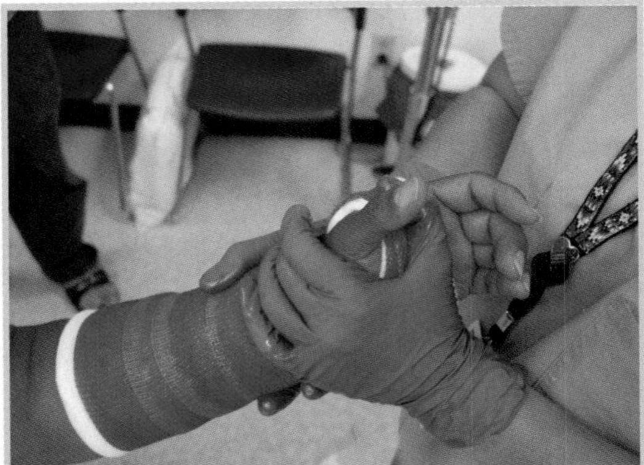

Step 12

Step 13. Mold the forearm into a rounded off rectangular shape instead of leaving it as a circle. This will conform to the natural shape of the arm and also prevent rotation of the radius and ulna in the cast.

- **PITFALL:** Use broad surfaces of your hands to mold the cast. Do not use the fingertips to mold the cast because this can leave dents and pressure points to the underlying structures.

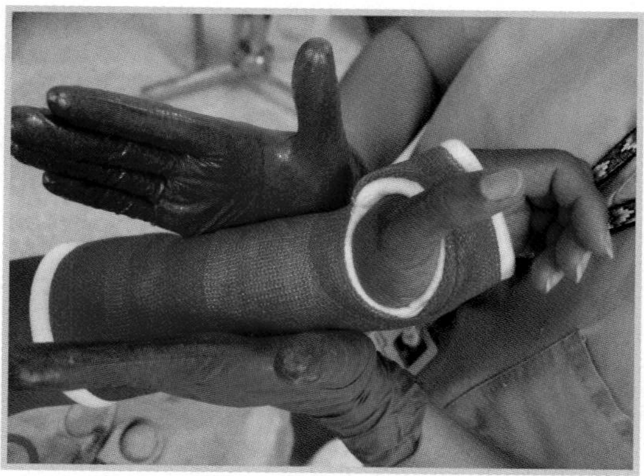

Step 13

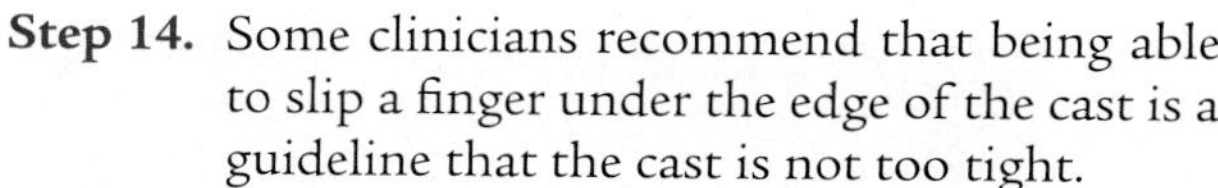

Step 14. Some clinicians recommend that being able to slip a finger under the edge of the cast is a guideline that the cast is not too tight.

Give the patient adequate follow-up instructions and precautions (see the section on patient education).

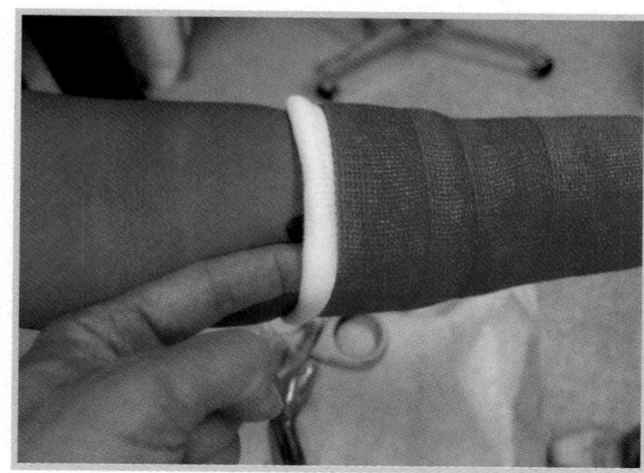

Step 14

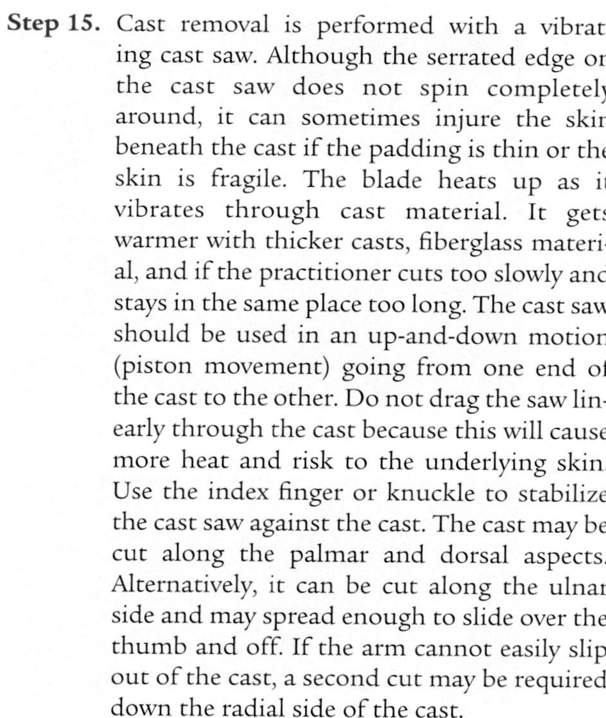

Step 15. Cast removal is performed with a vibrating cast saw. Although the serrated edge on the cast saw does not spin completely around, it can sometimes injure the skin beneath the cast if the padding is thin or the skin is fragile. The blade heats up as it vibrates through cast material. It gets warmer with thicker casts, fiberglass material, and if the practitioner cuts too slowly and stays in the same place too long. The cast saw should be used in an up-and-down motion (piston movement) going from one end of the cast to the other. Do not drag the saw linearly through the cast because this will cause more heat and risk to the underlying skin. Use the index finger or knuckle to stabilize the cast saw against the cast. The cast may be cut along the palmar and dorsal aspects. Alternatively, it can be cut along the ulnar side and may spread enough to slide over the thumb and off. If the arm cannot easily slip out of the cast, a second cut may be required down the radial side of the cast.

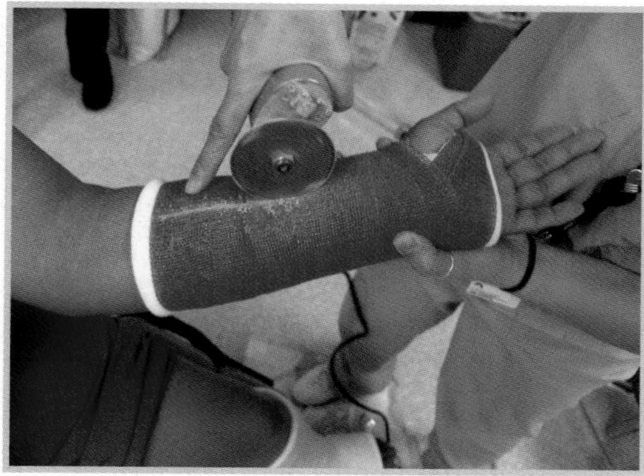

Step 15

Step 16. Spread the cast apart with cast spreaders.

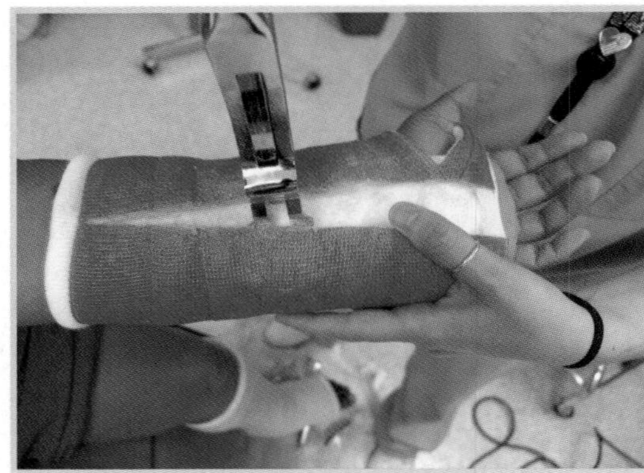

Step 16

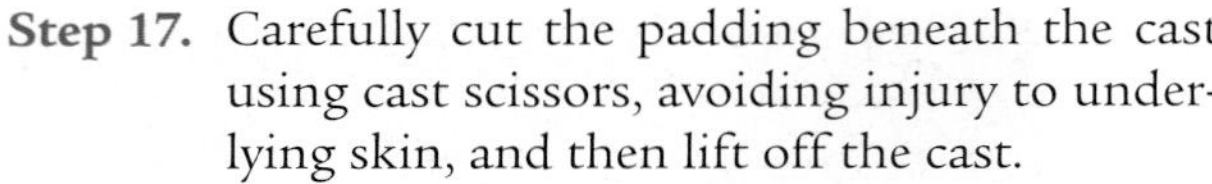

Step 17. Carefully cut the padding beneath the cast using cast scissors, avoiding injury to underlying skin, and then lift off the cast.

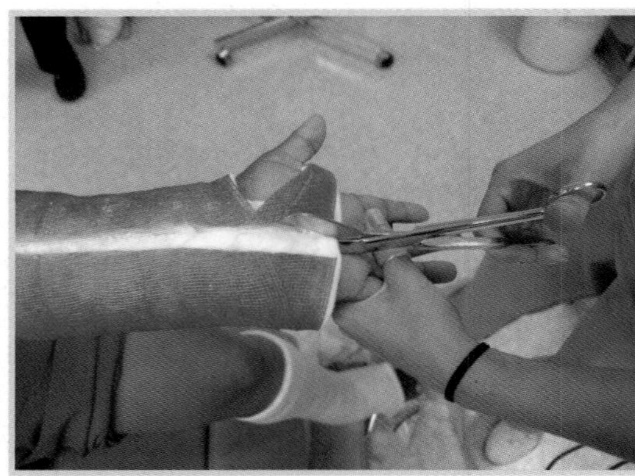

Step 17

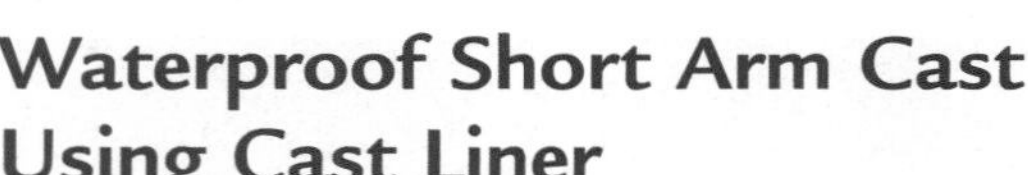

Waterproof Short Arm Cast Using Cast Liner

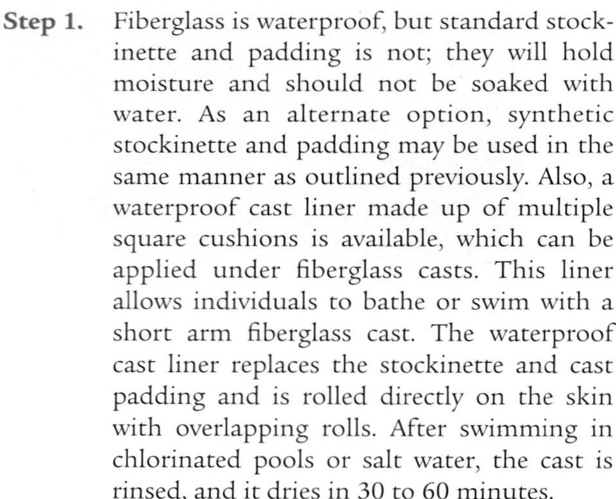

Step 1. Fiberglass is waterproof, but standard stockinette and padding is not; they will hold moisture and should not be soaked with water. As an alternate option, synthetic stockinette and padding may be used in the same manner as outlined previously. Also, a waterproof cast liner made up of multiple square cushions is available, which can be applied under fiberglass casts. This liner allows individuals to bathe or swim with a short arm fiberglass cast. The waterproof cast liner replaces the stockinette and cast padding and is rolled directly on the skin with overlapping rolls. After swimming in chlorinated pools or salt water, the cast is rinsed, and it dries in 30 to 60 minutes.

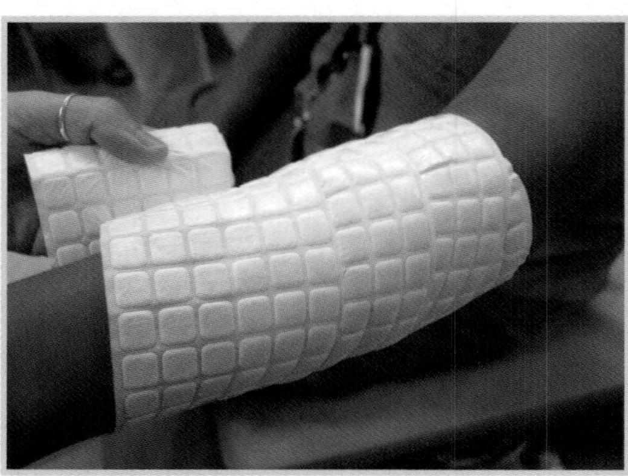

Step 1

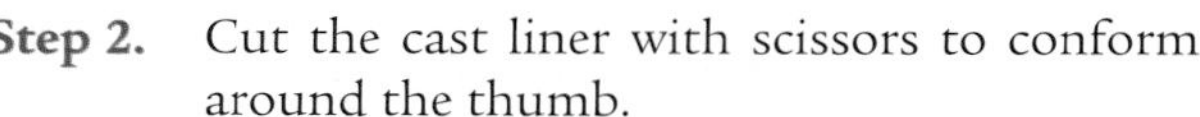

Step 2. Cut the cast liner with scissors to conform around the thumb.

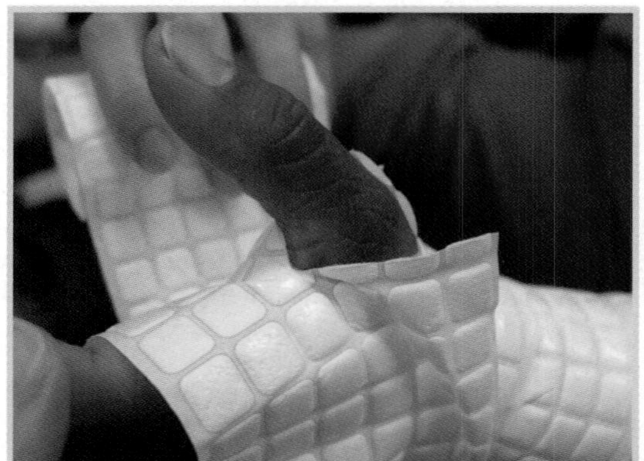

Step 2

Step 3. Cut the cast liner two squares' length from the end to form a padded edge to the cast before rolling the cast pad.

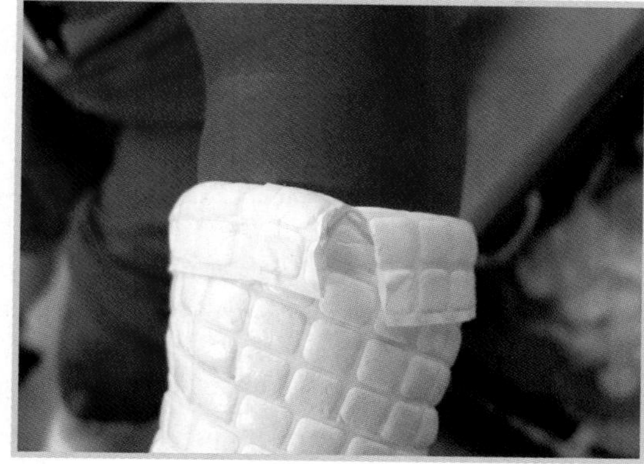

Step 3

Step 4. Place protective cutting strips along the anticipated lines where the cast will be cut off and allowing the colored edge to remain visible for cutting at the desired time. The fiberglass is then rolled on as described previously, incorporating the strips into the cast.

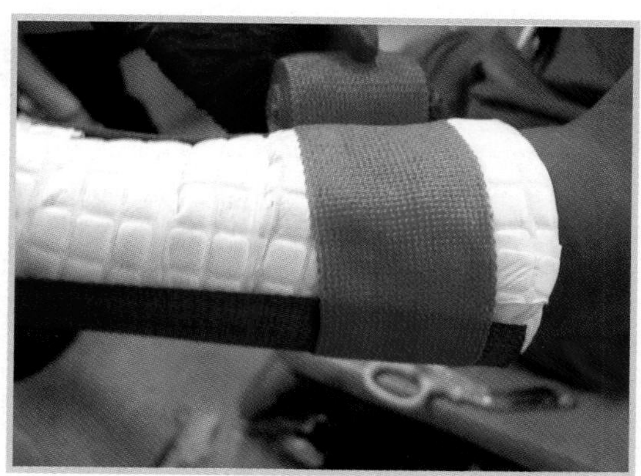

Step 4

Step 5. Cut the cast with the cast saw along the line of the protective strips, spread the cast with spreaders as before and use a scissors to cut the cast liner to remove.

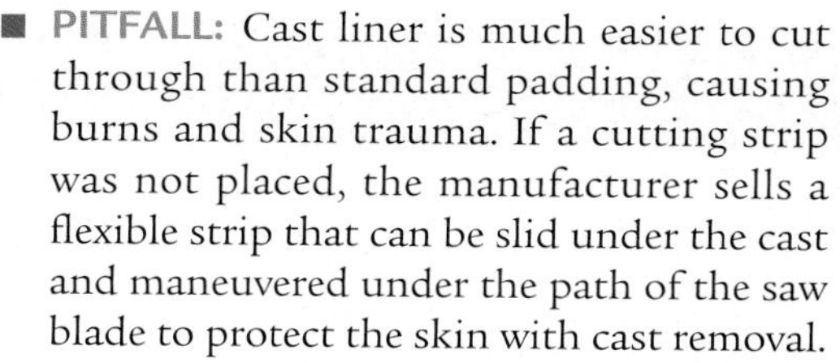

- **PITFALL:** Cast liner is much easier to cut through than standard padding, causing burns and skin trauma. If a cutting strip was not placed, the manufacturer sells a flexible strip that can be slid under the cast and maneuvered under the path of the saw blade to protect the skin with cast removal.

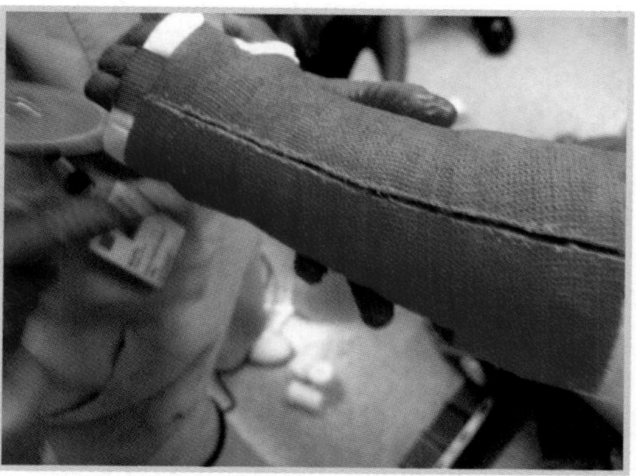

Step 5

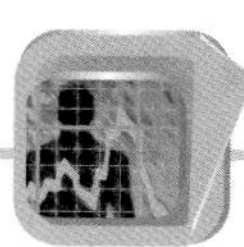

Complications

- Ischemia to the casted body part as a result of swelling of the extremity or the cast being applied to tightly
- Pressure ulcers due to a poorly padded or poorly fitting cast, especially at bony prominences
- Skin maceration if the cast gets wet and is not thoroughly dried out
- Skin damage from the patient inserting foreign objects into the cast or attempting to modify the cast

- Breakage of the cast as a result of misuse or inadequate structural strength as a result of inadequate overlapping of cast tape
- Failure to immobilize the area as a result of a poorly fitting cast

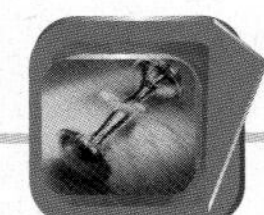

Pediatric Considerations

- Consider using a waterproof cast for ease of care and cleanliness.
- Active children may be harder on a cast, requiring earlier replacement if worn or damaged.
- Children are often frightened by the loud noise and vibration of the cast saw, so warning them and demonstrating against the practitioner's palm that the saw is not intended to cut skin can be helpful.

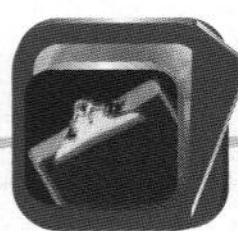

Postprocedure Instructions

Please see the patient education section. Advise the patient to elevate the arm as much as possible to avoid swelling on the first day of application. Additionally, if the cast becomes too tight, or if the patient has increasing pain in the arm, loss of sensation, or loss of circulation, or if a foreign body becomes lodged in the cast, the practitioner should not hesitate to remove the cast. After removing the cast, advise the patient to wash the area gently and not to aggressively scratch or abrade the area.

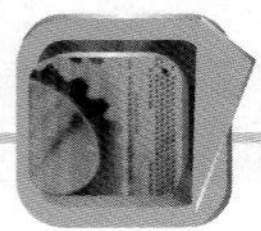

Coding Information and Supply Sources

These codes are used only for cast or splint reapplications during a follow-up period. The initial casting or splinting is considered part of the fracture management code. If no management code is reported, the cast application can be reported at the initial service. A supply code (99070) may be reported in addition to the cast code to help defray the cost of materials (estimated at $12 to $20 for plaster casts, $20 to $50 for fiberglass casts). Insurances including Medicaid may not cover the cost of materials.

CPT Code	Description	2008 Average 50th Percentile Fee	Global Period
29075	Short arm cast (elbow to finger), casting only	$189.00	0
29085	Gauntlet cast (hand and lower forearm), casting only	$194.00	0
26740	Global fee, closed treatment of metacarpophalangeal joint—no manipulation	$524.00	90
25500	Global fee, closed treatment of distal radial shaft fracture—no manipulation	$607.00	90
25530	Global fee, Ccosed treatment of ulnar shaft fracture—no manipulation	$588.00	90
25560	Global fee, closed treatment of radial and ulnar shaft fracture—no manipulation	$607.00	90

CPT is a registered trademark of the American Medical Association.
2008 average 50th Percentile Fees are provided courtesy of 2008 MMH-SI's copyrighted Physicians' Fees and Coding Guide.

The 2-, 3-, or 4-inch rolls of cotton or acrylic cast padding, cotton or acrylic stockinette, plaster bandages, and fiberglass cast tape can be ordered from these suppliers:

- DePuy OrthoTech, Tracy, CA. Web site: http://www.depuy.com
- Ray-Tek Inc. Fracture Management Supplies. Web site: http://www.ray-tek.com
- 3M Health Care, St. Paul, MN. Phone: 1-888-364-3577. Web site: http://www.3M.com/healthcare

Procel cast liner (formerly Gore cast liner) and De-flex Protective Strips can be ordered from

- W. L. Gore & Associates, Flagstaff, AZ. Phone: 1-800-528-8763. Web site: http://www.goremedical.com

Patient Education Handout

A patient education handout, "Short Arm Cast," can be found on the book's companion Web site.

The author would like to acknowledge Robert Fawcett, MD, for his review of the manuscript.

Bibliography

Hanel DP, Jones MD, Trumble TE. Wrist fractures. *Orthop Clin North Am.* 2002;33:35–57.

Killian JT, White S, Lenning L. Cast-saw burns: comparison of technique versus material versus saws. *J Pediatr Orthop.* 1999;19:683–687.

Kowalski KL, Pitcher JD Jr. Evaluation of fiberglass versus plaster of Paris for immobilization of fractures of the arm and leg. *Mil Med.* 2002;167(8):657–661.

Medley ES, Shirley SM, Brilliant HL. Fracture management by family physicians and guidelines for referral. *J Fam Pract.* 1979;8:701–710.

Phillips TG, Reibach AM. Diagnosis and management of scaphoid fractures. *Am Fam Physician.* 2004;70:879–884.

Shannon EG. Waterproof casts for immobilization of children's fractures and sprains. *J Pediatr Orthop.* 2005;25(1):56–59.

Spain D. Casting acute fractures, part 1: commonly asked questions. *Aust Fam Physician.* 2000;29:853–856.

Webb GR, Galpin RD. Fractures in the distal third of the forearm in children—comparison of short and long arm plaster casts for displaced fractures in the distal third of the forearm in children. *J. Bone Joint Surg Am.* 2006;88:9–17.

2008 MAG Mutual Healthcare Solutions, Inc.'s Physicians' Fee and Coding Guide. Duluth, Georgia. MAG Mutual Healthcare Solutions, Inc. 2007.

CHAPTER 111

The Short Leg Cast

Daniel L. Stulberg, MD, FAAFP

Associate Professor of Family and Community Medicine
University of New Mexico Health Sciences Center, Albuquerque, NM

Primary care practitioners frequently encounter fractures of a lower extremity. Improved commercial orthotic braces have reduced the need for short leg casts, but placement of short leg casts remain a useful procedure for treating many lower extremity fractures and musculoskeletal disorders in primary care practice. Open and significantly displaced fractures should be managed with orthopedic consultation. Simpler fractures that do not require reduction or surgical repair can often be managed by primary care practitioners. Immobilization is the major benefit of casting because it allows for stabilization and bone callus formation. Casts also provide pain relief, maintain position after reduction of a fracture, and protect the soft tissues surrounding the fracture site. Because casts are rigid and circumferential, they generally should not be applied immediately after a fracture. Fractures can produce a significant amount of bleeding and swelling, and the cast can compromise vascular flow to the tissues if significant swelling increases in the tissues beneath a rigid cast. Therefore, most lower extremity fractures should be splinted for at least 72 hours before cast placement is attempted.

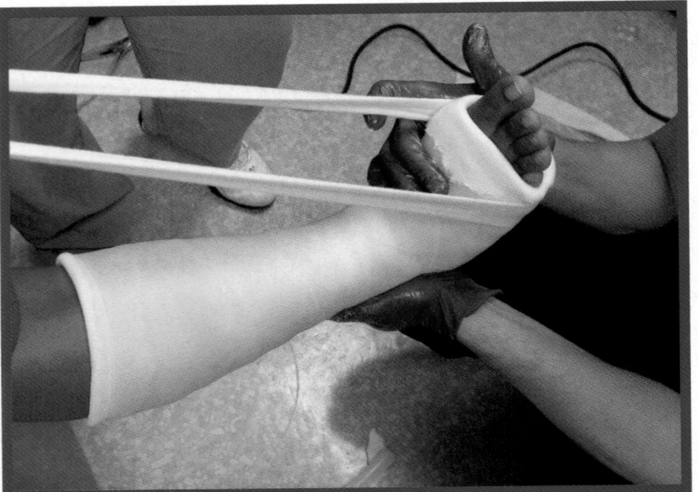

Plaster of Paris has been extensively used historically to achieve immobilization, is easy to use and inexpensive, but it is heavier than fiberglass. Walking short leg casts experience extensive stress from weight bearing. When composed of plaster, these casts require added splint material incorporated within the cast to enhance durability. Splint enhancement can also be incorporated within fiberglass casts, but the increased strength of the fiberglass material usually is adequate.

A waterproof cast liner (e.g., Procel; formerly Gore cast liner by W. L. Gore) made of rolls of multiple square cushions can be used in place of the stockinette and gauze beneath fiberglass casts. This cast liner allows individuals to shower, bathe, and swim when wearing the cast. Alternatively, synthetic stockinette and waterproof cast padding is also available. Both of these options can add to the cost of supplies, and some practitioners may add an additional fee to their patients for this option.

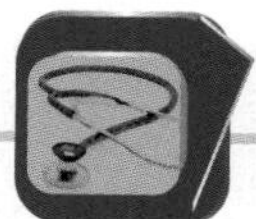

Equipment

- Cast material: fiberglass, three 3- or 4-inch rolls, or plaster, three 4- or 6-inch rolls based on patient size
- Stockinette: cotton or for waterproof casts—synthetic (3M Synthetic Cast Stockinette)
- Cast padding: Cotton (BSN Specialist Cotton Cast Padding) or either synthetic cast padding (3M Scotchcast Wet or Dry Cast Padding) or cast liner (Procel-Gore Cast Liner) for waterproof casts
- Nonsterile gloves
- Water basin
- Cast saw with vacuum attachment
- Cast spreader
- Bandage scissors
- A cut-resistant plastic strip (De-Flex Protective Strip) that provides protection from cuts and burns from cast saws during cast removal (optional if standard padding used); 1% lidocaine for use as local anesthetic as needed and for injection with corticosteroids

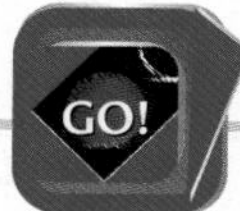

Indications

- Nondisplaced, stable ankle (unimalleolar) fractures
- Metatarsal fractures
- Proximal fifth metatarsal fractures, articular (avulsion; usually weight-bearing cast)
- Proximal fifth metatarsal fractures, nonarticular (Jones fractures; usually non-weight-bearing cast)
- Tarsal fractures (not talar neck fractures)
- Stable, nondisplaced distal fibular fractures
- High ankle sprain (torn distal tibiofibular ligament)
- Nondisplaced fractures of the body of the calcaneus

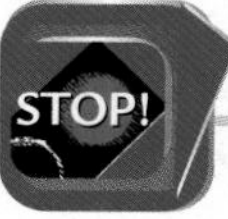

Contraindications

- Unfamiliarity with appropriate methods or techniques
- Fractures that are outside the expertise of the treating physician (best managed by specialty referral or surgical reduction or intervention)
- Improperly functioning equipment (e.g., cast saw)
- Infection in the tissues to be covered by the cast
- Open fractures

The Procedure

Step 1. When applying a cast, place the injured part in the position of function, unless alternate positioning is required by the clinical situation. The position of function for the foot is with the toes held horizontal and the ankle neutral in dorsiflexion and plantar flexion at 90 degrees to the lower leg, neutral in eversion

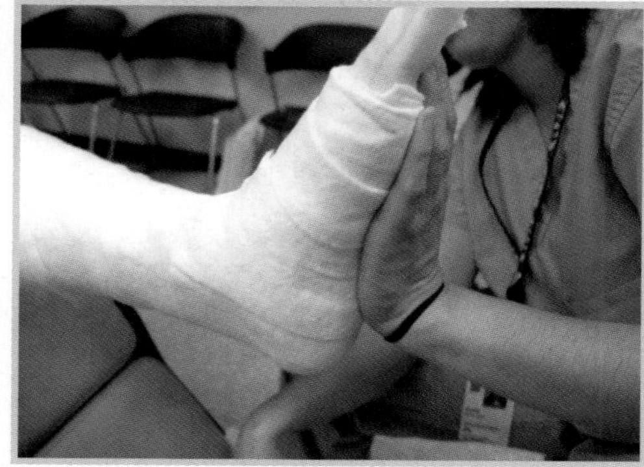

Step 1

and inversion. This positioning is critical to maintain throughout cast application. Pain, swelling, and fatigue may cause the patient to dangle their foot into plantar flexion.

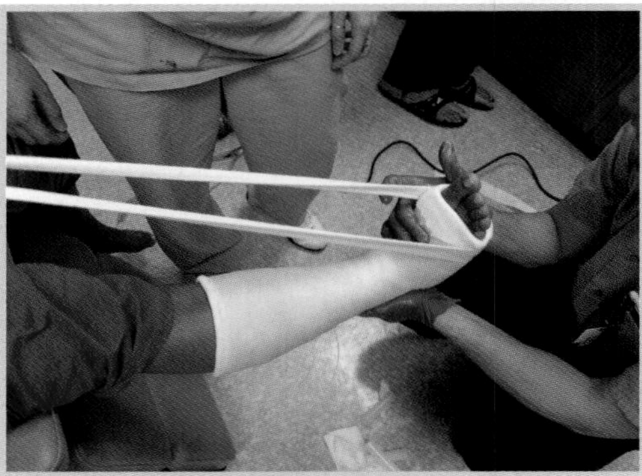

Step 2

Step 2. There are several techniques to assist in positioning. An assistant can grasp the toes during casting, the practitioner can wear a plastic apron and lean against the foot with the torso to maintain position of the foot while leaving the hands free to apply the cast, a strap can be held under the toes by the patient, or the patient can be placed prone and the knee flexed to 90 degrees, which allows gravity to help the foot stay at 90 degrees to the leg instead of plantar flexing.

- **PITFALL:** Do not let the foot plantar flex. Weeks in plantar flexion can cause significant shortening/contracture of the Achilles tendon.

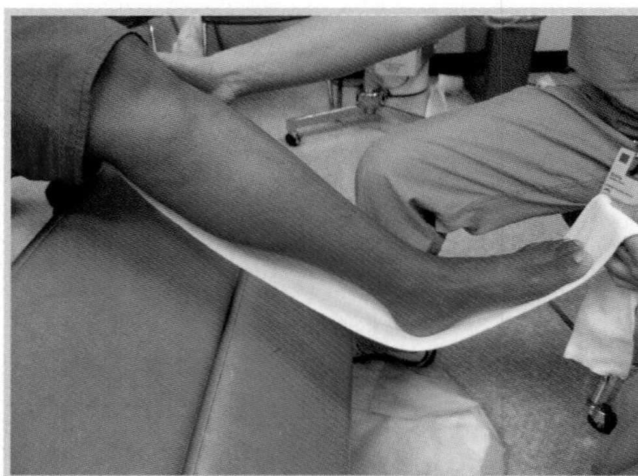

Step 3

Step 3. Measure the stockinette (typically a 3-inch stockinette) 2 inches beyond the end of the toes to the knee. The extra length helps to form smooth padded ends to the cast later in the procedure.

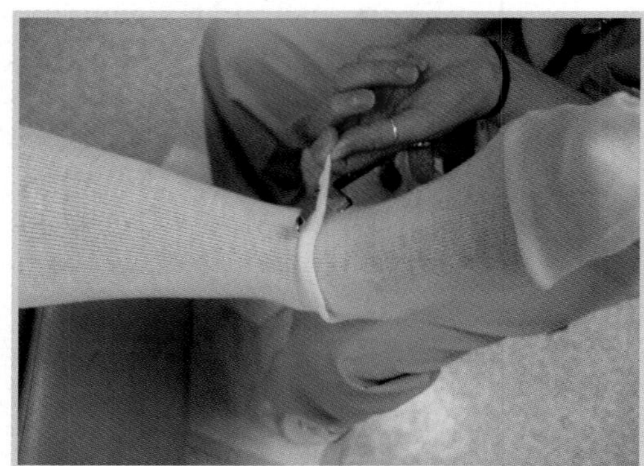

Step 4

Step 4. Cut away the overlapping stockinette where the dorsal foot meets the lower leg to avoid leaving any bunched-up stockinette against the skin.

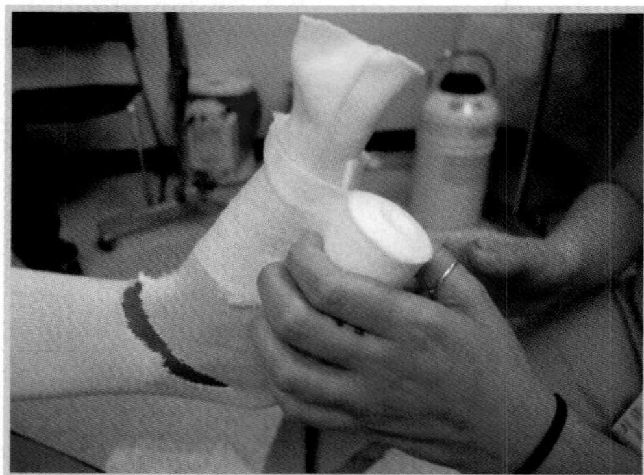

Step 5

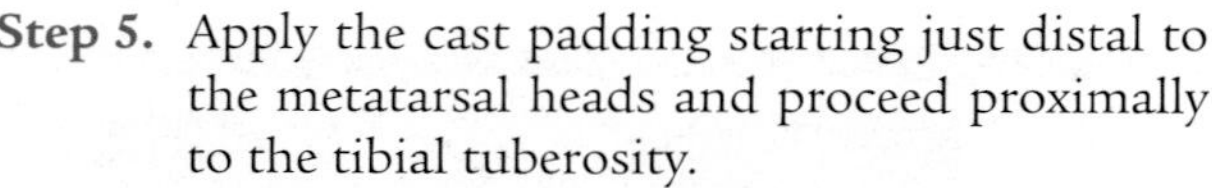

Step 5. Apply the cast padding starting just distal to the metatarsal heads and proceed proximally to the tibial tuberosity.

Step 6. Apply the cast padding to a double thickness by overlapping the roll 50% on each turn. Apply cast padding and cast material while keeping the roll flat against the patient. This is like unrolling carpet, with the bulk of the padding away from the patient. Doing the reverse would necessitate shifting the roll more from hand to hand. This allows the pad to roll on straight and not under too much tension.

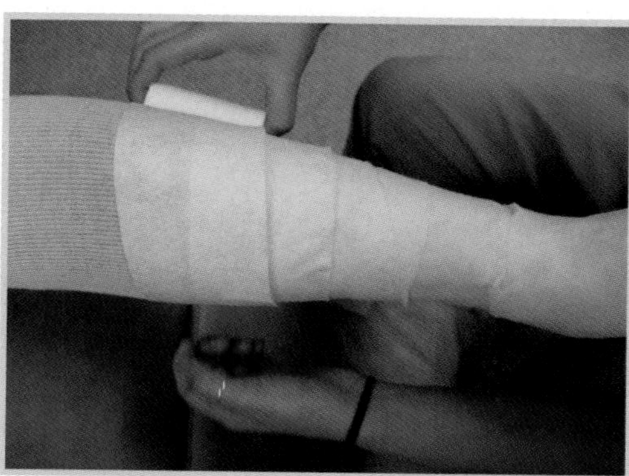

Step 6

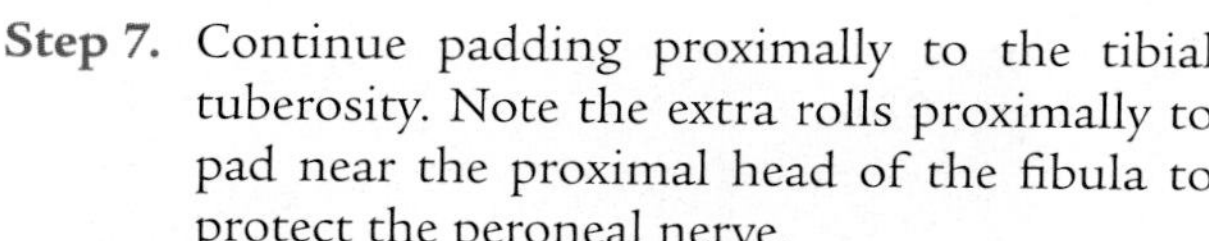

Step 7. Continue padding proximally to the tibial tuberosity. Note the extra rolls proximally to pad near the proximal head of the fibula to protect the peroneal nerve.

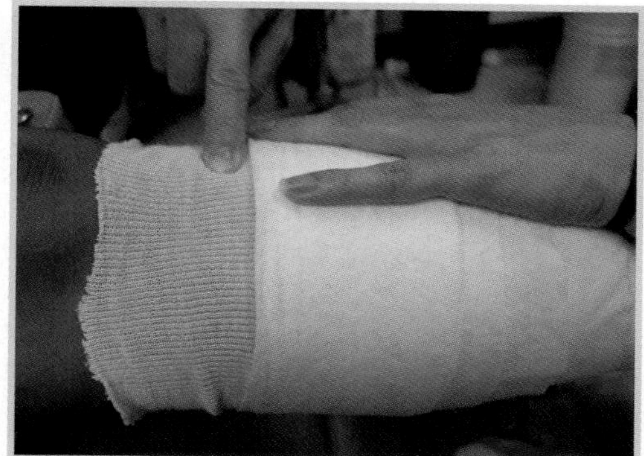

Step 7

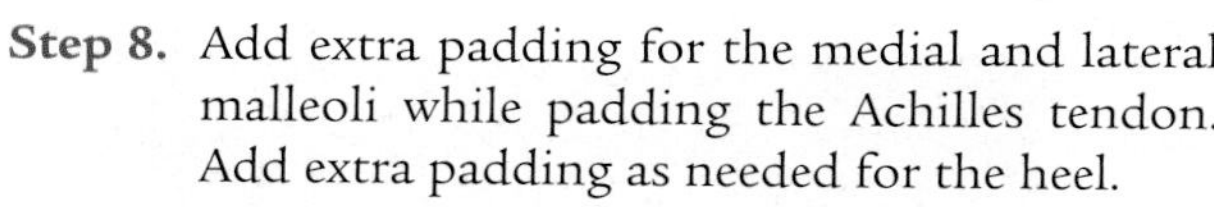

Step 8. Add extra padding for the medial and lateral malleoli while padding the Achilles tendon. Add extra padding as needed for the heel.

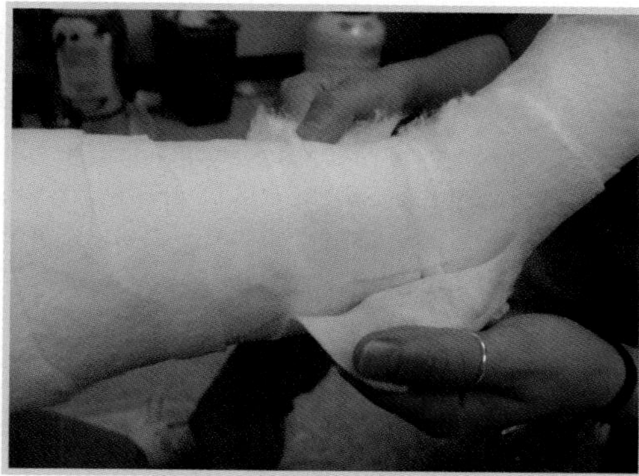

Step 8

Step 9. Add extra padding following the natural line of the metatarsal heads, angling slightly proximally from medial to lateral.

- **PITFALL:** Do not use too much padding, because this makes the cast too loose.

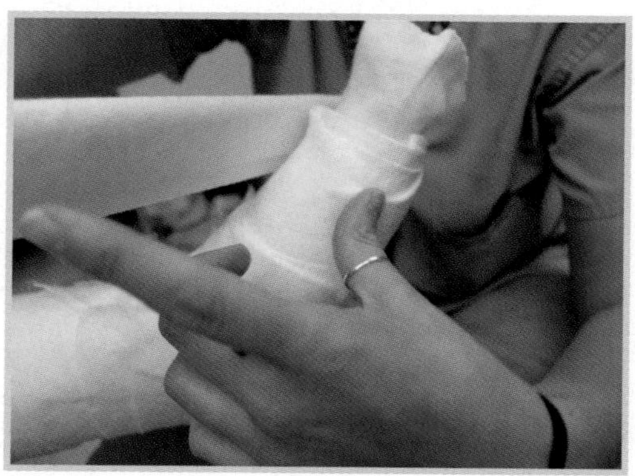

Step 9

Step 10. If desired, apply the De-flex protective strips down both sides of the cast at this time. See Chapter 110, applying a waterproof short arm cast with cast liner steps 1–5, for detailed instructions on applying a waterproof cast with Procel cast liner.

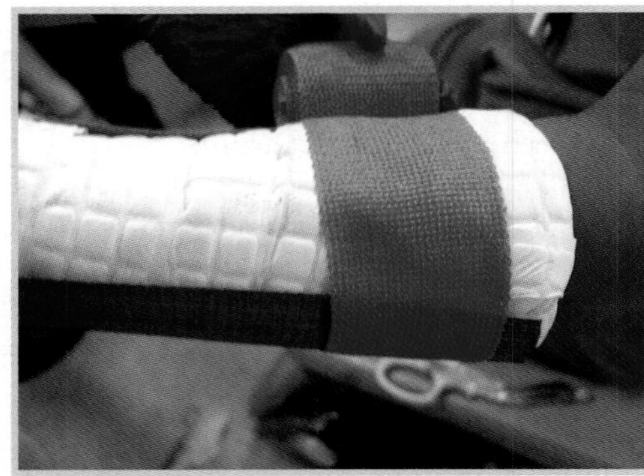

Step 10

Step 11. Place the plaster or fiberglass roll in lukewarm or room temperature water. Allow the plaster to sit in the water for a few seconds until the bubbling ceases. Remove the roll, and gently twist or gently squeeze the roll to remove excess water. Fiberglass can be applied without wetting if the clinician would like extra time for rolling it on or molding. The resin will react with ambient moisture in the air and harden in approximately 5 to 10 minutes.

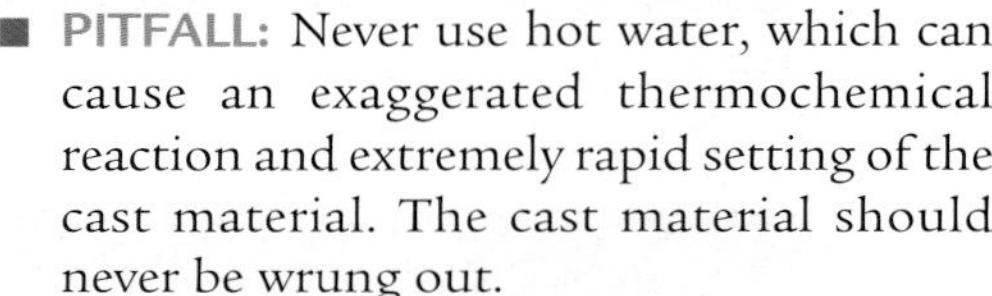

- PITFALL: Never use hot water, which can cause an exaggerated thermochemical reaction and extremely rapid setting of the cast material. The cast material should never be wrung out.

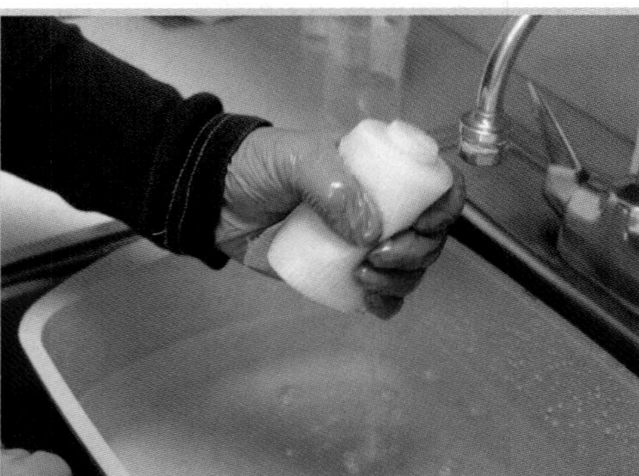

Step 11

Step 12. The fiberglass or plaster can be rolled starting either proximally or distally. The distal technique is described here. Start rolling the fiberglass just proximally to the distal edge of the padding (which was extended slightly beyond the metatarsal heads) to adequately support the metatarsal heads.

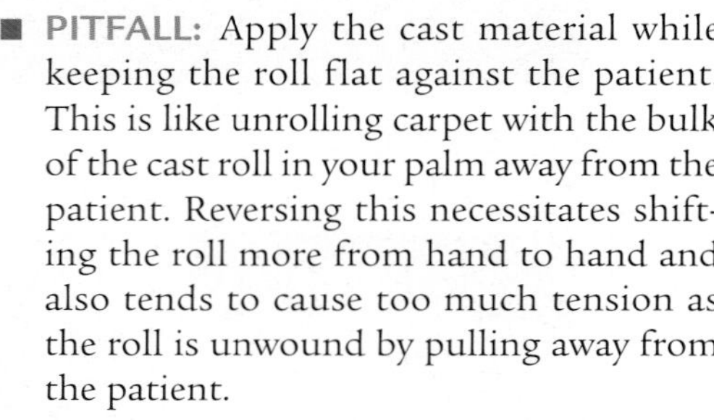

- PITFALL: Apply the cast material while keeping the roll flat against the patient. This is like unrolling carpet with the bulk of the cast roll in your palm away from the patient. Reversing this necessitates shifting the roll more from hand to hand and also tends to cause too much tension as the roll is unwound by pulling away from the patient.

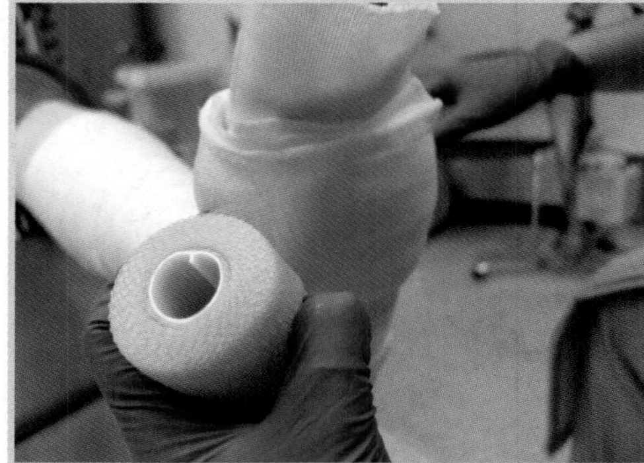

Step 12

Step 13. Roll the cast material with mild tension, applying it in similar fashion to the cast padding, from one end to the other. Overlap 50% of each prior roll, and continue rolling proximally up the leg.

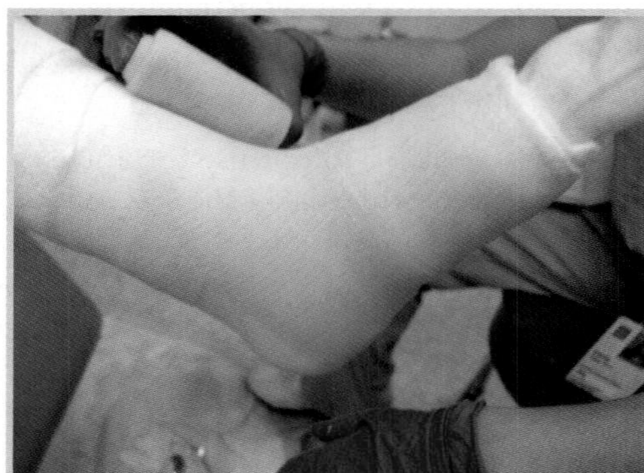

Step 13

Step 14. If plaster is used, apply the extra posterior splint material at this time if the cast will be a weight-bearing cast. Six-inch splint material that is about 0.25 inches thick is used for adults. Place the splint material from the metatarsal heads, over the back of the ankle, and up the posterior calf. Mold the splint so that it adheres and conforms to the first applied roll. Grasp the stockinette and pull it and the uncovered portion of cast padding over the rolled fiberglass to form nice padded ends to the cast. The distal aspect should be folded over to where it can support the metatarsal pads but allow flexion and extension of the toes. The upper portion of the cast should be well below the knee joint to allow flexion without impinging against the thigh and stop 1 to 2 fingerbreadths below the tibial tuberosity and 2 to 3 fingerbreadths below the fibular head.

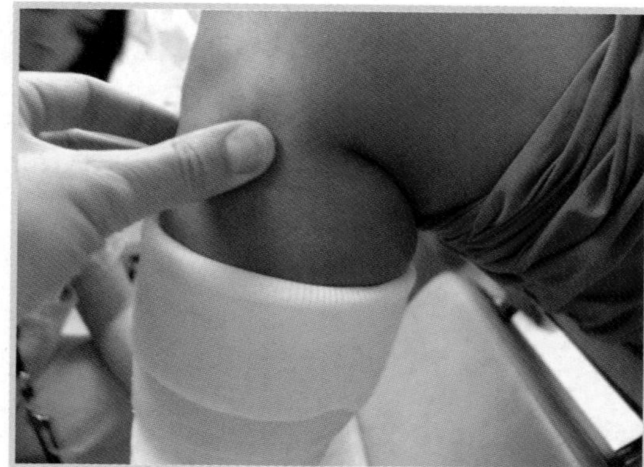

Step 14

- **PITFALL:** The ankle must be maintained in dorsiflexion to keep the 90-degree angle for the foot. The first roll of cast material is rapidly setting, and if the correct position is not maintained at this stage, the cast will maintain the foot in an incorrect position.
- **PITFALL:** A common and dangerous mistake is to apply the cast too high, so that the upper edge of the cast impinges on the peroneal nerve as it passes behind the fibular head. The upper edge of the cast must be well below the fibular head.

Step 15. Start the second roll of fiberglass, incorporating the folded-over stockinette.

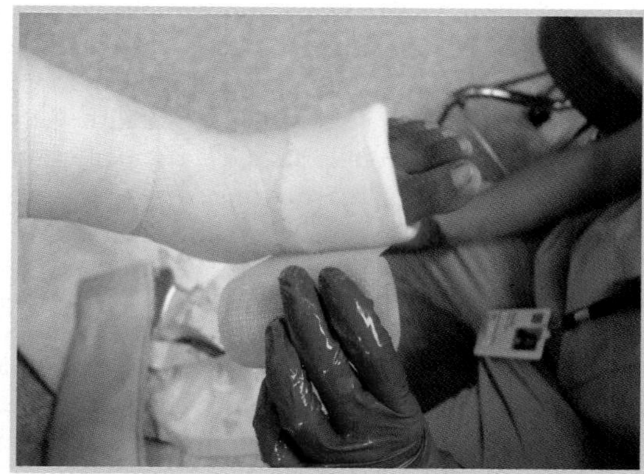

Step 15

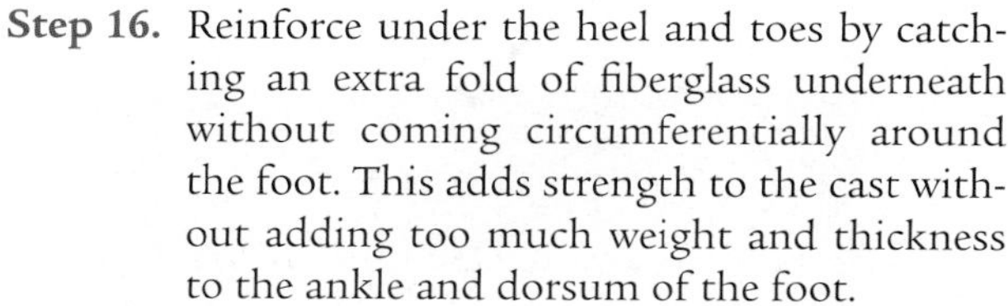

Step 16. Reinforce under the heel and toes by catching an extra fold of fiberglass underneath without coming circumferentially around the foot. This adds strength to the cast without adding too much weight and thickness to the ankle and dorsum of the foot.

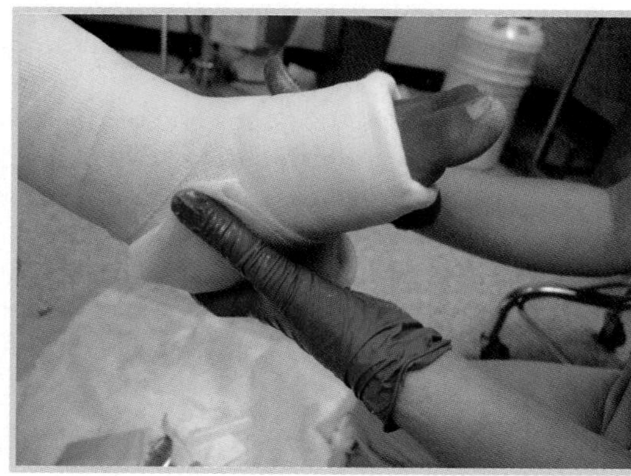

Step 16

Step 17. This extra fold is then incorporated into the cast and the roll is finished by rolling around the ankle and up the leg. If the practitioner is unable to roll up the leg to incorporate the stockinette and padding at the proximal cast, a third and last roll is used to finish off the upper leg and overlap it down to the ankle.

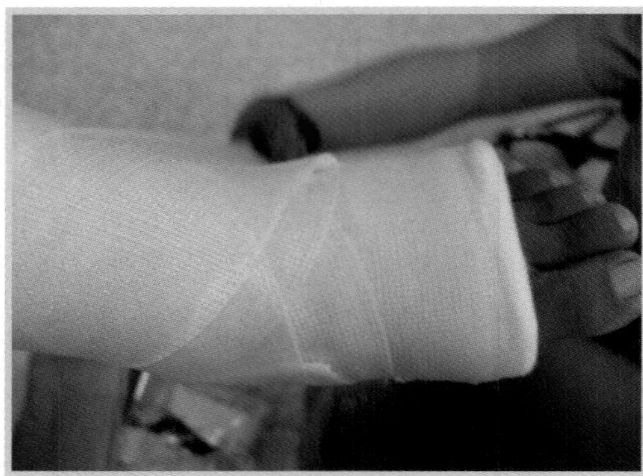

Step 17

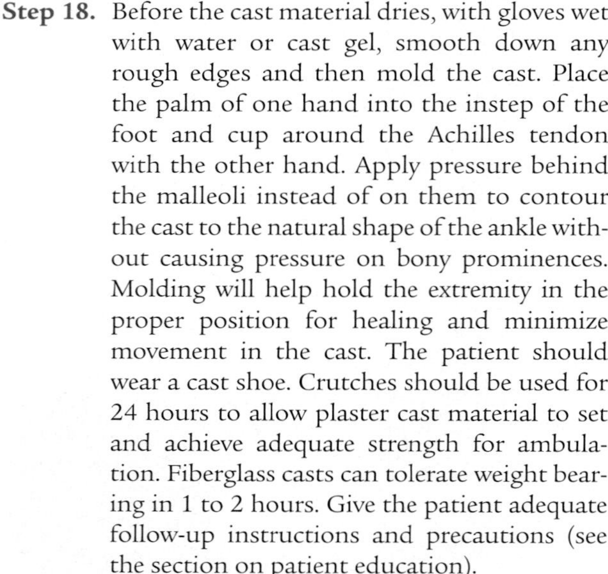

Step 18. Before the cast material dries, with gloves wet with water or cast gel, smooth down any rough edges and then mold the cast. Place the palm of one hand into the instep of the foot and cup around the Achilles tendon with the other hand. Apply pressure behind the malleoli instead of on them to contour the cast to the natural shape of the ankle without causing pressure on bony prominences. Molding will help hold the extremity in the proper position for healing and minimize movement in the cast. The patient should wear a cast shoe. Crutches should be used for 24 hours to allow plaster cast material to set and achieve adequate strength for ambulation. Fiberglass casts can tolerate weight bearing in 1 to 2 hours. Give the patient adequate follow-up instructions and precautions (see the section on patient education).

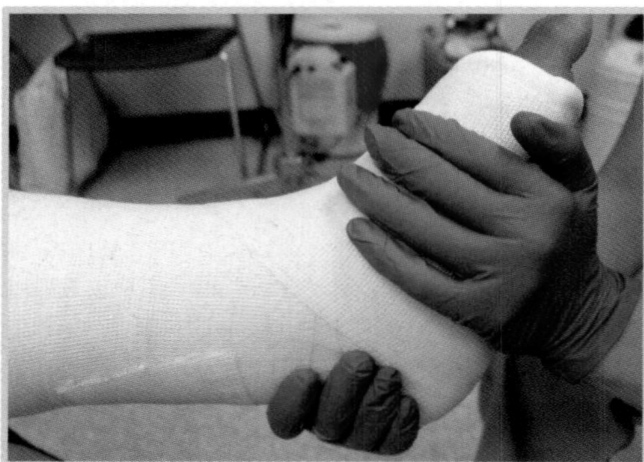

Step 18

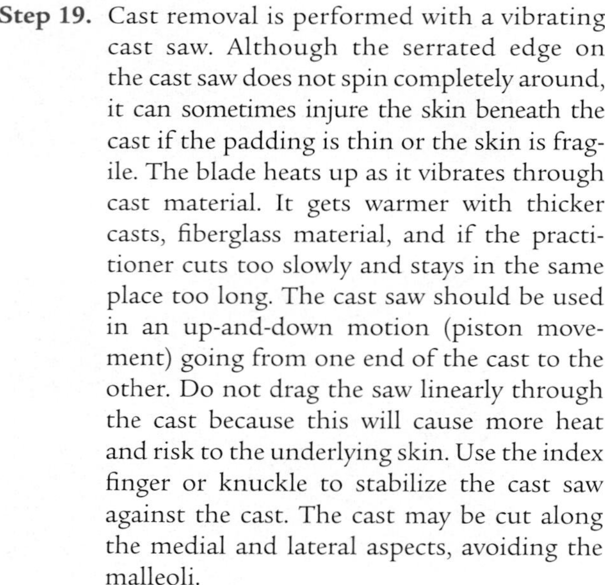

Step 19. Cast removal is performed with a vibrating cast saw. Although the serrated edge on the cast saw does not spin completely around, it can sometimes injure the skin beneath the cast if the padding is thin or the skin is fragile. The blade heats up as it vibrates through cast material. It gets warmer with thicker casts, fiberglass material, and if the practitioner cuts too slowly and stays in the same place too long. The cast saw should be used in an up-and-down motion (piston movement) going from one end of the cast to the other. Do not drag the saw linearly through the cast because this will cause more heat and risk to the underlying skin. Use the index finger or knuckle to stabilize the cast saw against the cast. The cast may be cut along the medial and lateral aspects, avoiding the malleoli.

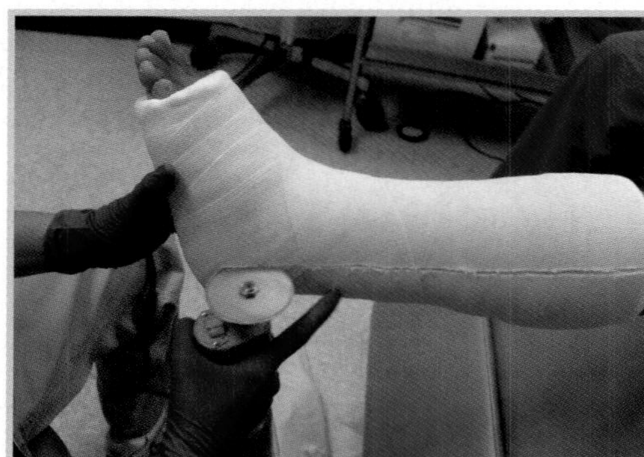

Step 19

Step 20. Spread the cast apart with cast spreaders.

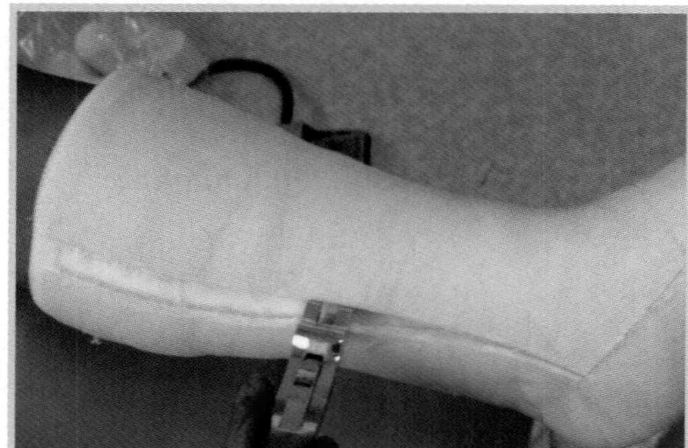

Step 20

Step 21. Carefully cut the padding beneath the cast using cast scissors, avoiding injury to underlying skin.

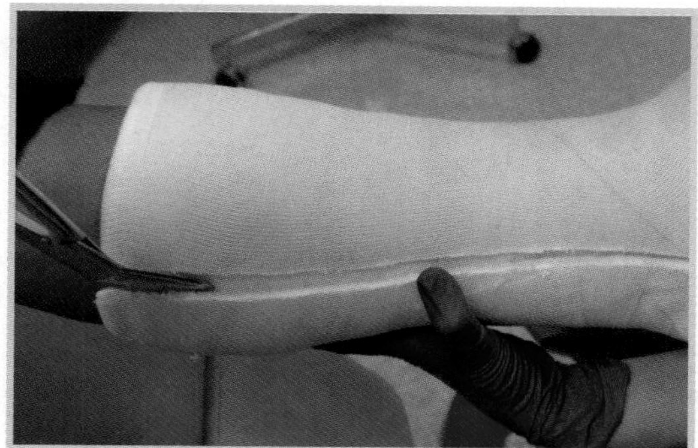

Step 21

Step 22. Separate and then lift off the cast.

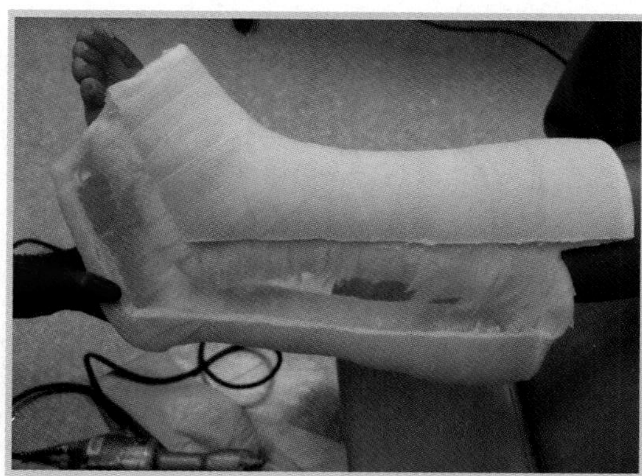

Step 22

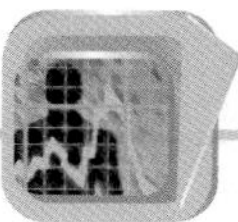

Complications

- Ischemia to the casted body part as a result of swelling of the extremity or the cast being applied to tightly
- Pressure ulcers attributable to a poorly padded or poorly fitting cast, especially at bony prominences
- Skin maceration if the cast gets wet and is not thoroughly dried out
- Skin damage from the patient inserting foreign objects into the cast or attempting to modify the cast
- Breakage of the cast as a result of misuse or inadequate structural strength due to inadequate overlapping of cast tape
- Failure to immobilize the area as a result of a poorly fitting cast

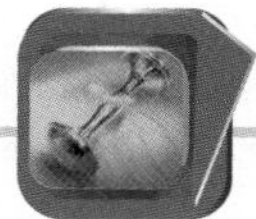

Pediatric Considerations

- Consider using a waterproof cast for ease of care and cleanliness.
- Active children may be harder on a cast, requiring earlier replacement if worn or damaged.
- Children are often frightened by the loud noise and vibration of the cast saw, so warning them and demonstrating against the practitioner's palm that the saw is not intended to cut skin can be helpful.

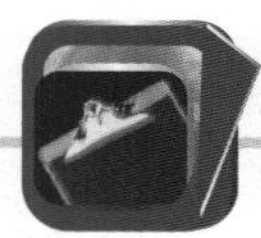

Postprocedure Instructions

Advise the patient to elevate the leg as much as possible to avoid swelling on the first day of application. Additionally, if the cast becomes too tight, if the patient has increasing pain in the foot or leg, loss of sensation, or loss of circulation, or if a foreign body becomes lodged in the cast, the practitioner should not hesitate to remove the cast. Apply a cast shoe for walking casts and advise the patient to wear the cast shoe with ambulation to prevent premature breakdown of the cast and also to give a gripping surface to diminish slipping and falling. After removing the cast, advise the patient to wash the area gently and not to aggressively scratch or abrade the area.

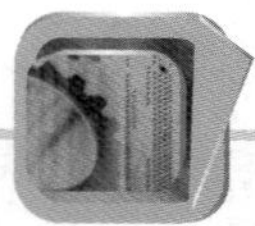

Coding Information and Supply Sources

The application codes are used only for cast or splint reapplication during a period of follow-up. The initial casting or splinting is considered part of the fracture management code. If no management code is reported, the cast application can be reported at the initial service. A supply code (99070) may be reported in addition to the cast code to help defray the cost of materials (estimated at $12 to $20 for plaster casts, $20 to $50 for fiberglass casts, and $5 to $12 for cast shoes). Insurance such as Medicaid may not cover the cost of materials.

CPT Code	Description	2008 Average 50th Percentile Fee	Global Period
27786	Global fee, closed treatment of distal fibular fracture—no manipulation	$686.00	90
28470	Global fee, closed treatment of metatarsal fracture—no manipulation	$686.00	90
29405	Cast application only: short leg cast, non-weight-bearing type	$254.00	0
29425	Cast application only: short leg cast, walking or ambulatory type	$279.00	0

CPT is a registered trademark of the American Medical Association.
2008 average 50th Percentile Fees are provided courtesy of 2008 MMH-SI's copyrighted Physicians' Fees and Coding Guide.

Instrument and Materials Ordering

Casting supplies, including rolls of cotton or acrylic cast padding, cotton or acrylic stockinette, plaster bandages, and fiberglass cast tape, can be ordered from these suppliers:

- DePuy OrthoTech, Tracy, CA. Web site: http://www.depuy.com
- Ray-Tek Inc. Fracture Management Supplies. Web site: http://www.ray-tek.com
- 3M Health Care, St. Paul, MN. Phone: 1-800-228-3957. Web site: http://www.3M.com/healthcare

Cast removal tools such as scissors, cast spreaders, and Stryker cast saws can be obtained from Applied Medical Service, Inc, Knoxville, TN. Web site: http://www.appliedmedicalinc.com.

Procel cast liner and De-flex protective strips can be ordered from W. L. Gore & Associates, Flagstaff, AZ. Phone: 1-800-528-8763. Web site: http://www.goremedical.com

Specific materials related to short leg casts include cast shoes from 3M, Inc., St. Paul, MN (phone: 1-888-364-3577; Web site: http://www.3m.com). Seal-tight cast covers, creating a waterproof seal using a nonlatex diaphragm that fits over the upper leg and attaches to a polyvinyl bag, allow daily bathing and showering while preventing water penetration. The acquisition cost is approximately $30 for a reusable cover, which can be obtained from Brown Medical Industries, Spirit Lake, IA (Web site: http://www.brownmed.com)

Patient Education Handout

A patient education handout, "Short Leg Cast," can be found on the book's companion Web site.

The author would like to acknowledge Robert Fawcett, MD, for his review of the manuscript.

Bibliography

Haley CA. Waterproof versus cotton cast liners: a randomized prospective comparison. *Am J Orthop.* 2006;35(3):137–140.

Hatch RL, Alsobrook JA. Diagnosis and management of metatarsal fractures. *Am Fam Physician.* 2007;76(6):817–826.

Killian JT, White S, Lenning L. Cast-saw burns: comparison of technique versus material versus saws. *J Pediatr Orthop.* 1999;19:683–687.

Kowalski KL, Pitcher JD Jr. Evaluation of fiberglass versus plaster of Paris for immobilization of fractures of the arm and leg. *Mil Med.* 2002;167(8):657–661.

LaBella CR. Common acute sports-related extremity injuries in children and adolescents. *CPEM.* 2007;8(1);31–42.

Steele PM, Bush-Joseph C, Bach B. Management of acute fractures around the knee, ankle, and foot. *Clin Fam Pract.* 2000;2:661–705.

2008 MAG Mutual Healthcare Solutions, Inc.'s Physicians' Fee and Coding Guide. Duluth, Georgia. MAG Mutual Healthcare Solutions, Inc. 2007.

CHAPTER 112

Lower Extremity Splinting

Jeff Harris, MD

Instructor of Family Medicine

Louisiana State University Health Science Center, Shreveport, LA

The five primary uses of splints are to immobilize fractures, dislocations, subluxations, sprains/strains, and painful joints. Secondarily, splints may be temporarily used to stabilize soft tissue injuries such as deep lacerations that cross joints. Splinting may be used as a definitive treatment in certain clinical situations such as de Quervain tenosynovitis.

Splints should be placed as soon as possible after the injury occurs. The immobilization of an extremity through splinting decreases pain and prevents further injury such as vascular injury, neurological compromise, and soft tissue injury. Ideally the splint should be left in place until the extremity has been fully and properly evaluated for more aggressive management such as surgery and/or casting, or until the fracture has healed. Splints remain the superior treatment in acute injury settings because they allow for swelling, which decreases the possibility of neurovascular compromise.

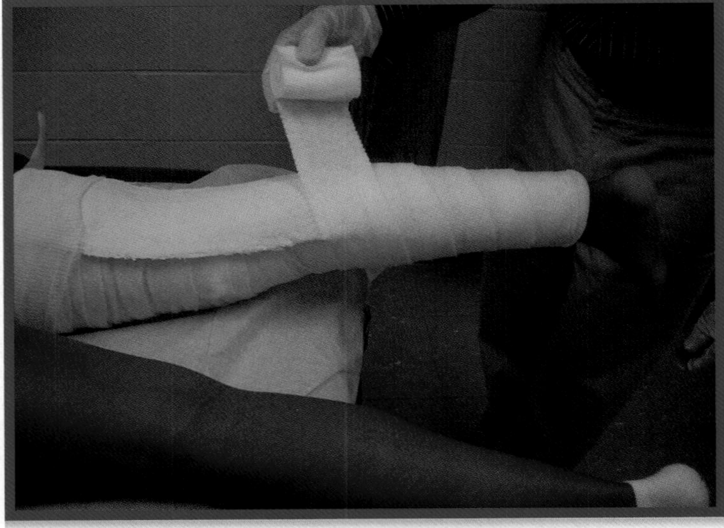

The knee splint is used to stabilize knee injuries and proximal tibia or fibula fractures. It is applied with the knee in full extension. The splint is placed from the posterior buttock down the posterior leg, knee, and calf to 3 inches above the level of the lateral malleolus. The posterior leg splint is used for distal leg, ankle, tarsal, and metatarsal fractures as well as ankle dislocations and severe sprains. It starts from the metatarsal heads on the plantar surface of the foot and extends up the back of the leg to the level of the fibular neck. These splints can be used along with a stirrup splint for unstable ankle fractures. The stirrup splint prevents eversion and inversion of the ankle joint. It is applied from below the medial side of knee and wrapped around the undersurface of the heel, then back up to the lateral side of the same knee. Stirrup splints, when used with a posterior leg splint, are better referred to as a *Sarmiento splint*. Buddy taping is used for phalangeal fractures of the toes. A small wadding of cotton is placed between the toes to prevent maceration. The fractured toe is secured to the adjacent toe with tape.

There are several types of splinting material available. Plaster splints consist of various width strips of a crinoline-type material impregnated with plaster of Paris, which crystallizes (hardens) after water is added. They are easier to mold and less expensive than other materials. However, they are more difficult to apply, are messy, are heavy, take longer to set, and are not water resistant (they get soggy when wet). Prefabricated splint rolls include 2-, 3-, 4-, and 6-inch rolls consisting of layers of fiberglass between polypropylene padding. These splints set more quickly, are lighter and stronger, and are water resistant. However, they are more expensive and difficult to mold. Air splints are preformed inflatable splints that are comfortable and indicated for ankle sprains but are not indicated for fractures or dislocations, and they are not discussed here.

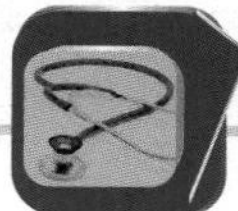

Equipment

- Stockinet
- Cast padding
- Splinting material
- Elastic bandage (e.g., Ace bandage)
- Adhesive tape
- Heavy scissors
- Room-temperature water
- Bucket
- Gloves
- Splinting material

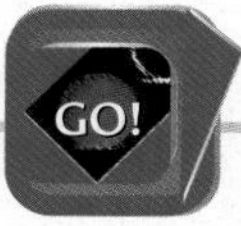

Indications

- To improve pain, decrease blood loss, reduce the risk for fat emboli, and minimize the potential for further neurovascular injury associated with fractures
- To improve pain associated with sprains
- To immobilize tendon lacerations
- To immobilize extremities associated with deep lacerations across joints
- To immobilize painful joints associated with inflammatory disorders

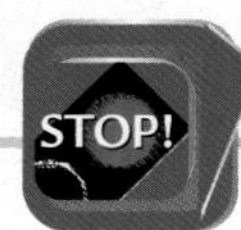

Contraindications

- Fractures that meet indication for emergent orthopedic surgical evaluation
- Open fractures
- Angulated fractures
- Displaced fractures
- Irreducible dislocations
- Neurovascular compromise

The Procedure

Knee Splint

Step 1. Prepare the patient by inspecting the skin for lacerations. Repair any injuries and clean any wounds before splinting. Prepare the stockinet by cutting it to fit the size of the leg being splinted. Allow 3 to 4 inches of extra material above and below the level of each end of the splint, which allows the ends of the stockinet to be folded back. Apply stockinet to limb.

- **PEARL:** Having the patient lie in the prone position on the examination table will make placing the splint an easier task.

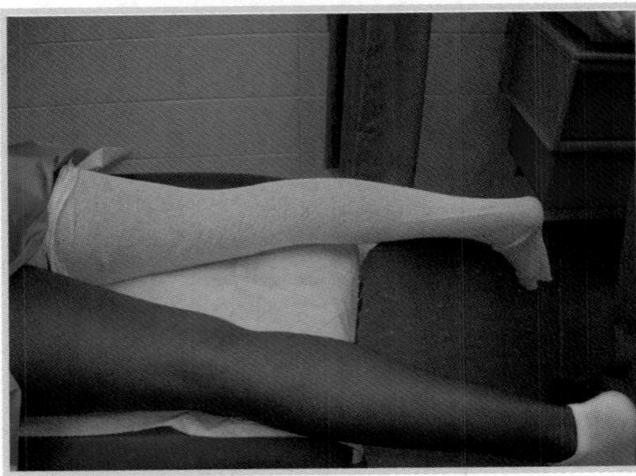

Step 1

Step 2. Roll the cast padding onto the leg, starting at the most distal end of the extremity and work proximally. The knee should be placed in full extension prior to wrapping to prevent kinks in the cast padding. Each layer should overlap the previous layer by about 50%.

- **PEARL:** Make sure to add extra cast padding at the most distal and proximal ends to avoid irritation to the ankle and buttock.
- **PEARL:** Use extra padding at sites of bony prominences and ends of splint to decrease the chance of pressure sores.
- **PEARL:** Cast padding should be rolled with the bulk of the material on top of the sheet adjacent to the skin. The rolling should be effortless.

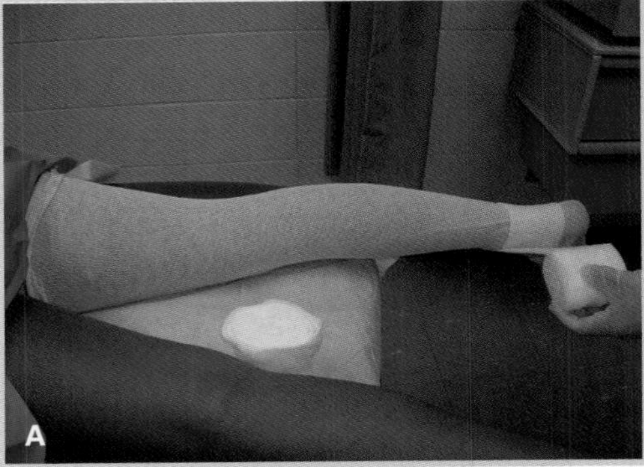

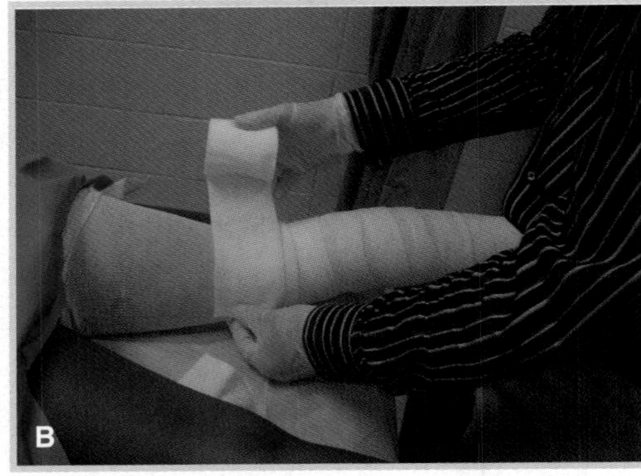

Step 2

Step 3. Prepare 10 to 15 sheets of plaster (which is enough for most lower extremity splints). Next, estimate the length needed by laying the splint sheets over the injured extremity. You may need to tear a small amount off one end of the splint sheets if the original length is too long.

- **PEARL:** Alternatively, when using fiberglass material, simply measure the extremity to be splinted. Unroll a length of fiberglass material, and accordion fold the material to the correct length. Then use scissors to cut the accordion fold away from the remaining roll.

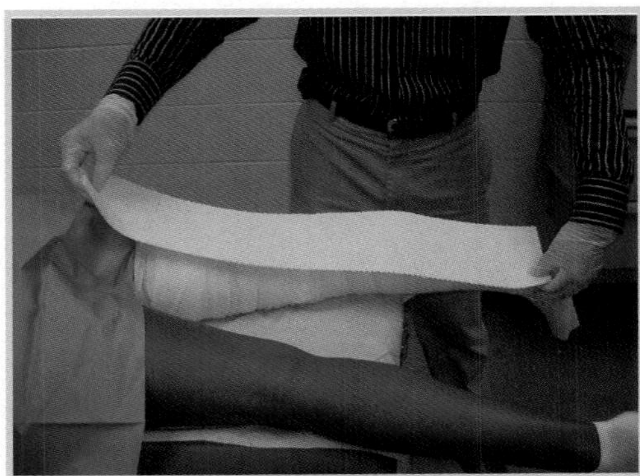

Step 3

Step 4. Immerse the splint material in room-temperature water. Squeeze out all the water and smooth the splint taking out all the wrinkles. Place the splint on the posterior side of the leg while immobilizing the patient's knee joint. It is applied from the posterior buttock down the posterior leg, knee, and calf to 3 inches above the level of the lateral malleoli.

- **PITFALL:** Never use hot water, which can cause an excessive thermochemical reaction and extremely rapid setting of the cast material. The cast material should never be wrung out.

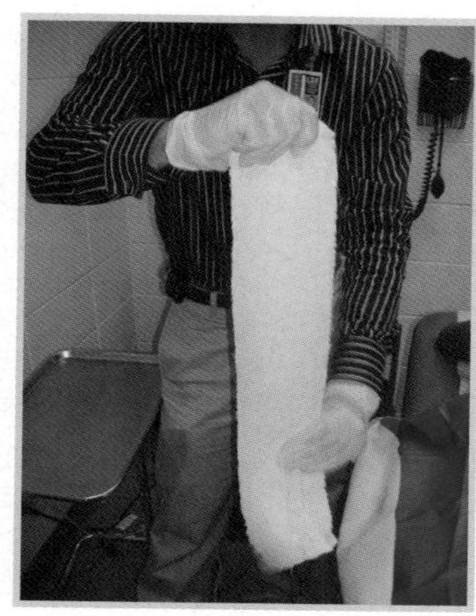

Step 4

Step 5. Roll the ends of the stockinet back over the splint, allowing a thick layer of padding at both ends to avoid irritations and lacerations from the splint material. Smooth and mold the splint as it sets.

- **PITFALL:** Always use the palms of your hands to smooth and mold the splint. Excessive use of the fingers can cause indentions in the splint, which can lead to pressure sores.

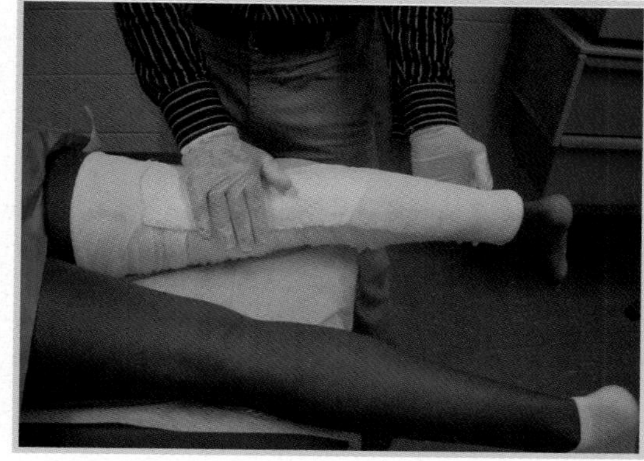

Step 5

Step 6. Secure the splint material with another single layer of cast padding. Mold the splint with the palm of your hand while keeping the extremity in full extension.

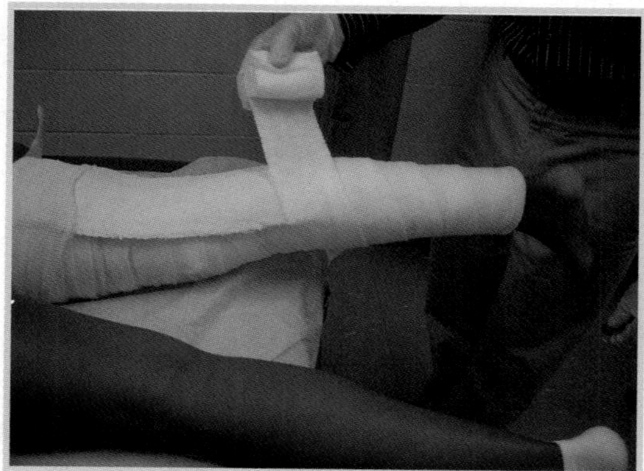

Step 6

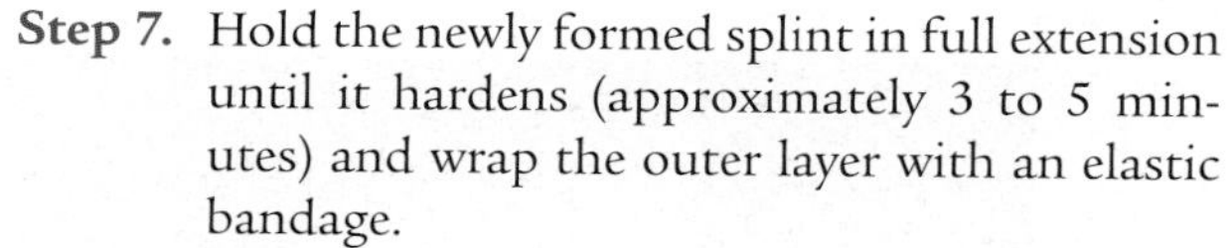

Step 7. Hold the newly formed splint in full extension until it hardens (approximately 3 to 5 minutes) and wrap the outer layer with an elastic bandage.

- **PITFALL:** Wrapping the elastic bandage too tightly could lead to vascular compromise and not allow for swelling.
- **PEARL:** Always allow for ankle and hip range of motion to prevent joint stiffness.

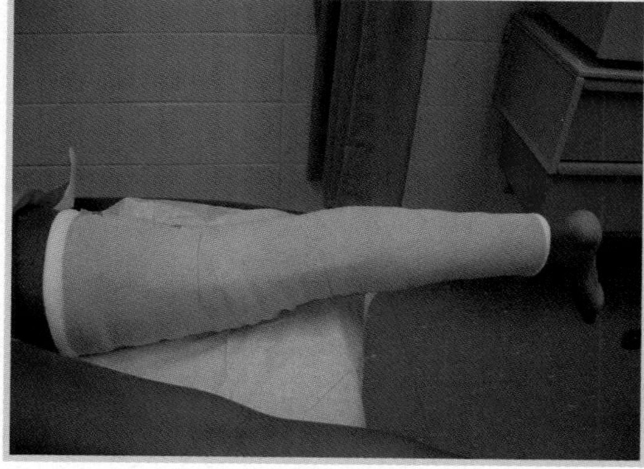

Step 7

Posterior Leg Splint

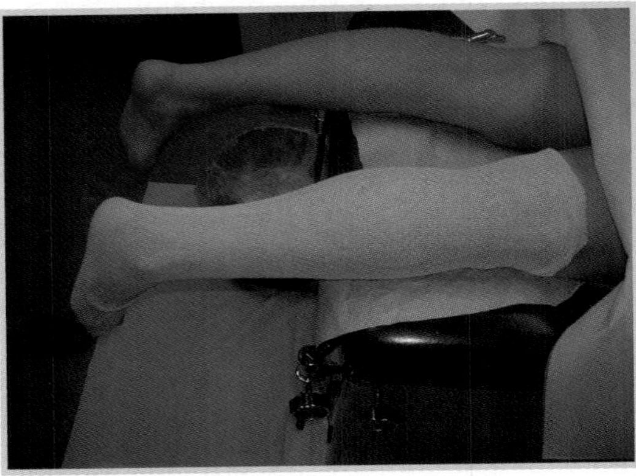

Step 1

Step 1. Begin by measuring, cutting, and placing the stockinet as discussed for the knee splint except this stockinet should be measured to incorporate the entire foot up the knee.

- **PEARL:** Having the patient lie in the prone position on the examination table will make placing the splint an easier task.

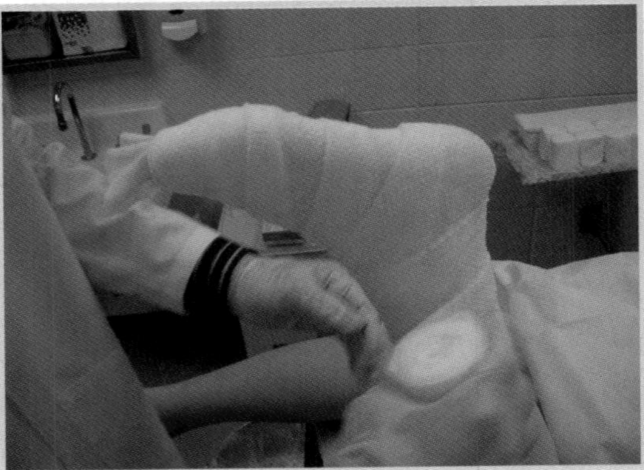

Step 2

Step 2. Next, place the cast padding. Start by wrapping the padding distally around the toes and work your way proximal until the knee is reached. The ankle should be placed in 90 degrees of dorsiflexion.

- **PITFALL:** Failing to place the ankle in 90 degrees of dorsiflexion will make it more difficult for your patient to regain range of motion once the splint is removed.
- **PEARL:** When immobilizing Achilles tendon injuries, the ankle should always be splinted in plantar flexion. Failing to splint an Achilles rupture in plantar flexion could allow tracking of the proximal portion of the tendon high into the leg, making surgical repair more difficult.

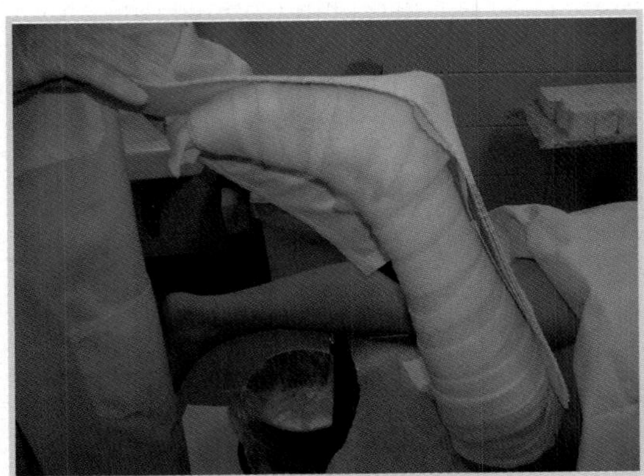

Step 3

Step 3. Measure the approximate length of plaster sheets. These should be long enough to be placed from metatarsal heads on the plantar surface of the foot and extend up the back of leg to the level of the fibular neck.

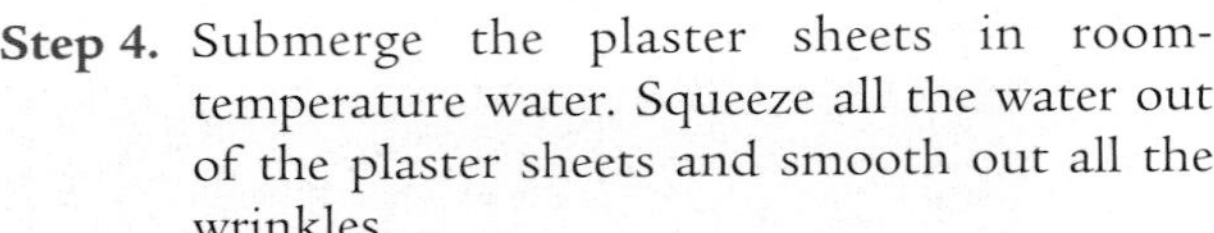

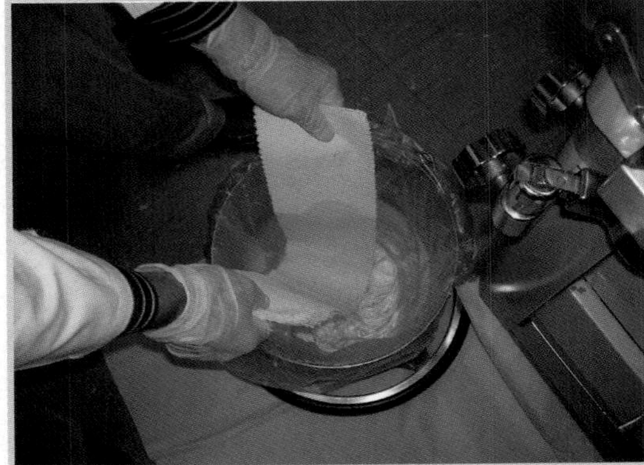

Step 4

Step 4. Submerge the plaster sheets in room-temperature water. Squeeze all the water out of the plaster sheets and smooth out all the wrinkles.

- **PITFALL:** Never use hot water, which can cause an excess thermochemical reaction and extremely rapid setting of the material. The splint material should never be wrung out.
- **PEARL:** Alternatively, when using fiberglass material, simply measure the extremity to be splinted. Unroll a length of fiberglass material, and accordion fold the material to the correct length. Then use scissors to cut the accordion fold away from the remaining roll.

Step 5. Mold the plaster sheets on the plantar surface of foot, posterior ankle, and leg.

- **PITFALL:** Always use the palms of your hands to smooth and mold the splint. Excessive use of the fingers can cause indentions in the splint, which can lead to pressure sores.

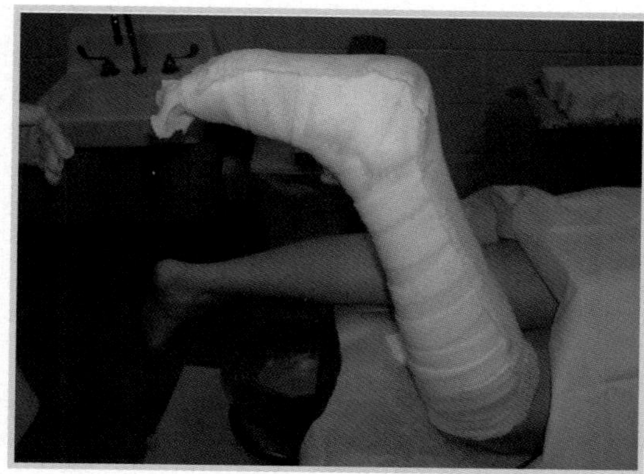

Step 5

Step 6. Roll both the distal and proximal ends of the stockinet back over the splint, allowing a thick layer of padding at both ends to avoid irritations and lacerations from the splint material. Secure the splint by wrapping a layer of cast padding around the entire outside of the splint. Wrapping should start at distal end of extremity and continue proximally to cover the entire splint.

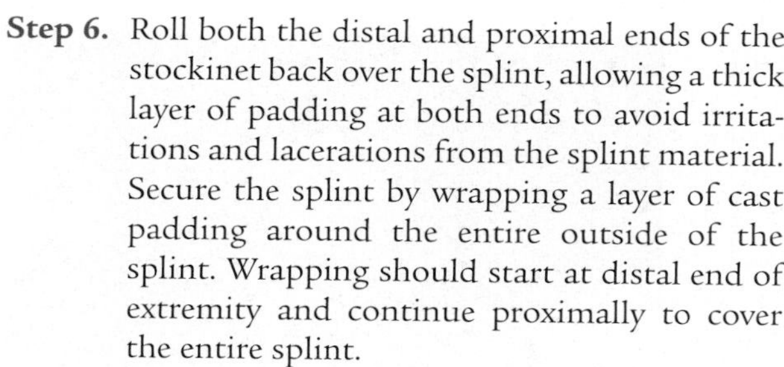

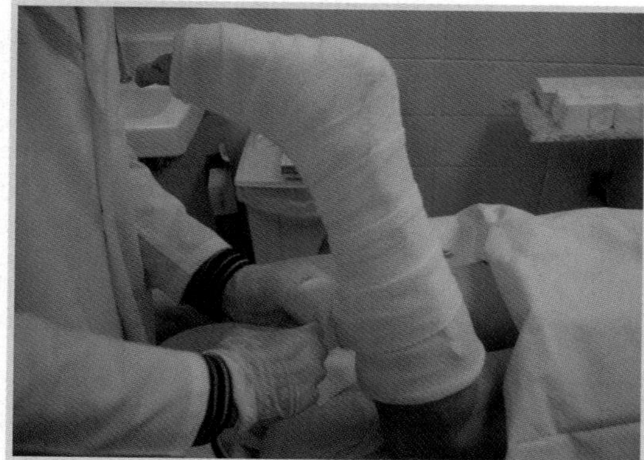

Step 6

Step 7. The splint should be molded with the ankle in approximate 90 degrees of dorsiflexion. Once the splint hardens, place an elastic bandage over the entire splint.

- **PEARL:** For unstable ankle fractures, this splint should be used in combination with a stirrup splint.

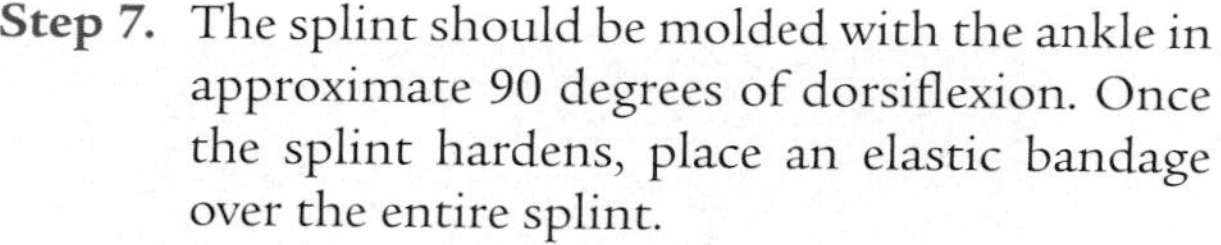

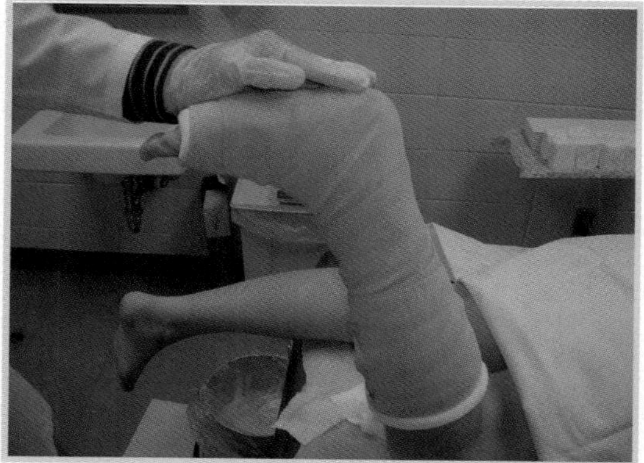

Step 7

Stirrup Splint

Step 1. Because this splint is most commonly used in combination with a posterior leg splint (Sarmiento splint), you should not have to reapply the stockinet and cast padding before placing this splint. Those steps should have taken place prior to placing the posterior leg splint.

- **PEARL:** Having the patient lie in the prone position on the examination table will make placing the splint an easier task.

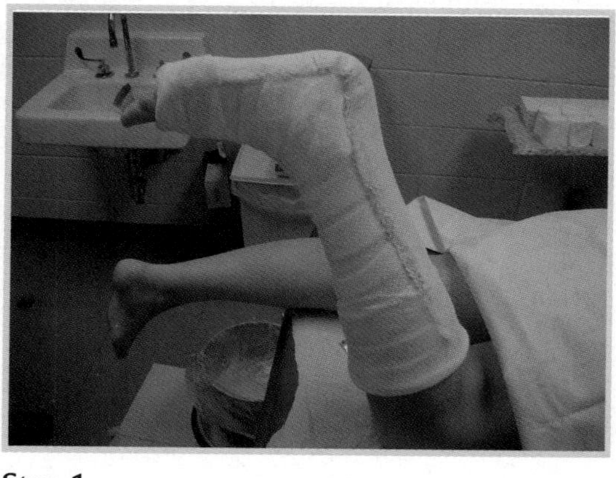

Step 1

Step 2. Measure the length of the plaster sheets against the patient's leg and tear or cut to length. The strips should be long enough to involve the leg from below the medial side of knee, wrap around the undersurface of the heel, and back up to the lateral side of the same knee.

- **PEARL:** This part of the splint is to prevent inversion and eversion of the ankle.
- **PEARL:** In some patients, the long splint material (5 inches × 30 inches) may not be long enough to reach from one side of the knee to the other. In this situation, you can measure and tear the material to cover from the medial side of knee to the lateral heel. Then measure and tear another piece to cover from the lateral side of the knee to the medial heel. When placing the splint, the two pieces should overlap at the undersurface of the heel.

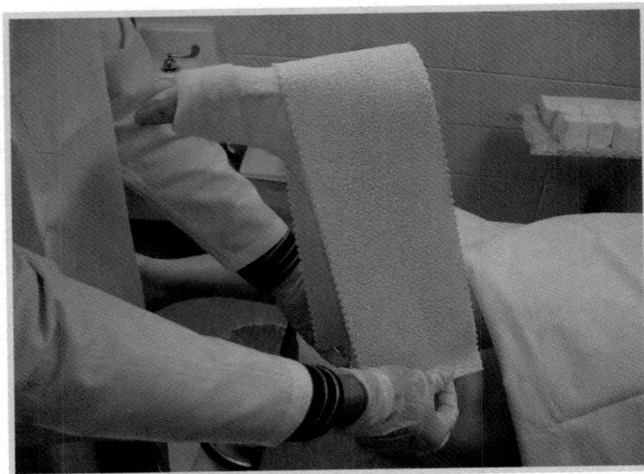

Step 2

Step 3. Submerge the plaster in room-temperature water, then squeeze out all the water and smooth out the wrinkles.

- **PEARL:** Alternatively, when using fiberglass material, simply measure the extremity to be splinted. Unroll a length of fiberglass material, and accordion fold the material to the correct length. Then use scissors to cut the accordion fold away from the remaining roll.

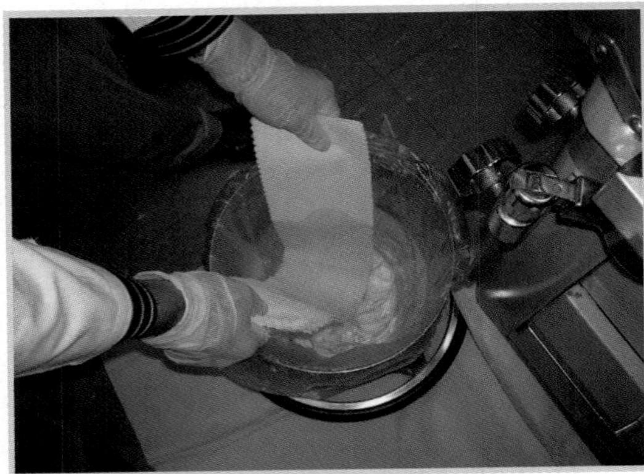

Step 3

Step 4. Mold the splint around the ankle to prevent inversion or eversion.

- **PITFALL:** Always use the palms of your hands to smooth and mold the splint. Excessive use of the fingers can cause indentions in the splint, which can lead to pressure sores.

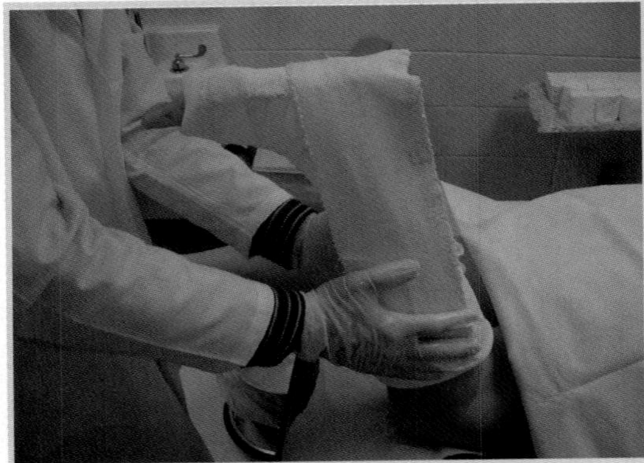

Step 4

Step 5. Roll both the distal and proximal ends of the stockinet back over the splint, allowing a thick layer of padding at both ends to avoid irritations and lacerations from the splint material. Wrap the outer layer of the splints with cast padding. Start by wrapping the padding distally around the foot and ankle and then work proximally. Starting distally around the foot and ankle will hold the splint in place while you prepare to finish the splint.

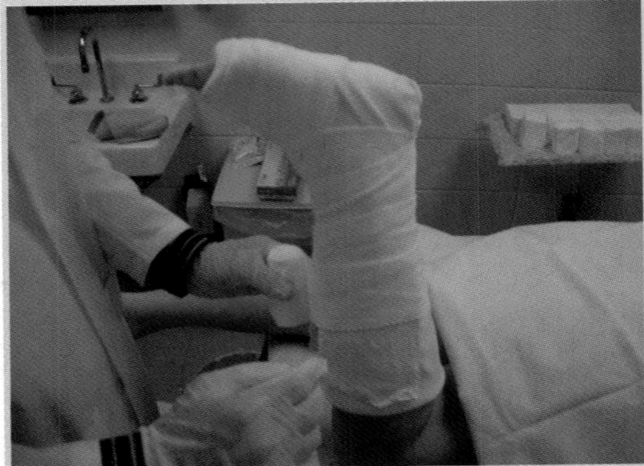

Step 5

Step 6. Once the splint hardens, finish by wrapping an elastic bandage over the entire splint.

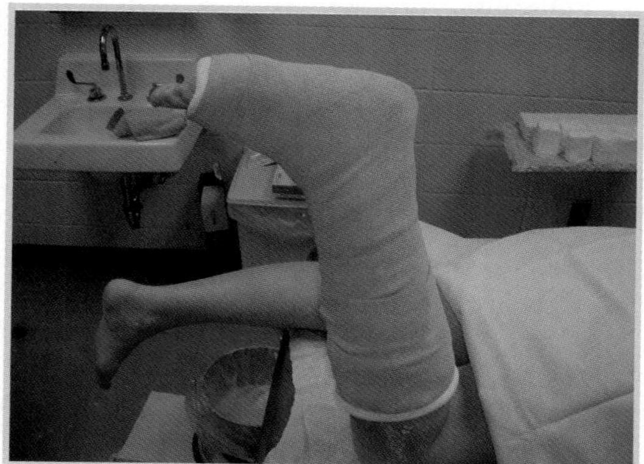

Step 6

Buddy Taping

Step 1. Start by folding a 3- × 3-inch cotton pad in half. Place the cotton pad or some other form of wadding between the affected and adjacent toe to prevent maceration. Tear a piece of tape, and secure the injured toe to the adjacent toe.

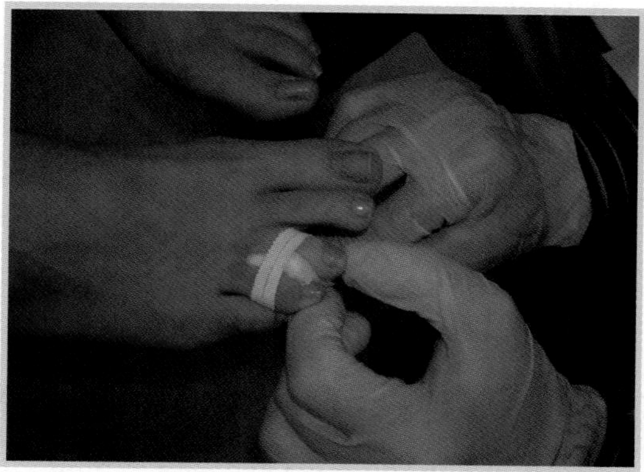

Step 1

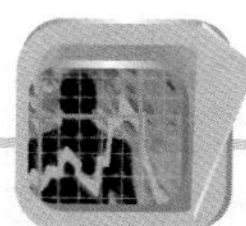

Complications

- Pressure sores result from insufficient padding over bony prominences or indentions in plaster from improper use of fingers to mold the splint or improper support of splint while hardening.
- Compartment syndrome occurs less commonly with splints than casts. Presenting signs of compartment syndrome include pain, pallor, paresthesias, paralysis, and lack of pulse. Avoid this by wrapping cotton padding with minimal pressure and minimize swelling with ice and elevation. Immediate splint removal and orthopedic consultation is required if compartment syndrome is suspected.
- Infection may occur if the patient places sharp instruments down the splint for scratching (e.g., a coat hanger). It is more common with open wounds present prior to splinting. The provider may prevent this complication by cleaning wounds well before splinting.
- Heat injury may result from plaster-generated heat during crystallizing. Reduce the risk of thermal injury by applying an appropriate amount of cotton padding and using room-temperature water.
- Joint stiffness may occur. Splinting the extremities in their position of function will reduce joint stiffness and make it easier to get range of motion back once the splint is removed. Avoid prolonged immobilization if possible.

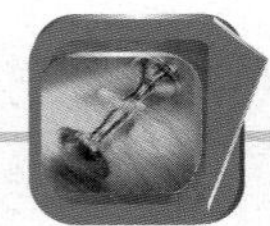

Pediatric Considerations

Children who present with swelling, immobility, pain with movement or palpation, anatomic deformity, discoloration, or crepitus should have radiographic studies. Immediate orthopedic consultation is needed for severe musculoskeletal injuries such as open fractures, evidence of neurovascular compromise, fractures and dislocations that cannot be easily reduced in the office or emergency department, or fractures that are displaced or too angulated to be splinted.

Patients with sprains need special attention because a sprain may represent a Salter-Harris type 1 injury that does not have any radiographic evidence of a fracture. Any patient who has tenderness over the physis (growth plate) should be presumed to have a Salter-Harris type 1 fracture and appropriate splinting should take place to immobilize the extremity. Be aware of tenderness to palpation at the injured site during the follow-up visit in 7 to 10 days. This could represent a nondisplaced Salter-Harris type 1 fracture, and additional follow-up radiographs should be ordered to confirm clinical suspicion. Rapid resolution (2 to 3 days) of tenderness after splinting implies the absence of a Salter-Harris type 1 fracture.

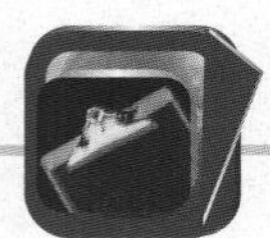

Postprocedure Instructions

Patients should be instructed to elevate and ice the extremity to minimize swelling. Ice can be applied using cold packs such as frozen bags of vegetables or ice bags for 15 to 20 minutes at a time for the first 48 hours. They should also be given instructions to not get the splint wet and not to remove it unless the provider has made it removable. Splints should be placed in a plastic bag while bathing to keep dry. Make sure the patient understands symptoms of neurovascular compromise. Patients should know to return if the splint gets wet or starts to come apart. They should also be instructed not to stick any objects (especially sharp objects such as hangers) down the splint to scratch. These recommendations should be given in writing as well as verbally.

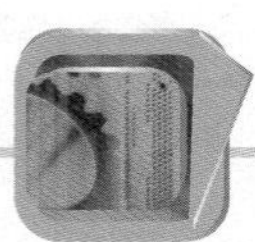

Coding Information and Supply Sources

CPT Code	Description	2008 Average 50th Percentile Fee	Global Period
29505	Long leg splint	$174.00	0
29515	Short leg splint	$146.00	0

CPT is a registered trademark of the American Medical Association.
2008 average 50th Percentile Fees are provided courtesy of 2008 MMH-SI's copyrighted Physicians' Fees and Coding Guide.

Suppliers

Plaster of Paris splinting material can be obtained from these suppliers:

- BSN medical. Web site: http://www.bsnmedical.com
- Specialized Medical Supplies Co. Ltd. Web site: http://www.specialized-medical/Plaster-of-Paris-slabs.htm

Fiberglass splinting material can be obtained from this supplier:

- 3M Health Care Professionals. Web site: http://www.3m.Com/product/information/scotchcast-custom-length-splint.html

Patient Education Handout

A patient education handout, "Splints," can be found on the book's companion Web site.

Bibliography

Bowker P, Powell ES. A clinical evaluation of plaster-of-Paris and eight synthetic fracture splinting materials. *Injury*. 1992;23:13–20.

Erick IM. Splinting. In: Yamamoto LG, Inada AS, Okamoto JK, et al., eds. *Case-Based Pediatrics for Medical Students and Residents*. Department of Pediatrics University of Hawaii John A. Burns School of Medicine; 2004. http://www.hawaii.edu/medicine/pediatrics/pedtext/s19c02.html.

Marshall PD, Dibble AK, Walters TH, et al. When should a synthetic casting material be used in preference to plaster-of-Paris? a cost analysis and guidance for casting departments. *Injury*. 1992;23:542–544.

Rowley DI, Pratt D, Powell ES, et al. The comparative properties of plaster of Paris and plaster of Paris substitutes. *Arch Orthel Orthop Trauma Surg*. 1985;103:402–407.

Principles of fractures and dislocations. In: Rockwood Jr CA, Green DP, Bucholz RW, eds. *Rockwood and Green Fractures in Adults,* 3rd ed. Philadelphia: Lippincott; 1991:25–27.

Smith G, Hart R, Tsai T. Fiberglass cast application. *Am J Emer Med*. 2005;23:347–350.

Lucas GL. General orthopaedics. In: Green WB, ed. *Essentials of Musculoskeletal Care*, 2nd ed. (IL): American Academy of Orthopaedic Surgeons, 2001:81–82.

2008 MAG Mutual Healthcare Solutions, Inc.'s Physicians' Fee and Coding Guide. Duluth, Georgia. MAG Mutual Healthcare Solutions, Inc. 2007.

CHAPTER 113

Upper Extremity Short Arm Splinting

Jeff Harris, MD
Instructor of Family Medicine
Louisiana State University Health Science Center, Shreveport, LA

Splinting plays a major role in the management of musculoskeletal injuries. Splints are used to temporarily immobilize fractures, subluxations/dislocations, sprains, or painful joints associated with inflammatory disorders. They also may be utilized to immobilize soft tissue injuries, such as deep lacerations that cross joints, until further evaluation and/or casting can be accomplished. Splinting may be used as a definitive treatment in certain clinical situations such as de Quervain tenosynovitis.

Immobilization of an extremity through splinting decreases pain and prevents further injuries, including vascular injury, neurological compromise, and soft tissue injury. A splint should be placed as soon as possible after the injury occurs. It should ideally be left in place until the injury has been fully evaluated, other therapy initiated, or until the injury is adequately healed. Splints allow for swelling, which decreases the possibility of neurovascular compromise. This makes them superior to casting in acute injury settings.

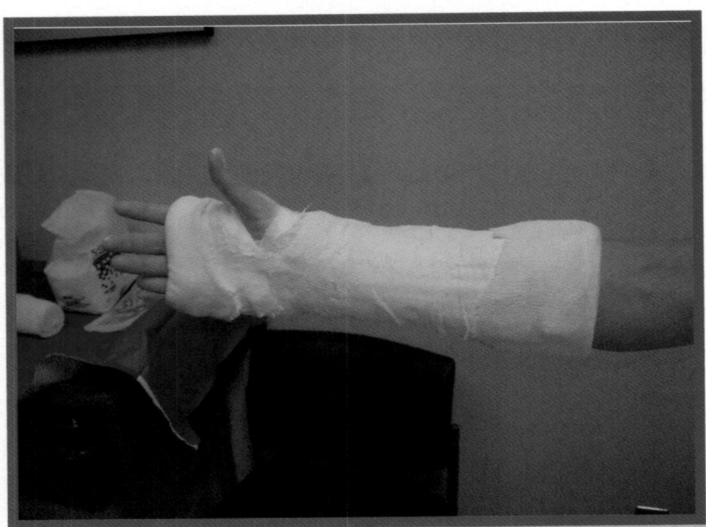

The volar splint is used to stabilize distal forearm and wrist fractures. It is applied from the volar palmar crease to a point that covers two thirds of the forearm. The ulnar gutter splint is used for phalange and metacarpal fractures and is most commonly used for boxer fractures. It starts at the distal interphalangeal (DIP) joint and covers the proximal two thirds of the forearm. The function of the ulnar gutter splint is to immobilize the ring and little finger. The thumb spica splint is used for scaphoid fractures, thumb phalanx fractures and/or dislocations, gamekeeper's thumb (skier's thumb), and de Quervain tenosynovitis. It starts at the DIP joint of the thumb (incorporating the thumb) and covers the proximal two thirds of radial forearm.

There are several types of splinting material available. Plaster splints consist of various width strips of a crinoline-type material impregnated with plaster of Paris or gypsum, which crystallize (harden) after water is added. Their advantage is that they are easier to mold and less expensive than other materials. However, they are more difficult to apply, are messy, are heavy, take longer to set, and are not water resistant (they get soggy when wet). Prefabricated splint rolls include 2-, 3-, 4-, and 6-inch rolls consisting of layers of fiberglass between polypropylene padding. These splints set more quickly, are lighter and stronger, and are water resistant. However, they are more expensive and difficult to mold. Air splints are preformed inflatable splints that are comfortable; they are indicated for ankle sprains but not for fractures or dislocations and are not discussed here.

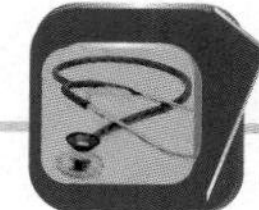

Equipment

- Stockinet
- Cast padding
- Splinting material
- Elastic bandage (e.g., Ace bandage)
- Adhesive tape
- Heavy scissors
- Room-temperature water
- Bucket
- Gloves
- Splinting material

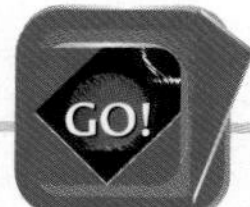

Indications

- To improve pain, decrease blood loss, reduce the risk for fat emboli, and minimize the potential for further neurovascular injury associated with fractures
- To improve pain associated with sprains
- To immobilize tendon lacerations
- To immobilize extremities associated with deep lacerations across joints
- To immobilize painful joints associated with inflammatory disorders (e.g., de Quervain tenosynovitis)

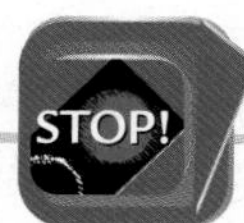

Contraindications

- Fractures that meet indications for emergent orthopedic surgical evaluation
- Open fractures
- Angulated fractures
- Displaced fractures
- Irreducible dislocations
- Neurovascular compromise

The Procedure

Volar Splint

Step 1. Prepare the patient by inspecting the skin for lacerations. Repair any injuries and clean any wounds before splinting. Prepare a stockinette by cutting it to fit the size of the limb being splinted. Allow 3 to 4 inches of extra material above and below the level of each end of the

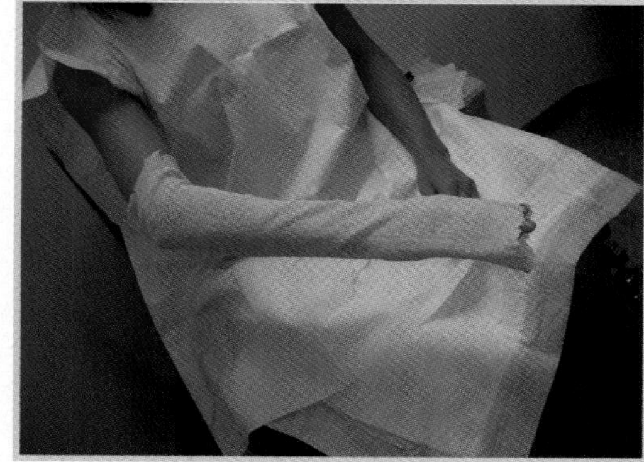

Step 1

splint, which allows the ends of the stockinet to be folded back. Apply the stockinet to limb.

Step 2. Make a small cut over the thumb area of the stockinet to allow the thumb to protrude through the stockinet.

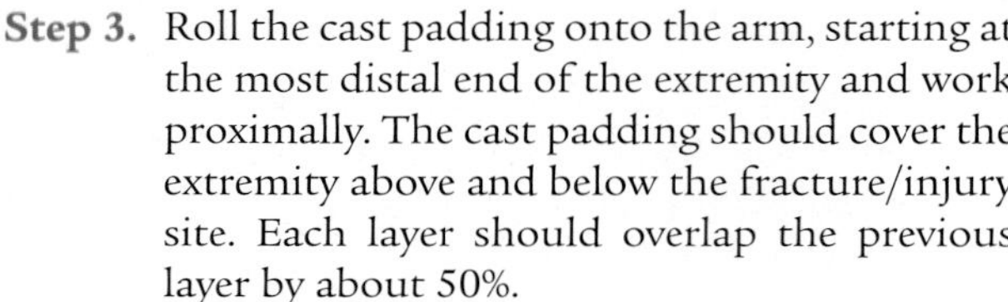

- **PITFALL:** Do not cut the patient's thumb while cutting the stockinet.

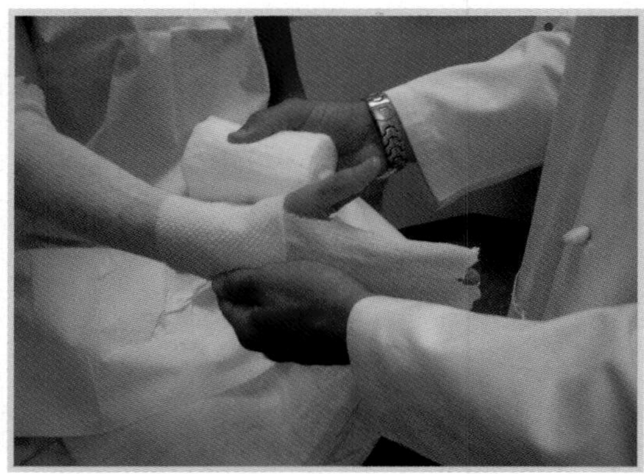

Step 2

Step 3. Roll the cast padding onto the arm, starting at the most distal end of the extremity and work proximally. The cast padding should cover the extremity above and below the fracture/injury site. Each layer should overlap the previous layer by about 50%.

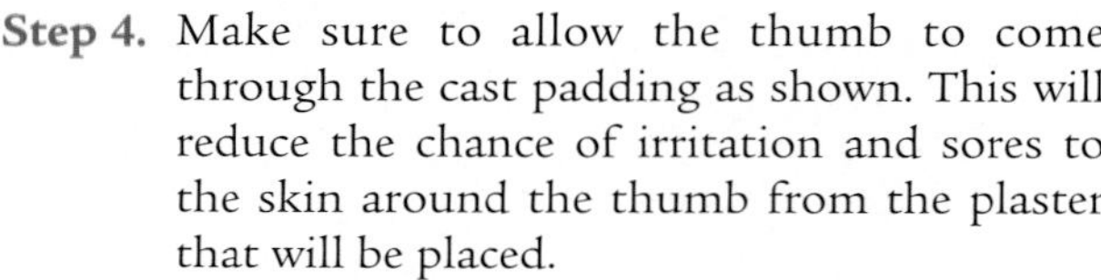

- **PEARL:** Make sure to add extra cast padding at the most distal and proximal ends to avoid irritation to the fingers and elbow.

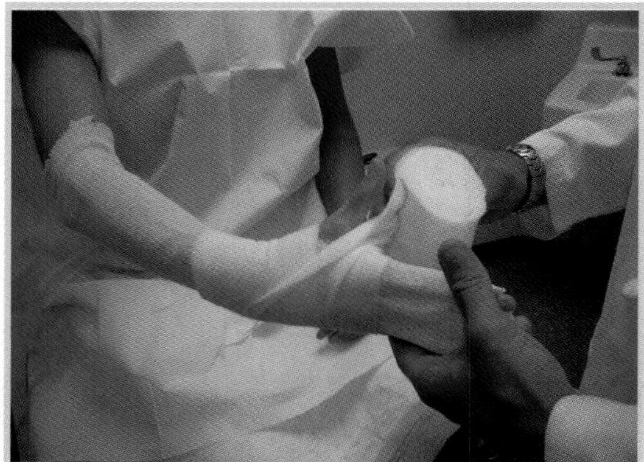

Step 3

Step 4. Make sure to allow the thumb to come through the cast padding as shown. This will reduce the chance of irritation and sores to the skin around the thumb from the plaster that will be placed.

- **PEARL:** Use extra padding at sites of bony prominences and ends of splint to decrease the chance of pressure sores.
- **PEARL:** Cast padding should be rolled with the bulk of the material on top of the sheet adjacent to the skin. The rolling should be effortless.

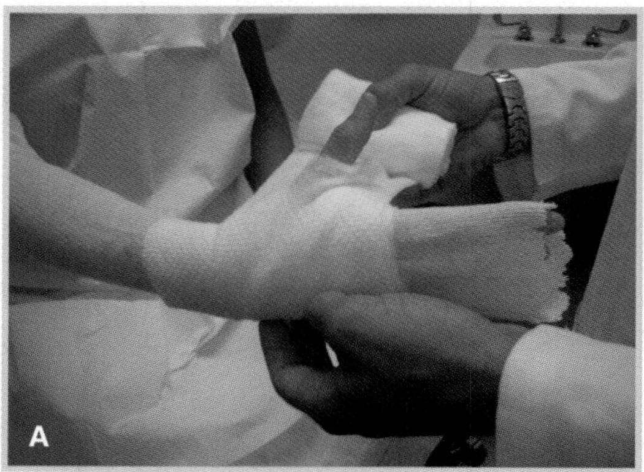

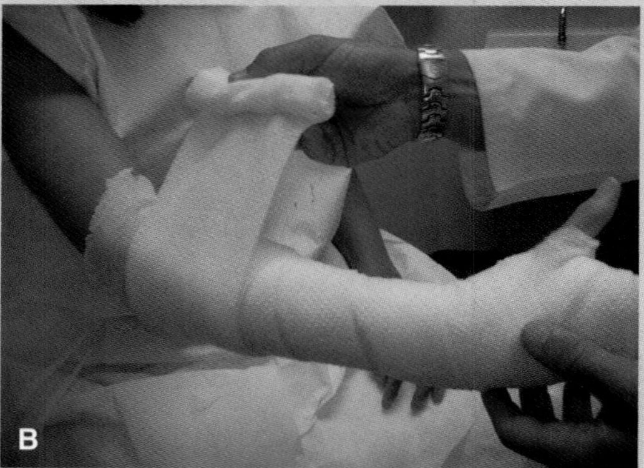

Step 4

Step 5. Prepare 8 to 10 sheets of plaster for most upper extremities splints. Next, estimate the length needed by laying the splint sheets over the injured extremity. You may need to tear a small amount off one end of the splint sheets if the original length is too long.

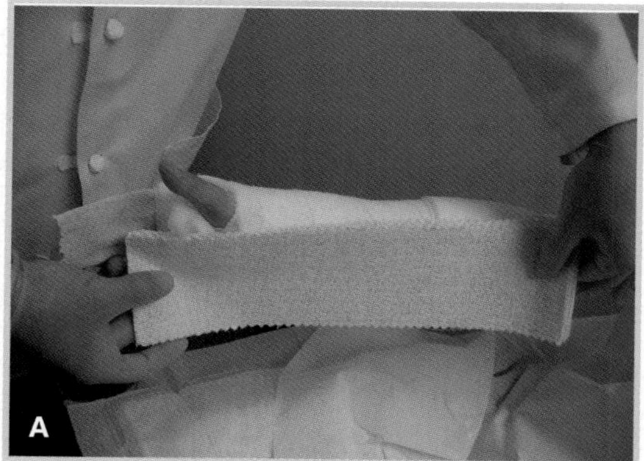

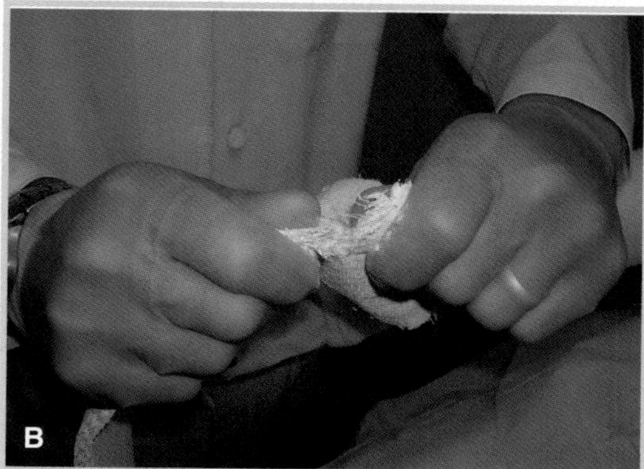

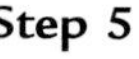

Step 5

Step 6. Tear out an area around the thumb to allow for a better fit.

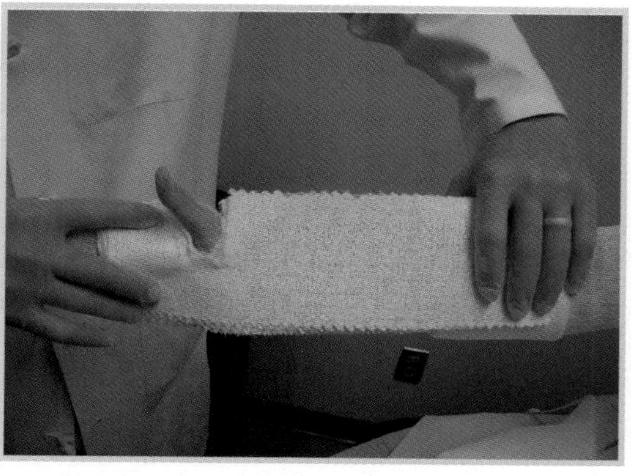

Step 6

Step 7. Alternatively, when using fiberglass material, simply measure the extremity to be splinted. Unroll a length of fiberglass material, and accordion fold the material to the correct length. Then use scissors to cut a notch for the thumb as described previously.

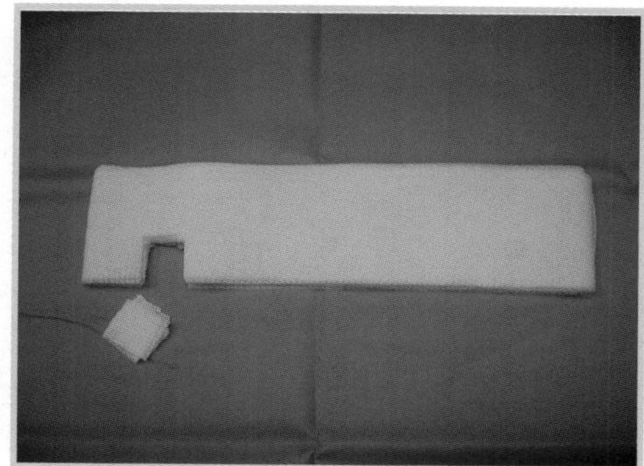

Step 7

Step 8. Immerse the splint material in room-temperature water. Squeeze out all the water and smooth the splint, taking out all the wrinkles. Place the splint on the radial side of the forearm while immobilizing the patient's joints above and below the fracture/injury site. It is applied from volar palmar crease to a point that covers two thirds of the forearm.

- **PITFALL:** Never use hot water, which can cause an excess thermochemical reaction and extremely rapid setting of the cast material. The cast material should never be wrung out.
- **PITFALL:** Always use the palms of your hands to smooth and mold the splint. Excessive use of the fingers can cause indentions in the splint, which can lead to pressure sores.

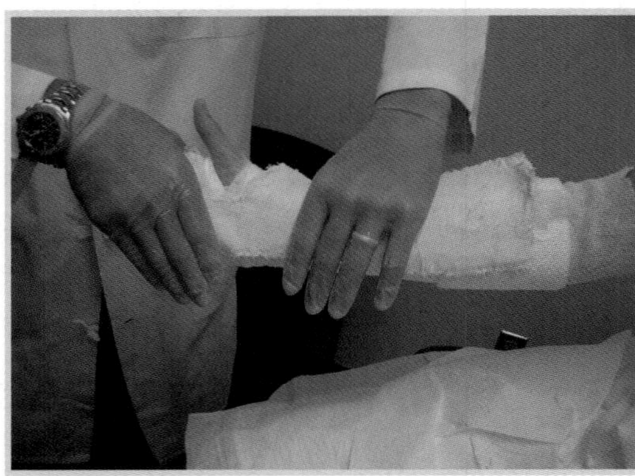

Step 8

Step 9. Roll the ends of the stockinet back over the splint, allowing a thick layer of padding at both ends to avoid irritations and lacerations from the splint material.

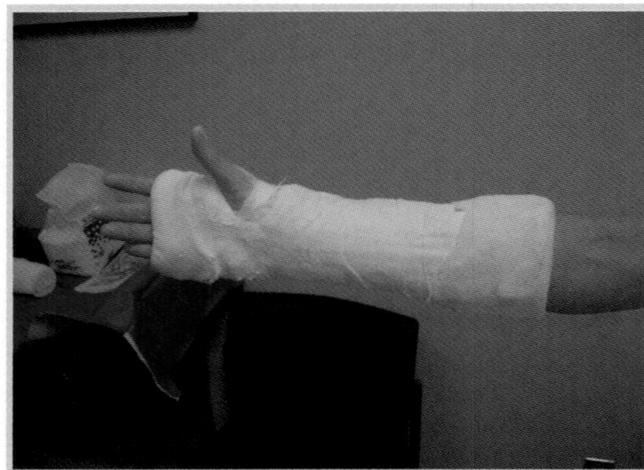

Step 9

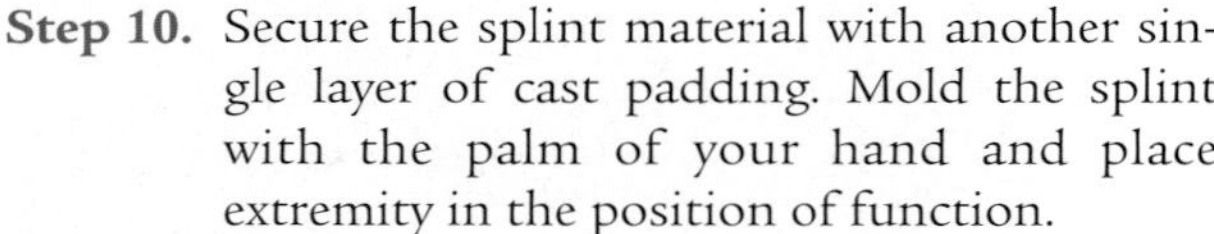

Step 10. Secure the splint material with another single layer of cast padding. Mold the splint with the palm of your hand and place extremity in the position of function.

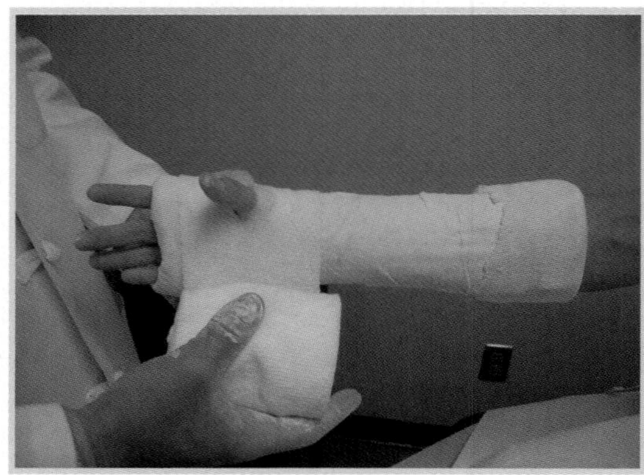

Step 10

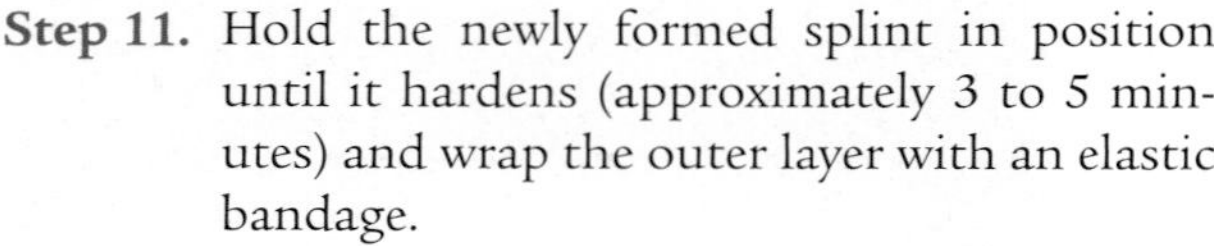

Step 11. Hold the newly formed splint in position until it hardens (approximately 3 to 5 minutes) and wrap the outer layer with an elastic bandage.

- **PITFALL:** Wrapping the elastic bandage too tightly could lead to vascular compromise and will not allow for swelling.
- **PEARL:** Always allow for finger and elbow range of motion.

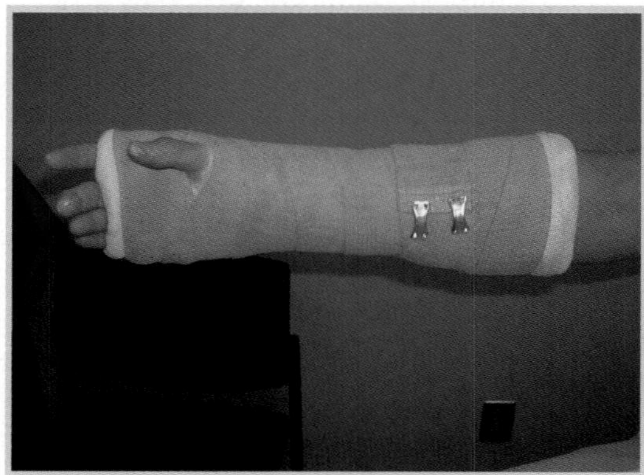

Step 11

Ulnar Gutter Splint

Step 1. Begin by measuring, cutting, and placing the stockinet as discussed for the volar splint. Cut the stockinet between the ring and little finger to allow wrapping of these fingers.

- **PEARL:** It may helpful to cut a slit in the stockinet between the ring and middle finger so that the splint only incorporates the little and ring finger, leaving the other three fingers free for motion.

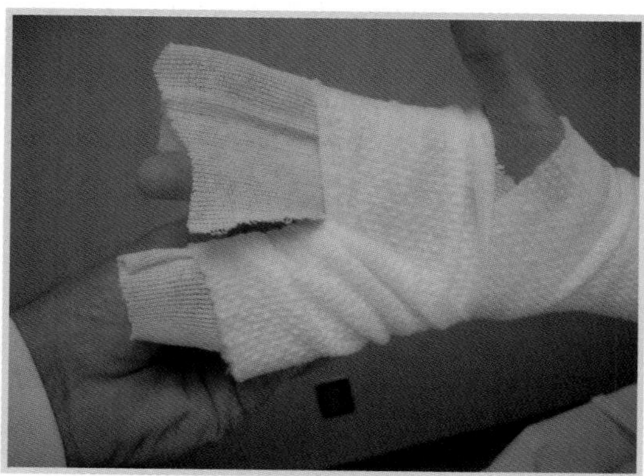

Step 1

Step 2. Next, place the cast padding by wrapping the padding around the ring and little finger, leaving the middle and pointer finger exposed. Work proximally toward the palm of hand, around the thumb, and up two thirds of the proximal forearm.

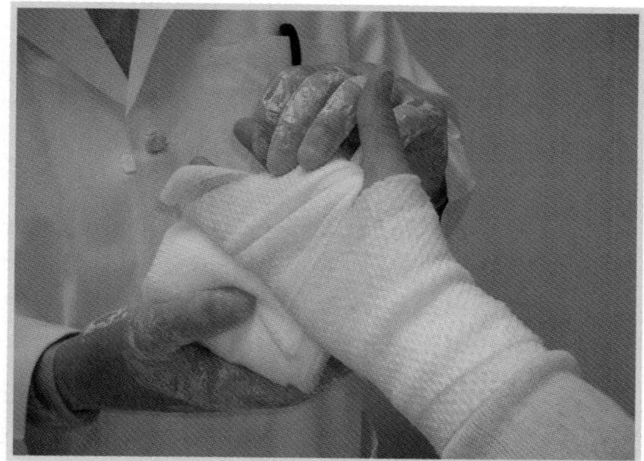

Step 2

Step 3. Measure the approximate length of plaster sheets. These should be long enough to involve the distal interphalangeal (DIP) joint and extend over two thirds of the proximal forearm.

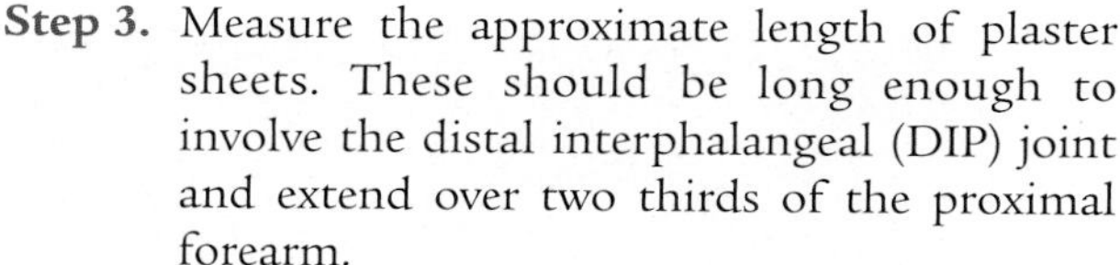

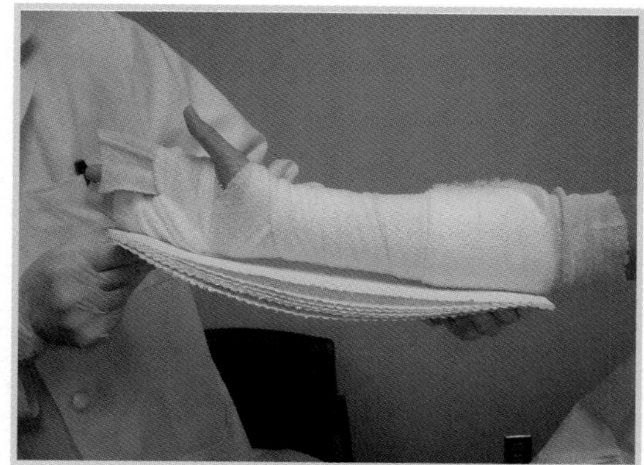

Step 3

Step 4. Tear a slit at one end of the plaster sheets so that it will be easier to form a mold around the ring and little finger, then submerge the plaster sheets in room-temperature water. Squeeze all the water out of the plaster sheets and smooth out all the wrinkles.

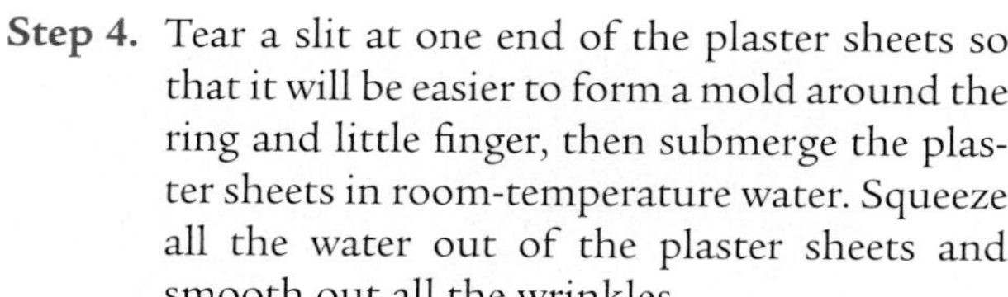

- **PITFALL:** Never use hot water, which can cause an excess thermochemical reaction and extremely rapid setting of the material. The splint material should never be wrung out.
- **PEARL:** Creating a slit in the plaster before wetting will make it easier to form a mold around the ring and little finger.

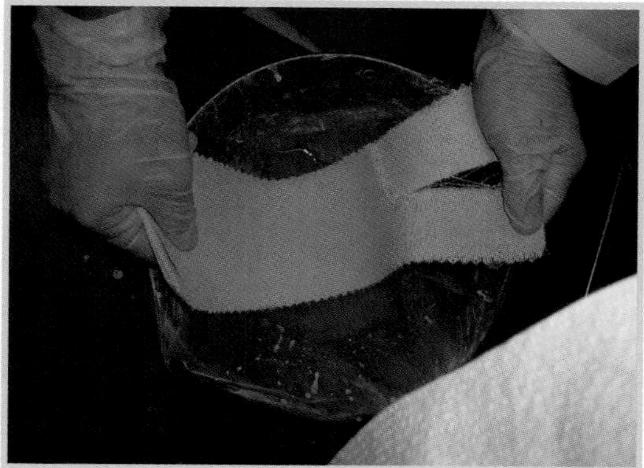

Step 4

Step 5. Alternatively, when using fiberglass material, simply measure the extremity to be splinted. Unroll a length of fiberglass material, and accordion fold the material to the correct length. Then use scissors to cut a slit at one end as described previously.

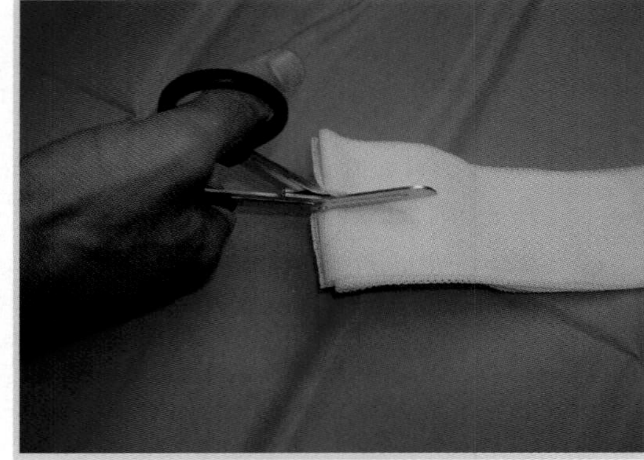

Step 5

Step 6. Mold the plaster sheets on the ulnar side of fingers, wrist, and forearm with the torn end distal. Immobilize the ring and little finger by wrapping the torn end of plaster around them.

- PITFALL: Always use the palms of your hands to smooth and mold the splint. Excessive use of the fingers can cause indentions in the splint, which can lead to pressure sores.

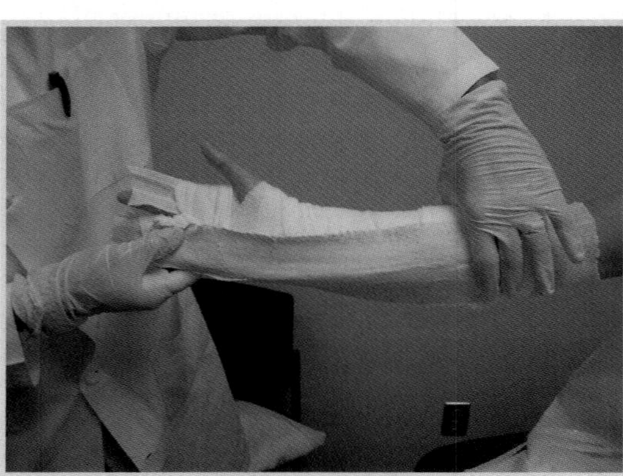

Step 6

Step 7. Secure the splint by wrapping a layer of cast padding around the entire outside of the splint. Wrapping should start at distal end of the extremity and continue proximally to cover the entire splint.

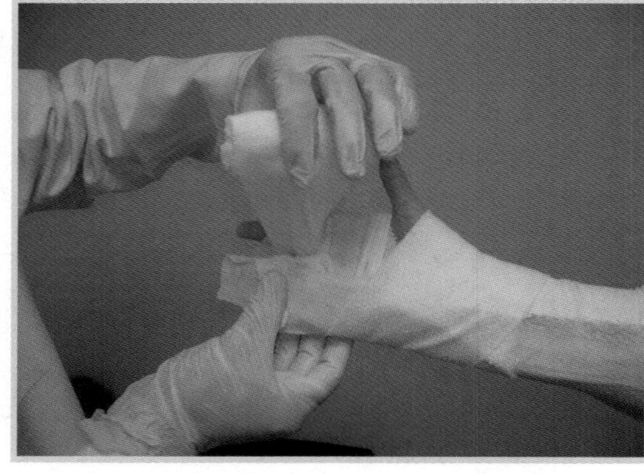

Step 7

Step 8. Roll both the distal and proximal ends of the stockinet back over the splint, allowing a thick layer of padding at both ends, which avoids irritations and lacerations from the splint material.

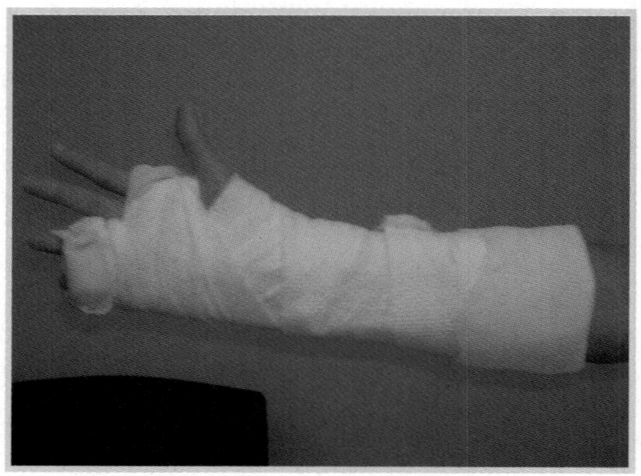

Step 8

Step 9. The splint should be molded with the metacarpophalangeal joint in approximate 70 degrees of flexion, the proximal interphalangeal (PIP) joint in 30 degrees of flexion, and the DIP joint in no more than 10 degrees of flexion. Once the splint hardens, place an elastic bandage over the entire splint.

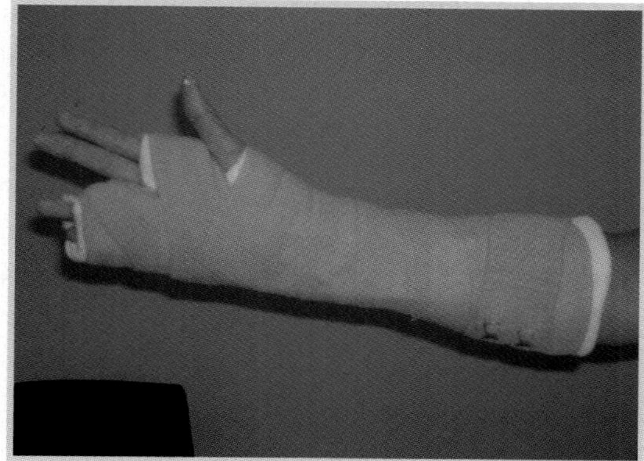

Step 9

Thumb Spica Splint

Step 1. Begin by measuring, cutting, and placing the stockinet as discussed for the volar splint. Place the cast padding as discussed for volar splint, but with this splint, wrap the thumb as well.

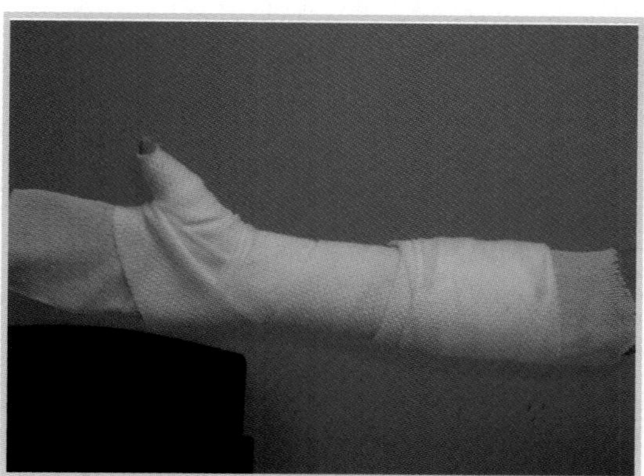

Step 1

Step 2. Measure the length of plaster sheets against the patient's arm and tear or cut to length. The strips should be long enough to involve the entire thumb and extend two thirds down the proximal forearm.

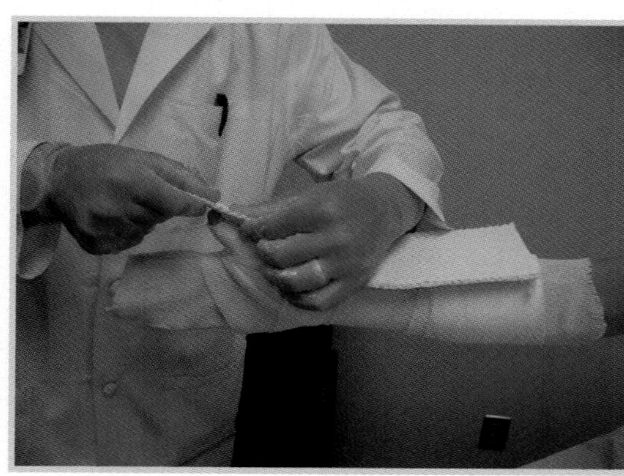

Step 2

Step 3. Make a 1- to 3-inch-long tear in one end of the plaster sheets so that the thumb can be wrapped and immobilized easier. Submerge the plaster in room-temperature water, then squeeze out all the water and smooth out the wrinkles.

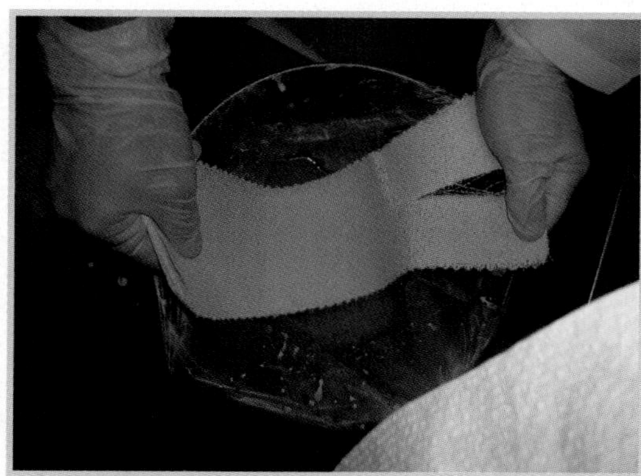

Step 3

Step 4. Alternatively, when using fiberglass material, simply measure the extremity to be splinted. Unroll a length of fiberglass material, and accordion fold the material to the correct length. Then use scissors to cut a slit at one end as described previously.

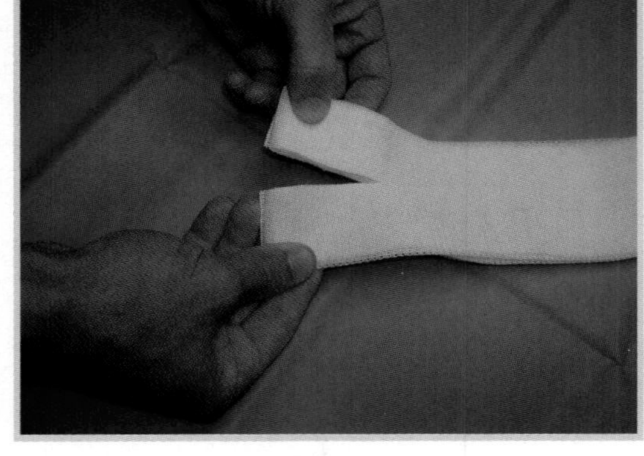

Step 4

Step 5. Mold the splint on the radial side of the extremity to be splinted.

- **PITFALL:** Always use the palms of your hands to smooth and mold the splint. Excessive use of the fingers can cause indentions in the splint, which can lead to pressure sores.

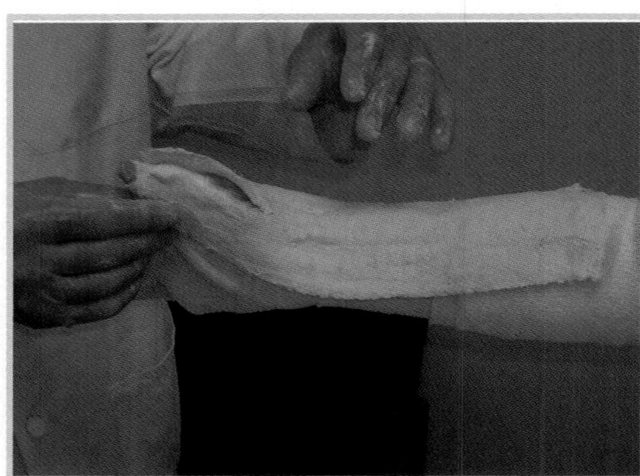

Step 5

Step 6. Form a mold around the thumb, allowing the thumb to remain in neutral or anatomical position.

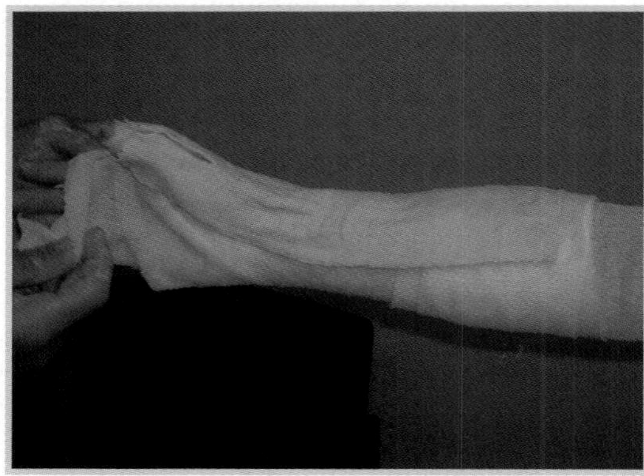

Step 6

Step 7. Wrap outer layer of the splint with cast padding. Start by wrapping the padding around the thumb and work proximally. This will hold the splint in place while you prepare to finish the splint.

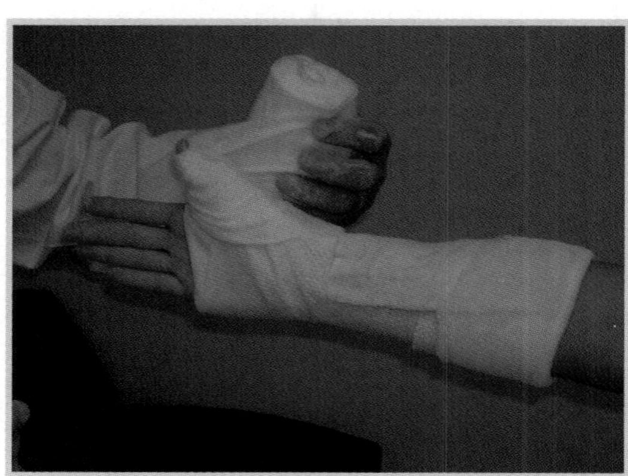

Step 7

Step 8. Roll both the distal and proximal ends of the stockinet back over the splint, allowing a thick layer of padding at both ends to avoid irritations and lacerations from the splint material.

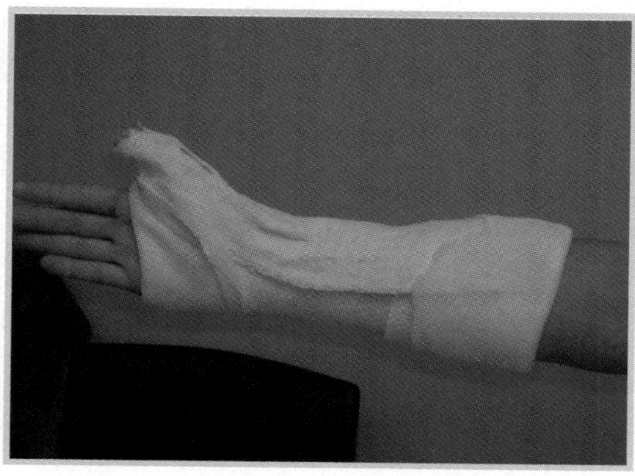

Step 8

Step 9. Once splint hardens, finish by wrapping an elastic bandage over the entire splint.

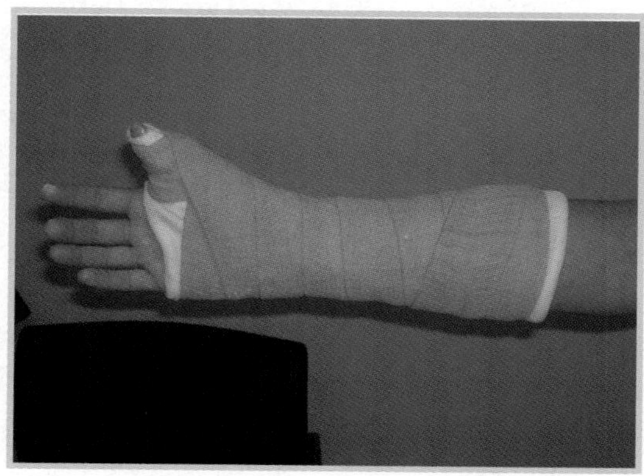

Step 9

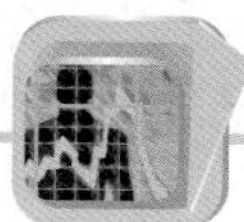

Complications

- Pressure sores result from insufficient padding over bony prominences or indentions in plaster from improper use of fingers to mold the splint or improper support of splint while hardening.
- Compartment syndrome occurs less commonly with splints than casts. Presenting signs of compartment syndrome include pain, pallor, paresthesias, paralysis, and lack of pulse. Avoid this by wrapping cotton padding with minimal pressure, and minimize swelling with ice and elevation. Immediate splint removal and orthopedic consultation is required if compartment syndrome is suspected.
- Infection may occur if the patient places sharp instruments down the splint for scratching (e.g., a coat hanger). It is more common with open wounds present prior to splinting. The provider may prevent this complication by cleaning wounds well before splinting.
- Heat injury may result from plaster-generated heat during crystallizing. Reduce the risk of thermal injury by applying an appropriate amount of cotton padding and using room-temperature water.
- Joint stiffness may occur. Splinting extremities in their position of function will reduce joint stiffness and make it easier to get range of motion back once the splint is removed. Avoid prolonged immobilization if possible.

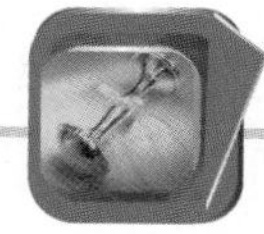

Pediatric Considerations

Children who present with swelling, immobility, pain with movement or palpation, anatomic deformity, discoloration, or crepitus should have radiographic studies.

Immediate orthopedic consultation is needed for severe musculoskeletal injuries such as open fractures, evidence of neurovascular compromise, fractures and dislocations that cannot be easily reduced in the office or emergency department, or fractures that are displaced or too angulated to be splinted.

Patients with sprains need special attention because they may have a Salter-Harris type 1 injury that does not have any radiographic evidence of a fracture. Any patient who has tenderness over the physis (growth plate) should be presumed to have a Salter-Harris type 1 fracture, and appropriate splinting should take place to immobilize the extremity. Be aware of tenderness to palpation at injured site during the follow-up visit in 7 to 10 days. This could represent a nondisplaced Salter-Harris type 1 fracture, and additional follow-up radiographs should be ordered to confirm clinical suspicion. Rapid resolution (2 to 3 days) of tenderness after splinting implies the absence of a Salter-Harris type 1 fracture.

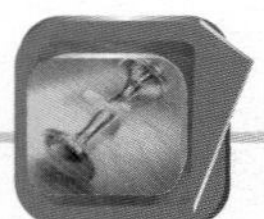

Postprocedure Instructions

Patients should be instructed to elevate and ice the extremity to minimize swelling. Ice can be applied using cold packs such as frozen bags of vegetables or ice bags for 15 to 20 minutes at a time for the first 48 hours. They should also be given instructions to not get the splint wet and not to remove it unless the provider has made it removable. Splints should be placed in a plastic bag while bathing to keep them dry. Make sure the patient understands symptoms of neurovascular compromise. Patients should know to return if the splint gets wet or starts to come apart. They should also be instructed not to stick any objects (especially sharp objects such as hangers) down the splint to scratch. These recommendations should be written as well as given verbally.

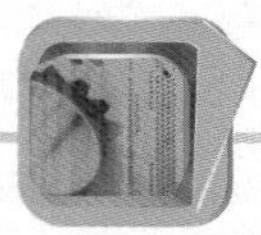

Coding Information and Supply Sources

CPT Code	Description	2008 Average 50th Percentile Fee	Global Period
29125	Short arm splint (forearm to hand)—static	$116.00	0
29130	Finger splint—static	$176.00	0

CPT is a registered trademark of the American Medical Association.
2008 average 50th Percentile Fees are provided courtesy of 2008 MMH-SI's copyrighted Physicians' Fees and Coding Guide.

Suppliers

Plaster of Paris splinting material can be obtained from these suppliers:

- BSN Medical. Web site: http://www.bsnmedical.com

Specialized Medical Supplies Co. Ltd. Web site: http://www.specialized-medical/Plaster-of-Paris-slabs.htm

Fiberglass splinting material can be obtained from this supplier:

- 1) 3M Health Care Professionals. Web site: http://www.3m.Com/product/information/scotchcast-custom-length-splint.html

Patient Education Handout

A patient education handout, "Splints," can be found on the book's companion Web site.

Bibliography

Bowker P, Powell ES. A clinical evaluation of plaster-of-Paris and eight synthetic fracture splinting materials. *Injury*. 1992;23:13–20.

Erick IM. Splinting. In: Yamamoto LG, Inada AS, Okamoto JK, et al., eds. *Case-Based Pediatrics for Medical Students and Residents*. Department of Pediatrics University of Hawaii John A. Burns School of Medicine; 2004. http://www.hawaii.edu/medicine/pediatrics/pedtext/s19c02.html

Marshall PD, Dibble AK, Walters TH, et al. When should a synthetic casting material be used in preference to plaster-of-Paris? a cost analysis and guidance for casting departments. *Injury*. 1992;23:542–544.

Rowley DI, Pratt D, Powell ES, et al. The comparative properties of plaster of Paris and plaster of Paris substitutes. *Arch Orthel Orthop Trauma Surg*. 1985;103:402–407.

Principles of fractures and dislocations. In: Rockwood Jr CA, Green DP, Bucholz RW, eds. *Rockwood and Green Fractures in Adults*. 3rd ed. Philadelphia: Lippincott; 1991:25–27.

Smith G, Hart R, Tsai T. Fiberglass cast application. *Am J Emer Med*. 2005;23:347–350.

Lucas GL. General orthopaedics. In: Green WB, ed. *Essentials of Musculoskeletal Care*, 2nd ed. (IL): American Academy of Orthopaedic Surgeons; 2001:81–82.

2008 MAG Mutual Healthcare Solutions, Inc.'s Physicians' Fee and Coding Guide. Duluth, Georgia. MAG Mutual Healthcare Solutions, Inc. 2007.

CHAPTER 114

Long Arm Splinting

Jeff Harris, MD
Instructor of Family Medicine
Louisiana State University Health Science Center, Shreveport, LA

The five primary uses of splints are to immobilize fractures, dislocations, subluxations, sprains/strains, and painful joints. Splints also may be temporarily used to stabilize soft tissue injuries such as deep lacerations that cross joints. Splinting may be used as a definitive treatment in certain clinical situations such as shoulder and clavicle injuries.

Splints should be placed as soon as possible after the injury occurs. The immobilization of an extremity through splinting decreases pain and prevents further injury such as vascular injury, neurological compromise, and soft tissue injury. Ideally the splint should be left in place until the extremity has been fully and properly evaluated for more aggressive management such as surgery and/or casting or until the fracture has healed. Splints remain the superior treatment in acute injury settings because they allow for swelling, which decreases the possibility of neurovascular compromise.

Figure-of-eight splints are prefabricated splints used for clavicle fractures. These splints are applied to the patient while the patient is standing with hands on the iliac crest. The patient's shoulders should be abducted while the splint is applied. Slings and swathes are used for shoulder and humeral injuries. The sling supports the weight of the shoulder, and the swathe holds the arm against the chest to prevent shoulder rotation. Sugar tong splints are for humeral shaft, forearm, and wrist fractures and can be divided into two categories. First, the proximal sugar tong, which is used for proximal humeral fractures, is applied from the axilla down around the elbow and up the arm to the lateral shoulder. Second, the distal sugar tong is used for wrist and forearm fractures. This splint extends from metacarpophalangeal joints on the dorsum of the hand along forearm, wraps around the back of the elbow to the volar surface, extending down to the midpalmar crease. This creates good immobilization of the wrist, forearm, and elbow. The long arm splint is also used for forearm and elbow injuries. These include those injuries involving the olecranon and radial head. Long arm posterior splints are not recommended for unstable fractures. These splints are applied from the palmar crease, wrapping around the lateral metacarpals, and extending up past the elbow to incorporate two thirds of the posterior arm.

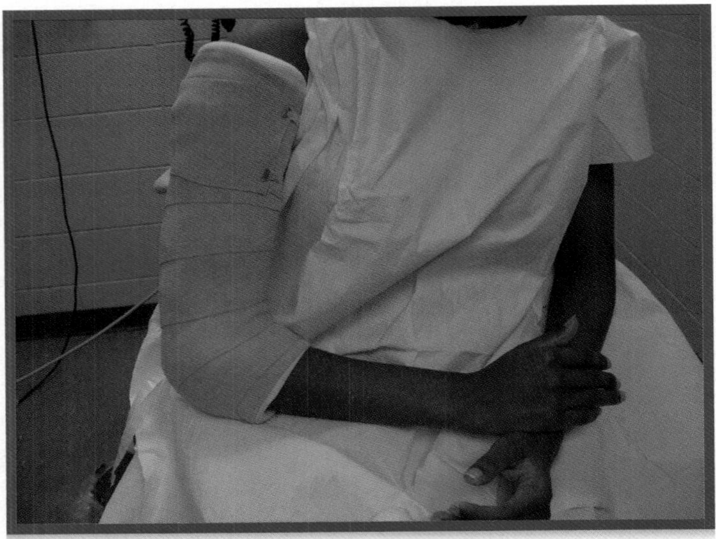

There are several types of splinting material available. Plaster splints consist of various width strips of a crinoline-type material impregnated with plaster of Paris, which crystallizes (hardens) after water is added. They are easier to mold and less expensive than other materials. However, they are more difficult to apply, are messy, are heavy, take longer to set, and are not water resistant (they get soggy when wet). Prefabricated splint rolls include 2-, 3-, 4-, and 6-inch rolls consisting of layers of fiberglass between polypropylene padding. These splints set more quickly, are lighter and stronger, and are water resistant. However, they are more expensive and difficult to mold. Air splints are preformed inflatable splints that are comfortable. They are indicated for ankle sprains but not for fractures or dislocations and are not discussed here.

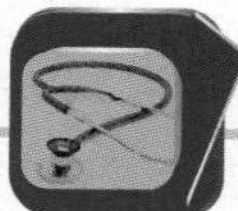

Equipment

- Stockinet
- Cast padding
- Splinting material
- Elastic bandage (e.g., Ace bandage)
- Adhesive tape
- Heavy scissors
- Room-temperature water
- Bucket
- Gloves
- Splinting material
- Prefabricated figure of eight
- Prefabricated sling and swath

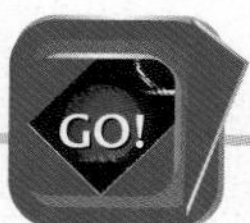

Indications

- To improve pain, decrease blood loss, reduce the risk for fat emboli, and minimize the potential for further neurovascular injury associated with fractures
- To improve pain associated with sprains
- To immobilize tendon lacerations
- To immobilize extremities associated with deep lacerations across joints
- To immobilize painful joints associated with inflammatory disorders

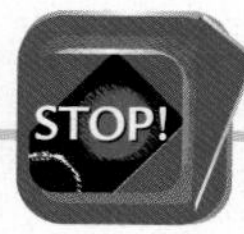

Contraindications

- Fractures that meet indications for emergent orthopedic surgical evaluation
- Open fractures
- Angulated fractures
- Displaced fractures
- Irreducible dislocations
- Neurovascular compromise

The Procedure

Figure of Eight

Step 1. Prepare the patient by having the patient stand with hands on the iliac crest and shoulders in the abduct position. Most figure-of-eight splints are prefabricated, and application is simple. Read the product information insert about the correct application process before applying the splint.

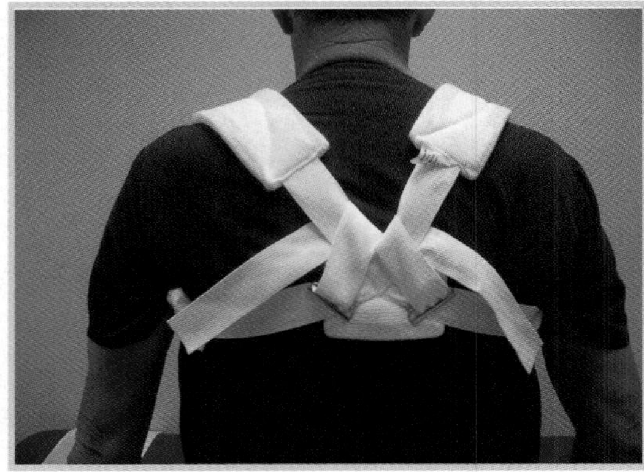

Step 1

Sling and Swath

Step 1. Apply the sling and swath with the patient standing. A prefabricated splint may be used or a splint may be constructed. Place the injured arm in the sling with the elbow at 90 degrees of flexion. Next, place the strap that is attached to the sling over the patient's head so that the weight of the arm is supported.

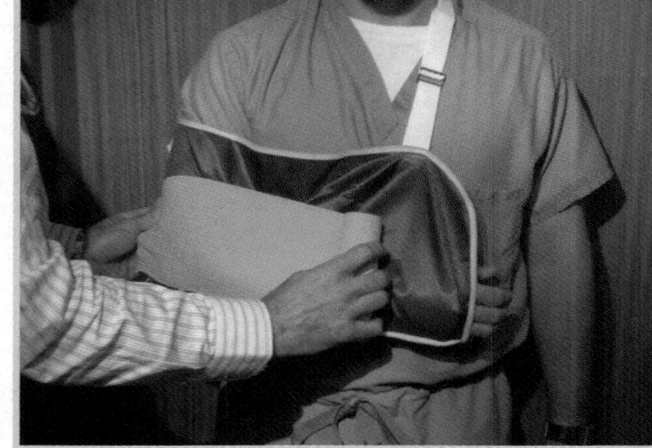

Step 1

Step 2. Apply the swath. This can be anything from an elastic bandage to a prefabricated swath. This is designed to hold the patient's affected arm (in the sling) against the body. The swath should wrap around the front and back of the sling, keeping the affected extremity against the midabdomen.

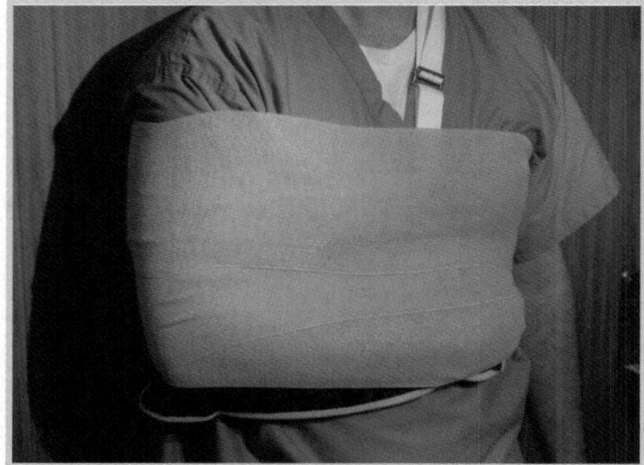

Step 2

Proximal Sugar Tong

Step 1. Prepare the patient by inspecting the skin for lacerations. Repair any injuries and clean any wounds before splinting. Prepare the stockinet by cutting it to fit the size of the arm being splinted. Allow 3 to 4 inches of extra material above and below the level of each end of the splint, which allows the ends of the stockinet to be folded back. Apply the stockinet to the limb.

- **PEARL:** Having the patient seated and arm slightly abducted will make placing the splint an easier task.

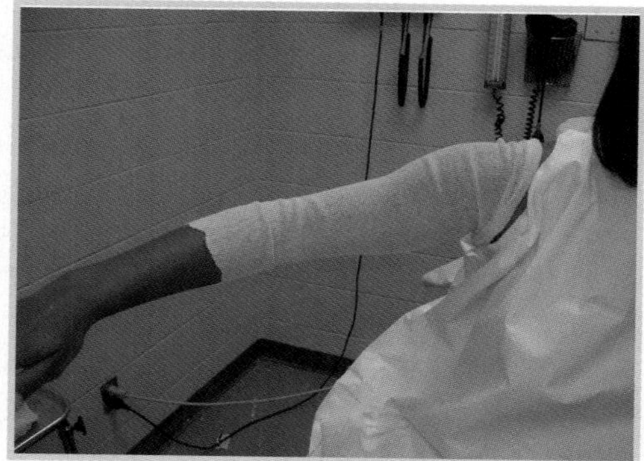

Step 1

Step 2. Roll the cast padding onto the arm, starting at the most distal end of the extremity, and work proximally. The elbow should be placed in 90 degrees of flexion prior to wrapping the cast padding. This will prevent kinks in the cast padding. Each layer should overlap the previous layer by about 50%.

- **PEARL:** Make sure to add extra cast padding at the most distal and proximal ends to avoid irritation to the elbow.
- **PEARL:** Use extra padding at sites of bony prominences and ends of splint to decrease the chance of pressure sores.
- **PEARL:** Cast padding should be rolled with the bulk of the material on top of the sheet adjacent to the skin. The rolling should be effortless.

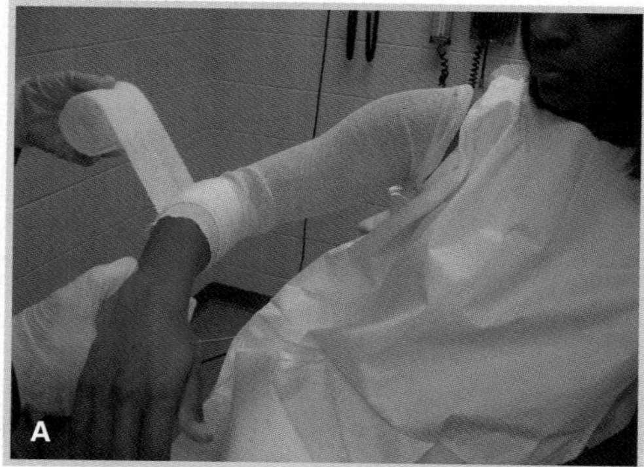

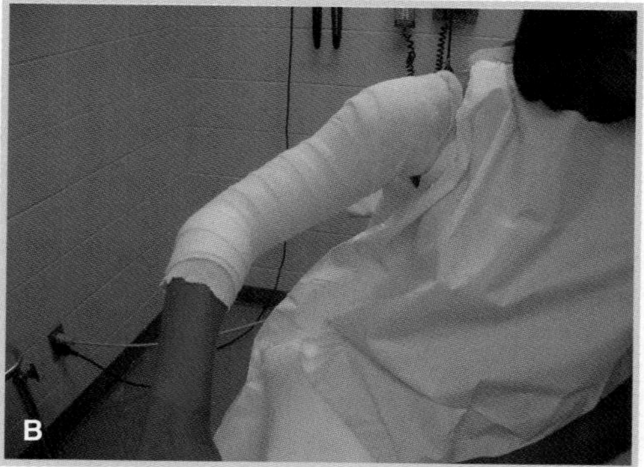

Step 2

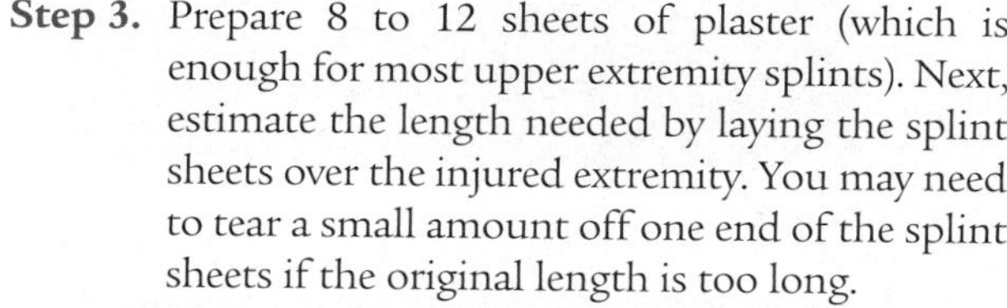

Step 3. Prepare 8 to 12 sheets of plaster (which is enough for most upper extremity splints). Next, estimate the length needed by laying the splint sheets over the injured extremity. You may need to tear a small amount off one end of the splint sheets if the original length is too long.

- **PEARL:** Alternatively, when using fiberglass material, simply measure the extremity to be splinted. Unroll a length of fiberglass material, and accordion fold the material to the correct length. Then use scissors to cut the accordion fold away from the remaining roll.

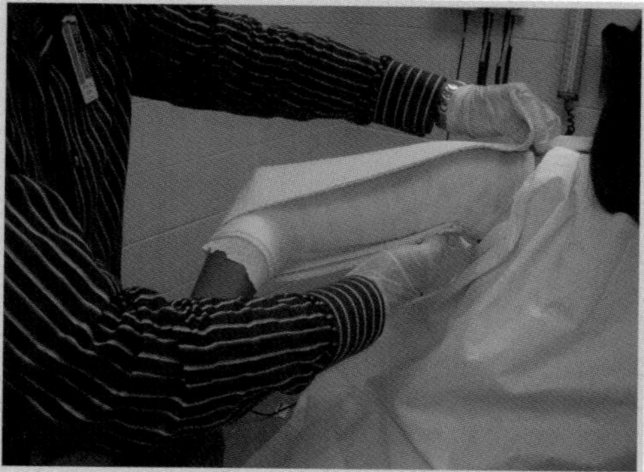

Step 3

Step 4. Immerse the splint material in room-temperature water. Squeeze out all the water, and smooth the splint, taking out all the wrinkles.

- **PITFALL:** Never use hot water, which can cause an excess thermochemical reaction and extremely rapid setting of the cast material. The cast material should never be wrung out.

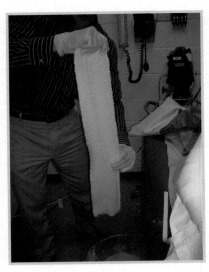

Step 4

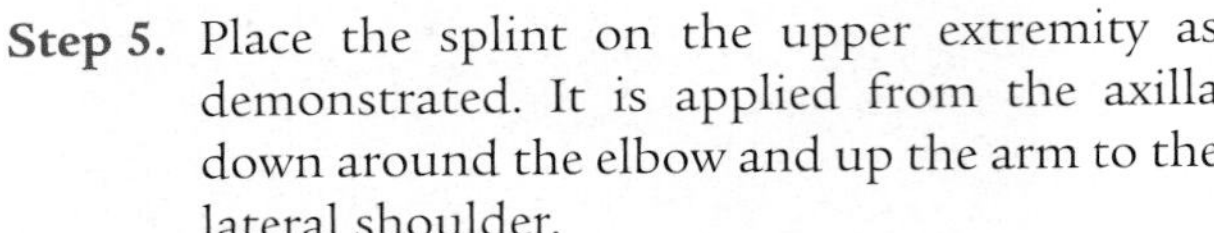

Step 5. Place the splint on the upper extremity as demonstrated. It is applied from the axilla down around the elbow and up the arm to the lateral shoulder.

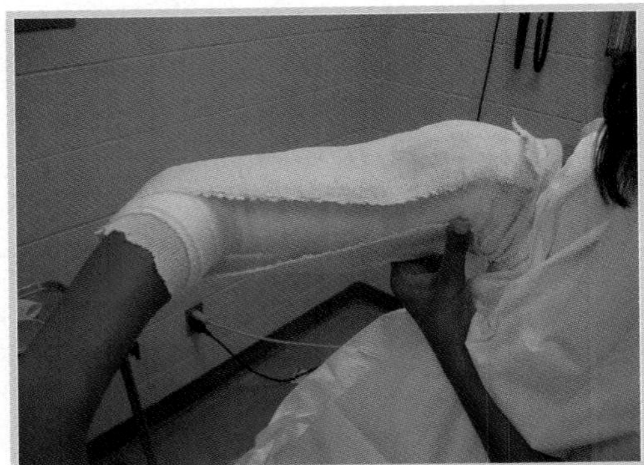

Step 5

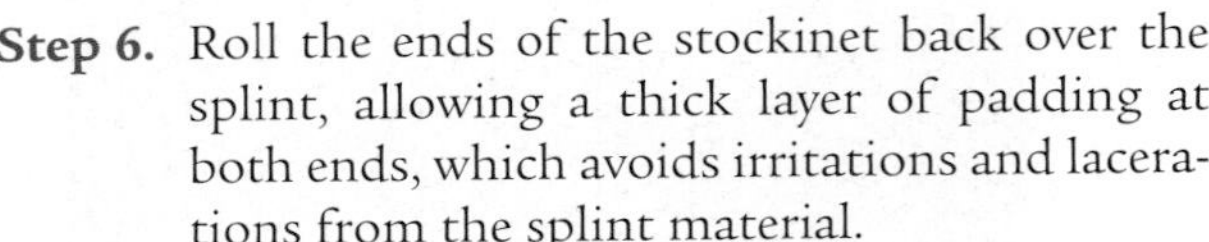

Step 6. Roll the ends of the stockinet back over the splint, allowing a thick layer of padding at both ends, which avoids irritations and lacerations from the splint material.

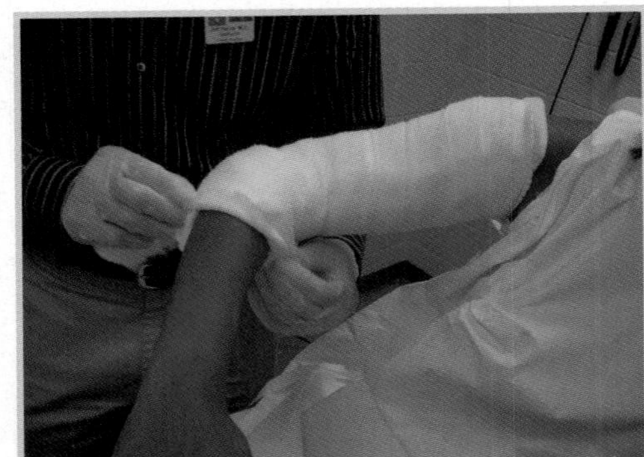

Step 6

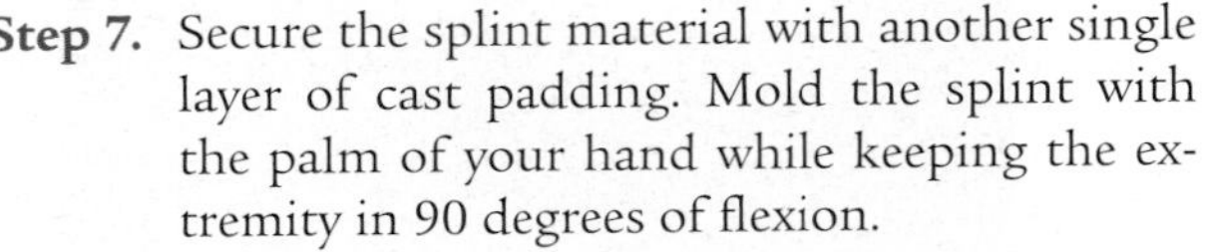

Step 7. Secure the splint material with another single layer of cast padding. Mold the splint with the palm of your hand while keeping the extremity in 90 degrees of flexion.

- **PITFALL:** Always use the palms of your hands to smooth and mold the splint. Excessive use of the fingers can cause indentions in the splint, which can lead to pressure sores.

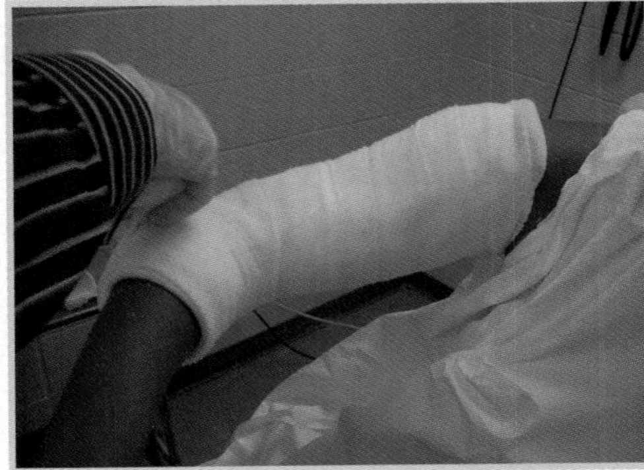

Step 7

Step 8. Hold the newly formed splint in 90 degrees of flexion until it hardens (approximately 3 to 5 minutes) and wrap the outer layer with an elastic bandage.

- **PITFALL:** Wrapping the elastic bandage too tightly could lead to vascular compromise and not allow for swelling.

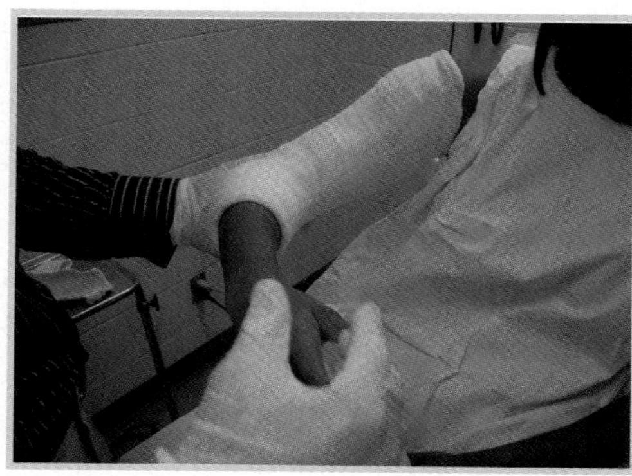

Step 8

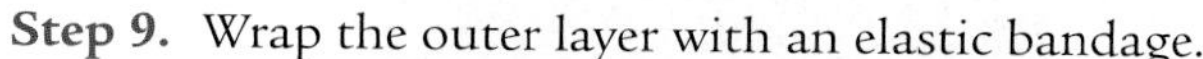

Step 9. Wrap the outer layer with an elastic bandage.

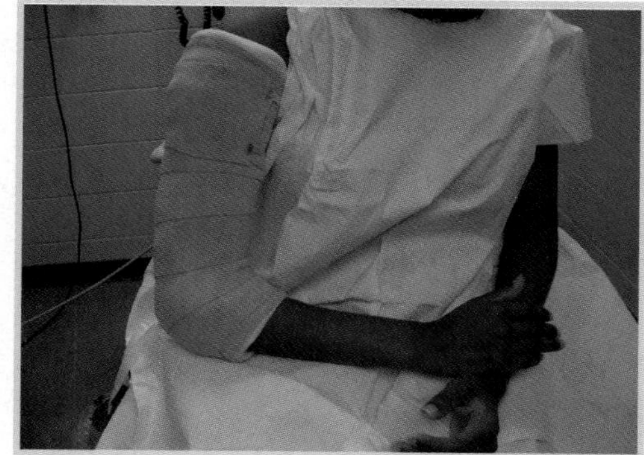

Step 9

Long Arm Posterior Arm Splint

Step 1. Begin by measuring, cutting, and placing the stockinet as discussed for the short arm splint, except that this stockinet should be measured to incorporate the entire arm up to the shoulder.

- **PEARL:** Having the patient lie in the prone position on the examination table will make placing the splint an easier task.

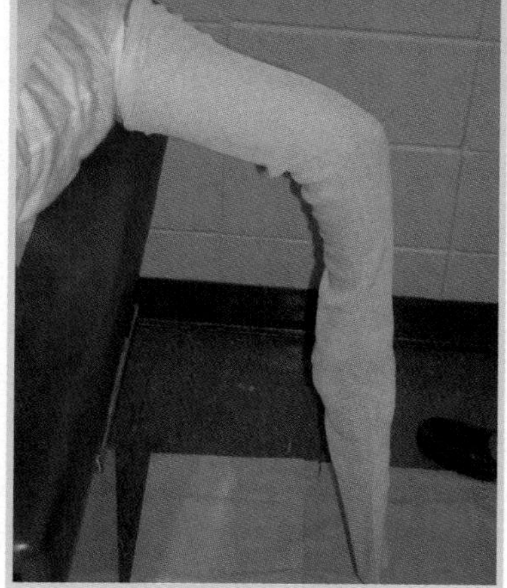

Step 1

Step 2. Make a small cut over the thumb area of the stockinet to allow the thumb to protrude through the stockinet.

- **PITFALL:** Do not cut the patient's thumb while cutting the stockinet.

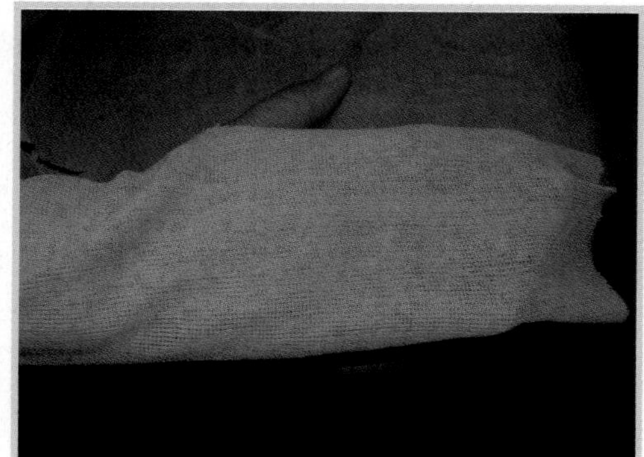

Step 2

Step 3. Roll the cast padding onto the arm, starting at the most distal end of the extremity, and work proximally. The cast padding should cover the extremity above and below the fracture/injury site. Each layer should overlap the previous layer by about 50%.

- **PEARL:** Make sure to add extra cast padding at the most distal and proximal ends as well as around the thumb to avoid irritation to the fingers and axillae.
- **PEARL:** Extra cast padding should be applied to the elbow to prevent irritation.
- **PITFALL:** Failing to place the elbow in 90 degrees of flexion will make it more difficult for your patient to regain range of motion once the splint is removed.

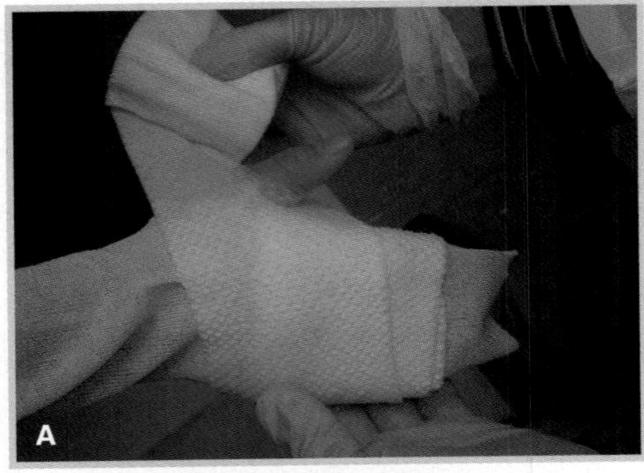

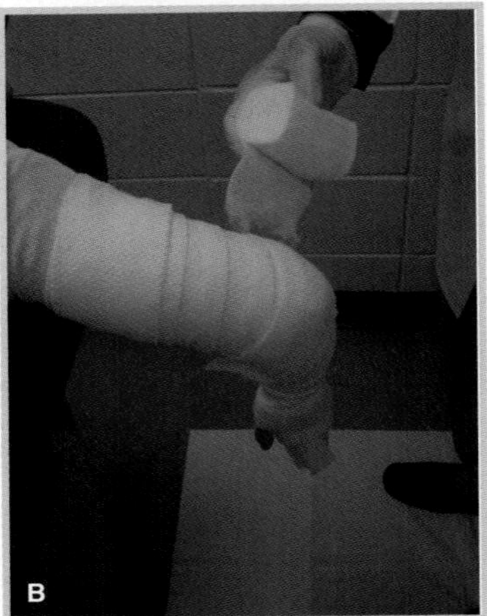

Step 3

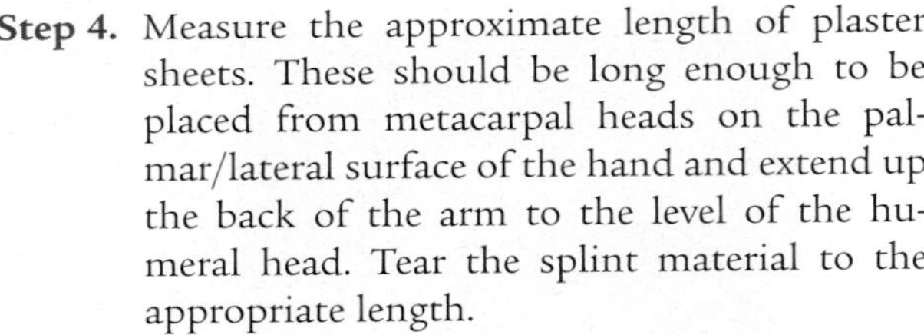

Step 4. Measure the approximate length of plaster sheets. These should be long enough to be placed from metacarpal heads on the palmar/lateral surface of the hand and extend up the back of the arm to the level of the humeral head. Tear the splint material to the appropriate length.

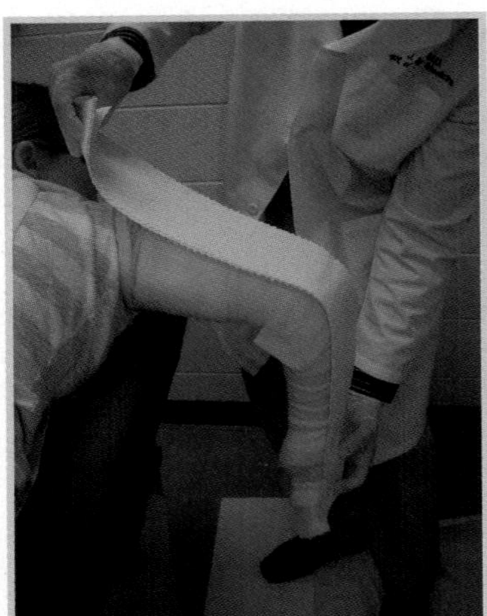

Step 4

Step 5. Submerge the plaster sheets in room-temperature water. Squeeze all the water out of the plaster sheets and smooth out all the wrinkles.

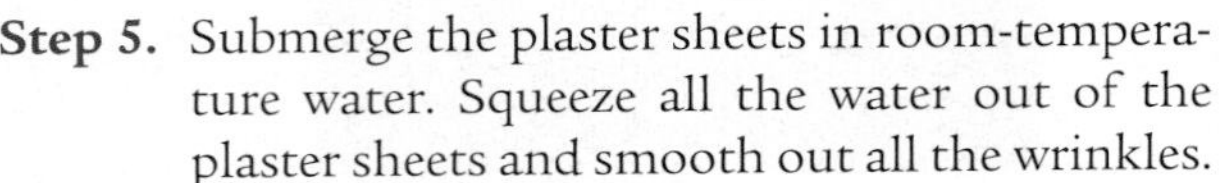

- **PITFALL:** Never use hot water, which can cause an excess thermochemical reaction and extremely rapid setting of the material. The splint material should never be wrung out.
- **PEARL:** Alternatively, when using fiberglass material, simply measure the extremity to be splinted. Unroll a length of fiberglass material, and accordion fold the material to the correct length. Then use scissors to cut the accordion fold away from the remaining roll.

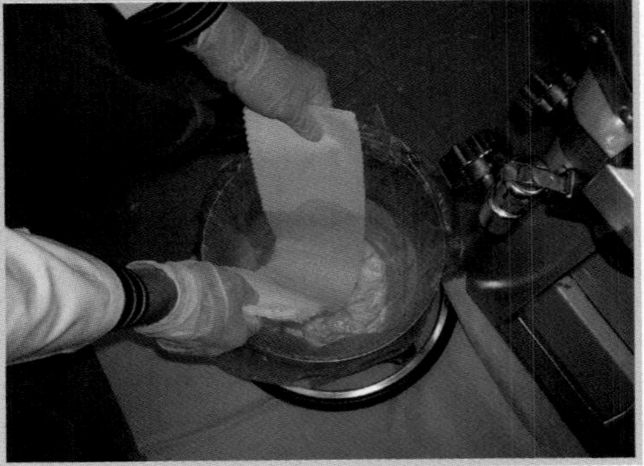

Step 5

Step 6. Mold the plaster sheets from the lateral palm, forearm, around the posterior elbow, and up to the level of the humeral head.

- **PITFALL:** Always use the palms of your hands to smooth and mold the splint. Excessive use of the fingers can cause indentions in the splint, which can lead to pressure sores.

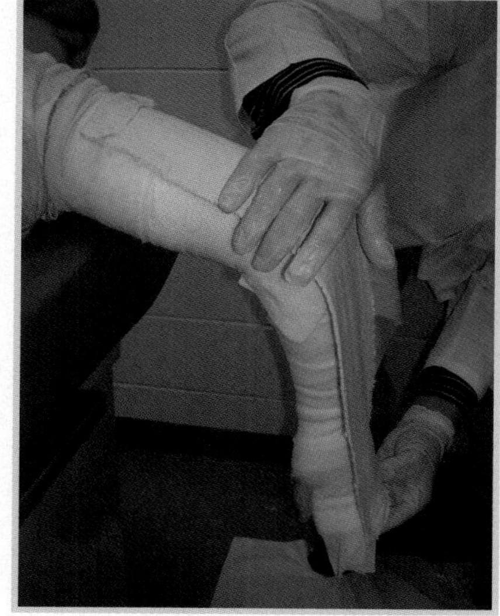

Step 6

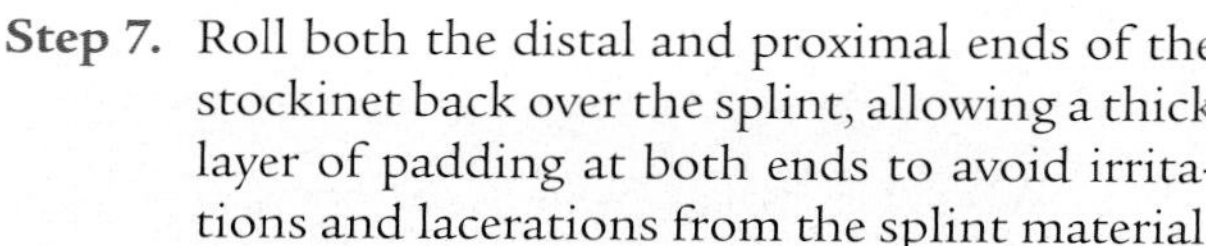

Step 7. Roll both the distal and proximal ends of the stockinet back over the splint, allowing a thick layer of padding at both ends to avoid irritations and lacerations from the splint material.

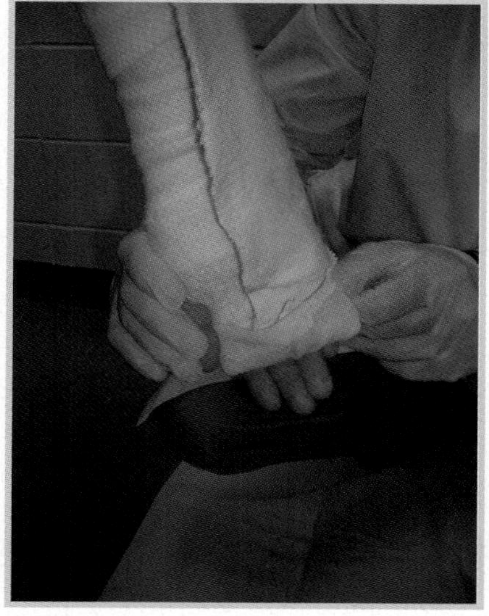

Step 7

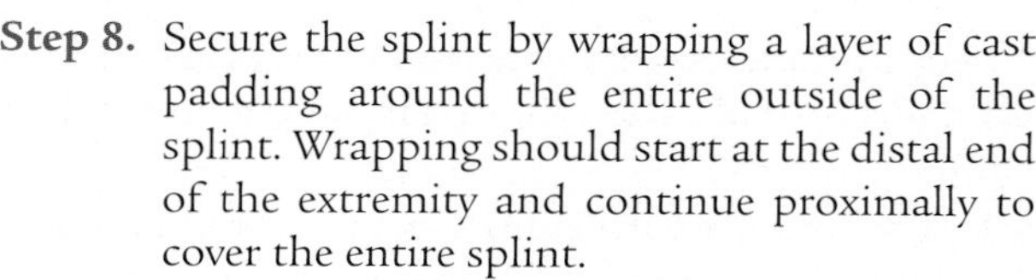

Step 8. Secure the splint by wrapping a layer of cast padding around the entire outside of the splint. Wrapping should start at the distal end of the extremity and continue proximally to cover the entire splint.

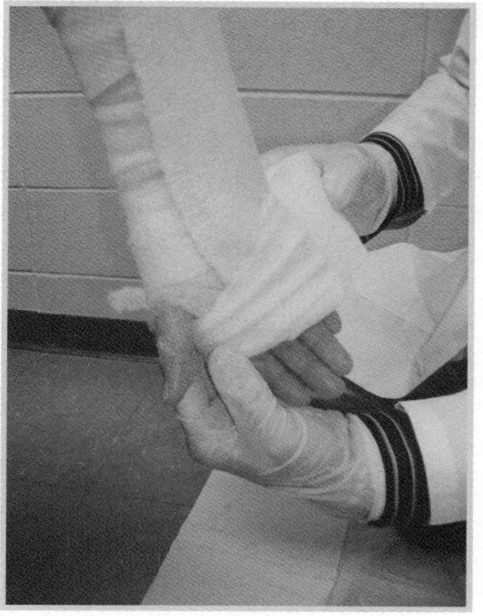

Step 8

Step 9. The splint should be molded with the elbow in approximate 90 degrees of flexion.

- **PEARL:** For unstable ankle fractures, this splint should be used in combination with a stirrup splint.

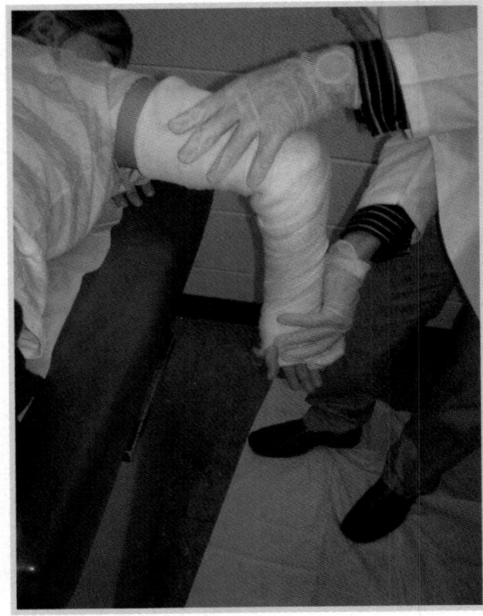

Step 9

Step 10. Once the splint hardens, place an elastic bandage over the entire splint.

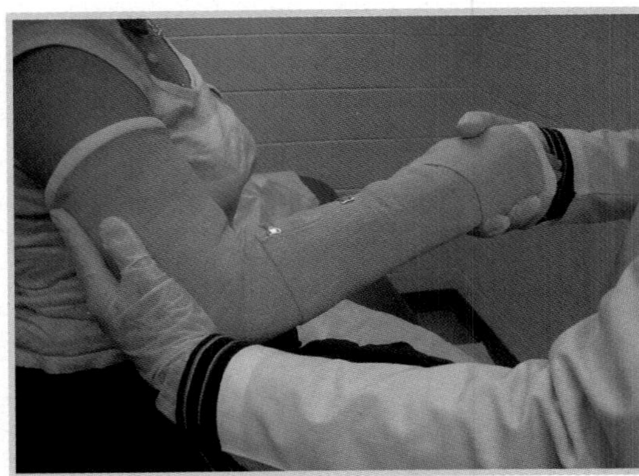

Step 10

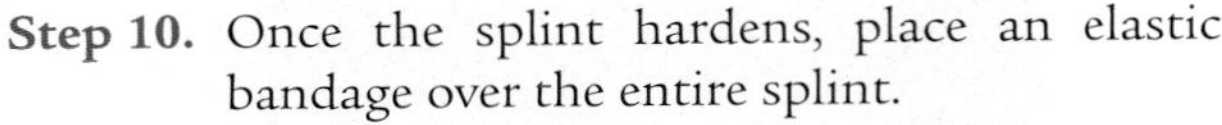

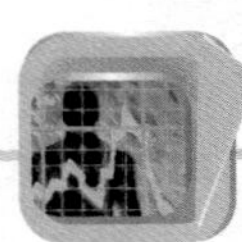

Complications

- Pressure sores result from insufficient padding over bony prominences or indentions in plaster from improper use of fingers to mold the splint or improper support of splint while hardening.
- Compartment syndrome occurs less commonly with splints than casts. Presenting signs of compartment syndrome include pain, pallor, paresthesias, paralysis, and pulselessness. Avoid this by wrapping cotton padding with minimal pressure, and minimize swelling with ice and elevation. Immediate splint removal and orthopedic consultation is required if compartment syndrome is suspected.
- Infection may occur if the patient places sharp instruments down the splint for scratching (e.g., a coat hanger). It is more common with open wounds present prior to splinting. The provider may prevent this complication by cleaning wounds well before splinting.
- Heat injury may result from plaster-generated heat during crystallizing. Reduce the risk of thermal injury by applying an appropriate amount of cotton padding and using room-temperature water.
- Joint stiffness may occur. Splinting the extremity in the position of function will reduce joint stiffness and make it easier to get range of motion back once the splint is removed. Avoid prolonged immobilization if possible.

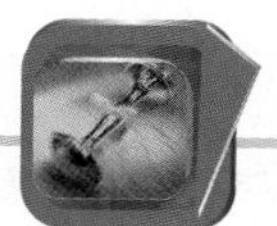

Pediatric Considerations

Children who present with swelling, immobility, pain with movement or palpation, anatomic deformity, discoloration, or crepitus should have radiographic studies. Immediate orthopedic consultation is needed for severe musculoskeletal injuries such as open fractures, evidence of neurovascular compromise, fractures and dislocations that cannot be easily reduced in the office or emergency department, or fractures that are displaced or too angulated to be splinted.

Patients with sprains need special attention because they may have a Salter-Harris type 1 injury that does not have any radiographic evidence of a fracture. Any patient who has tenderness over the physis (growth plate) should be presumed to have a Salter-Harris type 1 fracture, and appropriate splinting should take place to immobilize the extremity. Be aware of tenderness to palpation at the injured site during the follow-up visit in 7 to 10 days. This could represent a nondisplaced Salter-Harris type 1 fracture, and additional follow-up radiographs should be ordered to confirm clinical suspicion. Rapid resolution (2 to 3 days) of tenderness after splinting implies the absence of a Salter-Harris type 1 fracture.

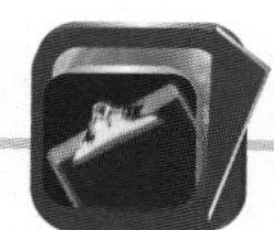

Postprocedure Instructions

Patients should be instructed to elevate and ice the extremity to minimize swelling. Ice can be applied using cold packs such as frozen bags of vegetables or ice bags for 15 to 20 minutes at a time for the first 48 hours. They should also be given instructions to not get the splint wet and not to remove it unless the provider has made it removable. Splints should be placed in a plastic bag while bathing to keep dry. Make sure the patients understand symptoms of neurovascular compromise. Patients should know to return if splint gets wet or starts to come apart. They should also be instructed not to stick any objects (especially sharp objects such as hangers) down the splint to scratch. These recommendations should be given in writing as well as verbally.

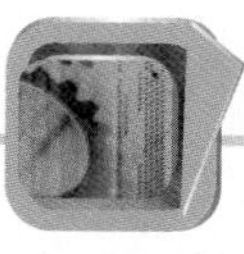

Coding Information and Supply Sources

CPT Code	Description	2008 Average 50th Percentile Fee	Global Period
29049	Long arm splint (shoulder to hand)	$163.00	0

Suppliers

Plaster of Paris splinting material can be obtained from these suppliers:

- BSN Medical. Web site: http://www.bsnmedical.com
- Specialized Medical Supplies Co. Ltd. Web site: http://www.specialized-medical/Plaster-of-Paris-slabs.htm

Fiberglass splinting material can be obtained from this supplier:

- 3M Health Care Professionals. Web site: http://www.3m.Com/product/information/scotchcast-custom-length-splint.html

Bibliography

Bowker P, Powell ES. A clinical evaluation of plaster-of-Paris and eight synthetic fracture splinting materials. *Injury*. 1992;23:13–20.

Erick IM. Splinting. In: Yamamoto LG, Inada AS, Okamoto JK, et al., eds. *Case-Based Pediatrics for Medical Students and Residents*. Department of Pediatrics University of Hawaii John A. Burns School of Medicine; 2004. http://www.hawaii.edu/medicine/pediatrics/pedtext/s19c02.html

Marshall PD, Dibble AK, Walters TH, et al. When should a synthetic casting material be used in preference to plaster-of-Paris? a cost analysis and guidance for casting departments. *Injury*. 1992;23:542–544.

Rowley DI, Pratt D, Powell ES, et al. The comparative properties of plaster of Paris and plaster of Paris substitutes. *Arch Orthel Orthop Trauma Surg*. 1985;103:402–407.

Principles of fractures and dislocations. In: Rockwood Jr CA, Green DP, Bucholz RW, eds. *Rockwood and Green Fractures in Adults,* 3rd ed. Philadelphia: Lippincott; 1991:25–27.

Smith G, Hart R, Tsai T. Fiberglass cast application. *Am J Emer Med*. 2005;23:347–350.

Lucas GL. General orthopaedics. In: Green WB, ed. *Essentials of Musculoskeletal Care*, 2nd ed. (IL): American Academy of Orthopaedic Surgeons; 2001:81–82.

2008 MAG Mutual Healthcare Solutions, Inc.'s Physicians' Fee and Coding Guide. Duluth, Georgia. MAG Mutual Healthcare Solutions, Inc. 2007.

CHAPTER 115

Trigger Finger Injection

E.J. Mayeaux, Jr., MD, DABFP, FAAFP

Professor of Family Medicine, Professor of Obstetrics and Gynecology
Louisiana State University Health Sciences Center, Shreveport, LA

Flexor tendon entrapment of the digits is a common condition encountered in primary care practice. This painful condition is known as a trigger finger, and it can produce locking of the finger in the position of flexion. Locking is released by forced extension of the digit, with or without applying pressure to the tendon at the metacarpal or metatarsal head. Release may be associated with a click that can be felt and occasionally heard. Although the fourth finger is most commonly involved, multiple fingers and the thumb also are commonly reported as trigger fingers. Tenderness is common but not always present. Most diagnoses are made from the classic physical findings.

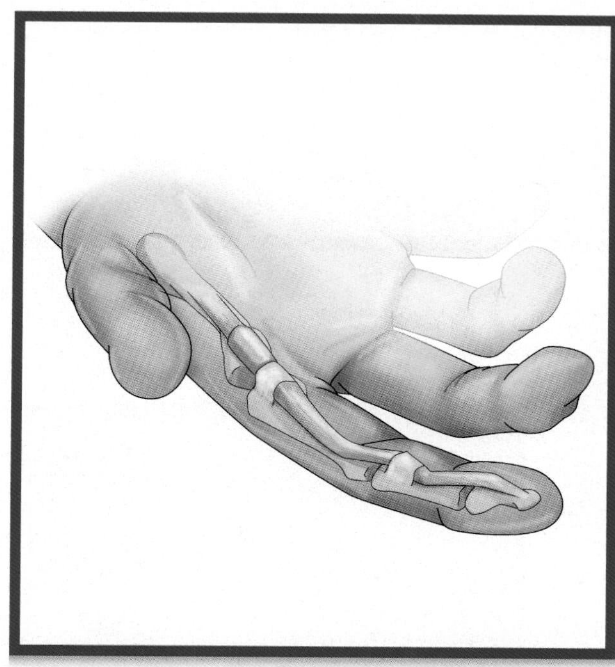

The problem with a trigger digit is mechanical. A nodular expansion of the tendon can develop, moving with finger motion and catching within the annular A1 pulley over the metacarpophalangeal joint. Alternately, the pulley can become too tight, constricting a normal-sized tendon. Trigger fingers occur in children, usually on the thumb, and probably represent a congenital discrepancy between the size of the tendon and that of the tendon sheath.

Trigger fingers were historically referred to as stenosing tenosynovitis, but histologic studies fail to document inflammation. Primary disease occurs more often in middle-aged women and is believed to develop from degenerative changes in the flexor tendons and A1 pulleys. Secondary trigger fingers develop from conditions that affect the connective tissues, such as rheumatoid arthritis, diabetes mellitus, and gout.

Currently, in an uncomplicated case of trigger digit the first-line therapy is still generally agreed to be tendon sheath injection with surgical release of the A1 pulley as second-line treatment. Corticosteroid injection (0.5 mL of triamcinolone [10 mg/mL] mixed with 0.5 to 1.5 mL of 1% lidocaine) can be highly successful, especially early in the course of the disorder. Injection is into the tendon sheath, not into the tendon itself. Steroid therapy may relieve discomfort and produces a cure in up to 85% of individuals with the disorder. If two or three injections fail to result in complete resolution, consultation with a hand surgeon should be sought.

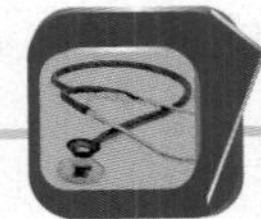

Equipment

- Syringes (1 or 3 mL), needles (25 or 27 gauge, 5/8 inch), and alcohol swabs are available from local surgical supply houses or pharmacies.
- Steroid solutions are available from manufacturers or local pharmacies. Celestone Soluspan (beta-methasone sodium) is produced by Schering-Plough (Kenilworth, NJ, www.schering-plough.com); Aristocort (triamcinolone diacetate) and Aristospan (triamcinolone hexacetonide) can be obtained from Baxter-Lederle (Deerfield, IL, www.baxter.com); and Depo-Medrol (methylprednisolone acetate) is available from Pharmacia Upjohn (Basking Ridge, NJ, www.pharmacia.com).
- A suggested tray for performing soft-tissue aspirations and injections is listed in Appendix I.
- Skin preparation recommendations appear in Appendix E.

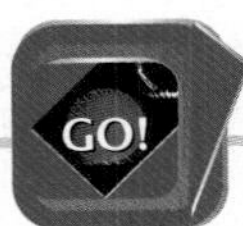

Indications

- Locking of flexor tendon of finger or thumb (i.e., flexor tendon entrapment syndrome)

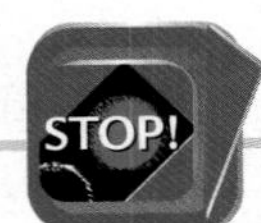

Contraindications (Relative)

- Failure to respond to multiple injections
- Uncooperative patient
- Bleeding diathesis
- Bacteremia or cellulitis of the palm or thumb
- Congenital trigger thumb in infants

The Procedure

Step 1. The fourth finger is commonly involved. The condition causes locking of the flexor tendon in a position of flexion.

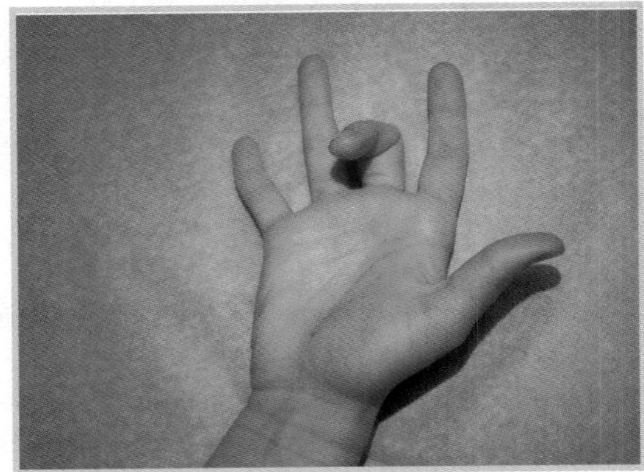

Step 1

Step 2. Place the supine hand flat on a firm surface. The correct insertion site generally is in the palm where the tendon crosses the distal palmar crease.

- **PITFALL:** Novice physicians frequently inject at the base of the digit (i.e., crease where the digit meets the palm). This is well above the metacarpophalangeal joint and above the A1 pulley. The joint can be palpated through the palm; it is at least 1 cm proximal to the crease at the base of the finger.

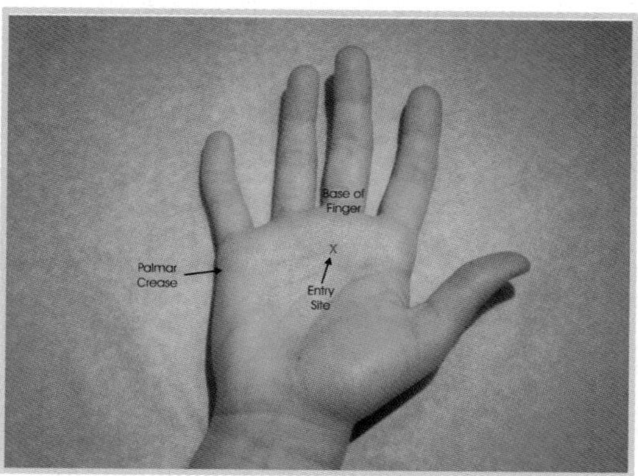

Step 2

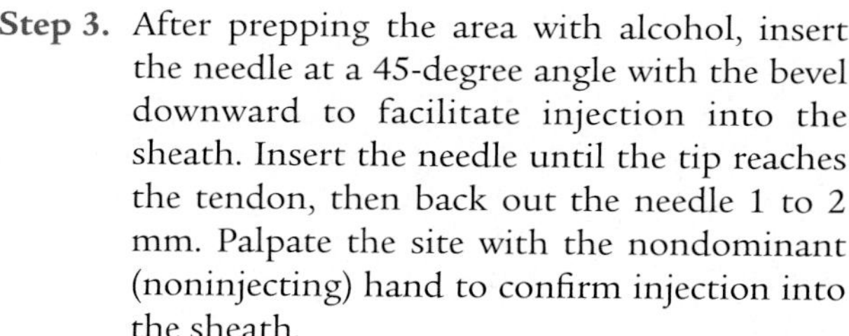

Step 3. After prepping the area with alcohol, insert the needle at a 45-degree angle with the bevel downward to facilitate injection into the sheath. Insert the needle until the tip reaches the tendon, then back out the needle 1 to 2 mm. Palpate the site with the nondominant (noninjecting) hand to confirm injection into the sheath.

- **PEARL:** The needle may enter the nodule with a distinct grating sensation. This may be verified by asking the patient to gently move the digit, and observing the needle move with the digit. The needle should be withdrawn very carefully until a give-way sensation is felt, indicating that the tip of the needle is in the sheath before injection.
- **PITFALL:** Topical ethyl chloride may be used preinjection if the patient is especially fearful of the needle stick.

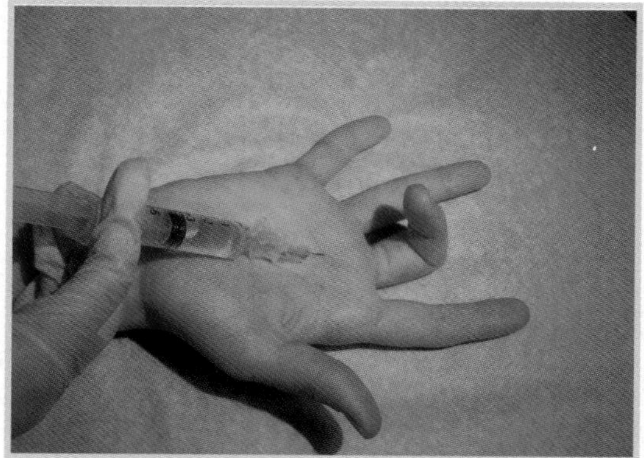

Step 3

Step 4. Move the finger immediately after injection to distribute the steroid. A bandage can be applied over the injection site. Nonsteroidal anti-inflammatory medication is prescribed for at least 72 hours to reduce the chance of postinjection flare (i.e., increased pain induced by the steroid crystals).

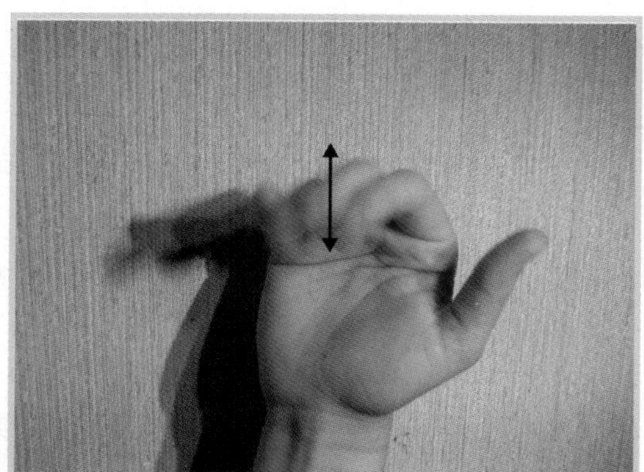

Step 4

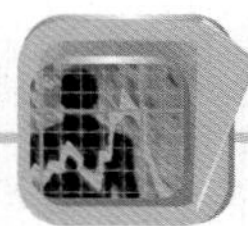

Complications

- Postinjection soreness
- Vasovagal syncope
- Local pain
- Needle breakage
- Skin infection
- Short-term increased tenderness
- Numbness in the digit due to local anesthetic coming into contact with a digital nerve
- Tendon rupture (rare)

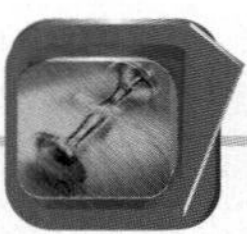

Pediatric Considerations

In infants, a nodule on the flexor pollicis longus tendon can be resected with excellent results. Corticosteroid injections are generally not helpful in pediatric cases of congenital trigger thumb.

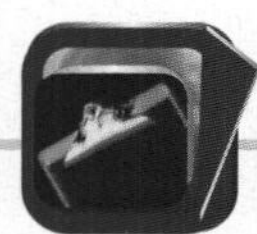

Postprocedure Instructions

Splinting is not used routinely after injection, although a hand splint is used by some providers. A second corticosteroid injection may be performed 3 to 4 weeks later if needed. If two or three injections fail to resolve the problem, consider referring the patient for surgical release. Have the patient watch for signs and symptoms of infection and bleeding. Any suggestion of infection or excessive bleeding should be reported to the physician immediately.

Inform the patient that some increased tenderness may be felt for a few days until the corticosteroid begins to have a significant effect. They may also have some numbness in the digit if some of the local anesthetic comes into contact with a digital nerve. This should resolve within a matter of hours. If there is prolonged numbness, signs of infection, or an inordinate amount of pain after the procedure, the patient should contact their provider.

Advise the patient to avoid using the injected fingers strenuously for the next few weeks to minimize the risk of postprocedure tendon rupture. The patient should be continued on a nonsteroidal anti-inflammatory drug or a cyclooxygenase-2 (COX-2) inhibitor if an oral nonsteroidal anti-inflammatory drug is needed.

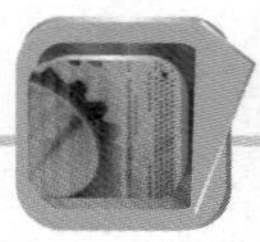

Coding Information and Supply Sources

CPT Code	Description	2008 Average 50th Percentile Fee	Global Period
20550	Injection of a tendon sheath or ligament	$140.00	0

CPT is a registered trademark of the American Medical Association.

2008 average 50th Percentile Fees are provided courtesy of 2008 MMH-SI's copyrighted Physicians' Fees and Coding Guide.

Patient Education Handout

Patient education handouts, "Trigger Finger" and "After Trigger Finger Injection" can be found on the book's Web site.

Bibliography

Akhtar S, Bradley MJ, Quinton DN, et al. Management and referral for trigger finger/thumb. *BMJ.* 2005;331(7507):30–33.

Anderson B, Kaye S. Treatment of flexor tenosynovitis of the hand ("trigger finger") with corticosteroids. *Arch Intern Med* 1991;151:153–156.

Brown JS. *Minor Surgery: A Text and Atlas,* 3rd ed. London: Chapman & Hall Medical; 1997:164–165.

Hollander JL. Arthrocentesis and intrasynovial therapy. In: McCarthy DJ, ed. *Arthritis,* 9th ed. London: Henry Kimptom Publishers; 1979:402–414.

Leversee JH. Aspiration of joints and soft tissue injections. *Prim Care,* 1986;13:579–599.

Moore JS. Flexor tendon entrapment of the digits (trigger finger and trigger thumb). *J Occup Environ Med.* 2000;42:526–545.

Nimigan AS, Ross DC, Gan BS. Steroid injections in the management of trigger fingers. *Am J Phys Med Rehabil.* 2006;85(1):36–43.

Owen DS, Irby R. Intra-articular and soft-tissue aspiration and injection. *Clin Rheumatol Pract.* 1986;2:52–63.

Reisdorf GE, Hadley RN. Treatment of trigger fingers and thumbs. In: Benjamin RB, ed. *Atlas of Outpatient and Office Surgery,* 2nd ed. Philadelphia: Lea & Febiger, 1994:92–96.

Rettig AC. Wrist and hand overuse syndromes. *Clin Sports Med.* 2001;20:591–611.

Saldana MJ. Trigger digits: Diagnosis and treatment. *J Am Acad Orthop Surg.* 2001;9:246–252.

Sheryl B, Fleisch BS, Lee DH. Corticosteroid injections in the treatment of trigger finger: A level I and II systematic review. *J Am Acad Orthop Surg.* 2007;15(3):166–171.

2008 MAG Mutual Healthcare Solutions, Inc.'s Physicians' Fee and Coding Guide. Duluth, Georgia. MAG Mutual Healthcare Solutions, Inc. 2007.

CHAPTER 116

Trigger Point Injection

E. J. Mayeaux, Jr., MD, DABFP, FAAFP

Professor of Family Medicine, Professor of Obstetrics and Gynecology
Louisiana State University Health Sciences Center, Shreveport, LA

Trigger points are discrete, focal, hyperirritable sites located within skeletal muscle. The points are painful on compression and can produce referred pain, referred tenderness, motor dysfunction, and autonomic phenomena. A "local twitch response" can usually be produced when firm "snapping" pressure is applied perpendicular to the muscle over the trigger point. Trigger points often accompany chronic musculoskeletal disorders.

An active trigger point often causes pain at rest and produces a referred pain pattern that is similar to the patient's pain complaint. This referred pain is felt not at the site of the trigger point origin, but remotely, and it is often described as spreading or radiating. Referred pain differentiates a trigger point from a tender point, which is associated with pain at the site of palpation only. A latent trigger point does not cause spontaneous pain but may restrict movement or cause muscle weakness. The patient commonly presents with muscle restrictions or weakness and may become aware of pain originating from a latent trigger point only when pressure is applied directly over the point.

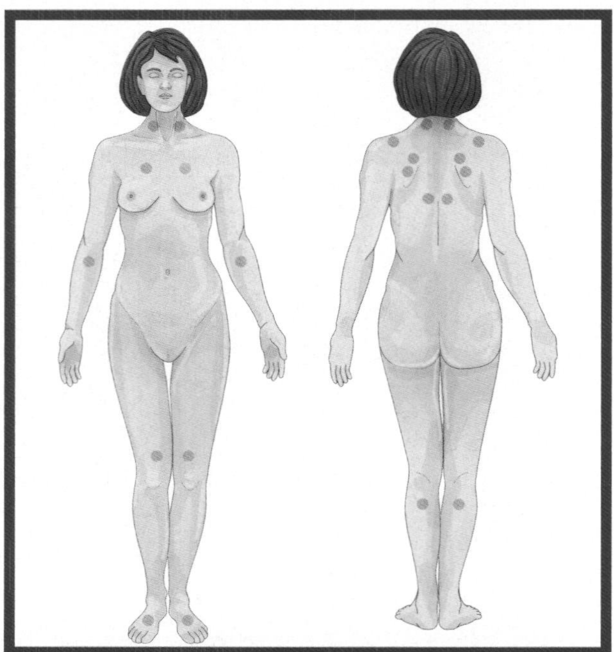

Acute trauma or repetitive microtrauma may lead to the development of a trigger point. Lack of exercise, prolonged poor posture, vitamin deficiencies, sleep disturbances, and joint problems may all predispose a patient to the development of microtrauma. Activities that produce repetitive stress on specific muscles may lead to trigger points. Acute sports injuries, repetitive stress, surgical scars, and tissues under tension after surgery also may predispose a patient to the development of trigger points.

Patients with trigger points often report regional, persistent pain that usually results in a decreased range of motion. Often, the postural muscles of the neck, shoulders, and pelvic girdle are affected. The pain may be related to muscle activity, or it may be constant. It is reproducible and does not follow a dermatomal or nerve root distribution. Joint swelling and neurologic deficits are generally absent on physical examination. In the head and neck region, myofascial pain syndrome with trigger points can manifest as tension headache, tinnitus, temporomandibular joint pain, eye symptoms, and torticollis.

Trigger points are diagnosed by palpation of a hard, hypersensitive nodule within a muscle. Localization of a trigger point is based on the examiner's sense of feel. Common locations of trigger points are shown in the figure. No laboratory test or imaging technique is helpful in diagnosing trigger points.

When treating myofascial pain syndromes, try to eliminate predisposing and perpetuating factors. Pharmacologic treatment includes analgesics, antidepressants, and cyclobenzaprine (Flexeril). Nonpharmacologic treatment modalities include massage, ultrasonography, application of heat or ice, diathermy, transcutaneous electrical nerve stimulation, ethyl chloride spray and stretch technique, and dry needling. These methods are more likely to require several treatments, and the benefits may not be fully apparent for days.

Trigger point injection with local anesthetic can effectively inactivate trigger points and provide prompt, symptomatic relief. It is a well-studied, effective, and commonly used treatment modality. It has a naloxone-reversible mechanism of action, suggesting an endogenous opioid system as a mediator for the decreased pain and improved physical findings after injection with local anesthetic. In comparative studies, dry needling was found to be as effective as injecting an anesthetic solution. However, soreness resulting from dry needling was found to be more intense and of longer duration than that experienced by patients injected with lidocaine.

An injectable solution of 1% lidocaine or 1% procaine typically is used, with or without a steroid such as triamcinolone (40 mg/mL) or dexamethasone (4 mg/mL). Diclofenac (Voltaren) and botulinum toxin type A (Botox) have been used, but these substances may have significant myotoxicity and are more expensive. Procaine has the distinction of being the least myotoxic of all local injectable anesthetics.

The patient's relief from the referred pain pattern measures the success of the injection. Reinjection of the trigger points is not recommended until the postinjection soreness resolves, usually after 3 or 4 days. If two or three previous attempts have been unsuccessful, do not continue injecting a site. Encourage patients to remain active, putting muscles through their full range of motion for a week after injection, but advise them to avoid strenuous activity, especially for 3 or 4 days.

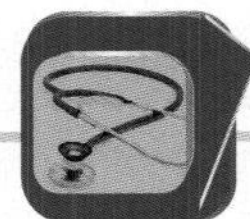

Equipment

- Common materials for trigger point injection include a 3- or 5-mL syringe, 1% lidocaine without epinephrine, or 1% procaine, triamcinolone (40 mg/mL), or dexamethasone (4 mg/mL), and 22-, 25-, or 27-gauge needles of various lengths.
- A suggested tray for performing soft tissue aspirations and injections is listed in Appendix I.
- Skin preparation recommendations appear in Appendix E.

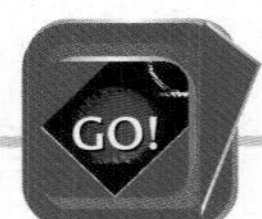

Indications

- Symptomatic trigger points

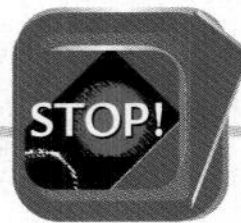

Contraindications

- Anticoagulation or bleeding disorders
- Aspirin ingestion within 3 days of injection
- Presence of local or systemic infection
- Allergy to anesthetic agents
- Acute muscle trauma
- Extreme fear of needles

The Procedure

Step 1. Place the patient in a comfortable position to assist with muscle relaxation. The prone or supine position is usually most effective and may also help to avoid injury if a vasovagal reaction occurs. Examine the patient for trigger points, especially in the areas where they most frequently occur.

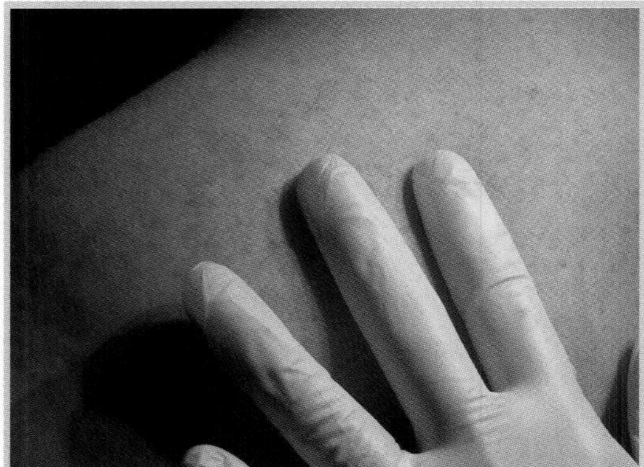

Step 1

Step 2. Cleanse the skin overlying the trigger point with alcohol. Use alternating pressure between the index and middle fingers to isolate the location of the trigger point (Figures A and B). Position the trigger point halfway between the fingers to keep it from sliding to one side during the injection (Figure C).

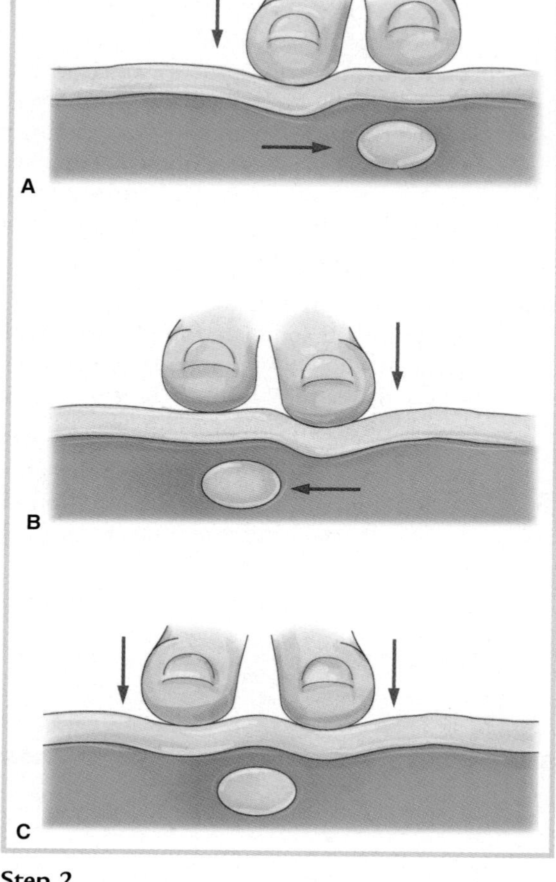

Step 2

Step 3. Using sterile technique, inject with the needle parallel to the fingers and away from the hand. Press firmly downward and apart with the fingers to maintain pressure for hemostasis and to ensure adequate tension of the muscle fibers to allow penetration of the trigger point. Choose a 23- to 25-gauge needle that is long enough to reach the trigger point; a 0.5- to 1.5-inch needle usually is adequate.

- **PITFALL:** Using a smaller-diameter needle may cause less discomfort, but it may be deflected away from a very taut muscular band.
- **PITFALL:** To minimize the risk of needle breakage, never insert the needle to its hub.
- **PEARL:** Before advancing the needle into the trigger point, warn the patient of the possibility of pain or muscle twitching when the needle enters the muscle.

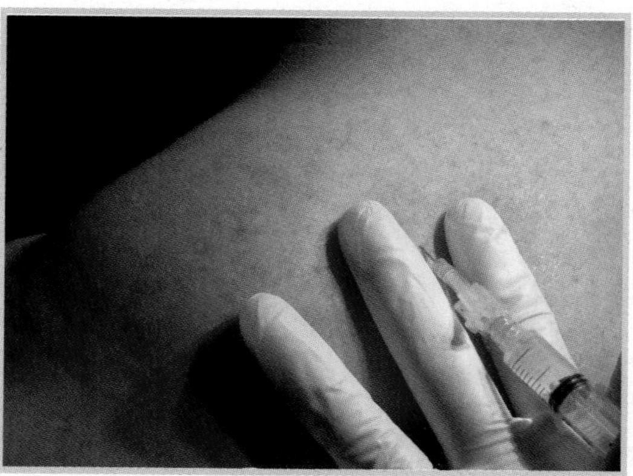

Step 3

Step 4. Insert the needle so that it may enter the trigger point at an angle of 30 degrees. Withdraw the plunger before injection to ensure that the needle is not within a blood vessel.

- **PITFALL:** To prevent the risk of pneumothorax, never aim a needle at an intercostal space.

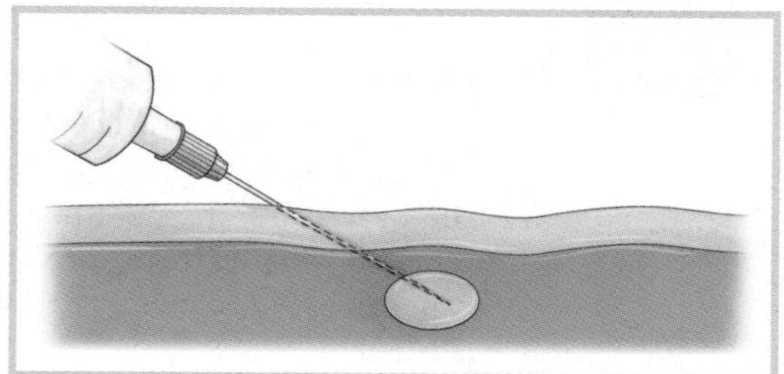

Step 4

Step 5. Inject a small amount (0.2 mL) of solution into the trigger point. Withdraw the needle to the level of the subcutaneous tissue, and then repeat the injection process superiorly, inferiorly, laterally, and medially until the local twitch response is eliminated or resisting muscle tautness is relieved. Immediately have the patient actively move each injected muscle through its full range of motion three times to stretch the injection site.

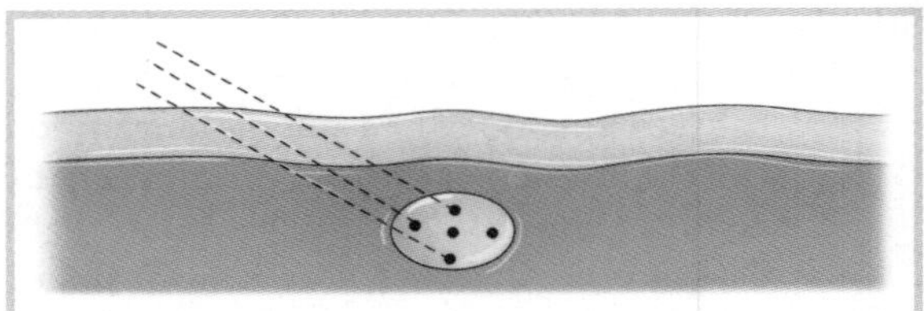

Step 5

Step 6. After injection, palpate the area for other trigger points. If some are found, they should be isolated and injected. Apply pressure to the injected area for 2 minutes to promote hemostasis. Apply an adhesive bandage.

- PITFALL: Failing to apply direct pressure for at least 2 minutes after injection makes hematoma formation much more likely.

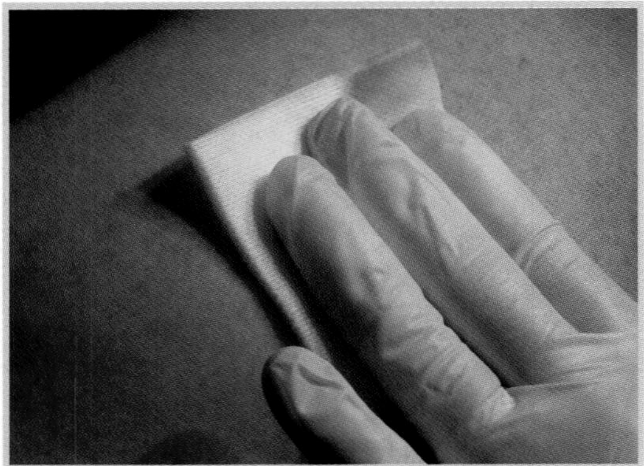

Step 6

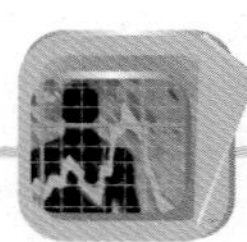

Complications

- Postinjection soreness (common).
- Vasovagal syncope.
- Local pain.
- Needle breakage.
- Hematoma formation.
- Skin infection.
- Entering or administering medication to an inappropriate or unintended area.
- Pneumothorax, which may be avoided by never aiming a needle at an intercostal space.
- Bleeding tendencies. Capillary hemorrhage increases postinjection soreness and ecchymosis. Have patients refrain from daily aspirin for at least 3 days before the procedure.

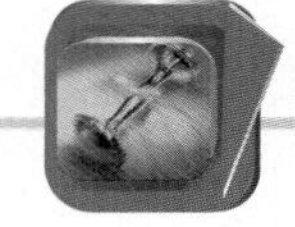

Postprocedure Instructions

Following the injections, it is often helpful to use ice on the injection sites. The injection itself is traumatic to the tissues and may result in swelling and edema. Icing the area reduces this inflammatory response. Explain to the patient that for the first 2 hours after the procedure, the pain may be completely relieved by the local anesthetic. This level of relief will abate after approximately 2 hours. By warning the patient in advance, the clinician can avoid many urgent phone calls. Pain relief will increase as the steroids exert their actions.

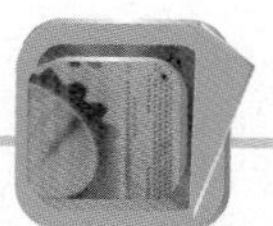

Coding Information and Supply Sources

CPT Code	Description	2008 Average 50th Percentile Fee	Global Period
20552	Injection, single or multiple trigger points, one or two muscle groups	$162.00	0
20553	Injection, single or multiple trigger points, three or more muscle groups	$173.00	0

Patient Education Handout

A patient education handout, "Trigger Point Injection," can be found on the book's companion Web site.

Bibliography

Alvarez DJ, Rockwell PG. Trigger points: diagnosis and management. *Am Fam Physician.* 2002;65:653–660.

Criscuolo CM. Interventional approaches to the management of myofascial pain syndrome. *Curr Pain Headache Rep.* 2001;5:407–411.

Elias M. Reduction of pain and EMG activity in the masseter region by trapezius trigger point injection. *Pain.* 1993;55:397–400.

Fine PG, Milano R, Hare BD. The effects of myofascial trigger point injections are naloxone reversible. *Pain.* 1988;32:15–20.

Fischer AA. Injection techniques in the management of local pain. *J Back Musculoskelet Rehabil.* 1996;7:107–117.

Fricton JR, Kroening R, Haley D, et al. Myofascial pain syndrome of the head and neck: a review of clinical characteristics of 164 patients. *Oral Surg Oral Med Oral Pathol.* 1985;60:615–623.

Garvey T, Marks MR, Wiesel SW. A prospective, randomized, double-blind evaluation of trigger-point injection therapy for low-back pain. *Spine.* 1989;14:962–964.

Han SC, Harrison P. Myofascial pain syndrome and trigger-point management. *Reg Anesth.* 1997;22:89–101.

Hong CZ. Lidocaine injection versus dry needling to myofascial trigger point: the importance of the local twitch response. *Am J Phys Med Rehabil.* 1994;73:256–263.

Hong CZ, Hsueh TC. Difference in pain relief after trigger point injections in myofascial pain patients with and without fibromyalgia. *Arch Phys Med Rehabil.* 1996;77:1161–1166.

Hopwood MB, Abram SE. Factors associated with failure of trigger point injections. *Clin J Pain.* 1994;10:227–234.

Ling FW, Slocumb JC. Use of trigger point injections in chronic pelvic pain. *Obstet Gynecol Clin North Am.* 1993;20:809–815.

McMillan A, Blasberg B. Pain-pressure threshold in painful jaw muscles following trigger point injection. *J Orofac Pain.* 1994;8:384–390.

Padamsee M, Mehta N, White GE. Trigger point injection: a neglected modality in the treatment of TMJ dysfunction. *J Pedod.* 1987;12:72–92.

2008 MAG Mutual Healthcare Solutions, Inc.'s Physicians' Fee and Coding Guide. Duluth, Georgia. MAG Mutual Healthcare Solutions, Inc. 2007.

CHAPTER 117

Wrist Ganglia Aspiration and Injection

Anne Boyd, MD
Assistant Professor, Department of Family Medicine
University of Pittsburgh School of Medicine
Director, Primary Care Sports Medicine Fellowship Program
UPMC Pittsburgh, PA
Scott Wissink, MD
Assistant Professor, Department of Orthopaedic Surgery
University of Pittsburgh Monroeville, PA

Ganglion cysts are common soft tissue tumors that arise from joint capsules or synovial sheaths of tendons. They can be mobile and vary in size. Ganglia occur at all ages, but roughly 70% appear in women between the ages of 20 and 40 years, with only approximately 15% in patients younger than 20 years. Women are affected three times as often as men. No predilection exists for the right or left hand, and occupation does not appear to increase the risk of ganglion formation. The dorsal and volar aspects of the wrist are the most common sites.

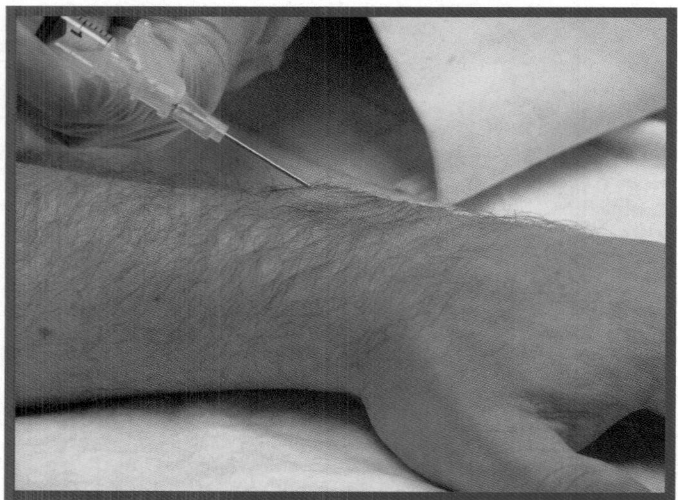

Ganglion cysts may be single- or multilobulated. They are smooth walled, translucent, and white. The content within a ganglion is clear and highly viscous mucin that consists of hyaluronic acid, albumin, globulin, and glucosamine. The cyst wall is made up of collagen fibers, and multilobulated cysts may communicate through a network of ducts. Ganglia may be obvious or occult. Obvious ganglia may slowly enlarge or develop suddenly after trauma. These ganglia often appear as firm, nontender, pea- to marble-sized lesions beneath the skin. Occult ganglia may compress superficial nerves and cause dull aching. Ganglia may also produce weakness and altered range of motion in the wrist and fingers. Imaging modalities such as ultrasonography or magnetic resonance imaging may help to identify suspected or occult ganglia.

Striking a dorsal wrist ganglion with a large Bible to rupture the cyst was a treatment used for centuries. Once the cyst ruptures, the body absorbs the fluid, and the lesion can be cured in approximately a third of individuals. This "Bible technique," however, carried with it a high recurrence rate as well as a significant risk of fracture and other injury to surrounding tissues. Today, a more controlled technique of aspiration with or without steroid injection has become the most commonly performed nonsurgical intervention for ganglia. A large-bore needle is placed within the ganglion to remove the thick, viscous fluid. Simple aspiration is associated with high rates of recurrence (>50%). Injection of corticosteroid after aspiration can help to shrink or resolve the lesions and reduces recurrences to between 13% and 50%.

Surgical intervention may be needed for recurrent or symptomatic lesions, but even surgical excision has recurrence rates >5% to 10%. Most ganglia in children resolve without intervention. The rate of spontaneous resolution in adults is not as high as that seen in children but is still significant enough to counsel patients about the option of observation.

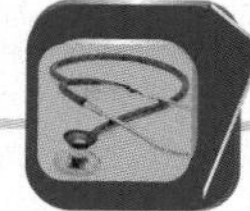

Equipment

- Needle (25 gauge, 1 inch long) on a 3-mL syringe with 2 mL of 1% lidocaine with epinephrine (for anesthesia)
- Needle (18 gauge, 1.5 inches long) on a 5 mL syringe (for aspiration)
- Methylprednisolone acetate (Depo-Medrol; 0.4 mL [10 mg]) and 1.6 mL of 1% lidocaine without epinephrine in a 3-cc syringe (for injection)

Ganglion cysts are best aspirated with 18-gauge, 1.5-inch needles. A hemostat may be used to exchange the injection syringe for the aspiration syringe. Needles, syringes, and ace wraps may be ordered from local surgical supply houses. Hemostats may be ordered from instrument dealers. A suggested tray for performing soft tissue aspirations and injections and ordering information are listed in Appendix I. Skin preparation recommendations appear in Appendix E.

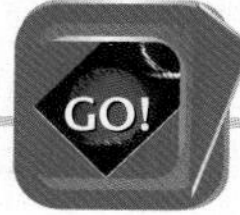

Indications

- Ganglia over the wrist that cause limitation of motion, pain, weakness, or paresthesias
- Externally draining ganglia or infectious concerns (no injection of steroid if suspect infection)
- Ganglia for which patients select nonsurgical intervention for cosmetic reasons

Contraindications (Relative)

- Uncooperative patients
- Ganglia overlying artificial joints
- Coagulopathy or bleeding diathesis
- Presence of septic arthritis or bacteremia

The Procedure

Step 1. After informed consent is obtained, hands are washed, materials are prepared, and gloves are applied. Position the patient so that the ganglion is exposed with the wrist supported. Swab the patient's skin with iodine or 70% ethanol (see Appendix E). Do not touch the injection site after swabbing.

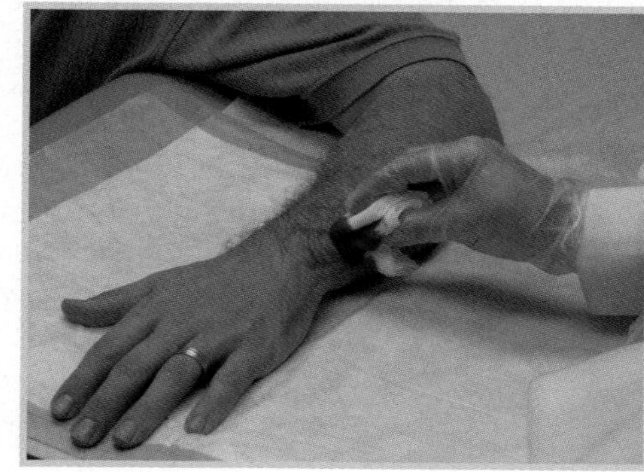

Step 1

- **PITFALL:** The location of the radial artery is particularly important in the assessment of volar wrist ganglia because they may be intimately associated with or adjacent to this vessel.

Step 2. Insert a 25-gauge, 1-inch needle on a 3-mL syringe, and inject approximately 2 mL of 1% lidocaine with epinephrine subcutaneously to create a small, superficially raised wheal.

- **PEARL:** Insertion of a large-bore needle for aspiration later in this procedure is painful. This pain is alleviated by prior intradermal injection of 1% lidocaine at the site where the aspiration needle is to be inserted.

Step 3. Enter the ganglion using an 18-gauge, 1.5-inch needle on a 5-mL syringe at an angle that provides optimal access to the cyst and comfort for the patient. Aspirate once in the cyst. The aspirating syringe will fill with thick, gel-like material.

Step 4. If, after aspirating, the provider chooses to inject a steroid solution, a hemostat or finger grasp can be used to stabilize the hub of the 18-gauge needle, which is already in place. Remove the gel-filled aspirating syringe from the needle, and attach the steroid-filled injecting syringe.

- **PITFALL:** Movement of the large needle when replacing syringes can make the procedure very uncomfortable and may dislodge the needle tip from inside the cyst.
- **PEARL:** Keep the needle tip immobile by maintaining a firm grasp on the needle hub, and by bracing (anchoring) the hand or hemostat holding the needle on the patient's wrist or forearm.

Step 5. Inject 0.4 mL (10 mg) of methylprednisolone acetate (Depo-Medrol) and 1.6 mL of 1% lidocaine without epinephrine through the 18-gauge needle into the ganglion. Apply pressure with a 4- × 4-inch gauze pad, clean the area with 70% ethanol, and apply a sterile bandage. Have the patient rest in the office for 20 to 30 minutes postinjection to ensure patient tolerability of the procedure and to review postprocedure instructions.

- **PITFALL:** Care must be taken to avoid the radial artery during injection of a volar wrist ganglion because injury to this vessel may potentially compromise circulation to the hand.

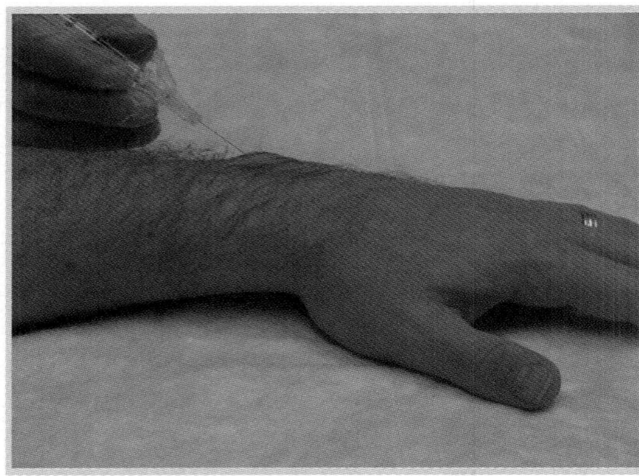

Step 2

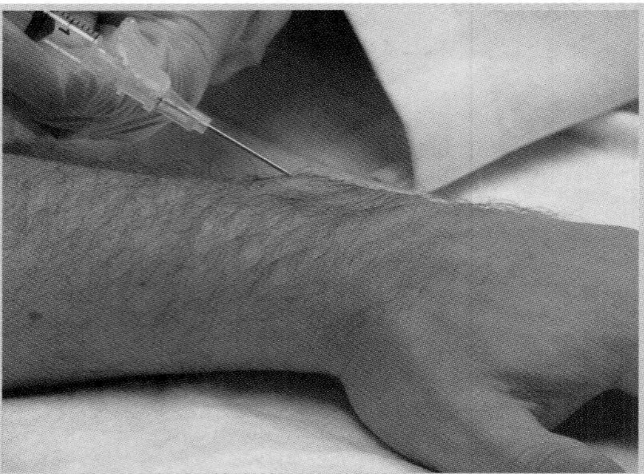

Step 3

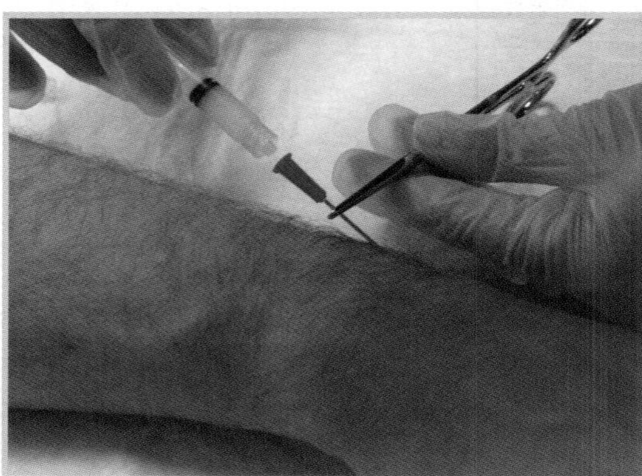

Step 4

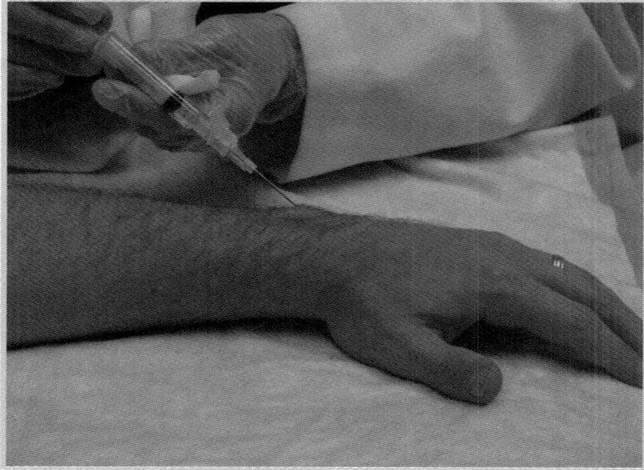

Step 5

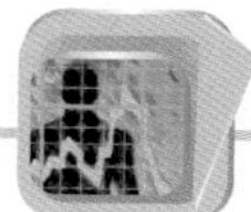

Complications

- Ganglion recurrence is the most common complication following treatment.
- Infection, bleeding, nerve and tendon injury, scarring, and vascular injury are possible.
- Joint stiffness and decreased range of motion may also occur.
- Skin and fat atrophy and thinning, as well as hypopigmentation are possible because of the superficial position of ganglia.
- Depending on anatomic location, injury to the superficial sensory branch of the radial nerve is a potential complication following dorsal ganglion injection, whereas injection of a volar ganglion can cause a radial artery injury.

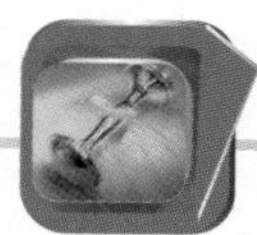

Pediatric Considerations

This condition rarely occurs in pediatric patients.

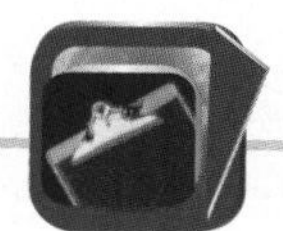

Postprocedure Instructions

Splinting and compression are advised after aspiration and injection. For the first 3 to 5 days, an elastic wrap may be used in combination with a volar splint to reduce pain and swelling. Mobilization is initiated after several days, and range-of-motion exercises are encouraged to restore wrist and finger mobility. The patient should return for re-evaluation within 1 week so the clinician can assess for re-accumulation of the fluid, any persistent drainage, or any signs of infection.

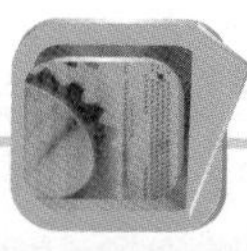

Coding Information and Supply Sources

CPT Code	Description	2008 Average 50th Percentile Fee	Global Period
20612	Aspiration and/or injection of ganglion cyst(s), any location	$135.00	0

ICD-9 Codes

Ganglion of joint	727.41
Ganglion of tendon sheath	727.42

Patient Education Handout

A patient education handout, "Ganglion Cyst," can be found on the book's companion Web site.

Bibliography

Griffin YG, ed. *Essentials of Musculoskeletal Care*, 3rd ed. Rosemont, IL: AAOS; 2005:362–367.
Ho PC, Griffiths J, Lo WN, et al. Current treatment of ganglion of the wrist. *Hand Surg.* 2001;6:49–58.

Hollister AM, Sanders RA, McCann S. The use of MRI in the diagnosis of an occult wrist ganglion cyst. *Orthop Rev*. 1989;18(11):1210–1212.

Pfenninger JL, Fowler GC. *Procedures for Primary Care*, 2nd ed. St. Louis (MO): Mosby; 2003: 1473–1499.

Rouzier P. *The Sports Medicine Patient Advisor: Ganglion Cyst and Ganglionectomy*, 1st ed. Amherst, MA: HBO & Company; 1999:251–254.

Wang AA, Hutchinson DT. Longitudinal observation of pediatric hand and wrist ganglia. *J Hand Surg Am*. 2001(26):599–602.

2008 MAG Mutual Healthcare Solutions, Inc.'s Physicians' Fee and Coding Guide. Duluth, Georgia. MAG Mutual Healthcare Solutions, Inc. 2007.

SECTION ELEVEN

PEDIATRICS

CHAPTER 118

Circumcision using Gomco Clamp and Dorsal Penile Block

E. J. Mayeaux Jr., MD, DABFP, FAAFP
Professor of Family Medicine, Professor of Obstetrics and Gynecology
Louisiana State University Health Sciences Center, Shreveport, LA

Circumcision is the most common procedure performed on male children younger than 5 years of age. The Gomco clamp is the instrument most commonly used in performing nonritual circumcision in the United States. It is designed to circumferentially crush a 1-mm band of foreskin, allowing hemostatic removal of the foreskin while protecting the glans from injury. The Gomco clamp is popular because of its ease of use and long safety record.

The Jewish faith ritual circumcision (Berit Mila) dates back 5,000 years to Abraham. This ceremony usually occurs on the eighth day of an infant boy's life and is usually performed by a ritual circumciser known as a mohel. Premature infants or infants who are ill may have the ceremony deferred until they are able to safely undergo circumcision. Checking with a local rabbi is a good way to find out about traditions and options for Jewish families.

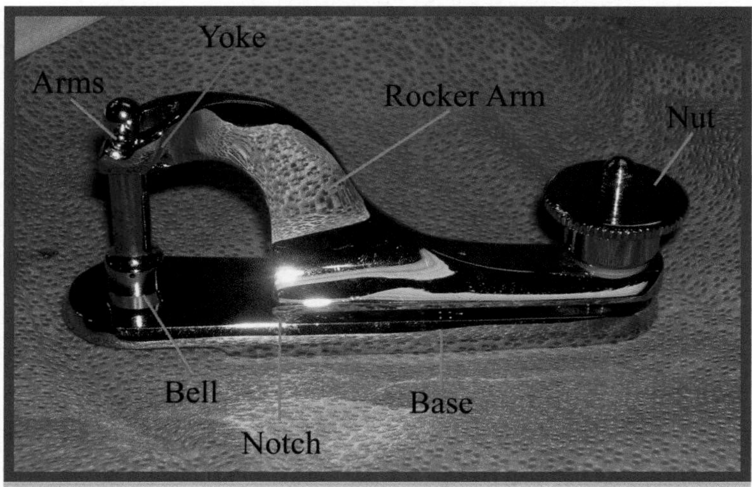

Infant feedings are suspended for 1 to 4 hours before the procedure to reduce the risk of aspiration. The infant is usually restrained in a molded plastic restraint device. Many infants urinate soon after being placed in the restraint, and the practitioner may have to move quickly to avoid the stream. An infant warmer should be considered if the room is cool.

Anesthesia is usually obtained using a dorsal penile nerve block. Multiple studies document a decrease in pain perceived by neonates during routine circumcision when a dorsal penile nerve block is used. A 1:10 mixture of 1% sodium bicarbonate and 1% lidocaine may decrease the pain caused by the acidic pH of the anesthetic solution. Dorsal penile nerve blocks have been performed since 1978 without any major complications reported in the literature. The most common problem associated with it is occasional failure to provide adequate analgesia. Minor complications such as local bruising, hematoma, and excessive bleeding at the injection site are rarely reported. The use of epinephrine is contraindicated in any procedure involving the penile shaft. Although topical prilocaine and lidocaine (i.e., EMLA cream) have been demonstrated to help, avoid the use of prilocaine in children younger than 1 month of age.

One of the most difficult parts of the procedure for novice practitioners is deciding how much foreskin to remove. Usually, about two thirds of the distal foreskin is removed. The amount of shaft skin that will remain after circumcision should be carefully assessed after the clamp is placed but before the screw is tightened. If it is necessary to adjust the amount of foreskin to be removed after the clamp is in place, disassemble the device, and pull the bell away from the base plate. If the foreskin is adjusted while the clamp and bell are still assembled, there is a risk that vessels between the foreskin and the underlying mucosa will be damaged and cause bleeding.

The penis should be inspected after the procedure for signs of bleeding or lack of union of the clamp line. Apply a dressing of petroleum jelly or petroleum gauze to the cut line, which may be removed in 12 to 24 hours. Most nurseries require that the infant urinate before undergoing circumcision, but barring complications during circumcision, this is probably not necessary. Warn parents that some swelling may occur, that a crust will often form on the incision line, and that small blood spots may be found in the diaper. Ask them to report any bloodstain greater than a quarter or any signs of infection. If soiled, the area may be gently cleaned with soap and water.

Rarely, the glans is not visible 30 minutes after the procedure. This indicates the presence of "concealed penis," which results from inadequate removal of foreskin or underlying mucosa. The penile shaft and glans are pushed back into the scrotal fat, and the penis is buried. There is no need for further procedure at this time as long as the baby is able to urinate without problems. However, a revision of the circumcision by a urologist may be necessary at a later time.

The decision on whether to offer circumcision for newborn males is controversial. The Task Force on Circumcision of the American Academy of Pediatrics in 2005 restated their position that newborn circumcision is not recommended and that the procedure is not essential to the child's current well-being. However, there is compelling evidence that newborn circumcision protects against penile cancer, local infection, phimosis, urinary tract infection, human papilloma virus (HPV) infection, and human immunodeficiency virus (HIV) infection. A recent study concludes that, overall, after adjusting for covariates, uncircumcised men have a more than threefold greater risk of contracting sexually transmitted infections (STIs) than circumcised men. The American Academy of Family Physicians recommends physicians discuss the potential harms and benefits of circumcision with all parents or legal guardians considering this procedure for their newborn son.

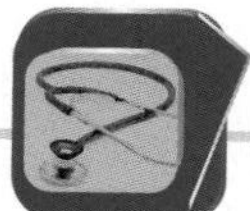

Equipment

- Blunt-edged probe
- Two or three small straight Kelly hemostats
- A scalpel
- Gomco clamps

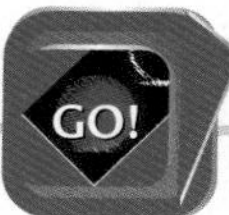

Indications

- Medical indications, including phimosis, paraphimosis, recurrent balanitis, extensive condyloma acuminata of the prepuce, and squamous cell carcinoma of the prepuce (all rare in neonates)
- Parental request
- Religious reasons

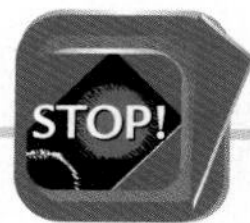

Contraindications

- Routine circumcision is contraindicated with the presence of urethral abnormalities such as hypospadias, epispadias, or megaurethra (i.e., foreskin may be needed for future repair or reconstruction).
- Less than 1 cm of penile shaft is visible when pushing down at the base of the penis (i.e., short penile shaft).
- Circumcision should not be performed until at least 12 hours after birth to ensure that the infant is stable. Circumcision in infants who are ill or premature should be delayed until they are well or ready for discharge from the hospital.
- Bleeding diathesis, myelomeningocele, significant prematurity, or imperforate anus.
- When there is a family history of a bleeding disorder, appropriate laboratory studies should be done to identify any bleeding abnormalities in the baby.

The Procedure

Step 1. Perform a dorsal penile nerve block by tenting the skin at the base of the penis and injecting 0.2 to 0.4 mL of 1% lidocaine (without epinephrine) as shown in Chapter 2. Consider the use of a restraint board/device to gently restrain the infant's legs during the procedure. Drape the baby's torso (but not head) with a fenestrated drape.

- **PEARL:** Some providers prefer a topical anesthetic cream (such as 2.5% prilocaine and 2.5% lidocaine [EMLA]) in place of a dorsal block.

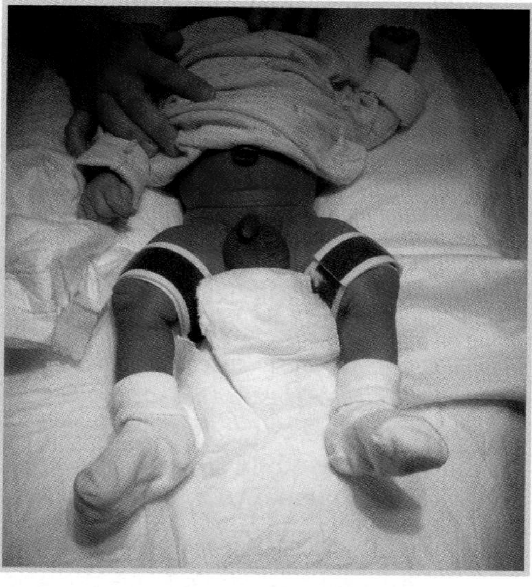

Step 1

- **PITFALL:** Anesthesia failure is often the result of failure to wait the necessary 5 minutes for the block to take effect. Avoid this problem by administering the block before draping the area, and then gently massage the area while waiting the 5 minutes required for maximum anesthetic effect.

Step 2. Clean the penis, scrotum, and groin area with povidone-iodine or chlorhexidine solution and sterilely drape the area. Inspect the infant for gross anatomic abnormalities. A pacifier dipped in 25% sucrose also appears to reduce infant discomfort.

- **PEARL:** Chlorhexidine may provide a better prep and be less irritating to tissues. See Appendix E.

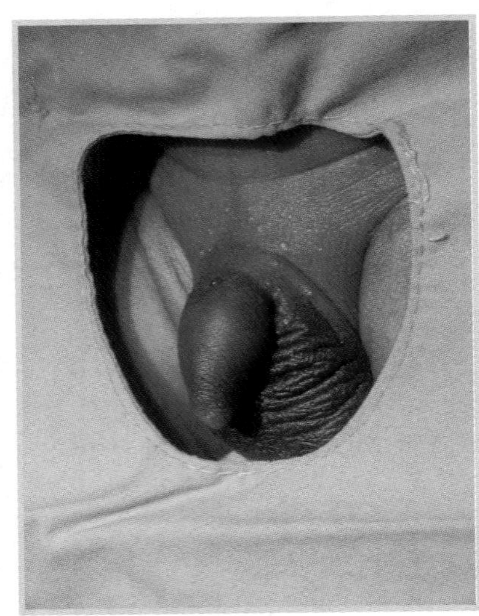

Step 2

Step 3. The size of the bell of the Gomco clamp used for the circumcision is selected based on the diameter of the glans (not the length of the penile shaft). The bell should be large enough to completely cover the glans penis without overly distending the foreskin.

- **PITFALL:** A bell that is too small will fail to protect the glans and may cause too little foreskin to be removed.
- **PITFALL:** Check the base, rocker arm, and bell of the Gomco clamp to make sure they all fit together. The bell and base from a 1.45-cm clamp will close but will not seal the skin properly if used with the rocker arm of a 1.3-cm set. Check to make sure that there are no defects in any of the parts.

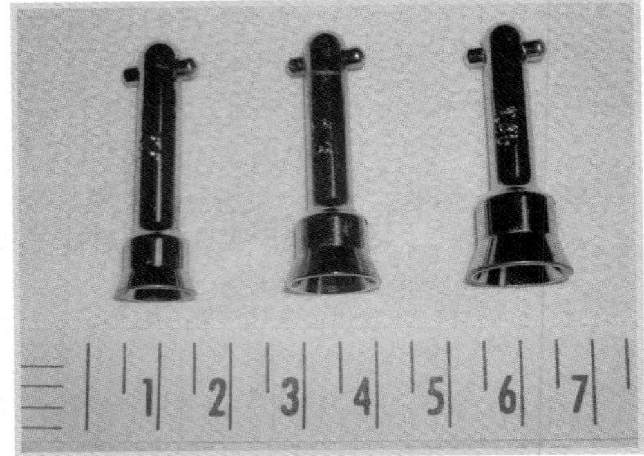

Step 3

Step 4. Grasp the end of the foreskin on either side of the dorsal midline at the 10 and 2 o'clock positions with two hemostats. Make sure to avoid the glans and the urethral meatus.

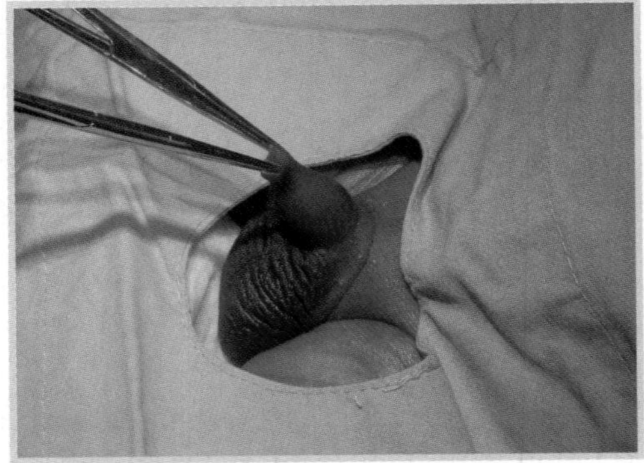

Step 4

Step 5. Carefully insert a closed hemostat or blunt probe into the preputial ring, and separate the foreskin from the glans down to the level of the corona. Slide the instrument down to the right and left sides to break up adhesions between the inner mucosal layer and the glans. Carefully avoid the ventral frenulum, because tearing it often causes bleeding.

- **PITFALL:** Failure to completely free mucosal adhesions from the glans is the most common reason for a poor cosmetic

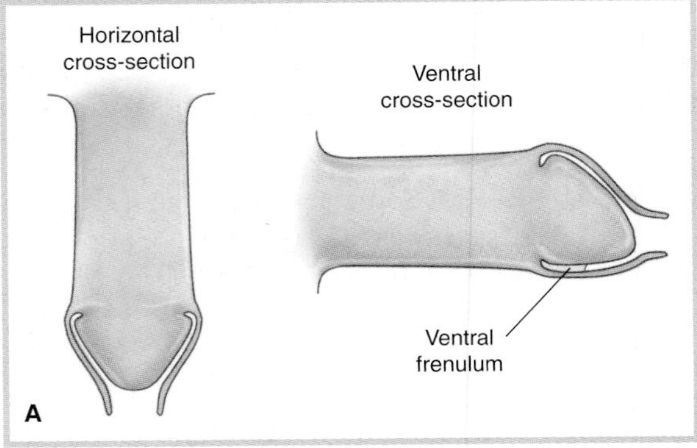

result. If the adhesions are not completely separated, not enough mucosa will be removed, and phimosis may result.

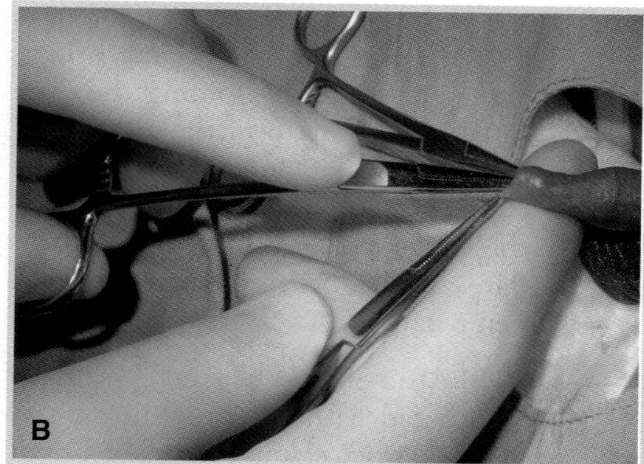

Step 5

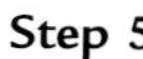

Step 6. Create a crush line on the dorsal aspect of the foreskin using a straight hemostat.

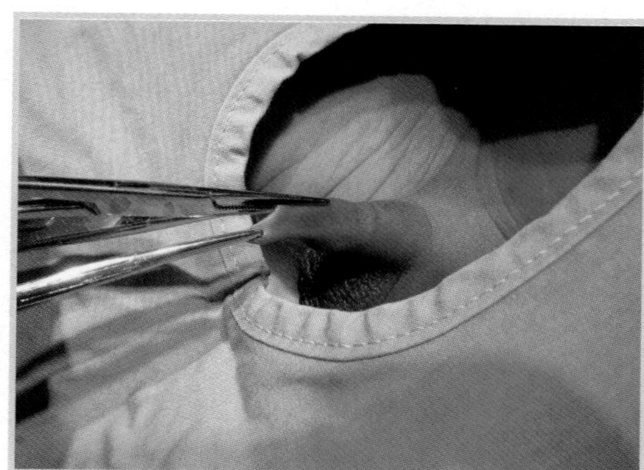

Step 6

Step 7. Cut the crushed skin with scissors, taking care to avoid the glans. The cut should proceed down the center of the crush line to avoid bleeding, which occurs if the cut strays laterally.

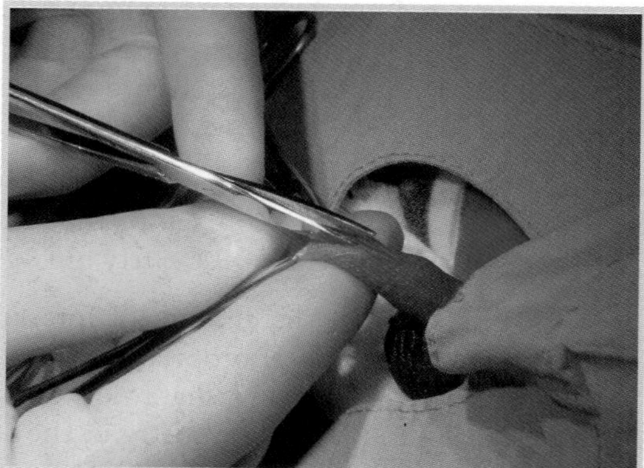

Step 7

Step 8. Finish breaking any remaining adhesions between the glans and foreskin all around the corona except at the frenulum. Examine the penis to make sure hypospadias or megameatus are not present.

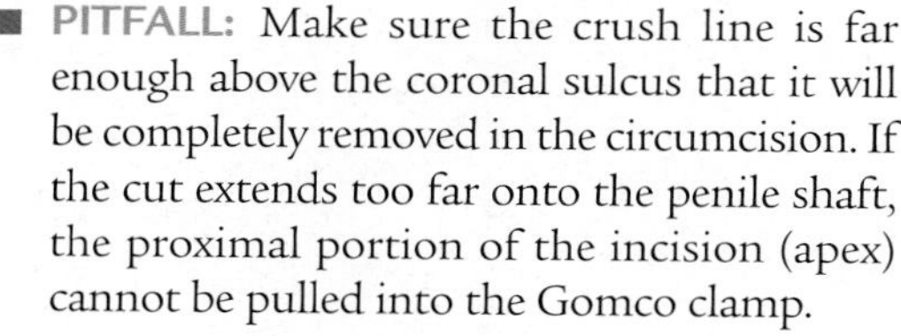

- PITFALL: Make sure the crush line is far enough above the coronal sulcus that it will be completely removed in the circumcision. If the cut extends too far onto the penile shaft, the proximal portion of the incision (apex) cannot be pulled into the Gomco clamp.
- PITFALL: If hypospadias or megameatus are present, terminate the procedure because any subsequent repair of these congenital anomalies may require the use of foreskin tissue.

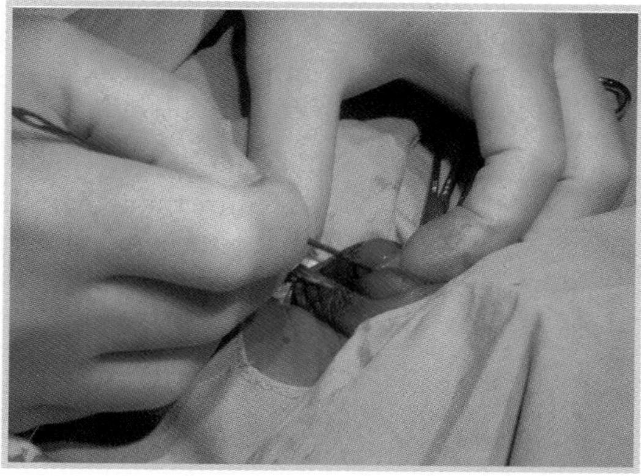

Step 8

Step 9. Insert the bell of the Gomco clamp under the foreskin and over the glans. Bring the two hemostats that are holding the edges of the foreskin together over the bell. Place an additional hemostat directly through the hole in the base plate. Then use the hemostat to draw the edges of the dorsal slit together over the flare of the bell, and remove the original hemostats.

- **PEARL:** Should bleeding occur, it is best to proceed with the procedure because once the Gomco clamp is in place, bleeding from the dorsal slit will stop.
- **PEARL:** If bleeding interferes with continuing the procedure, a hemostat can be used to create a second crush line overlying the area of bleeding.

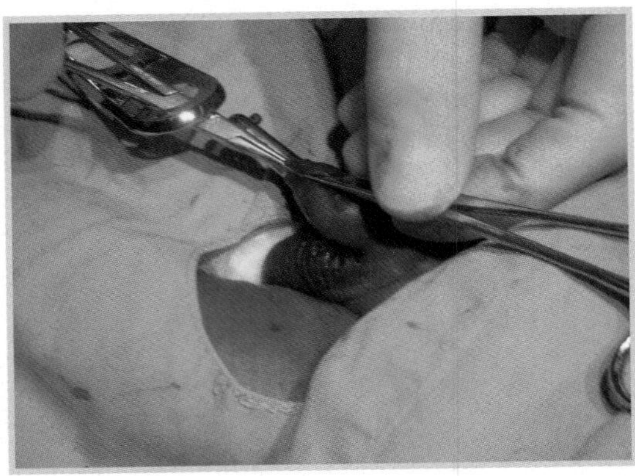

Step 9

Step 10. Pull the hemostat, foreskin, and stem of the bell through the hole in the base plate. Make sure that equal amounts of mucosa and foreskin are brought through the base plate.

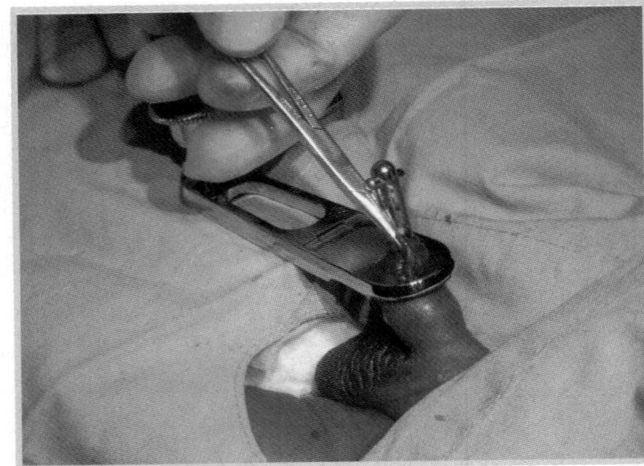

Step 10

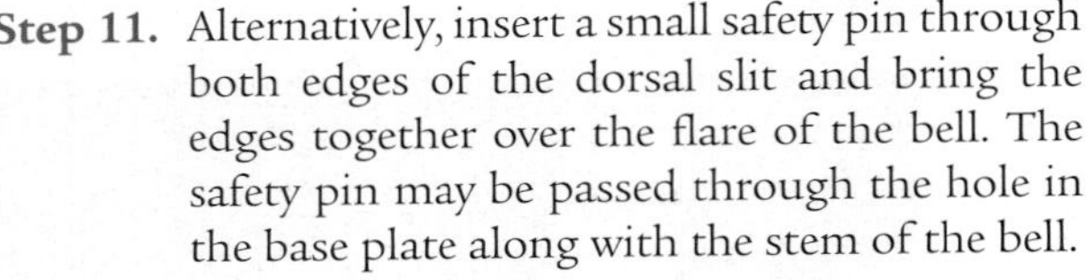

Step 11. Alternatively, insert a small safety pin through both edges of the dorsal slit and bring the edges together over the flare of the bell. The safety pin may be passed through the hole in the base plate along with the stem of the bell.

- **PITFALL:** Be careful not to cause inadvertent injury to yourself or the infant with the sharp end of the safety pin.

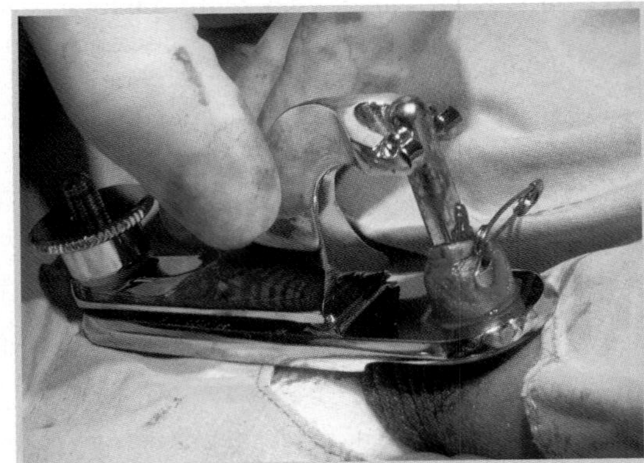

Step 11

Step 12. Determine if the amount of foreskin above the baseplate is appropriate for removal and that the remaining shaft skin is adequate. The amount and symmetry of the skin may still be adjusted at this time. The rocker arm of the Gomco clamp is then attached and brought around into the notch of the base plate. The arms of the bell are settled into the yoke, and the nut is tightened, crushing the foreskin between the bell and the base plate. Leave the clamp in place for 5 minutes.

- **PITFALL:** Make sure the apex of the dorsal slit is visible above the plate before putting the arms in the yoke and excising the foreskin.
- **PITFALL:** Make sure the rocker arm is well settled into the notch of the base plate. The clamp may be tightened outside of the notch, but it will not seal the skin well and will risk causing a degloving injury.

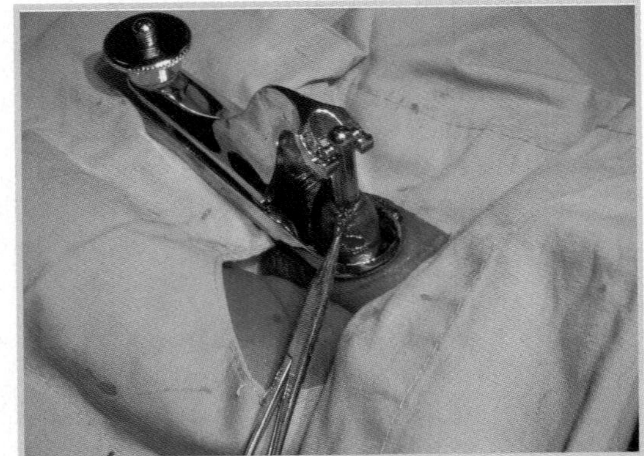

Step 12

Step 13. Place a scalpel blade flat against the base plate, and cut the top of the crush line.

- PITFALL: Cutting the foreskin at an angle into the base plate may disrupt the crush line and cause bleeding.
- PITFALL: Electrocautery should never be used with Gomco clamps, because the current could be transmitted to the entire penis via the metal clamp, and result in penile necrosis.

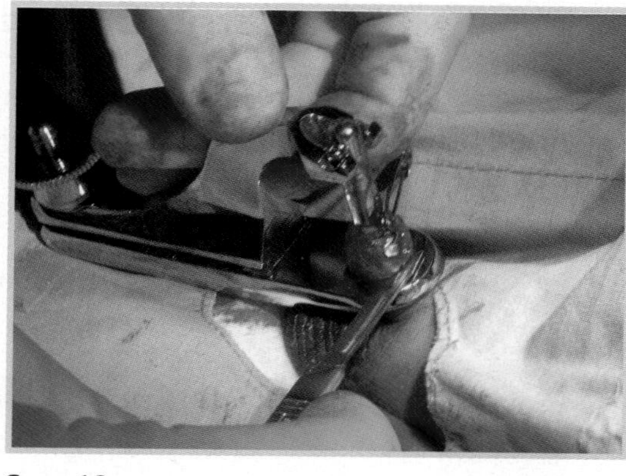

Step 13

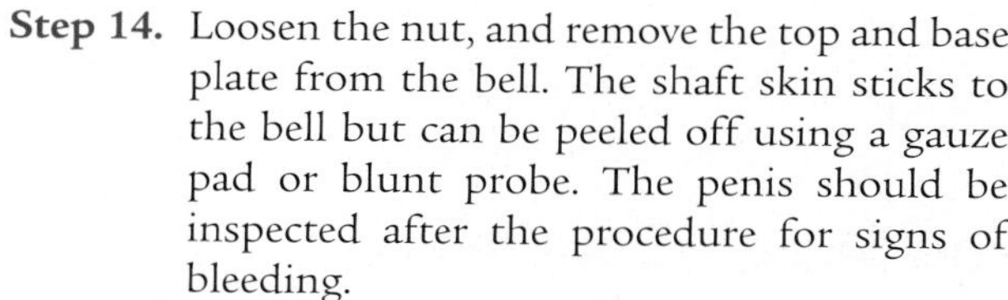

Step 14. Loosen the nut, and remove the top and base plate from the bell. The shaft skin sticks to the bell but can be peeled off using a gauze pad or blunt probe. The penis should be inspected after the procedure for signs of bleeding.

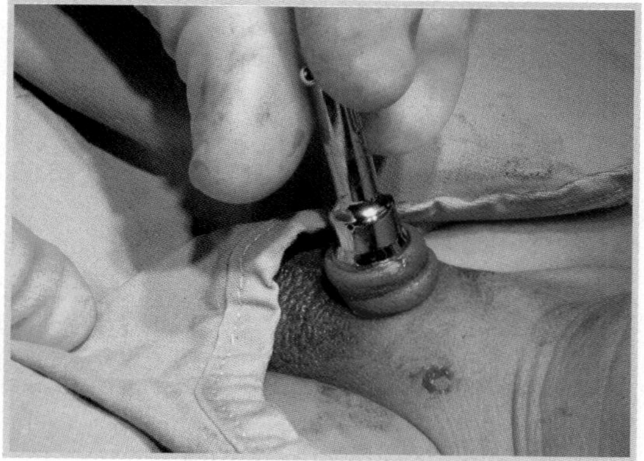

Step 14

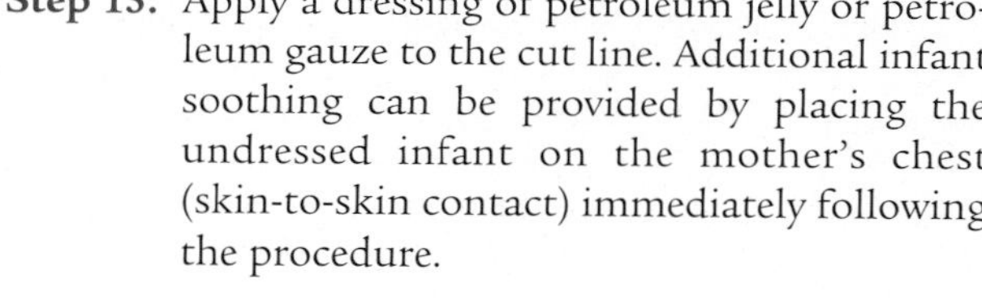

Step 15. Apply a dressing of petroleum jelly or petroleum gauze to the cut line. Additional infant soothing can be provided by placing the undressed infant on the mother's chest (skin-to-skin contact) immediately following the procedure.

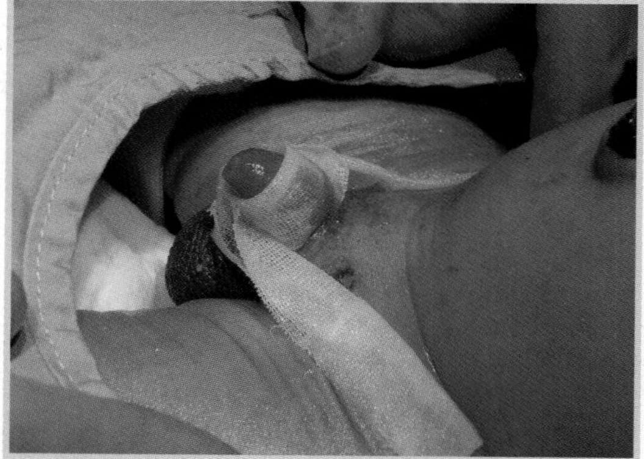

Step 15

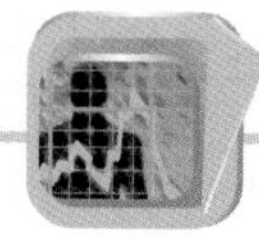

Complications

- Pain, infection, bleeding
- Phimosis or ring retention (urinary blockage secondary to swelling)
- Concealed penis
- Nonunion of skin crush line (degloving injury)
- Urethral stenosis, urethrocutaneous fistula, hypospadias and epispadias formation, necrotizing fascitis, penile amputation, and necrosis (all very rare)

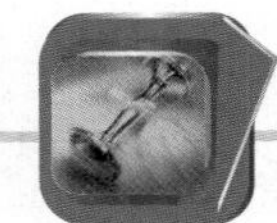

Pediatric Considerations

Children older than the age of 6 are dosed like adults except that the maximal dose is based on weight. The recommended maximum dose for lidocaine in children is 3 to 5 mg/kg, and 7 mg/kg when combined with epinephrine. Remember 1% lidocaine is 10 mg/mL. Children 6 months to 3 years have the same volume of distribution and elimination half-life as in adults. Neonates have an increased volume of distribution, decreased hepatic clearance, and doubled terminal elimination half-life (3.2 hours).

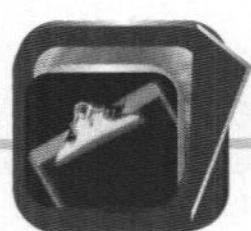

Postprocedure Instructions

- Patients may be bathed again within 24 hours after the procedure.
- Apply antibiotic ointment after each diaper change to prevent infections and adhesions.
- Report any signs of infection to your provider.

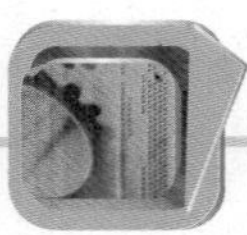

Coding Information and Supply Sources

CPT Code	Description	2008 Average 50th Percentile Fee	Global Period
54150	Circumcision using a clamp or other device	$427.00	0

CPT is a registered trademark of the American Medical Association.
2008 average 50th Percentile Fees are provided courtesy of 2008 MMH-SI's copyrighted Physicians' Fees and Coding Guide.
Note: CPT code 54152, "Circumcision using a clamp or other device, other than newborn," has been deleted. Use code 54150 for all circumcisions.

ICD Codes

Phimosis/paraphimosis	605
Routine circumcision	V50.2

Suppliers

- Gomco circumcision clamps may be obtained from Spectrum Surgical Instruments, 4575 Hudson Drive, Stow, OH 44224 (phone: 1-800-444-5644 or 330-686-4550; Web site: http://www.spectrumsurgical.com/catalog/instrument/circumcision.htm) or from Premier Medical Group Co. Ltd, P.O. Box 4132, Kent, WA 98032 (phone: 1-800-955-2774; Web site: http://premieremedical.safeshopper.com/).
- Restraint boards may be ordered from Olympic Medical Corp., 5900 First Avenue S., Seattle, WA 98108. Phone: 1-800-426-0353. Web site: http://www.natus.com/

Patient Education Handout

Two patient education handouts, "Deciding about Circumcision" and "Circumcision Aftercare," can be found on the book's companion Web site.

Bibliography

Anderson GF. Circumcision. *Pediatr Ann.* 1989;18:205–213.

Castellsagué X, Bosch FX, Muñoz N, et al. Male circumcision, penile human papillomavirus infection, and cervical cancer in female partners. *N Engl J Med.* 2002;346:1105–1112.

Fergusson DM, Boden JM, Horwood LJ. Circumcision status and risk of sexually transmitted infection in young adult males: an analysis of a longitudinal birth cohort. *Pediatrics.* 2006:118;1971–1977.

Fontaine P, Dittberner D, Scheltema KE. The safety of dorsal penile nerve block for neonatal circumcision. *J Fam Pract.* 1994;39:243–244.

Holman JR, Lewis EL, Ringler RL. Neonatal circumcision techniques. *Am Fam Physician.* 1995;52:511–518.

Lander J, Brady-Fryer B, Metcalf JB, et al. Comparison of ring block, dorsal penile nerve block, and topical anesthesia for neonatal circumcision. *JAMA.* 1997;278:2157–2162.

Laumann EO, Masi CM, Zuckerman EW. Circumcision in the United States: prevalence, prophylactic effects, and sexual practice. *JAMA.* 1997;277:1052–1057.

Lawler FH, Basonni RS, Holtgrave DR. Circumcision: a decision analysis of its medical value. *Fam Med.* 1991;23:587–593.

Mallon E, Hawkins D, Dinneen M, et al. Circumcision and genital dermatoses. *Arch Dermatol.* 2000;136:350–354.

Niku SD, Stock JA, Kaplan GW. Neonatal circumcision. *Common Problems Pediatr Urol.* 1995;22:57–65.

Peleg D, Steiner A. The Gomco circumcision: common problems and solutions. *Am Fam Physician.* 1998;58:891–898.

Tiemstra JD. Factors affecting the circumcision decision. *J Am Board Fam Pract.* 1999;12:16–20.

2008 MAG Mutual Healthcare Solutions, Inc.'s Physicians' Fee and Coding Guide. Duluth, Georgia. MAG Mutual Healthcare Solutions, Inc. 2007.

CHAPTER 119

Circumcision using the Mogen Clamp

E. J. Mayeaux, Jr, MD, DABFP, FAAFP
Professor of Family Medicine, Professor of Obstetrics and Gynecology
Louisiana State University Health Sciences Center, Shreveport, LA
Sandra M. Sulik MD, MS, FAAFP
Associate Professor Family Medicine
SUNY Upstate and St. Joseph's Family Medicine Residency, Fayetteville, NY

The Jewish people have practiced ritual circumcision for the last 4,000 years. The method to be used in ritual circumcision is not specified in the Torah or Bible. The Mogen clamp was invented in 1954 by Rabbi Harry Bronstein, a Brooklyn mohel (a Rabbi who performs circumcisions). For many years, it was used only in Jewish ritual circumcision in a ceremony called a *bris*. Now, providers are using the clamp more frequently in medical settings for newborn circumcision.

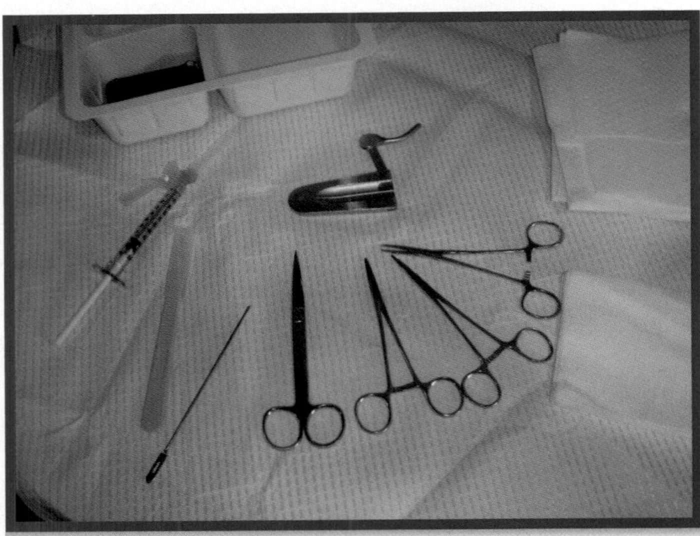

A properly working Mogen clamp will only open to 3.0 mm, minimizing the chance of trapping the glans. It locks closed with great force along a narrow crush line. Although commonly misperceived as a guillotine, it does not cut, it only crushes. In fact, "Mogen" is Yiddish for "shield," and the Mogen clamp shields the glans from the scalpel.

The Mogen clamp has a low incidence of complications, and the method requires few surgical instruments compared to other methods. The surgical time is short, typically <10 minutes for an experienced provider. There is good control of the amount of the prepuce removed, which allows the Mogen clamp to be used on a small penis. The inflammatory process usually starts to resolve by 72 hours.

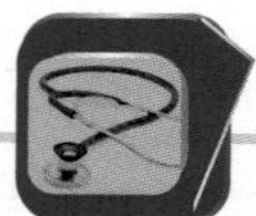

Equipment

- Blunt edged probe
- One or two small, straight Kelly hemostats
- A scalpel
- The Mogen clamp
- Scissors

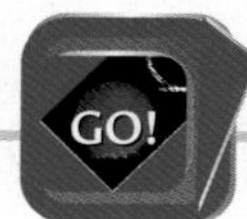

Indications

- Medical indications, including phimosis, paraphimosis, recurrent balanitis, extensive condyloma acuminata of the prepuce, and squamous cell carcinoma of the prepuce (all rare in neonates)
- Parental request
- Religious reasons

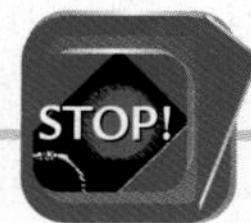

Contraindications

- Routine circumcision is contraindicated with the presence of urethral abnormalities such as hypospadias, epispadias, or megaurethra (i.e., foreskin may be needed for future repair or reconstruction).
- Less than 1 cm of penile shaft is visible when pushing down at the base of the penis (i.e., short penile shaft).
- Circumcision should not be performed until at least 12 hours after birth to ensure that the infant is stable. Circumcision in infants who are ill or premature should be delayed until they are well or ready for discharge from the hospital.
- Bleeding diathesis, myelomeningocele, significant prematurity, or imperforate anus.
- When there is a family history of a bleeding disorder, appropriate laboratory studies should be done to identify any bleeding abnormalities in the baby.

The Procedure

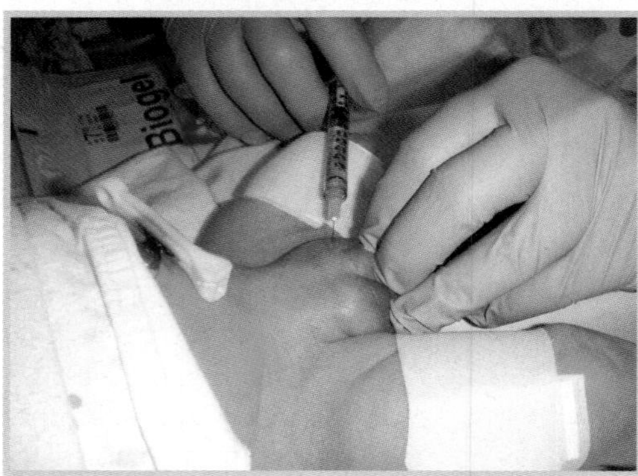

Step 1

Step 1. The first step in any circumcision is a dorsal ring block. Dorsal penile nerve block using about 1 mL of 1% lidocaine through a 30-gauge needle provides excellent anesthesia. Consider the use of a restraint board/device to gently restrain the infant's legs during the procedure. Drape the baby's torso (but not head) with a fenestrated drape.

- **PEARL:** Some providers prefer a topical anesthetic cream, such as 2.5% prilocaine and 2.5% lidocaine (EMLA) in place of a dorsal block.
- **PITFALL:** Anesthesia failure is often the result of failure to wait the necessary 5 minutes for the block to take effect. Avoid this problem by administering the block before draping the area, and then gently massage the area while waiting the 5 minutes required for maximum anesthetic effect.

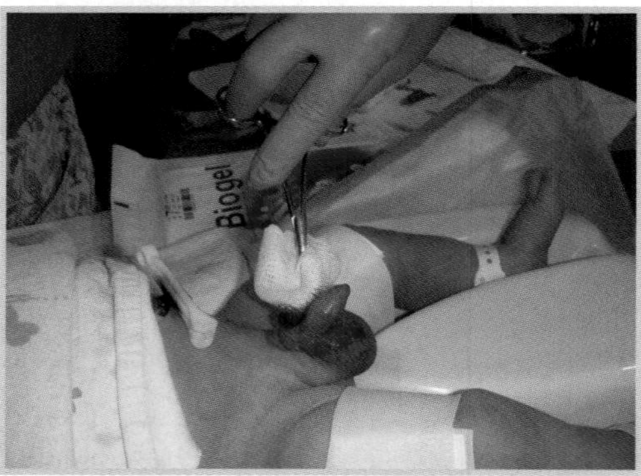

Step 2

Step 2. Clean the penis, scrotum, and groin area with Betadine or chlorhexidine solution and sterilely drape the area (see Appendix E). Inspect the infant for gross anatomic abnormalities. A pacifier dipped in 25% sucrose also appears to reduce infant discomfort.

- **PEARL:** Chlorhexidine may provide better preparation and be less irritating to tissues (see Appendix E).

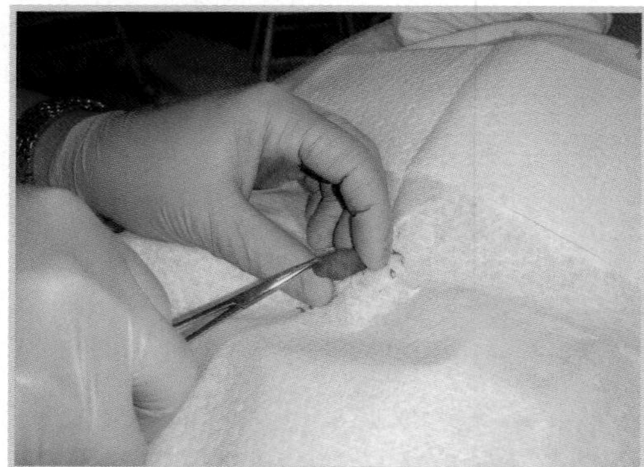
Step 3

Step 3. The dorsal tip of the foreskin is grasped with a fine hemostat for traction, and another fine hemostat or probe is used to open the plane between the glans and the foreskin all the way back to the corona. Take care keep the tip of the dissecting hemostat tenting the skin at all times. This keeps the hemostat out of the urethra. The ventral area is not dissected to avoid bleeding from the artery in the frenulum.

- **PITFALL:** Safeguard the frenulum by swinging the hemostat or probe right and left laterally not circularly.

Step 4. Placed another hemostat on the dorsal midline with its tip about 3 mm short of the corona and locked it in place to create a crush line.

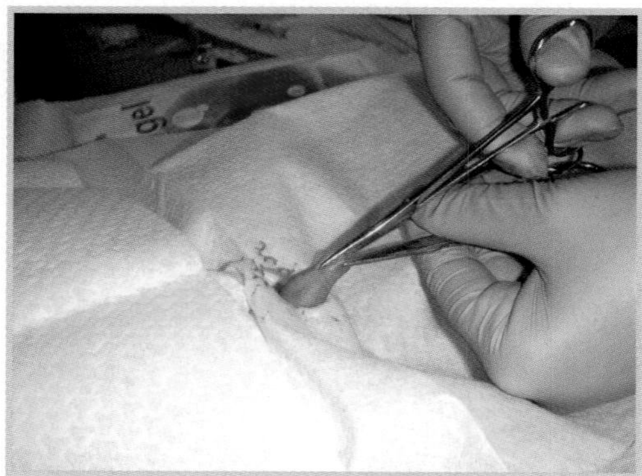

Step 4

Step 5. Cut the crushed skin with scissors, taking care to avoid the glans. The cut should proceed down the center of the crush line to avoid bleeding, which occurs if the cut strays laterally. Use the blunt probe to release any adhesions up to the corona, then gently pull the foreskin back over the glans.

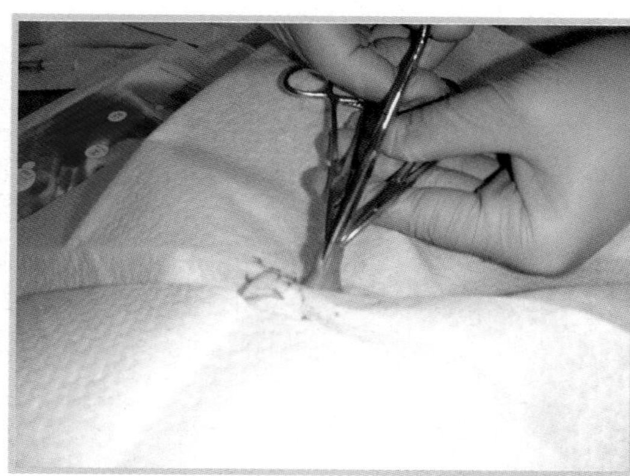

Step 5

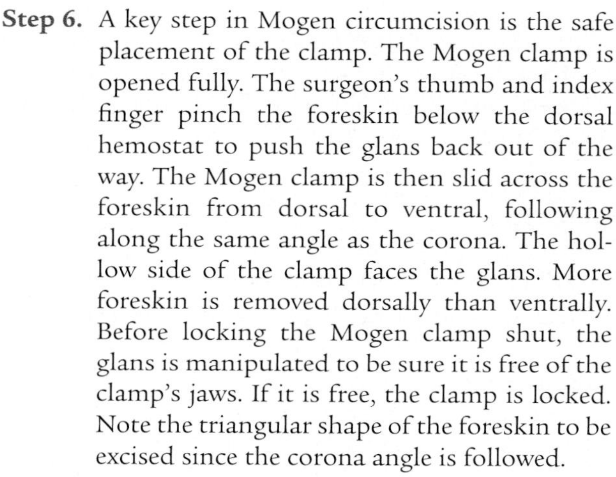

Step 6. A key step in Mogen circumcision is the safe placement of the clamp. The Mogen clamp is opened fully. The surgeon's thumb and index finger pinch the foreskin below the dorsal hemostat to push the glans back out of the way. The Mogen clamp is then slid across the foreskin from dorsal to ventral, following along the same angle as the corona. The hollow side of the clamp faces the glans. More foreskin is removed dorsally than ventrally. Before locking the Mogen clamp shut, the glans is manipulated to be sure it is free of the clamp's jaws. If it is free, the clamp is locked. Note the triangular shape of the foreskin to be excised since the corona angle is followed.

- **PEARL:** Clamps should be checked periodically to ensure that the opening is no more than 3.0 mm, and they should sent for repair or discarded if they do open wider.

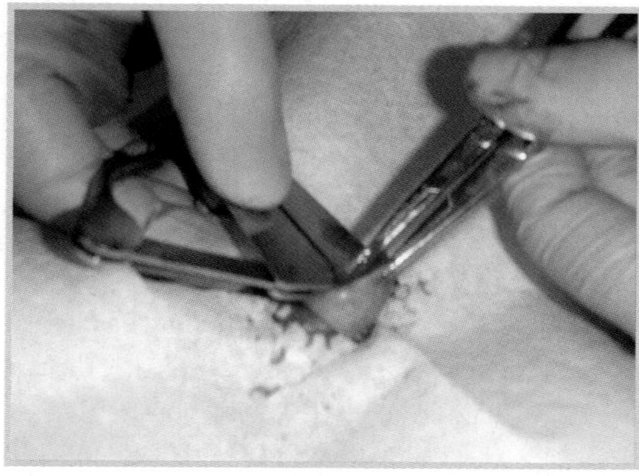

Step 6

Step 7. Once locked, the foreskin is excised flush with the flat surface of the clamp with a 10-blade scalpel. The clamp is left on for 1 minute to insure hemostasis, then unlocked and removed. The crush line covers the glans fully with penile shaft skin.

- **PEARL:** If the infant is more than 6 months old, the clamp should remain closed for no less than 5 minutes.
- **PITFALL:** If the clamp is removed prematurely, the crushed edges may separate and bleeding may occur. If this occurs, suture the skin margins, being careful to avoid deep sutures that might penetrate the glans, urethra, or corpus. If the whole edge separates, place quadrant sutures and close simple interrupted stitches.

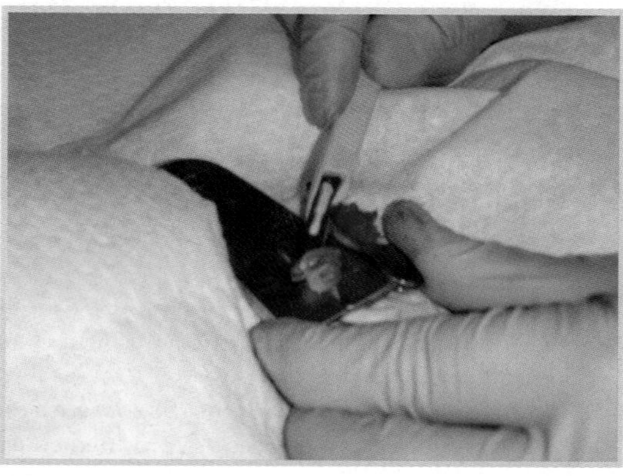

Step 7

Step 8. The glans is liberated by thumb traction at the 3 and 9 o'clock positions that pulls the crush line apart.

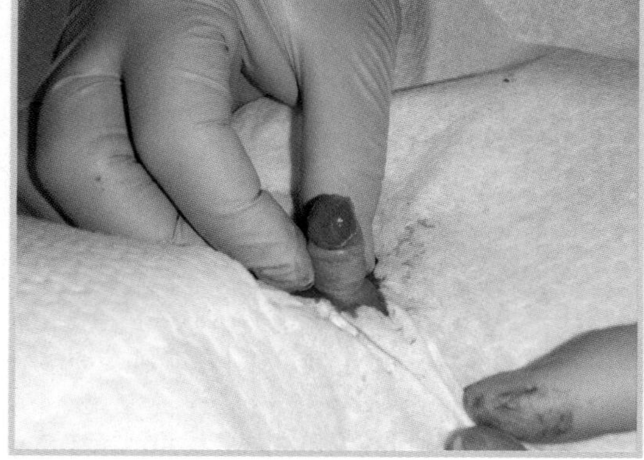

Step 8

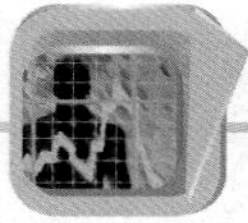

Complications

- Pain, infection, bleeding
- Phimosis or ring retention (urinary blockage secondary to swelling)
- Concealed penis
- Nonunion of skin crush line (degloving injury)
- Urethral stenosis, urethrocutaneous fistula, hypospadias and epispadias formation, necrotizing fascitis, penile amputation, and necrosis (all very rare)

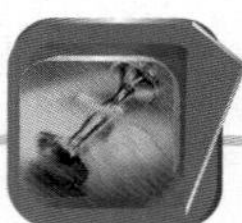

Pediatric Considerations

Children older than age 6 are given anesthesia like adults, except that the maximal dose is based on weight. The recommended maximum dose for lidocaine in children is 3 to 5 mg/kg, and 7 mg/kg when combined with epinephrine. Remember 1% lidocaine is 10 mg/mL. Children 6 months to 3 years have the same volume of distribution and elimination half-life as in adults. Neonates have an increased volume of distribution, decreased hepatic clearance and doubled terminal elimination half-life (3.2 hours).

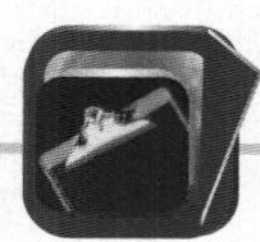

Postprocedure Instructions

- Patients may be bathed again within 24 hours after the procedure.
- Apply antibiotic ointment or petroleum jelly after each diaper change to prevent infections and adhesions.
- Report any signs of infection to your provider.

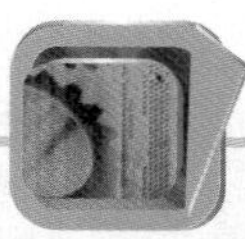

Coding Information

CPT Code	Description	2008 Average 50th Percentile Fee	Global Period
54150	Circumcision using a clamp or other device	$427.00	0

Note: CPT code 54152 – "Circumcision using a clamp or other device, other than newborn" has been deleted. Use code 54150 for all circumcisions.

2008 average 50th Percentile Fees are provided courtesy of 2008 MMH-SI's copyrighted Physicians' Fees and Coding Guide.

ICD-9 Codes

Phimosis/Paraphimosis 605, Routine circumcision V50.2

Suppliers

Clamps and instruments may be ordered from surgical supply houses such as:

- Spectrum Surgical Instruments Corp., 4575 Hudson Drive, Stow, OH 44224, Phone: 800- 444-5644; Web site: http://www.come-and-hear.com/editor/br-clamps/index.html.
- Surgicaltools.com, 404-A Walnut Avenue SE, Roanoke, VA 24014, Phone: 800-774-2040 Web site: http://www.surgicaltools.com.

Restraint boards may be ordered from:

- Olympic Medical Corp., 5900 First Avenue S., Seattle, WA 98108, Phone: 800-426-0353, Web site: http://www.natus.com

Bibliography

Holve RL, Bromberger PJ, Groveman HD, et al. Regional anesthesia during newborn circumcision: effect on infant pain response. *Clin Pediatr.* 1983;22:813–818.

Kaplan GW. Complications of circumcision. *Urol Clin North Am.* 1983;10:543–549.

Kaweblum YA, Press S, Kogan L, et al. Circumcision using the mogen clamp. *Clin Pediatr.* 1984;23:679–682.

Reynolds RD. Use of the Mogen clamp for neonatal circumcision. *Am Fam Phys.* 1996; 54:177–182.

Schlosberg C. Thirty years of ritual circumcisions. *Clin Pediatr.* 1971;10:205–209.

2008 MAG Mutual Healthcare Solutions, Inc.'s Physicians' Fee and Coding Guide. Duluth, Georgia. MAG Mutual Healthcare Solutions, Inc. 2007.

CHAPTER 120

Circumcision using the Plastibell Device

E. J. Mayeaux, Jr, MD, DABFP, FAAFP

Professor of Family Medicine, Professor of Obstetrics and Gynecology
Louisiana State University Health Sciences Center, Shreveport, LA

The practice of infant male circumcision predates recorded history. It is likely the most common operation in worldwide surgery. Throughout the world, millions of circumcisions are performed for religious and cultural reasons. Muslim and Jewish infants routinely undergo religious circumcision.

The Plastibell procedure was first introduced in the United States but has become the most common method of circumcision is England. It has more than 45 years of successful clinical use that has demonstrated its safety and effectiveness. The ligature minimizes bleeding and eliminates the need for postoperative dressings. The design of the Plastibell anchors the ligature securely, protects the glans, and allows for visual inspection through the device. Cosmetic results with the Plastibell are similar to other methods. A study in England by Palit et al. found 96% satisfaction rate with the use of this device.

The Plastibell device is supplied in individual presterilized packages. It comes in six sizes: 1.1, 1.2, 1.3, 1.4, 1.5, and 1.7 cm. Because it is disposable, it eliminates the need for sterilization required of stainless steel clamps. It also eliminates the potential problem of lost or mismatched parts that may occur with other systems. Determining the appropriate size of the device is important because a fit too small can cause tissue strangulation and necrosis, and one too large may result in too much foreskin being removed. The bell should be just large enough to completely cover the glans penis without overly distending the foreskin.

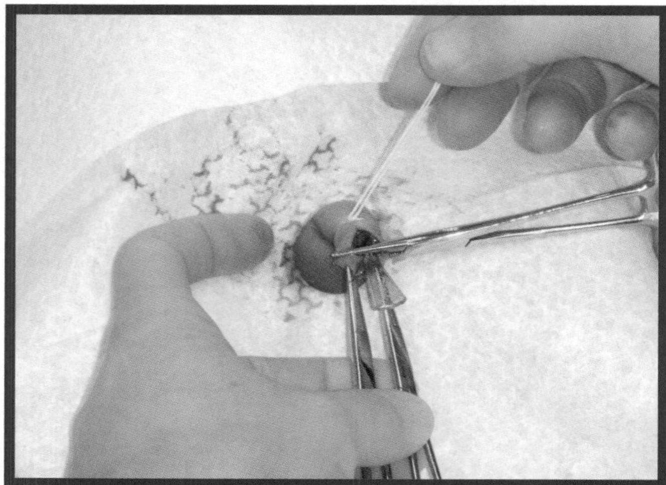

The shape of the handle is different for each size of the device. This makes it easy to identify different sizes by the shape of the handle. The handle allows for easy positioning of the bell. The ligature applied over the grooved bell completely cuts off circulation so there is no open wound to cause seepage. There is no need for dressings or special postoperative care. After the procedure is completed, the handle is easily snapped off. No part of the remaining bell projects beyond the glans to cause pressure or necrosis. Urination is unaffected, and the baby can be diapered in a normal way.

Plastibell complications are reported to be about 2% to 3%. Most complications are minor, related to bleeding. There has also been a report of a slight increase in infections compared with other methods. However, rare case reports of significant complications have been documented, including necrotizing fasciitis, urine retention, and ischemic necrosis of the glans.

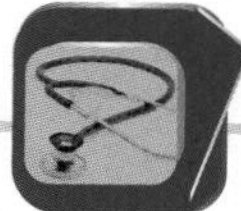

Equipment

- Sterile drape
- Two small forceps
- A probe
- A pair of scissors
- Prep materials (see Appendix E)
- The Plastibell device and ligature

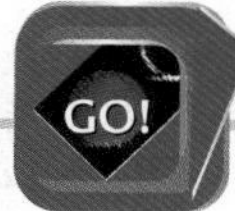

Indications

- Medical indications, including phimosis, paraphimosis, recurrent balanitis, extensive condyloma acuminata of the prepuce, and squamous cell carcinoma of the prepuce (all rare in neonates)
- Parental request
- Religious reasons

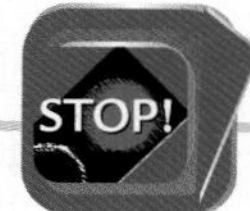

Contraindications

- Routine circumcision is contraindicated with the presence of urethral abnormalities such as hypospadias, epispadias, or megaurethra (i.e., foreskin may be needed for future repair or reconstruction).
- Less than 1 cm of penile shaft is visible when pushing down at the base of the penis (i.e., short penile shaft).
- Circumcision should not be performed until at least 12 hours after birth to ensure that the infant is stable. Circumcision in infants who are ill or premature should be delayed until they are well or ready for discharge from the hospital.
- Bleeding diathesis, myelomeningocele, significant prematurity, or imperforate anus.
- When there is a family history of a bleeding disorder, appropriate laboratory studies should be done to identify any bleeding abnormalities in the baby.

The Procedure

Step 1. Prep the area with alcohol, and inject with 1% lidocaine (without epinephrine) in a dorsal penile block (see Chapter 2). Consider the use of a restraint board/device to gently restrain the infant's legs during the procedure. Clean the penis, scrotum, and groin area with povidone-iodine or chlorhexidine solution, and sterilely drape the area (see Appendix E).

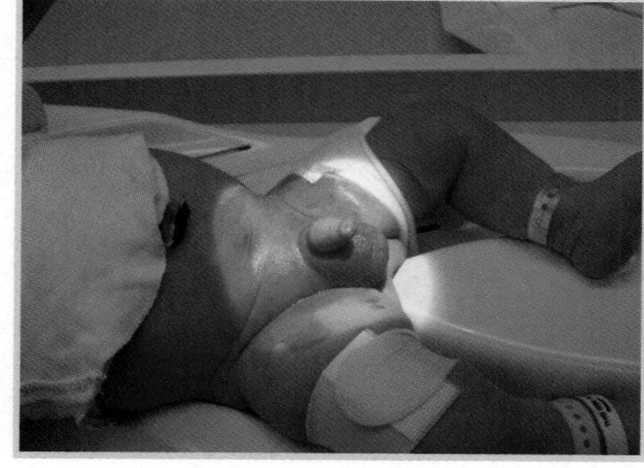

Step 1

Inspect the infant for gross anatomic abnormalities. Drape the baby's torso (but not head) with a fenestrated drape.

- **PEARL:** Some providers prefer a topical anesthetic cream (such as 2.5% prilocaine and 2.5% lidocaine [EMLA]) in place of a dorsal block.
- **PEARL:** Use a pacifier dipped in 25% sucrose to reduce infant discomfort and crying.
- **PITFALL:** Anesthesia failure is often the result of failure to wait the necessary 5 minutes for the block to take effect. Avoid this problem by administering the block before draping the area, and then gently massage the area while waiting the 5 minutes required for maximum anesthetic effect.

Step 2. Grasp the end of the foreskin on either side of the dorsal midline at the 10 and 2 o'clock positions with two hemostats. Make sure to avoid the glans and the urethral meatus.

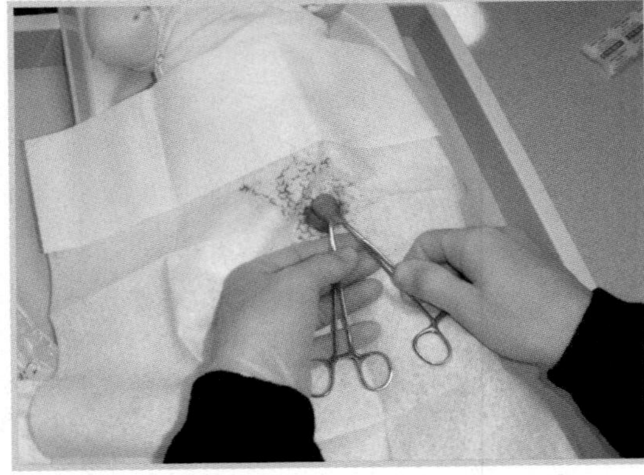

Step 2

Step 3. Carefully insert a closed hemostat or blunt probe into the preputial ring, and separate the foreskin from the glans down to the level of the corona. Slide the instrument down to the right and left sides to break up adhesions between the inner mucosal layer and the glans. Carefully avoid the ventral frenulum, because tearing it often causes bleeding. Create a crush line on the dorsal aspect of the foreskin using a straight hemostat.

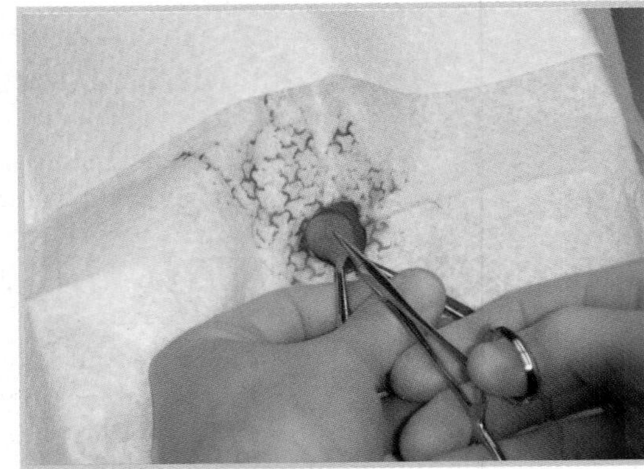

Step 3

Step 4. Cut the crushed skin with scissors, taking care to avoid the glans. The cut should proceed down the center of the crush line to avoid bleeding, which occurs if the cut strays laterally.

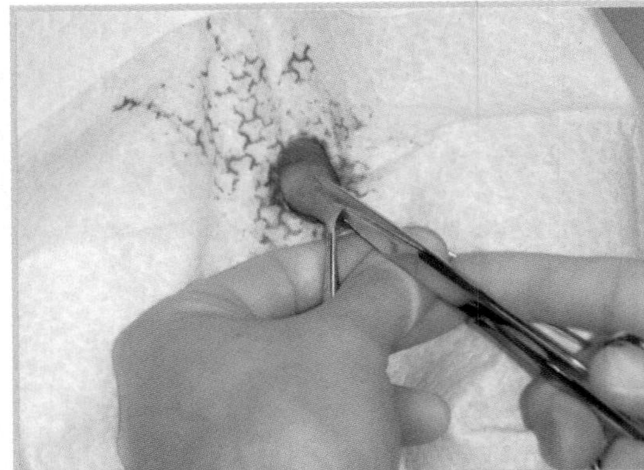

Step 4

Step 5. Finish breaking any remaining adhesions between the glans and foreskin all around the corona except at the frenulum. Examine the penis to make sure hypospadias or megameatus are not present. Select the proper size of Plastibell. The proper fit is a bell that fits halfway down on the glans. Place the Plastibell on the glans.

- **PITFALL:** Make sure the crush line is far enough above the coronal sulcus that it will be completely removed in the circumcision. If the cut extends too far onto the penile shaft, the proximal portion of the incision (apex) cannot be pulled into the clamp.
- **PITFALL:** If hypospadias or megameatus are present, terminate the procedure because any subsequent repair of these congenital anomalies may require the use of foreskin tissue.

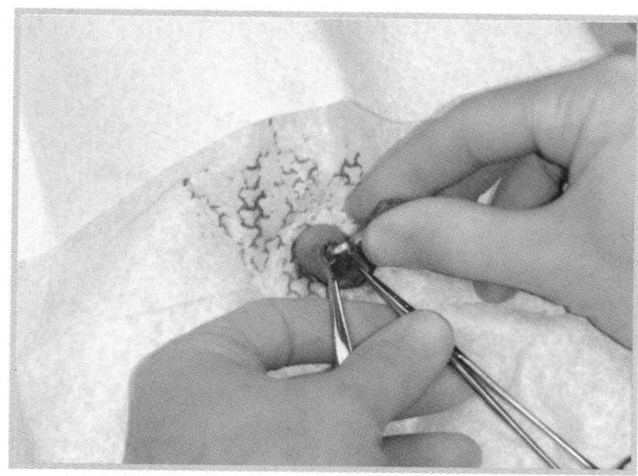

Step 5

Step 6. If the bell tends to slip out of the foreskin, cross the forceps or place an additional forceps across the top of the foreskin and handle of the Plastibell.

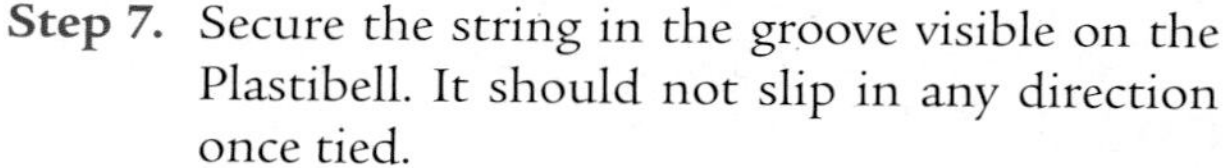

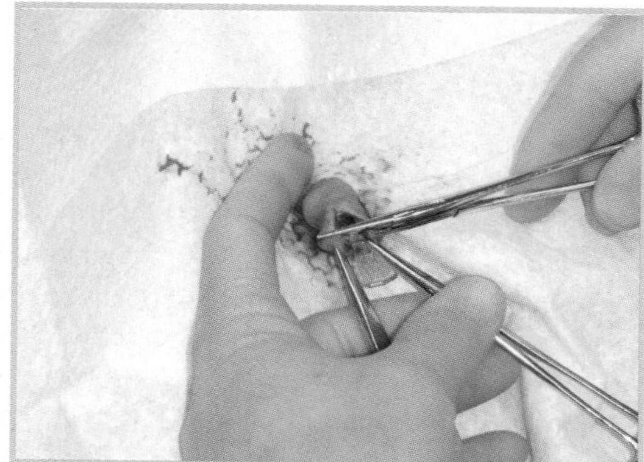

Step 6

Step 7. Secure the string in the groove visible on the Plastibell. It should not slip in any direction once tied.

- **PITFALL:** Improper placement of the ligature may increase bleeding complications.

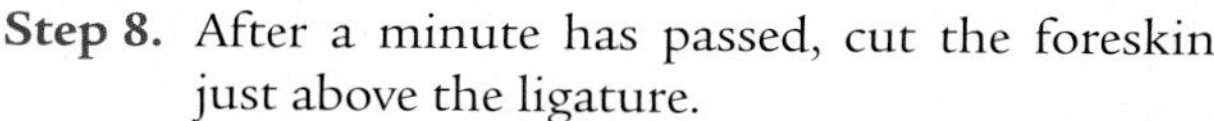

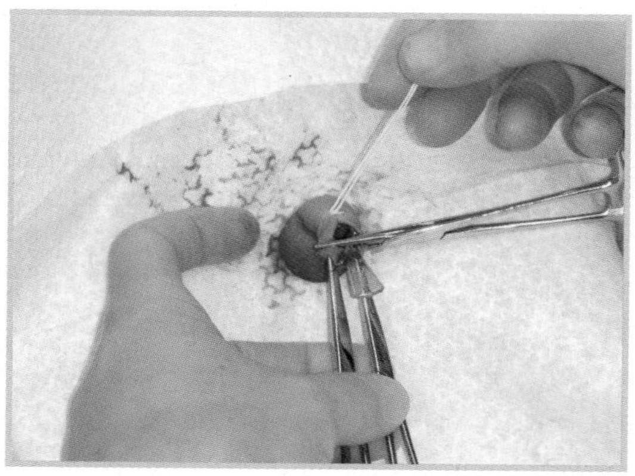

Step 7

Step 8. After a minute has passed, cut the foreskin just above the ligature.

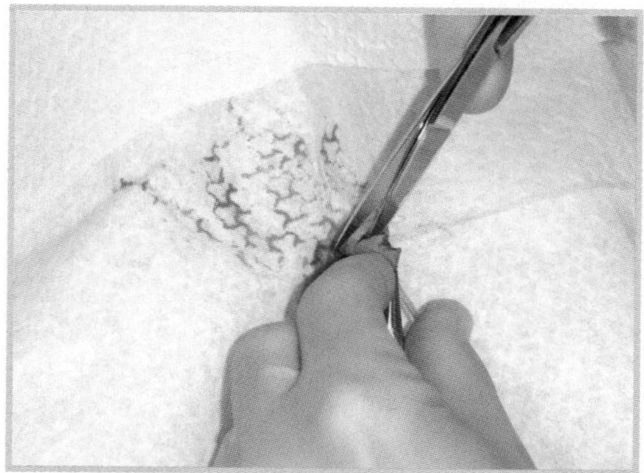

Step 8

Step 9. Snap off the handle, leaving the bell in position.

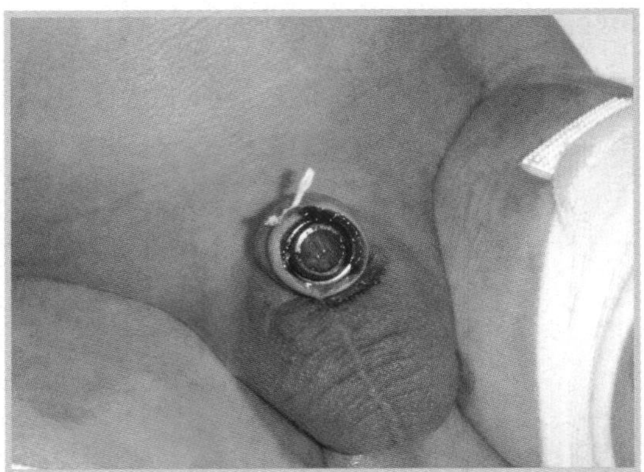

Step 9

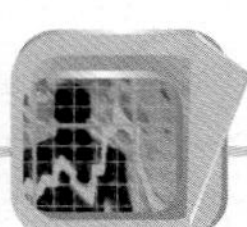

Complications

- Pain, infection, bleeding.
- Phimosis or ring retention (urinary blockage secondary to swelling).
- Urethral stenosis, urethrocutaneous fistula, hypospadias and epispadias formation, necrotizing fascitis, penile amputation, and necrosis (all very rare).
- Early separation.
- If the ring slips below the glans, it can result in venous congestion and necrosis.
- Ring migration/incomplete/delayed separation.
- Excess foreskin removed.

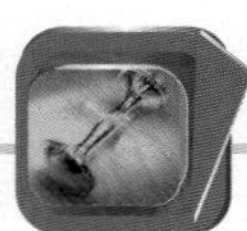

Pediatric Considerations

This procedure is only indicated in neonates. Older children and adults need to have circumcision performed in the operating room under general anesthesia.

Children older than 6 years are dosed like adults except that the maximal dose is based on weight. The recommended maximum dose for lidocaine in children is 3 to 5 mg/kg, and 7 mg/kg when combined with epinephrine. Remember that 1% lidocaine is 10 mg/mL. Children 6 months to 3 years have the same volume of distribution and elimination half-life as in adults. Neonates have an increased volume of distribution, decreased hepatic clearance, and doubled terminal elimination half-life (3.2 hours).

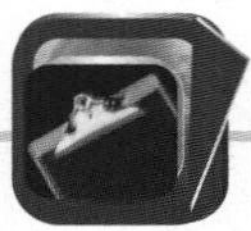

Postprocedure Instructions

Instruct the child's caregiver to bathe the infant the next day and to use a topical antibiotic such as Bacitracin or petroleum jelly on the glans and cut-line as a lubricant to keep penis from sticking to the diaper. Pain control is usually unnecessary for newborns, but acetaminophen may be used if desired. The skin under and distal to the ligature becomes dry and atrophic in 4 to 7 days. The ring should separate within two weeks.

Warn the baby's caregiver that some degree of swelling is expected, as well as a clear crust on the area. A small amount of blood also may normally be seen on the diaper. Active bleeding and blood spots larger than an inch should be reported to the provider. Also report if the Plastibell device has not fallen off within 12 days, if signs of infection develop, or if urination has not occurred within 1 day.

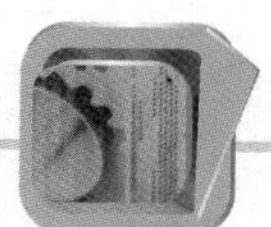

Coding Information and Supply Sources

CPT CODE	DESCRIPTION	2008 AVERAGE 50TH PERCENTILE FEE	GLOBAL PERIOD
54150	Circumcision using a clamp or other device	$427.00	0

CPT is a registered trademark of the American Medical Association.
2008 average 50th Percentile Fees are provided courtesy of 2008 MMH-SI's copyrighted Physicians' Fees and Coding Guide.

Supplies may be obtained from medical supply houses and at USA Hollister Incorporated, 2000 Hollister Drive, Libertyville, IL 60048 (phone: 1-800-323-4060; Web site: http://www.hollister.com).

Bibliography

al-Samarrai AY, Mofti AB, Crankson SJ, et al. A review of a Plastibell device in neonatal circumcision in 2,000 instances. *Surg Gynecol Obstet.* 1988;167(4):341–343.

Barrie H, Huntingford PJ, Gough MG. The Plastibell technique for circumcision. *Brit Med L.* 1965;2:273–275.

Gee WF, Ansell JS. Neonatal circumcision: a ten-year overview with comparison of the Gomco clamp and the Plastibell device. *Pediatrics.* 1976;58:824–827.

Palit V, Menebhi DK, Taylor I, et al. A unique service in UK delivering Plastibell circumcision: review of 9-year results. *Pediatr Surg Int.* 2007;23:45–48.

2008 MAG Mutual Healthcare Solutions, Inc.'s Physicians' Fee and Coding Guide. Duluth, Georgia. MAG Mutual Healthcare Solutions, Inc. 2007.

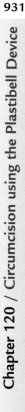

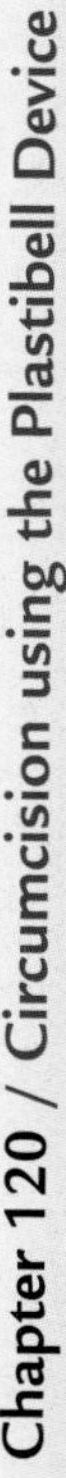

CHAPTER 121

Intraosseous Line Placement

Jennifer M. Springhart, MD
Assistant Professor of Clinical Emergency Medicine, Department of Emergency Medicine
Louisiana State University Health Sciences Center, Shreveport, LA

Intraosseous (IO) line placement is a skill that should be mastered by all physicians. In the setting of pediatric hypotension, peripheral vascular access may become difficult, or even impossible due to venous collapse. Placement of an IO may be a life-saving measure, as it is an extremely useful tool for the rapid infusion of intravenous fluids, blood, or medications. IO access requires less skill and practice than central line and umbilical line placement. With IO placement, access to the central circulation through veins in the marrow can be achieved in seconds. It should be considered after three failed attempts at peripheral venous access in the acutely ill child.

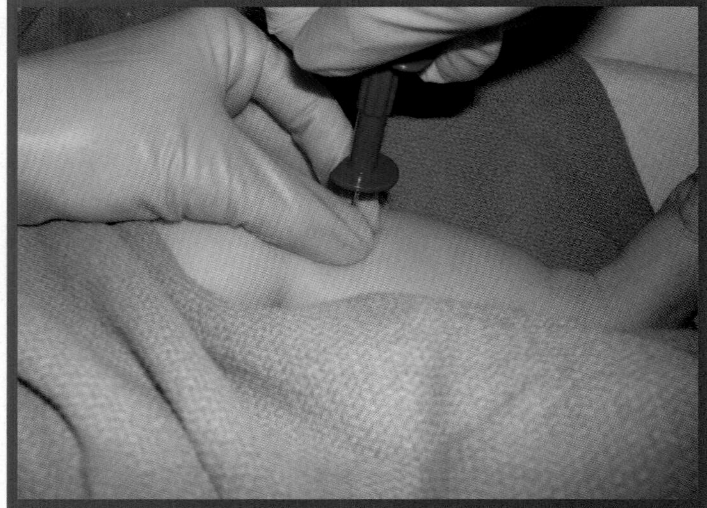

IO placement is most useful in neonates and children younger than 5 years of age because complete ossification of bones has not yet occurred, though it may be considered in adults as well. In children, the preferred site of infusion in the medial aspect of the proximal tibia. Other possible sites of infusion may include the distal femur, proximal hummers, ileum, or clavicle. In adults, the most common site of infusion is the medial malleolus, though the sternum may be considered as well.

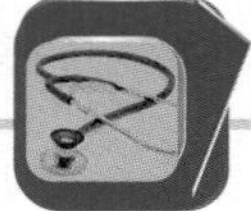

Equipment

- Sterile gloves
- Povidone-iodine (Betadine) or chlorhexidine gluconate (Hibiclens, others) solution. See Appendix E.
- Sterile drapes
- 3-cc syringe with 1% lidocaine for local anesthesia
- Disposable IO needle (16 or 18 gauge) that contains an inner stylet
- 10-cc syringe

- Sterile flush
- IV fluids and tubing

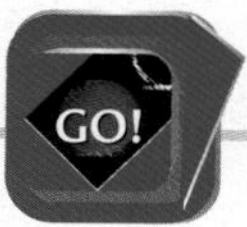

Indications

- Rapid vascular access in neonates and children for the infusion of IV fluids, blood, and medications

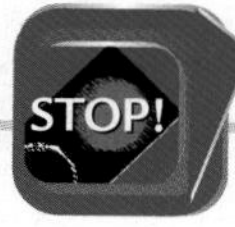

Contraindications

- Open tibial fracture
- Previous attempt on the same leg bone
- Overlying skin infection (relative)
- Osteogenesis imperfecta because of a higher likelihood of fractures occurring (relative)
- Osteopetrosis (relative)

The Procedure

Step 1. Obtain informed consent if caregiver or guardian if available. Identify proper puncture site approximately 2 cm below tibial tuberosity on medial surface of tibia.

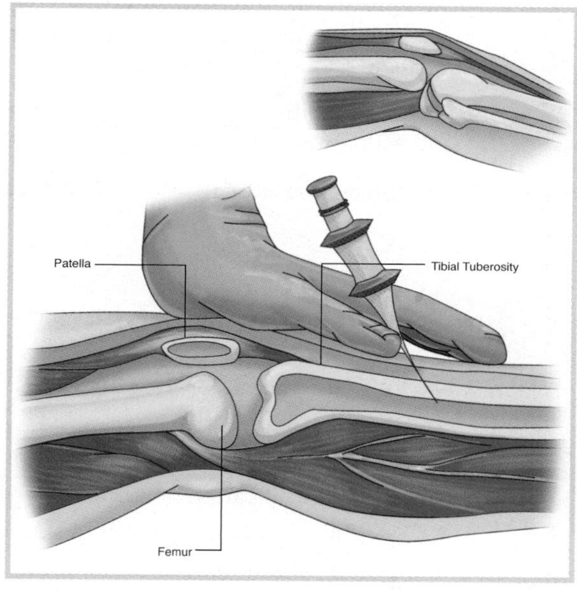

Step 1

Step 2. Prepare the skin with povidone-iodine or chlorhexidine solution, and drape the skin using sterile technique. Using 25-gauge (or less) needle attached to 3-cc syringe, anesthetize skin and subcutaneous tissue overlying puncture site. Insert the IO needle through the skin and underlying tissue. Stop when you reach the bone. Stabilize needle using your index finger and thumb.

- **PEARL:** If initial skin penetration is difficult, a small incision made with a scalpel may be necessary prior to insertion.

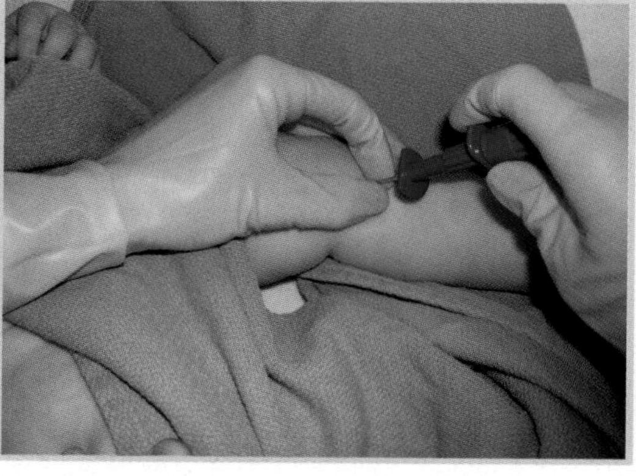

Step 2

- **PEARL:** The physician should not place his or her hand underneath the knee (popliteal fossa area.) This is a safety precaution to prevent possible lacerations and through-and-through penetration during insertion.

Step 3. Using the opposite hand, apply downward pressure and clockwise twisting motion of the palm of the hand; puncture the IO needle through cortex of tibia at a 30-degree angle. The bone will give way when you enter the marrow cavity. The needle should feel secure and nonmobile if placed properly.

- **PITFALL:** Be careful not to insert needle all the way through the cortex on the opposite side, as this puts the patient at risk for extravasation of fluid into the calf muscle and compartment syndrome.

Step 4. Carefully unscrew inner stylet of IO needle. Attach 10-cc syringe and aspirate for blood return (may be absent in shock). Attempt to flush 5 cc to 10 cc of fluid through the IO. Infusion should occur easily. Watch for extravasation in the surrounding tissues, including the calf muscle. Secure using tape and gauze.

- **PEARL:** Inability to aspirate blood does not indicate improper placement.

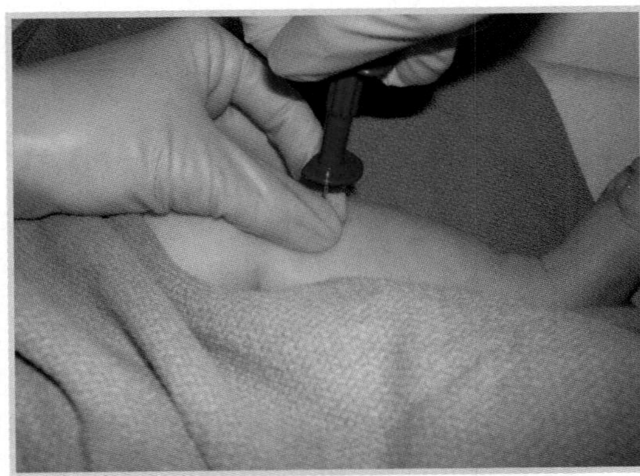

Step 3

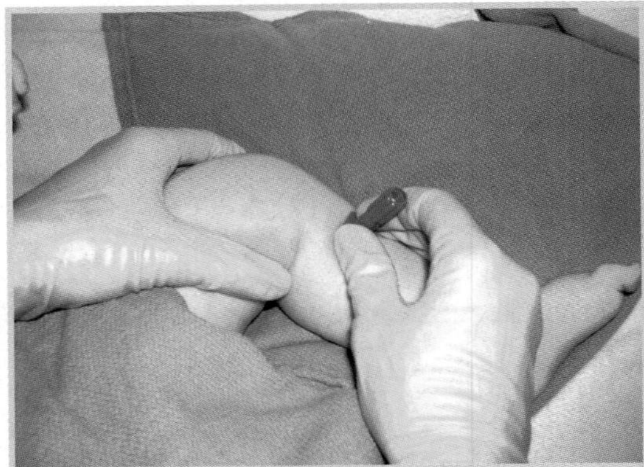

Step 4

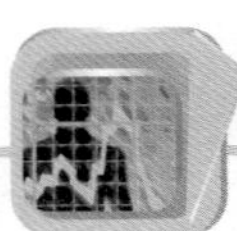

Complications

- Fracture of the tibia
- Growth plate disruption
- Hematoma
- Infiltration of surrounding tissues with extravasated fluids
- Cellulitis of overlying skin
- Osteomyelitis
- Fat emboli
- Compartment syndrome
- Muscle necrosis secondary to extravasation of hypertonic or caustic medications, such as sodium bicarbonate, dopamine, or calcium chloride.

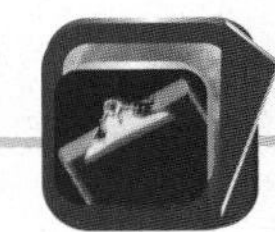

Postprocedure Instructions

After securing the IO line and stabilizing the patient, alternative sites of vascular access should be sought out. Ideally, the IO line should be removed within the first several hours after placement so as to decrease the likelihood of complications; however, it may be left in place for up to 72 hours if necessary. The infusion of IV antibiotics should begin immediately after the IO line is placed to prevent cellulitis of the leg and/or osteomyelitis.

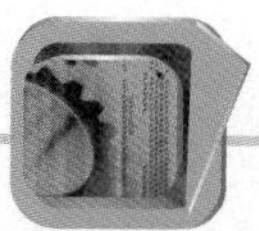

Coding Information and Supply Sources

CPT CODE	DESCRIPTION	2008 AVERAGE 50TH PERCENTILE FEE	GLOBAL PERIOD
36680	Intraosseous Line Placement	$252.00	0

2008 average 50th Percentile Fees are provided courtesy of 2008 MMH-SI's copyrighted Physicians' Fees and Coding Guide.

ICD-9 CODES

Hypovolemic shock	785.59
Dehydration	276.51
Hemorrhage	459.00

Supplies can be obtained from:

- EZ-IO needle. Vidacare Corporation, 722 Isom Road, San Antonio, TX 78216. Phone: 1-866-479-8500. Web site: http://www.vidacare.com/.
- Jamshidi needle. Baxter Healthcare Corp, One Baxter Parkway, Deerfield, IL 60015-4625. Phone: 1-800-422-9837. Web site: http://www.baxter.com/products/index.html.

Patient Education Handout

A patient education handout, "Intraosseous Line Placement" can be found on the book's Web site.

Bibliography

Abe KK, Blum GT, Yamamoto LG. Intraosseous is faster and easier than umbilical venous catheterization in newborn emergency vascular access models. *Am J Emerg Med.* 2000;18(2):126–129.

Berk WA, Sutariya B. Vascular access. In: Tintinalli JE, Kelen GD, Stapczynski JS. *Emergency Medicine A Comprehensive Study Guide.* New York: McGraw-Hill; 2004:130–131.

Gluckman W, Forti R, Lamba S. Intraosseous Cannulation. Available at: Emedicine.com. http://www.emedicine.com/ped/TOPIC2557.HTM. Accessed November 1, 2008.

Guy J, Haley K, Zuspan SJ. Use of intraosseous infusion in the pediatric trauma patient. *J Pediatr Surg.* 1993;28(2):158–161. Hodge D 3rd. Intraosseous infusions: a review. *Pediatr Emerg Care* 1985;1(4):215–218

Rosetti, VA, Thompson BM, Miller J. Intraosseous infusion: an alternative route of pediatric intravascular access. *Ann Emerg Med.* 1985;14(9):885–888.

Smith R, Davis N, Bouamra O. The utilisation of intraosseous infusion in the resuscitation of paediatric major trauma patients. *Injury* 2005;36(9):1034–1038; discussion 1039.

2008 MAG Mutual Healthcare Solutions, Inc.'s Physicians' Fee and Coding Guide. Duluth, Georgia. MAG Mutual Healthcare Solutions, Inc. 2007.

CHAPTER 122

Pediatric Sedation

Paul D. Cooper, MD
Assistant Professor of Clinical Pediatrics
Louisiana State University Health Sciences Center, Shreveport, LA

There are a number of reasons for sedating a child in medicine. Reduction or cessation of pain and/or anxiety is the most common grounds. In fact, The Joint Commission is so concerned about patient pain they recently designated pain as being the "fifth" vital sign. Sedation, especially in the outpatient setting, is used mainly to facilitate a better outcome for a procedure or an imaging study as well as to provide as comfortable an environment as possible for the patient. The levels of sedation are not exact states but rather a continuum from minimal sedation to deep sedation and general anesthesia. It is very easy for a child to slip into a deeper state of sedation, especially after anxiolysis has been achieved; therefore, great attention and care need to be exercised when sedating a pediatric patient. The overall goal is to adjust the sedation medication(s) in such a way as to provide adequate anxiolysis, sedation, and analgesia, but at a level that does not compromise respiratory or cardiovascular function (i.e. "deep enough but not too deep.") Table 122-1 describes the levels of pediatric sedation.

TABLE 122-1. Definitions of Levels of Pediatric Sedation

Minimal Sedation (anxiolysis)	Patients are conscious and can respond to verbal commands, but there may be impairment of cognitive function,
Moderate Sedation (formerly conscious sedation)	Patients are in a drug-induced state of depressed consciousness; however, patient is able to maintain airway patency and reflexes. Patient does respond to verbal commands with or without light stimulation/touch.
Deep Sedation	Patients are in a drug-induced state of depressed consciousness, and patient may or may not be able to maintain airway patency and reflexes. Patient responds to repeated verbal or painful stimulation.
General Anesthesia	Patients are in a drug-induced state where consciousness and responsiveness are lost and the ability of the patient to maintain ventilation independently may be lost. Cardiovascular function needs to also be closely monitored.

For a pediatric sedation procedure, it is important to have a provider who is trained in, and responsible for, the sedation procedure—not splitting their concentration between the sedation and the other procedure that requires sedation. The sedation provider should also be versed in methods to rescue the patient including advanced pediatric airway management. The provider may be the person administering the sedation; however, an independent support person must be present to document as above as well as monitor the patient's condition. For moderate sedation, it is strongly recommended to have an independent trained provider to administer the sedation and this is mandatory for sedation greater than moderate sedation.

When the patient arrives for the sedation/procedure, there are a number of important items that need to be addressed. First, always obtain an informed consent from the parent or guardian. Second, there are important minimum fasting periods before elective sedation. When clear liquids are ingested (e.g., water, oral electrolyte solutions, fruit juice, tea, coffee) 2 hours should elapse before sedation is attempted. That interval is extended to 4 hours for breast milk, 6 hours for infant formula or nonhuman milk, and 6 to 8 hours for solid food. Third, provide instructions and information to the person who will be responsible for taking care of the child after the sedation.

If a patient is being sedated for an imaging study, an immobilization device (i.e., a papoose board) may be considered for infants and small children. Most papoose boards are x-ray and magnetic resonance imaging safe, but be sure to confirm that this is the case with the one you are using.

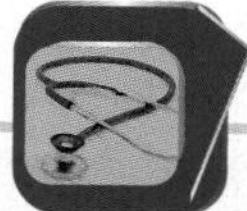

Equipment (SOAPME)

- S (suction)
- O (oxygen)
- A (Airway): Size-appropriate airway equipment, laryngoscope blades, endotracheal tubes, stylets, face mask, bag-valve-mask
- P (Pharmacy): Drugs for the sedation as well as emergency drugs including "rescue/ reversal" drugs).
- M (Monitors)
  - Blood pressure
  - Cardiorespiratory monitor
  - Expired carbon dioxide monitor
  - Pulse oximeter
- E (Equipment): An IV and possibly an emergency cart with medicines and defibrillator.

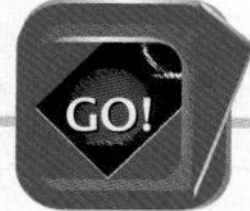

Indications

- Any procedure that elicits pain or anxiety. (This includes young children who need magnetic resonance imaging or computed tomography scans.)
- In an outpatient or non-operating room setting, patients who are in American Society of Anesthesiologists (ASA) Physical Status Classification Class I and II are usually acceptable patients (see Step 3).

Contraindications (Relative)

- Patients in ASA Class III-V (Table 122-2) require an experienced team for sedation, such as PICU staff or an anesthesiologist.
- For children with certain conditions such as a mediastinal mass, airway abnormalities (including tonsillar hypertrophy) and obstructive sleep apnea, the physician must weigh the risks of sedation versus the benefit of the procedure or imaging study.

The Procedure

Step 1. Review dietary precautions with the person who had been taking care of the child and confirm that the recommended time has elapsed since the last ingestion.

- PITFALL: Never prescribe a sedative medication for the parent to administer at home prior to the procedure.

MINIMUM FASTING PERIODS	
Clear liquids*	2 hours
Breast milk	4 hours
Formula and nonhuman milk	6 hours
Solid foods	6–8 hours

*Clear liquids include water, Pedialyte, fruit juice, tea, coffee, etc.

Step 2. Obtain IV access if required by the drugs and route of administration being planned. Although IV access is not mandatory for administration of all medications, it is strongly suggested to have IV access for any sedation in children.

- PITFALL: Because sedation is a continuum, it is in the best interest of the child to have IV access available, as in the event that the patient goes into a deeper state of sedation than intended or expected.

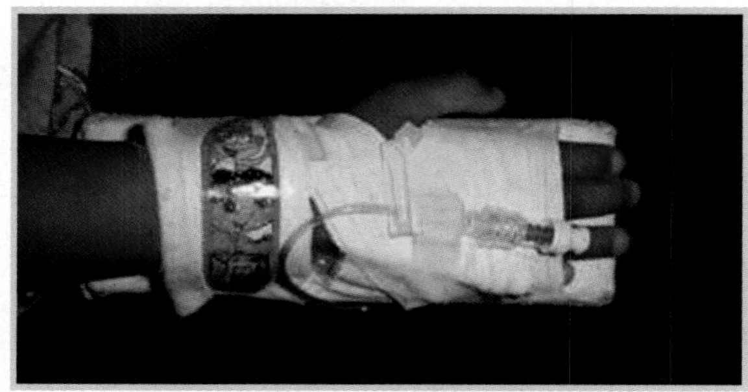

Step 2

Step 3. Before starting sedation, always document the patient's history and physical examination, including medical problems, prior surgeries, any history of anesthesia complications, allergies, and medicines. Also, document the patient's baseline mental status, baseline vitals, accurate weight, and ASA classification.

- PEARL: Do not forget about herbal medicines, as some may affect sedation drug half-life!

American Society of Anesthesiologists Physical Status Classification Physical Status Classification

Class I	A normally healthy patient
Class II	A patient with mild systemic disease (e.g., controlled reactive airway disease or asthma)
Class III	A patient with severe systemic disease (e.g., poorly controlled asthma or a child who is actively wheezing)
Class IV	A patient with severe systemic disease that is a constant threat to life
Class V	A moribund patient who is not expected to survive without the operation

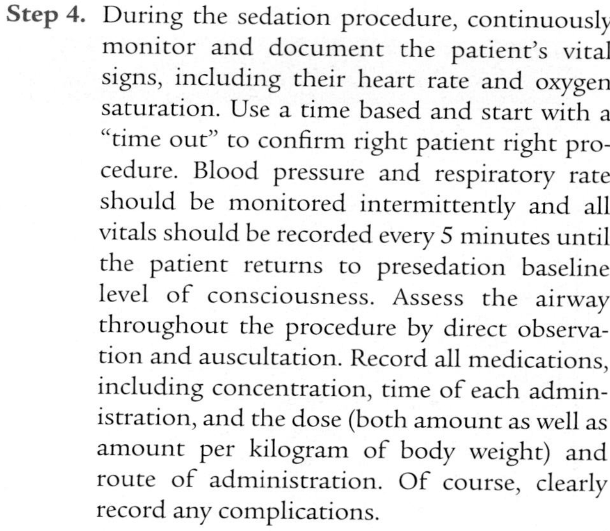

Step 4. During the sedation procedure, continuously monitor and document the patient's vital signs, including their heart rate and oxygen saturation. Use a time based and start with a "time out" to confirm right patient right procedure. Blood pressure and respiratory rate should be monitored intermittently and all vitals should be recorded every 5 minutes until the patient returns to presedation baseline level of consciousness. Assess the airway throughout the procedure by direct observation and auscultation. Record all medications, including concentration, time of each administration, and the dose (both amount as well as amount per kilogram of body weight) and route of administration. Of course, clearly record any complications.

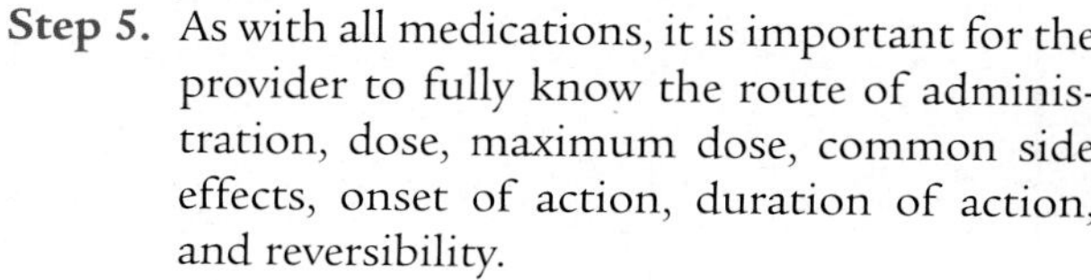

Step 5. As with all medications, it is important for the provider to fully know the route of administration, dose, maximum dose, common side effects, onset of action, duration of action, and reversibility.

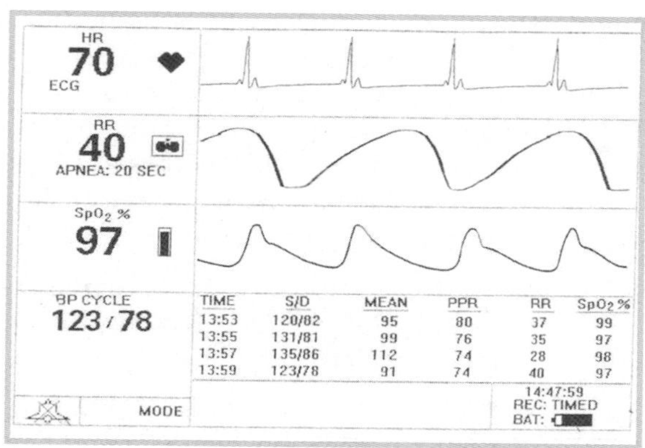

Step 4

Commonly Used Drugs and Their Properties

	Sedation/ Hypnosis	Analgesia	Anxiolysis	Reversible
Sedative-hypnotics				
Benzodiazepines	yes	no	yes	yes
Chloral hydrate	yes	no	no	no
Barbiturates	yes	no	no	no
Propofol*	yes	no	yes	no
Analgesics				
Topical agents	no	yes	no	no
Nonsteroidal anti-inflammatory drugs	no	yes	no	no
Opioids	yes	yes	no	yes
Dissociative Sedative				
Ketamine	yes	yes	yes	no

*Should be reserved in controlled settings, such as intensive care units and operating rooms.

Step 6. Use the minimum amount of medication necessary to adequately meet the goals of sedation, anxiolysis, and/or analgesia. It is also usually important to use the shortest acting medication(s) available both for expedient recovery as well as rescuing the patient from unintended deeper sedation.

- **PEARL:** Frequently used combinations include midazolam + fentanyl and ketamine + midazolam + atropine.
- **PITFALL:** Combining sedative drugs is helpful in sedation, but be careful because the side effects of respiratory and cardiovascular compromise may be potentiated with the use of multiple of drugs.
- **PITFALL:** The end of the procedure, especially a painful one, is not a time for the physician to be any less vigilant about monitoring the patient. Frequently, after the painful stimulus has been removed, the patient may progress into a deeper state of sedation.

Common Drugs and Doses

Drug	Route	Dose	Maximum Dose
Atropine*	IV/IM/SC	0.01 mg/kg/dose May repeat Q4-6hr	0.4 mg/dose
Chloral Hydrate	PO/PR	25–100 mg/kg/dose	1 g/dose (infant) 2 g/dose (child)
Fentanyl	IV/IM	1–2 mcg/kg/dose Q30–60min PRN	
Ketamine	IV	0.25–0.5 mg/kg	Rate of infusion should not exceed 0.5 mg/kg/min and should not be administered in <60 sec.
Midazolam 6 mo-5 yrs	IV	0.05–0.1 mg/kg/dose over 2–3 min. May repeat dose PRN in 2–3 min. intervals A total dose up to 0.6 mg/kg may be necessary for desired effect.	6 mg cumulative dose
Midazolam 6–12 y	IV	0.025–0.05 mg/kg/dose over 2–3 min. May repeat dose in 2–3 min intervals A total dose up to 0.4 mg/kg may be necessary for desired effect.	10 mg cumulative dose
Midazolam 13–16 y	IV	0.5–2 mg/dose over 2 min. May repeat dose in 2–3 min intervals Usual dose 2.5–5 mg	5 mg cumulative dose
Midazolam ≥6 mo**	PO	0.25–0.5 mg/kg/dose ×1	20 mg

IV, intravenously; IM, intramuscularly; PO, by mouth; PR, rectally; PRN, as needed; SC, subcutaneously

* The minimum dose of atropine is 0.1 mg/dose.

** Younger patients (6 months to 5 years) may require higher doses of 1 mg/kg/dose. Older patients (6 years to 15 years) may require only 0.25 mg/kg/dose.

Step 7. Reversal drugs may be used to rescue a patient who has become apneic. However, reversal drugs are not to be used just to "wake" the patient after the sedation is complete.

- **PITFALL:** Remember to monitor for the return of respiratory depression for at least 2 hours after administration of a reversal agent because the half-life of the reversal agent may be shorter than the sedation drug.

Rescue/Reversal Drugs

Drug	Route	Dose	Notes
Naloxone (opioid antagonist) Neonate, infant, child <20 kg	IV, SC, IM, ETT	0.1 mg/kg/dose. May repeat PRN Q2-3 min.	Short duration of action may call for multiple doses until the effects of the opioid have stopped.
Naloxone (opioid antagonist) Child >20 kg or >5 y	IV, SC, IM, ETT	2 mg/dose. May repeat PRN Q2-3 min	Will produce narcotic withdrawal syndrome in patients with chronic dependence.
Flumazenil (benzodiazepine antagonist)	IV	Initial dose: 0.01 mg/kg (max. dose: 0.2 mg) given over 15 sec, then 0.01 mg/ kg (max. dose: 0.2 mg) given Q1min to a max. total cumulative dose of 0.05 mg/kg or 1 mg, whichever is lower. May be repeated in 20 min up to a max. dose of 3 mg in 1 hr.	Does not reverse narcotics. Reversal effects of flumazenil (T1/2 approximately 1 hr) may subside before the effects of the benzodiazepine. May precipitate seizures in patients taking benzodiazepines or seizure control.

ETT, endotracheal tube; IM, intramuscularly; IV, intravenously; PRN, as needed; SC, subcutaneously.

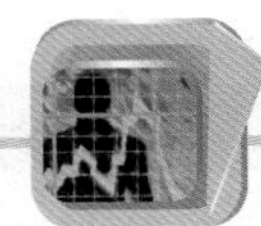

Complications

- The most common complication during pediatric sedation is to have the patient unintentionally progress into a state of sedation that is deeper than intended. Many of the drugs used depress respiratory drive and/or may precipitate airway compromise or obstruction. The first 5 to 10 minutes and the end of the procedure are two of the most critical times. At the beginning of a procedure, the provider is trying to get the procedure underway and may not have allowed enough time for the onset of action of the sedation medications before administering more. At the end of the procedure, after the painful stimulus has been removed, the patient may progress into a deeper state of sedation. Therefore, it is always important to remember the ABCs (Airway, Breathing, and Circulation) of life support as well as the reversal/antagonist drugs.
- Respiratory compromise: Hypoventilation, hypoxemia, apnea, airway obstruction
- Cardiovascular compromise: Hypotension and cardiopulmonary arrest, arrhythmia
- Seizures
- Allergic reactions/anaphylaxis
- Vomiting
- Hypothermia

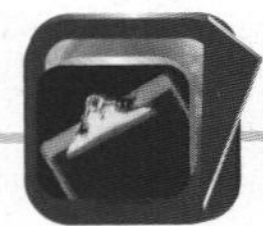

Postprocedure Instructions

After the procedure, the patient should be followed closely. The following are the recommended discharge criteria. Each criteria as well as the general condition of the patient needs to be documented as well as the time of discharge. A good "rule of thumb" is for the patient to be able to stay awake on his or her own for at least 30 minutes.

Recommended Discharge Criteria

- Cardiovascular function and airway patency are satisfactory and stable.
- The patient is easily aroused, and protective reflexes are intact.
- The patient can talk (if age appropriate).
- For a very young or handicapped child incapable of the usually expected responses, the presedation level of responsiveness or a level as close as possible to the normal level for that child should be achieved.
- Adequate hydration.

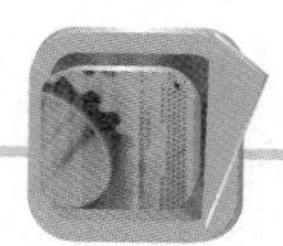

Coding Information and Supply Sources

CPT Code	Description	2008 Average 50th Percentile Fee	Global Period
99143	Moderate sedation services provided by the same physician performing the diagnostic or therapeutic service that the sedation supports, requiring the presence of an independent trained observer to assist in the monitoring of the patient's level of consciousness and physiological status: younger than 5 years of age, first 30 minutes intraservice time	$118.00	XXX
99144	Age 5 years or older, first 30 minutes intraservice time	$115.00	XXX
99145	each additional 15 minutes intraservice time (List separately in addition to code for primary service) Use 99145 in conjunction with 99143, 99144	$53.00	ZZZ
99148	Moderate sedation services provided a physician other than the health care professional performing the diagnostic or therapeutic service that the sedation supports; younger than 5 years of age, first 30 minutes intraservice time	$183.00	XXX
99149	Age 5 years or older, first 30 minutes intraservice time	$166.00	XXX
99150	Each additional 15 minutes intraservice time (List separately in addition to code for primary service) Use 99150 in conjunction with 99148, 99149	$64.00	ZZZ

XXX, global concept does not apply; ZZZ, code related to another service and is always included in the global period of the other service.

2008 average 50th Percentile Fees are provided courtesy of 2008 MMH-SI's copyrighted Physicians' Fees and Coding Guide.

Most of the drugs and equipment may be purchased from hospital supply sources.

Patient Education Handout

Two patient education handouts, "Before Pediatric Sedation" and "After Pediatric Sedation," can be found on the book's companion Web site.

Bibliography

American Society of Anesthesiologists. Practice guidelines for sedation and analgesia by non-anesthesiologists. *Anesthesiology.* 2002;96:1004.

Cote CJ, Wilson S. American Academy of Pediatrics Clinical Report: Guidelines for monitoring and management of pediatric patients during and after sedation of diagnostic and therapeutic procedures: an update. *Pediatrics.* 2006;118:2587.

Krauss, B, Green, SM. Procedural sedation and analgesia in children. *Lancet.* 2006;367:766.

Robertson J, Shilkofski N. Analgesia and Sedation. In: Custer JW, Rau RE Eds. *The Harriet Lane Handbook*, 17th ed. Philadelphia: Elsevier Mosby; 2006.

Robertson J, Shilkofski N. Formulary. In: Custer JW, Rau RE Eds. *The Harriet Lane Handbook*, 17th ed. Philadelphia: Elsevier Mosby; 2006.

2008 MAG Mutual Healthcare Solutions, Inc.'s Physicians' Fee and Coding Guide. Duluth, Georgia. MAG Mutual Healthcare Solutions, Inc. 2007.

CHAPTER 123

Suprapubic Bladder Catheterization

Jennifer M. Springhart, MD

Assistant Professor of Clinical Emergency Medicine

Department of Emergency Medicine

Louisiana State University Health Sciences Center, Shreveport, LA

Suprapubic bladder catheterization, or bladder tap, is a technique used typically in infants younger than 2 months of age to obtain sterile urine. This procedure is the true "gold standard" by which to guarantee a sterile specimen for culture and is recommended over urethral catheterization or urine bag placement.

Although this procedure may seem invasive in the short term, it may save the patient from undergoing unnecessary and expensive diagnostic tests and procedures in the future. Urine obtained via urethral catheterization or by "u-bag" is more likely to give false positive results, whereas urine obtained via a bladder tap approaches 100% sensitivity and specificity. The success of performing a bladder tap ranges from 23% to 90%; however, with the use of ultrasound guidance, the success rate approaches 100%. In general, this is a safe and easy procedure to perform, with very few risks involved.

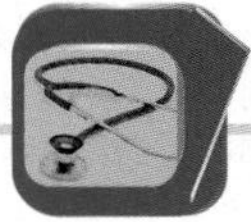

Equipment

- Needle (25 gauge, 1 inch long) attached to a 3-cc syringe
- Alcohol swab
- Sterile specimen container for urine transport
- Ultrasound and gel if available

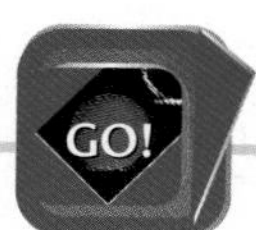

Indications

- To obtain a sterile urine specimen for urinalysis and/or culture
- To emergently relieve bladder pressure when urination and catheterization are not possible

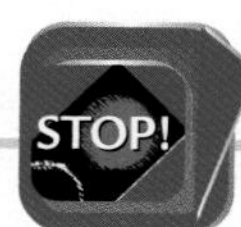

Contraindications (Relative)

- Bleeding disorder
- Abdominal distention
- Massive organomegaly

The Procedure

Step 1. Try to ensure that the infant has a full bladder (wait approximately 1 hour after voiding). Prep the area with alcohol, and allow it to dry. Have an assistant position and restrain the infant in the frog leg position.

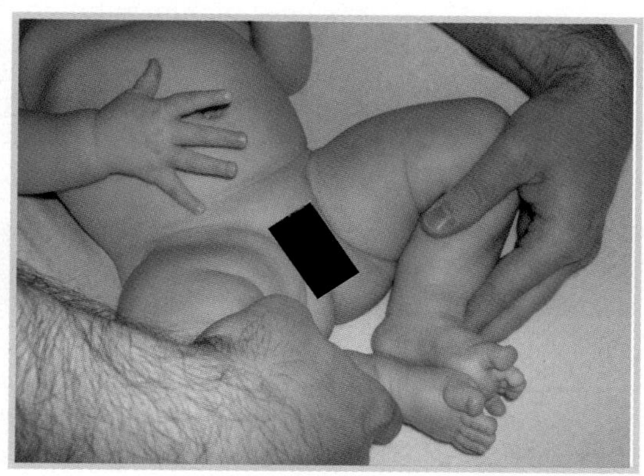

Step 1

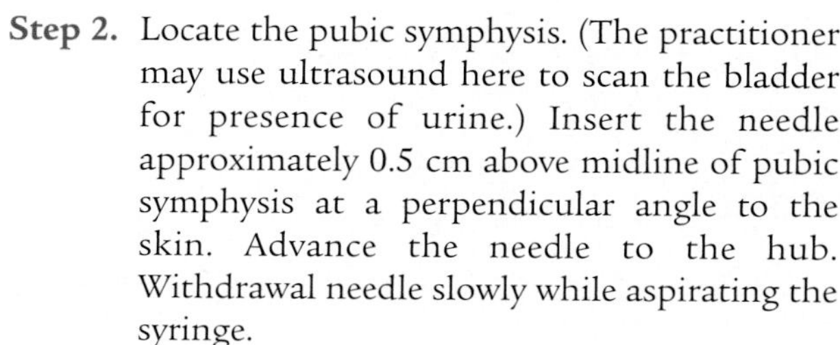

Step 2. Locate the pubic symphysis. (The practitioner may use ultrasound here to scan the bladder for presence of urine.) Insert the needle approximately 0.5 cm above midline of pubic symphysis at a perpendicular angle to the skin. Advance the needle to the hub. Withdrawal needle slowly while aspirating the syringe.

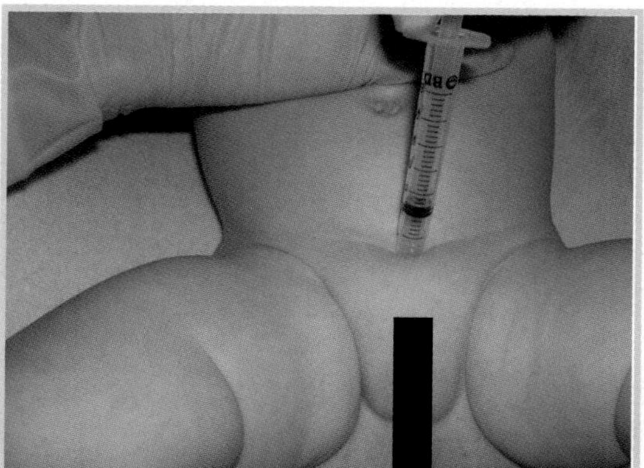

Step 2

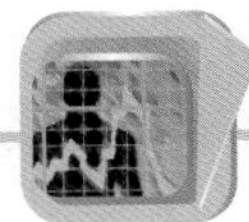

Complications

- Hematuria
- Bladder hematoma
- Vessel perforation (rare)
- Bowel perforation (rare and not usually significant)
- Abdominal wall abscess (rare)

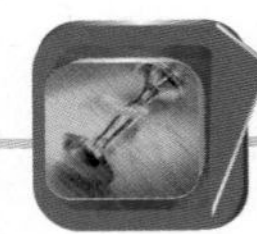

Pediatric Considerations

This procedure is most commonly performed in young children. Toddlers may have to be restrained in a "papoose board" for the procedure. Infants can usually be held by the parents or an assistant, and older children and adults can usually hold still enough for the procedure.

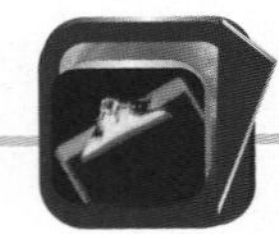

Postprocedure Instructions

Instruct the parents that there may be a small amount of hematuria noted in the diaper that day. There may be some very minor bleeding from the insertion site. The adhesive bandage may be removed later that same day.

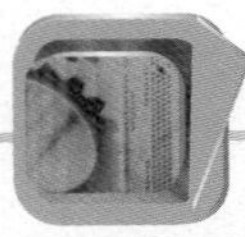

Coding Information and Supply Sources

CPT Code	Description	2008 Average 50th Percentile Fee	Global Period
51000	Suprapubic bladder tap	$162.00	0

ICD-9 Codes

Urinary tract infection of the newborn	771.82
Septicemia of the newborn	771.81

Patient Education Handout

A patient education handout, "Suprapubic Bladder Catheterization," can be found on the book's companion Web site.

Bibliography

Buys H, Pead L, Hallett R, et al. Suprapubic aspiration under ultrasound guidance in children with fever undiagnosed cause. *Br Med J.* 1994;308:690–692.

Downs S. Technical report: urinary tract infection in febrile infants and young children. *Pediatrics.* 1999;103(4):e54.

Hoberman A, Chao HP, Keller DM, et al. Prevalence of urinary tract infection in febrile infants. *J Pediatr.* 1993;123:17–23.

Lerner GR. Urinary tract infections in children. *Pediatr Ann.* 1994;23:463, 466–473.

2008 MAG Mutual Healthcare Solutions, Inc.'s Physicians' Fee and Coding Guide. Duluth, Georgia. MAG Mutual Healthcare Solutions, Inc. 2007.

APPENDIX A

Informed Consent

The principle of self-determination is the cornerstone of the American legal system. Rooted within this principle is the doctrine of informed consent, which posits that a competent individual or the individual's representative has the right to receive adequate information to form an intelligent decision regarding a proposed procedure. Although the information included in informed consent varies from state to state, the key component that must be included is information that a reasonable patient would need to know about the risks of a proposed procedure that might cause the patient not to undergo that treatment.

There are several key issues:

- The medical record is considered faithful documentation of what information was transmitted to the patient; the medical professional must provide complete notes.
- Courts assume that "if it's not written, it didn't happen."
- The physician's word that informed consent occurred is not sufficient. It must be documented in the medical record.
- All preoperative discussions about a procedure should be documented, including phone calls the night before a procedure.
- The name of the procedure, its indication, and the probable risks and benefits should be explained.
- There may be exceptions to the need to obtain informed consent, including emergency care when immediate treatment is required to prevent death or serious harm to the patient.

APPENDIX B

Lines of Least Skin Tension (Langer Lines)

When planning the layout of an excision, the longest part of the suture line is typically aligned with the lines of least skin tension (see Chapter 44). These lines run perpendicular to the long axis of the underlying musculature but are more complex on the face. Wounds that follow (parallel) these lines heal faster and are less likely to enlarge (i.e., hypertrophy or keloid).

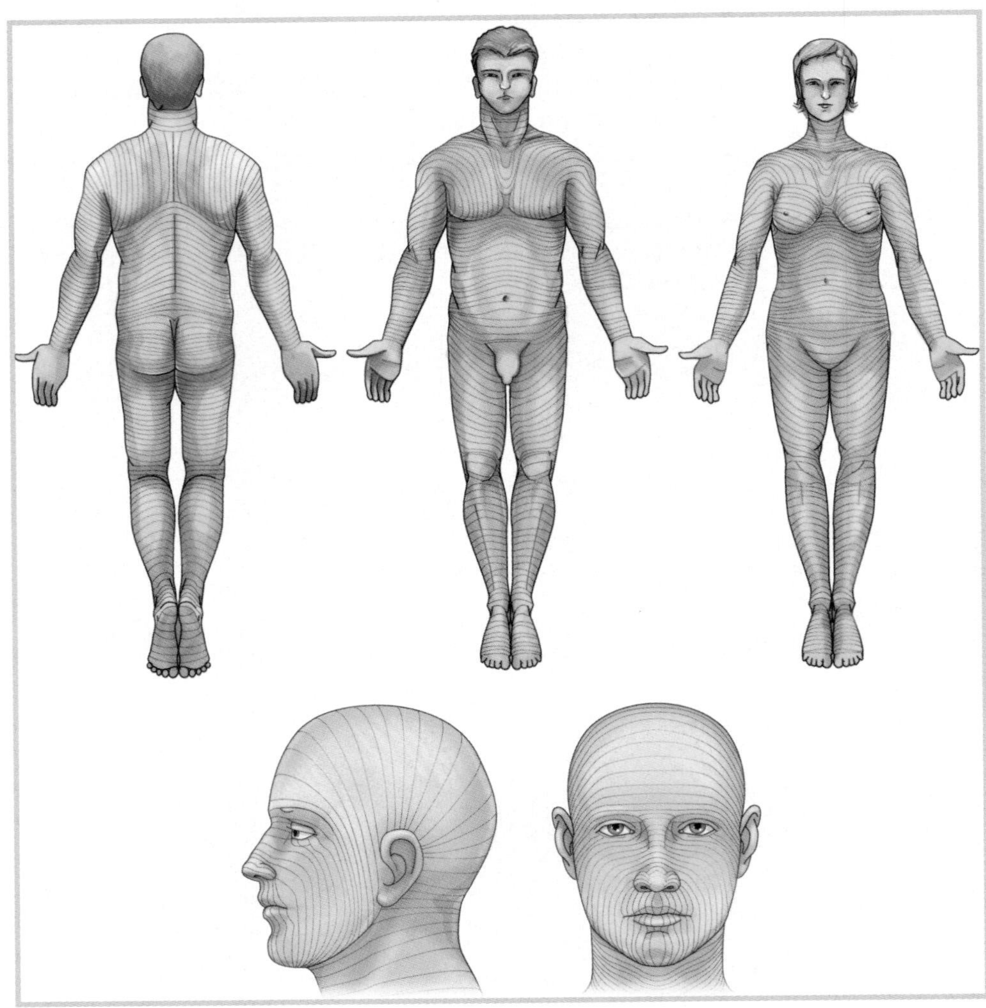

APPENDIX C

Bacterial Endocarditis Prevention Recommendations

Infectious endocarditis (IE) is a relatively uncommon, life-threatening disease that may result in substantial morbidity and mortality. Endocarditis usually develops in individuals with underlying structural cardiac defects (Table C-1) who develop bacteremia. Although bacteremia is common after many invasive procedures, only certain bacteria commonly cause endocarditis, and most cases of endocarditis are not attributable to an invasive procedure.

In 2007, the American Heart Association (AHA) published new guidelines for IE prevention that were unique because for the first time they were evidence-based. The new recommendations no longer recommend IE prophylaxis based solely on an increased lifetime risk of acquisition of IE. They noted that IE is much more likely to result from frequent exposure to random bacteremias associated with daily activities than from bacteremia caused by dental, gastrointestinal (GI) tract, or genitourinary (GU) tract procedures.

In patients with underlying cardiac conditions associated with the highest risk of adverse outcome from IE (Table C-1), IE prophylaxis for dental procedures may be reasonable, even though its actual effectiveness is unknown. Maintenance of optimal oral health and hygiene may reduce the incidence of bacteremia from daily activities and is probably more important than prophylactic antibiotics for a dental procedure to reduce the risk of IE. Antibiotic prophylaxis (Table C-2) is recommended for patients with the conditions listed in Table C-1 who undergo any dental procedure that involves the gingival tissues or periapical region of a tooth and for those procedures that perforate the oral mucosa. Dental procedures in which IE prophylaxis is not recommended are listed in Table C-3.

TABLE C-1. Cardiac Conditions Associated with the Highest Risk of Adverse Outcome from Endocarditis for which Prophylaxis with Dental Procedures Is Recommended

- Prosthetic cardiac valve
- Previous infectious endocarditis (IE)
- Congenital heart disease (CHD)
  - Unrepaired cyanotic CHD, including palliative shunts and conduits
  - Completely repaired congenital heart defect with prosthetic material or device, whether placed by surgery or by catheter intervention, during the first 6 months after the procedure
  - Repaired CHD with residual defects at the site or adjacent to the site of a prosthetic patch or prosthetic device (which inhibit endothelialization)
  - Cardiac transplantation recipients who develop cardiac valvulopathy

TABLE C-2. Infectious Endocarditis Prevention Antibiotic Regimens for Dental Procedures

		Regimen: Single Dose 30 to 60 min Before Procedure	
Situation	**Agent**	**Adults**	**Children**
Oral	Amoxicillin	2 g	50 mg/kg
Unable to take oral meds	Ampicillin **OR** cefazolin or ceftriaxone	2 g IM or IV 1 g IM or IV	50 mg/kg IM or IV 50 mg/kg IM or IV
Allergic to penicillins or ampicillin—oral	Cephalexin[a,b] **OR** clindamycin **OR** azithromycin or clarithromycin	2 g 600 mg 500 mg	50 mg/kg 20 mg/kg 15 mg/kg
Allergic to penicillins or ampicillin and unable to take oral medication	Cefazolin or ceftriaxone[b] **OR** clindamycin	1 g IM or IV 600 mg IM or IV	50 mg/kg IM or IV 20 mg/kg IM or IV

IM, intramuscular; IV, intravenous.
[a]Or other first- or second-generation oral cephalosporin in equivalent adult or pediatric dosage.
[b]Cephalosporins should not be used in an individual with a history of anaphylaxis, angioedema, or urticaria with penicillins or ampicillin.
Adapted from Dajani AS, Taubert KA, Wilson W, et al. Prevention of bacterial endocarditis. *JAMA* 1991;227:1794–1801, and Baltimore RS, Newburger JW, Strom BL, et al. Prevention of infective endocarditis: guidelines from the American Heart Association: a guideline from the American Heart Association Rheumatic Fever, Endocarditis, and Kawasaki Disease Committee, Council on Cardiovascular Disease in the Young, and the Council on Clinical Cardiology, Council on Cardiovascular Surgery and Anesthesia, and the Quality of Care and Outcomes Research Interdisciplinary Working Group. *Circulation* 2007;115. http://www.circulationaha.org. Accessed November 5, 2007.

Antibiotic prophylaxis is no longer recommended for any other form of congenital heart disease (CHD), except for the conditions listed in Table C-1. Antibiotic prophylaxis is recommended for procedures on the respiratory tract or infected skin, skin structures, or musculoskeletal tissue only for patients with underlying cardiac conditions associated with the highest risk of adverse outcome from IE (Table C-1). Antibiotic prophylaxis solely to prevent IE is *not* recommended for GU or GI tract procedures.

TABLE C-3. Dental Procedures for which Endocarditis Prophylaxis Is Not Recommended

- Routine anesthetic injections through noninfected tissue
- Dental radiographs
- Placement of removable prosthodontic or orthodontic appliances
- Adjustment of orthodontic appliances
- Placement of orthodontic brackets
- Shedding of deciduous teeth
- Bleeding from trauma to the lips or oral mucosa.

APPENDIX D

Recommended Margins for Removal of Neoplastic Skin Lesions

The primary goal of skin tumor excision is to completely remove the tumor while removing the minimal amount of normal skin. It is generally accepted that the microscopic margin of a malignant or premalignant lesion may extend beyond its visible or palpable edge. It is therefore recommended that a rim of normal-appearing tissue, or normal margin, be excised with the lesion in an attempt to minimize recurrences. Recommendations for surgical margins vary depending upon the type of lesion and the risk of local recurrence.

Surgical excision with appropriate margins is an effective, time-tested method for treating basal cell carcinomas (BCCs). When treating small BCCs that are located on lower-risk areas of the head and neck, trunk, and extremities and that lack aggressive histologic features, 4- to 5-mm margins are generally recommended to achieve cure rates of at least 95%. The cure rates are lower for higher-risk BCCs, such as lesions that are > 2 cm, have morpheaform morphology, are recurrent, or have aggressive histologic features on biopsy (Table D-1). Cure rates for tumors located on the lips, nose, paranasal or periocular region, ears, and scalp also are lower. Cure rates for these higher-risk BCCs can be improved substantially through the use of intraoperative margin evaluation (frozen sections) or Mohs micrographic surgery.

TABLE D-1. Features of "High-Risk" Basal Cell Carcinomas that May Benefit from Intraoperative Margin Evaluation or Mohs Micrographic Surgery

Location on high-risk areas (central face, eyelids, eyebrows, periorbital, nose, lips, chin, mandible, preauricular and postauricular skin/sulci, temple, ears, hands, or feet)
Size >10 mm in high-risk locations or >20 mm for other areas
Poorly defined borders by inspection or palpation
Recurrent lesions
Tumors at site of prior irradiation
Morpheaform, sclerosing, infiltrative, micronodular, or mixed subtypes
Presence of perineural spread
Basosquamous features

TABLE D-2. Features of "High-Risk" Squamous Cell Carcinomas that May Benefit from Intraoperative Margin Evaluation or Mohs Micrographic Surgery

Ill-defined borders
Diameter >2 cm
Poorly differentiated histologic subtype
Location on high-risk areas (central face, eyelids, eyebrows, periorbital, nose, lips, chin, mandible, genitalia, hands, and feet)
Recurrent tumors
Tumors that have invaded subcutaneous fat

A major difference between BCCs and squamous cell carcinomas (SCCs) is that SCCs can metastasize. When excising squamous cell carcinomas (SCC), both the type of lesion and the presence or absence of high-risk features must be considered in deciding on appropriate surgical margins (Table D-2). Well-defined, small (<2 cm) SCCs lacking any high-risk features require a 4-mm margin of normal tissue around the visible tumor to result in a 95% histologic cure rate. Primary SCCs that are ≥2 cm in diameter, are poorly differentiated on biopsy histology, in high-risk sites, or invade subcutaneous tissues require larger margins to achieve this level of histologic cure.

The basic approach to a suspicious pigmented cutaneous neoplasm consists of an initial biopsy and pathologic evaluation. If the lesion turns out to be a melanoma, a wide local excision of the tumor with surgical margins based on tumor depth should be performed. Intermediate-risk and high-risk melanomas may require additional measures, particularly sentinel lymph node biopsy. The sentinel lymph node should be considered before a wide local excision is performed. Patients with thin melanoma (primary tumor depth <1.0 mm) can be considered at low risk and treated solely with wide local excision. Patients with primary tumor depth >1.0 mm should be considered for a sentinel lymph node biopsy in addition to wide local excision. The use of Mohs micrographic surgery can optimize margin control in critical areas. For locally recurrent melanoma, and for critical anatomic sites, Mohs micrographic surgery may be especially helpful and has cure rates comparable to those of historical controls.

Bibliography

Bart RS, Schrager D, Kopf AW, Bromberg J, Dubin N. Scalpel excision of basal cell carcinomas. *Arch Dermatol.* 1978;114:739–742.

Brodland DG, Zitelli JA. Surgical margins for excision of primary cutaneous squamous cell carcinoma. *J Am Acad Dermatol.* 1992;27:241.

Huang CC, Boyce SM. Surgical margins of excision for basal cell carcinoma and squamous cell carcinoma. *Semin Cutan Med Surg.* 2004;23(3):167–173.

Kaufmann R. Surgical management of primary melanoma. *Clin Exp Dermatol.* 2000;25:476–481.

Wolf DJ, Zitelli JA. Surgical margins for basal cell carcinoma. *Arch Dermatol.* 1987;123:340.

APPENDIX E

Skin Preparation Recommendations

In this context, antiseptics are chemical agents primarily used to decrease the risk of infection in surgical wounds. Alcohol and iodophors have rapid action against bacteria but little persistent activity, whereas chlorhexidine is slower to act but persists on the stratum corneum. Most antiseptics are not suitable for open wounds because they may impede wound healing by direct cytotoxic effects.

Patient characteristics associated with an increased risk of surgical site infections include remote site infections, colonization, diabetes, cigarette smoking, systemic steroid use, obesity, extremes of age, poor nutritional status, and preoperative transfusion of certain blood products. Apply greater vigilance when performing office procedures on patients with these risk factors. Preoperative shaving for hair removal is associated with higher rates of surgical site infections. Clipping hair immediately before a surgical procedure has the lowest rates of associated infection and should be considered the preferred preparatory activity for hair removal.

Several effective antiseptic agents are available for preoperative skin preparation, including alcohol-containing products, the iodophors (e.g., povidone-iodine), and chlorhexidine gluconate.

- *Alcohol* is readily available, inexpensive, and the most rapid-acting skin antiseptic. It does not have any increased risk for the pregnant patient but must be allowed to dry completely to achieve a bacteriocidal effect. Drying also prevents any risk for ignition with use of electrocautery or lasers. Disadvantages include potential for spores to be resistant and potential for flammable reactions.
- *Iodophors* (Betadine, others) provide broad-spectrum coverage, are associated with lack of microbial resistance, and provide a bacteriostatic effect as long as they exist on the skin. They are effective against methicillin-resistant S aureus (MRSA) and *Enterococcus* species. Significant resistance to povidone-iodine has not been documented. They were formulated to be less irritating and allergenic than pure iodine solutions but are also less active. They require at least 2 minutes of contact to release free iodine, which exerts the antibacterial activity. Povidone-iodine absorption through mucous membranes has been linked to fetal hypothyroidism, although there are reports of contact dermatitis. They may also impair wound healing.
- *Chlorhexidine gluconate* (Hibaclens, others) offers broad-spectrum coverage against bacteria, yeast, and molds. It appears to provide greater reduction in skin microflora than povidone-iodine and remains active for hours after application. It does not have any increased risk for the pregnant patient. It should be used with caution around the eyes because of a risk for conjunctival irritation, keratitis, or corneal ulceration. It can cause ototoxicity if the patient has a perforated tympanic membrane.

For injections and superficial procedures, alcohol is adequate skin prep. For larger, full-thickness procedures, iodophors or chlorhexidine gluconate are usually preferred, typically applied in a spiral pattern that extends further outward with each application. The following recommendations are provided for applying skin preparation agents:

- Remove gross contamination from the skin, including soil, debris, or devitalized tissue.
- Apply the skin-cleansing agent in concentric circles, starting from the intended surgical site.
- Extend the area of skin cleansing to a wide enough area to cover the proposed operation, allowing for extension of the surgical field for the creation of additional incisions or drains.
- Do not rub or scrub the skin during application of the antiseptic agent. Damaging the skin during application can lead to increased surgical site infections.

Bibliography

Kaye ET. Topical antibacterial agents. *Infect Dis Clin North Am.* 2000;14:321–339.

Lio PA, Kaye ET. Topical antibacterial agents. *Infect Dis Clin North Am.* 2004;18(3):717–733.

Mangram AJ. Guidelines for prevention of surgical site infection, 1999: Centers for Disease Control and Prevention (CDC) Hospital Infection Control Practices Advisory Committee. *Am J Infect Control.* 1999;27:97–132.

Sweeney SM, Maloney ME. Pregnancy and dermatologic surgery. *Dermatol Clinics.* 2006;24(2):205–214.

2008 MAG Mutual Healthcare Solutions, Inc.'s Physicians' Fee and Coding Guide. Duluth, Georgia. MAG Mutual Healthcare Solutions, Inc. 2007.

APPENDIX F

Suggested Anesthesia Tray for Administration of Local Anesthesia and Blocks

The following items are placed on a nonsterile sheet covering the Mayo stand:

- Nonsterile gloves
- Skin preparation materials and gauze or swabs to apply them (see Appendix E)
- Syringe (5 or 10 mL)
- Needle (20 or 21 gauge, 1 inch long) for drawing anesthetic from the stock bottle
- Needle (25, 27, or 30 gauge, 1.5 inches or 1 inch long) for administering anesthetic
- Small pile of nonsterile 4- × 4-inch gauze
- Lidocaine hydrochloride (1%) with or without epinephrine (choice determined by procedure and site of administration)
- Antibiotic ointment and adhesive bandage if no procedure will follow at the injection site

All of the items are readily available through local pharmacies, hospital purchasing groups, or surgical supply houses.

Gloves, materials, and instruments can be ordered from the following sources:

- Robbins Instruments, Chatham, NJ. Web site: http://www.robbinsinstruments.com
- Sklar Instruments, West Chester, PA. Web site: http://www.sklarcorp.com.
- Surgical911.com, Old Saybrook, CT. Web site: http://www.surgical911.com
- Allegro Medical Supplies. Phone: 1-800-861-3211. Web site: http://www.allegromedical.com.
- VaxServe Scranton, PA. Phone: 1-800-752-9338. Web site: http://www1.vaxserve.com/.

APPENDIX G

Instruments and Materials in the Office Surgery Tray

The following instruments and materials are included in the suggested office surgery tray:

- No. 15 scalpel blade
- Skin preparation materials and gauze or swabs to apply them (see Appendix E)
- Scalpel blade with handle
- Webster needle holder
- Metzenbaum tissue scissors
- Straight iris scissors
- Adson forceps with teeth
- Adson forceps without teeth
- Two mosquito hemostats
- Two inches of 4- × 4-inch gauze
- Fenestrated disposable drape
- Needle (21 gauge, 1 inch long, bent into a skin hook)

These materials are dropped onto a sterile disposable drape laid across a metal stand. Anesthetic is applied with nonsterile gloves and a syringe that is not placed on the tray. Sterile gloves are then applied away from this sterile tray. Added to the tray are sterile suture materials (e.g., 4-0 nylon suture) that are required for the particular procedure.

Gloves, materials, and instruments can be ordered from the following sources:

- Robbins Instruments, Chatham, NJ. Web site: http://www.robbinsinstruments.com.
- Sklar Instruments, West Chester, PA. Web site: http://www.sklarcorp.com.
- Surgical911.com, Old Saybrook, CT. Web site: http://www.surgical911.com.
- Allegro Medical Supplies. Phone: 1-800-861-3211. Web site: http://www.allegromedical.com.
- VaxServe Scranton, PA. Phone: 1-800-752-9338. Web site: http://www1.vaxserve.com/.

APPENDIX H

Instruments and Materials in a Standard Gynecologic Tray

The following instruments and materials are included in the standard gynecologic tray:

- Gloves
- Graves metal speculum
- Tenaculum
- Uterine sound
- Ring or sponge forceps
- Basin with cotton balls and povidone-iodine
- Scalpel or scissors if needed
- Cervical dilators if needed

These items should be sterile for most procedures, except for removal of cervical polyps and treatment of Bartholin gland abscesses.

The instruments can be ordered from the following sources:

- Wallach Surgical Devices, Inc., Orange, CT. Phone: 1-800-243-2463; Web site: http://www.wallachsurgical.com.
- CooperSurgical, Trumbull, CT. Phone: 1-800-645-3760; Web site: http://www.coopersurgical.com.
- Delasco, Council Bluffs, IA. Web site: http://www.delasco.com.
- Robbins Instruments, Chatham, NJ. Web site: http://www.robbinsinstruments.com.
- Sklar Instruments, West Chester, PA. Web site: http://www.sklarcorp.com.
- Surgical911.com, Old Saybrook, CT. Web site: http://www.surgical911.com
- Allegro Medical Supplies. Phone: 1-800-861-3211. Web site: http://www.allegromedical.com.
- VaxServe Scranton, PA. Phone: 1-800-752-9338. Web site: http://www1.vaxserve.com/.

APPENDIX I

Suggested Tray for Aspiration and Injection Procedures

The following instruments and materials can be placed on a nonsterile sheet on the Mayo stand:

- Nonsterile gloves
- Fenestrated drape, if desired
- Skin preparation materials (see Appendix E) and gauze or swabs to apply them
- Two 10-mL syringes
- Needle (20 or 21 gauge, 1 inch long) for drawing up injecting solution
- Needle (21, 22, or 25 gauge, 1.25 inches long) for aspiration or injection
- Hemostat for stabilizing the needle when exchanging the medication syringe for the aspiration syringe
- Lidocaine hydrochloride (1%, without epinephrine) stock bottle (20 mL)
- Steroid of choice (e.g., triamcinolone [Kenalog] 40-mg/cc multiuse bottle for soft-tissue injection and 0.5 mL [20 mg] of methylprednisolone acetate [Depo-Medrol] and 2 mL of 1% lidocaine without epinephrine for joint injections)
- Adhesive bandage or sterile bandage

For intra-articular injections and certain soft-tissue injections, it may be preferable to use sterile gloves, drapes, and tray. An assistant should assist in drawing up the injecting solution to allow the practitioner to avoid contamination.

When using multiuse stock bottles, it is preferable to draw up the lidocaine first and then the steroid solution. This order prevents contamination of the lidocaine with steroid that may be on the needle. Lidocaine on the needle does not significantly alter the steroid solution.

Gloves, materials, and instruments can be ordered from the following sources:

- Robbins Instruments, Chatham, NJ. Web site: http://www.robbinsinstruments.com.
- Sklar Instruments, West Chester, PA. Web site: http://www.sklarcorp.com.
- Surgical911.com, Old Saybrook, CT. Web site: http://www.surgical911.com.
- Allegro Medical Supplies. Phone: 1-800-861-3211. Web site: http://www.allegromedical.com.
- VaxServe Scranton, PA. Phone: 1-800-752-9338. Web site: http://www1.vaxserve.com/.

APPENDIX J

Recommended Suture Removal Times

The following times for suture removal are approximate. Patient factors, such as age, presence of vascular or chronic disease, and nutritional status, influence healing times and suture removal times.

- Face: 3 to 5 days
- Neck: 5 to 7 days
- Scalp: 7 days
- Trunk: 10 to 14 days
- Upper extremity: 10 to 14 days
- Extensor surface of the hands: 14 days
- Lower extremity: 14 to 28 days

Consider earlier removal of single sutures that cause extra tension (such as a vertical mattress anchor) within a line of simple sutures to prevent suture marks ("Tram tracks" or "Frankenstein marks").

APPENDIX K

Recommendations for Endoscope Disinfection

The following recommendations are offered for disinfection of endoscopes:

- Every endoscopy should be performed with a clean, disinfected endoscope. The use of disposable-component systems (i.e., sheathed endoscopes) can provide an alternative to conventional chemical disinfection.
- Manual cleaning of the endoscope's surface, valves, and channels is the most important step for preventing the transmission of infections during endoscopy. Manual cleaning should occur immediately after each procedure to prevent drying of secretions or formation of a biofilm, both of which may be difficult to remove. The endoscope should be disassembled as much as possible and immersed in warm water and an enzymatic detergent, washed on the outside with disposable sponges or swabs, and brushed on the distal end with a small toothbrush. Valves should be removed and cleaned by brushing away adherent debris, and the hollow portions should be flushed with detergent solution. The biopsy-suction channel should be thoroughly cleaned with a brush that is appropriate for the instrument and channel size. Automatic washing devices can be used but do not replace manual cleaning.
- The scope should receive a high level disinfection with a disinfectant approved by the U.S. Federal Drug Administration (FDA; http://www.fda.gov/cdrh/ode/germlab.html). Many societies support the use of soaking the endoscope, valves, and all internal channels for at least 20 minutes in >2% glutaraldehyde at 20°C. The scope should be completely immersed, and all channels should be perfused. The newest multisociety guideline recommends phasing out nonimmersable scopes.
- Endoscope channels should be rinsed with water and then 70% alcohol, dried with compressed air, and hung vertically overnight to reduce bacterial colonization when the endoscopes are not in use.
- Accessories such as biopsy forceps should be mechanically cleaned and autoclaved after each use.

Bibliography

Axon AT. Working party report to the World Congresses: disinfection and endoscopy: summary and recommendations. *J Gastroenterol Hepatol.* 1991;6:23–24.

Multi-society guideline for reprocessing flexible gastrointestinal endoscopes. *Gastrointest Endosc.* 2003;58:1–8.

Nelson D. Newer technologies for endoscope disinfection: electrolyzed acid water and disposable-component endoscope systems. *Gastrointest Endosc Clin North Am.* 2000;10:319–328.

Spach DH, Silverstein FE, Stamm WE. Transmission of infection by gastrointestinal endoscopy and bronchoscopy. *Ann Intern Med.* 1993;118:117–128.

Tandon RK. Disinfection of gastrointestinal endoscopes and accessories. *J Gastroenterol Hepatol.* 2000;15(Suppl):S69–S72.

2008 MAG Mutual Healthcare Solutions, Inc.'s Physicians' Fee and Coding Guide. Duluth, Georgia. MAG Mutual Healthcare Solutions, Inc. 2007.

INDEX

Page numbers followed by *f* and *t* denote figure and table, respectively.